NUTRITION IN CRITICAL CARE

Nutrition in Critical Care

Gary P. Zaloga, M.D., F.A.C.P., F.A.C.N., F.C.C.M.
Professor of Anesthesia/Critical Care and Medicine
Bowman Gray School of Medicine
Wake Forest University
Winston-Salem, North Carolina

With 74 contributors

With 85 Illustrations

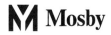 Mosby

St. Louis Baltimore Boston Chicago London Madrid Philadelphia Sydney Toronto

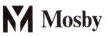
Mosby

Dedicated to Publishing Excellence

Publisher: George Stamathis
Executive Editor: Susan M. Gay
Developmental Editor: Sandra E. Clark
Project Manager: Nancy C. Baker
Project Supervisor: Carol A. Reynolds
Project Supervisor: Deborah Thorp
Proofroom Manager: Barbara M. Kelly
Designer: Carol A. Reynolds
Manufacturing Supervisor: Kathy Grone

Printed in the United States of America
Composition by Clarinda
Printing/binding by Maple-Vail

Mosby–Year Book, Inc.
11830 Westline Industrial Drive
St. Louis, Missouri 63146

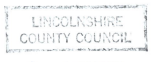

Library of Congress Cataloging in Publication Data
Nutrition in critical care / [edited by] Gary P. Zaloga.
    p.   cm.
    Includes bibliographical references and index.
    ISBN 1-55664-397-7
    1. Diet therapy. 2. Critically ill—
Nutrition. 3. Parenteral
  Nutrition. I. Zaloga, Gary P.
   [DNLM: 1. Critical Care. 2. Diet Therapy. 3. Enteral
Nutrition.
  WB 400 N9746 1993]
  RM217.N75 1993
  615.8′54—dc20
  DNLM/DLC   93-4836
  for Library of Congress   CIP

1 2 3 4 5 6 7 8 9 0 98 97 96 95 94

To Barbara and Stacey, for their love, understanding, and undying patience

CONTRIBUTORS

John C. Alverdy, M.D., F.A.C.S.
Associate Professor of Surgery
University of Chicago
Chicago, Illinois

Jeffrey Askanazi, M.D.
Mount Sinai School of Medicine
Mount Sinai Hospital
New York, New York

Timothy J. Babineau, M.D.
Instructor in Surgery
Assistant Director of Nutrition Support Service
Harvard Medical School
Deaconess Hospital
Boston, Massachusetts

Adrian Barbul, M.D., F.A.C.S.
Assistant Surgeon-in-chief
Sinai Hospital of Baltimore
Associate Professor of Surgery
Johns Hopkins Medical Institutions
Baltimore, Maryland

Nora Kizer Bell, Ph.D.
Dean
College of Arts and Sciences
Professor of Philosophy
University of North Texas
Denton, Texas

Bruce R. Bistrian, M.D., Ph.D.
Professor of Medicine
New England Deaconess Hospital
Harvard Medical School
Boston, Massachusetts

George L. Blackburn, M.D., Ph.D.
Associate Professor of Surgery
Director, Nutrition Support Service
Harvard Medical School
Deaconess Hospital
Boston, Massachusetts

Roy Blank, M.D.
Director, Metabolic Services
Presbyterian/Mercy Hospitals
Charlotte, North Carolina

Terri J. Blumeyer, P.A.-C.
Physician Assistant
Thorek Hospital and Medical Center
Chicago, Illinois

Lawrence J. Bortenschlager, M.D.
Associate Medical Director
Department of Critical Care Medicine
Methodist Hospital of Indiana
Indianapolis, Indiana

Diana Fullen Bowers, Ph.D., R.D., L.D.
Consulting Dietician
NMC Homecare
Columbus, Ohio

Rex Brown, Pharm.D.
Professor of Clinical Pharmacy
University of Tennessee at Memphis
Memphis, Tennessee

Angelo Chiareli, M.D.
Aiuto Corresposabile
Department of Plastic Surgery and Burn Unit School of
* Medicine*
University of Padua
Padua, Italy

Walter Jakob Chwals, M.D.
Associate Professor of Surgery and Pediatrics
Department of General Surgery
Bowman Gray School of Medicine
Winston-Salem, North Carolina

Fredric J. Cohen, M.D.
Department of Medicine
Bowman Gray School of Medicine
Winston-Salem, North Carolina

Brian J. Daley, M.D.
Senior Resident in Surgery
Mary Imogene Bassett
Cooperstown, New York

John M. Daly, M.D.
Professor of Surgery
Division of Surgical Oncology
University of Pennsylvania School of Medicine
Hospital of the University of Pennsylvania
Philadelphia, Pennsylvania

Diana S. Dark, M.D.
Associate Professor of Medicine
Division of Pulmonary Disease and Critical Care
  Medicine
UMKC School of Medicine
Kansas City, Kansas

Nicola D'Atellis, M.D.
Chief Resident in Anesthesiology
Department of Anesthesiology
Division of Critical Care Medicine
Albert Einstein College of Medicine
Montefiore Medical Center
Bronx, New York

Edwin A. Deitch, M.D.
Professor of Surgery
Department of Surgery
LSU Medical Center
Shreveport, Louisiana

Mark H. DeLegge, M.D.
Assistant Professor of Medicine
Section of Nutrition
Division of Gastroenterology
Medical College of Virginia Hospitals
Richmond, Virginia

Elisabeth M. Faber, Pharm.D.,
B.C.N.S.P.
Clinical Assistant Professor
College of Pharmacy
University of Illinois
Chicago, Illinois
Director, Nutrition Support Consult Service
Humana Hospital-Michael Reese
Chicago, Illinois

Josef E. Fischer, M.D., F.A.C.S., D.M.
(Hon)
Christian R. Holmes Professor and Chairman
Department of Surgery
University of Cincinnati Medical Center
Surgeon in Chief
University Hospital
Cincinnati, Ohio

Yuman Fong, M.D.
Department of Surgery
Memorial Sloan-Kettering Cancer Center
New York, New York

R. Armour Forse, M.D., Ph.D.
Associate Professor of Surgery
Director, Nutrition Support Service
Harvard Medical School
Boston, Massachusetts

Bruce Friedman, M.D., F.C.C.P.
Assistant Professor of Medicine and Anesthesia
Robert Wood Johnson School of Medicine
Director, Nutrition Support Services
Director, Intensive Care Unit
Cooper Hospital University Medical Center
Camden, New Jersey

Daniel L. Herr, M.S., M.D.
Assistant Professor
George Washington University
Medical Director, Surgical Intensive Care Unit
Medical Director, MedSTAR
Washington Hospital Center
Washington, D.C.

Loren F. Hiratzka, M.D.
Department of Surgery
Division of Cardiothoracic Surgery
The Jewish Hospital of Cincinnati
Cincinnati, Ohio

Barbara Hopkins, R.D., C.N.S.D.
Atlanta, Georgia

Moira Hurson, B.S.c., S.R.D.
Department of Surgery
Sinai Hospital and Johns Hopkins Medical Institutions
Baltimore, Maryland

Anita F. Jolly, M.S., R.D., C.N.S.D.,
L.D.
Marriott Health Care Services
Mid-Maine Medical Center
Waterville, Maine

Mitchell V. Kaminski, Jr., M.D., S.C.,
F.A.C.S., F.I.C.S., F.A.C.N.
Thorek Hospital and Medical Center
Clinical Professor of Surgery
University of Health Sciences
Chicago Medical School
Chicago, Illinois

David P. Katz, Ph.D.
Department of Anesthesia
Montefiore Medical Center
Bronx, New York

Donald F. Kirby, M.D., F.A.C.P.,
F.A.C.N., F.A.C.G.
Associate Professor of Medicine
Chief, Section of Nutrition
Division of Gastroenterology
Medical College of Virginia Hospitals
Richmond, Virginia

Ronald L. Koretz, M.D.
Professor of Medicine
UCLA School of Medicine
Los Angeles, California
Associate Chief
Division of Gastroenterology
Olive View Medical Center
Sylmar, California

Mark J. Koruda, M.D.
Assistant Professor
Department of Surgery
Chief, Gastrointerstinal Surgery
Associate Director of Adult Nutrition Support Service
University of North Carolina
Chapel Hill, North Carolina

Kenneth A. Kudsk, M.D.
Professor of Surgery
Director of Surgical Research
University of Tennessee
Memphis, Tennessee
Director of Nutrition Support Services
Director of Surgical Intensive Care Unit
Regional Medical Center
Memphis, Tennessee

Vladamir Kvetan, M.D.
Associate Professor of Anesthesiology and Medicine
Department of Anesthesiology
Division of Critical Care Medicine
Albert Einstein College of Medicine
Montefiore Medical Center
Bronx, New York

Sharon Lehmann, R.N., M.S.,
C.C.R.N., C.N.S.N.
Metabolic Nurse Consultant
Nutrition Support Service Team
Staff Nurse, Surgical ICU
University of Minnesota Hospital
Minneapolis, Minnesota

Gary M. Levine, M.D.
Professor of Medicine
Temple University School of Medicine
Head, Division of Gastroenterology and Nutrition
Albert Einstein Medical Center
Philadelphia, Pennsylvania

Robert D. Lindeman, M.D.
Professor and Chief
Division of Geriatric Medicine
Department of Medicine
University of New Mexico School of Medicine
Albuquerque, New Mexico

Calvin L. Long, Ph.D.
Corporate Director of Research
Baptists Medical Centers
Birmingham, Alabama

James M. Long III, M.D.
Senior Vice President
Medical Education and Research
Baptist Medical Centers
Birmingham, Alabama

Stephen F. Lowry, M.D.
Professor of Surgery
Director, Laboratory of Surgical Metabolism
Department of Surgery
Cornell University Medical College
New York, New York

Mark R. Mainous, M.D.
Assistant Professor of Surgery
Department of Surgery
LSU Medical Center
Shreveport, Louisiana

M. Molly McMahon, M.D.
Assistant Professor of Medicine
Mayo Medical School
Consultant
Division of Endocrinology, Metabolism, and Internal Medicine
Mayo Clinic and Mayo Foundation
Rochester, Minnesota

George Melnik, Pharm.D.
Clinical Assistant Professor
Audie L. Murphy Memorial Veterans' Hospital
College of Pharmacy
University of Texas at Austin
Clinical Pharmacy Programs
University of Texas Health Science Center at San Antonio
San Antonio, Texas

Gayle Minard, M.D.
Assistant Professor of Surgery
University of Tennessee
Memphis, Tennessee
Director of Surgical Intensive Care Unit
Veterans Affairs Medical Center
Memphis, Tennessee

Ernest E. Moore, M.D.
Chief, Department of Surgery
Denver General Hospital
Professor and Vice-Chairman
Department of Surgery
University of Colorado Health Science Center
Denver, Colorado

Frederick A. Moore, M.D.
Chief, Surgical Critical Care
Denver General Hospital
Associate Professor of Surgery
University of Colorado Health Science Center
Denver, Colorado

John E. Morley, M.D.
Geriatric Research, Education and Clinical Center
St. Louis VA Medical Center
Division of Geriatric Medicine
St. Louis University Medical School
St. Louis, Missouri

Christine A. Mowatt-Larrsen, Pharm.D.
Assistant Professor of Pharmacy Practice
Albany College of Pharmacy
Albany, New York

Michael S. Nussbaum, M.D, F.A.C.S.
Assistant Professor of Surgery, Physiology, and
  Biophysics
University of Cincinnati Medical Center
Cincinnati, Ohio

Marsha Orr, R.N., M.S., C.N.S.N.
Associate Director
Department of Parenteral and Enteral Nutrition
University of Cincinnati Medical Center
Cincinnati, Ohio

Linda Ott
Research Consultant
Department of Surgery
Division of Neurosurgery
University of Kentucky
Lexington, Kentucky

Michael D. Peck, M.D., Sc.D.
Associate Professor of Surgery
University of Miami School of Medicine
Miami, Florida

Susan K. Pingleton, M.D.
Professor of Medicine
University of Kansas Medical Center
Pulmonary and Critical Care Division
Kansas City, Kansas

Peter W. T. Pisters, M.D.
Department of Surgery
Memorial Sloan-Kettering Cancer Center
New York, New York

James Pomposelli, M.D., Ph.D.
Clinical Fellow in Surgery
Harvard Medical School
Boston, Massachusetts

Robert A. Rizza, M.D., Ph.D.
Professor of Medicine
Mayo Medical School
Consultant
Division of Endocrinology, Metabolism, and Internal
  Medicine
Mayo Clinic and Mayo Foundation
Rochester, Minnesota

Pamela R. Roberts, M.D.
Assistant Professor of Anesthesia/Critical Care
  Medicine
Bowman Gray School of Medicine
Wake Forest University
Winston-Salem, North Carolina

Richard J. Roche, M.D.
Assistant Professor of Medicine
Division of Geriatric Medicine
Department of Medicine
University of New Mexico School of Medicine
Albuquerque, New Mexico

Maurice E. Shils, M.D., Sc.D.
Adjunct Professor (Nutrition)
Department of Public Health Sciences
Bowman Gray School of Medicine
Winston-Salem, North Carolina;
Professor Emeritus of Medicine
Cornell University College of Medicine
New York, New York

Jian Shou, M.D.
Harrison Department of Surgical Research
University of Pennsylvania School of Medicine
Philadelphia, Pennsylvania

Luca Siliprandi, M.D.
Assistente
Department of Plastic Surgery and Burn Unit
School of Medicine
University of Padua
Padua, Italy

Pierre Singer, M.D.
Department of Intensive Care
Rambam Medical Center
Haifa, Israel

Bjorn Skeie, M.D.
Assistant Professor of Anesthesiology
Department of Anesthesiology
Ullevall Hospital
University of Oslo
Oslo, Norway

Michael Y. Suleiman, M.D.
Department of Anesthesia
Section on Critical Care
Bowman Gray School of Medicine
Wake Forest University
Winston-Salem, North Carolina

William A. Thompson III, M.D.
Clinical Research Fellow
Laboratory of Surgical Metabolism
Department of Surgery
Cornell University Medical College
New York, New York

Michael H. Torosian, M.D.
Associate Professor of Surgery
Division of Surgical Oncology
University of Pennsylvania School of Medicine
Hospital of the University of Pennsylvania
Philadelphia, Pennsylvania

Karl S. Ulicny, Jr., M.D.
Department of Surgery
Division of Cardiothoracic Surgery
The Jewish Hospital of Cincinnati
Cincinnati, Ohio

Charles Van Buren, M.D.
Department of Surgery
University of Texas Medical School
Houston, Texas

Robert Wolk, Pharm.D.
Coordinator, Nutrition Support Team
Department of Pharmacy
Tucson Medical Center
Tucson, Arizona

Byron Young, M.D.
Johnston-Wright Chair of Surgery
Division of Neurosurgery
University of Kentucky
Lexington, Kentucky

Gary P. Zaloga, M.D., F.A.C.P.,
F.A.C.N., F.C.C.M.
Professor of Anesthesia/Critical Care and Medicine
Bowman Gray School of Medicine
Wake Forest University
Winston-Salem, North Carolina

PREFACE

The supply of oxygen and nutrients to the tissues is important in the care of critically ill patients. Nutrients provide substrates for cellular energy, mineral homeostasis, and synthesis of vital proteins. They are essential for optimal organ function, and are required for wound repair, immune integrity, and cardiopulmonary function.

Optimal nutrition goes beyond the provision of calories and protein. The type and form of nutrient administration alters cellular metabolic activity and the response to injury. Specific nutrients are currently being used to improve wound healing and immune function, alter cytokine response, and protect organ integrity. Data from clinical studies suggest that optimal nutritional support can reduce infection rates and improve outcome (i.e., reduce mortality and hospital stay) in critically ill patients.

Our view of nutrition has changed dramatically over the past few years. We have learned to use the gut earlier, and have found major advantages of enteral over parenteral nutrition. The gut is believed to be a central organ for maintenance of immune function, and may act as a catalyst in the development of organ failure. In addition, the type of protein, lipid, and carbohydrate administered to patients alters the cellular response to critical illness and metabolic and organ function.

Nutrition in the critically ill hypermetabolic patient differs significantly from nutritional support in the ano-

retic, chronically ill, or healthy person. This book deals with nutritional support of critically ill patients. It discusses nutritional assessment, fuel metabolism, and macronutrient (i.e., protein, fat, carbohydrate, nucleic acid, mineral) and micronutrient (i.e., vitamins, trace element) metabolism. It addresses the route and timing of nutritional support, enteral feeding, parenteral nutrition, wound healing, inflammatory mediators, immunity, the gut barrier, bacterial translocation, and use of growth factors. Nutritional support of a number of common disease states treated in critical care units is discussed in separate chapters. These conditions include trauma, neuroinjury, sepsis, burns, gastrointestinal disease, respiratory and heart failure, renal failure, liver failure, AIDS, and diabetes mellitus.

We have assembled a large number of nutritional experts to address pertinent areas of critical care nutrition. Most are actively involved in research in their area of expertise. These authors have done a superb job of summarizing the available data and developing clinical recommendations based on the information. We thank them for their support of this worthy project.

Nutrition and metabolism are closely interrelated; each affects the other. Optimal nutritional and metabolic resuscitation is aimed at altering cellular response to improve or protect organ integrity and improve functional outcome. The large increase in our knowledge of nutrition and metabolic support over the past few years prompted the writing of this reference text. We hope the information will not only be useful in the clinical management of patients but will stimulate continued research into the benefits of nutrient modulation of critical illness. Nutrition research is evolving, and new discoveries rapidly appearing. I am reminded of a statement by Louisa May Alcott:

> Far away there in the sunshine are my highest aspirations. I may not reach them, but I can look up and see their beauty, believe in them, and try to follow where they lead.

Gary P. Zaloga, M.D.

CONTENTS

PART I

Principles of Nutrition in Critical Care

1

Importance of Nutrition for Critically Ill Patients

Maurice E. Shils, M.D., Sc.D.

Current status and problems

Improving current standard formulations

Critical care and nutrition education

"Sick. . . patients do not oblige their doctors by separating 'metabolic' from 'tissue pathology' states. . .; the whole problem must be solved together, not in sections" (Francis D. Moore).[1]

In his letter inviting me to prepare this introduction, Dr. Zaloga noted that despite the large influx of recent, important information applicable to nutrition/metabolic support of the critically ill patient, much of this information has not reached practicing clinicians taking care of such patients.

There are no doubt a variety of reasons for the lack of interest and awareness of the important roles of clinical nutrition in patient care, not only in the area of critical care but in medicine in general. A relatively poor level of nutrition education of medical students and house staff is the usual state of affairs in most medical schools; this issue is considered below. Another problem is the lack of orientation of many physicians in correlating clinical care with basic metabolic and pathophysiologic problems in patients. This is attribut-

able, in part, to a lack of training in the development of such concepts.

While the healing professions have long recognized the relationship between the wasting of the body and the presence of certain acute and chronic illnesses, the metabolic basis of these changes and their clinical implications have for the most part been developed only over the past 80 or so years. Newer developments in basic chemistry, biochemistry, physiology, nutrition, and technology have increasingly yielded information about the metabolic effects of disease processes. These, in turn, have stimulated interest in improving the nutritional status of the sick.

As the basis for understanding the current nutritional status and needs of the critically ill, it is useful to consider the status of total parenteral nutrition (TPN) at approximately decade intervals since World War II. A starting point is Robert Elman's work on parenteral nutrition in surgery.[2] Elman was a pioneer in his attempts to nourish sick patients intravenously. Although his book was published in 1947, it devoted primary attention to developments from the late 1930s to about 1945. As the result of the work of Warren Cox Jr. and his colleagues at the Mead Johnson Laboratories, a parenterally injectable casein hydrolysate was available to Elman and others. Glucose was given as either 5% or 10% solutions. The need for increased energy provision resulting from trauma and fever was recognized; however, the dependence on peripheral vein infusions with the problem of overhydration and the lack of a suitable intravenous fat preparation precluded meeting the total energy needs of the patient for prolonged periods.

A major concern at that time was to prove that intravenously administered amino acids in the form of the hydrolysate or as free amino acids (available for a short period at that time) were utilized for protein synthesis. This was adequately demonstrated for both types of preparations in adults and in pediatric patients by 1940. It was known that glucose infusions per se reduced the degree of negative nitrogen balance in postoperative patients as compared with saline infusion only. While glucose plus amino acids conserved still more body nitrogen, negative nitrogen balances were the rule for the relatively short periods (7 days or usually less) over which such parenteral infusions were given. Elman was aware that casein hydrolysate contained significant amounts of sodium, chloride, phosphate, sulfur, and smaller amounts of potassium, magnesium, iron, and copper. Potassium could be supplied as lactated Ringer's solution. Knowledge about the role of potassium in clinical states was in its infancy; very little was known about magnesium. When blood fibrin hydrolysate appeared later, its lack of phosphate was found to cause hypophosphatemia when given with large amounts of glucose in the absence of supplementary phosphate.

Some vitamins were available in parenteral form; recommendations were made only for dosages of thiamin, ribo-

flavin, niacin, and ascorbic acid. Trace elements were not mentioned; at the end of the 1930s, the only ones known to be essential for man were iron and iodide.

In uncontrolled nonrandomized clinical comparisons, Elman noted that postoperative surgical patients given glucose, saline, hydrolysate, and some vitamins lost less weight, maintained their serum albumin concentrations better, had less nitrogen loss, and ambulated more rapidly than those given saline and glucose. He regarded parenteral alimentation as a temporary expedient for both practical and theoretical reasons. He noted that there were "undoubtedly other as yet unknown substances in a full normal diet that are important for complete nourishment lasting for any length of time. Moreover, there may be unexplained physiologic advantages of the oral route as compared to the parenteral route."

The next guidepost in this brief review was the great teaching textbook authored by Francis D. Moore, *Metabolic Care of the Surgical Patient* published in 1959.[1] The period between this volume and that of Elman reflects a number of major advances in knowledge of disease-induced metabolic changes. These changes resulted, in part, from progress in endocrinology, electrolyte and fluid metabolism, radioisotope labeling, and clinical nutrition. Changes in body composition during malnutrition were elucidated in association with the concept of the metabolic importance of body cell mass.

It was clear that management of hypermetabolic states required protein and energy input above that of normal conditions. The use of percutaneous central catheters threaded from peripheral veins was advised, but only for 3 days. Major advances had been made concerning the needs of various electrolytes, including magnesium. All vitamins were now available, but Moore's recommendations for vitamin dosages in resting and semistarvation included only those for thiamin, riboflavin, niacin, pyridoxine, and pantothenic acid (all in relatively large amounts) plus vitamin K. There was no mention of trace element needs. Nitrogen equilibrium or even positive nitrogen balances were being achieved in some postoperative patients receiving shortterm parenteral nutrition.[3]

An intravenous fat preparation (intravenous Lipomul) was available at that time. Acute and chronic adverse reactions associated with its use were already apparent by 1957[4] and led to cessation of production by the early 1960s. This created a serious problem for the relatively few physicians in the United States who were attempting to maintain patients for prolonged periods on parenteral nutrition. Hypertonic glucose, by default, had to be the primary energy source for meeting hypercatabolic needs, and central venous catheters were rarely kept in place for periods of a week or more. The Swedish parenteral lipid emulsion Intralipid, which had been developed by Arvid Wretlind, had become widely available in Europe by 1963 but was not approved for general use in the United States and Canada until 1977.

The safety and efficacy, over longer periods, of parenteral nutrition solutions containing hypertonic glucose administered through indwelling central catheters were dramatically demonstrated in 1968 by Dudrick and associates in their initial reports of the use of parenteral nutrition in growing dogs and infants.[5] Their nutrient formula used in dogs included the recommended requirement for dogs of the National Research Council; hence it contained 13 vitamins and five essential trace elements plus cobalt. It was easier to provide all of these nutrients to dogs than to humans because there was no Food and Drug Administration (FDA)-approved commercial complete parenteral multivitamin formulation; therefore, combinations of different preparations were used in the patient studies.

Because there were no available trace elements available in parenteral form except iron and iodide, plasma was given as an interim substitute. The available vitamin formulation containing fat-soluble vitamins (MVI) was not only lacking four essential vitamins but also had its components in relatively high amounts. With the increasing duration of parenteral nutrition, this resulted in the appearance of some vitamin inadequacies and relatively high blood levels of other vitamins, particularly vitamin A. The lack of newer essential trace elements, particularly zinc and copper, meant that physicians and hospital pharmacists had to prepare their own sterile pyrogen-free solutions or else deny them to patients; the first approach created potential safety and regulatory problems but served the patients' needs; the second approach did neither, in which case depletion occurred in longer-term patients.

The Nutrition Advisory Group of the American Medical Association (AMA) recommended to the FDA in 1975 new multivitamin formulations for adult and pediatric use; these included all vitamins except vitamin K in the adult formula. The adult formulation was accepted by the FDA in 1979 and the pediatric formula in 1984; these became the standard formulations in the United States. Experience with these formulations has been satisfactory in avoiding obvious depletion or excess in adults and full-term and older children. However, it is apparent that the pediatric formulation must be revised to meet the needs of the very low−birth weight infant[6]; such a formulation is still not available. Following additional AMA recommendations, commercial intravenous solutions of zinc, copper, manganese, and chromium became available in late 1979. Solutions of selenite and molybdate became available later.

The other major change in formulations was the replacement of protein hydrolysate solutions by those composed of purified free amino acids.[7] This allowed the development of formulations for different clinical situations, ensured better quality control, and (unforeseen at the time) avoided aluminum-contaminated casein hydrolysates. The free amino acid solutions presented problems since they did not contain glutamate nor did they include cysteine and tyrosine, which are poorly soluble.

CURRENT STATUS AND PROBLEMS

Currently, those involved in providing special oral, enteral (tube), and/or parenteral nutrition can have a good degree of satisfaction in achievements in nutrition support. These include good survival outcomes in pregnant women dependent on long-term parenteral nutrition, improved outcome of the very low–birth weight infant, improved nutritional status of patients with a variety of serious malabsorption states (including long-term survival and a good quality of life for those with severe short-bowel syndromes), and improved survival and outcome of acutely ill patients with severe trauma, burns, and infections.

However, this satisfaction must be tempered by the recognition that particularly with regard to parenteral nutrition but also in some respects to enteral feeding, there are unresolved issues of varying degrees of clinical importance.

CAN CURRENT STANDARD FORMULATIONS BE IMPROVED?

There are a number of issues here. Are specific nutrients being given in excessive amounts, i.e., chromium and manganese? Is there still too much contamination with toxic minerals, i.e., aluminum? Are there nutrients and nonnutritional factors present in foods that will be beneficial if added to purified formulas? There is evidence reviewed in appropriate chapters of this

volume that favors the concept that amino acids not considered essential, e.g., glutamine and arginine, may be needed in additional amounts in hypercatabolic states. Should the current intravenous lipid formulations, which are high in long-chain polyunsaturated fats, be modified to include medium-chain fatty acids and ω-3 C20 polyunsaturated fatty acids? Should there be a lower fatty acid-to-phospholipid ratio? Will such lipid changes improve immune functions and decrease free cholesterol and lipoprotein X?

Can we reduce the incidence of hepatobiliary disease (i.e., hepatic cholestasis, fibrosis, and gallstones) associated with TPN beyond that achieved by avoiding excess calories? Is there a need for additional choline in the phospholipids of fat emulsions? Are there measures that will reduce biliary sludge? Can more be done to ensure better bone metabolism in long-term patients receiving parenteral nutrition beyond eliminating aluminum still further? Certainly, educating patients against cigarette smoking and the value of exercise and recommending estrogen or its equivalent to women may reduce the severity of osteoporosis.

Can hyperplasia of residual gut in patients with severe short-bowel syndrome be induced to a significantly greater degree than is currently possible? Certainly, parenteral feeding imposes increased risks, major expense, and a serious handicap. Successful small-bowel transplantation will be available to but a few in the foreseeable future. Optimally, current and future efforts to induce greater gut hyperplasia by the use of growth and other hormones and other agents will result in a significant increase in those able to be maintained on oral and/or tube feeding.

Perhaps the most important and intriguing issue concerns the need for better understanding and control of those metabolic factors that, in advanced cancer with cachexia, in acquired immunodeficiency syndrome (AIDS) with secondary infection, and in sepsis with organ failure, induce (1) a persistent inability of muscle to maintain an overall protein synthetic advantage, (2) abnormal fat loss, and (3) anorexia and other paraneoplastic events. *Can newer or improved measures of nutritional intervention help to prevent or reverse the changes that result in progressive wasting?* Or will the desired metabolic improvements depend entirely on new and more successful nonnutritional therapeutic modalities? Even in the latter event, a significant role for nutritional support will still be necessary to maintain such patients through the therapeutic period.

CRITICAL CARE AND NUTRITION EDUCATION

Many physicians appreciate the importance of nutrition as part of the overall care of patients (therapy), the prevention of disease, and maintenance of health. Despite this, the education of our medical students and house staff in this field continues to be woefully and generally inadequate. The main deficiency is a failure to develop the requisite sensitivity and essential knowledge throughout clinical training. Didactic lectures in particular and even case studies that are devoid of exposure to actual patient care problems are insufficient approaches. Critical care medicine combines a variety of interesting and important clinical challenges and the need for integrating a number of metabolic and therapeutic issues; these often bring nutrition into a meaningful focus for physicians in training. It is my opinion that physicians in the various aspects of critical care can and should play a major role in such an educational effort. To achieve this requires a consistent and planned effort to involve physicians trained in nutrition as an integral part of the teaching effort—preferably in conjunction with the hospital clinical nutrition team. The involvement of such a physician as a role model associated with other physicians in the field will help meet the concerns and actions implicit in Francis Moore's statement that opened this introduction and thus imprint in the students the importance of nutrition in their future practices.

REFERENCES

1. Moore FD: *Metabolic Care of the Surgical Patient.* Philadelphia, WB Saunders, 1959.
2. Elman R: *Parenteral Alimentation in Surgery With Special Reference to Problems and Amino Acids.* New York, Paul B. Hoeber, 1947.
3. Holden WD, Krieger, H, Levey S, et al: The effect of nutrition on nitrogen metabolism in the surgical patient. *Ann Surg* 1957; 146:563.
4. Levenson SM, Upjohn, HL, Sheehy TW: Two severe reactions following the long term infusion of large amounts of intravenous fat. *Metabolism* 1957; 6:807.
5. Dudrick SJ, Wilmore DW, Vars HM, et al: Long-term total parenteral nutrition with growth, development and positive nitrogen balance. *Surgery* 1968; 64:134.
6. Greene HL, Hambidge KM, Schanler R, et al: Guidelines for the use of vitamins, trace elements, calcium, magnesium, and phosphorus in infants and children receiving total parenteral nutrition. *Am J Clin Nutr* 1988; 48:1324, revised Dec 1990.
7. Winters RW, Heird WL, Dell RB: History of parenteral nutrition in pediatrics with emphasis on amino acids. *Fed Proc* 1984; 43:1407–1411.

2

Nutritional Assessment

Brian J. Daley, M.D.

Bruce R. Bistrian, M.D., Ph.D.

HISTORY OF NUTRITIONAL SUPPORT

Humans have recognized a relationship between eating and well-being for millennia, and the composition of the diet is even today assigned a causal role in health, illness, and temperament. Primitive cultures searched for and provided foods with alleged magical and healing properties to the sick and weak. Today, researchers and scientists seek specialized nutrients to circumvent disease and its sequelae and to prolong survival. Although today's goals are not radically different from those of our forebears, the recent understanding of the chemical basis of physiology has led nutrition support into the molecular arena. Substrates, or components of foods, rather than foods themselves are provided with specific metabolic implications that either in their original form or with minor chemical alterations after consumption and metabolism in various pathways can alter body function.

ROLE OF NUTRITIONAL ASSESSMENT

Nutritional assessment determines (1) who requires support to avoid or reduce protein/energy deficit–associated complications, (2) which mode of support to employ, (3) for what period, and

(4) how to gauge the effectiveness of the feeding regimen. Nutritional assessment has lagged scientifically behind metabolic research, mainly because strict clinical parameters that reliably define nutritional status have not been and probably will not be developed. Nutrition, the provision of nutrients, and malnutrition, the result of extended inadequate intake on body composition and function, have an impact on all body systems. Substantial biological variability exists in the individual response to starvation and critical illness. When the response to undernutrition is confounded by other disease processes, the effectiveness of many of the present markers and tests to predict the extent of malnutrition is limited.

Why should one even consider nutritional support? Malnutrition, even imprecisely defined, is associated with increased morbidity and mortality.[1, 2] Malnutrition is not confined to specific geographic areas or economically impoverished regions; 10% to 50% of hospitalized patients have been demonstrated to be undernourished by the same simple criteria,[3–5] although malnutrition in developed countries is overwhelmingly secondary to disease. Variability in the prevalence of malnutrition and the incidence of associated complications arises from the many and varied attempts to rigorously and objectively define malnutrition. This definition is made more difficult by the confusion of inadequate nutrient intake with the state that results. Although both have been called malnutrition, a better description of the pathophysiology results if the former is termed semistarvation and the latter, malnutrition. Semistarvation is best defined clinically as a deficit in protein or calories that leads to malnutrition and increased morbidity and mortality unless reversed. Such complications develop more rapidly in the setting of stress (7 to 10 days) than in the absence of the metabolic response to injury or infection (weeks to months). Refeeding of critically ill semistarved surgical patients with total parenteral nutrition (TPN) is effective in reducing complications[6, 7] and hospitalization costs,[8, 9] although it is less effective at reversing malnutrition. Malnutrition with semistarvation impairs wound healing, increases infectious susceptibility, fosters prolonged ventilatory dependence, and delays return to normal self-sufficient enteral intake.[10] State-of-the-art nutritional support that provides metabolic support, particularly in terms of acid-base status, euglycemia, and administration of essential vitamins and minerals, while avoiding overfeeding that can impair function of the reticuloendothelial system, is required to attain the positive effects of nutrition on outcome. Other research suggests that enteral nutritional support may provide additional benefits by trophic mucosal effects, blunting of hypermetabolism, and stimulation of physiologic absorptive pathways.[11, 12] Select amino acids (i.e., glutamine, arginine, branched-chain amino acids), lipids (i.e., short-chain, medium-chain, ω-3 long-chain, and structured triglycerides), and other nutrients (i.e., soluble fiber, nucleotides) are being investigated to see whether they improve various nutritional and immunologic parameters in the critically ill. These topics will be covered in detail elsewhere, but nutritional assessment is the first step in delivering these nutritional "magical and healing" agents.

Assessment methods have risen to the forefront of nutrition research because of the boom in testing equipment technology. Like many sophisticated therapies, efficient use is now measured by cost in relation to benefit. Given the ubiquitous impact of nutrition on clinical outcome, the search continues for an accurate and cost-efficient marker of malnutrition.

The most efficient and effective weapon in the nutrition support armamentarium is the clinician who possesses a thorough understanding of the metabolic responses to starvation and critical illness, as well as an appreciation for the tools of nutritional assessment. Until a definitive marker or criterion is elucidated to determine whom and/or how and when to feed, the intensivist must be able to assess, institute, and follow nutritional status by integrating many pieces of seemingly incongruous information. There are few if any gold standards in nutritional support; therefore assessment and reassessment rely on the clinical course. The delivery of nutritional support must fit within the confines of clinical care —*primum non nocere*. The efficacy of feeding regimens may not be recognizable by means other than what did *not* happen. This chapter will review metabolic states, discuss assessment tools, and it is hoped, educate the reader in the use of clinical findings as assessment parameters.

METABOLIC RESPONSE TO STARVATION AND INJURY

In the basic sense, nutrition encompasses the delivery of energy and structural substrates for the continued maintenance and function of the organism. In man, this is accomplished by a well-developed and sophisticated process, digestion, wherein foodstuffs are chemically degraded to a manageable and metabolically useful state. They are then absorbed by the intestine into the portal circulation and acted upon by the liver. The liver is the central metabolic regulator for energy synthesis or storage, production of functional and/or structural proteins, and numerous other essential processes. Decreased nutrient intake, malabsorption, or increased energy or protein needs lead to catabolism (consumption) exceeding anabolism (synthesis). The result is a loss of lean or functional tissue. The simplest measure of this loss of lean tissue is weight loss, although body weight

cannot fully describe the cause or composition of the weight loss. Both factors are important in measuring the impact and treatment of malnutrition.

The efficient utilization of energy substrates by various metabolic pathways, as well as the metabolic response to injury, has evolved over thousands of years. By taming his environment man has dramatically altered the etiology of inciting events such as starvation and critical illness. However, this period has been too brief in evolutionary terms for physiologic adaptation to occur.

The response to starvation and injury/infection is net catabolism of body substance for energy and substrate needs. In starvation, the body responds by metabolic adaptations that limit energy consumption and by catabolism. Essential organs (i.e., brain, liver, heart, kidney, etc.) are spared at the expense of skeletal muscle and connective tissue. During infection or critical illness, metabolic adaptation increases the catabolic rate to meet increased energy and protein needs. These changes attempt to increase function of the liver and immune system at the expense of the skeletal muscle and connective tissue.

Nutritionally, the body is composed of three compartments (Fig 2–1): fat-free mass consisting of lean tissue, extracellular water, and body fat. These three compartments, each containing a primary fuel, have a primary role in metabolism. Lean tissue, the metabolically active component, is composed of skeletal muscle, which is the labile protein pool for the body, and the liver, which contains the mobilizable carbohydrate glycogen. The second component, fat, is a vast form of stored energy, with little metabolic activity and minor structural function. The last component is the remaining extracellular aqueous fluid, into which glucose is largely assigned. The carbohydrate in this pool is quantitatively very small (20 g) but qualitatively very important. During normal

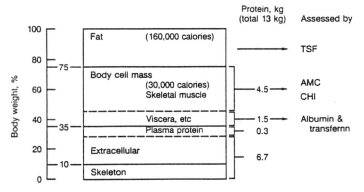

FIG 2–1.

Body composition and energy equivalence in a 70-kg reference subject. *TSF* = triceps skin fold; *AMC* = arm muscle circumference; *CHI* = creatinine height index. (From Bistrian BR: *J Am Diet Assoc* 1977; 71:393–397. Used by permission.)

metabolism, this pool functions to support the lean tissue by providing fuel and carrying away metabolic wastes. The mineral space (bone) is usually disregarded due to its limited metabolic role in response to starvation or injury.

Starvation

If one considers our paleolithic predecessors, the primary stimulus for man's response to starvation was based on the cyclic or seasonal supply of food. In time of plenty, carbohydrates were the primary fuel. This matched well with intake since carbohydrates were the largest component in the diet. Excess ingested energy was stored by the body in its densest form, fat. When resources became less plentiful, as during winter or drought, the body adapted to the reduced energy intake by consuming stored fat and reduced the rate of its metabolic machinery to decrease energy expenditure. Thus, the response to starvation was a beneficial one that protected lean tissue from catabolism as the body provided itself with energy from stored reserves.

The metabolic response to starvation (Table 2–1) is mediated by the potent hormone insulin. Insulin promotes glucose uptake into cells (for metabolism and glycogen storage), protein synthesis, and lipogenesis and reduces glycogenolysis, lipolysis, and proteolysis. During times of surfeit, insulin maintains

and renews lean tissue and stores excess energy. During starvation, because of decreased insulin levels, the metabolic processes are directed to mobilize fat, carbohydrate, and protein.

Physiologically, the response to starvation occurs in two phases. Initially, glycogen stores are consumed to provide glucose for mandatory glucose-burning tissues (i.e., brain, renal medulla, red blood cells). Carbohydrate stores provide only several days of energy; they are quite limited (300 to 500 g) and exhausted by 72 hours of fasting. If exogenous carbohydrate is not provided, further glucose is derived via gluconeogenesis from amino acids and glycerol released from labile protein stores in skeletal muscle (as opposed to visceral protein) and fat, respectively.

The second phase occurs when energy deprivation continues. Glucose is required for those tissues that cannot utilize other energy forms. The remaining tissue, particularly skeletal muscle, adapts to more efficiently burn free fatty acids. Protein for catabolism is prioritized; skeletal muscle protein is consumed preferentially. This is demonstrated by relatively normal serum protein levels and organ function despite the loss of fat and skeletal muscle. The metabolic response to starvation may continue for extended periods of time, with little health risk, until approximately 30% loss of the initial starting weight occurs. Weight loss is rapid

TABLE 2-1.

Metabolic Physiology

Characteristic Finding	Starvation (Marasmus)	Metabolic Response to Injury (Protein-Energy Malnutrition)
Energy needs	Decreased	Increased
Primary fuel (RQ*)	Lipids (0.75)	Mixed (0.85)
Insulin	Decreased	Increased (resistance)
Ketones	Present	Absent
Counterregulatory hormones	Basal	Increased
Total-body water	Decreased	Increased
Proteolysis	Decreased	Accelerated
Glycogenolysis	Increased	Accelerated
Lipolysis	Increased	Increased
Body stores		
Skeletal muscle	Reduced	Reduced
Fat	Reduced	Reduced
Visceral protein	Preserved	Increased liver/immune
Refeeding response	Net anabolism	None (unless reversed)
Weight (lean tissue) loss	Gradual	Accelerated
Typical setting	Chronic diseases (cardiac, COPD,* etc)	Hospitalized/ICU* patient

*RQ = respiratory quotient; COPD = chronic obstructive pulmonary disease; ICU = intensive care unit.

during the early part of starvation, but as the body adapts and reduces energy demands and fluid compartment shifts equilibrate, the rate of weight loss slows considerably. Approximately 25% of the weight loss in men and 33% in women is from lean tissue during prolonged starvation.

Providing enough energy and substrates, not only to halt catabolism but also to rebuild lean tissue, is the goal in refeeding a starved individual. To avoid complications, one must initially refeed judiciously. The structure and function of the heart, kidneys, gut, and other organ systems are diminished in a malnourished patient. Chronic undernutrition results in compensatory mechanisms that increase total-body water (TBW) and retain salt. Early nutritional replenishment should be aimed at gradual repletion with low fluid volume and salt load if refeeding edema or congestive heart failure is to be avoided. Additionally, the resynthesis of lean tissue consumes large quantities of potassium, phosphorus, magnesium, and other trace elements. Intrinsic stores of such elements may be severely depleted. Supplementation during refeeding is required to avoid serum levels that could potentially be fatal.

Critical Illness, Injury, and Infection

The metabolic response to injury (see Table 2-1) evolved as a system to improve the outcome from mild to moderate trauma or infection. Body water and salt are conserved to maintain euvolemia. The acute-phase response is launched to expand liver and immune system tissue volume so as to avoid or ameliorate infection and initiate wound repair. These metabolic events are energy demanding, particularly the protein synthetic and gluconeogenic components. With no expectation of external energy and with the anorexia of injury enforcing semistarvation, energy sources are provided from within.

The response to infection is similar qualitatively to the response to injury, with one important difference. The response to tissue injury is limited in duration in the absence of superimposed infection, whereas the response to infection continues until the infection is overcome. The response includes alterations in energy needs and production, limitation of intake by anorexia, decreased intestinal absorption, diversion of the synthetic machinery to produce immunoactive cells and hepatic structural and acute-phase proteins, and fever, which increases energy consumption on the order of 10% per degree Celsius rise. Again, energy must be provided from endogenous sources. The skeletal muscle and connective tissue components of lean body mass (LBM) bear the brunt of providing energy substrates and protein precursors.[13]

As with starvation, there are two physiologic phases to the metabolic response to injury/infection. The first phase is catabolism of stored sources: fat, labile proteins, and glycogen. Unlike starvation, this response is driven by a host of neuroendocrine and locally active mediators: adrenocorticotropic hormone (ACTH), growth hormone, catecholamines, cortisol, and glucagon. These hormones are collectively termed the counterregulatory hormones because their effects are opposite to insulin's. Glucose remains the preferred fuel for certain processes such as phagocytosis and anaerobic glycolysis. The counterregulatory hormones maintain the supply of glucose and result in hyperglycemia. These mediators drive net protein catabolism, with nitrogen losses of 20 to 30 g/day. Hepatic and immune tissues usually experience net anabolism. The goal is to provide energy and precursors to maintain the metabolic and immunologic response. Insulin is present in increased quantities, but many tissues, particularly skeletal muscle, are resistant to its action. Reversal of catabolism is not possible during severe stress (head and/or multiple trauma, burns, severe sepsis), even if maintenance or supraphysiologic quantities of nutrients are provided[14]; catabolism can only be halted when the factor responsible for the outpouring of the counterregulatory hormones is controlled. Weight and lean tissue loss is rapid and unremitting in the absence of feeding.

The physiologic changes occurring with the metabolic response to injury can be reproduced by cytokine infusion (interleukin-1 [IL-1] and tumor necrosis factor [TNF]).[15] In addition to increasing the other counterregulatory hormones,[16] IL-1 can specifically increase energy expenditure and enhance glucose use and lipolysis.[17] TNF appears to act uniquely on protein metabolism; it stimulates skeletal muscle proteolysis but net hepatic anabolism.[16] Other locally acting agents such as prostanoids (i.e., prostacyclins, prostaglandins, thromboxanes), leukotrienes, and endothelially active substances contribute to increased vascular permeability and altered vascular tone. New therapies are being aimed at manipulating these cytokines so as to alter the metabolic response to injury and improve the practice of nutritional support.

As in starvation, many of the responses characteristic of the metabolic response to injury/infection are beneficial to the host. Tissue sequestration of minerals and trace elements, especially iron, slow bacterial growth. The hyperglycemia of stress ensures that there is ample availability of this fuel, even during hypotension or in poorly perfused organs. Constitutional effects (i.e., anorexia, malaise) signal the host to reduce energy demands of the gut or skeletal muscle so that energy can be directed to the metabolic and repair responses.

For an uncomplicated trauma event such as with major surgery, the net catabolic phase lasts 24 to 72 hours and is followed by conversion to anabolism. In the convalescent anabolic phase, rebuilding of damaged or consumed lean tissue occurs and requires adequate energy and protein intake. On average, the previously well-nourished individual has a 7- to 10-day energy and protein reserve. If the catabolic response persists beyond that time because of the extent of the injury (i.e., major burns, severe trauma), complication(s), infection, or consecutive insults, the effects of cumulative protein losses on structure and function will have an adverse impact on morbidity and mortality for the individual. It is within this week-long window that either the inciting event must be terminated and catabolism reversed or nutritional support begun to avoid further complications.

It is with an understanding of these principles that clinical recommendations for the timing of nutritional support are based. For a severely injured patient whose course will surely extend beyond 7 days, feeding should begin once hemodynamic stability is achieved. For an individual who has undergone major surgery, a 5-day rule is used. If feeding has not resumed after 5 days, nutritional support should begin. If significant malnutrition is present on admission for major elective thoracoabdominal surgery (i.e., >15% weight loss; serum albumin, <3.5 g/dL), 7 days of nutritional repletion should be strongly considered prior to surgery and nutritional support restarted in the early postoperative period. For lesser degrees of pre-existing malnutrition/semistarvation and for emergent surgery, early postoperative feeding needs consideration.

In the setting of stress-induced catabolism, nutritional support is specifically tailored to the metabolic environment. The goal is to provide fluid and electrolytes, manage acid-base disorders, slow catabolism of functional and structural proteins, and provide sufficient precursors for the immune and wound response. Because sodium and fluid retention are maximized in critical illness and large volumes of crystalloid are used in resuscitation, TBW is increased. The fluid volume allowed for nutritional support is often limited below that needed for meeting full nutritional goals. During critical illness, only about half of the protein delivered is used for protein synthesis. The synthetic machinery is not prioritized for restoring lean tissue, but rather for supporting immunologic and hepatic synthesis and healing wounds. A significant proportion of administered protein is used for energy production. Protein-sparing therapy (about 1 g/kg) reduces catabolism of skeletal protein and supplies adequate precursors for the acute-phase response. The use of enteral feedings, even at minimally low rates, offers trophic effects for gut mucosa that may function to limit bacterial translocation as well as provide nutritional support.

METHODS OF NUTRITIONAL ASSESSMENT

The decision to intervene with nutritional support is relatively simple: either the acute event will terminate shortly and the patient resume eating, or the course will be protracted and support initiated. The patient with the "concentration camp" constitution or the patient with a chief complaint of significant unintentional weight loss is easily recognized as being at nutritional risk and requiring nutritional support. In general, even a well-nourished patient who has not begun eating by the fifth postevent day should begin nutritional support. A more difficult decision involves determining the method and formulation to employ. Nutritional deficits may also be disguised. These subtle cases, prominent in the obese and elderly or the anasarcous intensive care unit (ICU) patient, require specific nutritional assessment to determine risk.

The initial nutritional assessment should address three important issues. First, the quantity of lean tissue present and how ongoing processes or recent weight loss has had an impact on this important store of protein and energy should be assessed. Not only should the intensity of the current process be gauged, but the remaining reserve should also be estimated. Second, the temporal course of the nutritional deficit should be outlined. Has the weight loss been insidious over months, have there been remissions or cyclic weight changes, or has there been sudden and accelerated weight loss over the last few weeks? Finally, the natural history of the unsupported disease process must be considered. Is the event self-limited (i.e., long-bone fracture), easily treated (i.e., dehydration, urosepsis), or of low metabolic stress (i.e., coronary artery bypass); is the disease process wasting (i.e., acquired immunodeficiency syndrome [AIDS]); is surgical intervention a possibility (i.e., bowel obstruction/dysfunction, cancer); or is there a hypermetabolic state present (i.e., large burns, severe sepsis, head injury)? Understanding the metabolic milieu present and the driving forces allows one to fit nutritional care to the specific patient.

Assessment parameters encompass physical findings and measurements, laboratory evaluations, provocative or interactive functional tests, sophisticated metabolic and chemical analyses, and an ever-expanding list of new technologies. Several researchers have developed prognostic indices from which outcome conclusions can be drawn based on the extent of nutritional deficits. These indices may be employed to recognize marginal cases or to justify early intervention. In deciding upon which parameters to follow, one must deal with and understand the intricacies of each method. Each parameter may have implications beyond simple nutritional status alone. Just as nutritional status affects all body systems, nutritional support should not be aimed solely at one parameter or system.

Nutritional assessment is a dynamic, ongoing process. After deciding whether or not to feed a patient, clinical status determines the means. Critically ill patients usually have central intravenous access, which makes highly concentrated TPN an easy alternative. The majority of postsurgical patients should have enteral access, which can be ac-

complished by nasoenteral cannulation with feeding tubes. The gut is the preferred route for feeding in all patients. It is contraindicated only in those with intestinal obstruction, acute pancreatitis, or shock. Intolerance may occur at high feeding rates, but there may be benefit to even minimal enteral feeding rates. Less concentrated peripheral intravenous solutions are an alternative form of support for those patients who have no fluid constraints or need only a short period of support.

Assessment should establish protein and caloric goals for feeding, although they are often only partially achievable due to volume limits. Defining energy needs can be accomplished by simple estimates based on weight or weight/height and sex. Energy needs can be pursued more rigorously (by indirect calorimetry) if complications arise. Finally, assessment must judge efficacy of the therapy. In the critically ill, nutritional support therapy must attempt to maintain metabolic homeostasis and meet protein and calorie needs. Outcome is the best marker of optimal nutritional support in such patients, for no reliable short-term indicator exists.

In the intensive care setting, the most common findings upon which nutritional decisions will be based are initial weight/height, percent weight loss, and upper-arm anthropometry to assess body cell mass; caloric intake, past, present, and future, to assess the degree and duration of semistarvation; and serum albumin, leukocyte count, and differential to assess the degree and duration of stress.

History and Physical Examination

George Santayana said, "Those who cannot remember the past are condemned to repeat it."[18] In nutritional assessment, history gives the strongest indication of nutritional compromise prior to critical illness and is the best early indicator of nutritional risk. An unintentional weight loss of 5% in less than 1 month or 10% over 6 months should initiate a search for the cause of malnutrition. Weight loss of 20% is pathognomonic of severe protein energy malnutrition that will adversely affect the outcome from metabolic stress. Weight loss is an important prognostic indicator, with a 10-lb loss correlating with nearly a 20-fold increase in mortality among elective surgical patients.[19] Unfortunately, many critically ill patients will arrive in extremis, and accurate weights cannot be determined until after fluid resuscitation, thus blunting significant weight changes. Family members must then be questioned regarding weight loss, changes in clothing size, and other appropriate historical details.

Weight change does not faithfully reflect the changes in the body compartments. Additional factors in the history can often point to the cause for undernutrition and furnish the grounds for predicting the metabolic changes to be expected. Anorexia, limited food tolerances, dysphagia, nausea, vomiting, diarrhea, and changes in stool consistency are all important clues to ongoing processes that reduce energy/food intake, alter digestion/absorption, or foretell the likelihood of surgical intervention. Apathy, lethargy, and/or altered exercise tolerance can also be attributed to nutritional compromise.

Many nutritional deficiencies have physical manifestations that should be familiar to most observers (Table 2–2). Malabsorption may result in calcium or magnesium deficiency, and prolonged bleeding may be due to vitamin K deficiency. Physical examination can assess relative skeletal muscle mass in the upper part of the arm and quadriceps, and a quick pinch of the skin at these sites can indicate the amount of subcutaneous fat. Tests of muscle strength and endurance will be discussed later.

Subjective Global Assessment

Subjective global assessment (SGA) is a clinical technique to assess nutritional status by features of the history

TABLE 2–2.

Physical Findings in Nutritional Deficiencies

Deficiency	Finding
Protein/energy malnutrition (marasmus)	Muscle wasting, loss of subcutaneous fat, dull brittle hair
Kwashiorkor	Edema, moon facies
Essential fatty acid	Scaly dry skin
B vitamins	Glossitis, neurologic changes
Thiamin	Beriberi (peripheral neuropathy, cardiac failure)
Niacin	Pellegra (dermatitis, diarrhea)
B_{12}	Macrocytic anemia
Vitamin C	Scurvy-eczema, wound breakdown, multiorgan hemorrhages
Vitamin D	Ricketts, rachitic rosary
Vitamin E	Hemolysis
Vitamin K	Bleeding
Calcium	Tetany, paresthesias
Phosphorus	Weakness, confusion, seizures
Magnesium	Carpopedal spasm, lethargy
Iron	Pallor (anemia)
Iodine	Goiter (hypothyroidism)
Copper	Steely hair
Manganese	Dermatitis
Selenium	Myalgias, cardiomyopathy

and physical examination.[20] To remove the basis of nutritional assessment from laboratory tests, investigators sought to devise a scheme for rapid assessment based solely on clinical findings. After some revisions, a worksheet was devised that consisted of the history and physical findings. History deals with weight change, both recent and acute, dietary changes, gastrointestinal symptomatology, and activity level. This information is coordinated with the likely metabolic demands of the primary diagnosis. The physical examination does not rely on strict measurements or rigid documentation; rather it is the subjective impression of subcutaneous fat, muscle volume, and edema detected by palpation.

Patients are then assigned to one of the three classes of malnutrition: well nourished, moderate (or suspected) malnutrition, and severe malnutrition. The diagnosis is based not on a rigid scoring table but the subjective weighting of the factors by the clinician with accommodation for interactions between the findings. For example, weight loss is discounted if edema is present.

This technique has been tested for correlation with objective criteria, interobserver reproducibility, and predictive ability.[21] Statistical review found that the most important observations were weight loss, loss of fat stores, and loss of lean tissue. Other studies, however, have improved subjective assessments by adding an additional objective test, the serum albumin concentration, to improve diagnostic and predictive accuracy.[22, 23]

What role should SGA play in critical care assessment? The technique described is an excellent tool for obtaining the basic nutritional history and performing the physical examination. It can act as a reminder for the nutritionally naive physician to seek the answers to such questions and to further pursue the diagnosis. It is very "operator dependent" and relies on the clinical acumen of the rater. It emphasizes the important contribution that weight loss, fat loss, and muscle wasting play in predicting outcome. Additionally, SGA is very good at detecting the small fraction of patients who are at risk of severe malnutrition prior to a stressful event, such as major thoracoabdominal surgery. Unfortunately, SGA may miss patients with less obvious manifestations of undernutrition who are at risk for complications, as demonstrated in the recent Veterans Affairs Cooperative study.[24] Furthermore, in the intensive care situation it would seem to be of less utility than objective measures (such as fever, leukocytosis, bandemia, APACHE [Acute Physiology, Age, and Chronic Health Evaluation] scores) that define the presence and degree of metabolic stress.

Prognostic Indices

The object of nutritional assessment is to identify patients at risk for increased complications resulting from nutritional deficits and/or those in whom nutritional therapy potentially re-duces those risks. An objective documentation of risk would provide a criterion for instituting, following, and even terminating therapy. However, there are many objective measures purported to reflect nutritional status. These test many different body systems and functions, and each has its own predictive ability dependent on the population studied. Therefore, many researchers have developed equations or schedules based on several of these criteria in order to simplify the method of detection of risk and to improve diagnostic accuracy.

Valid markers or indices need to be simple, easy to obtain and apply, and more sensitive than specific. Early indices focused on single parameters such as weight loss or albumin and on simple application methods (i.e., single cutoff values). As testing became more sophisticated and complex and greater data pools were assembled, detailed mathematical and statistical analyses were developed.

The predictive ability of the prognostic indices is dependent upon the prevalence of malnutrition in the study population and the individual specificity and sensitivity of the test. The sensitivity and specificity can also be affected by the cutoff value for the parameter chosen. For example, when Studley's data are used, a change in the degree of weight loss from 20% to 15% reduces the specificity and accuracy by 50%.[25]

Moreover, these prognostic indices are not without other problems. The laboratory tests and diagnostic tests upon which they are based carry concerns regarding validity, accuracy, and applicability. The use of sophisticated formulas and intricate analysis makes clinical use difficult. The greatest concern arises in the application of specific equations derived from small populations, which tend to be more homogeneous, to the more heterogeneous majority (i.e., extrapolating from the particular to the general).

The earliest laboratory measurement

that received attention for its prognostic value was serum albumin. This marker was chosen after extensive experience with pediatric populations in lesser developed nations, where it defined the syndrome kwashiorkor. It has gained acceptance in hospitalized adults in developed countries because albumin is the most prevalent serum protein and is easily and routinely measured and because its level decreases in response to cytokines. Serum albumin remains one of the primary measures of nutritional status, although it is appreciated that low serum albumin levels better reflect recent injury than nutritional status. Many researchers have correlated serum albumin levels with the risk of surgical and nonsurgical mortality, and it is the standard against which other indices or markers are judged. Serum albumin is the best single assessment parameter for all patients and possibly the best assessment index when the incidence of malnutrition is low. Drawbacks to the use of albumin follow later in this chapter.

A number of other prognostic indices have also been reported. They include anthropometrics, serum proteins, blood cell counts, hand grip dynamometry, body composition analysis, and weight loss. Fortunately, one only needs to be acquainted with a few of the more stable indices.

Instant nutritional assessment (INA) predicts complication rates based on two common laboratory values—albumin and the total lymphocyte count. In an initial study in a general suburban hospital, abnormal values (albumin, <3.5 g/dL; lymphocyte count, <1500/mm^3) predicted increased mortality and increased complications in surgical patients.[26] However, when applying the INA to surgical ICU patients, who have greater incidences of abnormal values, the predictive ability was diminished.[27]

The prognostic nutritional index (PNI) is perhaps the most widely studied. It predicts the percent risk of postoperative complications in patients undergoing gastrointestinal surgery[28] but is of limited value for other clinical populations. This linear predictive equation is based on objective measurements of serum proteins, subcutaneous fat, and immunologic function:

$$PNI\ (\%\ risk) = 158\% - 16.6\ (alb) - 0.78\ (TSF) - 0.2\ (tfn) - 5.8\ (DSH)$$

where alb equals serum albumin in grams per deciliter, TSF equals triceps skin fold in millimeters, tfn equals serum transferrin in milligrams per deciliter, and DSH equals delayed skin hypersensitivity, which is assigned a value of 1 for anergy and 2 for reactive.

The PNI has been applied to several groups of surgical patients for validation[29] in prospective nonrandomized[30] and prospective randomized fashions.[31] Postoperative complications and mortality were reduced by preoperative nutritional support (i.e., at least 7 days of support). At issue in the validation of the PNI is the level at which sensitivity and specificity are maximal and the level at which nutritional support should be instituted.

Only in populations with a malnutrition incidence of at least 40% does the PNI exceed the accuracy of serum albumin alone.[21] Thus, the PNI may be useful in critically ill patients. With an adequate malnutrition prevalence, a PNI greater than 50 predicts mortality with an approximately 65% accuracy. It remains to be demonstrated whether improvement of the PNI by preoperative nutrition reduces complications. However, there is consensus that improvement of nutritional intake in patients with a high PNI improves postoperative outcome.

The hospital prognostic index (HPI) is based on a nonlinear discriminant function incorporating serum albumin, the presence or absence of sepsis and/or cancer, and delayed hypersensitivity. It was devised from an analysis of both medical and surgical patients. Several equations were calculated for predictive ability regarding anergy, sepsis (ongoing and subsequent), and survival[32]:

$$\text{Probability of survival} = 0.91 \, (\text{alb}) - 1.0 \, (\text{DSH}) - 1.44 \, (\text{SEP}) + 0.98 \, (\text{DIA}) - 1.09$$

where alb equals serum albumin in grams per deciliter, DSH equals delayed hypersensitivity where anergy = 2 and reactive = 1, SEP equals sepsis where no sepsis = 1 and septic = 2, and DIA equals diagnosis where cancer = 1 and noncancer = 2. The overall predictive value was 72%. Although the indices have not been widely employed or tested prospectively, serum albumin was the best single predictor of sepsis, anergy, and survival. It was contained in the functions evaluating all three outcomes.

The index of undernutrition (IOU) is based on the relative ranking of five nutritional markers (albumin, transferrin, midarm muscle and fat areas, and percent weight loss) from a series of 200 surgical patients. By using techniques from nonparametric statistics, a point schedule based on the percentile position of each marker was determined on a 100-point scale (five markers at 20 points each). A high point total has a greater likelihood of malnutrition. This technique was employed to create an index based on empirical data and distribution and to avoid constructing an index based on adverse outcome incidence[33] (Table 2–3). In applying the IOU prospectively, its predictive value was similar to the others indices re-

ported previously (68% accuracy). Malnutrition was well correlated with age, cancer diagnosis, hospital stay, and complications in general surgery patients. The IOU awaits further widespread use.

In summary, the use of an objective index is very appealing for nutritional assessment because it can provide a well-defined prognosis. All of the indices are based on combining two or more assays known to be affected by malnutrition, semistarvation, or metabolic stress. In general, they combine history (as percent weight loss), an assessment of body composition (as fat mass), a measure of protein dynamics (as serum proteins), and a functional test (as delayed hypersensitivity). In patient populations where malnutrition is prevalent and often obscured such as in the critically ill, indices have been demonstrated to be more accurate in predicting those patients at risk of complications than single assessment parameters have. In populations with a lower frequency of malnutrition, one or more of the parameters may cease to be relevant. Prognostic indices are, however, poor tools for gauging the efficacy of nutritional support because they are based on tests that are not rapidly responsive to refeeding. The important implication of prognostic indices is that a multisystem approach is needed for complete nutritional assessment due to the interaction of the three prime determinants of nutritional status—semistarvation, malnutrition, and metabolic stress.

TABLE 2–3.

Index of Undernutrition*

	Points				
Assay	0	5	10	15	20
Albumin (g/dL)	>3.5	3.1–3.5	2.6–3.0	2.0–2.5	<2.0
Transferrin (g/L)	>2.0	1.76–2.0	1.41–1.75	1.0–1.4	<1.0
Muscle area (%)	>80	76–80	61–75	40–60	<40
Fat area (%)	>70	56–70	46–55	30–45	<30
Weight lost (%)	0	0–10	11–14	15–20	>20

*Adapted from Hall JC: *JPEN* 1990; 14:582–587.

Laboratory Tests

The diagnosis and treatment of a disease is greatly simplified when a pathognomonic laboratory test exists. Unfortunately, no such parameter has or probably will be developed for nutritional assessment. Nutrition is only one of many factors that affect cell and organ function. Nevertheless, laboratory examination does have a role in nutritional assessment.

Visceral Proteins

Albumin is recognized as the standard for nutritional assessment. Differentiation of the two major forms of malnutrition depends on serum albumin levels. There is a long and productive history of albumin's role in nutritional assessment; it is a standard part of the initial laboratory profile, and low serum albumin levels are universally associated with a greater risk of complications. Why then is nutritional assessment not solely based on the serum albumin level?

Albumin is the most common serum protein and represents about two thirds of the total intravascular pool. It is water soluble and rapidly equilibrates within the bloodstream, where it is most densely concentrated; equilibration into the extracellular space (about 60% of the total pool) takes longer, but the plasma and extravascular pools are interchanged each day. Albumin is the major protein product of the liver and is secreted at a rate of about 200 mg/kg/day, equal to the daily consumption/degradation rate (or about 5% of the total-body albumin). The total albumin pool is 350 g for a 70-kg man. The albumin molecule has a biologic half-life of 20 days. Albumin acts to maintain intravascular oncotic pressure and to transport amino acids, fatty acids, enzymes, hormones, trace metals, and drugs in the plasma.

Because vascular permeability is altered and protein synthesis decreased with the metabolic response to injury, serum albumin levels fall precipitously.

Degradation/consumption of albumin is also increased, and albumin may be lost from sites such as the wound, gut, and kidney. The greatest change in albumin levels is due to redistribution between the intravascular and extracellular compartments, as a result of which about 80% of the albumin pool becomes extravascular. Therefore, a fall in albumin values is usually a better reflection of the metabolic response and its severity and duration than nutritional status per se.[34] Albumin is insensitive to short-term refeeding. Net synthesis does not occur until the catabolic signals remit, and its long half-life prevents acute changes from becoming readily apparent. In the hospitalized patient, additional interventions may also alter the albumin concentration: exogenous albumin infusion, fluid resuscitation, and other concomitant or consecutive insults (surgery, infection, etc.).

Other serum proteins with shorter half-lives such as transferrin, prealbumin, and retinol-binding protein (RBP) have been studied.[35] Transferrin, the serum transport protein for iron, has a half-life of 8 to 10 days. Transferrin also has prognostic value and is more likely to respond to nutritional repletion than albumin is, although this property has not been particularly useful in clinical practice. Baseline transferrin levels, however, are dependent on the iron status of the individual and can therefore be affected by blood loss and transfusion. Transferrin may be a good screening tool in population studies but is of less value for the individual patient.[36]

Prealbumin, with a half-life of 2 days, transports thyroxine in the plasma. It is predictive of nitrogen status as well as dietary carbohydrate intake and is responsive to short-term (7 days) nutritional repletion.[37] Prealbumin is susceptible to many of the same forces that affect albumin—distribution, synthesis, clearance, degradation rates, and comorbidities such as renal failure (the kidney is the major site of disposal).

RBP is a serum transport glycoprotein with a very short half-life (12 hours) and is itself carried by prealbumin. RBP is more responsive to short-term repletion than albumin is, yet it is altered by vitamin A levels and the carbohydrate concentration of the diet. Alteration of kidney function, the main catabolic site of RBP, leads to elevated serum levels. Baseline RBP levels and responses have not been consistent in malnutrition of different etiologies.

Other serum constituents, particularly acute-phase reactants, have also been examined as markers for nutritional status. All of these serum proteins are acutely affected by the state of metabolic stress,[38] and alterations in their levels are probably a better marker for the presence of an injury response than the nutritional state is. Although the identification of an injury response is an important factor in deciding whether nutritional support should be initiated, it can be done more easily, rapidly, economically, and reliably by other means. Restoration of depleted visceral protein levels by nutritional support, however, may be an effective measure of protein repletion under select conditions. However, comparative testing of these parameters has not indicated one parameter as being most effective.[39] The clinical value and cost-effectiveness of serum protein measurements other than albumin have not been established.

Nitrogen Excretion

For the human, an important chemical distinction exists in the composition of the various compartments and fuels metabolized by the body—only protein is composed of nitrogen. All of the nitrogen-containing wastes and by-products are derived from dietary protein. Thus, measuring nitrogen excretion is a method to assess protein nutriture, which constitutes the metabolically active and functional compartment of the body.

Skeletal muscle contains creatinine and creatine in relatively constant amounts. Since the dietary contribution is small in comparison to the skeletal muscle pool, measuring 24-hour creatinine production, which is derived from a constant percentage of creatinine metabolism, quantifies the skeletal muscle mass; decreased skeletal muscle mass reduces creatinine production. It is estimated that 18 to 20 kg of muscle is needed to produce 1 g of creatinine daily.[40] Dietary intake may contribute up to 20% of the creatinine excreted,[41] and creatinine kinetics may be altered in trauma and sepsis without changes in the skeletal muscle pool. Severe renal dysfunction that leads to increased nonurinary clearance (serum creatinine levels of 4 to 6 mg/dL) disrupts the correlation of creatinine excretion to lean tissue mass.[42]

An index of the loss of lean tissue is accomplished by calculating the creatinine height index (CHI). The CHI compares the actual measured value to an expected value of creatinine production from a normal individual of the same sex and height:

CHI = Measured creatinine/expected creatinine

where expected creatinine is ideal body weight (IBW) multiplied by 23 mg/kg for males or by 18 mg/kg for females.[43] A CHI of 80% reflects moderate wasting; a CHI of 60% indicates severe lean tissue loss and reflects an arm muscle circumference (AMC) measurement less than the 10th percentile. The collection of creatinine for 24 hours also provides data for an accurate measure of creatinine clearance.

Additional measurements of nitrogen in the urine may be used to infer protein balance. One gram of nitrogen represents 30 g of lean tissue. Dietary protein averages 16% nitrogen. Most nitrogen is lost in the urine as urea, and several methods to assay total urinary nitrogen exist. If one measures the urine urea nitrogen (UUN) and adds factors for nonurinary losses (2 g/day each for skin and stool losses), one can estimate the nitrogen lost in a day with reasonable accuracy. Nitrogen balance is nitrogen intake from the diet minus nitrogen lost:

$$NB = (\text{Dietary protein} \times 0.16)\\ - (\text{UUN} + 2 \text{ g stool} + 2 \text{ g skin})$$

Additionally, a catabolic index (CI) is derived from the same variables:

$$CI = \text{UUN} - [(0.5 \times \text{Dietary protein} \times 0.16)\\ + 3 \text{ g}]$$

This equation calculates the excess nitrogen created from catabolism of lean tissue for extraordinary energy needs by subtracting the estimated normal dietary nitrogen excretion (the second addend) from the measured excretion. No stress results in a CI less than or equal to zero, in moderate stress the CI is less than 5, and in severe stress it is greater than 5.[44]

Nitrogen balance can be used to estimate needs, assess therapy, and follow the metabolic status. A positive nitrogen balance is the goal of refeeding, but producing a positive balance must be done within the constraints of the clinical status. Protein supplied in quantities greater than 1.75 g/kg/day contributes solely to ureagenesis. A futile cycle may be created in which more protein is poured in to match the unused protein excreted. One may sense accomplishment by reaching a nitrogen balance, although this is a mirage because the nitrogen balance becomes increasingly inaccurate and falsely positive at high protein intakes. If counterregulatory hormones are orchestrating the metabolic response, net anabolism will not occur no matter what the nitrogen balance. For these reasons, nitrogen balances have little prognostic capability, although the more negative the balance is, despite adequate dietary protein (1.5 g/kg/day), the more catabolic the patient.

In patients with sources of extrarenal nitrogen losses (i.e., gastrointestinal fistulas, diarrhea), nitrogen loss is usually greater than assumed, although nitrogen stool losses greater than 2 g/day are uncommon. In patients with renal dysfunction, the increased blood urea pool and extrarenal urea losses must be accounted for:

$$NB = \text{Nitrogen in} - (\text{UUN} + 2 \text{ g stool} + 2 \text{ g skin}\\ + \text{BUN change})$$

where NB is nitrogen balance and blood urea nitrogen (BUN) change is TBW multiplied by the final minus the initial BUN values during the measurement period.[45]

Urine collections for nitrogen balance in the clinical setting are not a precise measurement but remain a useful tool in nutritional assessment even in the critically ill. They are fairly easy to obtain, although the completeness of the collection requires the determined cooperation of ancillary staff and may only be validated by serial collections or concordance of urinary creatinine levels. The metabolic milieu and level of catabolism are assessed by the amount of nitrogen generated in the urine. Providing adequate exogenous protein and calories will reduce the lean body catabolism, which can be followed by the UUN. Serial measurements should be performed on a weekly basis, primarily for assessment of the metabolic state.

It deserves reemphasis that the dietary goal in the setting of catabolic stress is to meet energy expenditure and provide protein at 1.5 g/kg/day of dry weight, whatever the resultant nitrogen balance. When stress remits, marked by declining fever, decreasing leukocyte counts, and improving nitrogen balance, consideration can be given to increasing the caloric intake to promote a positive energy and protein balance.

Body Composition
Division of the body into its compositional segments provides a means to uncover the effects of hidden malnutrition. Alterations in one functional component can be hidden by increases in the other components without significant

weight change. Repletion of the lean tissue compartment, which is normally hydrated, is the goal of nutritional support. Detecting changes in the size and composition of individual compartments may be used to diagnose malnutrition and judge the efficacy of support. Assessment of these compartments may be accomplished by several methods. The use of nitrogen and creatinine excreted in the urine has been discussed. Comparisons may be made to a normal distribution of humans of known status or composition by age, sex, and/or physical findings (weight for height, IBW tables) or by direct measurements such as skin fold thickness or precise elemental measurements.

Comparative Tables.—Data collected and tabulated from large groups of individuals are employed in an epidemiologic assessment of nutritional status. Collections of average weight for height and age are of little use for the individual and of even less value for the critically ill patient. Tables based on weight for height associated with mortality (Metropolitan Life Insurance Company tables) may be of more use since they have some prognostic value, but they are not based on age, need subjective assessment for frame size, include few ethnic variations, and are based on data from the past (>30 years). The equation for body mass index (BMI) normalizes for height and is an improvement for comparing diverse populations:

$$BMI = \text{Body weight (kg)/(height)}^2 \text{ (m)}$$

The BMI has only recently come int o favor, and its predictive value has been applied more to obesity rather than to undernutrition.

These comparative measures do have a descriptive value and can provide safe estimates for weight if no preresuscitation value was obtained. In the American population, marked deviation from the ideal weights is generally in the positive direction and indicative of the increasing prevalence of obesity. Obesity is important to diagnose, even in the critically ill patient, because its associated insulin resistance makes glucose control problematic and requires a deviation from normal nutritional goal estimation in terms of determining protein and calorie needs based on IBW rather than present weight.

Anthropometry.—Measurement of the midarm muscle circumference and triceps skin fold thickness has been used to define the skeletal muscle pool and the fat stores. Anthropometric measurements may be used in comparison to age and sex group normal values and in chronologic fashion individually. When making comparisons to normal distribution, similar problems arise as for weight-to-height records. Anthropometry is not temporally sensitive and may not detect changes when support periods are less than 1 month. Their principal value is to define the severely malnourished (i.e., under the 10th percentile), particularly in patients with increased TBW (ascites, edema). Skin fold thickness and arm circumference are easily, rapidly, and painlessly obtained and ready for immediate analysis. They require a trained technician since intermeasurement consistency is operator dependent. Costs and risks are minimal (no radiation or invasive procedure).

Half of body fat is subcutaneous in a normal healthy individual. The arm provides an easily accessible region for such measurements. The subcutaneous fat and arm circumference are used to calculate AMC based on a constant symmetrical distribution and simple geometric shape for fat, bone, and muscle, respectively. Although these assumptions are not precise measurements of these tissues (as correlated to computed tomography [CT] or ultrasound), the model does provide a reasonable range of accuracy,[46] and when compared with tables of normal individuals, these inherent errors are negated. Severe protein-energy malnutrition is defined by an AMC value less than the 10th percentile.

Arm muscle measurements have been correlated with other body composition assays. AMC correlated well with energy content and CHI but poorly with nitrogen balance or energy expenditure[47] for intuitively obvious reasons. Anthropometric measurements, as with all body composition analyses, are a static measure of tissue compartments. Unfortunately, this simple and inexpensive test is not sufficiently sensitive enough for assessing the efficacy of nutritional support. Skin fold thickness and AMC tables have not been established for the elderly, and there is no consideration for well-muscled individuals. The skin fold measurement should therefore not be extended to encompass the total-body fat pool. Anthropometric measurements are of value because they give immediate results, are more quantitative than subjective assessment, and can be of use when edema or ablative surgery has complicated body weight or other markers.

Chemical Analysis.—The physicochemical properties of the atoms that constitute the human body can be measured to precisely delineate the metabolically active mass, energy reserves, and fluid and mineral compartments of the body. The simple two-compartment model of body composition may now be expanded and configured by using data from measuring TBW and extracellular fluid (ECF) by isotope dilution methodology; total-body potassium (TBK) from whole-body ^{40}K γ-decay; various elemental minerals (Ca, Mg, P, Na, Cl, I, Cd) and total-body nitrogen from prompt γ-neutron activation; bone mineral and fat content by dual-photon absorptiometry; and total-body carbon from inelastic neutron scattering. Hydrodensitometry is widely used to determine body fat in competitive athletes but is not practical for the critically ill. The application of other biochemical principles, bioimpedance and bioconduc-

tance, await validation, although these techniques depend on normal hydration, a state that is invariably altered in the critically ill. These tests are research tools and difficult to apply to the critically ill because of both testing logistics and theoretical assumptions. Such tests are best employed to establish compositional relationships between more easily measured or obtained values. Moreover, findings from several clinical research trials with precise atomic compositional analyses confirm the present metabolic response hypothesis.

The use of tritiated water and a radioactive sodium isotope establishes TBW and the exchangeable sodium pool (^{Na}e). Other compositional compartments are derived from these values. LBM equals TBW divided by 0.73, a factor accounting for the measured water content of the lean tissue.[48] Body fat is simply body weight minus LBM. The ECF, calculated from the least-squares averaging of serial sodium isotope plasma concentrations, is used to determine intracellular fluid (ICF) by subtraction from TBW. Exchangeable potassium (^{K}e) can be derived from the aforementioned data or measured as TBK and, in addition, is a measure of body cell mass (BCM = LBM + extracellular mass [ECM]). To normalize for body size, the exchangeable sodium or potassium pools are divided by TBW. The latter technique does control to some extent for the hydrational disturbances in the critically ill patient but suffers from reliance on the assumption of a normal potassium/nitrogen ratio in lean tissue, which is known to be false. This technique is quite costly and requires further radiation exposures. Nevertheless, such distinctions are important when body composition methods are used to assess malnutrition and nutritional support efficacy.

Studies done in malnourished patients and controls revealed that weight loss, determined by the above methods, is due to body fat changes; LBM was not different between groups. However, the composition of the LBM in starved patients differed from the controls. BCM was reduced, with a concomitant increase in ECM.[49] Similar results were seen in postoperative patients, and an $^{Na}e/^Ke$ ratio less than 1.22 is representative of significant BCM loss and is therefore diagnostic of malnutrition.[50] In a malnourished patient, even short-term (i.e., 2 weeks) TPN led to increased BCM and decreased ECM.[51]

Other researchers have expanded the compartmental model and derived LBM-defining relationships to fit the increasing number of measurable elemental pools now available. Measuring total-body nitrogen by prompt γ-neutron activation and determining total-body calcium and chloride by delayed neutron activation can provide a compositional solution that is more appropriate when metabolic derangements exist, such as obesity and renal failure, than can TBK or dilutional methods.[52] Increased concern over bone mineralization has led to increased use of dual-photon absorptiometry, which can be employed to determine a mineral component for further detailed compositional analysis. In addition, fat compartment assessment is being evaluated with calibration of soft-tissue photon attenuation.

Relationships between body compartment and elemental composition have been derived from cadavers and noninstitutionalized volunteers. They are based on the assumption that the elemental and hydrational relationships are maintained in a steady state. Critically ill patients would not be described as being in a steady state. Measurement techniques also require equilibrium and often a sophisticated immobile machine. This prevents compositional measurement of most of the severely ill except in highly specialized and unique settings.[53] Also, the application of measurements, generalized to different age and ethnic groups, is not appropriate because compositional differences do exist.[54] Until further data accumulate, body compositional analysis of this com-plexity has little clinical utility in critical care nutritional assessment.

Functional Tests

Malnutrition represents a nutritional deficit that increases the risk of complications because the function of vital processes is impaired. The loss of tissue may forecast potential problems but does not measure functional status. As one recalls, there is relative, but not complete preservation of organ function during pure starvation. Most of the previous tests for assessment have focused on static quantities. Should not malnutrition and response to therapy be assessed by tests of tissue function rather than tissue volume?

Because of the intricacy and interaction of most organ systems, functional impairment is not easily assigned to one independent cause. Plasma protein synthesis may be viewed as an assessment of liver synthetic function, although, as discussed, the myriad of events surrounding that synthetic event do not solely relate to the level of nutritional status. Nitrogen excretion may be viewed as a measure of protein function in energy production, although it is more a function of the severity of the catabolic response and the amount of lean tissue. Immunologic function and skeletal muscle function are parameters that are frequently employed to assess nutrition because they are simple and readily available and have a direct link to outcome (i.e., susceptibility to infection and respiratory strength, respectively).

Immune Response

Testing immune function in malnourished patients is a sound idea because infectious complications are the root cause of morbidity and mortality in the critically ill. Immunologic function is altered by malnutrition.[55] Malnutrition affects almost every component of the immune response, including cell-mediated immunity, complement function, immunoglobulin synthesis, phagocytosis/killing function, and cytokine production. Malnutrition is the largest single cause for immunocompromise in the world. Reversal of malnutrition-induced immune defects should translate into reduced complications and improved survival.

Cellular immunity is perhaps the most sensitive component of undernutrition. Delayed cutaneous hypersensitivity testing is an easily performed and reliable test for cell-mediated immune function and correlates with host resistance to tumor, bacteria, and fungi. Following the intradermal injection of common recall antigens (i.e., *Candida*, mumps) the skin site is observed at 24 and 48 hours for a response. Induration greater than 5 mm is considered to represent intact immune function. Cutaneous anergy has been correlated with increased sepsis and mortality.[56] Anergy resulting from malnutrition can be corrected with nutritional support.[57]

Many nonnutritional factors also affect cellular immunity. The presence of an ongoing infection can alter the skin response, as can the presence of metabolic stress (response to injury, surgery). Numerous drugs, especially steroids, and chronic ailments such as liver and kidney diseases may result in anergy.[58] In light of the metabolic stress(es) and comorbidities present in the critically ill patient, it is difficult to ascribe skin anergy solely to nutritional status. Adequate nutritional support along with control of underlying disease is essential for delayed cutaneous hypersensitivity responses.

Lymphoid tissue such as the thymus, spleen, and lymph nodes is reduced in malnutrition. The number of lymphocytes in the periphery are also decreased by malnutrition. The lymphocyte count has been suggested as a "poor man's" test for immunocompetency.[59] However, lymphocyte counts are affected by many of the same factors that affect cell-mediated immune functions, particularly the stress response and therapeutic corticosteroids. Lymphocyte counts correlate best with undernutrition in marasmus where metabolic stress is absent. On the other hand, lymphocyte counts correlate poorly with nutritional status in critically ill patients, where metabolic stress and infection are common.

There is a reduced capacity to produce IL-1, a key mediator of fever and the metabolic stress response, in protein-malnourished animals[60] and patients.[61] This response is reversed by refeeding. Other concomitant responses to IL-1, such as leukocytosis and acute-phase protein production, are also suppressed with malnutrition.[62]

Muscle Strength

Skeletal muscle is the source of energy and synthetic precursors during the metabolic response to injury. Changes in skeletal muscle mass are assessed clinically by AMC, histologically by atrophy of fibers and Z-band degeneration, and metabolically by alterations in pH and electrolyte concentrations.[63] Electromyographic testing demonstrates an inability of malnourished muscle to maintain tetanic contractions, a slower relaxation rate, and a reduction in force generation. These changes occur before structural manifestations are apparent and result from reduced muscle glycogen, loss of phosphorylation capacity, and calcium accumulation.[64]

Reduced grip strength, measured by dynamometry, is correlated with an increased risk of postoperative complications.[65, 66] This method is rapid, inexpensive, and sensitive. It represents a good screening test for malnutrition.

Respiratory muscle function may be impaired by malnutrition. In those with protein depletion, as measured by body composition analysis, test results of respiratory muscle strength and function were depressed. Loss of respiratory muscle function predisposes to postoperative pneumonia and longer hospital stays.[67] Vital capacity may also hold promise as an assessment tool for malnutrition.

Functional tests (i.e., squeezing a dynamometer or performing pulmonary function tests) are difficult to perform in the critically ill patient. On the other hand, inspiratory muscle strength can be reasonably assessed, even in intubated patients. Subjective tests of muscle strength may also be useful and can be performed, for example, by simply having the patient squeeze the examiner's hand. Windsor and Hill suggest adding cough strength to the assessment of respiratory muscle function.[68] Our laboratory has experimented with measuring the work of breathing in ventilator-dependent patients. The oxygen cost of breathing represents the incremental change in oxygen consumption when going from full mechanical ventilatory support to spontaneous breathing.[69] This value, which is normally 3% of the energy expenditure, is associated with an inability to wean from mechanical ventilation when greater than 15%.[70]

Metabolic Cart

Nutritional assessment includes the prediction and/or estimation of protein and energy needs. The most accurate clinical method is to measure energy expenditure. Frequently, nutrition support services or ICU teams have indirect calorimeters at their disposal for precise energy expenditure measurements. Metabolic carts measure oxygen consumption and CO_2 production. They calculate the respiratory quotient and energy expenditure.

Basal energy expenditure (BEE) represents the resting basal metabolic rate. It is dependent on the size of lean tissue mass and is influenced by the metabolic milieu, fever, ambient temperature, the thermic effect of food, and activity. There are upward of 200 formulas for estimating energy expenditure. The most

frequent and widely used is the Harris-Benedict equation (HBE), which has good applicability in normal individuals:

HBE BEE = 66 + (13.7 × W) + (5 × H) − (6.8 × A) in males

665 + (9.6 × W) + (1.7 × H) − (4.7 × A) females

where W = weight in kilograms, H = height in centimeters, and A = age in years. The BEE is multiplied by factors for metabolic stress and activity level to arrive at an actual daily energy expenditure. Unfortunately, these equations predict well the average energy expenditure for normal patient populations but not the needs for individual critically ill patients.[71] On the other hand, indirect calorimetry is able to accurately measure two of the three major components of energy requirements—the basal metabolic rate and the thermogenic effect of feeding. The third component, activity, is trivial in comparison to the other two in the critically ill bedridden patient.

Indirect calorimetry is a labor-intensive test because a steady state is needed for accurate measurements. A complete assessment requires three to five measurements throughout the day to arrive at a daily average. Hyperventilation or hypoventilation may interfere with short-term CO_2 measurements, and high oxygen tensions reduce the sensitivity of the oxygen sensor. The practice of estimating the total energy needs by increasing the BEE by a stress/activity factor is questionable in the ICU patient.[72] The majority of patients are sedated, artificially ventilated, and expending energy at a rate determined by their response to injury/infection. To adjust the value of the BEE obtained directly from the metabolic cart by multiplying it by a stress or activity factor is folly. In a surgical intensive care population of elderly patients with complications from thoracoabdominal procedures, investigations have found that actual energy expenditure closely approximates the HBE BEE.[72] The HBE BEE or energy expenditure based upon weight (25 kcal/kg/day) both have about the same accuracy in predicting energy expenditure. However, the correlation of these methods with measured energy expenditure may be modest due to imprecision in measurements. When effort and time are used to obtain steady-state values for work-of-breathing analysis, the measured value of BEE by indirect calorimetry correlates closely with the HBE BEE.[73] We suggest initiating nutritional support by using estimates of energy expenditure based upon simple formulas. If clinical improvement does not occur (i.e., there are additional complications), then the labor-intensive and complex method for precise measurement of energy expenditure should be used.

MONITORING THERAPY

Nutritional assessment is a daily event in critically ill patients. It includes assessment of metabolic stress. Rapid clinical status changes warrant close observation and daily tailoring of nutritional support composition, mode of delivery, and volume of support. Nutritional support is aimed at maintaining the appropriate internal milieu in terms of metabolic homeostasis so as to facilitate effective resolution of the ongoing process without producing adverse consequences directly related to refeeding.

Intravascular and extracellular volumes are important considerations in critical care. There are shifts between fluid compartments coincident with the injury response, the need for diuresis, administration of fluids, and losses from wounds or ostomies. Electrolyte and mineral levels must be monitored and replaced. Nutrition provides an ideal means for replacing fluid and electrolytes, controlling acid-base disorders, and administering protein and energy substrates.

Nutritional Goals

To achieve the benefits of feeding, the critically ill patient should receive adequate protein and calories. Therapy is aimed at reducing protein catabolism while fostering whole-body protein synthesis. Protein requirements range from 1.0 to 1.5 g/kg/day.[74, 75] Nitrogen balance can be useful for adjusting protein intake. Protein requirements are decreased in patients with renal insufficiency, and protein intake may need to be restricted in patients with hepatic insufficiency.

Caloric goals may be estimated from the HBE or from weight (i.e., 25 kcal/kg/day for the older patient after elective surgery and 30 to 35 kcal/kg/day for the younger trauma patient). We recommend providing a mixed fuel system (i.e., carbohydrates and fats). Overfeeding, especially of carbohydrates but also of fats, can reduce the beneficial effects of nutritional support. Hyperglycemia resulting from large carbohydrate loads in the face of insulin resistance results in immunologic compromise.[76] Excessive carbohydrates can also impede weaning from mechanical ventilation[77] and lead to steatosis of the liver. Excessive administration of lipids, at greater than 50% of calories, can overload the reticuloendothelial system[78] and may impair alveolar gas exchange. Trials of preoperative TPN[23, 79] may have lacked benefit because of excessive feeding of carbohydrates and/or lipids. Due to underlying obesity and the high ω-6 fat intake of the American population, essential fatty acid deficiency is not a problem in short-term refeeding, although modest amounts of fat provided continuously can be helpful.

Nutritional goals should be set and therapy delivered to provide enough protein for synthesis of hepatic structural and acute-phase proteins and immunoactive cells and their paracrine messengers, wound repair, and limitation of catabolism. Caloric goals should just meet or slightly underestimate needs if complications attributable to overfeeding are to be avoided. Modest volumes of fat (about 20% of the total calories) and carbohydrates, with supplemental insulin if needed to control hyperglycemia, should be administered.

Most nutritional assessment tools are not sensitive enough to measure repletion on a daily or even weekly scale. The clinical course represents the best measure of nutritional support efficacy. Unfortunately, not all patients recover from their illness. In difficult or prolonged illness, where energy expenditure may be elevated secondary to an increased work of breathing or gastrointestinal and/or wound losses, the metabolic cart should be used to accurately measure energy expenditure. Final outcome is the ultimate assessment tool. It is hoped that aggressive nutritional support, instituted and revised daily, will eliminate protein-energy deficits as causative or contributing factors to poor outcomes.

Nutritional assessment should assess body composition, the presence and duration of semistarvation, and the degree and duration of metabolic stress to determine when nutritional support should be employed to reduce complication risks. A multifaceted approach is employed in assessing the critically ill patient. History and physical examination determine the pre-existing metabolism and nutritional status. They detect existing deficits and can be useful in predicting future metabolic stress and designing a nutritional support plan. Laboratory examination confirms these findings, provides an objective measure for risk assessment, and may be helpful in gauging therapeutic benefit. Tests of functional capacity can also detect deficits and be used to assess ongoing therapy. Current assessment methods are excellent for detecting the severely malnourished and the well-nourished patient. However, they are relatively poor at detecting borderline malnutrition. The best tool for uncovering clandestine nutritional deficits is a high index of suspicion and the liberal institution of nutritional support.

REFERENCES

1. Studley HO: Percentage of weight loss: A basic indicator of surgical risk in patients with chronic peptic ulcer. *JAMA* 1936; 106:458–460.
2. Cannon PR, Wissler RW, Woolridge RL, et al: The relationship of protein deficiency to surgical infection. *Ann Surg* 1944; 120:514.
3. Bistrian BR, Blackburn GL, Hallowell E, et al: Protein status of general surgical patients. *JAMA* 1974; 230:858–860.
4. Bistrian BR, Blackburn GL, Vitale J, et al: Prevalence of malnutrition in general medical patients. *JAMA* 1976; 235:1567–1570.
5. Willard MD, Gilsdorf RB, Price RA: Protein-calorie malnutrition in a community hospital. *JAMA* 1980; 243:1720–1722.
6. Muller JM, Keller HW, Brenner U, et al: Indications and effects of preoperative nutrition. *World J Surg* 1986; 10:53–63.
7. The Veteran Affairs Total Parenteral Nutrition Cooperative Study Group: Perioperative total parenteral nutrition in surgical patients. *N Engl J Med* 1991; 325:525–532.
8. Goel V, Detsky AS: A cost-utility analysis of preoperative total parenteral nutrition. *Int J Technol Assess Health Care* 1989; 5:183–194.
9. Askanazi J, Hensle TW, Stader PM, et al: Effect of immediate postoperative nutrition support on length of hospitalization. *Ann Surg* 1986; 203:236–239.
10. Mughal MM, Meguid MM: The effect of nutritional status on morbidity after elective surgery for benign gastrointestinal disease. *JPEN* 1987; 11:140–143.
11. Wilmore DW, Smith RJ, O'Dwyer ST, et al: The gut; a central organ after surgical stress. *Surgery* 1988; 104:917–923.
12. Daly JM, Bonau R, Stofberg P, et al: Immediate postoperative jejunostomy feeding: Clinical and metabolic results in a prospective trial. *Am J Surg* 1987; 139:198–206.

13. Scrimshaw NS: Effect of infection on nutrient requirements. *JPEN* 1991; 15:589–600.

14. Streat SJ, Beddoe AH, Hill GL: Aggressive nutritional support does not prevent protein loss despite fat gain in septic intensive care patients. *J Trauma* 1987; 27:262–266.

15. Pomposelli JJ, Flores EA, Bistrian BR: Role of biochemical mediators in clinical nutrition and surgical metabolism. *JPEN* 1988; 12:212–218.

16. Flores EA, Bistrian BR, Pomposelli JJ, et al: Infusion of tumor necrosis factor/cachectin promotes muscle catabolism in the rat; a synergistic effect with interleukin-1. *J Clin Invest* 1989; 83:1614–1622.

17. Tocco-Bradley R, Georgieff M, Jones CT, et al: Changes in energy expenditure and fat metabolism in rats infused with interleukin-1. *Eur J Clin Invest* 1987; 17:504–510.

18. Santayana G: *The Life of Reason,* vol 1, *Reason in Common Sense.* In Beck EM, ed: *Familiar Quotations by John Bartlett,* ed 14. Boston, 1968, Little, Brown, p 866.

19. Seltzer MH, Slocum BA, Cataldi-Betcher EI, et al: Instant nutritional assessment: Absolute weight loss and surgical mortality. *JPEN* 1982; 6:218–221.

20. Detsky AL, McLaughlin JR, Baker JP, et al: What is subjective global assessment of nutritional status? *JPEN* 1987; 11:8–13.

21. Baker JP, Detsky AS, Wesson D, et al: Nutritional assessment: A comparison of clinical judgment and objective measurements. *N Engl J Med* 1982; 306:969–972.

22. Detsky AS, Baker JP, O'Rourke K, et al: Predicting nutrition-associated complications for patients undergoing gastrointestinal surgery. *JPEN* 1987; 11:440–446.

23. Pettigrew RA, Hill GL: Indicators of surgical risk and clinical judgment. *Br J Surg* 1986; 73:47–51.

24. The Veterans Affairs Total Parenteral Nutrition Cooperative Study Group: Perioperative total parenteral nutrition in surgical patients. *N Engl J Med* 1991; 325:525–532.

25. Dempsey DT, Mullen JL: Prognostic value of nutritional indices. *JPEN* 1987; 11(suppl):109–114.

26. Seltzer MH, Bastidas JA, Cooper DM, et al: Instant nutritional assessment. *JPEN* 1979; 3:157–159.

27. Seltzer MH, Fletcher HS, Slocum BA, et al: Instant nutritional assessment in the intensive care unit. *JPEN* 1981; 5:70–72.

28. Mullen JL, Buzby GP, Waldman MT, et al: Prediction of operative morbidity and mortality by preoperative nutritional assessment. *Surg Forum* 1979; 30:80–82.

29. Buzby GP, Mullen JL, Hobbs CL, et al: Prognostic nutritional index in gastrointestinal surgery. *Am J Surg* 1980; 139:160–167.

30. Mullen JL, Buzby GP, Matthews DC, et al: Reduction of operative morbidity and mortality by combined preoperative and postoperative nutritional support. *Ann Surg* 1980; 192:604–613.

31. Smith RC, Hartemink R: Improvement of nutritional measures during preoperative parenteral nutrition in patients selected by the prognostic nutritional index: A randomized controlled trial. *JPEN* 1988; 12:587–591.

32. Harvey KB, Moldawer LL, Bistrian BR, et al: Biologic measures for the formulation of a hospital prognostic index. *Am J Clin Nutr* 1981; 34:2013–2022.

33. Hall JC: Use of internal validity in the construct of an index of undernutrition. *JPEN* 1990; 14:582–587.

34. Klein S: The myth of serum albumin as a measure of nutritional status. *Gastroenterology* 1990; 99:1845–1846.

35. Shetty PS, Watrasiewicz KE, Jung RT, et al: Rapid-turnover transport proteins: An index of subclinical protein-energy malnutrition. *Lancet* 1979; 2:230–232.

36. Roza AM, Tuitt D, Shizgal HM: Transferrin: A poor measure of nutritional status. *JPEN* 1984; 8:523–528.

37. Tuten MB, Wogt S, Dasse F, et al: Utilization of prealbumin as a nutritional parameter. *JPEN* 1985; 9:709–711.

38. Rem J, Saxtrup-Nielsen O, Brandt MR, et al: Release mechanisms of postoperative changes in various acute phase proteins and immunoglobulins. *Acta Chir Scand* 1980; 502:51–56.

39. Borras M, Peterson O, Knox L, et al: Serum proteins and outcome in surgical patients. *JPEN* 1982; 6:585.

40. Forbes GB, Bruining GJ: Urinary creatinine excretion and lean body mass. *Am J Clin Nutr* 1976; 29:1359–1366.

41. Bleiler RE, Schedl HP: Creatinine excretion: Variability and relationships to diet and body size. *J Lab Clin Med* 1962; 59:945–955.

42. Jones JD, Burnett PC: Creatinine metabolism in humans with decreased renal function: Creatinine deficit. *Clin Chem* 1974; 20:1204–1212.

43. Bistrian BR, Blackburn GL, Sherman M, et al: Therapeutic index of nutritional depletion in hospitalized patients. *Surg Gynecol Obstet* 1975; 141:512–516.

44. Bistrian BR: A simple technique to estimate the severity of stress. *Surg Gynecol Obstet* 1979; 148:675–678.

45. Smith LC, Mullen JL: Nutritional assessment and indications for nutritional support. *Surg Clin North Am* 1991; 71:449–457.

46. Heymsfield SB, Olafson RP, Kutner MH, et al: A radiographic method of quantifying protein-calorie undernutrition. *Am J Clin Nutr* 1979; 32:693–702.

47. Heymsfield SB, Casper K: Anthropometric assessment of the adult hospitalized patient. *JPEN* 1987; 11(suppl):36–41.

48. Pace H, Rathbun EN: Studies in body composition III. The body water and chemically combined nitrogen in relation to fat content. *J Biol Chem* 1945; 158:685–689.

49. Shizgal HM: The effect of malnutrition on body composition. *Surg Gynecol Obstet* 1981; 152:22–26.

50. Forse RA, Shizgal HM: The assessment of malnutrition. *Surgery* 1980; 88:17–24.

51. Shizgal HM: Nutritional assessment and body composition. *JPEN* 1987; 11(suppl):42–47.

52. Cohn SH, Vaswani AN, Yasumura S, et al: Improved models for determination of body fat by in vivo neutron activation. *Am J Clin Nutr* 1984; 40:255–259.

53. Hill GH: Body composition research: Implications for the practice of clinical nutrition. *JPEN* 1992; 16:197–218.

54. Cohn SH, Abesamis C, Zanzi I, et al: Body elemental composition: A comparison between black and white adults. *Am J Physiol* 1977; 232:419–422.

55. Chandra RK: Interactions of nutrition, infection and immunity. Immunocompetence in nutritional deficiency, methodological considerations, and intervention strategies. *Acta Paediatr Scand* 1979; 68:137–144.

56. Meakins JL, Pietsch JB, Bubenick O, et al: Delayed hypersensitivity: Indicator of acquired failure of host defenses in sepsis and trauma. *Ann Surg* 1977; 186:241–250.

57. Bistrian BR, Sherman M, Blackburn GL, et al: Cellular immunity in adult marasmus. *Arch Intern Med* 1977; 137:1408–1411.

58. Twomey P, Ziegler D, Rombeau J: Utility of skin testing in nutritional assessment: A critical review. *JPEN* 1982; 6:50–58.

59. Seltzer MH, Bastidas JA, Cooper DM, et al: Instant nutritional assessment. *JPEN* 1979; 3:157–159.

60. Hoffman-Goetz L, Kluger MJ: Protein deficiency: Its effects on body temperature in health and disease states. *Am J Clin Nutr* 1979; 32:1423–1427.

61. Keenan RA, Moldawer LL, Yang RD, et al: An altered response by peripheral leukocytes to synthesize and release leukocyte endogenous mediator in critically ill, protein-malnourished patients. *J Lab Clin Med* 1982; 100:844–857.

62. Drabik MD, Schnure FC, Mok KT, et al: Effect of protein depletion and short-term parenteral refeeding on host responses to interleukin 1 administration. *J Lab Clin Med* 1987; 109:509–516.

63. Russel DM, Walker PM, Leiter LA, et al: Metabolic and structural changes in skeletal muscle during hypocaloric dieting. *Am J Clin Nutr* 1984; 39:503–513.

64. Jeejeebhoy KN: Bulk or bounce—The object of nutritional support. *JPEN* 1988; 12:539–549.

65. Klidjian AM, Foster KJ, Kammerling RM, et al: Relation of anthropometric and dynamometric variables to serious postoperative complications. *BMJ* 1980; 281:899–901.

66. Hunt DR, Rowlands BJ, Johnston D: Hand grip strength—A simple prog-

nostic indicator in surgical patients. *JPEN* 1985; 9:701–704.

67. Windsor JA, Hill GL: Risk factors for postoperative pneumonia. The importance of protein depletion. *Ann Surg* 1988; 208:209–214.

68. Windsor JA, Hill GL: Weight loss with physiologic impairment. A basic indicator of surgical risk. *Ann Surg* 1988; 207:290–296.

69. Lewis WD, Chwals W, Benotti PN, et al: Bedside assessment of work of breathing. *Crit Care Med* 1988; 16:117–122.

70. Shikora SA, Bistrian BR, Borlase BC, et al: Work of breathing: A reliable indicator of weaning and extubation. *Crit Care Med* 1990; 18:157–162.

71. Makk LJK, McClave SA, Creech PW, et al: Clinical application of the metabolic cart to the delivery of total parenteral nutrition. *Crit Care Med* 1990; 18:1320–1327.

72. Hunter DC, Jaksic T, Lewis D, et al: Resting energy expenditure in the critically ill: Estimation versus measurement. *Br J Surg* 1988; 75:875–878.

73. Hernandez E, Bistrian B, Swails W, et al: Indirect calorimetry in critically ill ventilator dependent patients: Energy expenditure and work of breathing. *Crit Care Med* 1992; 20(suppl):107.

74. Shaw JHF, Wildbore M, Wolfe RR: An integrated analysis of glucose, fat, and protein metabolism in severely traumatized patients: Studies in the basal state and the response to total parenteral nutrition. *Ann Surg* 1987; 209:66–72.

75. Wolfe RR, Goodenough RD, Burke JF, et al: Response of protein and urea kinetics in burn patients to different levels of protein intake. *Ann Surg* 1979; 197:163–171.

76. Rayfield EJ, Ault MJ, Keusch GT, et al: Infection and diabetes: The case for glucose control. *Am J Med* 1982; 72:439–450.

77. Delafosse B, Bouffard Y, Viale JP, et al: Respiratory changes induced by parenteral nutrition in post-operative patients undergoing inspiratory pressure support ventilation. *Anesthesiology* 1987; 66:393–399.

78. Seidner DL, Mascioli EA, Istfan NW, et al: The effects of long chain triglyceride emulsions on reticuloendothelial system function in humans. *JPEN* 1989; 13:614–619.

79. Muller JM, Keller V, Brenner V, et al: Indications and effects of preoperative parenteral nutrition. *World J Surg* 1986; 10:53–63.

3

Fuel Metabolism

James M. Long III, M.D.

Calvin L. Long, Ph.D.

Energetics of biologic fuels	**Effects of exogenous fuel substrates**
Changes of metabolism during critical illness	**Protein requirements**

Metabolism of fuel substrates is important in homeostasis during critical illness or following severe injury. Before the introduction of total parenteral nutrition (TPN) in the mid-1960s and the ensuing surge of research interest in clinical nutrition and metabolic processes, resuscitation and support of critically ill patients focused primarily on measuring physiologic indices such as vital signs, arterial blood gases, central venous pressure, and cardiac output. Treatment was generally directed at correcting abnormal indices toward normal. More recently, understanding of fuel and protein metabolism has resulted in more precise support of metabolic processes, the prevention of body wasting, which has long been recognized as characteristic of critical illness, and a decrease in morbidity and mortality in some patient groups. This chapter examines the metabolism of endogenous and exogenous fuels that are involved in energy homeostasis during rest and critical illness.

ENERGETICS OF BIOLOGIC FUELS

The energy substrates that fuel the metabolic machinery of the human body are carbohydrates, fats, and proteins. The potential energy of these substrates and the energy actually consumed are expressed as kilocalories. Normally when ingested, these substrates are oxidized to produce energy with heat as a by-product or are converted to potential energy in the form of adenosine triphosphate (ATP). In this process approximately 50% of the calories are dissipated as heat, which represents relative "inefficiency" in the transfer of energy (Fig 3–1). The stored energy (ATP) is then used to fuel the basic body machinery and to provide for physical, or external, work. Approximately 65% of energy expenditure is for internal work, and 35% is for external work.

Carbohydrate, fat, and protein are oxidized at different rates under different metabolic and clinical conditions. In ad-

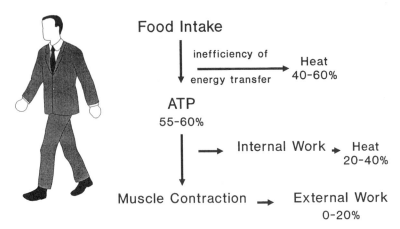

FIG 3–1.
Efficiency of energy transfer in humans. *ATP* = adenosine triphosphate.

dition, specific tissues show preferences for particular fuels (Table 3–1). Red and white blood cells, renal medulla, brain, skeletal muscle, intestinal mucosa, fetal tissues, and malignancies utilize predominantly glucose. Liver, renal cortex, cardiac muscle, and resting skeletal muscle primarily use fatty acids, while cardiac muscle, renal cortex, skeletal muscle, and brain can also use ketone bodies for fuel.

Body composition studies show that male human beings are composed of 40% organic material, 55% water, and 5% minerals. In the female, organic compounds account for 45% of the body weight, and the water content is slightly less than in the male (approximately 50%), the difference attributable to a greater percentage of body weight as fat, which is stored in its anhydrous form. The mineral content is about the same for both males and females (5%). The energy content of the body, however, varies substantially from composition by weight (Table 3–2).[1] Fat typically represents 85% of the stored fuel in the body and is an excellent form of energy storage for highly mobile creatures because it is anhydrous, lightweight, and calorie dense (containing 9 kcal/g). Sixteen kilograms of adipose tissue can yield 141,000 kcal of energy from oxidation, which means that a 70-kg man theoreti-

TABLE 3–1.

Fuels of Individual Tissues*

Source	Tissue
Glucose	RBC, WBC, renal medulla, brain, skeletal muscle (exercise), malignant tumors, fetal tissues, intestinal mucosa
Free fatty acids	Liver, kidney cortex, cardiac muscle, skeletal muscle
Ketone bodies	Cardiac muscle, renal cortex, skeletal muscle, brain
Other energy sources	
Amino acids (minor)	
Lactate (from glucose)	
Glycerol (minor)	

*From Krebs HA: *Enzyme Reg* 1972; 10:397–420. Used by permission.

TABLE 3–2.

Normal Fuel Composition*

Fuel	Amount (kg)	Calories (kcal)
Tissue		
Fat (adipose triglyceride)	15	141,000
Protein (mainly muscle)	6	24,000
Glycogen (muscle)	0.150	600
Glycogen (liver)	0.075	300
Total		165,900
Circulating fuels		
Glucose (extracellular fluid)	0.020	80
Free fatty acids (plasma)	0.0003	3
Triglycerides (plasma)	0.003	30
Total		113

*From Cahill GF Jr: *N Engl J Med* 1970; 282:668–675. Used by permission.

cally has enough adipose to live 60 to 70 days under total starvation in the absence of significant stress or complications. Indeed, this theory has been substantiated from records of prisoners of war and more recently from observations in Belfast, Ireland, when protestors died after almost 60 days of voluntary starvation.

Although weight loss may be a sign of significant catabolism, gradual loss of approximately 10% of body weight has very little effect on physical performance and no significant health implications. Loss of 25% to 30% of body weight, however, can be life-threatening, especially when major illness or injury is superimposed on total starvation.[2, 3]

In normal man carbohydrate, primarily as glycogen, and fat in adipose tissue are the two main fuels used to maintain homeostasis during brief periods of resting starvation. The amount of glycogen in muscle and liver and the extracellular glucose together provide less than 1000 kcal in a 70-kg man. Although glucose is immediately available from glycogenolysis and gluconeogenesis to supply the nervous system, renal medulla, granulation of tissue, erythrocytes, and leukocytes (Fig 3–2), glycogen is rapidly

depleted during the first 18 to 24 hours of starvation, and the body then becomes dependent primarily on adipose and protein stores.[4]

After glycogen depletion during fasting, fat provides the greatest number of calories and free fatty acids to all except the glucose-dependent tissues. Under hormonal control, fatty acids are mobilized, as the plasma free fatty acid concentration is elevated after 24 hours of fasting. This stimulates increased fatty acid uptake and oxidation by the liver, heart, skeletal muscles, and other tissues. These tissues lose most of their capacity to oxidize glucose even though plasma glucose levels are not depressed. The increased supply of free fatty acids stimulates the conversion of two-carbon fragments by the liver into ketone bodies, specifically acetoacetic and β-hydroxybutyric acids. Furthermore, the biosynthesis of fatty acids is almost completely curtailed during even a short period of fasting.

Body proteins are mobilized and catabolized to provide glucose to meet the needs of glucose-dependent tissues in addition to providing amino acids for the synthesis of acute-phase proteins. Body protein and its constituent amino

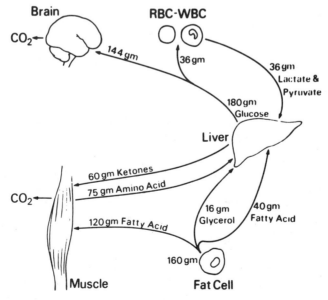

FIG 3–2.
Substrate distribution in fasting man. (Adapted from Cahill GF Jr: *N Engl J Med* 1970; 282:668–675.)

acids should not, however, be considered a long-term fuel reserve, because these compounds represent important structural and functional components of the body. When catabolized under stressful conditions such as trauma, sepsis, or prolonged starvation, total-body protein depletion can occur along with loss of structural integrity. In practice, protein depletion in excess of 20% is not compatible with life, the terminal event most often resulting from infection secondary to immunologic compromise. Overall, the homeostatic process will compromise body tissues as necessary to sustain cell function literally up to the point of structural or functional collapse.

Glucose production from gluconeogenesis in normal subjects is approximately 180 g/day.[5] Cahill measured the use of glucose after 24 hours of fasting by arteriovenous differences across the brain and found that approximately 80% of the total oxidation occurred in the brain.[1] The remainder was metabolized by other glucose-dependent tissues. Approximately 75 g of amino acids is released by the muscles for gluconeogenesis, along with lactate and glycerol. Ketogenesis, which is initially at a low rate, increases during 5 weeks of starvation to the point that 80% of the energy needs of the brain are met by ketone bodies. This endocrine-controlled adaptation to use of ketone bodies results in protein sparing in normal man even in the face of decreased carbohydrate intake.

The endocrine milieu, characterized by the dominance of catecholamines and glucagon over insulin, favors the mobilization of fuel and is facilitated by hypoglycemia during resting starvation. Epinephrine enhances glycogenolysis and lipolysis, and glucagon further stimulates the breakdown of glycogen. Fat mobilization from adipose tissue during fasting is probably enhanced by a decrease in insulin, which inhibits lipase and allows intracellular hydrolysis of triglycerides. In addition, hypoglyce-mia decreases the production of L-α-glycerophosphate, a rate-limiting substrate in the conversion of free fatty acids to triglycerides. The milieu of hormones and enzymes that facilitate increased levels of free fatty acids and fatty acyl coenzyme A (acyl-CoA) in tissues regulates lipid synthesis by inhibition of acyl-CoA carboxylase.

Several mechanisms are involved in the reduced capacity of various tissues to catabolize glucose. Low insulin levels decrease the rate of glucose translocation from extracellular fluid into skeletal muscle, heart, and other tissues. Increased free fatty acid levels inhibit enzymes such as hexokinase, phosphofructokinase, pyruvate kinase, and pyruvate dehydrogenase, which are necessary to metabolize glucose. These glycolytic enzymes decrease so dramatically that only brain, renal medulla, and erythrocytes remain capable of metabolizing glucose.

Although fatty acids are the dominant fuel in long-term starvation, some tissues continue to require glucose as fuel, and the only endogenous source of glucose is gluconeogenesis from mobilized amino acids. Relatively low insulin levels induced by fasting permit the release of amino acids from skeletal muscles. The high glucagon-to-insulin ratio, along with epinephrine, promotes increased gluconeogenesis from amino acids as well as from glycerol, lactate, and pyruvate (which are derived from muscle, adipose tissue, and anaerobic glycolysis through the Embden-Meyerhof pathway).

Fasting man expends about 1800 kcal/day while consuming approximately 160 g of fat, 180 g of glucose, and 75 g of amino acids. The contribution of muscle protein to this homeostatic process in normal fasting man has been studied by radioisotopes.[6] Following an overnight fast, protein synthesis has been estimated to be from 2.5 to 3.0 g/kg/day, and protein breakdown exceeds synthesis by the equivalent of urinary nitrogen losses. Muscle contribution to whole-body protein breakdown, as measured by 24-hour urinary excretion of 3-methylhistidine, is estimated to be 0.5 to 0.7 g/kg/day, or about 25% of whole-body protein turnover in normal subjects. The reduction in metabolic rate associated with simple starvation has been related to a decrease in lean body mass. Although retention of lean body mass is enhanced by adaptive mechanisms, erosion of nitrogen cannot be reduced below approximately 2 to 3 g/day in the average adult.

One technique for elucidation of fuel metabolism that has proved useful experimentally and clinically is indirect calorimetry. During oxidation of metabolic fuels oxygen is consumed, high-energy phosphate bonds are produced, and carbon dioxide and heat are liberated (Fig 3–3). Both ventilation and circulation are obviously necessary to maintain the flow of substrate and soluble gases to and from tissue. The rates of oxygen consumption and carbon dioxide production therefore reflect tissue metabolism and allow a calculation of energy expenditure. The ratio of carbon dioxide produced to oxygen consumed is the respiratory quotient (RQ), which allows an estimation of the composition of fuels being burned. Although oxidation of protein substrate represents about 15% to 20% of the total daily calories in the fuel mixture, the RQ of protein substrate is midway between fat and carbohydrate such that it can be ignored during the use of mixed-fuel substrates.

This so-called nonprotein RQ is 0.71 for the oxidation of fatty acids and 1.0 for the oxidation of glucose. A nonprotein RQ of 0.845 suggests that equal amounts of fatty acids and glucose are being oxidized. The Lusk table derived from measurements of substrate oxidation in animals provides the relationship between nonprotein RQ and the corresponding percentage of the two fuels oxidized.[7] The table also provides the energy equivalents of oxygen for the calculation of calories expended.

Oxygen consumption in the normal adult is about 250 mL/min with a minute ventilation of 6 L. The concentration of oxygen decreases from 20.95% in inspired air to almost 16.95% in expired air. The uptake of oxygen varies significantly among various tissues in normal man (Table 3–3).[8] The four organs that consume the greatest amount of oxygen are the liver, brain, heart, and kidney, which collectively amount to only 5% to 6% of body weight but account for more than 70% of the oxygen consumption and hence the resting energy expenditure (REE). In contrast, skeletal muscle, which makes up almost 40% of the body weight, accounts for only 18% of the oxygen consumption and energy expenditure. Physical activity would, of course, greatly increase the energy expenditure of skeletal muscle.

REE results essentially from involuntary, or internal, work, as depicted in Figure 3–3, and may be defined clinically as energy expenditure measured in the morning while awake, at rest, and in the postabsorptive state. REE is usually expressed as calories per day or calories

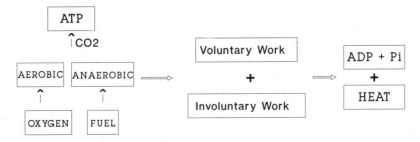

FIG 3–3.
Summation of whole-body metabolic rates by indirect calorimetry. *ADP* = adenosine triphosphate; *ADP* = adenosine diphosphate; *Pi* = inorganic phosphate.

TABLE 3-3.

Distribution of Oxygen Use in Major Body Organs in a Resting Man*

Organ	Oxygen Consumption (mL)	Resting Metabolism (%)
Liver (+ Splanchnic)	67	27
Brain	47	19
Kidneys	14	7
Heart	26	10
Skeletal muscles	45	18
Remainder	48	19
Total	280	100

*Adapted from Brožek J, Grande F: *Hum Biol* 1955; 27:24.

per kilogram per minute. REE is similar to the basal metabolic rate (BMR). However, since the BMR is measured while the patient is asleep by using an open-circuit method, REE is approximately 10% higher than the BMR.[9]

CHANGES IN METABOLISM DURING CRITICAL ILLNESS

Metabolically, critical illness is characterized by an increased resting metabolic expenditure and increased urinary nitrogen loss, both of which correlate with the severity of the illness. These hormone-mediated responses result either primarily or secondarily in an increase in protein catabolism. The association of injury with a catabolic response was made more than 60 years ago by Cuthbertson, who reported increased urinary nitrogen losses after fractures of long bones.[10, 11] In 1924, DuBois found energy expenditures to range from 20% to 60% above normal during acute infections.[12]

The metabolic rate in critically ill patients can be calculated by indirect calorimetry, from a measurement of the oxygen consumption, as in normal subjects. The closed-circuit method utilizes a spirometer filled with oxygen from which flow is directed to the lungs through a face mask or mouthpiece. The expired air is directed back into the spirometer through a carbon dioxide ab-

sorber. The decrease in volume in the spirometer during a measured time period represents the amount of oxygen consumed, from which calorie expenditure can be calculated. The open-circuit method uses unidirectional flow of air through one-way valves, and expired air is collected for a specific time in a Douglas bag. The volume and composition of the expired gas are measured. Oxygen consumption and carbon dioxide production are calculated from the difference between room air and the expired gas. Using either method, investigators have developed equations for predicting REE in normal men and women. The Harris-Benedict equation predicts REE from weight, height, age, and sex.[13] Although this equation does not precisely define energy expenditures, it is useful to estimate calorie requirements.[14]

The Douglas bag technique proved difficult to use in critically ill patients because they were often disoriented, anxious, and occasionally comatose. In order to circumvent these problems, a system for continuous breath analysis using the open-circuit method was developed by Kinney, Long, and others.[15, 16] Expired air from a ventilated head canopy was directed to gas analyzers, thus eliminating the need for a face mask or mouthpiece. C.L. Long used this canopy system to study numerous patients with varying severities of injury.[17, 18] REE was usually measured early in the morning after an overnight fast with minimal stimulation by the clinical staff. The extent of hypermetabolism was consistently related to the severity of stress as summarized in Figure 3-4, where REE is expressed as a percentage of normal. The metabolic rates typically peak 3 to 7 days after injury, in contrast to simple starvation, which results in a decrease in REE. Benedict demonstrated a decrease of 30% in total energy expenditure during a 30-day fast.[19]

Injured, septic, and burned patients are hypercatabolic and show dramatically high urinary nitrogen losses. In addition, decreased nutrient intake result-

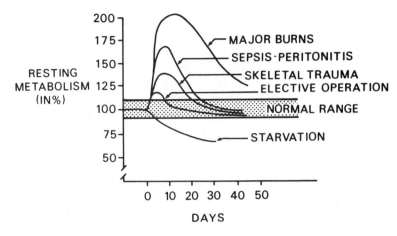

FIG 3—4.
Effect of various stresses on resting metabolic expenditure in hospitalized patients. The mean percentage of increase above normal in resting energy expenditure for hospitalized patients is shown. The normal range is indicated by the *shaded area.*

ing from diminished appetite or an inability to eat adds starvation to the picture. When starvation is superimposed on injury or critical illness, the metabolic responses do not permit the protein sparing and decrease in energy expenditure characteristic of starvation in normal man. On the contrary, urinary nitrogen losses increase with the severity of injury or illness (Fig 3—5) and

peak in about 5 to 7 days.[17] Those patients who were hypercatabolic and catabolized endogenous protein at rates approaching 30 g of nitrogen per day (430 mg N/kg) lost about 1.5% of lean body mass every day. Normal nitrogen losses are about 7 to 10 g/day.

In contrast to starvation in normal man, critically ill patients often have hyperglycemia and glycosuria, classically

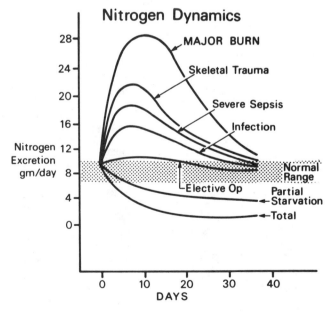

FIG 3—5.
Starvation vs. injury. The increase in urinary nitrogen loss with time is shown for various groups of hospitalized patients. The normal range is indicated by the *shaded area.* (Adapted from Long CL: *JPEN* 1979; 3:452—456.) Used by permission.

referred to as "diabetes of injury," resulting from glucose intolerance and some degree of insulin resistance. Early after injury, energy expenditure decreases during what Cuthbertson described as the "ebb" phase after injury.[20] This phase is characterized by increased production of adrenocorticotropic hormone (ACTH), cortisol, epinephrine, and norepinephrine, the latter as evidence of increased activity of the sympathetic nervous system. This neuroendocrine response causes rapid mobilization of glucose with resulting hyperglycemia. The second, or "flow," phase is characterized by increases in both the metabolic rate and protein catabolism.

The hyperglycemic response following trauma and sepsis results from an increased production relative to the utilization of glucose. Elevated blood glucose levels result from glycogenolysis and gluconeogenesis, the latter coming primarily from a breakdown of alanine and glutamine in the liver. To elucidate posttraumatic hyperglycemia, C.L. Long et al. studied glucose kinetics in human subjects after elective operations, after major injury, and during sepsis by using labeled glucose and a three-pool model (Fig 3–6).[5, 21, 22] The production of glucose by the liver was found to be 1.89 mg glucose/kg/min in normal subjects, almost 59% of which was oxidized. When normal subjects received glucose infusions in amounts equivalent to hepatic glucose production rates, glucose production decreased to some extent, thus confirming a feedback mechanism to control hepatic glucose production in normal man.

Glucose production in patients with trauma and sepsis was increased to 3.06 mg/kg/min, and about 58% of the glucose was oxidized.[5, 21, 22] Septic and burn patients showed glucose production of 4.43 mg/kg/min, double the control values, and about 56% of the glucose was oxidized.[22] Although the absolute rate of glucose oxidation increased in trauma, septic, and burn patients, the percentage of glucose oxidized was not altered significantly. The turnover of glucose was significantly increased after stress, even though these patients were considered to be glucose intolerant and insulin resistant. These observations have been confirmed recently by Shaw et al.,who observed that the rate of glucose oxidation in septic patients receiving glucose infusions was higher than in normal controls and the

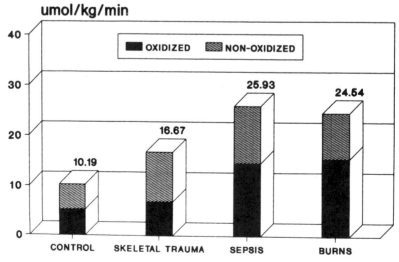

FIG 3–6.

Comparison of glucose production rates in sepsis, trauma, and burns vs. controls. Glucose disposal by oxidative and nonoxidative pathways is shown in control subjects and injured patients. (From Long CL: *Nutr Res* 1993, in press. Used by permission.)

percentage of expired carbon dioxide derived from glucose oxidation was higher in septic patients as compared with normal volunteers.[23] Normalizing glucose infusion to the rate of glucose oxidation made no difference in either group. In 1991, Wolfe et al. concluded that contrary to their previous studies, they were unable to identify a defect in carbohydrate oxidation after burn injury.[24]

The increased glucose production and oxidation after trauma and during sepsis are considered to be obligatory for host survival. During critical illness gluconeogenesis persists continuously and is not curtailed by the infusion of glucose, as measured by the conversion of labeled alanine to glucose by Long et al. (Fig 3–7).[25] In a normal control, 15% of the labeled alanine was converted to glucose. When control subjects were given glucose infusions, the conversion was almost completely curtailed. A similar response was observed during enteral feeding. In the septic patient, conversion of labeled alanine to glucose was not suppressed by infusions of exogenous glucose. This study of septic patients and another of trauma patients suggested that gluconeogenesis cannot be totally suppressed during hypermetabolism in critically ill patients.[26] This hypothesis was corroborated by further studies that showed that gluconeogenesis was not completely suppressed even at 6 mg glucose/kg/day (600 g glucose per day for a 70-kg man)[25–27] (Fig 3–8). Shaw et al. showed that gluconeogenesis was suppressed but that oxidative deamination of amino acids was not suppressed.[23] These studies effectively establish that critically ill patients are unable to adapt to starvation and that this obligatory catabolism adversely affects body protein mass.

Measurement of whole-body protein synthesis and breakdown following injury by using isotopes revealed increases in both synthesis and breakdown, but breakdown was faster.[6] The net difference between synthesis and breakdown of protein is reflected, of

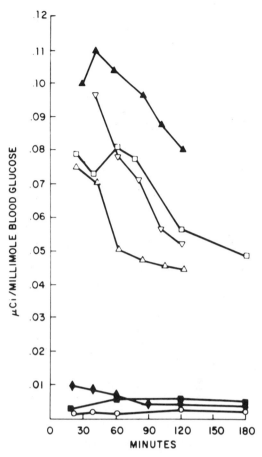

FIG 3–7.
Effect of glucose intake on gluconeogenesis. The specific activity of blood glucose from ^{14}C-alanine is depicted during fasting and intravenous or oral alimentation in control patients (□), (■), (○), and (♦) and in septic patients (△) and (▽). (From Long CL, et al: *Metabolism* 1976; 25:193–201. Used by permission.)

course, by increased nitrogen excretion in the urine. For example, the control patients had a mean postabsorptive synthesis rate of 2.8 g protein/kg/day and a mean breakdown rate of 3.3 g protein/kg/day, a 14% difference reflecting a net urinary nitrogen loss of 5.6 g of nitrogen. Trauma patients showed synthesis rates of 4.0 g protein/kg/day and breakdown rates of 5.6 g protein/kg/day, a 40% difference reflecting 18 g of urinary nitrogen loss.[28] Studies in other septic and critically ill patients gave similar results.[29, 30] Excretion of 3-methylhistidine is also increased significantly in patients during febrile episodes and following trauma and re-

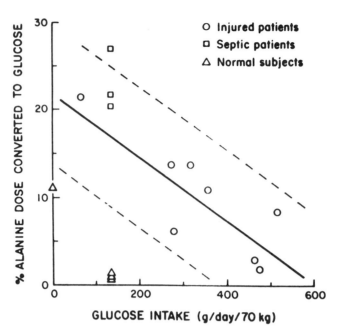

FIG 3–8.
Effect of glucose intake on gluconeogenesis. (Data for injured patients and for the regression line and 95% confidence limits *(dotted lines)*. (From Elwyn DH: *Ann Surg* 1980; 191:40–46. Used by permission.)

flects increased muscle protein breakdown in man.[31, 32] Studies of peripheral and visceral components of whole-body protein breakdown by using 3-methylhistidine excretion and stable isotopes showed that muscle contributed 40% in males and 33% in females during the catabolic phase after trauma.[31, 33]

Preservation of whole-body protein during catabolism has been questioned. Studies of whole-body protein kinetics in trauma patients showed that infusion of a 3% amino acid solution did not modulate protein breakdown, even though trauma patients showed more severe negative nitrogen balance than controls.[6] The nitrogen balance was less negative, however, than that for trauma patients receiving only 5% glucose. Since excretion of 3-methylhistidine was not decreased by amino acid infusion, the authors concluded that protein synthesis was enhanced without a change in the protein breakdown rate. Similar studies in adult burn patients by Wolfe et al. showed that intake of protein substrate increased the protein

synthesis rates but did not affect the catabolic rate.[29] Shenkin et al. also studied protein catabolism after trauma by measuring nitrogen balance and 3-methylhistidine excretion.[34] One group of trauma patients received 3200 kcal of glucose alone, and another similar group received 3200 kcal of glucose plus 24 g of nitrogen per day as amino acids. During 8-day study periods, nitrogen balance was only positive in the group receiving amino acids and glucose, but both groups of patients showed similar excretion of 3-methylhistidine (Fig 3–9). These findings suggest that amino acids are an important component of nutrition support to stimulate protein synthesis, even if protein catabolism is not appreciably curtailed.

Fuel utilization is, however, quite sensitive to even small amounts of carbohydrate intake. Gamble showed that healthy adults decreased urinary nitrogen excretion to half the fasting values during consumption of 100 g of glucose per day.[35] In other studies, the same amount of glucose suppressed gluconeo-

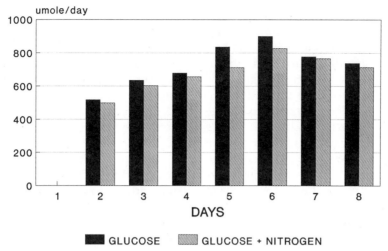

FIG 3-9.
Effect of total parenteral nutrition *(TPN)* on muscle protein breakdown measured by 3-methylhistidine. The effect of 3200 kcal of glucose per day or 3200 kcal of glucose per day + 24 g of nitrogen per day on muscle protein breakdown in trauma as measured by 3-methylhistidine excretion is shown. (Adapted from Shenkin AN: *J Am Clin Nutr* 1980; 33:2119–2117. Used by permission.)

genesis and ketogenesis in malnourished patients (Fig 3–10).[36] After 3 days without glucose intake following trauma, burn injury, and sepsis, plasma total ketone bodies were depressed to approximately one third of the concentrations found in control subjects.[37–41] When glucose intake was resumed after

the 3 days, plasma ketones levels were further depressed. Plasma insulin and glucose concentrations were greater in the trauma group, and free fatty acid levels were slightly depressed.

Glucose infusion spares protein presumably by reducing the demand for glucose from gluconeogenesis. All of the

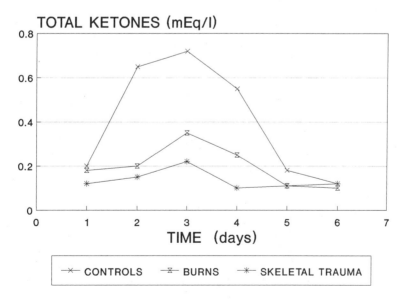

FIG 3-10.
Fasting total ketones after trauma. A comparison between trauma, burn, and control subjects of changes in total plasma ketone bodies during a 3-day fast (days 1 to 3) and 3 days of carbohydrate intake (days 4 to 6) is shown. Total ketones are the sum of acetoacetate and 3-hydroxybutyrate. (From Birkhahn RH, Long CL, Fitkin DL, et al: *J Trauma* 1981; 21:513–519 and from Abbott WC, et al: *JPEN* 1985; 9:153–158. Used by permission.)

glucose infused, however, is not oxidized. Burke et al. reported that the rate of glucose oxidation plateaued at 50% of the Vco_2 in a group of burn patients receiving glucose at 5 to 6 mg/kg/min.[42] The RQ increased to 1.0, and when higher rates of glucose were infused, the RQ increased above 1.0. In 1971, Long et al. reported glucose oxidation rates of 52% of the turnover rate in control and trauma patients in a postabsorptive state.[5, 22] The percentage of Vco_2 from direct oxidation of glucose was 29% in both groups. Infusion of 2 mg glucose/kg/min increased glucose oxidation to 61% of the glucose turnover with a 31% contribution to Vco_2. When Elwyn et al. infused glucose at rates from 2 to 6 mg/kg/min in trauma patients, the rate of glucose oxidation was considerably less than the infusion rate.[27] Peak glucose oxidation occurred at 6 mg/kg/min but amounted to only 50% of the infused glucose at any level of glucose infused. More recently, Long et al. reported that glucose oxidation was not impaired in severely injured and septic patients receiving TPN with glucose as the sole nonprotein calorie source at levels of glucose intake of 6 mg/kg/min.[43] The oxidation rate was about 50% of the turnover rate. Septic patients, trauma patients, and normal controls produced 55% to 60% of the Vco_2 from the direct oxidation of glucose. The RQ values were all greater than 1.0. The observation of a plateau of 50% to 60% of Vco_2 from glucose oxidation calculated by using isotopes is in disagreement with the 80% calculated from nonprotein RQ values by indirect calorimetry.

The availability of intravenous fat emulsions for clinical use with parenteral nutrition introduced the opportunity to study the relative metabolic effects of carbohydrate and fat as calorie sources in moderately to severely stressed patients receiving isonitrogenous parenteral feeding. J. M. Long et al.[44] reported that glucose infusion in amounts up to the measured or estimated REE resulted in protein sparing.

In larger amounts, glucose did not further spare protein, and hyperglycemia resulted. Only when insulin was given for hyperglycemia did nitrogen excretion decrease further. In that study, fat infusion did not exert a protein-sparing effect at any level of fat or glucose infusion. Exogenous fat emulsion appeared to function similarly to endogenous fat stores but did not enhance protein sparing. Similarly designed studies in normal and stressed animals by Souba et al. showed that the protein-sparing effect of glucose was blunted by stress. During stress fat did not spare protein at all.[45] Reports by Jeejeebhoy and others suggested that fat appeared to spare protein in minimally stressed patients, but a mechanism to explain this observation has not emerged.[46] Brennan et al. suggested that the apparent protein-sparing effect of fat emulsion could be attributed to glycerol, which is a constituent of the fat emulsion and is released by hydrolysis of triglycerides.[47]

Despite some limitation of protein sparing, mixed-fuel substrates do offer several advantages over glucose alone in septic and injured patients. Askanazi et al. reported that 14 septic, injured patients had RQ calculations of 0.90 when glucose calories equaled or slightly exceeded the resting metabolic energy (RME).[48] The unstressed control group had an RQ of 1.05 with intakes of glucose 1.34 times their REE. They concluded that injured man appeared to utilize endogenous fat stores preferentially as an energy resource. A problem with the study, however, was that the range of REE values was so great (1.35 to 2.25) that the mean values did not truly represent a typical patient. A similar objection may be made to the conclusion of Stoner and Little, who used indirect calorimetry and a sepsis score to document decreased glucose oxidation in septic patients.[49] If their maximum glucose infusion rate (40 kcal/m^2/hr or 4.8 mg/kg/min) is compared with their maximum metabolic rate (5.74 kcal/m^2/hr or 6.95 mg/kg/min), an

RQ of less than 1.0 would have been expected. Presumably the RQ in both studies would have been 1.0 or greater if the glucose infusion rates had been greater than the resting or total energy needs of the patients.

To evaluate the amount of glucose required in excess of REE to produce an RQ of 1.0 or greater, C.L. Long et al. reported that hypermetabolic septic patients given increasing loads of glucose up to 12 mg/kg/min showed increasing RQ values, which reached approximately 1.0 at 6 mg glucose/kg/min, a value also reported by Burke et al. for burn patients.[42, 43] Increasing glucose infusion above 6 mg/kg/min resulted in RQ values greater than 1.0. At very high glucose loads REE values were significantly increased above controls, a reflection of lipogenesis, which was confirmed by RQ values of approximately 1.4. The relationship between infused glucose and REE was also evaluated by Merrick et al. in a group of colorectal cancer patients receiving a glucose-based TPN regimen.[50] Glucose loading had a minimal thermogenic effect until the intake exceeded the patient's measured RME by 30% to 50%. These results are similar to those of Elwyn et al., who showed that severely depleted patients receiving glucose-based TPN did not increase RME during negative energy balance.[27] When energy intake reached 30% above energy expenditure, the RQ increased to 1.0 with no increase in oxygen consumption. When glucose calories exceeded REE by 100%, both oxygen consumption and RQ increased by 14% to 20%. In septic patients, Giovannini et al. showed an RQ of 1.0 when glucose was infused at a rate of 1.33 times the metabolic rate.[51] The preponderance of data suggests that hypermetabolic patients do not have a defect in glucose oxidation, but they do reach a point of maximum glucose oxidation that occurs at an intake of approximately 6 mg/kg/min.

The plateau of direct oxidation of glucose at 50% to 60% of Vco_2 is in dis-

agreement with studies using indirect calorimetry that suggest that at an RQ of 1.0 all glucose is being oxidized. This discrepancy may be explained by lipogenesis of the unoxidized glucose. The conversion of excess glucose to lipid occurs at an RQ of 8.6, and the net gas exchange from the oxidation of glucose, protein, and fat and lipid synthesis is unity, thus an RQ of 1.0. On the assumption that 24-hour urinary urea losses define protein needs based on the principle of balance, the stoichiometric equivalent of CO_2 from such protein losses was about 20% of the Vco_2 in the above patients. Since glucose oxidation provided 60% of the Vco_2 and protein oxidation provided 20% of the Vco_2, the percentage from lipid oxidation must be 20%. This also suggests triglyceride cycling during glucose infusions. Lipid synthesis during infusions of glucose at rates commonly employed in glucose-based TPN has been shown to occur. Nordenström et al. showed a linear decline in free fatty acid oxidation with increasing rates of glucose infusion in injured and septic patients.[52] When the infused glucose intake equaled the measured metabolic rate, the net fat oxidation fell to 17% of the RME. Triglyceride recycling was also shown to be affected significantly by high rates of glucose infusion even though the rate of fatty acid oxidation was diminished.[43, 52–54] Glucose infusions may suppress lipid oxidation in both normal and stressed patients, but glucose does not appear to suppress recycling of lipid. This cycling of lipid may have an impact on metabolic rates.

Critically ill patients are consistently hyperglycemic during the "flow" phase after injury. This may be due to insulin resistance in the liver and skeletal muscle. The RME is increased, as is urinary nitrogen excretion. Despite hyperglycemia, gluconeogenesis persists and is unresponsive to infusions of glucose at rates approaching the daily energy needs of the patient. Furthermore, hyperglycemia prevents the formation of ketone bodies, further preventing the critically ill patient from adapting to starvation and thereby sparing body protein.

During hypermetabolism and hypercatabolism a balanced nutrition regimen stimulates protein synthesis, thus decreasing net protein breakdown. This effect diminishes the erosion of lean body mass without significantly changing the metabolic rate. Although the fuel preferences of various tissues may be slightly modified during critical illness, the V_{CO_2} from direct oxidation of glucose plateaus at 60% of intake in both normal individuals and critically ill patients.[43] As noted above, the protein contribution to the V_{CO_2} is 20% in injured and septic patients, and oxidation of lipid accounts for the remaining 20% of the V_{CO_2}. These observations serve as a basis for recommendations of a fuel mixture for the nutritional care of critically ill patients.

EFFECTS OF EXOGENOUS FUEL SUBSTRATES

When energy substrates are ingested or infused in amounts exceeding the rate of oxidation, the excess will be converted to glycogen or lipid. Since the oxidation and storage processes require work, measurement of oxygen consumption and carbon dioxide production may be used to estimate the optimal energy intake at a time when maintenance, not storage, is the primary goal. Fuel intake, up to the level of metabolic expenditure, does not increase REE. Moreover, the increase in REE observed when energy intake exceeds requirements may well be due to the work of storage. The energy cost for storage is about 5% to 10% for excess carbohydrate, 1.4% to 4.6% for storage of excess lipid, and 20% to 30% for storage of excess protein.[55] After excess carbohydrate has repleted glycogen stores, the energy cost of conversion of excess glucose to lipid is even greater and reaches

approximately 21% to 30% in patients reported by Askanazi,[48] Merrick,[50] and MacFie and their colleagues.[56]

These studies suggest that glucose calories should not exceed the REE or cause an RQ of 1.0 or greater. Energy intake must be adjusted, however, on the basis of hypermetabolism. Clinical guidelines for energy requirements of critically ill patients were developed by C. L. Long et al.[43] (Table 3–4). The injury or stress factors indicate an increase over predictions by the Harris-Benedict equation. Again, the severity of injury determined the extent of hypermetabolism and hence the energy requirements.

In addition to the REE, the activity level of the patient must be considered when estimating actual energy needs. C. L. Long et al. reported that daily activities resulted in an average energy increase of 20% above REE. They recommended that ambulatory patients receive 30% more than their predicted or measured requirements to fully satisfy the energy cost of daily activity.[57]

If measurement of REE is not feasible, a regression equation such as the Harris-Benedict formula may be used. Adjustments are then based on the injury factor for a particular severity of illness of injury and the activity factor (Table 3–4).[17] Since the injury factors represent maximal or peak responses, the injury factors must be reduced as the patient recovers. Although specific guidelines for energy requirements during convalescence have not been precisely defined, energy expenditure usually approaches normal as nitrogen losses return to preinjury levels. Even though small amounts of extra calories are usually tolerated well, glucose overloading should be avoided to prevent the potential metabolic complications resulting from hyperglycemia, excess lipogenesis, or excess CO_2 production.

The optimal ratio of carbohydrate and fat in parenteral nutrition mixtures remains somewhat controversial. The requirement for essential fatty acid (EFA)

TABLE 3-4.

Total Daily Energy and Protein Needs*

Estimation of energy requirements

Various approaches are used to evaluate the total calories required. The methods described consider the individual's age, weight, height, sex, and additional factors that have an influence on energy requirements. The guidelines set forth herein are based on estimates of the injury and activity factors previously discussed. The following equations predict the approximate total daily energy expenditure *(TDE)* by multiplying BMR (Harris-Benedict equation) by an activity and an injury factor. Approximate zero energy balance and weight maintenance can be achieved by matching energy intake to the TDE.

TDE for men (kcal/day) = $(66.47 + 13.75W + 5.0H - 6.76A) \times$ (Activity factor) $\times$ (Injury factor)

TDE for women (kcal/day) = $(655.10 + 9.56W + 1.85H - 4.68A) \times$ (Activity factor) $\times$ (Injury factor);

where W = weight (kg), H = height (cm), A = age (yr)

Activity Factor		Injury Factor	
Confined to bed	1.2	Surgery	
Out of bed	1.3	Minor	1.0-1.1
		Major	1.1-1.2
		Infection	
		Mild	1.0-1.2
		Moderate	1.2-1.4
		Severe	1.4-1.8
		Trauma	
		Skeletal	1.2-1.35
		Head injury with steroid therapy	1.6
		Blunt	1.15-1.35
		Burns (body surface area)	
		Up to 20%	1.0-1.5
		20% to 40%	1.5-1.85
		Over 40%	1.85-1.95

*From Long CL: The energy and protein requirements of the critically ill patient, in Wright RA, Heymsfield S (eds): *Nutritional Assessment.* St Louis, Mosby–Year Book, 1984.

is usually 4% to 5% of the daily energy intake and can be met easily by most oral diets and supplements. Prior to the availability of fat emulsions, TPN patients received all nonprotein calories as glucose, but now EFA requirements can be met by two to three 500-mL units of 10% fat emulsion weekly. In addition, fat can provide 30% to 50% of the nonprotein calories without adversely affecting protein metabolism in most patients.

Regardless of the nonprotein calorie source, both normal and stressed patients show enhanced retention of nitrogen when given adequate calories. Rutten et al. gave a TPN formula with a fixed calorie-to-nitrogen ratio of 150:1 and showed that nitrogen balance occurred at 1.7 times the REE predicted by the Harris-Benedict formula.[58] Spanier and Shizgal showed that lean body mass increased in patients receiving 57 kcal/kg/day but not 38 kcal/kg/day.[59] Elwyn et al. reported a linear relationship between nitrogen balance and calorie intake in malnourished patients receiving a constant nitrogen intake.[60] Nitrogen balance remained dependent on calorie intake even when infused calories exceeded energy expenditure. Peters and Fischer evaluated a similar group of malnourished patients receiving 1.5 g protein/kg/day and found that nitrogen balance was achieved at 41 kcal/kg/day, which represented a calorie-to-nitrogen ratio of 163:1.[61] C. L. Long et al. reported nitrogen balance at a calorie-to-nitrogen ratio of 138:1 in septic patients when calories were provided at 1.5 times the RME.[62]

In general, most clinicians agree that mixed-fuel TPN regimens are as effective as all-glucose regimens for most patients. Jeejeebhoy et al. reported that nitrogen balance was similar between regimens in which all calories were glucose or 83% were lipid and only 17% were glucose.[46] MacFie et al. provided gastroenterologic patients with either all-glucose or 50% lipid regimens and found that total-body nitrogen measured by in vivo neutron activation was slightly improved in patients who received the mixed-fuel substrate.[63] On the other hand, Paradis et al. reported that the lean body mass of malnourished patients did not change regardless of the calories infused.[64] Shizgal and Forse, using an isotope dilution technique, found that a mixed-fuel regimen repleted body cell mass at only one fourth the rate of the all-glucose regimen over a 2-week period in a mixed patient population.[65] Nitrogen balance has been reported to be equally well maintained by glucose calories or 50:50 glucose-lipid systems.[66, 67]

To fine-tune the planning of a fuel mixture beyond what can be done by using nitrogen retention, C. L. Long et al. have suggested the use of substrate flux and oxidation, as referred to above.[43] Glucose oxidation contributed 60% to the V_{CO_2} in normal subjects, trauma patients, septic patients, and cancer patients at glucose infusion rates of 5 to 6 mg/kg/min. This observation seemed to be independent of stress. If this premise is accepted, the logical conclusion, therefore, was to use glucose to provide 60% of the V_{CO_2}. The stoichiometric equivalent of CO_2 generated from protein represented by urinary nitrogen was between 15% and 20% of the V_{CO_2} in normal and stressed patients, respec-

tively. To make up the difference, lipid should be provided to cover 20% to 25% of the V_{CO_2}. The recommendation for composition of the nutrient mixture should be 20% protein, 20% lipid, and 60% glucose. This proposal results in feeding similar amounts to that previously recommended, namely, up to 30% of nonprotein calories as fat without adversely affecting protein metabolism.[46]

PROTEIN REQUIREMENTS

Protein requirements are usually estimated from nitrogen balance, which reflects the overall metabolism of protein in the body. Clinically, 24-hour urine excretion of urea nitrogen can be determined and adjusted to total urinary nitrogen excretion by adding 4 g to cover skin and fecal losses. Urinary urea excretion is directly related to the severity of illness or injury. Normally, without nitrogen intake, urinary nitrogen loss is approximately 100 mg N/kg body weight. Mild hypercatabolism results in a loss of 200 mg N/kg body weight. Alternatively, nitrogen can be estimated from known or estimated energy requirements by applying a ratio of 150 kcal/g N. Conversely, if nitrogen losses are known, the ratio may predict caloric needs.

C. L. Long showed that urinary nitrogen losses vary with illness and gradually return toward normal during convalescence (see Fig 3–5).[17, 18] Estimation of the nitrogen balance every 3 or 4 days can help with modulation of nitrogen intake to achieve a goal of 4 to 7 g N per day positive balance. Despite diligent efforts to achieve a positive nitrogen balance, even very large intakes of protein substrate rarely result in a positive nitrogen balance in critically ill, hypermetabolic patients. Nevertheless, if calorie and protein requirements can be estimated and provided, body protein synthesis will increase, and lean body mass will be protected from the ravages of unbridled consumption that occurs to meet exaggerated energy expenditure. Often, a return of positive nitrogen balance indicates that stress is abating and that the patient's metabolic processes are returning to normal.

REFERENCES

1. Cahill GF Jr: Starvation in man. *N Engl J Med* 1970; 282:668–675.
2. Studley HO: Percentage of weight loss: A base indicator of surgical risk in patients with chronic peptic ulcer. *JAMA* 1936;106:458.
3. Wilmore DW: Energy and energy balance, in Wilmore DW (ed): *The Metabolic Management of the Critically Ill.* New York, Plenum Publishing Corp, 1977.
4. Moore FD: Energy and the maintenance of the body cell mass. *JPEN* 1980; 4:228–259.
5. Long CL, Spencer JL, Kinney JM, et al: Carbohydrate metabolism in normal man and the effect of glucose infusion. *J Appl Physiol* 1971; 31:102–109.
6. Long CL: The modulation of protein turnover by nutritional intervention in the critically ill patient, in Gruber D, Walker RI, MacVitte TJ, et al (eds): *The Pathology of Combined Injury and Trauma.* Boston, Academic Press, 1987.
7. Lusk G: *The Elements of the Science of Nutrition,* ed 4. Philadelphia, WB Saunders, 1928.
8. Brozek J, Grande F: Body composition and basal metabolism in man: Correlation analysis versus physiological approach. *Hum Biol* 1955; 27:24.
9. Long CL, et al: Comparison of metabolic expenditures awake and during sleep. *JPEN* 1979; 3:502.
10. Cuthbertson DP: Observations on disturbance of metabolism produced by injury to the limbs. *Q J Med* 1932; 25:233–246.
11. Cuthbertson DP, Tilstone WJ: Metabolism during the post injury period. *Adv Clin Chem* 1969; 12:1–55.
12. DuBois E: *Basal metabolism in Health and Disease.* New York, Lea & Febiger, 1924.
13. Harris JA, Benedict FG: *A Biometric Study of Basal Metabolism in Man.* Washington, DC, Carnegie Institute, Publication No 270, 1919.
14. Benedict FG: Basal metabolism data on normal men and women (series II) with some considerations on the use of prediction standards. *J Physiol* 1928; 85:607.
15. Kinney JM, Morgan AP, Dominguez JF, et al: A method for continuous measurement of gas exchange and expired radioactivity in acutely ill patients. *Metabolism* 1978;85:607.
16. Long CL, Carlo MA, Schaffel N, et al: A continuous analyzer for monitoring respiratory gases and expired radioactivity in clinical studies. *Metabolism* 1979; 28:320–332.
17. Long CL: The energy and protein requirements of the critically ill patient, in Wright, RA, Heymsfield S (eds): *Nutritional Assessment.* Boston, Blackwell, 1984, pp 157–181.
18. Long CL: Metabolic response to injury and illness: Estimation of energy and protein needs from indirect calorimetry and nitrogen balance. *JPEN* 1979; 3:452–456.
19. Benedict FG: *A Study of Prolonged Fasting.* Washington, DC, Carnegie Institute, *Publication No 203,* 1915.
20. Cuthbertson DP: Post-shock metabolic response. *Lancet* 1942; 1:433–437.
21. Howard JM: Studies of the absorption and metabolism of glucose following injury. The systemic response to injury. *Ann Surg* 1955; 141:321–326.
22. Long CL, Spencer JL, Kinney JM, et al: Carbohydrate metabolism in man: Effect of elective operations and major injury. *J Appl Physiol* 1971; 31:110–116.
23. Shaw JHF, Kien S, Wolfe RR: Assessment of alanine, urea, and glucose interrelationships in normal subjects and in patients with sepsis with stable isotopic tracers. *Surgery* 1985; 97:557–567.
24. Wolfe RR, et al: Isotopic evaluation of the metabolism of pyruvate and related substrates in normal adult volunteers and severely burned children: Effect of dichlorate and glucose infusion. *Surgery* 1991; 110:54–67.
25. Long CL, Kinney JM, Geiger JW: Nonsuppressibility of gluconeogenesis by glucose in the septic patient. *Metabolism* 1976; 25:193–201.

26. Long CL, Schiller WR, Geiger JW, et al: Gluconeogenic response during glucose infusions in patients following skeletal trauma or sepsis. *JPEN* 1978; 22:619–625.

27. Elwyn DH, Kinney JM, Jeevanandam M, et al: Influence of increasing carbohydrate intake on glucose kinetics in injured patients. *Ann Surg* 1979; 190:117–127.

28. Long CL, Jeevanandam M, Kim BM, et al: Whole body protein synthesis and catabolism in septic patients. *Am J Clin Nutr* 1977; 30:1340–1344.

29. Wolfe RR, Goodenough RD, Burke JF, et al: Response of protein and urea kinetics in burn patients to different levels of protein intake. *Ann Surg* 1983; 197:163–171.

30. Kien CL, Young VR, Rohrbaugh DK, et al: Increased rates of whole body protein synthesis and breakdown in children recovering from burns. *Ann Surg* 1978; 187:383–391.

31. Long CL, Birkhahn RH, Geiger JW, et al: Contribution of skeletal muscle in elevated rates of whole body protein catabolism in adult normal subjects and during malnutrition, sepsis, and skeletal trauma. *Metabolism* 1981; 30:765–776.

32. Long CL, Haverberg LN, Young VR, et al: Metabolism of 3-methylhistidine in man. *Metabolism* 1975; 24:929–935.

33. Long CL, Dillard DR, Bodzin JH, et al: Validity of 3-methylhistidine excretion as an indicator of skeletal muscle protein breakdown in humans. *Metabolism* 1988; 37:844–849.

34. Shenkin A, Neuhäuser M, Bergström, et al: Biochemical changes associated with severe trauma. *J Am Clin Nutr* 1980; 33:2119–2127.

35. Gamble JL: Physiological information gained from studies on the life raft ration. *Harvey Lect* 1947; 42:247–273.

36. Gil FM, Gump PM, Starker J, et al: Splanchnic substrate balance in malnourished patients during parenteral nutrition. *Am J Physiol* 1985; 248:409–419.

37. Birkhahn RH, Long CL, Fitkin DL, et al: A comparison of the effects of skeletal trauma and surgery on ketosis of starvation in man. *J Trauma* 1981; 21:513–518.

38. Abbott WC, Schiller WR, Long CL, et al: The effect of major thermal injury on plasma ketone body levels. *JPEN* 1985; 9:153–158.

39. Beisel WR, Wannemacher RW: Gluconeogenesis, ureagenesis, and ketogenesis during sepsis. *JPEN* 1980; 4:277–285.

40. Clowes GH Jr, O'Donnell TF, Blackburn GL, et al: Energy metabolism and proteolysis in traumatized and septic man. *Surg Clin North Am* 1976; 56:1169–1184.

41. Wannemacher RW Jr, Pace JG, Beall RA, et al: Role of the liver in regulation of ketone body production during sepsis. *J Clin Invest* 1979; 64:1565–1572.

42. Burke JF, Wolfe RR, Mullany CJ, et al: Glucose requirements following burn injury: Parameters of optimal glucose infusion and possible hepatic and respiratory abnormalities following excessive glucose intake. *Ann Surg* 1979; 190:274–285.

43. Long CL, Nelson KM, Akin JM Jr, et al: A physiologic basis for the provision of fuel mixtures in normal and stressed patients. *J Trauma* 1990; 30:1077–1086.

44. Long JM, Wilmore DW, Mason AD, et al: Effect of carbohydrate and fat intake on nitrogen excretion during total intravenous feeding. *Ann Surg* 1977; 185:417-422.

45. Souba WW, Long JM, Dudrick SJ: Effect of stress and diet on nitrogen excretion in growing rats. *JPEN* 1979; 3:34.

46. Jeejeehboy KN, Anderson GH, Nakhooda AF, et al: Metabolic studies in total parenteral nutrition with lipid in man. *J Clin Invest* 1976; 57:125–136.

47. Brennan MF, Moore FD: An intravenous fat emulsion as a nitrogen sparer: comparison with glucose. *J Surg Res* 1973; 14:501.

48. Askanazi J, Carpenter YA, Elwyn DH, et al: Influence of total parenteral nutrition on fuel utilization in injury and sepsis. *Ann Surg* 1980; 191:40–46.

49. Stoner HB, Little KN: The effect of sepsis on the oxidation of carbohydrate and fat. *Br J Surg* 1983; 70:32–35.

50. Merrick HW, Long CL, Grecos GP, et al: Energy requirements for the cancer patient and the effect of total parenteral nutrition. *JPEN* 1988; 12:8–14.

51. Giovannini I, Boolderini G, Castagneto M, et al: Respiratory quotient and patterns of substrate utilization in human sepsis and trauma. *JPEN* 1983;7:226–230.

52. Nordenström J, Carpentier YA, Askanazi J, et al: Free fatty acid mobilization and oxidation during total parenteral nutrition in trauma and infection. *Ann Surg* 1983; 198:725–735.

53. Carpentier YA, Askanazi J, Elwyn DH, et al: Effects of hypercaloric glucose infusions on lipid metabolism in injury and sepsis. *J Trauma* 1979; 19:649–654.

54. Jeevanandam M, Grote-Holman AE, Chikenji T, et al: Effects of glucose on fuel utilization and glycerol turnover in normal and injured man. *Crit Care Med* 1990; 18:125–135.

55. Himms-Hagen J: Cellular thermogenesis. *Annu Rev Physiol* 1976; 38:315–351.

56. MacFie J, Holmfield JHM, King RFG, et al: Effect of the energy source on changes in energy expenditure and respiratory quotient during total parenteral nutrition. *JPEN* 1983; 7:1–5.

57. Long CL, Kopp K, Kinney JM: Energy demands during ambulation in surgical convalescence. *Surg Forum* 1969; 20:93–94.

58. Rutten P, Blackburn GL, Flatt JP, et al: Determination of optimal hyperalimentation infusion rate. *J Surg Res* 1975; 18:477–483.

59. Spanier AH, Shizgal HM: Caloric requirements of the critically ill patient receiving intravenous hyperalimentation. *Am J Surg* 1977; 133:99–104.

60. Elwyn DH, Gump FE, Munro HN, et al: Changes in nitrogen balance in depleted patients with increasing infusions of glucose. *Am J Clin Nutr* 1979; 32:1597–1611.

61. Peters C, Fischer JE: Studies on calorie to nitrogen ratio for total parenteral nutrition. *Surg Gynecol Obstet* 1980; 151:1–8.

62. Long CL, Crosby F, Geiger JW, et al: Parenteral nutrition in the septic patient: Nitrogen balance, limiting plasma amino acids, and calorie to nitrogen ratios. *Am J Nutr* 1976; 29:380–391.

63. MacFie J, Smith RC, Hill GL, et al: Glucose or fat as a nonprotein energy source. *Gastroenterology* 1981; 80:103–107.

64. Paradis C, Spanier AH, Shizgal HM, et al: Total parenteral nutrition with lipid. *Am J Surg* 1979; 135:164–171.

65. Shizgal HM, Forse A: Protein and calorie requirement with total parenteral nutrition. *Ann Surg* 1980; 95:562–569.

66. Kirkpatrick JR, Dahn M, Lewis L: Selective versus standard hyperalimentation. *Am J Surg* 1980; 92:562–569.

67. Nordenström J, Askanazi J, Elwyn DH, et al: Nitrogen balance during total parenteral nutrition. *Ann Surg* 1983; 197:27–33.

PART II

Specific Proteins

Proteins

4

Intact Proteins, Peptides, and Amino Acid Formulas

Gary P. Zaloga, M.D.

Protein is essential for normal cellular function and integrity. It is required for the manufacture of vital cell components including enzymes and structural proteins. Protein is also essential for the manufacture of hormones, cytokines, neuromodulating substances, and other cellular messengers. As such, protein is required for normal cardiovascular function, muscle contraction, immune response, synthesis of hepatic and other essential proteins, healing, growth, recovery from illness, and maintenance of health.

The body contains endogenous stores of protein (i.e., muscle, skin, liver) that it can mobilize to supply needed nitrogen when exogenous supplies are limited. A healthy individual is estimated to have approximately 100 g of surplus nitrogen available for mobilization. Once this limit is exceeded, nitrogen continues to be mobilized. However, mobilization occurs at the expense of normal organ structure or function. Despite adequate nitrogen stores, it remains unclear whether such stores can supply adequate nitrogen to all organ systems under severe stress (i.e., critical illness). There may be limitations in the supply of specific protein components (i.e., glutamine, arginine, biogenic amines) during critical illness.

The body is dependent upon the supply of exogenous protein for normal physiologic function. In this chapter, we discuss the role of the gut in digestion and absorption of protein, the concept of biogenic amines, the importance of enteral administration of protein, and the effect of protein form on organ function.[1] We have attempted to include both animal and human studies in our discussion and to develop guidelines for using protein formulas in nutritional therapy.

TERMINOLOGY

Protein is available in three major forms: free amino acids, peptides or hydrolyzed protein, and intact protein. The use of terms such as elemental or nonelemental are confusing since elemental is frequently applied to both amino acids and peptides. In addition, elemental frequently suggests low fat and no fiber. We prefer to refer to formulas with descriptive terminology such as amino acid based, peptide based, intact protein, low fat, or fiber containing.

DIGESTION AND ABSORPTION OF PROTEIN

Most dietary nitrogen is ingested in the form of intact protein. The digestibility of various proteins differs. For example, plant proteins are less digestible than animal proteins.[2] A high proline and phosphorus content (i.e., glutens) also increases resistance to digestion. Thus, all proteins are not equal. Some are better digested and better absorbed than others.

Endogenous proteins (i.e., secretions from salivary glands, stomach, intestine, biliary tract, pancreas) (20 to 30 g/day) and desquamated cells from the small intestine (30 g/day) may constitute 30% to 50% of the total protein that enters the intestinal lumen each day.[3] Most of these proteins are digested and absorbed (in normal individuals). Some proteins (i.e., intrinsic factor) are resistant to digestion. Endogenous protein losses represent a significant source of protein loss in patients with abnormal digestion/absorption. Protein-losing enteropathies may account for significant protein losses in critically ill patients.

Protein digestion consists of three major phases: a gut lumen phase, a brush border phase, and a cytoplasmic phase. Protein digestion is initiated by acid proteases in the stomach (gut lumen phase). The major group of proteolytic enzymes consists of pepsins. Pepsins are secreted as pepsinogens that are activated in the presence of acid. Gastric proteolysis requires an acidic pH (<5) and is impaired in patients receiving agents that alkalinize the stomach. Gastric hydrolysis produces a mixture of peptides and a few amino acids. Although gastric digestion of protein plays a limited role in protein digestion in normal individuals, peptic digestion enhances intestinal protein absorption in patients with pancreatic insufficiency.[4]

In normal situations, gastric emptying and not hydrolysis is rate limiting in the absorption of protein.[5] Thus, in normal individuals, there is little benefit to using predigested protein formulas. Most protein is absorbed in the proximal portion of the bowel because of the slow and controlled emptying of the stomach. However, when control of gastric emptying is lost (i.e., postpyloric feeding tubes), the entire length of the small intestine may not be sufficient for complete absorption of dietary protein.[5] In these situations, hydrolyzed protein can be more completely absorbed than amino acids or intact proteins. Delayed gastric emptying (common in many critically ill patients) may also decrease the assimilation rate of protein by limiting flow of nutrients to the intestinal absorptive surface. Factors that decrease gastric emptying include critical illness, hyperosmolality, hypo-osmolality, high fat content, high fiber content, and acidic duodenal pH. Delayed gastric emptying can be overcome by placing feeding tubes in a postpyloric position. In addition, increased intestinal transit (i.e., hypermotility) can limit nutrient absorption.

Digested protein products are potent stimuli for the release of cholecystokinin (CCK), which in turn stimulates the secretion of pancreatic enzyme precursors. Pancreatic proteases are secreted in the form of proenzymes. They are activated by enterokinase, a brush border enzyme that is stimulated by trypsinogen and released from the brush border by bile acids. Trypsin (from trypsinogen) activates other pancreatic proproteases and releases more trypsin from trypsinogen. This process results in a mixture of endopeptidases (i.e., trypsin, chymotrypsin, elastase) and exopeptidases (i.e., carboxypeptidases A and B). These enzymes digest proteins to peptides and amino acids.[6, 7] Small oligopeptides are not further hydrolyzed in the gut lumen because they are not suitable substrates for pancreatic proteolytic enzymes. These processes of protein digestion will be limited in situations of pancreatic insufficiency and loss of membrane-bound enzymes (i.e., following infection, gut atrophy, mucosal damage).

The time required for complete in vitro digestion of protein to free amino acids by the successive actions of pepsin, trypsin, and erepsin is measured in days rather than hours.[8] Thus, most protein must be absorbed from peptide rather than in amino acid form. In the proximal portion of the jejunum, peptides account for 60% to 70% of luminal amino nitrogen. This percentage falls to 50% in the distal part of the small bowel.[9, 10] The remainder of hydrolysis occurs through the action of membrane (i.e., brush border) and cytoplasmic (i.e., intracellular) peptidases. Normally, only 3% to 5% of ingested nitrogen escapes absorption and is excreted in the stool. Incomplete assimilation of amino acid nitrogen may be due to peptide bonds resistant to digestion or excess transit times.

The number of peptidases found in the enterocyte (brush border and cytoplasm) is large. Enterokinase is found in the brush border and converts trypsinogen to trypsin. Other brush border enzymes include endopeptidases and aminopeptidases (brush border phase of digestion). The hydrolytic activity of

these peptidases is primarily for tetrapeptides and higher peptides. Hydrolase activity is small for peptides of shorter length (i.e., dipeptides and tripeptides), which can be absorbed intact. Many brush border enzymes are induced by substrate and enzyme activity decreases when luminal nutrients are absent (i.e., starvation, total parenteral nutrition).

Peptides larger than three amino acids are hydrolyzed extracellularly by brush border enzymes. Dipeptides and tripeptides can be absorbed intact. There are a large number of dipeptidases and tripeptidases in the enterocyte (cytoplasmic phase of digestion). Although it was once thought that most dipeptides and tripeptides were cleaved intracellularly, it is now apparent that some small peptides escape intracellular hydrolysis and reach the blood intact.

Amino acids are absorbed by multiple specific transport systems that are sodium dependent. Amino acid absorption is primarily performed by enterocytes at the top third of the villus. Protein may also be absorbed in the dipeptide and tripeptide forms.[7, 11, 12] Currently, it is believed that most protein is absorbed in the peptide form but that most protein enters the portal circulation as free amino acids (70%). Some amino acids are absorbed from the intestinal lumen more rapidly in the form of peptides than when presented as an equimolar mixture of free amino acids.[11, 13, 14] At least one distinct sodium-requiring transport system for dipeptides and tripeptides has been described.[15]

There are numerous cases in which small peptides have been demonstrated to cross the intestine and enter the circulation intact.[6, 16, 17] The passage of intact peptides across the intestine reflects the extracellular and intracellular digestibility of the peptide as well as the availability of peptide transport systems. Gardner[18] perfused rat small intestine with hydrolyzed protein and estimated that up to 30% of the amino nitrogen reaching the serosal surface of the intestine was in the form of peptides. Webb[19] measured amino acid and peptide levels in the portal vein following a mixed meal in calves. The investigators reported that approximately 70% of the amino acids entering the portal blood were in the form of peptides (molecular weight, 300 to 1500).

The importance of peptide digestibility is further supported by the intact absorption of peptides with blocked amino terminals. These include N-benzoyl-L-tyrosyl-p-aminobenzoic acid, luteinizing hormone releasing hormone (LHRH, a decapeptide) and thyrotropin releasing hormone (TRH, a tripeptide).[6] Both hypothalamic peptides contain a pyroglutamyl residue at the amino terminus and are resistant to peptidase hydrolysis.

After transport across the intestinal wall, amino acids are degraded, metabolized to other amino acids, incorporated into proteins, or released into the portal blood. Luminal amino acids are utilized more readily for intestinal protein synthesis than are intravenous amino acids.[20] These processes are relatively independent of hormonal regulation. Glutamine, the only amino acid consistently consumed by the small intestine, is a major source of energy for the gut and is an important source of ammonia. The colon absorbs water, electrolytes, sugars, and fiber degradation products but not protein products. Thus, protein that reaches the colon is lost from the body.

DISORDERS OF DIGESTION/ABSORPTION

There is a reduction in the formation of peptides from dietary protein in patients with pancreatic insufficiency, celiac disease, congenital enterokinase deficiency, trypsinogen-trypsin deficiency, and other diseases that disrupt pancreatic secretion or intestinal brush border integrity. Many patients with critical illnesses following shock, trauma, resus-

citation, and sepsis may have altered digestive capabilities. Altered digestion may result from pancreatic insufficiency, altered brush border integrity, diminished mucus secretion, and atrophy of enterocytes. In addition, gut atrophy from a lack of luminal nutrients (i.e., starvation, total parenteral nutrition) may impair digestive functions. Patients with disorders of nutrient digestion benefit from the administration of nutrients in an optimally absorbable form.

Diffuse diseases of the intestinal mucosa such as celiac disease reduce amino acid and peptide absorption. In celiac disease, amino acid absorption is affected more than peptide absorption.[21-23] Nitrogen retention is significantly higher in patients with Crohn's disease who are receiving peptide-based diets as compared with amino acid–based diets.[24] Amino acid absorption is also decreased in patients with pancreatic insufficiency and renal failure. Peptide absorption in these patients is not significantly altered.[4, 25-27]

Gut absorption is impaired in patients following trauma. Using D-xylose absorption tests, we found that 60-minute D-xylose levels were significantly lower in patients following trauma than in normal individuals (14 ± 6 vs. 46 ± 4 mg/dL). Interestingly, levels were similar in patients with and without diarrhea. These patients had significantly less diarrhea when fed with peptide vs. intact protein diets.

The gut is very sensitive to the effects of malnutrition. Hypoplasia and hypofunction develop rapidly. Starvation and protein deprivation reduce amino acid absorption in human volunteers[28] and animals.[29] Protein-calorie malnutrition secondary to jejunoileal bypass for obesity also reduces jejunal absorption of amino acids.[30] Dipeptide absorption remains normal in many of these patients. Patients with cystinuria and Hartnup's disease have selective disorders of amino acid transport. Protein malnutrition does not develop in these patients because of intact peptide transport.[11] To date, no genetic defect of peptide transport has been described. Owing to the physiologic importance of peptide transport in assimilating dietary protein, such a defect is felt to be incompatible with life.

PROTEIN QUALITY

Protein quality depends upon the amino acid profile. The most commonly used method for evaluating the quality of a specific protein is determination of its biological value (BV). This is a measure of nitrogen retained and is expressed as nitrogen retained divided by nitrogen absorbed. The lower the BV, the greater the amount of protein required to achieve nitrogen equilibrium. For example, lactalbumin plus methionine has a BV of 130; whole egg, 100; cow's milk, 90; fish, 85; beef, 76; soybeans, 75; and casein, 72.[31] Enteral nutrition with protein in the form of free amino acids results in poor nitrogen retention. Much of the ingested nitrogen is converted to urea and excreted rather than retained for protein synthesis.[32, 33] The BV of peptides exceeds intact protein, which in turn exceeds amino acids.[33]

Although many nutritional formulas contain peptides and amino acids, there are significant differences in the content (i.e., quantity) and quality of both free amino acids and peptides in these diets. Current formulas contain from 20% to 70% peptides. The peptide chain lengths and need for further digestion vary. In addition, the sequences of peptides differ depending upon the source of protein or proteins utilized (i.e., whey, casein, soy, lactalbumin, meat) and the degree and type of hydrolysis employed (i.e., controlled vs. noncontrolled). Controlled hydrolysis utilizes specific enzymes (i.e., trypsin, chymotrypsin) that cleave the proteins at well-defined points. Uncontrolled hydrolysis (i.e., acid) cleaves at random and is poorly reproducible. The specific types and quantities of peptides can affect absorption, biological activity, nitrogen retention, and the overall metabolic response. For example, sodium and water absorption is stimulated with casein and lactalbumin hydrolysates but not fish protein hydrolysates.[34] In addition, protein hydrolysates with higher concentrations of small peptides have greater stimulatory effects on sodium and water absorption than do formulas containing lower peptide concentrations.[35, 36]

There are four major factors that have an influence on amino acid assimilation from protein hydrolysates.[36, 37] These are the starter protein, the amino acid sequence of constituent peptides in the hydrolysate, the enzymes used in hydrolysis, and the chain length of peptides in the hydrolysate. In the absence of pancreatic secretions, hydrolysates of higher molecular weight are absorbed slower than lower–molecular-weight peptides.[35, 36]

BIOGENIC AMINES

Classic theories of protein digestion and absorption assert that proteins are completely digested within the intestine so that only free amino acids enter the circulation. However, accumulating evidence indicates that digested fragments of proteins (i.e., peptides) cross the small intestine and access peripheral tissue via the systemic circulation. Diseases that affect the integrity, permeability, and digestive capacity of the small intestine alter the ability of peptides to enter the circulation. The known potent biological activities of small peptides (i.e., picogram quantities) suggest that many small peptides derived from dietary proteins may play a role in regulating physiologic processes. These peptides may act as neurotransmitters and release hormones and cytokines.

A variety of amino acids and small

peptides have been shown to have biological activity in excess of their nutrient value. Small peptides have been observed to traverse the intestine and end up in the plasma.[38-40] Studies in man and animals have shown beyond doubt that the transmucosal passage of many molecules larger than amino acids, in small but significant quantities, is possible.[8, 38-49] Examples include glycyl-glycine,[40, 42, 43] Gly-Pro,[40] Gly-Phe,[40] TRH,[39] LHRH,[38] carnosine,[40, 44] insulin,[47] vasopressin, albumin,[48] hydroxyproline peptides,[45, 49] immunoglobulins in colostrum, ferritin, polyethylene glycol, polyvinylpyrrolidone, benzoyl-tyrosyl-p-aminobenzoic acid, and many other small peptides.[8, 46] The absorption of nitrogen in the form of small peptides plays a major role in nitrogen absorption. However, most of the absorbed nitrogen is probably exported into the portal vein in the form of amino acids. Despite this, the entry of small peptides into the circulation is of great potential pathophysiologic significance and merits further investigation.

The passage of intact peptides across the intestine is a reflection of the nature of the parent proteins. Soy and casein hydrolysates result in greater peptide absorption than do muscle digests.[46] The quantity of peptides passing the intestine intact is debated. Some investigators believe that little peptide enters the circulation intact and that most nitrogen absorbed in peptide form enters the circulation as amino acids. The difficulty in quantitating the amount of peptide that enters the circulation intact stems from the difficulty in assaying for absorbed peptides and variations in transport of different peptides. Gardner[46] perfused rat small intestines with hydrolyzed proteins and estimated that up to 30% of the amino nitrogen reaching the serosal surface of the intestine during absorption was peptide bound. Subsequently, Gardner et al.[50] confirmed these findings in an in vivo model. Webb[51] assayed for arterial venous differences of amino acids and peptides across the gastrointestinal tract of calves following a mixed meal. Large quantities of peptide amino acids appeared in the portal blood, and the investigators reported that more than 70% of the amino acids appearing in portal blood were in the peptide fraction. Their molecular weights were between 300 and 1500. These authors also reported that the liver and hindlimb removed these small peptides from the circulation.[51, 52] In addition, intravenous dipeptides have been utilized to maintain body nitrogen economy.[53] Thus, it appears that a significant quantity of luminal peptides escape hydrolysis, cross the intestine intact, and are utilized for nitrogen economy.

Peptides absorbed from the gastrointestinal tract can exert biological actions. Oral administration of LHRH (p-Glu-His-Trp-Ser-Tyr-Gly-Leu-Arg-Pro-Gly) and an LHRH metabolite (i.e., p-Glu-His-Trp) stimulate the release of luteinizing hormone (LH).[38] Ten micrograms of oral LHRH increased plasma LH by 451%, and 1 mg of oral LHRH increased plasma LH 1448%. Oral TRH (cyclo-Glu-His-Pro) stimulates the release of TSH.[39] The oral dose required for maximal thyroid-stimulating hormone (TSH) release was 40 times the intravenous dose. In addition to stimulating the release of TSH from the pituitary gland, TRH also possesses significant hypertensive[54, 55] and neuromodulating activity.[56] Interestingly, common foods and nutritional supplements contain the bioactive peptide cyclo(His-Pro).[57, 58] This peptide is the active form of TRH. A number of peptides have been isolated from digested food and demonstrate opiate-like activity.[59, 60] These peptides appear to act on gut luminal receptors and act as exogenous regulators of gastrointestinal motility, gut permeability, and gut hormone release.[59-61] One such peptide is β-casomorphin (Tyr-Pro-Phe-Pro-Gly-Pro-Ile). β-Caso-morphin decreases small-bowel electrical activity, enhances sodium and chloride absorption, and modulates bowel permeability.[61, 62] It is currently under evaluation for the treatment of diarrhea.

A large number of other small peptides have been discovered that produce significant biological effects (Table 4–1)[63–67] Met-enkephalin is a pentapeptide that modulates immune reactions.[63, 64] It alters antibody responses, delayed cutaneous hypersensitivity responses, and allograft rejection. Met-enkephalin has been shown to reverse the age-related decline in immune function.[64] Recent studies in our laboratory indicate that small peptides produced in the diet have the capability of altering cardiovascular function, renal function, and wound healing. Histidine-methionine stimulates growth hormone release in some acromegalics,[66] thus suggesting the presence of pituitary receptors for the peptide in growth hormone–producing tumors. Arg-Gly-Asp forms a component of the cell attachment site for microbes. This peptide has been used to antagonize the adherence of *Candida albicans* to subendothelial binding sites.[67] There are

TABLE 4–1.

Biologically Active Peptides

Peptide	Bioactivity
LRH* (p-Glu-His-Trp-Ser-Tyr-Gly-Leu-Arg-Pro-Gly)	Releases LH* and FSH*
p-Glu-His-Trp	Releases LH and FSH
TRH* (cyclo-Glu-His-Pro)	Releases TSH and prolactin, neuromodulator, vasoactive
Cyclo-His-Pro	Same as TRH
Met-enkephalin	Immunomodulatory
Carcinine (β-alanylhistamine)	Lowers blood pressure, positive inotrope
His-Met	Growth hormone release in acromegalics
Arg-Gly-Asp	Microbe cell attachment site
Met-Leu-Phe	Leukocyte chemoattractant
Tyr-Pro-Phe-Val-Glu-Pro-Ile	β-Casomorphin; opiate activity
Tyr-Pro-Phe	Opiate activity
Tyr-Arg	Releases Met-enkephalin

*LRH = luteinizing hormone releasing hormone; LH = luteinizing hormone; FSH = follicle-stimulating hormone; TRH = thyrotropin releasing hormone.

many other peptides with biological activities. The potential biological effects of these peptides when administered enterally and the implications for nutritional therapy remain to be explored.

The parent protein used in nutritional formulas can alter physiologic/metabolic functions. Different proteins may produce their effects through production of biogenic peptides with different activities. For example, the immune responses of mice fed lactalbumin hydrolysates are significantly greater than those of mice fed casein hydrolysates.[68] Immune function is also better in mice fed a diet containing casein vs. legume protein.[69] Blood pressure is lower in individuals consuming vegetable vs. meat proteins.[70] Small intestinal transit time is enhanced with soy protein as compared with casein.[71] Finally, the glomerular filtration rate and renal plasma flow are significantly higher in humans receiving animal vs. vegetable protein diets.[72]

Arginine is a biogenic amine that is important for protein synthesis, especially in connective tissue.[73, 74] Although arginine is considered a nonessential amino acid in adults, dietary arginine deficiency impairs protein synthesis and healing during stress. These effects are reversed with arginine. Thus, many consider arginine to be a semiessential amino acid in that arginine requirements exceed synthesis capacity during stress. Recently, supplementation with large doses of arginine (i.e., 1% to 3% of nonprotein calories) has been shown to improve wound healing[73–76] and enhance lymphocyte blastogenesis.[73, 74, 76–80]

Glutamine, a "nonessential" amino acid that forms an important component of proteins and functions as a nitrogen carrier and energy source,[73, 81] is consumed by replicating cells and is important for maintenance of gastrointestinal integrity.[73, 81, 82] Glutamine deficiency is associated with gut atrophy during stress. Large doses of glutamine have been shown to prevent gut atrophy, maintain bowel integrity, and prevent bacterial translocation following various insults (i.e., methotrexate [MTX], radiation injury, lack of luminal nutrients). Thus, many would also consider glutamine to be semiessential. It appears that both arginine and glutamine possess specific biological activity beyond their "nutrient" value. The optimal dose and optimal form (i.e., amino acid, peptide) for delivery of these amino acids remain to be determined. In addition, specific diseases that might benefit from the administration of these amines needs to be defined.

In summary, small peptides and amines have been known for many years to be important cellular messengers and neurohumoral modulators throughout the body. It is now recognized that small peptides with biological activity can enter the circulation intact via the gastrointestinal tract. It is also recognized that small peptides have biological effects locally on the gut. This has spurred research efforts into the possibility of enteral administration of biogenic amines. The implications for the nutritional/metabolic treatment of patients is clear and exciting.

STUDIES OF ORGAN FUNCTION

Gastrointestinal Tract

Because of the existence of a dual system for protein absorption (i.e., amino acid and peptide), experiments have been conducted to determine whether the form of protein (i.e., amino acids, peptides, intact protein) alters absorption. Numerous investigators have demonstrated improved protein absorption from the gastrointestinal tract when protein is administered in the form of peptides (i.e., protein hydrolysates) as opposed to amino acids.[8, 13, 29, 83–87] Chain length affects peptide absorption. Some investigators report that peptides with three or fewer amino acids are absorbed faster than peptides of longer length.[85] Others have failed to

confirm these findings.[88, 89] In addition, some have claimed that the absorptive advantage of peptides disappears when they are administered as part of a mixed meal.[90] The net transmembrane flux of nutrients has been examined by using the isolated ileal loop technique in animals.[91, 92] The administration of hydrolyzed protein, as part of enteral nutrition, results in slightly better absorption when compared with amino acids or intact protein in normal animals.

It is clear that peptides play a major role in the absorption of protein. However, overall the absorptive benefits of peptide diets over amino acid or intact protein diets appear to be marginal in the normal unstressed gut. Thus, we favor the use of intact protein–based nutritional formulas in normal individuals. These formulas are cheaper than amino acid– or peptide-based formulas and have the capacity to generate intraluminal peptides through normal digestive process.

On the other hand, during hypermetabolic stress (i.e., critical illness, sepsis, trauma, surgery) and diseases of the gastrointestinal tract, there may be an absorptive advantage to peptide-based feeding solutions. With the isolated ileal loop technique, peptide diets were better absorbed when compared with amino acid or intact protein diets in fluid-resuscitated hypo-oncotic animals.[91, 92] In fact, amino acid– and intact protein–based formulas resulted in net secretion. A formula containing 50% small peptides was better absorbed than a formula containing 20% small peptides. Gut absorption was also examined in animals following the administration of endotoxin[93] and the chemotherapeutic agent 5-fluorouracil (5-FU).[94] Gut absorption was higher on a peptide diet following endotoxin administration than on an amino acid diet.[93] After 5-FU, diarrhea developed in 80% of the animals fed chow (a solid complex fiber–based diet)[94] and in all animals given an amino acid–based formula. Diarrhea developed in only 32% of animals fed a high-peptide formula. Following burn injury, diarrhea developed in 50% of animals fed an amino acid–based diet vs. only 20% of animals fed an intact protein diet.[95] We believe that these animals maintained the capacity to digest the intact protein to peptides. The resultant endogenously hydrolyzed protein diet was better absorbed when compared with the amino acid diet.

These animal studies have been extended to humans. Ziegler et al.[96] reported better amino acid absorption from a peptide vs. intact protein diet in 12 intensive care patients following abdominal surgery. The insulin response was also greater in the patients receiving the peptide diet. Amino acid peripheral bioavailability[97] was evaluated in 11 patients following gastrointestinal surgery. Amino acid absorption (area under the curve) was assessed following the administration of a protein hydrolysate or intact protein formula in a randomized crossover design. Amino acid peripheral bioavailability was significantly better with the protein hydrolysate diet. Cosnes et al.[98] measured protein absorption in six patients with high jejunostomies (i.e., short bowel) following intestinal resection. Residual jejunum ranged from 90 to 150 cm. Patients were randomized to three 3-day feedings of an intact protein, peptide, or mixed peptide–intact protein diet. Nitrogen absorption was significantly increased with the peptide diets vs. the whole-protein diet. In addition, a peptide-based diet decreased stool output in critically ill and irradiated patients when compared with an intact protein diet.[99–101] We performed a prospective randomized trial of a peptide diet vs. an intact protein diet in patients early following traumatic injury.[102] Diarrhea developed in 40% of patients receiving the intact protein formula vs. 0% receiving the peptide diet. In previous studies, we have found a 50% incidence of diarrhea when these patients were fed an amino acid–based diet. A peptide diet has also been reported to be better tolerated than an amino acid diet (i.e., nausea, vomiting, diarrhea, abdominal distention) in postoperative patients.[103]

Reicht et al.[104] measured nitrogen absorption in healthy subjects (using multilumen tubes) fed whey or hydrolyzed whey protein. When an occluding balloon was used to exclude gastric and pancreatic secretions, only the hydrolyzed whey was absorbed. The intact protein resulted in a net luminal gain of nitrogen (i.e., secretion). When no occluding balloon was used, both protein solutions were absorbed. However, absorption was greater with the hydrolyzed protein (6.1 vs. 2.3 g/hr/30 cm). These data suggest that protein absorption is greater in patients fed into the proximal part of the jejunum with peptide vs. intact protein diets.

Amino acid absorption is impaired in patients with celiac sprue,[21–23] Hartnup's disease,[8] pancreatitis,[4, 25] chronic renal failure,[26] and starvation.[28–30, 105, 106] Despite decreases in amino acid absorption, many of these patients maintain adequate peptide absorption. Following pancreatectomy,[27] a protein hydrolysate was also better absorbed than an intact protein diet. Peptide transport systems appear to be more resistant to disease processes than amino acid transport. The degree of amino acid vs. peptide absorption in critically ill or injured patients has not been fully evaluated.

The gut may serve as a portal of entry for bacteria responsible for sepsis and organ failure during critical illness. The form of protein in the diet can affect gut mass and function. Amino acid–based diets are associated with gut atrophy when compared with more complex diets containing intact protein and peptides.[107–112] In one study,[111] peptides were found to have a trophic effect and resulted in higher gut mass than either an amino acid diet or chow diet. Following 60% small-bowel resection, gut mass, glucose uptake, and amino acid uptake are higher in animals receiving hydrolyzed protein as compared with animals receiving intact protein.[113] Intact protein diets also maintain better small-bowel mass when compared with amino acid–based diets following burn injury in animals.[95]

Intestinal integrity is better maintained with a hydrolyzed protein diet vs. a regular diet in animals following hemorrhage.[114] Bacterial translocation has also been reported to be higher in animals fed amino acid–based diets vs. peptide or intact protein diets.[107, 112, 115–118] Shou et al.[107] fed mice a regular chow diet, free amino acid diet, peptide-based diet, or polypeptide-based diet for 7 days. Bacterial translocation occurred in 67% of the mice fed amino acids, 20% of those fed polypeptides, 13% of those fed peptides, and 6.6% of the mice fed chow. Amino acid–based diets have been shown to impair macrophage tumor cytotoxicity when compared with intact protein diets.[116] Bacterial translocation to the mesenteric lymph nodes was higher in animals fed an amino acid–based diet for 7 days vs. regular chow (75% vs 0%).[112] The animals fed the elemental diet also had poorer macrophage function (i.e., superoxide production, *Candida albicans* killing). Endotoxin challenge results in greater translocation, increased bacteremia, greater release of tumor necrosis factor, and higher mortality in animals fed an amino acid–based formula vs. standard rat chow.[118] Animals fed a peptide-based diet, when compared with chow, do not demonstrate an increased incidence of translocation following endotoxin administration.[119]

Hypotension not only decreases gut blood flow and alters the gut barrier, but leads to bacterial translocation/sepsis.[114, 120, 121] Ischemic necrosis of the intestinal mucosa has been reported in various states of critical illness (i.e., sepsis, hemorrhage, burns). We have reported higher mortality rates in animals receiving amino acid–based formulas after hemorrhage when compared with peptides or intact protein–based formulas.[122] Bounous et al.[114] reported higher mortality after hemorrhage and mesenteric artery clamping in animals fed oral regular diets vs. hydrolyzed protein diets. Higher mortality was associated with greater intestinal and extraintestinal pathology.

Amino acid–based formulas have been associated with higher mortality in animals treated with high-dose MTX vs. peptide or intact protein diets.[117, 123, 124] Mortality following MTX administration in animals was reduced in parallel with the substitution of polypeptides for amino acids in the diet.[123] The effect of diet on 5-FU toxicity has also been studied. A peptide diet, when compared with an intact protein diet, protected the intestinal mucosa against injury[125] and maintained better body weight and albumin levels[125–127] after 5-FU administration. Diarrhea was less in rats fed a peptide diet following 5-FU administration vs. an amino acid diet or control diet.[128] On the other hand, mortality, diarrhea, and positive blood cultures increased in animals treated with 5-FU as one advanced from a chow diet to intact protein–, peptide-, and finally amino acid–based diets.[129, 130] Humans with malignancies treated with 5-FU maintain better weight and gut integrity on a peptide diet when compared with regular food.[131] Peptide-based diets improve intestinal function and survival in animals subjected to radiation injury.[132–134] Mucosal cell regeneration has been reported to be enhanced in animals fed protein hydrolysates instead of intact protein diets during irradiation.[135] A peptide diet was also associated with reduced gastrointestinal toxicity in patients following abdominal irradiation,[101] whereas an amino acid diet had no effect.[136] Beer et al,[137] reported better nitrogen utilization with a peptide vs. an amino acid diet in patients with radiation enteritis (and chronic diarrhea).

Recently, small peptides have been shown to modulate bowel permeability and protein leakage.[61, 138] Gut permeability was assessed in animals by using[51] Cr-labeled ethylenediamine tetraacetic acid (EDTA) clearance.[61] Gut permeability was increased following fluid resuscitation and the production of a hypoalbuminemic state. This increase in gut permeability was prevented by infusing the gut with a specific peptide, β-casomorphin, during fluid resuscitation.[61] These data suggest that specific peptides produced in the gut lumen through protein digestion can modulate permeability of the bowel mucosa. Intestinal integrity was also evaluated in 14 critically ill patients by measuring leakage of α_1-antitrypsin into the stool.[138] In a prospective randomized study, stool α_1-antitrypsin levels were lower (i.e., integrity improved) in patients fed an enteral peptide-based diet vs. an intact protein diet. Peptide-based diets have also been reported to decrease protein leakage into the gastrointestinal tract and improve intestinal morphology in patients with radiation-induced gut injury[139] and inflammatory bowel disease.[140]

We conclude that there is little absorptive advantage of peptide-based diets over intact protein–based diets in patients with intact digestive/absorptive functions. Patients with intact digestion can generate physiologically active peptides from intact protein in their guts. We believe that there are advantages to the use of peptide-based formulas in patients with impaired digestion or amino acid transport. However, there are few available data to support the use of amino acid–based formulas over intact protein or peptide formulas.

Liver Function

The liver is an important organ for maintenance of immunologic competence (i.e., synthesis of immune-related proteins, reticuloendothelial system function), synthesis of vital proteins, and processing of endogenous waste products. Liver dysfunction is common during critical illness and is associated with a poor prognosis. Maintenance of hepatic integrity is associated with improved outcome.

The effect of diets on hepatic function is an area of intense interest. Parenteral nutrition is associated with a rise in hepatic enzyme levels and a decrease in hepatic function.[141–143] When compared with parenteral nutrition, enteral nutrition is less frequently associated with hepatic alterations. However, the composition of enteral diets may also affect hepatic function. Lipid is deposited in the livers of animals fed diets containing amino acids and low fat (<5%).[144] The liver lipid content ranged from 3% to 5% in animals fed a complex fiber diet (i.e., chow), intact protein diet, or peptide-based diet. On the other hand, the liver lipid content ranged from 9% to 10% in animals fed amino acid/low-fat diets. Liver lipid deposition partially relates to the high-carbohydrate/low-fat ratio of the diet and is frequently associated with hepatic dysfunction. Recently, hepatic function, as measured by cytochrome P-450 activity and hepatic drug clearance, was evaluated in animals fed various diets.[145] Hepatic function was reduced by 40% to 50% in animals fed amino acid/low-fat diets vs. diets containing intact protein or peptides and moderate fat (approximately 30% to 35%). Impairment of liver function was felt to relate to both the use of amino acids as the protein source and the low fat content of the diet.

We recently evaluated the effect of enteral diet composition on liver function in animals following hemorrhage. Enteral nutrient administration protected the liver from injury when compared with the enteral administration of saline.[146] In another study,[122] we assessed liver function by bile acid levels. Liver function deteriorated in animals fed intact protein– and amino acid–based enteral diets following hemorrhage. It remained intact in animals fed a peptide-based diet. Liver function has also been reported to worsen in MTX-treated animals fed amino acid–based diets vs. animals fed polypeptide-based diets.[123] In addition, thermal injury results in lower liver weights, albumin levels, and transferrin concentrations in animals fed amino acid–based diets vs. intact protein diets.[95]

We evaluated liver function (by using retinol-binding protein, prealbumin, and transferrin) in trauma patients fed intact protein– vs. peptide-based diets in two prospective randomized studies.[102, 147] In both studies, we found a significant improvement in hepatic protein levels in patients randomized to the peptide diets. Improved visceral protein synthesis appears to result from faster resolution of the systemic inflammatory response to injury. Ziegler et al.[97] also reported improved visceral protein responses (i.e., albumin, transferrin, retinol-binding protein) with a peptide vs. intact protein diet in intensive care unit (ICU) patients following abdominal surgery. In an additional but nonrandomized trial in trauma patients no differences in prealbumin or transferrin responses were found when comparing an intact protein with a peptide diet.[148] Dietscher et al.[149] randomized acutely ill patients to a peptide or intact protein diet for 7 days. Albumin and prealbumin levels increased more on the peptide diet. However, the number of patients studied was small, and the differences between groups did not meet statistical significance at the $P = 0.05$ level. Ford and colleagues[150] randomized patients to small-bowel feeding with an amino acid vs. intact protein diet following abdominal surgery. Serum prealbumin levels improved similarly in both groups. Retinol-binding protein, transferrin, and albumin concentrations were also found to improve to a greater extent in nursing home patients fed a peptide diet vs. an amino acid–based diet.[151]

Overall, we believe that peptide-based diets can better support liver function in critically ill patients when compared with intact protein- and amino acid-

based diets. Diets containing amino acids and low fat are associated with significant impairment of hepatic function. Again, we do not believe that there is any benefit of peptide-based diets over intact protein diets in patients with normal digestion/absorption who can generate bioactive peptides in their gut lumina.

Endocrine/Hormonal Responses

Peptides are known to be regulators of neurohumoral secretion. Examples include TRH, corticotropin-releasing hormone, and endogenous opioids. TRH is secreted as a tripeptide (Glu-His-Pro) and metabolized to an active dipeptide (i.e., cyclo-His-Pro). These peptides are absorbed via the gastrointestinal tract and have been shown to stimulate the release of TSH. TRH is an example of a small peptide that is bioactive when administered via the gastrointestinal tract. Studies under way suggest that peptide-based enteral formulas contain a large variety of small peptides that possess bioactivity.

Gut hormones are important for the maintenance of gut integrity (i.e., intestine, liver, pancreas). These hormones are secreted into the portal circulation where they stimulate growth and repair of the gut. Gut hormone secretion is stimulated by enteral but not parenteral feeding. The most important factor for their stimulation is the presence of luminal nutrients. The form of protein can also affect gut hormone secretion. Glucagon secretion is greater when stimulated by enteral peptides as compared with enteral amino acids.[13] In addition, gastrin release is greater with intact protein vs. amino acid diets.[152]

We recently evaluated the response of somatomedin C (i.e., insulin growth factor 1 [IGF-1]) to dietary manipulation.[108] IGF-1 is a major growth factor in the body that is responsible for body growth and repair. Levels of IGF-1 were higher in animals fed a peptide-based diet vs. an intact protein– or amino acid–based diet. Levels of the growth factor were lowest in animals receiving amino acid/low-fat diets and correlated with their body growth.

In summary, available data suggest that the peptides contained in enteral feeding formulas can gain access to the circulation and have bioactivity. We believe that the poor "hormonal" response to amino acid–based diets (which have no potential of producing bioactive peptides) is responsible for their lower nutritional performance when compared with peptide- and intact protein–based diets.

NITROGEN UTILIZATION AND GROWTH

It is well established that the quantity of dietary protein has an influence on nitrogen utilization and growth/repair. Recent investigations have centered upon the effect of the form of dietary protein on these parameters.

Normal and malnourished animals grow faster when fed isocaloric isonitrogenous formulas containing peptides vs. intact protein or amino acids.[33, 108] Growth was lowest with amino acid–based diets. Following abdominal surgery, growth was found to be highest with an intact protein diet and lowest with an amino acid–based diet.[153] Growth was intermediate with a peptide-based diet. In pancreatic-deficient rats, growth was significantly greater on the peptide diet when compared with the intact protein– or amino acid–based diet.[153] Following thermal injury, body mass was lower on an amino acid–based diet vs. an intact protein diet.[95] The intact protein diet maintained better body weight, muscle mass, jejunal mucosal weight, liver weight, and visceral protein levels.

The metabolic rate following burn injury is also affected by the form of nitrogen in the diet.[154] There is a progressive increase in metabolic rate as one switches from an intact whey protein diet to an amino acid mixture of the same pattern as whey protein to an intravenous formulation given intragastrically. Thus, these data suggest that both the "quantity" and the form of nitrogen affect the hypermetabolic response.

Peptide-based diets stimulate faster wound healing after abdominal surgery in rats as compared with amino acid–based diets.[155] Peptide-based diets are associated with higher levels of IGF-1[108] and better nitrogen retention[33, 156] when compared with the other diets. Net dietary protein utilization is also better in pancreatic ligated rats when fed a peptide-based diet vs. an amino acid–based diet.[156]

Nitrogen utilization has also been compared in patients with radiation enteritis who received amino acid/low-fat and peptide/low-fat diets.[157] Nitrogen absorption and balance were better with the peptide diet than the amino acid diet. Protein balance studies performed in patients with Crohn's disease also revealed better nitrogen balance with a peptide diet (4.4 g/day) vs. solid food (2.8 g/day) or an amino acid–based diet (0.5 g/day).[24] Children with Crohn's disease and growth failure demonstrate improved growth when switched from a regular diet to a peptide-containing diet.[158] Improved nitrogen retention with peptide-based diets has also been confirmed in postoperative cancer patients[159] and in primates.[160] There was a more rapid increase in plasma amino acid concentrations and a decrease in luminal nitrogen in ICU patients receiving a peptide diet vs. an intact protein diet.[96] These data suggest that protein is better utilized when supplied as peptides vs. amino acids.

OUTCOME

Few studies have evaluated the effect of diet (especially protein form) on outcome parameters. Trocki et al.[95] evaluated the effect of an amino acid diet vs. an intact protein diet on survival from burn injury. Animals fed the intact protein diet demonstrated better survival. The intact protein diet was also associated with better weight maintenance, better muscle mass, better gut and liver mass, and higher circulating levels of visceral proteins. On the other hand, Langlois et al.[161] reported improved survival in animals fed amino acid vs. chow diets following burn injury.

Survival is higher in animals fed intact protein or peptide diets when compared with amino acid–based diets following MTX administration,[117, 123, 124, 162] 5-FU,[129, 130] and hemorrhage.[122] Sitren et al.[162] assessed mortality following MTX treatment in mice fed diets differing in protein source (i.e., casein or soy). Loose stool occurred in 60% of the casein group vs. 0% of the soy group. The soy-fed group maintained better body weight and had higher survival rates (60% vs. 20%). The difference in outcome may have resulted from differences in peptide products generated during protein digestion. This group[162] also assessed the outcome in MTX-treated mice fed diets containing free amino acids, hydrolyzed casein, whole casein, and soy protein. The mortality rate was 100% with amino acids, 60% with intact casein, 0% with hydrolyzed casein, and 0% with soy protein. In radiation injury studies, animals fed protein hydrolysates have better survival rates than do animals fed regular diets or intact protein diets.[132–134]

Jones et al.[163] evaluated the effect of an amino acid diet vs. an intact protein diet on patient recovery from illness and mortality in a prospective randomized study of 70 patients. The amino acid diet was associated with poorer recovery and higher mortality. Meredith et al.[102] evaluated the effect of an intact protein diet vs. a peptide diet in patients with multiple trauma. Patients receiving the peptide diet had less diarrhea, greater increases in visceral protein levels, and a shorter hospital stay. Cerra et al.[164] compared two amino acid diets and a peptide-based diet in surgical patients.

However, the study was not randomized, and patients received different quantities of protein. Patients who received a higher nitrogen:calorie ratio did better. No conclusions could be made regarding the effect of protein form on clinical variables.

FUTURE STUDIES

Although protein quantity has been long recognized to be of major nutritional importance, less investigation has been directed at protein quality. Accumulating data suggest that the dietary protein form can alter metabolic responses. There is a need for both experimental and clinical studies evaluating the effect of protein formulation on gut absorption, tolerance (i.e., diarrhea), gut integrity and bacterial translocation, immune function, infectious complications, organ function, growth, wound repair, hospital stay, and survival. Studies should be performed on a variety of models that reproduce different types and degrees of stress (i.e., burn, trauma, surgery, respiratory failure, malignancy). There is also a need for studies evaluating the effect of protein form on basic biological mechanisms related to immunocompetence, cytokine production, growth factor production, hormonal responses (especially anabolic and catabolic), vasoregulation, growth, and repair. In addition, there is a need for prospective randomized clinical trials evaluating the suitability and effectiveness of enteral products containing different forms of protein (i.e., amino acids, peptides, intact protein) on outcome variables (i.e., organ function, sepsis, hospital stay, survival).

THERAPEUTIC IMPLICATIONS

An important consideration in enteral nutrition is the choice of nitrogen source. The available choices are free amino acids, peptides, or intact proteins. Intact proteins and larger peptides (greater than three amino acids) require digestion for absorption. A knowledge of the source and form of protein is important when prescribing diets for individuals with defects in protein digestion or absorption.

We believe that the form of protein in the diet can affect absorption, gut integrity, hormonal and metabolic responses, and organ function. The gastrointestinal tract evolved over millions of years to digest, process, and absorb protein. Accumulating evidence suggests that the ability to generate peptides in the gut lumen has metabolic advantages (Table 4–2). Diets that lack this capacity (i.e., amino acid based) are generally associated with poorer metabolic and organ responses. Patients with a diminished capacity to digest intact protein to peptides may benefit from peptide-based enteral diets. This information is exciting and offers opportunities for improved patient outcome. The idea that bioactive peptides can be administered through the gastrointestinal tract has numerous implications for improved patient care.

Although we have concentrated on the protein component of nutritional formulas in this review, it is important to realize that carbohydrate and fat also have an impact on metabolic/nutritional responses. In addition, the supplementation of enteral formulas with specific nutrients (i.e., glutamine, arginine, nucleic acids) may also have significant benefit. It is our belief that the optimal composition of the diet for improved patient outcome will be both disease and time dependent. A day may come when we possess the knowledge to match nutrient intake to a specific disease state and then alter that intake depending upon the phase of the patient's illness.

REFERENCES

1. Zaloga GP: Physiologic effects of peptide-based enteral formulas. *Nutr Clin Pract* 1990; 5:231.
2. Gardner MG: L-Amino acid and peptide absorption from partial digests of proteins in isolated small intestine. *J Physiol (Lond)* 1978; 284:83.
3. Freeman HH, Kim YS: Digestion and absorption of proteins. *Annu Rev Med* 1978; 29:99.
4. Curtis KJ, Gaines HD, Kim YS: Protein digestion and absorption in rats with pancreatic duct occlusion. *Gastroenterology* 1979; 74:1271.
5. Koretz RL, Meyer JH: Elemental diets—Facts and fantasies. *Gastroenterology* 1980; 78:393.
6. Gardner MG: Intestinal assimilation of intact peptides and proteins from the diet—a neglected field. *Biol Rev* 1984; 59:289.
7. Matthews DM, Adibi SA: Peptide absorption. *Gastroenterology* 1976; 71:151.
8. Matthews DM: Intestinal absorption of peptides. *Physiol Rev* 1975; 55:537.
9. Nixon SE, Mawer GE: The digestion and absorption of proteins in man. I. The site of absorption. *Br J Nutr* 1970; 24:227.
10. Nixon SE, Mawer GE: The digestion and absorption of proteins in man. II. The form in which digested protein is absorbed. *Br J Nutr* 1970; 24:241.
11. Matthews DM: Intestinal absorption

TABLE 4–2.

Benefits of Peptides in Nutritional Support

Gastrointestinal
  Improved absorption, less diarrhea
  Stimulation of gut mass, prevention of atrophy
  Maintenance of gut integrity, prevention of bacterial
    translocation
Liver function
  Maintenance of hepatic function
  Improved visceral protein synthesis
Endocrine
  Improved secretion of trophic gut hormones
  Improved IGF-1* production
Nitrogen utilization
  Improved nitrogen balance
  Improved growth
  Improved wound healing
Outcome
  Improved survival in experimental models, i.e.,
    hemorrhage, burn, chemotherapy, radiation

*IGF-1 = insulin growth factor 1.

of peptides. *Physiol Rev* 1975;
55:537.

12. Brinson RR, Hanumanthu SK, Pitts
WM: A reappraisal of the peptide-
based formulas: Clinical applications.
Nutr Clin Pract 1989; 4:211.

13. Rerat A, Nunes CS, Mendy F, et al:
Amino acid absorption and production of pancreatic hormones in non-
anesthetized pigs after duodenal infusions of a milk enzymatic hydrolysate
or of free amino acids. *Br J Nutr*
1988; 60:121.

14. Sleisenger MH, Kim YS: Protein digestion and absorption. *N Engl J Med*
1979; 300:659.

15. Matthews DM, Gundy RW, Taylor E,
et al: Influx of two dipeptides glycyl-
sarcosine and ʟ-glutamyl-ʟ-glutamic
acid into hamster jejunum in vitro.
Clin Sci Mol Med 1979; 56:15.

16. Bouillin DJ, Crampton RF, Heading
CE, et al: Intestinal absorption of dipeptides containing glycine phenylalanine, proline, β-alanine, or histidine
in the rat. *Clin Sci Mol Med* 1973;
45:849.

17. Adibi SA, Kim YS: Peptide absorption
and hydrolysis, in Johnson LR (ed):
*Physiology of the Gastrointestinal
Tract.* New York, Raven Press, 1981,
p 1073.

18. Gardner MG: Absorption of intact
peptides—Studies on transport of
protein digests and dipeptides across
rat small intestine in vitro. *Q J Exp
Physiol* 1982; 67:629.

19. Webb KE: Amino acid and peptide absorption from the gastrointestinal
tract. *Fed Proc* 1986; 45:2268.

20. Hirschfield JS, Kern F: Protein starvation and the small intestine. III. Incorporation of orally and intraperitoneally administered ʟ-leucine-4,5-³H into
intestinal mucosal proteins of protein-
deprived rats. *J Clin Invest* 1969;
48:1224.

21. Matthews DM, Adibi SA: Peptide absorption. *Gastroenterology* 1976;
71:151.

22. Adibi SA, Fogel MR, Agrawal RM:
Comparison of free amino acid and
dipeptide absorption in the jejunum
of sprue patients. *Gastroenterology*
1974; 67:586.

23. Silk DBA, Kumar PJ, Perrett D, et al:
Amino acid and peptide absorption in
patients with coeliac disease and dermatitis herpetiformis. *Gut* 1974;
15:1.

24. Smith JL, Arteaga C, Heymsfield SB:
Increased ureagenesis and impaired
nitrogen use during infusion of a synthetic amino acid formula. *N Engl J
Med* 1982; 306:1013.

25. Milla PJ, Kilby A, Rassam UB, et al:
Small intestinal absorption of amino
acids and a dipeptide in pancreatic
insufficiency. *Gut* 1983; 24:818.

26. Sterner G, Lindberg T, Denneberg T:
Small intestinal absorption of glycine
and glycyl-glycine in patients with
chronic renal failure. *Acta Med Scand*
1983; 213:375.

27. Steinhardt HJ, Wolf A, Jakober B, et
al: Nitrogen absorption in pancreatec-
tomised patients: Protein versus protein hydrolysate as substrate. *J Lab
Clin Med* 1989; 113:162.

28. Adibi SA, Allen ER: Impaired jejunal
absorption rates of essential amino
acids induced by either dietary caloric
or protein deprivation in man. *Gastroenterology* 1970; 59:404.

29. Li MT, Matthews DM: Effects of dietary restriction and protein deprivation on intestinal absorption of protein digestion products in the rat. *Br
J Nutr* 1972; 28:443.

30. Fogel MR, Ravitch MM, Adibi SA: Absorption and digestive function of the
jejunum after jejunoileal bypass for
treatment of human obesity. *Gastroenterology* 1976; 71:729.

31. MacBurney MM, Russell C, Young LS:
Formulas, in Rombeau JL, Caldwell
MD (eds): *Clinical Nutrition—Enteral
and Tube Feeding* ed 2. Philadelphia,
WB Saunders, 1990, p. 149.

32. Smith JL, Arteaga C, Heymsfield SB:
Increased ureagenesis and impaired
nitrogen use during infusion of a synthetic amino acid formula. *N Engl J
Med* 1982; 306:1013.

33. Poullain MG, Cezard JP, Roger L, et
al: Effect of whey proteins, their oligo-
peptide hydrolysates, and free amino
mixtures on growth and nitrogen retention in fed and starved rats. *JPEN*
1989; 13:382.

34. Silk DBA, Fairclough PD, Clark ML, et al: Use of a peptide rather than free amino nitrogen source in chemically defined "elemental" diets. *JPEN* 1980; 4:548.
35. Keohane PP, Grimble GK, Brown B, et al: Influence of protein composition and hydrolysis method on intestinal absorption of protein in man. *Gut* 1985; 26:907.
36. Grimble GK, Keohane PP, Higgins BE, et al: Effect of peptide chain length on amino acid and nitrogen absorption from two lactalbumin hydrolysates in normal human jejunum. *Clin Sci* 1986; 71:65.
37. Grimble GK, Silk DBA: The nitrogen source of elemental diets—an unresolved issue? *Nutr Clin Pract* 1990; 5:227.
38. Amoss M, Rivier J, Guillemin R: Release of gonadotropins by oral administration of synthetic LRF or a tripeptide fragment of LRF. *J Clin Endocrinol Metab* 1972; 35:175.
39. Bowers CY, Schally AV, Enzmann F, et al: Porcine thyrotropin releasing hormone is (pyro)-Glu-His-Pro (NH2). *Endocrinology* 1970; 86:1143.
40. Boullin DJ, Crampton RF, Heading CE, et al: Intestinal absorption of dipeptides containing glycine, phenylalanine, proline, beta-alanine or histidine in the rat. *Clin Sci Mol Med* 1973; 45:849.
41. Gardner MG: Intestinal assimilation of intact peptides and proteins from the diet—a neglected field? *Biol Rev* 1984; 59:289.
42. Adibi SA: Intestinal absorption of dipeptides in man: Relative importance of hydrolysis and intact absorption. *J Clin Invest* 1971; 50:2266.
43. Newey H, Smyth DH: The intestinal absorption of some dipeptides. *J Physiol* 1959; 145:48.
44. Perry TL, Hansen S, Tischler B, et al: Carnosinemia: A new metabolic disorder associated with neurological disease and mental defect. *N Engl J Med* 1967; 227:1219.
45. Hueckel HJ, Rogers QR: Prolylhydroxyproline absorption in hamsters. *Can J Biochem* 1972; 50:782.
46. Gardner MLG: Absorption of intact peptides: Studies on transport of protein digests and dipeptides across rat small intestine in vitro. *Q J Exp Physiol* 1982; 67:629.
47. Danforth E, Moore RO: Intestinal absorption of insulin in the rat. *Endocrinology* 1959; 65:118.
48. Warshaw Al, Walker WA, Isselbacher KJ: Protein uptake by the intestine: Evidence for absorption of intact macromolecules. *Gastroenterology* 1974; 66:987.
49. Prockop DJ, Keiser HR, Sjoerdsma A: Gastrointestinal absorption and renal excretion of hydroxyproline peptides. *Lancet* 1962; 2:527.
50. Gardner MLG, Lindbland BS, Burston D, et al: Transmucosal passage of intact peptides in the guinea-pig small intestine in vivo: A reappraisal. *Clin Sci* 1983; 64:433.
51. Webb KE: Amino acid and peptide absorption from the gastrointestinal tract. *Fed Proc* 1986; 45:2268.
52. McCormick ME, Webb KE: Plasma free, erythrocyte free and plasma peptide amino acid exchange of calves in steady state and fasting metabolism. *J Nutr* 1982; 112:276.
53. Furst P, Albers S, Stehle P: Dipeptides in clinical nutrition. *Proc Nutr Soc* 1990; 49:343.
54. Zaloga GP, Chernow B, Zajtchuk R, et al: Diagnostic dosages of protirelin (TRH) elevate blood pressure by noncatecholamine mechanisms. *Arch Intern Med* 1984; 144:1149.
55. Koskinen LOD: Effect of low intravenous doses of TRH, acid-TRH and cyclo(his-Pro) on cerebral and peripheral blood flows. *Br J Pharmacol* 1986; 87:509.
56. Holaday JW, Bernton EW: Protirelin (TRH)—A potent neuromodulator with therapeutic potential. *Arch Intern Med* 1984; 144:1138.
57. Hilton CW, Prasad C, Vo P, et al: Food contains the bioactive peptide, Cyclo(His-Pro). *J Clin Endocrinol Metab* 1992; 75:375.
58. Hilton CW, Prasad C, Svec F, et al: Cyclo(his-Pro) in nutritional supplements. *Lancet* 1990; 1:1455.
59. Morley JE, Levine AS, Yamada T, et al: Effect of exorphins on gastrointes-

tinal function, hormonal release, and appetite. *Gastroenterology* 1983; 84:1517.

60. Zioudrou C, Streaty RA, Klee WA: Opioid peptides derived from food proteins: The exorphins. *J Biol Chem* 1979; 254:2446.

61. Brinson RR, Pitts WM, Benoit J: Effect of β-casomorphin, a casein hydrolysate derivative, on intestinal permeability in volume expanded hypoproteinemic rats. *JPEN* 1990; 14(suppl):10.

62. Hautefeuille M, Brantl V, Dumontier AM, et al: In vitro effects of β-casomorphins on ion transport in rabbit ileum. *Am J Physiol* 1986; 250:92.

63. Jankovic BD, Maric D: In vivo modulation of the immune system by enkephalins. *Intern J Neurosci* 1990; 51:167.

64. Maric D, Jankovic BD: Immunorestorative activity of methionine-enkephalin in senescence. *Intern J Neurosci* 1990; 51:185.

65. Brotman DN, Flancbaum L, Kang YH, et al: Positive inotropic effect of carcinine in the isolated perfused guinea pig heart. *Crit Care Med* 1990; 18:317.

66. Wantanobe H, Sasaki S, Sone K, et al: Paradoxical response of growth hormone to peptide histidine methionine in acromegaly: Comparison with the effects of thyrotropin-releasing hormone and vasoactive intestinal peptide. *J Clin Endocrinol Metab* 1991; 72:982.

67. Klotz SA, Smith RL: *Candida albicans* adherence to subendothelial extracellular matrix and matrix components is inhibited by arginine-glycine-aspartic acid peptides (abstract). *Clin Res* 1990; 38:13.

68. Bounous G, Kongshavn PAL: Influence of dietary proteins on the immune system of mice. *J Nutr* 1982; 112:1747.

69. Martinez JA, Macarulla MT, Marcos R, et al: Nutritional outcome and immunocompetence in mice fed on a diet containing raw field beans (*Vicia faba*, var. *minor*) as the source of protein. *Br J Nutr* 1992; 68:493.

70. Rouse IL, Beilin LJ: Vegetarian diet and blood pressure. *J Hypertens* 1984; 2:231.

71. Hara H, Nishikawa H, Kiriyama S: Different effects of casein and soyabean protein on gastric emptying and small intestinal transit after spontaneous feeding of diets in rats. *Br J Nutr* 1992; 68:59.

72. Kontessis P, Jones S, Dodds R, et al: Renal, metabolic and hormonal responses to ingestion of animal and vegetable proteins. *Kidney Int* 1990; 38:136.

73. Zaloga GP: Nutrition and prevention of systemic infection. *Crit Care State Art* 1991; 12:31.

74. Barbul A: Arginine: Biochemistry, physiology, and therapeutic implications. *JPEN* 1986; 10:227.

75. Seifter E, Rettura G, Barbul A, et al: Arginine—an essential amino acid for injured rats. *Surgery* 1978; 84:224.

76. Barbul A, Fishel RS, Shimazu S, et al: Intravenous hyperalimentation with high arginine levels improves wound healing and immune function. *J Surg Res* 1985; 31:328.

77. Barbul A: Arginine and immune function. *Nutrition* 1990; 6(suppl):53.

78. Barbul A, Wasserkrug HL, Seifter E, et al: Immunostimulatory effects of arginine in normal and injured rats. *J Surg Res* 1980; 29:228.

79. Barbul A, Wasserkrug HL, Sisto DA, et al: Thymic and immune stimulatory actions of arginine. *JPEN* 1980; 4:446.

80. Barbul A, Sisto DA, Wasserkrug HL, et al: Arginine stimulates immune responses in healthy humans. *Surgery* 1981; 90:244.

81. Souba WW, Smith RJ, Wilmore DW: Glutamine metabolism by the intestinal tract. *JPEN* 1985; 9:608.

82. Proceedings of an international glutamine symposium: Glutamine metabolism in health and disease—Basic science and clinical aspects. *JPEN* 1990; 14(suppl):39.

83. Crampton RF, Gangolli SD, Simson P, et al: Rates of absorption by rat intestine of pancreatic hydrolysates of proteins and their corresponding amino acids. *Clin Sci* 1971; 41:409.

84. Lis MT, Crampton RF, Matthews DM: Effect of dietary changes on intestinal

absorption of L-methionine and L-methionyl-L-methionine in the rat. *Br J Nutr* 1972; 27:159.

85. Grimble GK, Rees RG, Keohane PP, et al: Effect of peptide chain length on absorption of egg protein hydrolysates in the normal human jejunum. *Gastroenterology* 1987; 92:136.

86. Hara H, Funabiki R, Iwata M, et al: Portal absorption of small peptides in rats under unrestrained conditions. *J Nutr* 1984; 114:1122.

87. Craft IL, Geddes D, Hyde CW, et al: Absorption and malabsorption of glycine and glycine peptides in man. *Gut* 1968; 9:425.

88. Hegarty JE, Fairclough PD, Moriarty KJ, et al: Effects of concentration on in vivo absorption of a peptide containing hydrolysate. *Gut* 1982; 23:304.

89. Moriarty KJ, Hegarty JE, Fairclough PD, et al: Relative nutritional value of whole protein, hydrolysed protein, and free amino acids in man. *Gut* 1985; 26:694.

90. Raimundo AH, Grimble GK, Rees RG, et al: The effect of carbohydrate and fat on the absorption of amino acids and peptides in the normal human small intestine. *JPEN* 1989; 13(suppl):9.

91. Granger DN, Brinson RR: Intestinal absorption of elemental and standard enteral formulas in hypoproteinemic (volume expanded) rats. *JPEN* 1988; 12:278.

92. Brinson RR, Pitts VL, Taylor AE: Intestinal absorption of peptide enteral formulas in hypoproteinemic (volume expanded) rats: A paired analysis. *Crit Care Med* 1989; 17:657.

93. Brinson RR: The effect of peptide-based diets on the intestinal microcirculation in a rat model. *Nutr Clin Pract* 1990; 5:238.

94. Plumb JA, Gardner MLG: Can elemental diets reduce the intestinal toxicity of 5-fluorouracil? *JPEN* 1983; 7:351.

95. Trocki O, Mochizuki H, Dominioni L, et al: Intact protein versus free amino acids in the nutritional support of thermally injured animals. *JPEN* 1986; 10:139.

96. Ziegler F, Ollivier JM, Cynober L, et al: Efficacy of enteral nitrogen support

in surgical patients: Small peptides vs non-degraded proteins. *Gut* 1990; 31:1277.

97. Ziegler F, Nitenberg G, Coudray-Lucas C, et al: Influence of the form of nitrogen supply on amino acid (AA) peripheral bioavailability (PB) and insulin secretion during post-operative enteral nutrition (EN). *JPEN* 1993; 17(suppl):32.

98. Cosnes J, Evard D, Beaugerie L, et al: Improvement in protein absorption with a small-peptide based diet in patients with high jejunostomy. *Nutrition* 1992; 8:406.

99. Brinson RR, Kolts BE: Diarrhea associated with severe hypoalbuminemia: A comparison of a peptide-based chemically defined diet and standard enteral alimentation. *Crit Care Med* 1988; 16:130.

100. Brinson RR, Curtis WD, Singh M: Diarrhea in the intensive care unit: The role of hypoalbuminemia and the response to a peptide-based, chemically defined diet. *J Am Coll Nutr* 1987; 6:517.

101. Bounous G, Le Bel E, Shuster J, et al: Dietary protein during radiation therapy. *Strahlentherapie* 1975; 149:476.

102. Meredith JW, Ditesheim JA, Zaloga GP: Visceral protein levels in trauma patients are greater with peptide diet than intact protein diet. *J Trauma* 1990; 30:825.

103. Ortiz C, Candau P, Arock M, et al: A comparative post-operative study—an enteral solution based on small peptides compared to an enteral solution based on free amino acids. *Gastroenterol Clin Biol* 1985; 9:182.

104. Reicht G, Petritsch W, Eherer A, et al: Jejunal protein absorption of whey protein and its hydrolysate. *JPEN* 1992; 16(suppl):25.

105. Vazquez JA, Morse EL, Adibi SA: Effect of starvation on amino acid and peptide transport and peptide hydrolysis in humans. *Am J Physiol* 1985; 249:563.

106. Lis MT, Crampton RF, Matthews DM: Effect of dietary changes on intestinal absorption of L-methionine and L-methyl-L-methionine in the rat. *Br J Nutr* 1972; 27:159.

107. Shou J, Ruelaz EA, Redmond HP, et

al: Dietary protein prevents bacterial translocation from the gut. *JPEN* 1991; 15(suppl):29.

108. Zaloga GP, Ward KA, Prielipp RC: Effect of enteral diets on whole body and gut growth in unstressed rats. *JPEN* 1991; 15:42.

109. Janne P, Carpentier Y, Willems G: Colonic mucosal atrophy induced by a liquid diet in rats. *Dig Dis Sci* 1977; 22:808.

110. Morin CL, Ling V, Bourassa D: Small intestinal and colonic changes induced by a chemically defined diet. *Dig Dis Sci* 1980; 25:123.

111. Birke H, Thorlacus-Ussing O, Hessov I: Trophic effect of dietary peptides on mucosa in the rat bowel. *JPEN* 1990; 14(suppl):26.

112. Shou J, Minnard E, Motyka L, et al: Interleukin-4 reduces chemically-defined diet (CDD) induced bacterial translocation in mice. *JPEN* 1992; 16(suppl):24.

113. Vanderhoff JA, Grandjean CJ, Burkley KT, et al: Effect of casein versus casein hydrolysate on mucosal adaptation following massive bowel resection in infant rats. *J Pediatr Gastroenterol Nutr* 1984; 3:262.

114. Bounous G, Sutherland NG, McArdle AH, et al: The prophylactic use of an "elemental" diet in experimental hemorrhagic shock and intestinal ischemia. *Ann Surg* 1967; 166:312.

115. Alverdy JC, Aoys E, Moss GS: Total parenteral nutrition promotes bacterial translocation from the gut. *Surgery* 1988; 104:185.

116. Shou J, Redmond HP, Leon P, et al: Elemental diet impairs macrophage responsiveness to endotoxin in mice. *JPEN* 1991; 15(suppl):23.

117. Shou J, Lieberman MD, Hofmann K, et al: Dietary manipulation of methotrexate-induced enterocolitis. *JPEN* 1991; 15:307.

118. Jones WG, Minei JP, Barber AE, et al: Elemental diet promotes spontaneous bacterial translocation and alters mortality after endotoxin challenge. *Surg Forum* 1989; 40:20.

119. White KG, Dickerson RN, Markoroff KL, et al: Elemental liquid diet does not facilitate bacterial translocation in normal or endotoxin-stressed animals. *J Am Coll Nutr* 1990; 9:530.

120. Sori AJ, Rush BF, Lysz TW, et al: The gut as a source of sepsis after hemorrhagic shock. *Am J Surg* 1988; 155:187.

121. Koziol J, Rush BF, Smith SM, et al: Occurrence of bacteremia during and after hemorrhagic shock. *J Trauma* 1988; 28:10.

122. Zaloga GP, Knowles R, Ward K, et al: Total parenteral nutrition (TPN) increases mortality after hemorrhage. *Crit Care Med* 1991; 19:54.

123. McAnena OJ, Harvey LP, Bonau RA, et al: Alteration of methotrexate toxicity in rats by manipulation of dietary components. *Gastroenterology* 1987; 92:354.

124. Harvey LP, McAnena OJ, Mehta BM, et al: Reversibility of elemental liquid diet–induced methotrexate toxicity by refeeding with chow. *JPEN* 1987; 11:119.

125. Bounous G, Hugon J, Gentile JM: Elemental diet in the management of the intestinal lesion produced by 5-fluorouracil in the rat. *Can J Surg* 1971; 14:298.

126. Bounous G, Maestracci D: Use of an elemental diet in animals during treatment with 5-fluorouracil. *Cancer Treat Rep* 1976; 60:17.

127. Bounous G, Maestracci D: Use of an elemental diet in animals during treatment with 5-fluorouracil. *Cancer Treat Rep* 1976; 60:17.

128. Plumb JA, Gardner MLG: Can elemental diets reduce the intestinal toxicity of 5-fluorouracil? *JPEN* 1983; 7:351.

129. Stanford JR, King D, Carey L, et al: The adverse effects of elemental diets on tolerance for 5-FU toxicity in the rat. *J Surg Oncol* 1977; 9:493.

130. Bounous G, Papeau R, Regoli D: Enhanced 5-FU mortality in rats eating defined formula diets. *Int J Clin Pharmacol* 1978; 16:265.

131. Bounous G, Gentile JM, Hugon J: Elemental diet in the management of the intestinal lesion produced by 5-fluorouracil in man. *Can J Surg* 1971; 14:312.

132. Hugon JS, Bounous G: Elemental diet in the intestinal lesions produced by radiation in the mouse. *Can J Surg* 1972; 15:18.

133. Pageau R, Lallier R, Bounous G: Systemic protection against radiation. I.

Effect of an elemental diet on hematopoietic and immunologic systems in the rat. *Radiat Res* 1975; 62:357.

134. Pageau R, Bounous G: Systemic protection against radiation. II. Increased intestinal radioresistance in rats fed a formula-defined diet. *Radiat Res* 1977; 71:622.

135. Beitler MK, Mahler PA, Yamanaka WK, et al: The effect of the hydrolytic state of dietary protein on post-irradiation morbidity and mucosal cell regeneration. *Int J Radiat Oncol Biol Phys* 1987; 13:385.

136. Brown MS, Buchman RB, Karran SJ: Clinical observations on the effects of elemental diet supplementation during irradiation. *Clin Radiol* 1980; 31:19.

137. Beer WH, Fan A, Halsted CH: Clinical and nutritional implications of radiation enteritis. *Am J Clin Nutr* 1985; 41:85.

138. Anderson WMD, Brinson RR, Conrad SA, et al: Intestinal protein loss during enteral alimentation in critically ill patients. *JPEN* 1990; 14(suppl):24.

139. Bounous G: Elemental diets in the prophylaxis and therapy for intestinal lesions: An update. *Surgery* 1989; 105:571.

140. Steinhardt HJ, Payer E, Henn B, et al: Effect of whole protein vs hydrolyzed protein on nitrogen economy and intestinal protein loss. *Gastroenterology* 1988; 94:433.

141. Robertson JFR, Garden OJ, Shenkin A: Intravenous nutrition and hepatic dysfunction. *JPEN* 1986; 10:172.

142. Lindor KD, Fleming CR, Abrams A, et al: Liver function values in adults receiving total parenteral nutrition. *JAMA* 1979; 241:2389.

143. Lambert JR, Thomas SM: Metronidazole prevention of serum liver enzyme abnormalities during total parenteral nutrition. *JPEN* 1985; 9:501.

144. Young EA, Cioletti LA, Traylor JB, et al: Gastrointestinal response to oral versus gastric feeding of defined formula diets. *Am J Clin Nutr* 1982; 35:715.

145. Knodell RG: Effects of formula composition on hepatic and intestinal drug metabolism during enteral nutrition. *JPEN* 1990; 14:34.

146. Zaloga G, Black KW, Prielipp R: Enteral feeding minimizes liver damage following hemorrhage. *Chest* 1991; 100(suppl):135.

147. Zaloga GP, Meredith JW, Roberts P, et al: Improved hepatic protein responses with hydrolyzed protein versus intact protein diets following trauma. *Crit Care Med* 1992; 20(suppl):94.

148. Mowatt-Larssen CA, Brown RO, Wojtysiak SL, et al: Enteral nutrition efficacy and tolerance: Comparison of peptide with standard formulas. *JPEN* 1991; 15(suppl):32.

149. Dietscher JE, Foulks C, Smith R: Effect of elemental and polymeric formula on visceral proteins and nitrogen balance (N) in acutely ill patients. *JPEN* 1993; 17(suppl):31.

150. Ford EG, Hull SF, Jennings M, et al: Clinical comparison of tolerance to elemental or polymeric enteral feedings in the postoperative patient. *J Am Coll Nutr* 1992; 11:11.

151. Feller A, Rudman D, Caindec N: Comparison of nutritional efficacy of peptamin and vivonex TEN elemental diets in elderly tube fed subjects. *JPEN* 13(suppl):12.

152. Sircar B, Johnson LR, Lichtenberger LM: Effect of chemically defined diets on antral and serum gastrin levels in rats. *Am J Physiol* 1980; 238:376.

153. Imondi AR, Stradley RP: Utilization of enzymatically hydrolyzed soybean protein and crystalline amino acid diets by rats with exocrine pancreatic insufficiency. *J Clin Invest* 1974; 104:793.

154. Alexander JW: Nutrition and infection. *Arch Surg* 1986; 121:966.

155. Roberts P, Black K, Zaloga G: Peptide-based enteral diets improve wound healing after abdominal surgery in rats. *JPEN* 1993; 17(suppl):32.

156. Monchi M, Vaugelade P, Vaissade P, et al: Net protein utilization after duodenal infusion of small peptides or free amino acids. *JPEN* 1991; 15(suppl):29.

157. Beer WH, Fan A, Halsted CH: Clinical and nutritional implications of radiation enteritis. *Am J Clin Nutr* 1985; 41:85.

158. Polk DB, Hattner JAT, Kerner JA: Improved growth and disease activity after intermittent administration of a

defined formula diet in children with Crohn's disease. *JPEN* 1992; 16:499.

159. Meguid MM, Landel AM, Terz JJ, et al: Effect of elemental diet on albumin and urea synthesis: Comparison with partially hydrolyzed protein diet. *J Surg Res* 1984; 37:16.

160. Albina JE, Jacobs DO, Melnik G, et al: Nitrogen utilization from elemental diets. *JPEN* 1985; 4:548.

161. Langlois P, Williams HB, Gurd FN: Effect of an elemental diet on mortality rates and gastrointestinal lesions in experimental burns. *J Trauma* 1972; 12:771.

162. Sitren HS, Johns LG, Solomon PL: Modulation of methotrexate (MTX) toxicity by protein source in solid diets and in enteral formulas. *JPEN* 1993; 17(suppl):32.

163. Jones NJM, Lees R, Andrews J, et al: Comparison of an elemental and polymeric enteral diet in patients with normal gastrointestinal function. *Gut* 1983; 24:78.

164. Cerra FB, Shronts EP, Raup S, et al: Enteral nutrition in hypermetabolic surgical patients. *Crit Care Med* 1989; 17:619.

5

Branched-Chain Amino Acids

Nicola D'Atellis, M.D.

Bjorn Skeie, M.D.

Vladamir Kvetan, M.D.

The branched-chain amino acids (BCAAs) valine, leucine, and isoleucine have metabolic properties and metabolic effects that may be unique in several aspects. First, their initial metabolism occurs mainly in the periphery, particularly in skeletal muscle rather than the liver. Surprisingly, this may be of particular importance, not so much for muscle, but for other tissues and organs in the body. Second, one or more of the BCAAs may exert a specific regulatory effect on the rates of protein degradation and synthesis in skeletal muscle. Third, BCAAs are transported into brain tissue via the same carrier that transports the aromatic amino acids (AAAs). Competition for entry into the brain between BCAAs and aromatic acids may have an influence on the rate of synthesis of some monoamine neurotransmitters and therefore the level of such neurotransmitters. In this way BCAAs could affect behavior.

The various metabolic effects of BCAAs suggest that they might have therapeutic uses that are pharmacologic in addition to being components of complete mixtures of amino acids for protein synthesis. Beneficial effects of

BCAA-enriched solutions have been demonstrated in the treatment of hepatic failure with encephalopathy and in chronic renal failure. Their effects in hepatic encephalopathy along with their effects on the respiratory drive and appetite suggest that BCAAs stimulate the central nervous system (CNS). The use of mixtures enriched with BCAAs has not clearly been shown to improve nitrogen balance in injured or septic patients. However, nitrogen balance may be an insensitive index for the beneficial effects of BCAA supplementation in such patients. Further studies of protein metabolism in the stressed state are required, with special emphasis on the role of muscle metabolism in immune function via provision of glutamine for lymphocytes, macrophages, and tissue repair cells. The variability in clinical results obtained in different studies could be explained on the basis of factors that affect the conversion of BCAAs to glutamine. Hence, future research should consider whether patients are "responders" as opposed to "nonresponders" to BCAA administration. Analysis of all patients as one population in a disease state such as sepsis may obscure a benefit to certain subsets. Recently, the possibility of providing increased glutamine to stressed patients (as L-alanyl-L-glutamine) as part of parenteral nutrition has been raised.[1] This may have an important impact on the clinical utility of BCAAs in stress and septic states. The standard balanced amino acid solutions used in intravenous nutrition contain 19% to 25% BCAAs, whereas the commercially available BCAA-enriched solutions have about 45% of the amino acids as BCAAs. In this chapter, we discuss the metabolism, metabolic effects, and clinical utility of BCAA solutions.

METABOLISM

Source of Amino Acids

Amino acids are obtained from protein in the diet. Approximately 100 g/day of amino acids is consumed as part of the average Western diet. In normal healthy, well-fed subjects, about 300 g/day of tissue protein is hydrolyzed (approximately 5 g/kg) and replaced by newly synthesized protein. About 50 g is required for production of digestive juices and 20 g for the cells of the small intestine that are lost during normal digestion. Approximately 100 g/day of protein turns over in the gastrointestinal tract.[2, 3] An estimated 15% to 20% of the basal metabolic rate is due to protein turnover.[3] It is particularly interesting that the turnover of individual proteins varies enormously. Protein degradation is necessary to prevent the accumulation of abnormal and potentially harmful proteins and peptides. The concentration of a protein can be changed more rapidly by modifications in the rates of synthesis or degradation if it has a rapid turnover rate. Amino acids are generally considered to be either incorporated into protein or transaminated and their carbon skeletons oxidized.[4] However, amino acids also act as precursors for many other very important compounds in the body, and the high turnover rates of some proteins ensure that amino acids are available (under normal conditions) for the formation of these components.[5]

Amino Acid Degradation

The final stage in the oxidation of amino acids occurs through the reactions of the tricarboxylic acid (TCA) cycle. Many amino acids are also precursors for glucogenesis. Since there are a large number of amino acids, there are a large number of processes by which they are converted into common metabolic intermediates. A recent review details amino acid metabolism in man.[6] Before intracellular metabolism can occur, amino acids must be transported from the interstitial space across the cell membrane. Amino acid transport requires the presence of a carrier system in the cell membrane. The intracellular concentrations of amino acids may be considerably greater than those in the bloodstream, so the transport of amino acids into most if not all cells is an active process, usually but not always associated with the operation of a Na^+ ion pump. There are at least seven different carriers, with overlapping specificity for the different amino acids; these are known as the A, ASCP, L, L7, dicarboxylate, N, and beta-systems.

Central Role of Transdeamination

The dextroamino acids are deaminated by an amino acid oxidase that catalyzes a nonequilibrium reaction. Natural amino acids are deaminated by transamination followed by oxidative deamination via glutamate dehydrogenase. The transdeamination process provides metabolic economy. By means of a small number of near-equilibrium reactions, most amino acids can be maintained in equilibrium with their corresponding keto acids and with each other (Fig 5–1). Such an interrelationship would not be possible with a nonequilibrium deamination system. Furthermore, having a common amino acid (glutamate) to which most others are related by transamination requires fewer specific enzymes for interconversion than if separate enzymes were required for transamination between each pair of amino acids. Further economy is

achieved since glutamate is reversibly deaminated and oxidized by glutamate dehydrogenase and oxygenated nicotinamide adenine nucleotide (NAD^+) to give L-ketoglutamate, ammonia, and reduced nicotinamide adenine dinucleotide (NADH). This near-equilibrium transdeamination system provides a simple mechanism for maintaining fairly constant concentrations of both amino and keto acids despite variations in the magnitude and direction of the flux through the transdeamination system. There are at least seven processes that feed reactants into or out of the transdeamination system (Fig 5–2). The rates of these various processes control the magnitude and direction of the flux through the transdeamination system.

Some important metabolic consequences of the integration achieved through this transdeamination system can be seen by following the changes that occur when the rate of one or more of the related processes is altered. Two examples are given. First, during the ingestion of excess protein (in a mixed diet), the rate of amino acid supply from the intestine (process 1; Fig 5–2) is increased, and any amino acids not required for the synthesis of protein (process 3) will produce keto acids that can be oxidized or converted to carbohydrate and lipid (processes 4, 5, and 6). Second, during starvation, the rate

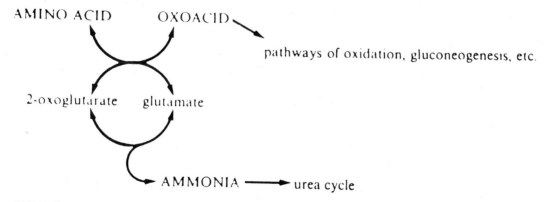

FIG 5–1.

Transdeamination of amino acids. This pathway is used in reverse for synthesis of amino acids. From Newsholme EA, Leech AR: Biochemistry for the Medical Sciences, Chichester, UK, 1983, John Wiley & Sons.

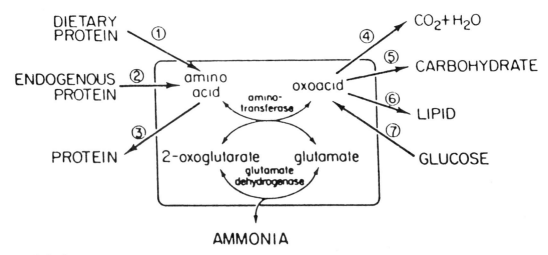

FIG 5–2.
Central role of transdeamination reactions: 1) Digestion and absorption; 2) protein degradation in the tissues; 3) protein synthesis; 4) oxidation; 5) gluconeogenesis or glyconeogenesis; 6) lipid synthesis (via acetyl-CoaA); glycolysis, etc. From Newsholme EA, Leech AR: Biochemistry for the Medical Sciences, Chichester, UK, 1983, John Wiley & Sons.

of degradation of body protein (process 2) exceeds the rate of protein synthesis (process 3), and the available amino acids are converted to keto acids. However, because of inhibition of pyruvate oxidation (process 4) and lipid synthesis (process 6), the keto acids are converted preferentially to glucose (in the liver) for use by the brain. This account of the integration of the various aspects of amino acid metabolism is somewhat oversimplified, but it illustrates the principles that can be applied to the changes that occur in amino acid metabolism under different conditions.

Branched-Chain Amino Acid Metabolism

BCAAs are transported into cells via a specific carrier termed the large neutral amino acid carrier (L system). Within the cell, BCAAs are transaminated to form keto acids (BCKAs) by two enzyme transaminases that probably catalyze near-equilibrium reactions. Each BCKA then undergoes oxidative decarboxylation, a process that is catalyzed by a single enzyme, and the reaction is a nonequilibrium one. The product is the acyl coenzyme A (acyl-CoA) derivative with one less carbon (Fig 5–3). There-

after, the pathways resemble those for fatty acid oxidation and lead to end products that can enter the TCA cycle. The end products of valine and isoleucine metabolism are succinyl-CoA. Leucine yields acetoacetate and acetyl-CoA. The BCAA aminotransferase (BCAAT) is widely distributed among tissues. The enzyme activity per gram has been found to be high in heart and kidney, intermediate in skeletal muscle, and lowest in liver.[7–9] The liver is believed to play almost no role in the transamination of BCAAs. The metabolism of most other amino acids, including the AAAs (e.g., tyrosine, tryptophan), is initiated in the liver and is therefore dependent on hepatic function.

The BCKAs formed by transamination of BCAAs are the substrates for oxidative decarboxylation, the second enzymatic step in the pathway of BCAA degradation. The BCKA concentrations in most tissues rarely exceed the dissociation constant of the Michaelis-Menten constant (K_m) for the BCKA dehydrogenase (BCKAD); therefore, the rate of degradation of BCAAs in vivo is mainly controlled through changes in the concentrations of the substrates for the BCAAT reaction.[8]

The BCAAs are transaminated (by

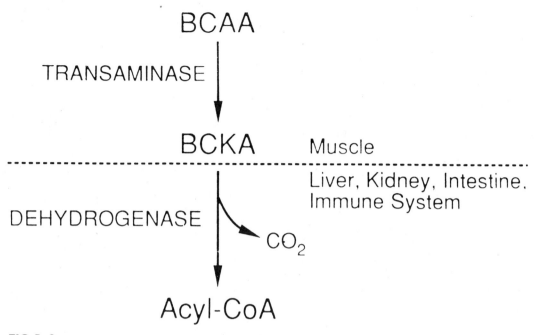

FIG 5–3.
Catabolism of BCAA. From Madsen DC: Branched-chain amino acids: Metabolic roles and clinical applications. In Johnson IDA, editor: Advances in Clinical Nutrition, Hague, Netherlands, 1982, MTP Press.

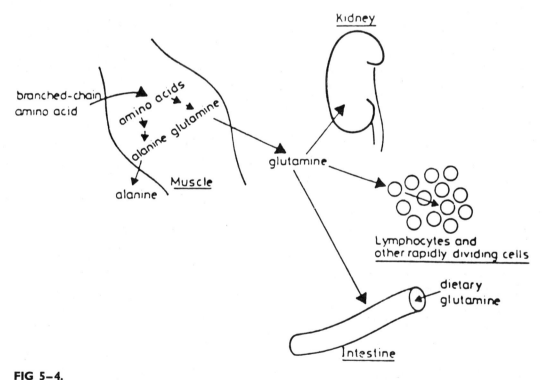

FIG 5–4.
Relationship between glutamine production in muscle and glutamine utilization in various tissues. The flux-generating step for glutamine utilization in kidney, lymphocytes, and intestine may be in muscle; thus, glutamine metabolism can be considered as a branched metabolic pathway which is initiated in muscle and is complete in several other tissues. The clinical implications of this relationship may be considerable. From Ardawi MS, Newsholme EA: Metabolism in lymphocytes and its importance in the immune response, Essays Biochem 21:1, 1985.

leucine and valine aminotransferase enzymes), and the resultant keto acids are oxidatively decarboxylated by a single mitochondrial enzyme, 2-oxoisovalerate dehydrogenase. The key regulatory enzyme for this pathway in muscle is the 2-oxoisovalerate dehydrogenase, which exists in two forms, active and inactive. They are interconverted by phosphorylation and dephosphorylation reactions. Phosphorylation leads to inactivation. It is important to note that, at least in skeletal muscle of the rat, the enzyme is almost totally in the inactive form. Hence, in rat skeletal muscle, BCAAs that are taken up from the bloodstream or released endogenously from muscle protein are transaminated, and most of the keto acids are then released into the bloodstream. The keto acids are then metabolized by other tissues that possess an active dehydrogenase, i.e., tissues in which the enzyme exists in the dephosphorylated form (e.g., liver, heart, kidney). Previous reports that muscle tissue could convert the carbons of BCAAs into CO_2 or alanine[10, 11] were based on studies in diaphragm muscle in which a high proportion of the dehydrogenase is in the active form. This emphasizes the danger of extrapolating results in the diaphragm to other skeletal muscle. In human skeletal muscle, a higher proportion of the dehydrogenase is in the active form. Thus, some BCAAs can be metabolized within the muscle, and only a small part is released as keto acids.

These findings lead to the suggestion that BCAAs that are taken up by skeletal muscle in the rat are used primarily for nitrogen transfer, via transamination, for the formation of alanine and glutamine (Fig 5–4). However, the oxidation of some keto acids indicates that in human skeletal muscle BCAAs provide some energy as well as nitrogen. Nevertheless, the fact that little oxidation occurs in rat muscle suggests, to the present authors, that transfer of nitrogen to glutamine is the key physiologic process in skeletal muscle rather than the generation of energy.

Branched-Chain Amino Acid Metabolism in Muscle

Important findings in different areas of amino acid metabolism that have been made over the last quarter of a century allow for a new theory concerning the physiologic importance of BCAA metabolism and glutamine formation and release in muscle. In the 1960s it was established that the liver plays a quantitatively major role in the uptake and utilization of most dietary amino acids with exception of the BCAAs, which are taken up primarily by the periphery,[12] and glutamate, aspartate, and especially glutamine (*plus* asparagine), which are utilized by the absorptive cells of the small intestine.[13, 14] Although muscle takes up BCAAs, it releases alanine and glutamine. In the postabsorptive state, 60% of the amino acids released are composed of alanine plus glutamine. Furthermore, adding BCAAs to the incubation medium of an isolated rat muscle increases the rate of formation and release of alanine and glutamine.[15]

These observations lead to the suggestion that the nitrogen and some carbon of the BCAAs can be used to synthesize alanine and glutamine in muscle.[10, 11] In addition, at least in the rat, BCAAs are transaminated, but normally not further metabolized since the key enzyme controlling their rate of oxidation (2-oxoisovalerate dehydrogenase) is almost totally in the inactive form in skeletal muscle in most conditions.[16, 17] Hence, it appears that rat muscle takes up BCAAs primarily to use their nitrogen for the formation of glutamine and alanine. Consequently, BCAA utilization by muscle in conditions such as injury, sepsis, and burns can no longer be considered an energy source (at least in the rat). The primary role of BCAAs is as a nitrogen intermediary. However, this role does not exclude the use of these amino acids as an energy source under certain conditions.[18, 19]

CLINICAL UTILITY

Branched-Chain Amino Acids in Metabolic Stress States

It has been established that surgery, trauma, sepsis, or burns result in a negative nitrogen balance and that this is due largely to an increased net rate of skeletal muscle breakdown.[20] The degree of the catabolic response depends on the severity and duration of the trauma or stress.[21] After an uncomplicated surgical procedure in an otherwise healthy patient, the catabolic response persists for about 1 week with net nitrogen loss. These mild nitrogen losses are well tolerated and readily replaced by subsequent oral feedings. By contrast, a fasting patient with severe trauma or sepsis catabolizes considerably more lean body mass and fat. The metabolic response can be viewed as a means for mobilization of body protein, fat, and carbohydrate so as to maintain optimal metabolic conditions for wound repair and host defense when dietary intake is limited or absent. The increased availability of plasma amino acids occurs predominantly at the expense of skeletal muscle protein.[22] Gluconeogenesis is increased even in the presence of high plasma levels of glucose. Fatty acids are mobilized from adipose tissue and are used for the energy needs of cardiac, skeletal, and respiratory muscles. Despite the hyperglycemia and the hyperinsulinemia, the muscles of a stressed patient use fatty acids instead of glucose. This is an important role for the glucose/fatty acid cycle; it allows glucose to be spared for tissues that specifically require it, such as the CNS, immune system, and healing wounds. The hormonal changes of stress include increased levels of adrenal glucocorticoids, glucagon, and catecholamines.[23, 24] It is of interest to note that the response is probably mediated by afferent nervous pathways and by cytokines such as interleukin-1.[25, 26]

Increased plasma levels of AAAs are usually observed in septic patients and may result from hepatic dysfunction induced by the septic process.[27, 28] The plasma concentrations of BCAAs are generally normal or slightly elevated in the early stages of sepsis, but with increasing time and severity BCAA concentrations tend to fall below normal.[27, 29, 30] Therefore, in both liver failure and severe sepsis, changes in the plasma levels of AAAs and BCAAs result in an increase in the AAA/BCAA concentration ratio.[31-34] If the change in this ratio is severe, it may result in encephalopathy, which is sometimes seen in severe sepsis and identical to that seen with hepatic encephalopathy. Septic patients with encephalopathy have increased mortality rates as compared with those without encephalopathy.[35] It has been hypothesized that many metabolic encephalopathies (i.e., hepatic, septic, uremic, hypercapnic) may share this common mechanism.[34, 36] Therefore, changes in the ratio of AAAs to BCAAs, similar to those seen in hepatic encephalopathy, may be useful in evaluating the severity of sepsis and may be subject to therapy with BCAA-enriched solutions.[37] In fact, several animal and human studies have indicated beneficial effects when BCAA solutions are used for trauma, injury, and sepsis.[38] BCAAs may also serve as fuels to promote the synthesis of muscle and visceral protein[39] and reduce the breakdown of muscle protein.[40]

Glutamine Formation

Under metabolic stress, muscle and plasma concentrations of glutamine decrease, yet the rate of glutamine release by skeletal muscle is increased.[41-43] Furthermore, the isolated epitrochlearis muscle releases glutamine at a greater rate from thermally injured rats than from control animals. The maximum ac-

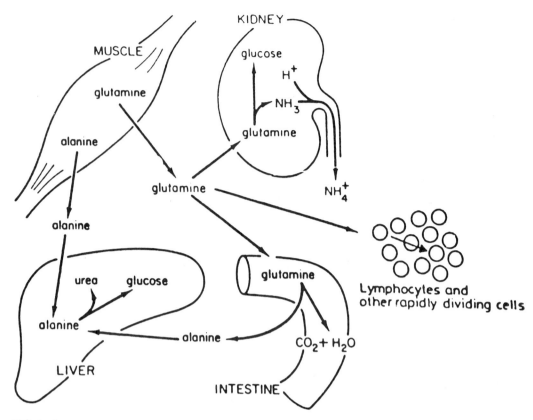

FIG 5–5.
Interrelationship of organs in glutamine metabolism. From Skeie B, Kuetan V, Gil K et al: Branch-chain amino acids: Their metabolism and clinical utility, Crit Care Med 18:549–71, 1990.

tivity of glutamine synthetase is increased by at least 50% in injured animals. Increased net rates of protein degradation in muscle may provide BCAAs within muscle that donate their nitrogen for the synthesis of glutamine in the muscle. After release by muscle, glutamine is used by cells of the immune system, cells involved in tissue repair, and those used by the kidney to combat acidosis (Fig 5–5). More specifically, the increased net rate of protein degradation in skeletal muscle may be essential for providing glutamine for the markedly increased number of cells involved in cell division (e.g., lymphocytes, fibroblasts, endothelial cells) and for ammonia formation in the kidney.

Why should glutamine requirements increase further in conditions of sepsis, trauma, burns, or surgery? In all of these conditions, the number of im-

mune and repair cells is increased. In addition, cellular metabolic "activity" is also increased. A greater rate of glutaminolysis is required to provide substrate for optimal metabolic control and energy production. In the skeletal muscle of man, BCAAs are metabolized to keto acids. Oxidation of the keto acids provides cellular energy. BCAAs provide nitrogen for the synthesis of glutamine, which is utilized by cells of the immune system. Metabolism of glutamine to glutamate, aspartate, and lactate provides precursors for hepatic gluconeogenesis. Nonetheless, the primary role for muscle BCAA metabolism is to provide nitrogen for the formation of glutamine, which is then used by cells of the immune and repair systems. This hypothesis explains why there is such a large increase in protein degradation in skeletal muscle during injury, sepsis, and burns. This muscle protein degradation is essential for the survival of the animal.

Muscle concentrations of glutamine are considerably lower in patients who do not survive severe abdominal sepsis in comparison to those who do survive. In addition, the rates of muscle protein degradation appear to be higher in non-surviving patients.[44] Plasma levels of glutamine and cytokines have been measured in patients undergoing major and minor abdominal surgery. Significant decreases in plasma glutamine levels correlate with elevated interleukin-6 levels after major surgery.[45] Decreased glutamine levels may contribute to immunosuppression following major surgery. Release of glutamine by the lung increases markedly in hyperdynamic septic patients after surgery, but not in elective general surgical patients without sepsis. This release is paralleled by that of alanine.[46] Experimental data suggest that skeletal muscle and lung contribute roughly equally to the maintenance of blood glutamine and alanine levels.[47] An understanding of the role of BCAAs and glutamine in the maintenance of immune function following injury and critical illness may improve our ability to support the immune response.

Rationale

The use of BCAAs to decrease muscle catabolism in injured and septic patients was based on the in vitro observation that BCAAs inhibited muscle protein degradation and stimulated muscle protein synthesis. Studies with isolated rat diaphragm[48-50] and perfused rat muscle,[51] heart,[52, 53] and liver[54-57] found that leucine stimulated protein synthesis and decreased the rate of protein degradation. However, in these studies, valine and isoleucine given alone had little effect on protein turnover, whereas the BCKA analogues were more effective than BCAAs.[52, 58] These observations suggest that infusion of solutions containing BCAAs may de-crease the nitrogen wasting associated with trauma, surgery, sepsis, or burns. In addition, BCAAs may improve muscle glutamine levels for use by the immune system, intestine, and kidney.

BCAA-enriched solutions (45%) increase the rate of hepatic protein synthesis[54-56] and acute-phase proteins in critically ill and septic patients. These proteins may be important in host defense mechanisms against infection; thus the administration of solutions containing a high proportion of BCAAs may improve the chances of survival for such patients via this mechanism.[59-62] BCAAs may also correct the increase in the AAA/BCAA concentration ratio in sepsis and thus could be helpful in preventing metabolic encephalopathy.

Several animal studies indicate that the use of BCAA solutions in injured and septic animals improves nitrogen balance. The most optimistic results have been found in studies where the effects of BCAAs have been compared with those obtained with hypocaloric infusions of energy substrates alone (i.e., dextrose) or with isonitrogenous infusions of alanine. One study compared hepatic protein synthesis rates in three groups of septic rats that received infusions of dextrose alone, a balanced amino acid solution, or a BCAA-enriched solution.[63] All solutions were isocaloric, and the amino acid solutions were isonitrogenous. There were no differences in hepatic protein synthesis rates among the three groups. The negative nitrogen balance seen in the dextrose-infused animals was reversed to the same degree by the two different amino acid solutions. This study failed to support the use of BCAA-enriched solutions over standard BCAA solutions. Conceivably, the ratio of the individual BCAA or the amount of leucine was inadequate for a significant nitrogen sparing effect.[64]

In recent years, many studies of the efficacy of BCAAs on protein metabolism

TABLE 5–1.

Studies of Nitrogen Balance with BCAA Supplementation in Patients with Surgical Stress and Sepsis

Study	Patient Profile	Control/Study BCAA, %	Preferred Therapy	Remarks
Freund[114]	Laparotomy	0/22 0/33 0/100	BCAA	5% dextrose as calorie source All BCAA concentrations supported nitrogen retention equally
Bower[65]	ICU/Septic	25/45	BCAA (marginal benefit)	No difference in outcome 25% calories as fat
Daly[66]	Gastrectomy/ileal conduit	25/45	NS*	Dextrose 5%; no fat
Cerra[67]	Laparotomy/	4 groups with	BCAA	Increased nitrogen-retention with increasing BCAA doses, effect started at 0.5/BCAA/day
Cerra[68]	Surgery/multi-trauma/sepsis	25/45	BCAA	BCAA: 0.7 g/kg/day Improved nitrogen-retention at the end of the 7-day study with BCAA Improved immunologic function?
Cerra[69]	Laparotomy/	15.5/50	BCAA	35 kcal/kg/day (dextrose 25%)
Pelosi[70]	Multiple trauma	25/43	BCAA	10-day study
Nuwer[72]	ICU	25/43	BCAA	7-day study Improved immunologic tests
Bonau[64]	Cystectomy	0/25	?	More positive nitrogen-balance with BCAA 25% and 45% (high leucine) than BCAA 45% (low leucine)
van der Wounde[73]	ICU	19/45	NS	4-day study 30 kcal/kg/day; lipid 30%
van Way[74]	ICU	25/45	NS	14-day study
Okada[71]	Gastrectomy: subtotal (87 pts)	22/36	NS	40 kcal/kg/day; no fat Nitrogen-balance positive after 3 days with BCAA and after
	total (86 pts)		BCAA	6 days standard solution (total gastrectomy)
Jimenez-Jimenez[111]	Sepsis/Peritonitis	22.5/45	BCAA	
Sandstedt[112]	GI surgery	0/45	NS	Balanced AA solution with adequate energy has optimal nitrogen-sparing effect
Vente[113]	Multiple trauma/sepsis	15.6/50.2	NS	Mortality did not differ. Pre-Albumin levels increased in BCAA group. Nitrogen-balance not more efficient in BCAA

in catabolic patients have been carried out (Table 5–1). Most studies deal with patients with severe stress or sepsis resulting from trauma or major operations. The overall conclusions are clouded by the variability of stress, the number of septic patients included, and the relatively small number of patients. In a prospective, randomized trial, infusion of a standard amino acid solution was compared with two BCAA solutions, one of which was enriched primarily with valine, whereas the other was enriched with leucine.[65] The study contained 37 patients who received an isocaloric, isonitrogenous dextrose solution infused within 24 hours of the onset of major surgery, injury, or sepsis. Marginal improvement in nitrogen retention was demonstrated in the BCAA-fed groups, but cumulative nitrogen retention was not improved. The patients receiving the leucine-enriched solution appeared to maintain a higher rate of hepatic protein synthesis since the plasma concentration of short-turnover proteins was higher. However, there were no differences in outcome. When cystectomy and ileal conduit were the surgical insult, there was no difference in the cumulative nitrogen balance when comparing 25% and 45% BCAA solutions. Other studies suggest an advantage for BCAAs.[66-70] In a prospective, controlled trial of the nutritional effects of BCAA-enriched solutions in surgical patients with gastric cancer, the group receiving a solution high in BCAAs demonstrated a statistically significant improvement in nitrogen balance on days 2 and 3 after total gastrectomy.[71] A significant increase in the absolute lymphocyte count and delayed cutaneous hypersensitivity occurred in patients receiving BCAA-enriched solutions,[68, 72] as did significant increases in short—half-life plasma proteins such as transferrin and prealbumin.[65, 68] Several noncontrolled studies in postoperative patients who received hypercaloric nutritional support supplemented with BCAAs have reported nitrogen sparing effects, but other studies have not found any difference in nitrogen retention between solutions containing standard or high contents of BCAAs.[73, 74]

Most of the studies showing promotion of nitrogen balance with enriched BCAA solutions have not used a balanced substrate for nonprotein caloric support, although a balanced total parenteral nutrition (TPN) regimen itself can lead to positive nitrogen balance.[75] In one study where a balanced substrate for nonprotein caloric support was used (carbohydrate:lipid calorie ratio, 7:3), no significant difference was found in nitrogen balance when a 44.6% BCAA solution was compared with standard TPN (19% BCAAs).[73] The lack of difference in this study may be due to effective utilization of lipid as a fuel source by both groups. Conceivably, there is an increased dependence on lipids as a fuel source in patients with sepsis as compared with those without sepsis.[76] On the other hand, with a mixed fuel source, a BCAA-enriched regimen was associated with a rapid rise in fibrin, transferrin, ceruloplasmin, and α-antitrypsin, as well as platelets.[77] These data suggest that perhaps nitrogen balance alone is a poor index of the success or failure of nutritional support in stress conditions.

Branched-Chain Amino Acids in Hepatic Failure

Several factors contribute to the compromised nutritional status of patients with severe chronic liver disease: poor diet or reduced intake secondary to anorexia, malabsorption, hypercatabolism, and dietary protein restriction. Of all the factors currently known to have an influence on liver regeneration (steroids, triiodothyronine, insulin, glucagon, and other factors), nutrition is the easiest to manipulate. Parenteral feeding permits selective delivery of necessary nutrients and is therefore attractive in this setting. However, the administration of adequate amounts of nutrients to these patients is made difficult by the presence of profound metabolic alterations that impair substrate utilization. In compromised hepatic function, the peripheral plasma levels of glucagon and insulin are elevated, probably because of decreased rates of hepatic degradation.[78] This hyperglucagonemia has also been correlated with portosystemic shunting,[78] and it is likely that the increased insulin results from the same mechanism. The increase in glucagon level is greater than that of insulin. A reduced insulin activity similar to that observed in type II diabetes mellitus has also been reported.[79] The net result is a decreased insulin:glucagon ratio, which favors catabolism.

Skeletal muscle proteolysis associated with cirrhosis liberates BCAAs.[80] Thus, in cirrhotic patients there is an increased rate of muscle protein degradation coupled with impaired liver function. The result is a profound alteration of the plasma amino acid profile, which probably plays a key role in the pathogenesis of hepatic encephalopathy. These changes are also responsible for the protein intolerance and resultant encephalopathy seen in patients with liver failure. At the same time, there are alterations in the supply and utilization of fat and carbohydrates as energy substrates.[79] Impaired glucose and fat utilization is responsible for the energy deficiency and the hypercatabolic state that characterizes advanced cirrhosis.

Plasma Amino Acids and Hepatic Encephalopathy

Hepatic encephalopathy is a neuropsychiatric syndrome associated with acute or chronic parenchymal liver disease and is due to failure of the liver to remove an endogenously produced toxic substance or substances from the circulation. The observations that protein and certain other nitrogenous substances in the colon exacerbate hepatic encephalopathy whereas broad-spectrum antibiotics such as neomycin cause significant amelioration suggest an intestinal origin for the causative substance(s).

Hepatic failure is also associated with considerable changes in the plasma concentrations of amino acids, and much attention has been given to the possible role of amino acid changes in the patho-

genesis of the encephalopathy.[81] One hypothesis suggests that accumulation of "false" neurochemical transmitters is important in the pathogenesis of hepatic encephalopathy. Several biogenic amines, primarily octopamine and phenylethanolamine (both metabolites of tyrosine and phenylalanine), can be stored in nerve terminals and replace the true neurotransmitters norepinephrine and dopamine.

The serum levels of the AAAs (phenylalanine, tyrosine, and tryptophan) are elevated considerably, whereas levels of BCAAs are markedly reduced.[82] The increase in the levels of AAAs is thought to be due to reduced hepatic metabolism. Since the BCAAs are metabolized by muscle, there is a decrease in the BCAA concentration relative to the AAAs. Decreases in the levels of BCAAs may also be facilitated by hyperinsulinemia (resulting from decreased hepatic insulin clearance), which would enhance BCAA uptake into muscle. Since BCAAs compete with AAAs for entry into the brain, these changes would result in increased brain entry of the AAAs, especially tryptophan. Brain levels of serotonin (5-hydroxytryptamine [5-HT]) and other neurotransmitters might increase. These compounds may contribute to the hepatic encephalopathy and coma of hepatic failure. Although the reduced ratio of BCAAs to large neutral amino acids has been confirmed in cirrhosis, there appears to be no difference in the ratio between patients with and without hepatic encephalopathy.[83]

If this hypothesis for the cause of hepatic coma is correct, treatments that reduce the rate of brain serotonin (5-HT) formation might be of use (Fig 5–6). Since increased brain serotonin formation is thought to be due to an increase in the tryptophan level in the brain, treatments that normalize the plasma amino acid pattern, such as infusions of BCAAs, were attempted.[84, 85] Although the initial results of such treatments were encouraging, more recent studies

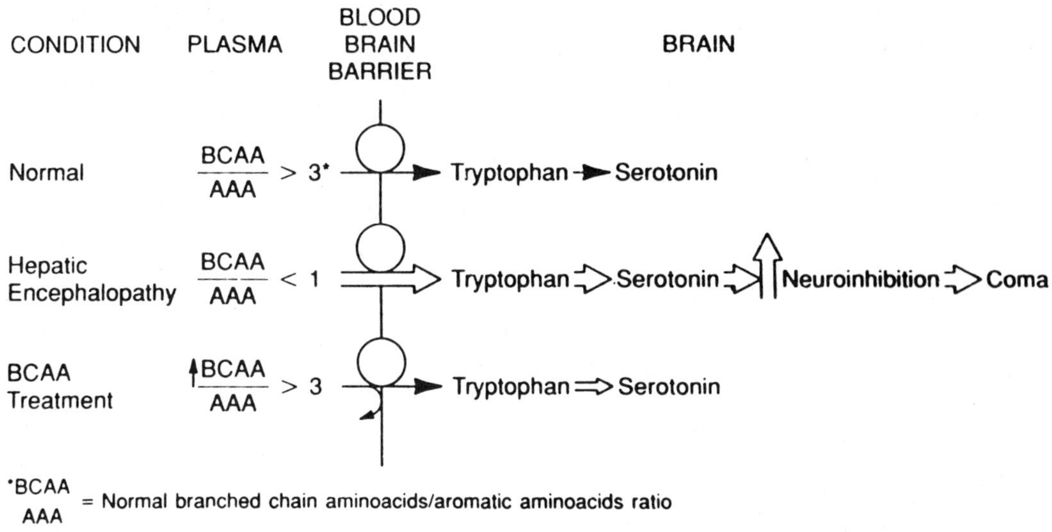

| CONDITION | PLASMA | BLOOD BRAIN BARRIER | BRAIN |

Normal $\dfrac{BCAA}{AAA} > 3^*$ Tryptophan → Serotonin

Hepatic Encephalopathy $\dfrac{BCAA}{AAA} < 1$ Tryptophan ⇒ Serotonin ⇒ Neuroinhibition ⇒ Coma

BCAA Treatment $\uparrow\dfrac{BCAA}{AAA} > 3$ Tryptophan ⇒ Serotonin

$^*\dfrac{BCAA}{AAA}$ = Normal branched chain aminoacids/aromatic aminoacids ratio

FIG 5–6.
Overall scheme of the BCAA : AAA ratio in health, hepatic coma, and postulated results of treatment. (Reproduced with permission from Alexander WF, Spindel E, Harty RF, et al: The usefulness of branched-chain amino acids in patients with acute or chronic hepatic encephalopathy. Am J Gastroenterol 84:91, 1989.)

including randomly assigned control groups have been unable to demonstrate significant benefits.[86] Before testing in man, solutions enriched in BCAAs underwent extensive testing in dogs and monkeys.[87, 88] An end-to-side portocaval shunt offered a model of hepatic encephalopathy with an amino acid pattern similar to that seen in man with hepatic failure. The results clearly indicated that a BCAA-enriched solution was superior to amino acid solutions with standard BCAA content in achieving positive nitrogen balance and normalizing neurologic symptoms.[88–90] Encouraged by these promising reports, numerous anecdotal studies were published in which BCAA-enriched amino acid solutions were given with hypertonic dextrose to patients with liver disease[91] and produced dramatic effects on arousal from encephalopathy and on the improvement of consciousness in cirrhotic patients. Conclusions of efficacy, however, cannot be drawn from these uncontrolled reports. In a disease as variable as hepatic failure, only randomized and prospective studies can be accepted as showing efficacy.

There have been seven controlled, randomized clinical studies[79] using intravenous BCAAs in patients with acute hepatic encephalopathy.[92–98] As can be seen in Table 5–2, disagreement concerning their efficacy for reducing mortality and improving encephalopathy ex-

TABLE 5–2.

Studies of BCAA on Mental Recovery and Mortality in Hepatic Encephalopathy

Study	No. of Patients	Control Treatment	Preferred Treatment	
			Encephalopathy	Mortality
Rossi-Fanelli[92]	34	Lactulose	ND	ND
Fiaccadori[94]	48	Lactulose	BCAA	ND
Cerra[95]	75	Neomycin	BCAA	BCAA
Strauss[97]	29	Neomycin	BCAA	ND
Michel[96]	47	Standard amino acids	ND	ND
Wahren[93]	50	Glucose	ND	ND
Volstrup[98]	65	Glucose	ND	ND

ists. It should be emphasized that in most of these studies the control group did not receive any amino acids or protein. The first randomized controlled trial of BCAA therapy in acute hepatic encephalopathy tested the efficacy of BCAA administration to patients with severe hepatic encephalopathy.[92] Forty patients with hepatic encephalopathy were randomly assigned to receive oral lactulose with hypertonic dextrose or 60 g of BCAAs in isoenergetic hypertonic dextrose. Patients were treated for at least 4 days. Wake-up occurred in 70% of the patients receiving BCAAs and in 47% of those who received lactulose, but the difference was not statistically significant. Intravenous BCAAs were thus found to be at least as effective as lactulose in reversing hepatic coma. Blood BCAA levels in patients receiving BCAAs were increased at the time of mental recovery as compared with control values before initiation of therapy, but they subsequently returned to baseline when treatment was discontinued despite continued improvement in mental state. There were no changes in blood amino acid levels in patients receiving lactulose and no difference in survival. Nitrogen balance studies were not available. In another trial, patients were randomized to three groups: group A received lactulose alone plus hypertonic dextrose, group B received a BCAA-enriched solution with hypertonic dextrose, and group C received both lactulose and the BCAA–hypertonic dextrose mixture.[94] Sixty-two percent of the patients in group A, 94% in group B, and 100% in group C "came out of coma" after 7 days of therapy. Treatments B and C were significantly better than treatment A. In a U.S. multicenter trial, 75 patients received either oral neomycin and a 25% dextrose solution intravenously or an isocaloric dextrose solution enriched with BCAAs.[95] Wake-up time was significantly shorter and nitrogen balance better in the BCAA-dextrose group as compared with the neomycin-dextrose group. Survival was improved in the group receiving BCAA-dextrose: 85% as

opposed to 55% in the neomycin-dextrose group. The improved survival may, however, be a result of the nutritional support of these patients with severe illness rather than the BCAA mixture in itself.

These studies seem to indicate that BCAAs are of value in the treatment of hepatic encephalopathy when given with hypertonic dextrose as an energy source. Patients in hepatic coma awoke at least as quickly in response to the administration of BCAAs and hypertonic dextrose solution as they did in response to the conventional treatment (i.e., starvation and neomycin-lactulose therapy). Both regimens worked much more quickly than placebo.[92, 94, 95, 97]

The exceptions to this trend have used fat as the major energy source[93, 96] and have failed to show that BCAA-enriched solutions are preferable to a standard amino acid solution in hepatic encephalopathy. No difference in the rate of awakening was found between a group receiving a conventional amino acid solution and one receiving a 35% BCAA mixture.[96] In both groups, 60% of the energy was given as fat. A multicenter study conducted in France and Sweden also failed to confirm any efficacy for the BCAA solution.[93] Fifty patients with cirrhosis and acute hepatic encephalopathy were randomized to receive 5 days of either 30 kcal/kg/day of amino acid–free TPN or isocaloric TPN with 40 g of BCAAs per day added. The study demonstrated clinical improvement in hepatic encephalopathy in 56% of the patients receiving the BCAA-enriched solution with glucose and fat, but this was not significantly different from the 48% improvement in the control group receiving the isoenergetic solution of glucose and fat. Fifty percent of the energy was given as fat. Mortality was not significantly different between the two groups.

It is clear from the trials under review that BCAA enrichment does not further deteriorate hepatic encephalopathy and that arousal is as fast or faster in a larger proportion of the patients than in a control group receiving conventional treatment.[99, 100] In only one study did the control group receive isonitrogenous amounts of a conventional amino acid mixture[96]; no difference was observed between the two amino acid mixtures. Therefore, it can be concluded that parenteral amino acid solutions allow a wake-up response that is favorable or better than that with conventional treatment. It is not certain, however, that this is due to the BCAA content of the amino acid mixtures. The studies to date do not permit an unqualified conclusion in favor of the use of BCAA solutions for patients with hepatic encephalopathy. Although a beneficial effect on mental status is demonstrable, the impact on mortality is discrepant across the trials. Given the uncertainty about effects on mortality and the short follow-up times in all studies, a further confirmatory randomized controlled trial with longer follow-up periods is warranted. A meta-analysis of five randomized controlled studies published in 1989 showed a highly significant improvement in mental recovery from high-grade encephalopathy with BCAA-enriched solutions. However, the uncertainty about effects on mortality and the short-term follow-up times in all studies require that randomized controlled trials with longer follow-up periods be performed.[100]

The primary goal of nutritional support in hepatic failure should be to prevent further injury to liver cells and promote their regeneration. When examining amino acid requirements, the approach in a nonencephalopathic patient would be to start with a relatively low intake of a standard amino acid solution at 0.6 g/kg of body weight per day (14% to 23% BCAAs) and to increase it stepwise until a goal of between 1.2 and 1.5 g/kg of body weight per day is obtained, provided that encephalopathy does not occur. Should encephalopathy develop, a BCAA-enriched formula could be substituted to provide 50% of the total amino acid mixture. If, on the other hand, the patient is encephalopathic at

the outset, evidence would support the initial use of a BCAA-enriched solution together with overall attention to general nutritional, metabolic, and electrolyte requirements. Since no evidence exists at present to suggest that the BCAA-enriched formula should be continued after encephalopathy subsides, conversion to a standard formula should be attempted.[101]

Chronic Renal Failure

Chronic renal failure, like portosystemic encephalopathy, is characterized by subnormal concentrations of plasma BCAAs and their keto acids.[102] The mechanism is not fully understood but may reflect increased peripheral uptake of BCAAs,[103] perhaps mediated by insulin. Although evidence is lacking that these abnormalities are harmful, attempts to correct them in hopes of improving protein nutrition have been undertaken by several investigators.[104–107]

When balanced supplements of essential amino acids or supplements containing increased proportions of BCAAs were given to patients with chronic renal failure, plasma levels of BCAAs did not increase significantly[102, 108–110] despite clinical improvement. These amino acid supplements appeared to counteract the development of secondary hyperparathyroidism and retard the progression of chronic renal failure.[106] Whether BCAAs or their keto acids were responsible for these important effects is unknown. The lowering of the urea production rate by BCAAs[107] may also be of benefit in renal failure.

EFFECTS OF BRANCHED-CHAIN AMINO ACIDS ON TRYPTOPHAN-RELATED FUNCTIONS

This section will discuss the importance of plasma amino acid levels on the concentration of brain amines and their possible neurophysiologic and behavioral importance. Since the entry of tryptophan into the brain is affected by BCAAs because of competition for the carrier for transit through the blood-brain barrier, we will focus on tryptophan and 5-HT. Relevant aspects of metabolic control logic, 5-HT synthesis in the brain, regulation of amino acid levels, and transport of amino acids into the brain were reviewed by us in detail elsewhere.[118]

Nerve cells communicate with one another via synapses. Although transient changes in electrical potential convey information along the axons of nerve cells, the transmission of such information across synapses is brought about chemically by neurotransmitters. An increasing number of compounds (>40) are believed to function as neurotransmitters in the CNS, including the catecholamines (noradrenaline, dopamine); acetylcholine; the amino acids glutamate, aspartate, glycine, and taurine; the amines 5-HT and 4-aminobutyrate; and many peptides.[119] Accordingly, in addition to being neurotransmitters in their own right, amino acids are also precursors for many of the neurotransmitters (e.g., the catecholamines, 5-HT, histamine, and the peptide neurotransmitters). The brain concentrations of neurotransmitters can be influenced by tissues outside the brain and concentrations of their precursors in the blood. These neurotransmitters include 5-HT, the catecholamines (i.e., norepinephrine and dopamine), histamine, and glycine. For example, an increased concentration of tryptophan in plasma can increase the level in the brain. This will, in turn, increase the rate of synthesis and the brain concentration of 5-HT and thus increase the rate or amount of release of the neurotransmitter into the synapse and cause a change in behavior. BCAAs compete for the same carrier system as tryptophan and can alter brain tryptophan levels. The precise behavioral change may depend on the area(s) in the brain in which a change in 5-HT levels occurs.

Sleep

A substantial amount of evidence indicates that 5-HT neurons are involved in the control of sleep. Controlled studies indicate that tryptophan administration can increase sleep duration or drowsiness in normal subjects. Differences in the results obtained in various studies can usually be attributed to differences in the dose of tryptophan or the degree of insomnia of the subjects. In subjects with "mild insomnia" or in normal subjects with long latencies, the results appear to be almost always positive. However, in entirely normal subjects or in patients with more severe insomnia, the results are mixed and less clear. Our recent studies of infusion of BCAA-enriched solutions during sleep under full polysomnographic and respiratory monitoring in normal subjects and in patients with chronic renal failure associated with sleep disturbance show increased nocturnal ventilation and normalization of rapid eye movement (REM) sleep in the latter population.[120, 121] The possibility that BCAA-enriched solutions may be of benefit in patients with other disease processes associated with sleep apnea (i.e., severe heart failure, acute myocardial ischemia, severe chronic lung disease) needs to be explored in controlled studies.

Exercise and Fatigue

One of the possible mechanisms of fatigue, the physiologic equivalent of the inability to maintain power output, is an increase in cerebral levels of 5-HT as outlined in Fig 5–7. The mechanism of central fatigue[122] could consist, in part, of increased conversion of tryptophan to 5-HT. During exercise, elevation of blood catecholamine levels results in fatty acid mobilization and an increase in their plasma concentrations. The blood fatty acid concentration could be increased sufficiently, because of discoordination of the rate of fatty acid mobilization and oxidation in a setting of

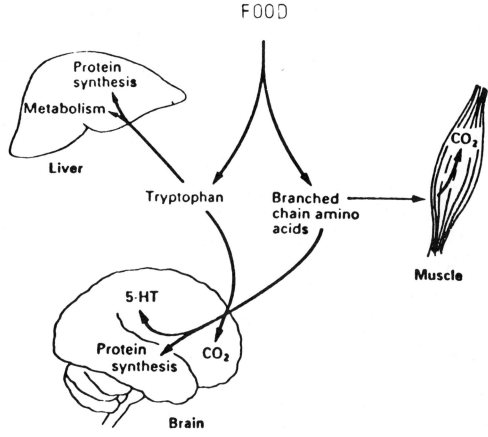

FIG 5–7.
The relationship between plasma tryptophan and branched-chain amino acids in relation to 5-HT formation in the brain. From Newsholme E, Calder P, Yaqoob P: The regulatory, informational and immunodulatory roles of fat fuels, Am J Clin Nutr 57:(suppl)7385–515, 1993.

detraining or hypoglycemia, to result in an increase in plasma concentrations of free tryptophan. Tryptophan is bound to plasma albumin and exists in equilibrium with its free form, which can be changed by increased plasma free fatty acid concentrations because of binding of fatty acids to albumin. An increase in plasma fatty acid concentrations above 1 mmol/L accompanied by a decrease in plasma concentrations of BCAAs because of increased muscle uptake during exercise could result in an increased free tryptophan-to-BCAA ratio. Tryptophan and BCAAs enter the brain on the same amino acid carrier. Thus, an increase in the tryptophan-BCAA ratio could increase tryptophan entry into the brain. An increase in brain tryptophan concentrations results in an increase in the rate of formation of 5-HT.

Moderate exercise has been found to cause significant decreases in the plasma concentrations of BCAAs but no change in the total (free plus that bound to albumin) concentration of tryptophan in some studies.[123] The plasma concentration of free tryptophan measured in marathon runners increased 2.4-fold during the race, probably because of a pronounced elevation in the concentration of plasma free fatty acids. The resulting increase in the plasma concentration of the free tryptophan: BCAA ratio should increase the rate of synthesis of 5-HT in the brain. An elevated concentration of 5-HT in specific areas of the brain may be responsible, at least in part, for the development of physical or mental fatigue during prolonged exercise. Recent studies suggest[124] that oral supplementation with

BCAA solutions improves performance in marathon runners (in terms of fatigue and mental alertness). In addition, whereas short-term high-intensity exercise increases plasma glutamine concentrations, overtraining results in low glutamine levels and immune dysfunction. These effects are preventable by BCAA ingestion. Implications for improving cardiopulmonary reserve such as are required during weaning need to be explored.

Appetite, Food Intake, and Gastric Emptying

The relationship between plasma and brain amino acid patterns and feeding behavior demonstrates suppression of food intake when serotonin receptors have been activated directly or indirectly.[125] An increase in food intake resulting from an inhibition of 5-HT metabolism or a blockade of receptors has also been reported.[126] Manipulation of 5-HT metabolism can produce changes in food intake, food preferences, and body weight. It may be possible to increase appetite and food intake by infusing BCAA-enriched solutions. The hypothesis is that elevated plasma levels of BCAAs will decrease the transport of tryptophan across the blood-brain barrier. The resulting decreased 5-HT activity in brain may decrease the anorexic action of 5-HT.

TPN with standard amino acid solutions reduces appetite and food intake in normal subjects by an amount that closely compensates for the infused calories; this effect seems to be primarily due to glucose rather than fat.[127] This loss in appetite and food intake may prolong the transition from intravenous to oral feeding in patients who need nutritional support. When BCAA-enriched parenteral nutrition was compared with standard amino acid solutions, the suppression of appetite was greatly attenuated in normal subjects.[128]

Another possible mechanism for the effect of BCAA solutions on appetite in addition to alterations in brain 5-HT levels may be the accelerated gastric emptying that we have seen in subjects receiving BCAA-enriched parenteral solutions vs. conventional amino acid solutions.[129] BCAAs may enable patients to maintain and spontaneously increase their caloric intake and to accelerate conversion from parenteral to enteral nutrition. The effect of changes in gastric emptying on other aspects of patient care such as the risk of pulmonary aspiration has not been explored.

Respiration and Cardiopulmonary Reserve

Infusion of a standard amino acid solution stimulates ventilation.[130] The ventilatory response following amino acid infusion exceeds the increase in metabolic rate, which suggests that amino acids specifically increase ventilatory drive. The responses of the ventilatory drive do not parallel the changes in Vo_2 but instead parallel the change in the ratio of tryptophan to the amino acids that compete with tryptophan for transport across the blood-brain barrier. This decrease in the ratio of tryptophan to its competitors for uptake (Val + Leu + Ile + Tyr + Phe) led to the hypothesis that the increased ventilatory sensitivity was mediated through inhibition of central 5-HT synthesis resulting from a rise in the level of amino acids that oppose tryptophan uptake across the blood-brain barrier. Changing the amino acid profile and infusing a solution consisting primarily of BCAAs (85%) further increased the ventilatory response to CO_2 inhalation.[131]

To separate the central, potentially 5-HT–dependent effect on respiration from the peripheral muscle effects of BCAAs, we studied the contractility and fatigue of isolated rat diaphragm exposed to solutions containing different amino acid profiles. The studies to date suggest that leucine but not valine or isoleucine directly increases contractility and recovery from fatigue of respiratory muscle in vitro.[132] It seems that BCAAs increase the central respiratory drive, which may be detrimental in high-output states but beneficial in apnea states, and may provide direct positive contractile effects on respiratory muscles.

The effect of exogenous amino acid administration on cardiac metabolism and physiology has been partially studied. Some amino acids such as glutamate (the only amino acid with positive arteriovenous differences in the coronary circulation) and aspartate have found a role in clinical metabolic cardioprotection. The role of BCAAs in the regulation of cardiac protein metabolism has been demonstrated, with leucine having been shown to primarily inhibit protein degradation. Infusion of BCAAs in patients with coronary artery disease demonstrated preferential uptake of BCAAs over other essential amino acids accompanied by a change of the normally negative cardiac protein balance to a neutral balance. These effects occurred without a change in coronary blood flow or myocardial oxygen consumption.[133] BCAAs regulate cardiac protein synthesis and act as preferred energy substrates. BCAAs may have protective effects on the ischemic myocardium, and some studies evaluating the effect in the setting of global ischemia in the energy-depleted heart suggest enhanced myocardial protection.[134] In a model of sepsis-induced myocardial depression, the administration of a balanced BCAA mixture demonstrated a beneficial effect in maintaining systolic properties and improving coronary blood flow.[135] While suggestive, the effects of BCAAs on integrated cardiopulmonary respiratory function are not sufficiently clear to recommend their clinical use without further studies.

The BCAAs have some unique metabolic characteristics; their uptake occurs mainly in the muscle rather than in the liver so that muscle can obtain nitrogen for the formation of glutamine. One or more BCAAs may exert specific

regulatory effects on the rates of protein degradation and synthesis in some tissues, including muscle and liver. In addition, BCAAs can compete with AAAs for entry into the brain. A major role for the increased net rates of protein degradation in muscle during metabolic stress may be to provide amino acids, especially the BCAAs that donate nitrogen for the synthesis of glutamine. Glutamine, after release by the muscle, is essential for the functioning of immune system cells, for cells involved in tissue repair, for small-bowel integrity, and for the kidney to combat acidosis. This hypothesis explains why there is such a large increase in protein degradation in skeletal muscle during injury, sepsis, and burns and indicates that it is an adaptive process and should not be considered necessarily detrimental to the patient.

It is apparent that only a few therapeutic uses of BCAA-enriched mixtures have been firmly established, even though the unique metabolic effects of the BCAAs, in vivo as well as in vitro, suggest that they might be effective in a variety of disorders. This suggests that our interpretation of the metabolism of these amino acids may be oversimplified. Beneficial effects of BCAA-enriched solutions have been shown in the treatment of hepatic failure with encephalopathy and in chronic renal failure. Their effects in hepatic encephalopathy, when considered with the effects on respiration and appetite, suggest that stimulation of CNS function occurs. The use of mixtures enriched with BCAAs has not been clearly shown to improve nitrogen balance in injured or septic patients; nitrogen balance may, however, be an insensitive index of the beneficial effects of BCAAs in such patients. Further studies of protein metabolism in the stressed state are required, with special regard to the role of muscle and its metabolism on the immune system (via provision of glutamine for lymphocytes, macrophages, and tissue repair cells). The variability in clinical results could be explained on the basis of factors that affect the conversion of BCAAs to glutamine. Future research should consider whether there may be some patients who are "responders" as opposed to "nonresponders" to BCAA administration. Analysis of all patients as one population in a disease state such as sepsis may obscure a benefit to certain subsets. The experience in providing glutamine to stressed patients as part of parenteral nutrition is reviewed elsewhere in this book.

Amino acid concentrations in plasma can have an influence on neurotransmitter levels in the brain and affect behavior. Few studies, however, have been performed to evaluate the interaction between increased BCAA levels and CNS effects. An augmented respiratory drive has been observed during the infusion of BCAA-enriched solutions. BCAA-enriched solutions as part of a TPN regimen have prevented TPN-related reduction in food intake and appetite and thus may be of importance in shortening the transition from intravenous to oral feeding and increasing the total energy intake in patients receiving intravenous feeding as a supplement to oral feeding.

Many controversies regarding the metabolism and use of BCAAs in clinical practice still exist. Most TPN regimens contain quantities of BCAAs that approximate those in an average Western diet. Therefore, the question is not whether to provide BCAAs but rather whether BCAAs given in higher amounts than normal are useful to achieve suggested metabolic and pharmacologic effects. Satisfactory evaluation of such therapies may require a better and more profound metabolic knowledge of BCAA metabolism in muscle and perhaps other tissues, glutamine metabolism in several different types of cells, behavioral assessment of nutritional modification, and the role of hormones, lymphokines, and cytokines in the integration of interorgan nitrogen redistribution.

REFERENCES

1. Stehle P, Zander J, Mertes N, et al: Effect of parenteral glutamine peptide supplements on muscle glutamine loss and nitrogen balance after major surgery. *Lancet* 1989; 1:231.
2. Young VR, Munro HN: N'-methylhistidine and muscle protein turnover. An overview. *Fed Proc* 1978; 37:2291.
3. Waterlow JC, Jackson AA: Nutrition and protein turnover in man. *Br Med Bull* 1981; 37:5.
4. Young VR, Meguid M, Meredith, et al: Recent developments in knowledge of human amino acid requirements, in Waterlow JC, Stephen JML (eds): *Nitrogen Metabolism in Man.* London, Applied Sciences, 1981, pp 133–153.
5. Newsholme EA, Crabtree B: Substrate cycles in metabolic regulation and in heat regulation. *Biochem Soc Symp* 1976; 41:61.
6. Rosenberg LE, Scriver CR: Disorders of amino acid metabolism, in Bondy PK, Rosenberg LE (eds): *Metabolic Control and Disease,* ed 8. Philadelphia, WB Saunders, 1980, pp 583–776.
7. Khatra BS, Chawla RK, Sewell CW, et al: Distribution of branched-chain alpha–keto acid dehydrogenases in primate tissues. *J Clin Invest* 1977; 59:558.
8. Ichihara A, Koyama E: Transaminase of branched chain amino acids. I. Branched chain amino acids—α-ketoglutarate. *J Biochem* 1966; 59:160.
9. Cappuccino CC, Kadowaki H, Knox WE: Assay of leucine aminotransferase in rat tissues and tumors. *Enzyme* 1978; 23:328.
10. Goldstein L, Newsholme EA: The formation of alanine from amino acids in diaphragm muscle of the rat. *Biochem J* 1976; 154:555.
11. Snell K: Muscle alanine synthesis and hepatic gluconeogenesis. *Biochem Soc Trans* 1980; 8:205.
12. Miller LL: The role of the liver and the non-hepatic tissues in the regulation of free amino acid levels in the blood, in Holden JT (ed): *Amino Acid Pools: Distribution, Formation, and Func-*

tion of Free Amino Acids Amsterdam, Elsevier, 1962, pp 708–721.

13. Windmueller HG, Spaeth AE: Uptake and metabolism of plasma glutamine by the small intestine. *J Biol Chem* 1974; 249:5070.

14. Hanson PJ, Parsans DS: The utilization of glucose and production of lactate by in vitro preparations of rat small intestine. Effects of vascular perfusion. *J Physiol* 1976; 255:775.

15. Goldberg AL, Demartino G, Chang TW: Release of gluconeogenic precursors from skeletal muscle, in *Proceedings of the FEBS 11th Annual Meeting.* Copenhagen, 1978, pp 347–358.

16. Wagenmakers AJ, Schepens JT, Veldhuizen JA, et al: The activity state of the branched chain 2-oxo acid dehydrogenase complex in rat tissues. *Biochem J* 1984; 220:273.

17. Wagenmakers AJ, Veerkamp JH: The effect of starvation on branched-chain 2-oxo acid oxidation in rat muscle. *Nutrition* 1984; 219:253.

18. Vary TC, Siegel JH, Zechnich A, et al: Pharmacological reversal of abnormal glucose regulation, BCAA utilization, and muscle catabolism in sepsis by dichloroacetate. *J Trauma* 1988; 28:1301.

19. Vary TC, Siegel JH, Tall BD, et al: Inhibition of skeletal muscle protein synthesis in septic intra-abdominal abscess. *J Trauma* 1988; 28:981.

20. Cuthbertson DP: Post-shock metabolic response. *Lancet* 1942; 1:433.

21. Kinney JM, Duke JH Jr, Long CL, et al: Tissue fuel and weight loss after injury. *J Clin Pathol* 1970; 23(suppl 4):65.

22. Kinney JM, Elwyn DH: Protein metabolism and injury. *Annu Rev Nutr* 1983; 3:433.

23. Kinney JM, Elwyn DH: Protein metabolism and injury. *Annu Rev Nutr* 1983; 3:433.

24. Shamoon H, Hendler R, Sherwin RS: Synergistic interaction among antiinsulin hormones in the pathogenesis of stress hyperglycemia in humans. *J Clin Endocrinol Metab* 1981; 52:1235.

25. Clowes GH, George BC, Villee CA, et al: Muscle proteolysis induced by a circulating peptide in patients with sepsis or trauma. *N Engl J Med* 1983; 308:545.

26. Powanda MC, Beisel WR: Hypothesis: Leukocyte endogenous mediator/endogenous pyrogen/lymphocyte activating factor modulates the development of nonspecific and specific immunity and affects nutritional status. *Am J Clin Nutr* 1982; 35:762.

27. Weber FL Jr, Reiser BJ: Relationship of plasma amino acids to nitrogen balance and portal-systemic encephalopathy in alcoholic liver disease. *Dig Dis Sci* 1982; 27:103.

28. Cerra FB, Siegel JH, Border JR, et al: The hepatic failure of sepsis: Cellular versus substrate. *Surgery* 1979; 86:409.

29. Rossi-Fanelli F, Freund H, Krause R, et al: Induction of coma in normal dogs by the infusion of aromatic amino acids and its prevention by the addition of branched chain amino acids. *Gastroenterology* 1982; 83:664.

30. Berl S, Takagaki G, Clarke DD, et al: Metabolic compartments in vivo: Ammonia and glutamine acid metabolism in brain and liver. *J Biol Chem* 1962; 237:2562.

31. Freund HR, Ryan JA Jr, Fischer JE: Amino acid derangements in patients with sepsis: Treatment with branched chain amino acid rich infusions. *Ann Surg* 1978; 188:423–430.

32. Cerra FB, Siegel JH, Coleman B, et al: Septic autocannibalism. A failure of exogenous nutritional support. *Ann Surg* 1980; 192:570.

33. James JH, Hodgman JM, Funovics JM, et al: Brain tryptophan. Plasma free tryptophan and distribution of plasma neutral amino acids. *Metabolism* 1976; 25:471.

34. Jeppsson B, Freund HR, Gimmon Z, et al: Blood brain barrier derangement in sepsis: Cause of septic encephalopathy. *Am J Surg* 1981; 141:136.

35. Sprung CL, Peduzzi PN, Shatney CN, et al: Veterans Administration Systemic Cooperative Group. The impact of encephalopathy and physiologic derangements in the sepsis syndrome. *Crit Care Med* 1990; 18:801.

36. Unger RH: Glucagon and the insulin:glucagon ratio in diabetes and other catabolic illnesses. *Diabetes* 1971; 20:834.

37. Sprung CL, Cerra FB, Freund HR, et

al: Amino acid alterations and encephalopathy in the sepsis syndrome. *Crit Care Med* 1991; 19:753–757.

38. Delany HM, Teh E, Dwarka B, et al: Infusion of enteral vs. parenteral nutrients using high-concentration branch-chain amino acids: Effect on wound healing in postoperative rat. *JPEN* 1991; 15:464–468.

39. Platell C, McCauley R, McCulloch R, et al: Influence of glutamine and branched chain amino acids on the jejunal atrophy associated with parenteral nutrition. *J Gastro Hepatol* 1991; 6:345–349.

40. Blackburn GL, Desai SP, Keenan RA, et al: Clinical use of branched chain amino acid enriched solutions in the stressed and injured patient, in Walser M, Williamson JR (eds): *Metabolism and Clinical Implications of Branched Chain Amino Acids and Ketoacids: Proceedings of the International Symposium on Metabolism and Clinical Implications of Branched Chain Amino and Ketoacids, Charleston, SC, 1980.* New York, Elsevier, 1981, pp 521–539.

41. Munro HN: Hormones and the metabolic response to injury. *N Engl J Med* 1979; 300:41.

42. Greig PD, Baker JP, Jeejeebhoy KN: Metabolic effects of total parenteral nutrition. *Annu Rev Nutr* 1982; 2:179.

43. Furst P, Albers S, Stehle P: Stress induced intracellular glutamine depletion. The potential use of glutamine containing peptides in parenteral nutrition. *Clin Nutr* 1987; 17:117.

44. Roth E, Funovics J, Muehlbacker F, et al: Metabolic disorder in severe abdominal sepsis: Glutamine deficiency in skeletal muscle. *Clin Nutr* 1982; 1:25.

45. Parry-Billings M, Baigrie RJ, Lamont PM, et al: Effects of major and minor surgery on plasma glutamine and cytokine levels. *Arch Surg* 1992; 127:1237–1240.

46. Plumley DA, Souba WW, Hautamaki RD, et al: Accelerated lung amino acid release in hyperdynamic septic surgical patients. *Arch Surg* 1990; 125:57–61.

47. Plumley DA, Austgen TR, Salloum RM, et al: Role of the lungs in maintaining amino acid homeostasis. *JPEN* 1990; 14:569–573.

48. Fulks RM, Li JB, Goldberg AL: Effects of insulin, glucose, and amino acids on protein turnover in rat diaphragm. *J Biol Chem* 1975; 250:290.

49. Buse MG, Reid SS: Leucine. A possible regulator of protein turnover in muscle. *J Clin Invest* 1975; 56:1250.

50. Tischler ME, Desautels M, Goldberg AL: Does leucine, leucyl tRNA, on some metabolite of leucine regulate protein synthesis and degradation in skeletal and cardiac muscle. *J Biol Chem* 1982; 257:1613.

51. Li JB, Jefferson LS: Influence of amino acid availability on protein turnover in perfused skeletal muscle. *Biochim Biophys Acta* 1978; 544:351.

52. Chua B, Siehl DL, Morgan HE: Effect of leucine and metabolites of branched chain amino acids on protein turnover in heart. *J Biol Chem* 1979; 254:8358.

53. Chua B, Siehl DL, Morgan HE: A role of leucine in regulation of protein turnover in working rat hearts. *Am J Physiol* 1980; 239:510.

54. Sakamoto A, Moldawer LL, Usui S, et al: In vivo evidence for the unique nitrogen sparing mechanism of branched chain amino acid administration. *Surgery* 1979; 30:67.

55. Freund HR, James JH, Fischer JE: Nitrogen sparing mechanisms of singly administered branched chain amino acids in the injured rat. *Surgery* 1981; 90:237.

56. Sakamoto A, Moldawer LL, Bothe A Jr, et al: Are the nitrogen sparing mechanisms of branched chain amino acid administration really unique? *Surg Forum* 1980; 31:99.

57. Poso AR, Wert JJ Jr, Mortimore GE: Multifunctional control of amino acids of deprivation induced proteolysis in liver. Role of leucine. *J Biol Chem* 1982; 257:1214.

58. Sapir DG, Owen OE, Pozefsky T, et al: Nitrogen sparing induced by a mixture of essential amino acids given chiefly as their ketoanalogues during prolonged starvation in obese sub-

jects. *J Clin Invest* 1974; 54:974.

59. Bower RH, Muggia Sullam M, Vallgren S, et al: Branched chain amino acid enriched solutions in the septic patient. A randomized, prospective trial. *Ann Surg* 1986; 203:13.

60. Clowes GH Jr, Randall HT, Cha CJ: Amino acid and energy metabolism in septic and traumatized patients. *JPEN* 1980; 4:195.

61. Nuwer N, Cerra FB, Shronts EP, et al: Does modified amino acid total parenteral nutrition alter immune response in high level surgical stress? *JPEN* 1983; 7:521.

62. Sax HC, Talamini MA, Fischer JE: Clinical use of branched chain amino acids in liver disease, sepsis, trauma, and burns. *Arch Surg* 1986; 121:358.

63. Pedersen P, Shujun L, Hasselgren PO, et al: Administration of balanced or BCAA-enriched amino acid solution in septic rats. *Ann Surg* 1988; 201:714.

64. Bonau RA, Ang SD, Malayappa J, et al: High-branched chain amino acid solutions: Relationship of composition of efficacy. *JPEN* 1984; 8:622.

65. Bower RH, Muggia Sullam M, et al: Branched-chain amino acid enriched solutions in the septic patient. A randomized, prospective trial. *Ann Surg* 1986; 203:13.

66. Daly JM, Mihranian MH, Kehoe JE, et al: Effects of postoperative infusion of branched chain amino acids on nitrogen balance and forearm muscle substrate flux. *Surgery* 1983; 94:151.

67. Cerra FB, Mazuski J, Teasley K, et al: Nitrogen retention in critically ill patients is proportional to the branched chain amino acid load. *Crit Care Med* 1983; 11:775.

68. Cerra FB, Mazuski JE, Chuter E, et al: Branched chain metabolic support: A prospective, randomized, double-blind trial in surgical stress. *Ann Surg* 1984; 199:286.

69. Cerra FB, Upson D, Angelico R, et al: Branched chains support postoperative protein synthesis. *Surgery* 1982; 92:192.

70. Pelosi G, Proietti R, Magalini SL, et al: Anticatabolic properties of branched chain amino acids in trauma. *Resuscitation* 1983; 10:153.

71. Okada A, Mori S, Totsuka M, et al: Branched-chain amino acids metabolic support in surgical patients: A randomized, controlled trial in patients with subtotal or total gastrectomy in 16 Japanese institutions. *JPEN* 1988; 12:332.

72. Nuwer N, Cerra FB, Shronts EP, et al: Does modified amino acid total parenteral nutrition alter immune-response in high level surgical stress? *JPEN* 1983; 7:521.

73. van der Wounde P, Morgan RE, Kosta JM, et al: Addition of branched-chain amino acids to parenteral nutrition of stressed critically ill patients. *Crit Care Med* 1986; 14:685.

74. van Way CW, Moore EE, Allo M, et al: Comparison of total parenteral nutrition with 25 percent and 45 percent branched chain amino acids in stressed patients. *Am Surg* 1985; 51:609.

75. Kirkpatrick JR, Dahn M, Lewis L: Selective versus standard hyperalimentation: A randomized prospective study. *Am J Surg* 1981; 141:116.

76. Nanni GA, Siegel JH, Coleman B, et al: Increased lipid fuel dependence in the critically ill septic patient. *J Trauma* 1984; 24:14.

77. Chiarla C, Siegel JH, Kidd S, et al: Inhibition of post-traumatic septic proteolysis and ureagenesis and simulation of hepatic acute-phase protein production by branched-chain amino acid TPN. *J Trauma* 1988; 28:1145.

78. Sherwin R, Joshi P, Hendler R, et al: Hyperglucagonemia in Laënnec's cirrhosis. The role of portal systemic shunting. *N Engl J Med* 1974; 290:239.

79. Riggio O, Merli M, Cangiano C, et al: Glucose intolerance in liver cirrhosis. *Metabolism* 1982; 31:6.

80. Marchesini G, Zoli M, Angiolini A, et al: Muscle protein break down in liver cirrhosis and the role of altered carbohydrate metabolism. *Hepatology* 1981; 1:294.

81. James JH, Ziparo V, Jeppsson B, et al: Hyperammonaemia, plasma amino acid imbalance, and blood brain amino acid transport: A unified

theory of portal systemic encephalopathy. *Lancet* 1979; 2:772.

82. Okuno M, Nagayama M, Takai T, et al: Postoperative total parenteral nutrition in patients with liver disorders. *J Surg Reg* 1985; 39:93.

83. Morgan MY, Milsom JP, Sherlock S: Plasma ratio of valine, leucine and isoleucine to phenylalanine and tyrosine in liver disease. *Gut* 1978; 19:1068.

84. Fischer JE, Baldessarini RJ: False neurotransmitters and hepatic failure. *Lancet* 1971; 2:75.

85. Fischer JE, Rosen HM, Ebeid AM, et al: The effect of normalization of plasma amino acids on hepatic encephalopathy in man. *Surgery* 1976; 80:77.

86. Walser M: Therapeutic aspects of branched chain amino and keto acids. *Clin Sci* 1984; 66:1.

87. Smith AR, Rossi-Fanelli F, Ziparo V, et al: Long-term sampling of intraventricular CSF in the unanesthetized monkey and dog. *J Surg Res* 1979; 26:69.

88. Smith AR, Rossi-Fanelli F, Ziparo V, et al: Alterations in plasma and CSF amino acids, amines and metabolites in hepatic coma. *Ann Surg* 1978; 187:343.

89. Fisher JE, Funovics JM, Aguirre A, et al: The roles of plasma amino acids in hepatic encephalopathy. *Surgery* 1975; 78:276.

90. Smith AR, Rossi-Fanelli F, Ziparo V, et al: Alterations in plasma and CSF amino acids, amines and metabolites in hepatic coma. *Ann Surg* 1978; 187:343.

91. Okada A, Kamata S, Kim CW, et al: Treatment of hepatic encephalopathy with BCAA-enriched amino acid mixture, in Walser M, Williamson R (eds): *Metabolism and Clinical Implications of Branched Chain Amino and Ketoacids.* New York, Elsevier, 1981, pp 447–452.

92. Rossi-Fanelli F, Riggio O, Cangiano C, et al: Branched chain amino acids vs lactulose in the treatment of hepatic coma: A controlled study. *Dig Dis Sci* 1982; 27:929.

93. Wahren J, Denis J, Desurmont P, et al: Is intravenous administration of branched chain amino acids effective in the treatment of hepatic encephalopathy? A multicenter study. *Hepatology* 1983; 3:475.

94. Fiaccadon F, Ghinelli F, Pedretti G, et al: Branched chain amino acid enriched solutions in the treatment of hepatic encephalopathy: A controlled trial, in Capocaccia L, Fischer JE, Rossi-Fanelli F (eds): *Hepatic Encephalopathy in Chronic Liver Failure.* New York, Plenum, 1984, p 323.

95. Cerra FB, Cheung NK, Fischer JE, et al: Disease specific amino acid infusion (F080) in hepatic encephalopathy: A prospective, randomized, double-blind, controlled trial. *JPEN* 1985; 9:288.

96. Michel H, Bories P, Aubin JP, et al: Treatment of acute hepatic encephalopathy in cirrhosis with a branched chain amino acids enriched versus a conventional amino acids mixture. *Liver* 1985; 5:282.

97. Strauss E, dos Santos WR, da Silva EC, et al: Treatment of hepatic encephalopathy: A randomized clinical trial comparing a branched-chain enriched amino acid solution to oral neomycin. *Nutr Supp Serv* 1986; 6:18.

98. Vistrup H, Gluud C, Hardt F, et al: Branched chain enriched amino acids versus glucose treatment of hepatic encephalopathy. A double-blind study of 65 patients with cirrhosis. *J Hepatol* 1990; 10:291–296.

99. Rossi-Fanelli F, Cangiano C, Cascino A, et al: Branched chain amino acids in the treatment of hepatic encephalopathy, in Capocaccia L, Fisher JE, Rossi-Fanelli F (eds): *Hepatic Encephalopathy in Chronic Liver Failure.* New York, Plenum, 1984, pp 335–344.

100. Naylor CD, O'Rourke K, Detsky AS, et al: Parenteral nutrition with branched-chain amino acids in hepatic encephalopathy. A meta-analysis. *Gastroenterology* 1989; 97:1033–1042.

101. Blackburn GL, O'Keefe SJD: Nutrition in liver failure. *Gastroenterology* 1989; 97:1049.

102. Walser M: Conservative management of the uremic patient, in Brenner B,

Rector FC (eds): *The Kidney*, ed 2. Philadelphia, WB Saunders, 1981, pp 2383–2424.

103. Tizianello A, Deferrari G, Garibotto G, et al: Branched-chain amino acid metabolism in chronic renal failure. *Kidney Int* 1983; 16(suppl):17.

104. Alvestrand A, Ahlberg M, Furst P, et al: Clinical experience with amino acid and keto acid diets. *Am J Clin Nutr* 1980; 33:1654.

105. Mitch WE, Abras EA, Walser M: Long-term effects of a new ketoacid amino acid supplement in patients with chronic renal failure. *Kidney Int* 1982; 22:48.

106. Walser M: Nutritional support in renal failure: Future directions. *Lancet* 1983; 1:340.

107. Walser M, Lund P, Ruderman NB, et al: Synthesis of essential amino acids from their ketoanalogues by perfused rat liver and muscle. *J Clin Invest* 1973; 52:2865.

108. Marchesini G, Zoli M, Dondi C, et al: Anticatabolic effect of branched chain amino acid enriched solutions in patients with liver cirrhosis. *Hepatology* 1982; 2:420.

109. McGhee A, Henderson JM, Millikan WJ Jr, et al: Comparison of the effects of hepatic acid and a casein modular diet on encephalopathy, plasma amino acids, and nitrogen balance in cirrhotic patients. *Ann Surg* 1983; 197:288.

110. Fischer JE: Amino acids in hepatic coma. *Dig Dis Sci* 1982; 27:97.

111. Jimenez-Jimenez FJ, Ortiz Leyba C, Morales Mendez S, et al: Variations in plasma amino acids in septic patients subjected to parenteral nutrition with a high proportion of branched-chain amino acids. *Nutrition* 1992; 8:237–244.

112. Sandstedt S, Jorfelt L, Larsson J: Randomized, controlled study evaluating effects of branched chain amino acids and alpha-ketoisocaproate on protein metabolism after surgery. *Br J Surg* 1992; 79:217–220.

113. Vente JP, Soeters PB, von Meyenfeldt MF: Prospective randomized double-blind trial of branched chain amino acid enriched versus standard parenteral nutrition solutions in trauma-

tized and septic patients. *World J Surg* 1991; 15:128–132.

114. Freund H, Hoover MC, Atamian S, et al: Infusion of the branched chain amino acids in postoperative patients. *Am Surg* 1979; 190:18.

115. Newsholme EA, Leech AR: *Biochemistry for the Medical Sciences*. Chichester, UK, John Wiley & Sons, 1983, pp 382–442.

116. Madsen DC: Branched-chain amino acids: Metabolic roles and clinical applications, in Johnston IDA (ed): *Advances in Clinical Nutrition*. The Hague, The Netherlands, MTP Press, 1982, pp 3–23.

117. Ardawi MS, Newsholme EA: Metabolism in lymphocytes and its importance in the immune response. *Essays Biochem* 1985; 21:1.

118. Skeie B, Kvetan V, Gil K, et al: Branch-chain amino acids: Their metabolism and clinical utility. *Crit Care Med* 1990; 18:549–571.

119. James JH, Hodgman JM, Funovics JM, et al: Brain tryptophan, plasma free tryptophan and distribution of plasma neutral amino acids. *Metabolism* 1976; 25:471.

120. Kirvela O, Thorpy M, Takala J, et al: Respiratory and sleep patterns during nocturnal infusions of branched chain amino acids. *Acta Anaesthesiol Scand* 1990; 34:645–648.

121. Soreide E, Skeie B, Kirvela O, et al: Branched chain amino acid in chronic renal failure patients: Respiratory and sleep effects. *Kidney Int* 1991; 40:539–543.

122. Newsholme E, Calder P, Yaqoob P: The regulatory, informational and immunomodulatory roles of fat fuels. *Am J Clin Nutr* 1993; 57(suppl):738–751.

123. Blomstrand E, Celsing F, Newsholme EA: Changes in plasma concentrations of aromatic and branched-chain amino acids during sustained exercise in man and their possible role in fatigue. *Acta Physiol Scand* 1988; 133:115.

124. Parry-Billings M, Budgett R, Koutedakis Y, et al: Plasma amino acid concentrations in the overtraining syndrome: Possible effects on the immune system. *Med Sci Sports & Exerc* 1992; 24:1353–1358.

125. Harper AE, Peters JC: Amino acid signals and food intake and preference: Relation to body protein and metabolism. *Experientia Suppl* 1983; 44:107.

126. Blundell JE: Serotonin and appetite. *Neuropharmacology* 1984; 23:1537.

127. Gil KM, Skeie B, Kvetan V, et al: Parenteral nutrition and oral intake: Effect of glucose and fat infusions. *JPEN* 1991; 15:426–432.

128. Gil KM, Skeie B, Kvetan V, et al: Parenteral nutrition and oral intake: Effect of branched-chain amino acids. *Nutrition* 1990; 6:291–295.

129. Bursztein-DeMyttenaere S, Gil K, Heymsfield S, et al: Postabsorptive control of food intake in healthy humans (abstract). *FASEB J* 1988; 2:1795.

130. D'Attellis N, Bursztein SA, Kvetan V, et al: Beneficial effects of intravenous branched chain amino acids on gastric emptying. *Clin Nutr* 1988; 8:73.

131. Takala J, Askanazi J, Weissman C, et al: Changes in respiratory control induced by amino acid infusions. *Crit Care Med* 1988; 16:463.

132. Yamada H, Kvetan V, Ohta Y, et al: Effect of individual branched chain amino acids on contractility and fatigue of diaphragm (abstract). *Anesthesiology* 1990; 73:258.

133. Young LH, McNulty PH, Morgan C, et al: Myocardial protein turnover in patients with coronary artery disease: Effect of branched chain amino acid infusion. *J Clin Invest* 1991; 87:554–560.

134. Schwalb H, Izhar U, Yaroslavsky E, et al: The effect of amino acids on the ischemic heart. Improvement of oxygenated crystalloid cardioplegic solution by an enriched branched chain amino acid formulation. *J Thorac Cardiovasc Surg* 1989; 98:551–556.

135. Freund HR, Dann EJ, Burns F, et al: Systolic properties of normal septic isolated rat hearts. *Arch Surg* 1985; 120:483–488.

6

Arginine

Adrian Barbul, M.D.

Moira Hurson, B.Sc., S.R.D.

Arginine biochemistry and physiology	Arginine and wound healing
Arginine and hormone secretagogue activity	Arginine and immune function
Arginine and posttraumatic nitrogen metabolism	Clinical recommendations

It is generally accepted that adequate nutritional support is an essential component in the successful treatment of the critically ill patient. Nutritional intervention affects how the hospitalized patient responds to infection, injury, and neoplasia. In the past two decades the concept of nutrition support for the hospitalized patient has evolved considerably. The aim of most therapeutic nutritional regimens is to maintain a positive nitrogen balance in order to preserve or restore lean body tissue. More recently interest has focused on the use of various nutrients, solely or as part of a complete nutritional regimen, to modulate the immune system and positively enhance patient outcome. In particular, the amino acids arginine and glutamine, the ω-6 and ω-3 fatty acids, metals such as iron and zinc, and certain vitamins including A, C, and E have all been shown to possess a number of important immune-modulating properties. Among these dietary factors,

the amino acid arginine has been found to possess a number of extremely useful and unique effects on immune function, posttraumatic nitrogen metabolism, and wound healing. All of these effects, coupled with relative safety, make the use of arginine attractive for the care of traumatized or seriously ill patients.

ARGININE BIOCHEMISTRY AND PHYSIOLOGY

Arginine, a dibasic amino acid, is considered to be a dietary conditionally dispensable amino acid.[1] Arginine is synthesized endogenously from ornithine via citrulline as a result of interorgan reactions. The quantities produced, sufficient to maintain muscle and connective tissue mass, may be less than that required for optimal protein biosynthesis and growth. In times of immaturity and severe stress such as sepsis, trauma, and nitrogen overload, endogenous synthesis of arginine is insufficient to meet the increased demands that increased protein turnover requires. Therefore, in such situations arginine is an indispensable amino acid for optimal growth and maintenance of a positive nitrogen balance[2-4] (Fig 6-1).

Arginine is a normal constituent of numerous body proteins and is associated with a variety of essential reactions of intermediary metabolism. The intestinal absorption of arginine involves a transport system shared with lysine, ornithine, and cysteine. This system is energy and sodium dependent and has substrate specificity. Arginine, ornithine, and lysine also share a common uptake and transport system in the brain, leukocytes, erythrocytes, and fibroblasts.[5]

Arginine serves as a vehicle for the transport, storage, and excretion of nitrogen. The transamidation between arginine and glycine results in guanidinoacetic acid, which is further methylated to form the high-energy phosphagen creatine phosphate. The reversible release of fumaric acid by dismutation of argininosuccinic acid further links arginine metabolism with cellular energetics via the tricarboxylic acid cycle. Arginine and its metabolite ornithine are also utilized for polyamine biosynthesis, an important requirement for cellular division (Fig 6-1).

The urea cycle represents the major metabolic pathway for ammonia detoxification, and arginine plays a key regulatory role within this cycle (Fig 6-1).[6] Any condition that increases the demand for ammonia detoxification is

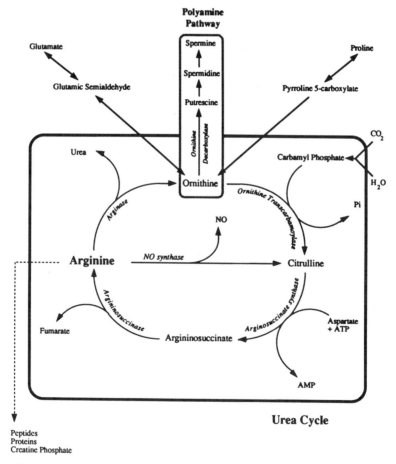

FIG 6-1.

Schematic representation of the major metabolic cycles of arginine. *NO* = nitric oxide.

likely to increase arginine requirements. Approximately twice as much ornithine and four times as much citrulline are needed to achieve the same degree of protection against hyperammonemia as that provided by arginine.

Recently, L-arginine has been shown to be the unique substrate for the production of the biological effector molecule nitric oxide (NO). This important pathway has been shown to be present in many tissues and cells including endothelium, brain, inflammatory cells (lymphocytes, macrophages, neutrophils, mast cells), platelets, and hepatocytes.[7] NO, which is pharmacologically and chemically identical to endothelial-derived relaxing factor (EDRF), is a recently identified biological effector molecule. In addition to its role in vasodilatation, NO is a putative neurotransmitter and cytotoxic effector molecule. NO is formed by oxidation of one of two identical terminal guanidino groups of L-arginine by the enzyme NO synthase (provisionally EC 1.14.13.39), a dioxygenase of which there are at least two identified isoforms. The enzyme has been found in almost all tissue types examined and occurs in all animal species from mammals, reptiles, and birds to the horseshoe crab.[8-11] The latter animal has survived unchanged during 500 million years of evolution, thus indicating that the generation of NO is one of the oldest phylogenetically preserved regulatory systems. Both isoforms of NO synthase have been identified as flavoproteins,[12-14] each containing flavine adenine dinucleotide and flavine adenine mononucleotide, and both are inhibited by diphenyleneiodonium, a flavoprotein inhibitor.[15]

NO synthase type I is cytosolic, expressed constitutively, and activated by Ca^{2+}/calmodulin.[16] Following stimulation by various agonists, the generation of NO by this isoform is quantitatively smaller in both amount and duration than that of NO synthase type II.[8] NO synthase I has been identified in the brain,[16-18] lung,[19] retina,[20] adrenal glands,[21] platelets,[22] endocardial cells, vascular endothelial cells,[23, 24] skeletal muscle, spleen, and skin.[25]

NO synthase type II has been cloned[26, 27] and identified as two 125- to 135,000-kd monomer proteins that form a 250,000 kd dimer.[14, 28] The enzyme is inducible by endotoxins, exotoxins, and/or cytokines and is found in macrophages,[29-31] Kuppfer cells,[32] parenchymal liver cells,[33, 34] neutrophils,[35] fibroblasts,[36] chondrocytes,[37] and smooth muscle cells.[38] Mouse macrophage NO synthase II shares 51% homology with the rat cerebellar NO synthase I.[27] Like NO synthase I, macrophage NO synthase II contains binding sites for both flavine adenine dinucleotide and reduced nicotinamide adenine dinucleotide phosphate (NADPH).[26, 27] It is soluble and has an absolute requirement for tetrahydrobiopterin and possibly for Mg^{2+} and reduced thiols such as dithiothreitol or glutathione.[39] The induction of this isoform is inhibited by glucocorticoids,[40-42] transforming growth factor β1, 2, and 3,[43] interleukin-4 (IL-4), and IL-10.[44] These compounds have no inhibitory activity on the formation of NO once the enzyme is expressed.

There are still many questions regarding the physiology of NO synthesis and its alterations in different pathologic states. There is no evidence, as of yet, that exogenous arginine, even in large doses, modulates the rate of synthesis of NO (for one possible exception see the next section). Conversely, plasma and tissue levels of arginine are usually high enough to meet the demands of the NO synthase enzyme in health. The two exceptions noted thus far involve the local wound environment, where arginine levels are very low,[45] and the atherosclerotic vessel, where once again low arginine concentrations may be responsible for the lack of endogenous vasodilatation.[46] A great deal of current research is focusing on modulating NO synthase activity, whether endogenous or induced by different disease states.

ARGININE AND HORMONE SECRETAGOGUE ACTIVITY

Increased plasma levels of arginine lead to enhanced secretion of several hormones including insulin, glucagon, growth hormone, prolactin, and adrenal catecholamines[5] (Table 6–1). While arginine is not the only amino acid that stimulates the release of these hormones, it is certainly the most potent.

The strong endocrine secretagogue action of arginine occurs via largely unexplained mechanisms that appear to be linked to cholinergic activity. This fact and the recent demonstration of NO synthase immunoreactivity and functional activity in several secretory organs suggest that NO is involved in arginine-induced hormone secretion. For example, both L-arginine and L-ornithine are potent insulotrophic agents.[47] The depolarizing activity of these two cationic amino acids has been proposed to account for their ability to stimulate insulin release.[48] However, this explanation is insufficient to account for all of the insulin release. In vivo, pancreatic NO is produced in response to D-glucose, L-arginine, or tolbutamide, a hypoglycemic drug.[49, 50] As opposed to this constitutive NO synthesis, large NO production is induced by IL-1β,[51] probably by intrapancreatic macrophages and endothelial cells. This mechanism has been implicated in the pathologic damage found in autoimmune insulitis, characteristic of type I diabetes mellitus. Inhibition of constitutive NO production by N-monomethylarginine (a competitive inhibitor of arginine for NO synthase) reduces insulin secretion in response to L-arginine. Inhibition of inducible NO synthesis by N-monomethylarginine is effective in reducing the onset of streptozotocin-induced diabetes.[52]

NO synthase immunoreactivity and functionality have also been located in the adrenal gland.[21] NO modulates adrenal medullary vasodilatation and may increase the release of adrenal hormones during increased perfusion. In addition, L-arginine,[53] as well as other agents that increase intracellular cyclic guanosine monophosphate (cGMP) levels such as NO, stimulates catecholamine release from the adrenal gland.[54, 55] Endogenously formed NO facilitates the release of adrenaline[56] in the rabbit.

Since L-arginine causes the release of so many other hormones by cholinergic actions, it is reasonable to speculate that NO may be involved in the secretion of other hormones such as pituitary growth hormone and prolactin. The lack of NO synthase immunoreactivity in the anterior pituitary is given as evidence against this possibility. However, a form of the enzyme that does not react with NO synthase type I may be present there.

Increased NO synthesis may be the mechanism by which arginine leads to enhanced hormone secretion. This would be one of the first known instances whereby exogenous arginine directly regulates levels of NO synthesis, whether by the constitutive or the inducible NO synthase systems.

ARGININE AND POSTTRAUMATIC NITROGEN METABOLISM

Based on the concept that nutritional requirements posttrauma approximate those of a growing rather than those of

TABLE 6–1.

Endocrine Secretagogue Effects of Arginine

Pituitary gland
  Growth hormone
  Prolactin
Pancreas
  Insulin
  Glucagon
  Somatostatin
  Pancreatic polypeptide
Adrenal gland
  Catecholamines
  Aldosterone
Brain
  Vasopressin

an adult organism, Seifter has shown that arginine is required for the survival and weight gain of mildly injured rats.[4] Animals subjected to either partial starvation or bilateral closed femoral fractures have improved nitrogen retention when given amino acid mixtures containing a larger proportion of arginine.[57, 58]

Healthy elderly human volunteers demonstrate increased nitrogen retention following supplementation with 30 g of arginine aspartate (17 g of free arginine) for 2 weeks.[59] Clinically, arginine given alone or in conjunction with complete nutritional support has been shown to reduce nitrogen loss in postoperative patients. Thus, elective surgical patients given 30 g/day of arginine hydrochloride intravenously for the first 3 days postcholecystectomy had a 60% reduction in urinary nitrogen excretion.[60] Following major abdominal surgery for gastrointestinal malignancies, patients receiving immediate enteral feedings supplemented with 25 g of arginine had a mean positive nitrogen balance when compared with glycine-supplemented controls.[61]

Supplemental ornithine also increases nitrogen retention following surgery in humans.[62, 63] Because ornithine cannot replace arginine for nutritional requirements,[64] this similar mode of action on nitrogen balance suggests a similar pharmacologic mechanism. The amounts of arginine and ornithine required to achieve the above effects are in excess of those achieved by normal nutritional means and represent a pharmacologic dose.

ARGININE AND WOUND HEALING

Successful wound healing is the cornerstone of recovery following surgical procedures. Nearly half of all postoperative morbidity involves wound complications.[65] One of the most common problems encountered among critically ill patients is a delay in the efficiency of wound healing. In particular, the elderly are more prone to certain wound healing complications, including abdominal wound dehiscence and bowel anastomosis breakdown. Both animal and human experimental evidence demonstrates that arginine can positively modulate the wound healing process, mainly by enhancing wound collagen deposition.

The role of arginine in wound healing was demonstrated first in studies of animals placed on arginine-deficient diets. When such animals are subjected to the minor trauma of a dorsal skin incision and closure, they have increased postoperative weight loss and increased mortality when compared with rats fed a similar defined diet containing arginine. Furthermore, the arginine deficiency results in decreased wound breaking strength and wound collagen accumulation (Fig 6-2).[4] Subsequently, we noted that chow-fed rats (which are not arginine deficient) given 1% arginine HCl supplementation also have enhanced wound breaking strength and collagen synthesis when compared with chow-fed controls (Fig 6-2).[4] A similar enhancement of both these wound healing parameters was observed in parenterally fed rats given an amino acid mixture containing high doses (7.5 g/L) of arginine.[66] Mature or old rats fed a diet supplemented with a combination of both arginine and glycine also have an enhanced rate of wound collagen deposition when compared with controls.[67] The effect of arginine on wound healing in rats is dependent on the presence of an intact hypothalamic-pituitary axis since hypophysectomized rats, whether or not treated with growth hormone, do not demonstrate any beneficial effects on wound healing when given arginine supplementation.[68]

Two studies have been carried out in healthy human volunteers examining the effect of arginine supplementation on collagen accumulation. Young healthy human volunteers (25 to 35

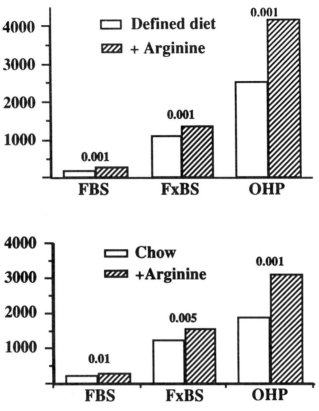

FIG 6–2.
Effect of arginine on wound healing in rats. *Top panel,* effect of arginine deficiency (defined diet) on wound healing; *Bottom panel,* effect of 1% arginine supplementation on wound healing. *FBS* = fresh wound breaking strength (grams); *FxBS* = formaldehyde-fixed wound breaking strength (grams); *OHP* = hydroxyproline (μg/100 mg of polyvinyl alcohol sponge inserted).

years old) were found to have significantly increased wound collagen deposition following oral supplementation with either 30 g of arginine aspartate (17 g of free arginine) or 30 g of arginine HCl (24.8 g of free arginine) daily for 14 days (Fig 6–3).[69] In a subsequent study of healthy aged humans (67 to 82 years old), daily supplements of 30 g of arginine aspartate for 14 days resulted in significantly enhanced collagen and total protein deposition at the wound site when compared with placebo controls. There was no enhanced production of DNA in the wounds of the arginine-supplemented subjects, thus suggesting that the effect of arginine was not mediated by an inflammatory mode of action (Fig 6–4).[59] In this study, arginine supplementation had no effect on the rate of epithelialization of a superficial skin

defect, further suggesting that the main effect of arginine on wound healing is to enhance wound collagen deposition.

Gains in breaking strength during the first weeks of healing are directly related to new collagen synthesis. An early progressive gain in tensile strength is an important factor in determining the competence of surgical incisions. Previous studies suggest that an increased deposition of collagen early in the wound healing process correlates with an increase in wound strength. Thus, arginine supplementation may result in an improvement in wound strength as a consequence of enhanced collagen deposition.

The T-cell–dependent immune system has been shown to have an important role in the regulation of wound healing.[70] T lymphocytes are necessary

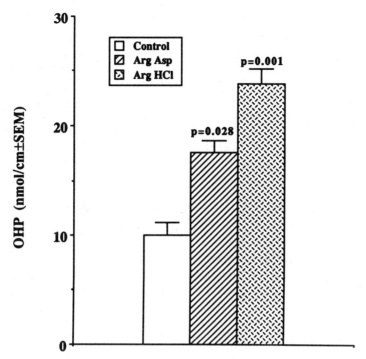

FIG 6–3.

Effect of 2 weeks of arginine supplementation on hydroxyproline *(OHP)* accumulation in subcutaneously implanted polytet-rafluoroethylene catheters in young human volunteers. Each group of 12 volunteers received placebo syrup (control), 30 g of arginine asparate *(Arg Asp)* or 30 g of arginine HCl *(Arg HCl)* for 2 weeks.

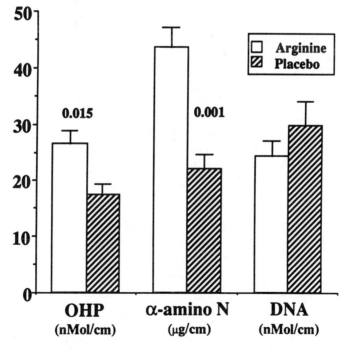

FIG 6–4.

Effect of arginine on wound healing parameters in healthy elderly human volunteers. The hydroxyproline *(OHP)*, total α-amino nitrogen *(α-amino N)*, and DNA accumulation in subcutaneously implanted polytetrafluoroethylene catheters were measured at the end of 2 weeks. Controls *(n* = 15) received a placebo syrup, while the arginine-treated group *(n* = 30) received 30 g of arginine asparate in double-blind fashion.

for the progression and orderly outcome of the normal wound healing process. Activated T lymphocytes are capable of recruiting, expanding, and activating the fibroblasts that are primarily responsible for this repair process.[71] Perhaps the effect of arginine in enhancing T-cell function (vide infra) may also underlie its beneficial effects on wound collagen accumulation and/or maturation.

ARGININE AND IMMUNE FUNCTION

Depressed immune responsiveness is a prominent feature of critical surgical illness, significant trauma, and burn injury. It has become apparent that less catastrophic traumatic insults, including elective moderate surgical operative procedures, also induce significant alterations in immune competence. Changes in the functional ability of the immune system have also been observed with the aging process. Alterations in the T-cell population have been observed, with a decrease in overall numbers and a shift in the proportions of subpopulations toward a predominance of the Ts/c subset. These alterations in immune function are reflected as a decreased proliferative capacity in older animals and humans in response to a challenge with mitogenic and allogeneic target cells. There is evidence that the addition of posttraumatic immune suppression to the coexisting decrease in immunity contributes to morbidity and mortality in elderly patients.

In animals, thymic involution is one of the hallmarks of stress, injury, and aging. Because the thymus plays a critical role in T-cell—mediated immune responses, thymic involution is likely to represent a deleterious aspect of the general reaction to stress and injury.

Arginine, given in large doses, possesses numerous beneficial effects on the immune system, particularly on the thymus-dependent and T-cell—dependent immune reactions (Table 6–2). Additionally, arginine plays a key role in the metabolic intracellular activity of lymphocytes. In vitro, there is an absolute requirement for arginine for the normal growth of lymphocytes.[71, 72] In vivo, this requirement for arginine can be substituted for by citrulline but not by ornithine. If the cultures are carried out in an arginine-free media, the mitogenic response of lymphocytes to phytohemagglutinin (PHA) and concanavalin A (Con A) is reduced by 60% to 80%, while RNA and protein synthesis is diminished by approximately 25%.[73, 74] Arginine is also required for the effective induction of cytotoxic T-cell function in vitro.[75] All of these parameters of lymphocyte function are restored at a media concentration of 0.04mM arginine; further increases in arginine concentration do not result in any further enhancement in response. The adult human

TABLE 6–2.

Immune Effects of Arginine*

Action (Increased)	Animals	Humans
Mitogenic response of lymphocytes		
Health	Yes	Yes
Injury/stress	Yes	Yes
Allograft rejection	Yes	ND
T cells, mitogenic reactivity, and DTH responses in immunocompromised host	Yes†	Yes‡
Antitumor cytotoxicity in vitro	Yes	Yes
Antitumor responses in vivo	Yes	ND
Response to sepsis	Yes	ND

*ND = not done; DTH = delayed-type hypersensitivity.
†Athymic nude animals.
‡Human immunodeficiency virus infected.

plasma arginine concentration ranges from 0.04 to 0.1mM. Some of the in vitro arginine requirements for optimal lymphocyte proliferation relate to the induction of NO synthesis following mitogenic stimulation. This is supported by the fact that NO donors, such as S-nitroso-acetyl penicillamine or sodium nitroprusside, can totally substitute for arginine.[72]

In animals, arginine supplementation leads to an increase in thymic weight and minimizes the thymic involution that normally occurs with injury.[76] Subsequently, it was demonstrated that the gain in thymic weight is due to a significant increase in the number of lymphocytes present in the thymic glands. This increase in the number of thymic gland lymphocytes is accompanied by a significant enhancement of the lymphocyte blastogenic response to mitogens.[77, 78]

In healthy humans, arginine supplementation (15 to 30 g/day) stimulates peripheral blood mononuclear cell responses to the mitogens Con A, PHA, and pokeweed mitogen (PWM) and to allogeneic target cells[59, 69, 79] (Table 6–3). An increase in the activity of these parameters is thought to correlate with enhanced T-cell function in vivo. This enhanced mitogenic response of peripheral blood mononuclear cells is noted in both healthy young and old human subjects supplemented with arginine. In aged humans and rodents, arginine restores plasma levels of thymulin, a

thymic hormone, to values found in younger subjects.[80] This effect may underlie the enhanced T-cell function noted with arginine supplementation.

In injured animals, arginine is capable of abrogating the deleterious effects of trauma on T-cell responses or of restoring thymic-mediated function earlier than in controls.[58, 66, 76, 77] Following a 30% total–body surface area, third-degree burn, guinea pigs supplemented with 1% to 2% arginine have enhanced immune responses as assessed by increased delayed hypersensitivity responses to dinitrofluorobenzene or diminished abscess formation following Staphylococcus aureus inoculation.[81] In rats subjected to lethal peritonitis, survival rates were greatly increased by arginine administered either intragastrically or intravenously.[82]

A reversal of the alterations in T-cell function associated with trauma or surgery has been demonstrated in patients fed enteral diets rich in arginine.[61] Arginine-supplemented patients undergoing major abdominal operations for gastrointestinal malignancies had increased in vitro immune responses. These responses correlated with decreased wound infection rates and decreased length of hospital stay.[83] Additionally, moderately stressed intensive care unit patients given an enteral diet containing large amounts of arginine demonstrated preservation or enhancement of T-lymphocyte blastogenesis.[84] In children with severe burn injuries,

TABLE 6–3.

Effect of Arginine Supplementation on Peripheral Blood Mononuclear Cell Responses to Mitogens in Different Patient Populations

Subjects	Concanavalin A		Phytohemagglutinin	
	Prearginine	Postarginine	Prearginine	Postarginine
Healthy	58	217*	84	307*
Postoperative	45	88*	94	145*
Intensive care unit		+172%†		+68%†
Human immunodeficiency virus infected	5	15*	28	75*

*Stimulation index.
†Percent change from baseline.

maintenance of normal plasma levels of arginine correlates with parameters of enhanced host immune and nutritional status.[85] Subsequently, the administration of an enteral diet supplemented with arginine was shown to result in reduced rates of wound infections and shortened hospital stay in a small group of young burned patients.[86] In a preliminary study, patients infected with the human immunodeficiency virus (HIV) showed a significant enhancement of the mitogenic responses to Con A and PHA following a 2-week dietary arginine supplementation[87] (see Table 6–3).

The exact mechanism whereby arginine stimulates T-cell function is not known. As mentioned above, thymic hormone secretion is enhanced by arginine. In athymic nude mice, arginine increases the number of T cells and enhances their response to mitogens in vitro, and this results in the acquisition of delayed hypersensitivity responses in vivo.[88] This suggests that arginine can enhance T-cell maturation and differentiation at extrathymic sites independent of functioning thymus.

Ornithine also exhibits strong thymotrophic activity.[89] Since both arginine and ornithine are precursors for polyamine synthesis and polyamines are required for heightened cellular proliferation, one could speculate that this is a possible mechanism of action; however, experimental data suggest that the thymotrophic effects of arginine and ornithine are not mediated directly via polyamine synthesis. Seifter et al. have suggested that the thymic effects may be related to the pituitary secretagogue activity of the two basic amino acids.[4] Further supporting this hypothesis is the requirement for an intact hypothalamic-pituitary axis for arginine to exert its immune effects.[90] The arginine-induced release of prolactin and growth hormone is possibly the most important in terms of its immunologic effects. Recent evidence indicates that prolactin has a direct effect on both cellular and humoral immunity. Lymphocytes have been shown to both produce and respond to prolactin. Part of the in vivo immune effects of arginine may be due to its ability to elevate serum prolactin levels.[91] Receptors for growth hormone are found on both monocytes and lymphocytes.[92] Growth hormone has been shown to potentiate the activity of lymphocytes, natural killer cells, and cytotoxic T lymphocytes in vitro and to enhance lectin-induced T-cell proliferation and IL-2 synthesis in vivo.[93, 94] All of the above actions of growth hormone can be replicated by arginine administration, strongly supporting the hypothesis that enhanced pituitary hormone secretion may underlie, at least in part, the mechanism of action of arginine on the immune system.

CLINICAL RECOMMENDATIONS

As can be seen, arginine possesses numerous pharmacologic actions that can have great potential benefit in clinical practice. Although the animal experimental data are compelling, there is need for continued clinical studies in order to better define the role of arginine in the care of patients. Since large doses of arginine are relatively safe and well tolerated and have mild or no untoward effects, there is the danger that there will be indiscriminate application of arginine in a variety of conditions where it may be ineffectual at best or harmful at worst. The need to define the role and use of arginine for wound healing, in states of diminished immune function, or as part of anticancer therapy is critical. The minimal effective dosage in human clinical practice has not been fully defined. The plea for careful studies is not meant to hinder the application of arginine in clinical practice, but it is meant as a call for judicious and scientific usage. Such application should result in arginine playing an important role in the nutritional and pharmacologic management of patients.

REFERENCES

1. Rose WC: The nutritive significance of the amino acids and certain related compounds. *Science* 1937; 86:298–300.

2. Rose WC: Amino acid requirements of man. *Fed Proc* 1949; 8:546–552.

3. Nakagawa I, Takahashi T, Suzuki T, et al: Amino acid requirements of children: Minimal needs of tryptophan, arginine, histidine based on nitrogen balance method. *J Nutr* 1963; 80:305–310.

4. Seifter E, Rettura G, Barbul A, et al: Arginine: An essential amino acid for injured rats. *Surgery* 1978; 84:224–230.

5. Barbul A: Arginine: Biochemistry, physiology and therapeutic implications. *JPEN* 1986; 10:227–238.

6. Fahey JL: Toxicity and blood ammonia rise resulting from intravenous amino acid administration in man: The protective effect of L-arginine. *J Clin Invest* 1957; 36:1647–1655.

7. Moncada S, Higgs EA (eds): *Nitric Oxide From Arginine: A Bioregulatory System.* New York, Elsevier, 1990.

8. Moncada S, Palmer RM, Higgs EA: Nitric oxide: Physiology, pathophysiology, and pharmacology. *Pharmacol Rev* 1991; 43:109–142.

9. Miller V, Vanhoutte P: Endothelium-dependant relaxation in isolated blood vessels of lower vertebrates. *Blood Vessels* 1986; 23:411–425.

10. Sung YJ, Hotchkiss JH, Auistic RE, et al: L-Arginine–dependent production of a reactive nitrogen intermediate by macrophages of a uricotelic species. *J Leukoc Biol* 1991; 50:49–56.

11. Radomski MM, Martin JF, Moncada S: Synthesis of nitric oxide by the haemocytes of the American horseshoe crab *(Limulus polyphemus). Philos Trans R Soc Lond [Biol]* 1991; 334:129–133.

12. Mayer B, John M, Heinzel B, et al: Brain nitric oxide synthase is a biopterin- and flavin-containing multifunctional oxido-reductase. *FEBS Lett* 1991; 288:187–191.

13. Stuehr D, Cho HJ, Kwon NS, et al: Purification and characterization of the cytokine-induced macrophage nitric oxide synthase: an FAD- and FMN-containing flavoprotein. *Proc Natl Acad Sci U S A* 1991; 88:7773–7777.

14. Hevel JM, White KA, Marletta MA: Purification of the inducible murine macrophage nitric oxide synthase. *J Biol Chem* 1991; 266:22789–22791.

15. Stuehr DJ, Fasehun OA, Kwon NS, et al: Inhibition of macrophage and endothelial cell nitric oxide synthase by diphenyleneiodonium and its analogs. *FASEB J* 1991; 5:98–103.

16. Bredt DS, Snyder SH: Isolation of nitric oxide synthetase, a calmodulin-requiring enzyme. *Proc Natl Acad Sci U S A* 1990; 87:682–685.

17. Knowles RG, Palacios M, Palmer RMJ, et al: Formation of nitric oxide from L-arginine in the central nervous system: A transduction mechanism for stimulation of the soluble guanylate cyclase. *Proc Natl Acad Sci U S A* 1989; 86:5159–5162.

18. Förstermann U, Schmidt HHHW, Pollock JS, et al: Enzymes synthesizing guanylate cyclase–activating factors in endothelial cell, neuroblastoma cells, and rat brain. *J Cardiovasc Pharmacol* 1991; 17(suppl):57–64.

19. Mayer B, Böhme E: Ca^{2+}-dependent formation of an L-arginine–derived activator of soluble guanylate cyclase in bovine lung. *FEBS Lett* 1989; 256:211–214.

20. Venturini CM, Knowles RG, Palmer RMJ, et al: Synthesis of nitric oxide in the bovine retina. *Biochem Biophys Res Commun* 1991; 180:920–925.

21. Palacios M, Knowles RG, Palmer RMJ, et al: Nitric oxide from L-arginine stimulates the soluble guanylate cyclase in adrenal glands. *Biochem Biophys Res Commun* 1989; 165:802–809.

22. Radomski MW, Palmer RM, Moncada S: An L-arginine/nitric oxide pathway present in human platelets regulates aggregation. *Proc Natl Acad Sci U S A* 1990; 87:5193–5197.

23. Palmer RM, Moncada S: A novel citrulline-forming enzyme implicated in the formation of nitric oxide by vascular endothelial cells. *Biochem Biophys Res Commun* 1989; 159:348–352.

24. Mülsch A, Bassenge E, Busse R: Nitric oxide synthesis in endothelial cytosol: Evidence for a calcium-dependent and a calcium-independent mechanism.

Naunyn Schmiedebergs Arch Pharmacol 1989; 340:767–770.

25. Salter M, Knowles RG, Moncada S: Widespread tissue distribution, species distribution and changes in activity of Ca^{2+}-dependent and Ca^{2+}-independent nitric oxide synthases. *FEBS Lett* 1991; 291:145–149.

26. Lyons CR, Orloff GJ, Cunningham JM: Molecular cloning and functional expression of an inducible nitric oxide synthase from a murine macrophage cell line. *Proc Natl Acad Sci U S A* 1992; 267:6370–6374.

27. Xie Q, Cho HJ, Calaycan J, et al: Cloning and characterization of inducible nitric oxide synthase from mouse macrophages. *Science* 1992; 256:225–228.

28. Yui Y, Hattori R, Kosuga K, et al: Purification of nitric oxide synthase from rat macrophages. *J Biol Chem* 1991; 266:12544–12547.

29. Stuehr DJ, Marletta MA: Induction of nitrite/nitrate synthesis in murine macrophages by BCG infection, lymphokines, or interferon-γ. *J Immunol* 1987; 140:518–525.

30. Hibbs JB, Taintor RR, Vavrin Z: Macrophage cytotoxicity: Role for L-arginine deiminase and imino nitrogen oxidation to nitrite. *Science* 1987; 235:473–476.

31. Marletta MA, Yoon PS, Iyengar R, et al: Macrophage oxidation of L-arginine to nitrite and nitrate: Nitric oxide is an intermediate. *Biochemistry* 1988; 27:8706–8711.

32. Billiar TR, Curran RD, Stuehr DJ, et al: An L-arginine–dependent mechanism mediates Kupffer-cell inhibition of hepatocyte protein synthesis in vitro. *J Exp Med* 1989; 169:1467–1472.

33. Curran RD, Billiar TR, Stuehr DJ, et al: Hepatocytes produce nitrogen oxides from L-arginine in response to inflammatory products of Kupffer cells. *J Exp Med* 1989; 170:1769–1774.

34. Knowles RG, Merrett M, Salter M, et al: Differential induction of brain, lung and liver nitric oxide synthase by endotoxin in the rat. *Biochem J* 1990; 270:833–836.

35. McCall TB, Boughton-Smith NK, Palmer RMJ, et al: Synthesis of nitric oxide from L-arginine by neutrophils. Release and interaction with superoxide anion. *Biochem J* 1989; 261:293–296.

36. Werner FG, Werner ER, Fuchs D, et al: Tetrahydrobiopterin-dependent formation of nitrite and nitrate in murine fibroblasts. *J Exp Med* 1990; 172:1599–1607.

37. Stadler J, Stefanovic-Racic M, Billiar TR, et al: Articular chondrocytes synthesize nitric oxide in response to cytokines and lipopolysaccharide. *J Immunol* 1991; 147:3915–3920.

38. Busse R, Mülsch A: Induction of nitric oxide synthase by cytokines in vascular smooth muscle cells. *FEBS Lett* 1990; 275:87–90.

39. Stuehr DJ, Kwon NS, Nathan CF: FAD and GSH participate in macrophage synthesis of nitric oxide. *Biochem Biophys Res Commun* 1990; 168:558–565.

40. DiRosa M, Radomski M, Carnuccio R, et al: Glucocorticoids inhibit the induction of nitric oxide synthase in macrophages. *Biochem Biophys Res Commun* 1990; 172:1246–1252.

41. Radomski MW, Palmer RM, Moncada S: Glucocorticoids inhibit the expression of an inducible, but not the constitutive, nitric oxide synthase in vascular endothelial cells. *Proc Natl Acad Sci U S A* 1990; 87:10043–10047.

42. Knowles RG, Salter M, Brooks SL, et al: Anti-inflammatory glucocorticoids inhibit the induction by endotoxin of nitric oxide synthase in the lung and aorta of the rat. *Biochem Biophys Res Commun* 1990; 172:1042–1048.

43. Förstermann U, Schmidt HHHW, Kohlhaas KL, et al: Induced RAW 264.7 macrophages express soluble and particulate nitric oxide synthase: Inhibition by transforming growth factor-b. *Eur J Pharmacol* 1992; 225:161–165.

44. Nathan C: Nitric oxide as a secretory product of mammalian cells. *FASEB J* 1992; 6:3051–3064.

45. Albina JE, Mills CD, Barbul A, et al: Arginine metabolism in wounds. *Am J Physiol* 1988; 254:459–467.

46. Drexler H, Zeiher AM, Meinzer K, et al: Correction of endothelial dysfunction in coronary microcirculation of hyper-

cholesterolemic patients by L-arginine. *Lancet* 1991; 338:1546–1550.

47. Floyd JCJ, Fajans SS, Conn JW, et al: Stimulation of insulin secretion by amino acids. *J Clin Invest* 1966; 45:1487–1502.

48. Sener A, Blachier F, Rasschaert J, et al: Stimulus-secretion coupling of arginine-induced insulin release: Comparison with histidine-induced insulin release. *Endocrinology* 1989; 127:107–113.

49. Laychock SG, Modica ME, Cavanaugh CT: L-Arginine stimulates cyclic guanosine 3′,5′-monophosphate formation in rat islets of Langerhans and RINm5F insulinoma cells: Evidence for L-arginine: Nitric oxide synthase. *Endocrinology* 1991; 129:3043–3052.

50. Schmidt HHHW, Warner TD, Ishii K, et al: Insulin secretion from pancreatic B cells caused by L-arginine–derived nitrogen oxides. *Science* 1992; 255:721–723.

51. Welsh N, Eizirik DL, Bendtzen K, et al: Interleukin 1β–induced nitric oxide production in isolated rat pancreatic islets requires gene transcription and may lead to inhibition of the Krebs cycle enzyme aconitase. *Endocrinology* 1991; 129:3167–3173.

52. Lukic ML, Stosic GS, Ostojic N, et al: Inhibition of nitric oxide generation affects the induction of diabetes by streptozocin in mice. *Biochem Biophys Res Commun* 1991; 178:913–920.

53. Imms FJ, London DR, Neame RLB: The secretion of catecholamines from the adrenal gland following arginine infusion in the rat. *J Physiol (Lond)* 1969; 200:55–56.

54. Dohi T, Morita K, Tsujimoto A: Effect of sodium azide on catecholamine release from isolated adrenal gland and on guanylate cyclase. *Eur J Pharmacol* 1983; 94:331–335.

55. O'Sullivan AJ, Burgoyne RD: Cyclic GMP regulates nicotine-induced secretion from cultured bovine adrenal chromaffin cells: Effects of 8-bromo-cyclic GMP, atrial natriuretic peptide, and nitroprusside (nitric oxide). *J Neurochem* 1990; 54:1805–1808.

56. Halbrügge T, Lutsh K, Thyen A, et al: Role of nitric oxide formation in the regulation of haemodynamics and the release of noradrenaline and adrenaline. *Naunyn Schmiedebergs Arch Pharmacol* 1991; 344:720–727.

57. Steffe CH, Wissler RW, Humphreys EM, et al: Studies in amino acid utilization V: The determination of minimum dietary essential amino acid requirements in protein depleted adult male albino rats. *J Nutr* 1950; 40:483–497.

58. Barbul A, Sisto DA, Wasserkrug HL, et al: Metabolic and immune effects of arginine in post-injury hyperalimentation. *J Trauma* 1981; 21:970–974.

59. Kirk SJ, Regan MC, Holt D, et al: Arginine stimulates wound healing and immune function in aged humans. *Surgery*, in press.

60. Elsair J, Poey J, Issad H, et al: Effect of arginine chlorhydrate on nitrogen balance during the three days following routine surgery in man. *Biomedicine* 1978; 29:312–317.

61. Daly J, Reynolds J, Thom A, et al: Immune and metabolic effects of arginine in the surgical patient. *Ann Surg* 1988; 208:512–523.

62. Leander U, Furst P, Vesterberg K, et al: Nitrogen sparing effect of ornicetil in the immediate postoperative state: Clinical biochemistry and nitrogen balance. *Clin Nutr* 1985; 4:43–51.

63. Wernerman J, Hammarqvist F, von der Decken A, et al: Ornithine-alpha-ketoglutarate improves skeletal muscle protein synthesis as assessed by ribosome analysis and nitrogen use after surgery. *Ann Surg* 1987; 206:674–678.

64. Levenson SM, Rettura G, Barbul A, et al: Citrulline replaces arginine as a dietary essential in rats; ornithine does not. *Fed Proc* 1980; 726:2421.

65. Bucknall T: Factors affecting wound healing, in Bucknall T, Ellis H (eds): *Wound Healing for Surgeons*. London, Bailliere Tindall, 1984, pp 42–74.

66. Barbul A, Fishel RS, Shimazu S, et al: Intravenous hyperalimentation with high arginine levels improves wound healing and immune function. *J Surg Res* 1985; 38:328–334.

67. Chyun J, Griminger P: Improvement of nitrogen retention by arginine and glycine supplementation and its relation to collagen synthesis. *J Nutr* 1984; 114:1697–1704.

68. Barbul A, Rettura G, Levenson SM, et al: Wound healing and thymotropic effects of arginine: A pituitary mechanism of action. *Am J Clin Nutr* 1983; 37:786–794.

69. Barbul A, Lazarou S, Efron DT, et al: Arginine enhances wound healing in humans. *Surgery* 1990; 108:331–337.

70. Regan MC, Barbul A: Regulation of wound healing by the T cell–dependent immune system, in Janssen H, Rooman R, Robertson JIS (eds): *Wound Healing*. Petersfield, England, Wrightson Biomedical, 1991, pp 21–31.

71. Eagle H: Amino acid metabolism in mammalian cell cultures. *Science* 1959; 130:432–437.

72. Efron D, Kirk SJ, Regan MC, et al: Nitric oxide generation from L-arginine is required for optimal peripheral blood lymphocyte DNA synthesis. *Surgery* 1991; 110:327–334.

73. Chisari FV, Nakamura M, Milich DR, et al: Production of two distinct and independent hepatic immunoregulatory molecules by the perfused rat liver. *Hepatology* 1985; 5:735–743.

74. Her-Lin S, Huang MH, Han SH, et al: The mechanism of inhibitory effects of liver extract on lymphocyte proliferation: II. Inhibition of DNA, RNA, and protein synthesis and their relationship to the effects of metabolic inhibitors. *Clin Exp Immunol* 1988; 72:228–232.

75. Moriguchi A, Mukai K, Hiroaka I, et al: Functional changes in human lymphocytes and monocytes after in vitro incubation with arginine. *Nutr Res* 1987; 7:719–729.

76. Barbul A, Rettura G, Levenson SM, et al: Arginine: A thymotropic and wound healing promoting agent. *Surg Forum* 1977; 28:101–103.

77. Barbul A, Wasserkrug HL, Seifter E, et al: Immunostimulatory effects of arginine in normal and injured rats. *J Surg Res* 1980; 29:228–235.

78. Barbul A, Wasserkrug HL, Sisto DA, et al: Thymic and immune stimulatory actions of arginine. *JPEN* 1980; 4:446–449.

79. Barbul A, Sisto DA, Wasserkrug HL, et al: Arginine stimulates lymphocyte immune responses in healthy humans. *Surgery* 1981; 90:244–251.

80. Fabris N, Mocchegiani E: Arginine-containing compounds and thymic endocrine activity. *Thymus* 1992; 19(suppl):21–30.

81. Saito H, Trocki O, Wang S, et al: Metabolic and immune effects of dietary arginine supplementation after burn. *Arch Surg* 1987; 122:784–789.

82. Madden HP, Breslin RJ, Wasserkrug HL, et al: Stimulation of T cell immunity enhances survival in peritonitis. *J Surg Res* 1988; 44:658–663.

83. Daly JM, Lieberman MD, Goldfine J, et al: Enteral nutrition with arginine, RNA, and omega-3 fatty acids in patients after operation: Immunologic, metabolic, and clinical outcome. *Surgery* 1992; 112:56–67.

84. Cerra FB, Lehman S, Konstantinides N, et al: Effect of enteral nutrient on in vitro tests of immune function in ICU patients: A preliminary report. *Nutrition* 1990; 6:84–87.

85. Alexander JW, MacMillan BG, Stinnett JD, et al: Beneficial effects of aggressive protein feeding in severely burned children. *Ann Surg* 1980; 192:505–517.

86. Alexander JW, Gottschlich M: Nutritional immunomodulation in burn patients. *Crit Care Med* 1990; 18(suppl):149–153.

87. Barbul A: Arginine and immune function. *Nutrition* 1990; 6(suppl):51–62.

88. Kirk SJ, Regan MC, Wasserkrug HL, et al: Arginine enhances T cell responses in athymic nude mice. *JPEN* 1992; 16:429–432.

89. Barbul A, Rettura G, Levenson SM, et al: Thymotropic actions of arginine, ornithine and growth hormone (abstract 282). *Fed Proc* 1978; 37:264.

90. Barbul A, Rettura G, Prior E, et al: Supplemental arginine, wound healing and thymus: Arginine-pituitary interaction. *Surg Forum* 1978; 29:93–95.

91. Kirk SJ, Regan MC, Wasserkrug HL, et al: Inhibition of prolactin secretion reduces the T cell immunostimulatory effects of arginine. *Surg Forum* 1991; 42:3–5.

92. Kiess W, Butenandt O: Specific growth hormone receptors on human peripheral mononuclear cells. Reexpression, identification, and characterization. *J Clin Endocrinol Metab* 1985; 60:740–746.

93. Davila DR, Breif S, Simon J, *et al:* Role of growth hormone in regulating T-dependant immune events in aged, nude, and transgenic rodents. *J Neurosci Res* 1987; 18:108–116.

94. Snow EC, Feldbush TL, Oakes JA: The effects of growth hormone and insulin upon MLC responses and the generation of cytotoxic lymphocytes. *J Immunol* 1981; 126:161–164.

7

Glutamine

Jian Shou, M.D.

Presently, glutamine is one of the most intensely investigated amino acids in the field of nutrition support. The occurrence of free glutamine in certain plants has been known for about 100 years, while its presence in proteins was demonstrated in the early part of this century. Krebs first reported glutamine synthesis from glutamate and ammonia in rabbit and guinea pig kidney in 1935.[1] Less than a decade later, Van Slyke et al. discovered that glutamine was the main source of urinary ammonia in acidosis. This latter observation suggested that in addition to its role as a protein constituent, glutamine might also play a significant role in the metabolic process.[1] Eagle demonstrated the importance of glutamine as a nutritional substrate for mammalian cells in culture.[2] Since then, supplementary glutamine is added to almost all cell and tissue culture media.

Glutamine is the most abundant amino acid in blood and tissue. It serves mainly as an ammonia scavenger and as an amide nitrogen or amino nitrogen donor for the biosynthesis of a number of important metabolites.[3] Because glutamine can be synthesized in many tissues, it is traditionally considered a nonessential amino acid, and thus common parenteral nutrition formulas are not supplemented with glutamine. In critical illness, however, glutamine metabolism is significantly altered, and the degree of change in metabolism has been correlated with the severity of disease.[4] There is an increasing body of evidence demonstrating the importance of glutamine as a respiratory fuel for various tissues, especially during stressed states such as injury, sepsis, total parenteral nutrition (TPN) feeding, and the presence of tumors.[5, 6]

BIOCHEMISTRY AND PHYSIOLOGY

The general structure of amino acids includes a central carbon atom alpha (α) bound to a carboxylic acid group, an α-amino acid group, and a hydrogen atom. The α-carbon atom also binds a side-chain group that defines each of the 20 common amino acids. Glutamine is one of these amino acids but has an amide group (NH_2) besides an α-ammonia (NH_3^+) (Fig 7–1).[7] This characteristic of glutamine contributes to its important role as a nitrogen transporter that carries nitrogen between the tissues and splanchnic organs.[5, 6]

Glutamine metabolism relies on two major enzyme systems. Cytosolic glutamine synthetase catalyzes the synthesis of glutamine from glutamate and ammonia. Intramitochondrial glutaminase catalyzes the hydrolysis of glutamine to glutamate and ammonia. In most tissues, one or the other enzyme activity predominates; this characterizes the organ as a glutamine donor or consumer. Skeletal muscle is a major glutamine donor with a high glutamine synthetase activity. In contrast, the jejunum is a major glutamine consumer with a higher glutaminase activity. The liver, unlike most tissues, which are either

predominantly glutamine consumers or producers, can change from donor to consumer depending on physiologic requirements.[5, 6]

The glutamine carbons, as a metabolic fuel, are oxidized to carbon dioxide in the tricarboxylic acid (TCA) cycle with production of adenosine triphosphate (ATP) in mammalian tissues. The glutamine nitrogens are metabolized first to glutamate and then to alanine, citrulline, and proline (Fig 7–2).[6] In all cells, glutamate and then to alanine, citrulline, and proline (Fig 7–2).[6] In all cells, glutamine is a precursor that donates nitrogen atoms for the synthesis of glutamine plays a role in acid-base balance as the most important substrate for renal ammoniagenesis. In the liver, it can serve as a gluconeogenic substrate and is an important end product in ammonia-trapping pathways. Important regulatory roles for glutamine include increasing protein synthesis and decreasing protein degradation in skeletal muscle while stimulating glycogen synthesis in the liver.[3, 8–10]

Glutathione is a tripeptide consisting of glutamate, cysteine, and glycine.[11] One important function of glutathione is as an oxygen free radical scavenger protecting tissues from free radical–related injury.[12] It has been demonstrated that glutathione is necessary for lymphocyte proliferation and macrophage functions.[13] Glutathione biosynthesis is mainly limited by the substrate cysteine, while the glutamate portion of the molecule is derived from glutamine.[12] Recently it has been reported that supplementation of glutamine can increase liver and intestinal tissue glutathione levels in animals, which may have significant clinical application.[12, 14]

The physiologic functions of glutamine are summarized as follows:

1. Major portion of the amino acid pool
2. Important metabolic fuel for many tissues

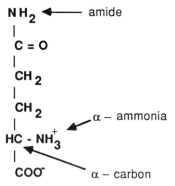

$$NH_2 \longleftarrow \text{amide}$$
$$|$$
$$C = O$$
$$|$$
$$CH_2$$
$$|$$
$$CH_2$$
$$| \longleftarrow \alpha - \text{ammonia}$$
$$HC - NH_3^+$$
$$|$$
$$COO^- \quad \alpha - \text{carbon}$$

FIG 7–1.
Structure of glutamine.

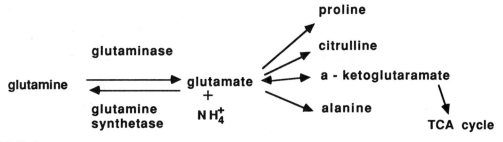

FIG 7–2.
Glutamine metabolism in the intestinal epithelial cell. Glutamine is metabolized similarly whether it enters the cell from the lumen or from the blood. Two thirds of glutamine carbons are oxidized to carbon dioxide in the tricarboxylic acid (TCA) cycle. The glutamine nitrogens are released into the portal blood as ammonia, citrulline, alanine, and proline. The ammonia and alanine are extracted mainly by the liver. The citrulline is used by the kidneys for arginine synthesis. (Adapted from Souba WW et al: JPEN 1990; 14(suppl 4):90–93.)

3. Important precurser for biosynthesis
4. Factor that increases protein synthesis and gluconeogenesis
5. Source of renal ammonia production
6. Efficient nitrogen and carbon transporter
7. Inhibitory factor in protein degradation
8. Possible precurser of glutathione synthesis

INTERORGAN GLUTAMINE FLOW: BASAL (POSTABSORPTIVE) STATE

The intestinal tract is the principal organ of glutamine uptake.[8] Most of the glutamine uptake occurs in the small intestine epithelial cells (enterocytes), which have a high glutaminase activity. The small intestine in laboratory animals can extract 20% to 30% of blood glutamine during each circulation. Data from patients undergoing elective abdominal surgery demonstrate that the human gastrointestinal tract can extract 12% to 13% of circulating glutamine. The intestinal microflora is not involved in the absorptive process since glutamine uptake is the same in germ-free and conventional rats.[5, 6] Recently, the glutamine transport system across the brush border and basement membrane of the epithelial cell has been characterized in the small intestine of

dogs and humans and appears to be predominantly an Na^+-dependent pathway.[15, 16]

Lung flux measurements in rats demonstrate that the lungs export large amounts of glutamine in the postabsorptive state. The lungs along with skeletal muscle are the most important organs of net glutamine release. Lung parenchyma contains the enzyme glutamine synthetase and continuously extracts ammonia and glutamate from the pulmonary circulation and converts these to glutamine.[17]

The liver plays a central regulatory role in interorgan glutamine metabolism because of its ability to act as a glutamine donor or consumer as required.[6, 18] Two types of hepatocytes have been distinguished in the functional units of liver acini. The periportal hepatocytes are those near the sinusoidal inflow and contain glutaminase and enzymes for urea synthesis (urea cycle). The perivenous hepatocytes are those near the sinusoidal outflow and contain glutamine synthetase. The portal blood flows through periportal hepatocytes first and then passes through the perivenous hepatocytes to the hepatic vein. The glutaminase in periportal hepatocytes is different from the one in other tissues because it is not inhibited by its product glutamate but instead requires ammonia, its other product, as an essential activator (feedforward). Ammonia activates the glutaminase enzyme system of the periportal cells, which results in the production of ammonia. The ammonia produced from liver glutamine metabolism and the portal blood ammonia together activate urea synthesis, in which the glutaminase serves as an "ammonia signal amplifer." The perivenous cells, on the other hand, act as downstream scavengers and convert ammonia to glutamine. The major regulatory advantage arising from this structure and functional heterogeneity is that ammonia flux through the urea cycle in the periportal compartment can be varied and even exceed ureagenesis without the threat of hyperammonemia. This is because glutamine synthesis in perivenous hepatocytes acts as an effective "backup system" for ammonia detoxification.[6, 18]

In a healthy host, the activities of these two systems are balanced, and overall, the liver consumes only a small amount of glutamine in the postabsorptive state. Relatively high portal glutamine and alanine and low ammonia levels favor liver ureagenesis, while relatively low portal glutamine and alanine and high ammonia levels activate glutamine synthesis such that portal ammonia is the main regulatory factor in liver glutamine metabolism. In addition, the glutamine transport system in the hepatocyte membrane regulates liver glutamine metabolism by controlling glutamine entry into cells.[6, 18] This structural and functional heterogeneity is established mainly in rats, but there is enough evidence to suggest that the situation is similar in human liver.[19]

Lymphocytes and macrophages demonstrate high glutaminase activity and can utilize a significant amount of glutamine, especially during lymphocyte proliferation.[5, 6] Glutamine is essential for lymphocyte proliferation in response to antigen in vitro, while physiologic levels of glutamine are necessary for macrophage phagocytosis.[20-22] It is speculated that the high degree of glutamine uptake in some tissues such as intestine may be due in part to a high lymph content.[6] Animal studies have shown that the brain and heart can release small amounts of glutamine into the circulation, while the kidney utilizes small amounts of glutamine in the postabsorptive state.[5, 6]

Figure 7–3[23] summarizes glutamine flow in the postabsorptive state. Skeletal muscle, lung, and liver are the central organs in glutamine homeostasis. Skeletal muscle contains as much as 80% of the total-body amino acid pool,

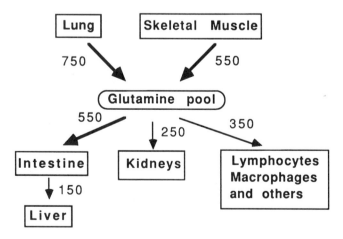

FIG 7–3.

Interorgan glutamine flow (net flux rates, nmol/100 g/min) in the postabsorptive rat. Glutamine homeostasis is maintained by the net rates of uptake and release by various organs. The major organs of net glutamine release are the lung and skeletal muscle, although the brain and heart also produce small amounts. The intestine is the major organ of glutamine uptake, with smaller amounts consumed by the kidneys, liver, lymphocytes/macrophages, and adipocytes. (Adapted from Souba WW et al: *JPEN* 1990; 14(suppl 4): 90–93.)

and 60% of the amino acid nitrogen released is in the form of glutamine and alanine. Lung is another major glutamine donor. The intestine is the major glutamine consumer. Glutamine provides a major portion of the energy required by enterocytes. The enterocyte mitochondrial glutaminase rapidly hydrolyzes glutamine, and the ammonia produced in the process diffuses into the portal blood. Once it reaches the liver, the ammonia can enter the urea cycle or be diverted to glutamine synthesis before reentering the systemic circulation. This makes the intestine an ideal site for glutamine metabolism.[3, 5, 6]

INTERORGAN EXCHANGE OF GLUTAMINE: PATHOLOGIC STATES AND GLUTAMINE SUPPLEMENTATION

Starvation

The normal arterial glutamine concentration is maintained in a dog model of short-term starvation. Glutamine uptake by the intestine remains constant or is increased, and the liver becomes a glutamine donor. There is, in addition, a reduced output of alanine from glutamine catabolism and an increase in ammonia production by the intestine. This leads to an increased portal blood ammonia load, which in turn causes an increase in the activity of perivenous hepatocyte glutamine synthetase. Associated with the increase in glutamine synthesis and decrease in urea production is an increase in renal utilization of glutamine and release of alanine. The net effect of this adaptative process is to reduce skeletal muscle protein catabolism in order to meet the glutamine requirements of the intestine and kidney.[6, 24] Glutamine solution infusion in starved dogs results in a 20% rise in arterial glutamine concentration; most of the glutamine infused is taken up by the visceral organs, with liver uptake accounting for 60% and the kidneys and intestine accounting for the rest.[24]

Metabolic Acidosis

Arterial glutamine levels are decreased in both animal models and patients subjected to chronic metabolic acidosis.[6, 25] The kidney becomes the major organ of glutamine consumption, the liver becomes a glutamine donor, and the intestine effectively decreases glutamine uptake. This adaptation process meets the glutamine needs of the kidney. In the acidotic state the portal blood profile (relatively low in glutamine and alanine and high in ammonia) serves as a stimulus for hepatic glutamine synthetase activity with a decrease in urea production. This is thought to be a more energy-efficient process.[25]

Welbourne studied the effect of a 0.49% (weight per volume [w/v]) glutamine-supplemented liquid elemental diet and an identical glutamine-free diet in a rat chronic acidosis model. The arterial blood glutamine levels were not changed. There was, however, peripheral tissue utilization of enteral glutamine as evidenced by a fivefold rise in urinary glutamine excretion and an increase in hepatic glutamine concentration. Intestinal glutamine uptake and hepatic glutamine release were significantly increased, while hindquarter muscle glutamine release was decreased. Creatinine excretion was also significantly elevated in the glutamine-supplemented group. These findings indicate that enteral glutamine supplementation is able to maintain cellular reserves, decrease proteolysis, and enhance organ function in metabolic acidosis.[26]

Trauma

Elective abdominal surgery is associated with a reduction in arterial glutamine and muscle glutamine levels in animals and humans.[6, 23] Figure 7–4[23] demonstrates the changes in glutamine metabolism after trauma. Glutamine uptake by the intestine is augmented, and its glucose consumption declines.

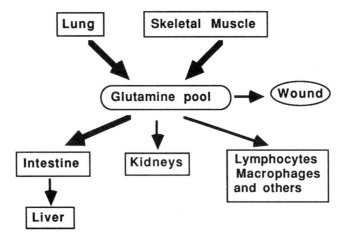

FIG 7–4.
Interorgan glutamine flow following surgical trauma in the rat. Lung and skeletal muscle glutamine efflux is accelerated to provide substrate for the intestine, kidneys, liver, lymphocytes/macrophages, and wound. (Adapted from Souba WW et al: *JPEN* 1990; 14(suppl 4):90–93.)

There is also an increase in glutamine consumption by the liver. The net release of glutamine by muscle and lung significantly increases. Glutamine is also consumed by healing wounds. These changes in glutamine metabolism are thought to be regulated by stress hormones such as glucocorticoids, glucagon, and catecholamines rather than by dietary depletion of glutamine in trauma patients. In the dog model undergoing elective surgery, an increase in adrenal glucocorticoid production and pancreatic glucagon output are noted.[6] A triple-hormone infusion of adrenaline, cortisol, and glucagon (simulating surgical stress) depresses the glutamine concentration after 6 hours.[27] Elective surgery results in a decrease in muscle glutamine levels 12 hours after surgery.[28] Starvation alone causes a reduction in muscle glutamine content after 3 days.[29] This decrease cannot be prevented by glutamine-free nutritional supplementation.[30] Dexamethasone treatment in animals increases intestinal glutamine uptake by more than twofold, while portal blood flow remains unchanged[31]; intestinal glutaminase activity is also elevated.[32] The treatment also results in a marked increase in glutamine efflux from muscle in association with a fall in intracellular gluta-

mine.[33] The administration of glucagon reduces circulating glutamine levels by 25% in healthy dogs; this is mainly due to a significant increase in hepatic and intestinal glutamine uptake.[34] The reduced intestinal glucose uptake and increased hepatic glutamine consumption noted in the dog model may provide more substrate for hepatic gluconeogenesis and protein and nucleotide synthesis in response to surgical trauma.[5, 6] In patients with major burn injury, plasma glutamine levels have been documented to be two thirds lower than normal levels, and these low levels have persisted for more than 3 weeks after injury.[20] Similar observations have been made in postoperative patients.[35, 36]

Sepsis and Endotoxemia

The alterations in interorgan glutamine flow that occur during sepsis and endotoxemia share similarities and differences with the changes that characterize surgical stress (Fig 7–5).[23] Muscle glutamine depletion generally tends to be more severe and of longer duration. Muscle glutamine release is markedly accelerated, and glutamine synthetase activity nearly doubles during endotoxemia.[23] During endotoxemia, lung glutamine efflux increases within

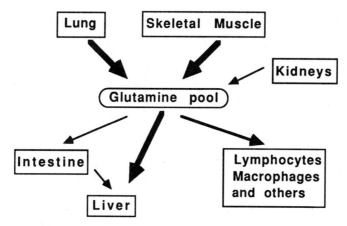

FIG 7–5.
Interorgan glutamine flow during sepsis/endotoxemia in the rat. Endotoxin further accelerates skeletal muscle and lung glutamine release. The kidneys cease consuming glutamine and actually release a net amount of glutamine into the renal vein. Intestinal glutamine uptake is diminished in endotoxin-treated rats and in septic patients. The liver and possibly cells of the immune system may be major glutamine consumers during severe infection. (Adapted from Souba WW et al: *JPEN* 1990; 14(suppl 4):90–93.)

the first 2 hours, but this augmented output ceases when macroscopic evidence of adult respiratory distress syndrome (ARDS) develops in the lung.[23] In contrast to surgical stress, sepsis and endotoxemia inhibit the intestinal utilization of circulating and luminal glutamine in both experimental animal models and clinical studies.[5, 6, 23] Reduced intestinal glutamine absorption is due to a reduction in intestinal glutaminase activity.[37] Mucosal cell glutamine transport is also impaired in septic patients and in the endotoxemic rat model.[38] Other changes noted in endotoxemia include an increase in intestinal glucose uptake and utilization, a tenfold increase in hepatic glutamine uptake because of an increase in hepatic blood flow, and a higher rate of glutamine extraction.[5, 6, 23] The reduced intestinal glutamine utilization may be mediated by cytokines produced during sepsis.[39]

Inoue et al.[40] compared the effect of a 1.5% glutamine–supplemented TPN solution with a glutamine-free TPN formula in an *Escherichia coli* peritonitis model. Rats were fed the respective solutions for 7 days and then received a dose of *E. coli* (5×10^5 colony-forming units per 200 g of body weight) by direct intraperitoneal injection. Glutamine-

supplemented TPN–fed rats had a significantly better survival rate (92.1%) than glutamine-free TPN–fed rats (44.7%). Glutamine supplementation maintains the glutamine pool during sepsis, and this may help the host overcome such metabolic stresses. Yoshida et al.[41] reported that TPN-fed rats showed significant histologic damage in the jejunum and ileum (with lower mucosal protein synthesis) 24 hours after receiving an intravenous injection of *E. coli*. TPN supplemented with 2% glutamine attenuated these changes and significantly increased protein synthesis of the intestinal mucosa of septic rats. In vitro studies suggest that glutamine can significantly increase protein synthesis in rat enterocytes obtained 16 hours after the rats received a septic challenge (cecal ligation and puncture).[42]

Ardawi et al.[43, 44] further reported that besides improving survival in a rat cecal ligation and puncture model, glutamine-enriched TPN significantly increased the rate of glutamine utilization in the intestine, which was diminished during sepsis. Glutamine-enriched TPN also reduced the loss of intracellular glutamine in skeletal muscle and increased the protein and RNA content of liver and muscle. Also noted in glutamine-supplemented TPN—fed animals was an increase in the rate of incorporation of leucine and tyrosine into liver and muscle proteins in vitro and a decrease in the rate of muscle tyrosine release.[44]

Advanced Malignant Disease

Tumors are fast-growing tissues with a high glutamine requirement.[45] As tumor growth proceeds, its glutamine requirements will exceed that of the intestine, and the tumor becomes the major glutamine consumer in animal models.[46] The host can readily become glutamine deficient, and this deficiency may contribute to the cachexia and anorexia of the tumor-bearing state.[5, 6, 47] The blood glutamine level falls in the tumor-bearing host. The liver becomes a net glutamine donor, and intestinal uptake significantly decreases (Fig 7—6). There is a decrease in hepatic glutaminase activity and an increase in the hepatic glutamine level. The increased intrahepatic glutamine concentration and reduced circulating glutamine level lead to an increased intracellular-blood glutamine concentration gradient. This effectively drives glutamine out of the hepatocyte and into the circulation.[47] In addition, the cell membrane glutamine transport system favors glutamine transport out of the cell. These changes result in a reduced host tissue utilization of glutamine to meet the tumor's glutamine demands.[47]

Maintaining the nutritional status of a patient with advanced malignant disease is a major clinical challenge. Advanced malignant disease is associated with a state of partial glutamine depletion. A major concern with glutamine supplementation to the tumor-bearing host is the possibility that this may also stimulate tumor growth because tumor cells are active glutamine consumers. Popp et al. demonstrated that the rate of neoplastic growth varies directly with the caloric and protein infusion rate in MCA sarcoma—bearing rats.[48] Depletion of glutamine and asparagine (required by MCA tumor cells in vitro) or their direct precursors (glutamate or aspartate) reduced tumor growth when compared with TPN containing these amino acids. Currently none of these amino acids are found in commercially available TPN solutions.[49] Administration of the glutamine antimetabolite acivicin also slows MCA tumor growth.[50] Conversely, two enteral feeding studies using the MCA sarcoma and a rat mammary carcinoma model indicate that the provision of glutamine does not stimulate tumor growth but can improve the host's nutritional status.[51, 52] Glutamine significantly in-

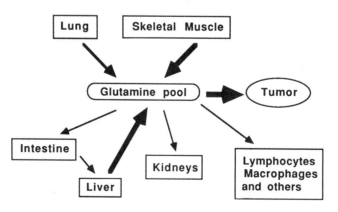

FIG 7—6.
Interorgan glutamine flow in the tumor-bearing host. The liver, joining the lung and muscle, becomes a glutamine donor. The intestine significantly decreases glutamine uptake. Glutamine is spared from visceral organs to meet the demands of the tumor.

creases the intestinal glutaminase levels but does not affect tumor glutaminase.[51]

Austgen et al.[49] evaluated the effects of glutamine-supplemented TPN in the MCA sarcoma–bearing rat with small (tumor weight <5% of body weight) and large (tumor weight, 10% of body weight) tumor burdens. The growing MCA tumor has a high glutamine requirement, and consequently an imbalance in interorgan glutamine flow with partial glutamine depletion develops when the tumor weight approaches 8% to 10% of body weight.[46] Providing 20% of TPN protein as glutamine for 7 days caused a significant increase in arterial glutamine levels and maintained skeletal muscle intracellular glutamine concentrations. Concurrently, hindquarter glutamine fractional release increased nearly threefold in the glutamine-enriched TPN animals, but there was no change in carcass weight, tumor weight, tumor DNA content, or tumor glutaminase activity. While DNA flow cytometric analysis could not demonstrate any change in growth fraction, the ratio of aneuploid to diploid cells in the tumor mass increased by 20% in animals receiving glutamine. The fact that increased arterial glutamine did not increase the tumor glutaminase activity during glutamine supplementation suggests that the tumor may be less sensitive to exogenous glutamine–induced metabolic changes as compared with the glutamine-depleted host. In skeletal muscle, the provision of glutamine increased the muscle cytoplasmic glutamine concentration even greater than the arterial glutamine concentration. This study suggests that the provision of glutamine-supplemented TPN may be beneficial to the tumor-bearing host by restoring the glutamine pool and maintaining muscle glutamine efflux without significantly affecting tumor growth and/or tumor glutamine metabolism. The effect of glutamine supplementation in patients with advanced malignant disease remains to be defined.

GLUTAMINE AND INTESTINE-RELATED INFECTIONS

The passage of small numbers of bacteria across the intact epithelial surface of the intestine is a natural process that normally does not cause disease. Once bacteria enter the lamina propria, they are actively phagocytized and killed by macrophages and neutrophils.[53] In almost all stressed states, including malnutrition, trauma/burn injury, sepsis, chemotherapy, radiation therapy, gastrointestinal cancer, small-bowel obstruction, and TPN and enteral feeding of chemically defined diets, there is some degree of intestinal mucosal atrophy, mucosal barrier dysfunction, overgrowth of intestinal microflora, and decreased local immunity to bacteria. Bacteria normally resident in the lumen can readily cross the intestinal mucosa through the lamina propria to mesenteric lymph nodes or other systemic organs in large numbers.[53–64] In burn injury, the number of viable bacteria cultured from mesenteric lymph nodes can increase 1,000-fold.[53] This process, defined as intestinal bacterial translocation, is considered to be an important cause of infectious complications and to contribute to multiple organ system failure.[64]

The intestine is the principal organ of glutamine metabolism. Glutamine is thought to protect the intestinal mucosa in stressed states by acting as a principal fuel for enterocytes, whose requirements increase under these circumstances.[65] Additional glutamine may be necessary for DNA, RNA, and protein synthesis, which are also increased in stressed states and wound healing. Finally, glutamine supplementation significantly increases the intestinal glutathione level,[49] which is thought to be an important protective mechanism against tissue injury. In normal animals fed a regular chow diet, glutamine supplementation has demonstrated little effect on intestinal mucosa (Shou et al., unpublished data). However, a lack of glutamine may account for intestinal atrophy and sequential bacterial translocation when glutamine depletion occurs in critical illness or when regular TPN and chemically defined enteral diets lacking in glutamine are used.[5, 6]

Windmueller et al. demonstrated that rat intestine can metabolize parenteral glutamine as efficiently as enteral glutamine.[66] The effect of enteral and parenteral supplementation of glutamine on intestine structure and function has been widely studied in animal models. Several studies indicate that the addition of glutamine (2% glutamine w/v) to TPN solutions and chemically defined liquid enteral diets can prevent parenteral or enteral nutrition–induced mucosal atrophy. Glutamine supplementation can preserve the normal intestinal mucosal weight, DNA/RNA, protein content, and architecture, all of which are associated with a decrease in the rate of bacterial translocation in different experimental animal models.[63, 67–71] Glutamine upregulates the intestinal glutaminase activity and increases the intestinal glutamine transport through the brush border.[71] There is a dose-response relationship between the increase in intestinal DNA content and the uptake of glutamine.[69] Alverdy et al.[72] demonstrated that TPN results in a significant decrease in bile secretory IgA, which is considered to be an important first line of defense against bacterial invasion from the lumen. Secretory IgA neutralizes endotoxin, prevents bacterial adherence to epithelium, and opsonizes bacteria for phagocytosis. In the rat, the biliary secretory IgA accounts for 60% of the total secretory IgA in the lumen. Glutamine supplementation of TPN solutions can increase biliary IgA levels to normal, which may contribute to a decrease in bacterial translocation.[73]

There are, however, some differences between the results produced by various studies. Studies by Jacobs et al. indicate that more than 1% (W/V) glutamine supplementation in parenteral nutri-

tion solutions is necessary to produce significant trophic effects.[68] Grant et al. reported that both 1% and 2% gulamine–enriched TPN affect intestinal structure in a similar rat model.[70] Barber et al. reported that 2% glutamine–enriched TPN can prevent the loss of bowel mass during TPN feeding but failed to demonstrate any protection against bacterial translocation in a rat model.[74]

In 2% glutamine–enriched parenteral nutrition solutions, glutamine accounts for about 20% to 30% of the total amino acids, while glutamine only accounts for about 5% of the total protein in normal chow diets. In our laboratory, TPN containing physiologic levels of glutamine (5% of TPN amino acid) fails to demonstrate any effect on rat intestine (Shou et al., unpublished data). Work by Burrin et al. also indicates that parenteral glutamine supplementation at physiologic levels does not influence small intestinal growth and development in infant piglets.[75] It appears that glutamine supplementation produces its trophic effects via a pharmacologic action rather than simply by physiologic nutritional repletion.

Dietary glutamine supplementation for the prevention of chemotherapy- and radiotherapy-induced enterocolitis has also been studied in animal models. The administration of a chemically defined glutamine-free enteral diet and a dose of methotrexate (20 mg/kg) in rats causes mucosal atrophy, degeneration, and necrosis, which are associated with bacterial and endotoxin translocation to the portal and lymphatic system and lead to sepsis and death. No deaths are observed when rats fed a normal chow diet receive similar doses of methotrexate. The glutamine-supplemented diet results in an increased cellularity of the intestinal mucosa and decreased bacterial/endotoxin translocation. This is associated with a significantly decreased mortality rate from 100% to 76%.[76] Shou et al.[62] compared a glutamine-enriched defined diet with a polypeptide-based identical enteral diet in the same animal model. A polypeptide-based diet prevented methotrexate toxicity and resulted in a 0% mortality rate as compared with a 75% mortality rate in the glutamine-supplemented group. Less than 5% of the amino acids in the peptide diet are glutamine, which suggests that polypeptides protect the intestine through some mechanism that is far more effective than that of glutamine. In another model, rats fed glutamine-enriched TPN received a toxic dose of 5-fluorouracil (5-FU). These animals demonstrated greater mean jejunal villus height, increased mucosal DNA content, and higher intestinal glutaminase activity as compared with animals fed a glutamine-free TPN regimen. In addition, nitrogen balance in the glutamine-enriched TPN fed animals was significantly improved.[76, 77]

A major side effect of abdominal and pelvic radiation is injury to the small bowel. Abdominal radiation in rats results in enteritis that is characterized by a loss of mucosal cellularity, mucosal degeneration and necrosis, bacterial translocation, sepsis, and death.[78, 79] Rats fed a glutamine-enriched oral diet prior to radiotherapy demonstrate accelerated intestinal mucosal healing, greater intestinal glutaminase activity and intestinal glutamine uptake, decreased bacterial translocation, and improved survival.[78–80] Interestingly, a glutamine-enriched parenteral solution failed to demonstrate the same benefits in a similar model.[81]

In small-bowel transplantation, mucosal atrophy of the transplanted intestinal segment and sequential bacterial translocation-induced infection frequently occur. Frankel et al.[82] and Schroeder et al.[83] reported in a rat syngeneic small-bowel transplant model that glutamine and glutamine-containing dipeptide-supplemented TPN significantly preserved mucosal structure and function of the transplanted segment. Furthermore, bacterial translocation was significantly decreased.[84] A similar study in an allogeneic graft model is needed to assess the value of clinical application since glutamine supplementation may affect the immune response.

In addition, massive small-bowel resection results in a decrease in intestinal glutaminase activity and glutamine utilization in a rat model.[85] Glutamine-enriched (2%) TPN after small-bowel resection significantly improves small-bowel growth and function.[86] On the other hand, Vanderhoof et al. reported that using a 5% (W/V) glutamine–supplemented enteral diet had a detrimental effect on small intestinal mucosa following the resection.[87]

GLUTAMINE SUPPLEMENTATION AND IMMUNE FUNCTION

It is postulated that postinjury glutamine depletion plays a significant role in posttrauma macrophage suppression.[20] Physiologic levels of glutamine are needed for normal rat peritoneal macrophage phagocytosis in vitro.[20] Additional glutamine in the media can enhance the phagocytosis and cytotoxicity of these macrophages (Shou et al., unpublished data). Studies in our laboratory indicate that pulmonary alveolar macrophage and peritoneal macrophage phagocytosis and killing of Candida albicans are impaired in rats fed a glutamine-free TPN formula as compared with rats fed a normal chow diet. This TPN-induced impairment can be reversed by glutamine-enriched TPN (Shou et al., unpublished data). Yoshida et al. report that glutamine-enriched TPN is also beneficial for lymphocyte proliferation in septic rats.[88]

GLUTAMINE SUPPLEMENTATION AND LIVER INJURY

In the rat, infusion of excess carbohydrate calories leads to the development of hepatic steatosis, which is associated with an elevated portal insulin/glucagon ratio. Glutamine-enriched TPN in this rat model can effectively prevent the development of hepatic steatosis. This effect may be due to glutamine stimulation of glucagon secretion and lowering of the portal insulin/glucagon ratio, which can increase the liver's ability to export lipid. Glutamine-enriched enteral elemental diets also attenuate the gain in liver weight and fat content after massive small-bowel resection. These findings are consistent with studies showing that exogenous glutamine can regulate pancreatic endocrine function.[6]

Hong et al.[12, 14] compared glutamine-enriched TPN with glutamine-free TPN in a number of rat liver injury models. Acetaminophen toxicity causes hepatic glutathione depletion, hepatic necrosis, and death. Glutamine-supplemented animals are resistant to the fall in plasma glutathione levels, and hepatic glutathione stores are rapidly replenished, resulting in significantly less liver injury and improved survival after acetaminophen challenge.[12] In another animal model evaluating 5-FU toxicity, glutamine-enriched TPN significantly increases plasma, liver, and jejunal glutathione levels and is associated with improved animal survival.[14]

The administration of *Corynebacterium parvum* causes extensive recruitment and activation of hepatic macrophages. When a small dose of endotoxin is given to primed animals, the elaboration of oxygen free radicals and tumor necrosis factor results in massive hepatic necrosis. The provision of glutamine-supplemented TPN preserves hepatic glutathione stores, attenuates the degree of oxidant stress, and results in significantly less liver damage.[89]

CLINICAL APPLICATION

Glutamine is actively involved in and mediates many basic energy and nitrogen metabolic functions in normal and pathologic states. During normal conditions, tissues use various sources of energy and nitrogen. During critical illness, the host undergoes dramatic metabolic adaptations to meet the high energy and nitrogen demands of the pathologic state. A major portion of these metabolic adaptations are through glutamine metabolism. Glutamine appears to be a unique amino acid in that it serves as a preferred respiratory fuel for rapidly dividing cells such as enterocytes and lymphocytes, as a regulator of acid balance through the production of urine ammonia, as a carrier of nitrogen between tissues, and as an important precursor of nucleic acids, nucleotides, amino sugar, and proteins. During stress, the body's requirements for glutamine appear to exceed the individual's ability to produce sufficient amounts of this animo acid.[3, 90] The classification of glutamine as a nonessential amino acid has been challenged by the fact that marked declines in both the plasma and body tissue concentrations of glutamine often occur in the setting of catabolic disease states in animal models and humans.[3, 90] During glutamine depletion, vital tissues such as lymphocytes and macrophages are deprived of sufficient fuel to properly function, which may increase the severity of illness and delay recovery. Glutamine supplementation in stressed animals has several benefits that may help the host overcome metabolic stress. Thus, glutamine is a conditionally essential nutrient. Provision of glutamine through enteral or parenteral routes in critically ill patients may enhance the host's metabolic status and augment recovery.[3, 89]

SAFETY OF GLUTAMINE SUPPLEMENTATION

Traditional parenteral formulas lack glutamine. On the other hand, glutamine is present in most enteral diets at relatively low levels. These low levels may meet normal physiologic requirements but are probably inadequate when glutamine demands increase in states such as sepsis, trauma, etc.[5, 6] The reason for eliminating glutamine from TPN solutions is that glutamine is relatively unstable and breaks down to ammonia and glutamate, both of which are toxic to patients (especially those with compromised liver function).[5, 6] Clinical trials demonstrate that therapeutic supplementation of glutamine (0.28 and 0.57 g/kg/24 hr) in TPN solutions is well tolerated and devoid of central nervous system toxicity in healthy humans.[91, 92] Glutamine-enriched TPN increases plasma glutamine levels by 25% and does not significantly increase plasma ammonia and glutamate.

An additional reservation regarding glutamine is its use in the tumor-bearing host because it might stimulate tumor growth (since many tumors are major glutamine consumers). However, the present evidence demonstrates that glutamine-enriched nutrition does not accelerate tumor growth and may be beneficial to host muscle and intestinal glutamine metabolism. Despite the fact that glutamine in solution is hydrolyzed in a relatively short time at room temperature, it appears that its breakdown is negligible if added to the diet mixture immediately before its administration[6] or if the solution is kept at 4° C until use.[93] Another option is to use glutamine-containing short peptides. Jiang et al. reported that alanine-glutamine or glycine-glutamine dipeptide–enriched TPN was as effective as glutamine-enriched TPN but that the dipeptides were stable in solution after 121° C sterilization.[94]

CLINICAL STUDIES

A decreased free glutamine concentration in skeletal muscle is a reproducible and reliable sign of whole-body protein catabolism. It is commonly observed after trauma and elective surgery.[30, 35, 36, 95, 96] The fall may be profound in severely ill intensive care unit patients and is correlated with increased mortality.[4] Hammarqvist et al.[36] studied the effects of glutamine-enriched TPN and glutamine-free TPN feeding in elective surgical patients. Twenty-two patients undergoing elective abdominal surgery were randomized to receive TPN with glutamine (0.285 g/kg of body weight/24 hr) or glutamine-free TPN for 3 days following surgery. The amount of glutamine supplemented was calculated from the reduction in plasma glutamine levels. Quadriceps femoris muscle biopsy specimens were taken before surgery and on the third postoperative day to study intracellular amino acid profiles. The postoperative decrease in intracellular free glutamine concentration was less pronounced with glutamine supplementation. In addition, the daily nitrogen balance from postoperative days 1 to 3 and the cummulative nitrogen balance were significantly improved. Another clinical study using alanine-glutamine dipeptide–enriched TPN supported this observation.[35] Hammarqvist et al.[30] demonstrated that branched-chain amino acid (BCAA) solutions did not attenuate the fall in tissue or blood glutamine levels,[30] thus indicating the importance of direct glutamine supplementation.

Care should be taken, however, with glutamine supplementation in trauma patients with head injury. Glutamate is one of the major metabolites of glutamine. Endogenous glutamate is considered to be one of the most common neurotransmitters in the fast excitatory synapses in the central nervous system. Its excitotoxic properties are increasingly cited to explain some of the brain damage linked with hypoxia and ischemia. An excessive release of glutamate could, either directly or indirectly, activate receptors on the postsynaptic neuron and cause ion influxes accompanied by the entry of water, which could lead to acute swelling of dendrites. In addition, calcium influx deregulates calcium homeostasis, and could lead to cell death.[97, 98] Despite the fact that glutamine-enriched TPN is well tolerated without evidence of toxicity in healthy humans,[91, 92] it is unclear whether exogenous glutamine and glutamate have excitotoxic effects on the central nervous system of patients with head injury.

Bone marrow transplantation is being increasingly used in the treatment of hematologic malignancies. Patients undergoing bone marrow transplantation consistently lose body protein because of the catabolic effects of chemotherapy. Total-body irradiation and gastrointestinal toxicity often limit the ingestion of enteral nutrients. Infectious complications still remain a major cause of morbidity in these patients. Proper parenteral nutrition attenuates protein loss and may prevent malnutrition-related complications. Recently, several clinical trials have demonstrated that parenteral nutrition is associated with an increased incidence of infectious complications in allogeneic bone marrow transplantation patients receiving chemotherapy with or without irradiation. Furthermore, markedly negative nitrogen balance persists in these patients despite the provision of standard nutritional support.[99, 100]

Ziegler et al.[99] evaluated the effect of glutamine-enriched parenteral nutrition in a prospective trial in bone marrow transplantation patients. Forty-five adults receiving allogeneic bone marrow transplants for hematologic malignancies received either glutamine-supplemented (0.57 g/kg/24 hr) TPN ($n = 24$) or glutamine-free TPN ($n = 21$) after transplantation. The glutamine-supplemented patients were clinically similar to the controls at entry. Nitrogen and calorie intake was similar in both groups. Nitrogen balance, measured from day 4 to day 11 after transplantation, was improved in the glutamine-supplemented patients as compared with controls. Clinical infection developed in significantly fewer glutamine-supplemented patients (3/24 vs. 9/21, $P = .041$), and the incidence of micro-

bial colonization was significantly reduced. Hospital stay was also shorter in those patients receiving glutamine supplementation (29 ± 1 vs. 36 ± 2; $P = .017$).

In another trial,[100] the same authors reported a 20% extracellular water expansion in patients ($n = 10$) receiving glutamine-free parenteral nutrition and standard bone marrow transplantation. Clinical infections developed in five out of ten patients. The fluid expansion in infected patients was significantly greater than in noninfected patients. In contrast, the extracellular fluid compartment in patients ($n = 10$) receiving glutamine-supplemented parenteral nutrition and standard bone marrow transplantation procedures did not change, and no clinical infections developed in these patients. In this particular model of catabolic stress, the fluid retention and expansion of the extracellular fluid compartment commonly observed after standard TPN could be attenuated by administering glutamine-supplemented intravenous feeding. Glutamine supplementation also protected these patients from septic complications. All patients in these trials lacked evidence of glutamine-related toxicity.[98, 99]

Glutamine is the most abundant amino acid in blood and tissue and actively serves as an important intermediate in energy and nitrogen metabolism. It is also a necessary fuel for intestinal mucosal cells. In stressed states, the host breaks down skeletal muscle and other tissues to release energy and nitrogen in the form of glutamine, alanine, and other amino acids to meet the increasing metabolic demands of vital organs. If the stress exceeds the metabolic adaptation process, glutamine depletion occurs and further exhausts host energy and nitrogen stores as well as organ function. Supplementation with exogenous glutamine by both the enteral and/or parenteral route can preserve the host's energy and nitrogen stores, help the host overcome the metabolic stress of critical illness, reduce associated complications, and facilitate the recovery process. In this way, glutamine may be a direct and efficient nutrient for the nutritional support of critically ill patients. The information to date suggests that in addition to providing adequate nutrition, glutamine supplementation is beneficial to the stressed host. The use of glutamine supplementation in the tumor-bearing host or head-injured patient still needs further research to evaluate its possible benefits.

REFERENCES

1. Krebs H: Glutamine metabolism in the animal body, in Mora J, Palacios R (eds): *Glutamine: Metabolism, Enzymology, and Regulation.* New York, Academic Press, 1980, pp 319–329.
2. Eagle H: Nutritional needs of mammalian cells in tissue culture, *Science* 1935; 122:501–504.
3. Smith RJ: Glutamine metabolism and its physiologic importance. *JPEN* 1990; 14(suppl 4):40–44.
4. Roth E, Funovics J, Muhlbacher F, et al: Metabolic disorders in severe abdominal sepsis: Glutamine deficiency in skeletal muscle. *Clin Nutr* 1982; 1:25–41.
5. Souba WW: The gut as a nitrogen-processing organ in the metabolic response to critical illness. *Nutr Supp Serv* 1988; 8:15–22.
6. Souba WW: Glutamine: A key substrate for the splanchnic bed. *Annu Rev Nutr* 1991; 11:285–308.
7. Mehler AH: Amino acid metabolism I: General pathways, in Devlin TM (ed): *Textbook of Biochemistry With Clinical Correlations.* New York, Wiley-Liss, 1992, pp 480–481.
8. Souba WW, Smith RJ, Wilmore DW: Glutamine metabolism by the intestinal tract. *JPEN* 1985; 9:608–617.
9. Windmueller HG: Glutamine utilization by the small intestine. *Adv Enzymol* 1982; 53:202.
10. Windmueller HG, Spaeth AE: Respiratory fuels and nitrogen metabolism in vivo in small intestine of fed rat. *J Biol Chem* 1980; 255:107–112.
11. Mehler AH: Amino acid metabolism II: Metabolism of the individual amino acids, in Devlin TM (ed): *Textbook of Biochemistry With Clinical Correlations.* New York, Wiley-Liss, 1992, pp 522–525.
12. Hong RW, Round JD, Helton WS, et al: Glutamine preserves liver glutathione after lethal hepatic injury. *Ann Surg* 1991; 215:114–119.
13. Robinson MK, Rodrick ML, Jacobs DO: Glutathione depletion in rats impairs T-cell and macrophage immune function. *Arch Surg* 1993; 128:29–35.
14. Hong RW, Helton WS, Round JD, et al: Glutamine supplemented TPN preserves hepatic glutathione and improves survival following chemotherapy. *Surg Forum* 1990; 76:9–11.
15. Bulus NM, Abumrad NN, Ghishan FK: Characteristics of glutamine transport in dog jejunal brush border membrane vesicles. *Am J Physiol* 1989; 257:80–85.
16. Said HM, Voorhis K, Ghishan FK, et al: Transport characteristics of glutamine in human intestinal brush border membrane vesicles. *Am J Physiol* 1989; 256:240–245.
17. Souba WW, Herskowitz K, Pulmley DA: Lung glutamine metabolism. *JPEN* 1990; 14(suppl 4):68–70.
18. Haussinger D: Liver glutamine metabolism. *JPEN* 1990; 14(suppl 4):56–62.
19. Moormann AFM, Vermeulen JLM, Charles R: Localization of ammonia metabolizing enzymes in human liver: Ontogenesis of heterogeneity. *Hepatology* 1989; 9:367–372.
20. Parry-Billings M, Evans J, Calder PC, et al: Does glutamine contribute to immunosuppression after major burns? *Lancet* 1990; 336:523–525.
21. Wallace C, Keast D: Glutamine and macrophage function. *Metabolism* 1992; 41:1016–1020.
22. Newsholme EA, Parry-Billing M, Phil D: Properties of glutamine release from muscle and its importance for the immune system. *JPEN* 1990; 14(suppl 4):63–67.
23. Souba WW, Austgen TR: Interorgan glutamine flow following surgery and infection. *JPEN* 1990; 14(suppl 4):90–93.

24. Abumrad NN, Yazigi N, Cersosimo E, et al: Glutamine metabolism during starvation. *JPEN* 1990; 14(suppl 4):71–76.
25. Welbourne T, Joshi S: Interorgan glutamine metabolism during acidosis. *JPEN* 1990; 14(suppl 4):77–85.
26. Welbourne TC: Enteral glutamine spares endogenous glutamine in chronic acidosis. *JPEN* 1993; 17(suppl):23.
27. Wernerman J, Botta D, Ali MR, et al: The effect of stress hormones upon the intracellular concentration of free amino acids in skeletal muscle. *Clin Nutr* 1982; 1:25–41.
28. Essen P, Werverman J, Ali MR, et al: Changes in concentrations of free amino acids in skeletal muscle during 24 hr immediately following elective surgery. *Clin Nutr* 1988; 7(suppl):67.
29. Vinnars E, Bergstrom J, Furst P: Effects of starvation on plasma and muscle amino acid concentration in normal subjects. *Clin Nutr* 1988; 7(suppl):62.
30. Hammarqvist F, Wernerman J, Vinnars E: The effects of postoperative total parenteral nutrition including a BACC enriched amino acid supply upon the concentrations of free amino acids in skeletal muscle. *Clin Nutr* 1987; 6(suppl):14.
31. Souba WW, Smith RJ, Wilmore DW: Effect of glucocorticoids on glutamine metabolism in visceral organs. *Metabolism* 1985; 34:450–456.
32. Fox AD, Kripke SA, Berman JM, et al: Dexamethasone administration induces increased glutaminase specific activity in the jejenum and colon. *J Surg Res* 1988; 44:391–396.
33. Muhlbacher F, Kapadia CR, Colpoys MF, et al: Effects of glucocorticoids on glutamine metabolism in skeletal muscle. *Am J Physiol* 1984; 247:75–83.
34. Geer RJ, Williams PE, Lairmre T, et al: Glucogon: An important stimulator of gut and hepatic glutamine metabolism. *Surg Forum* 1987; 38:27–29.
35. Stehle P, Mertes N, Puchatein CH, et al: Effect of parenteral glutamine peptide supplements on muscle glutamine loss and nitrogen balance after major surgery. *Lancet* 1989; 1:231–233.
36. Hammarqvist F, Wernerman J, Ali R, et al: Addition of glutamine to total parenteral nutrition after elective abdominal surgery spares free glutamine in muscle, counteracts the fall in muscle protein synthesis, and improves nitrogen balance. *Ann Surg* 1989; 209:455–461.
37. Souba WW, Herskowitz K, Klimberg VS, et al: The effect of sepsis and endotoxemia on gut glutamine metabolism. *Ann Surg* 1990; 211:543–551.
38. Salloum RM, Copeland EM, Souba WW: Brush border transport of glutamine and other substrates during sepsis and endotoxemia. *Ann Surg* 1991; 213:401–410.
39. Souba WW, Copeland EM: Cytokine modulation of Na^+-dependent glutamine transport across the brush border membrane of monolayers of human intestinal Caco-2 cells. *Ann Surg* 1992; 215:536–545.
40. Inoue Y, Grant JP, Snyder PJ: Effect of glutamine-supplemented intravenous nutrition on survival after *Escherichia coli*–induced peritonitis. *JPEN* 1993; 17:41–46.
41. Yoshida S, Leskiw MJ, Schluter MD, et al: Effect of total parenteral nutrition, systemic sepsis, and glutamine on gut mucosa in rats. *Am J Physiol* 1992; 263:368–373.
42. Higashiguchi T, Frederick JA, Zamir O, et al: Effect of glutamine on protein synthesis in isolated enterocytes from septic rats. *Surg Forum* 1992; 78:26–28.
43. Ardawi MS: Effects of glutamine-enriched total parenteral nutrition on septic rats. *Clin Sci* 1991; 81:215–222.
44. Ardawi MS: Effect of epidermal growth factor and glutamine-supplemented parenteral nutrition on the small bowel of septic rats. *Clin Sci* 1992; 82:573–580.
45. Sauer LA, Stayman JW, Dauchy RT: Amino acid, glucose, and lactic acid utilization in vivo by rat tumor. *Cancer Res* 1982; 42:4090–4097.
46. Chen MK, Austgen TR, Klimberg S, et al: Tumor glutamine use exceeds intestinal glutamine use in cachectic tumor-bearing rats. *Surg Forum* 1990; 76:12–14.
47. Souba WW, Strebel FR, Bull JM, et al:

Interorgan glutamine metabolism in the tumor-bearing rat. *J Surg Res* 1988; 44:720–726.

48. Popp MB, Enrione EB, Wagner SC, et al: Influence of total nitrogen, asparagine, and glutamine on MCA tumor growth in the Fischer 344 rat. *Surgery* 1988; 104:152–160.

49. Austgen TS, Dudrick PS, Sitren H, et al: The effects of glutamine-enriched total parenteral nutrition on tumor growth and host tissues. *Ann Surg* 1992; 215:107–113.

50. Chance IL, Cao L, Fischer JE: Insulin and acivicin improve host nutrition and prevent tumor growth during total parenteral nutrition. *Ann Surg* 1988; 208:524–531.

51. Klimbarg SV, Souba WW, Salloum RM, et al: Glutamine-enriched diets support muscle glutamine metabolism without stimulating tumor growth. *J Surg Res* 1990; 48:319–323.

52. Bartlett D, Torosian M: Effect of oral glutamine on tumor and host growth. *J Surg Oncol,* 1993, in press.

53. Alexander JW, Peck MD: Future prospects for adjunctive therapy: Pharmacologic and nutritional approaches to immune system modulation. *Crit Care Med* 1990; 18(suppl):159–164.

54. Berg RD, Garlinton AW: Translocation of certain indigenous bacteria from the gastrointestinal tract to the mesenteric lymph nodes and other organs in a gnotobiotic mouse model. *Infect Immun* 1979; 23:403–411.

55. Berg RD, Wommack E, Deitch EA: Immunosuppression and intestinal bacterial overgrowth synergistically promote bacterial translocation. *Arch Surg* 1988; 123:1359–1364.

56. Alverdy JC, Aoy S, Moss GS: Total parenteral nutrition promotes bacterial translocation from gut. *Surgery* 1988; 104:185–190.

57. Alverdy JC, Aoy S, Moss GS: Effect of commercially available chemically defined liquid diets on the intestinal microflora and bacterial translocation from the gut. *JPEN* 1990; 14:1–6.

58. Jones WG, Minei JP, Baber AE et al: Elemental diet promotes spontaneous bacterial translocation and alters mortality after endotoxin challenge. *Surg Forum* 1990; 40:20–22.

59. Jones WG, Minei JP, Barber AE, et al:

Bacterial translocation and intestinal atrophy after injury and burn wound sepsis. *Ann Surg* 1990; 211:399–405.

60. Deitch EA, Winterton J, Berg RD: Effect of starvation, malnutrition, and trauma on the gastrointestinal tract flora and bacterial translocation. *Arch Surg* 1987; 122:1019–1024.

61. Shou J, Redmond HP, Leon P, et al: Elemental diet alters macrophage function in mice. *J Surg Res* 1991; 51:192–196.

62. Shou J, Lieberman MD, Hoffmann KP, et al: Dietary manipulation of methotrexate-induced enterocolitis. *JPEN* 1991; 15:307–312.

63. Shou J, Ruelaz EA, Redmond HP, et al: Dietary protein prevents bacterial translocation from intestine. *JPEN* 1991; 15(suppl):29.

64. Alexander JW: Nutrition and translocation. *JPEN* 1990; 14(suppl 5):170–174.

65. Windmueller HG: Glutamine utilization by the small intestine, in Fleischen S, Pocker L (eds): *Advances in Enzymology.* San Diego, Academic Press, 1982, pp 202–237.

66. Windmueller H, Spaeth AE: Intestinal metabolism of glutamine and glutamate from the lumen as compared to glutamine from blood. *Arch Biochem Biophys* 1975; 171:662–672.

67. Hwang TL, O'Dwyer, Smith RJ, et al: Preservation of small bowel mucosa using glutamine-enriched parenteral nutrition. *Surg Forum* 1986; 73:56–59.

68. Jacobs DO, Evans DA, Mealy K, et al: Combined effects of glutamine and epidermal growth factor on the rat intestine. *Surgery* 1988; 104:358–364.

69. O'Dwyer, Smith RJ, Hwang TL, et al: Maintenance of small bowel mucosa with glutamine-enriched parenteral nutrition. *JPEN* 1989; 13:579–585.

70. Grant JP, Snyder PJ: Use of L-glutamine in total parenteral nutrition. *J Surg Res* 1988; 44:506–513.

71. Klimberg VS, Souba WW, Sitren H, et al: Glutamine-enriched total parenteral nutrition supports gut metabolism. *Surg Forum* 1989; 75:175–177.

72. Alverdy J, Chi HS, Sheldon GF: The effect of parenteral nutrition on gas-

trointestinal immunity. *Ann Surg* 1985; 202:681–684.

73. Burke DJ, Alverdy JC, Aoys E, et al: Glutamine-supplemented total parenteral nutrition improves gut immune function. *Arch Surg* 1989; 124:1396–1399.

74. Barber AE, Jones WG II, Minel JP, et al: Glutamine or fiber supplementation of a defined formula diet: Impact on bacterial translocation, tissue composition, and response to endotoxin. *JPEN* 1990; 14:335–343.

75. Burrin DG, Shulman RJ, Storm MC, et al: Glutamine or glutamic acid effects on intestinal growth and disaccharidase activity in infant piglets receiving total parenteral nutrition. *JPEN* 1991; 15:262–266.

76. Rombeau JL: A review of the effects of glutamine-enriched diets on experimentally induced enterocolitis. *JPEN* 1990; 14(suppl 4):100–105.

77. O'Dwyer ST, Scott T, Smith RJ: 5-Fluorouracil toxicity on small intestinal mucosa but not white blood cells is decreased by glutamine (abstract). *Clin Nutr* 1987; 35:367.

78. Souba WW, Klimberg VS, Copeland EM: Glutamine nutrition in the management of radiation enteritis. *JPEN* 1990; 14(suppl 4):106–108.

79. Karatzas T, Scopa S, Tsoni I, et al: Effect of glutamine on intestinal mucosal integrity and bacterial translocation after abdominal radiation. *Clin Nutr* 1991; 10:199–205.

80. Klimberg VS, Salloum RM, Kasper M, et al: Oral glutamine accelerates healing of the small intestine and improves outcome after whole abdominal radiation. *Arch Surg* 1990; 125:1040–1045.

81. Scott TE, Moellman JR: Intravenous glutamine fails to improve gut morphology after radiation injury. *JPEN* 1992; 16:440–444.

82. Frankel WL, Zhang W, Afonso J, et al: Glutamine enhancement of structure and function in transplanted small intestine in the rat. *JPEN* 1993; 17:47–55.

83. Schroeder P, Schweizer E, Blomer, et al: Glutamine prevents mucosal injury after small bowel transplantation. *Transplant Proc* 1992; 24:1104.

84. Zhang W, Frankel WL, Singh A, et al: Glutamine improves structure and function in orthotopic small bowel transplantation in the rat. *Transplantation*, 1993, in press.

85. Klimberg VS, Souba WW, Salloum RM, et al: Intestinal glutamine metabolism after massive small bowel resection. *Am J Surg* 1990; 159:27–33.

86. Gouttebel MC, Astre C, Briand D, et al: Influence of *N*-acetylglutamine or glutamine infusion on plasma amino acid concentrations during the early phase of small bowel adaption in the dog. *JPEN* 1992; 16:117–121.

87. Vanderhauf JA, Blackwood DJ, Mohammadpour H, et al: Effects of oral supplementation of glutamine on small intestinal mucosa mass following resection. *JPEN* 1992; 11:223–227.

88. Yoshida S, Hikida S, Tanaka Y, et al: Effect of glutamine supplementation on lymphocyte function in septic rats. Unpublished paper.

89. Hong RW, Robinson MK, Round JD, et al: Glutamine protects the liver following *Corynebacterium parvum*/endotoxin–induced hepatic necrosis. *Surg Forum* 1991; 77:1–1.

90. Lacey JM, Wilmore DW: Is glutamine a conditionally essential amino acid? *Nutr Rev* 1990; 40:297–300.

91. Lowe DK, Benfell K, Smith RJ, et al: Safety of glutamine-enriched parenteral nutrition solutions in humans. *Am J Clin Nutr* 1990; 52:1101–1106.

92. Zieglar TR, Benfell K, Smith RJ, et al: Safety and metabolic effects of L-glutamine administration in humans. *JPEN* 1990; 14(suppl 4):137–146.

93. Khan K, Hardy B, Elia M: The stability of L-glutamine in total parenteral nutrition solutions. *Clin Nutr* 1991; 10:193–198.

94. Jiang ZM, Wang LJ, Qi Y, et al: Comparision of parenteral nutrition supplemented with L-glutamine or glutamine dipeptides. *JPEN* 1993; 17:134–141.

95. Vinnars E, Bergstrom J, Furst P: Influence of the postoperative state on the intracelullar free amino acids in human muscle tissue. *Ann Surg* 1972; 182:665–671.

96. Askanazi J, Faust P, Michelsen CB, et al: Muscle and plasma amino acids

after injury: Hypocaloric glucose vs. amino acids after injury. *Ann Surg* 1980; 191:465–472.

97. Pujol R, Rebillard G, Puel JL, et al: Glutamine neurotoxicity in the cochlea: A possible consequence of ischaemic or anoxic conditions during ageing. *Acta Otolaryngol Suppl (Stockh)* 1990; 476:32–36.

98. Auer RN: Excitotoxic mechanisms, and age-related susceptibility to brain damage in ischaemia, hypoglycemia and toxic mussel poisoning. *Neurotoxicology* 1991; 12:541–546.

99. Ziegler TR, Young LS, Benfell K, et al: Clinical and metabolic efficacy of glutamine-supplemented parenteral nutrition after bone marrow transplantation: A randomized, double-blind, controlled study. *Ann Intern Med* 1992; 116:821–828.

100. Schelting MR, Young LS, Benfell K, et al: Glutamine enriched intravenous feedings attenuate extracellular fluid expansion after a standard stress. *Ann Surg* 1991; 214:385–393.

8

Albumin Supplementation: Starling's Law as a Guide to Therapy and Literature Review

Mitchell V. Kaminski, Jr., M.D.

Terri J. Blumeyer, P.A.-C.

Albumin as a major index of nutritional status

Hypoproteinemia as a cause of edema

Physiology of edema

Starling's equation

$P_c - P_{if}$

$\pi_c - \pi_{if}$

Q_{lymph}

Kf

σ

Recognition and treatment of hyperoncotic edema

Critical literature review

Use of albumin for intravascular expansion

Albumin administration based on empirical formula

Studies titrating albumin by hemodynamic stabilization

Albumin in patients with pulmonary insufficiency

Albumin in patients undergoing open heart surgery

Albumin in patients with thermal injury

Albumin in patients with cirrhosis

Albumin and nutrition

Albumin administration and enteral feeding tolerance

Albumin administration in patients receiving total parenteral nutrition

ALBUMIN AS A MAJOR INDEX OF NUTRITIONAL STATUS

The serum albumin level is the best index of nutritional status as it relates to outcome.[1-4] Patients whose serum albumin level is below 3.5 g/dL have consistently higher morbidity rates. The morbidity associated with these patients includes an increased rate of infection, length of hospital stay, time on a ventilator, time in the intensive care unit, cost, and most significantly, mortality. As the albumin drops from 3.5 to 3.0 g/dL, there is a 15% increase in morbidity and mortality. For patients whose

143

serum albumin concentration is less than 2.0 g/dL, morbidity and/or mortality approach 100%.

Malnutrition can be manifested as either kwashiorkor or marasmus. In fact, hypoproteinemic patients may appear otherwise well nourished. They are suffering from the hypoalbuminemic type of malnutrition known as the adult kwashiorkor-like syndrome. In the natural setting, kwashiorkor is found in populations where dietary carbohydrate and fat are abundant but protein intake is minimal.[5, 6] Conversely, marasmus results from the deprivation of both protein and calories. In marasmus, visceral proteins are maintained while somatic proteins are consumed. In fact, weight loss secondary to simple starvation is initially not associated with a decrease in circulating proteins. This is because amino acids from the somatic protein compartment (i.e., muscle and carcass) support the turnover of visceral proteins. It is not until end-stage marasmus that somatic proteins no longer support the visceral protein compartment and visceral protein concentrations also decrease. This is the most severe form of malnutrition (i.e., marasmus-kwashiorkor mix).[6]

These conditions are also found in the clinical setting. For example, the provision of carbohydrate without amino acids suppresses growth hormone, raises insulin, and lowers glucagon concentrations, all of which predispose to the development of visceral protein deficits. In fact, overfeeding a patient nonprotein calories can produce obesity while suppressing visceral proteins.

Another clinical variable that suppresses visceral protein synthesis is inflammation. Tumor necrosis factor, interleukin-1, and interleukin-6 are inflammatory mediators that directly depress albumin synthesis.[7-9] An infected patient consuming a carbohydrate meal, whether intravenously or enterally, is prone to the development of the hypoalbuminemic type of malnutrition.

HYPOPROTEINEMIA AS A CAUSE FOR EDEMA

The focus of this chapter, however, has little to do with serum albumin levels as they relate to the nutritional assessment. This chapter deals with albumin as the major component of total protein. Total protein produces colloid osmotic pressure. When nutritional status deteriorates to a point that circulating proteins can no longer sustain a colloid pressure capable of holding fluid in the circulation, hypo-oncotic edema will develop[10-12] and can be clinically significant. Corporal edema is associated with the development of pressure ulcers.[13, 14] Hypoproteinemia is associated with intestinal edema. Intestinal edema negatively affects luminal absorption and results in diarrhea. Recently, there has been evidence that intestinal edema associated with hypoproteinemia compromises the tensile strength of an intestinal anastomosis.[15] Finally, if profound hypoproteinemia is pillared with an elevated wedge pressure, interstitial fluid flow can overwhelm lymphatic clearance and result in pulmonary edema.[16] This produces a rather typical radiologic appearance that can be misinterpreted as adult respiratory distress syndrome (ARDS). In fact, this could be referred to as a pseudo–leaky membrane, or pseudo-ARDS. It is amenable to correction by bringing the Starling forces into homeostasis.

Physiology of Edema

The relationship of colloid in the circulation to intracapillary pressure and interstitial fluid flow was described almost a century ago. The equation published by Starling has stood the test of time. With an understanding of the principles governing fluid/space dynamics, there should be no controversy regarding the use of colloid or crystalloid during resuscitation or nutritional support.

Although excellent work has been done by reliable investigators, it seems that the Starling equation has been either neglected or misunderstood during the interpretation of results. There are three additional physiologic concepts to mention before discussing Starling's equation. These three concepts were developed by van't Hoff, Gibbs-Donnan, and Landis and Pappenheimer.[11, 17] In summary, the principles are that a particle in solution that cannot cross a semipermeable membrane will draw water to itself, thus creating a gradient. The magnitude of this gradient is effected by the number of particles in solution, not the size of the particles. Therefore, since protein molecules in the circulation do not easily cross the semipermeable membrane of the cell, each of those molecules contributes equally to the oncotic gradient across the end-capillary membrane. Albumin, globulin, and fibrinogen compose total protein. It is total protein and not albumin alone that produces the oncotic gradient pulling fluid into the circulation, thereby maintaining circulating volume. Finally, oncotic pressure becomes osmotic pressure as the negative charges surrounding the protein molecules attract sodium, which in turn holds water. This property gives an extra boost to the *oncotic* pressure and is the reason why COP is known as colloid *osmotic* pressure.

There have been a number of reviews of Starling's equation in the literature.[18-21] The goal of this chapter is to leave the reader with the ability to interpolate Starling's equation into the clinical setting and guide the use of albumin supplementation. To exercise this skill, we will review a number of clinical categories where work has been published that fueled the colloid-vs.-crystalloid controversy.

Starling's Equation

$$J_v = Kf[(P_c - P_{if}) - \sigma(\pi_c - \pi_{if})] - Q_{lymph}$$

Interstitial fluid flow is governed by a number of forces (Fig 8–1).

$P_c - P_{if}$

Pressure within the lumen of a blood vessel is designated P_c. That pressure in the corpus is reflected by the central venous pressure (CVP). Within the lung, it is reflected by the pulmonary capillary wedge pressure (PCWP). This pressure pushes fluid across the membrane into the interstitial space. Since the interstitium also has a pressure, P_{if} opposes P_c. Taken together, they are known as the hydrostatic pressure.

$\pi_c - \pi_{if}$

π_c is the COP generated by total protein within the capillary. The weight of a fibrinogen molecule is 490,000 daltons. Globulins are approximately 150,000 daltons, and albumin is the smallest at 69,000 daltons. Therefore, 1 g of albumin will have approximately twice the oncotic pull as 1 g of globulin and about five times the pull as the same amount of fibrinogen. Albumin makes up approximately 60% of circulating proteins. Thus, it is the most populous protein.

There is, of course, protein in the interstitial fluid (π_{if}). In fact, 60% of the total-body albumin in a healthy individual is found in the interstitial space. However, at the border between the end-capillary and the interstitial space, the concentration of protein in the circulation is many times higher than the protein found in the interstitial fluid. Therefore, a patient with a normal serum total protein level (π_c) and a normal CVP (P_c) will have an interstitial fluid pressure of − 7 mm Hg. Thus, these tissues are physiologically dry. This gives them structural strength and integrity. It also minimizes the distance solutes

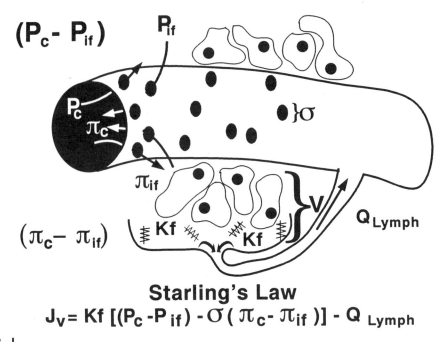

Starling's Law

$$J_v = Kf\,[(P_c - P_{if}) - \sigma(\pi_c - \pi_{if})] - Q_{Lymph}$$

FIG 8–1.

Schematic representation of Starling's law, where J_v = net volume fluid flow; Kf = filtration coefficient; P_c = capillary hydrostatic pressure; P_{if} = interstitial fluid hydrostatic pressure; σ = reflection coefficient; π_c = capillary COP; π_{if} = interstitial fluid COP; and Q_{lymph} = lymph flow.

have to diffuse to bathe, feed, and oxygenate cells.

Q_{lymph}

Lymph channels are the "back door" of tissue perfusion. Their primary function is to carry protein and solute back into the circulating volume. It is through the lymphatic system that protein will translocate from interstitial fluid reserves into the circulating volume to maintain a favorable COP/CVP or COP/PCWP gradient. Only after interstitial protein reserves have been depleted and can no longer support a loss of circulating proteins will π_c fall below P_c. This derangement in homeostasis favors a flux of fluid across the semipermeable membrane into the interstitial space that can overwhelm lymphatic clearance and result in interstitial edema.

Kf

Kf, the filtration coefficient, describes the resistance to flow across the gel sol matrix in the interstitial space. Thus, it is affected by depletion of π_{if}. As albumin reserves are translocated from the interstitial space into the circulating volume to maintain homeostatic pressure, the gel-sol matrix becomes "less gel," and interstitial fluid flow increases. The net effect might be called a pseudo–leaky membrane since σ is not affected.

σ

The pore membrane size is termed σ. Every tissue in the body has a different pore membrane size, for example, severe hypoproteinemia will not result in edema of the liver. The liver manufactures albumin and allows it to leave and enter the sinusoidal space without interference. In order to have hepatomegaly secondary to Starling's forces, the CVP must be significantly elevated. On the other hand, the endothelial junctions within the lung are relatively tight. This is supplemented by an active lymphatic system being continually massaged during respiration. Hypoproteinemia must therefore be coupled with elevated PCWPs in order to create enough interstitial fluid flow for lymphatic drainage to be overwhelmed. On the other hand, damage to a membrane that alters σ will produce a "true" leaky membrane.

Recognition and Treatment of Hypo-oncotic Edema

In summary, there are overlapping factors that can result in clinically significant edema. They include elevated hydrostatic pressure, low COP, and altered membrane pore size and lymphatic flow. A relatively new concept in the interpolation of Starling's law into the clinical setting is our appreciation for Kf, that is, resistance of the gel-sol matrix to interstitial fluid flow. Kf decreases as total-body visceral protein status decreases.

A clinician who understands Starling's equation should assign an adjective to describe the finding of edema. Edema should be reported as either hydrostatic, hypo-oncotic, σ or lymphedema. Potentiating combinations such as hydrostatic and hypo-oncotic edema also exist.

The average intensive care unit is capable of measuring central venous and wedge pressures. In fact, these pressures can be maintained at a given level by controlling the fluid intake vs. output as long as there is adequate colloid pressure. On the other hand, if profound hypoproteinemia is allowed to develop and colloid pressure falls below hydrostatic pressure, infused fluid will no longer be effectively held in the circulation. In nonacute resuscitation, hypoproteinemia can be corrected by simply adding albumin to the total parenteral nutrition (TPN) solution. However, albumin should never be administered to simply raise serum albumin levels. It should be clear that albumin is added to raise the total protein concentration. The goal of adding colloid is to restore adequate colloid pressures and prevent or recover clinically significant interstitial edema.

CRITICAL LITERATURE REVIEW

Much of the controversy on the use of colloid vs. crystalloid is really not a controversy at all. The origin of a perceived controversial finding may be more attributable to an interpretation of the data based on too strict a definition of the question asked by the study. To some extent, this represents the classic error of overlooking the forest because of careful observation of the tree. We will limit our review to work reported in humans. The categories were defined in a paper by Erstad et al.[22]

Use of Albumin for Intravascular Expansion

There are a number of papers that studied the use of albumin in the emergency setting to expand circulating volume. In fact, one of the more frequently cited studies is by Lucas et al.[23] This group aggressively administered albumin by protocol to patients with hemorrhage who were healthy prior to admission. In addition to having normal visceral protein reserves within the interstitial space, all patients were given whole blood and fresh frozen plasma, which provided on average an additional 300 g of albumin. They were then randomized to receive either more albumin or crystalloid. This resulted in a colloid osmotic pressure of 24 cm of water in patients who were in the control group and 29 cm of water in patients who received albumin (normal COP, 32 to 38 cm H_2O). No difference between the groups would be expected because the colloid pressures were not allowed to drop to clinically significant ranges.

Two other uncontrolled reports administered albumin to patients whose COP dropped below 15 mm Hg (normal COP, 24 to 28 mm Hg).[24, 25] In the lymphatic channel–rich lung, 15 mm Hg can be an adequate colloid pressure if the wedge pressure is kept within low normal ranges, which it was. Thus, we again see papers that are well done.

However, they fail to observe patients with clinically significant altered COP. The broad conclusion that the administration of albumin or crystalloid makes no difference is thus flawed if it is applied to patients beyond the parameters of the studies.

Albumin Administration Based on Empirical Formula

A number of studies[26-30] administered albumin per protocol. Unfortunately, these reports are again characterized by the use of whole blood or the administration of colloid to patients who basically did not need it. To exemplify, in a study by Skillman et al,[26] the treatment group received 1 g/kg of 25% albumin and 1 L of 5% albumin in saline, but both study and control patients received 3 L of whole blood during surgery. Further, all patients were given electrolytes and albumin postoperatively. It is no surprise that there was no difference between the two groups.

Studies Titrating Albumin by Hemodynamic Stabilization

The paper by Stein et al.[31] compared the use of crystalloid vs. colloid resuscitation with a goal of keeping the pulmonary artery diastolic pressure below 25 mm Hg or the PCWP below 22 mm Hg. Resuscitation was also stopped if dyspnea and moist rales developed. The starting total protein level was not recorded. Therefore, the status of Kf and π_{if} cannot be determined. The group that received crystalloid had a 70% incidence of pulmonary edema vs. a 25% incidence for the colloid group. This is a helpful study in that it suggests that elevated PCWP should also be avoided.

The error of not recording the total protein at the time of resuscitation is noted throughout most studies. Starling's equation is multifactorial. For example, five manuscripts looked at patients undergoing laparotomy following acute trauma. We could presume that given the usual age group and status of patients entering the trauma unit, these patients had adequate protein reserves and circulating proteins prior to injury. The amount of whole blood lost was not recorded. Thus, it is difficult to interpret the results of being in the crystalloid or colloid group during resuscitation.[32-36]

On the other hand, Rockow et al. did report colloid vs. wedge pressure.[37] It was noted that a COP of 14.7 mm Hg in the saline-treated group was significantly less than the COP of 21.5 mm Hg and 23.5 mm Hg in the albumin- and hetastarch-treated groups, respectively. Pulmonary edema was found in 22% of the patients in the albumin and hetastarch groups at 24 hours vs. 87% in the saline-treated group. Once again, the importance of maintaining a favorable COP/PCWP gradient was illustrated.

Albumin in Patients With Pulmonary Insufficiency

A number of papers discussed the use of albumin in patients with pulmonary insufficiency.[38-42] The patients studied had respiratory insufficiency secondary to chronic obstructive pulmonary disease. This is a significant extraneous variable affecting the interpolation of Starlings law. In a study by Skillman et al.,[38] patients were given ethacrynic acid or albumin plus ethacrynic acid, but π_c was not reported. The amount of pulmonary inflammation that could affect σ was not mentioned. Similarly, in the paper by Metildi et al.,[42] patients were given either lactated Ringer's solution (LR) or LR plus 50 g of albumin per liter "when hemodynamic instability occurred" (not defined). During the 48 hours of the study, there were no significant differences between the colloid and crystalloid groups in PCWP or COP. However, without starting pressures, one cannot make a meaningful interpretation of their results.

Albumin in Patients Undergoing Open Heart Surgery

Several papers examined the use of albumin during various time points in the management of patients undergoing open heart surgery.[43–47] In a paper by Hallowell et al.,[43] whole blood was given as needed to maintain circulatory stability and hematocrit. On the other hand, whole blood is not usually available today. If a patient bleeds whole blood and receives only crystalloid and packed cells in return, the patient in essence is undergoing plasmapheresis. A patient entering the operating room for an elective procedure can probably tolerate the loss of approximately half of the total-body albumin. Acute edema will not develop if the translocation of interstitial albumin back into circulating volume restores a favorable COP/PCWP gradient. In the study by Hallowell and associates, group 1 patients received 127 g of albumin vs. 66 g in group 2. The amount of albumin provided by blood products, however, was approximately the same for both groups. Data that would indicate that these patients were at risk for either hypo-oncotic or hydrostatic edema were not provided. There was no difference between the groups in terms of the need for respiratory support, creatinine levels, length of stay, or mortality. The difference between 127 g of albumin plus blood products vs. 66 g of albumin plus blood products in patients who may not have a colloid deficit is probably insignificant and accounts for the comparable results between groups. In another report by Sade et al.,[44] patients received either hydroxy/ethel starch, albumin, or LR as a priming solution for cardiopulmonary bypass. If the π_c and π_{if} of patients being placed on cardiopulmonary bypass are not depleted and blood loss is either not significant or replaced with whole blood, no difference in outcome would be expected. In addition, this study allowed the use of red blood cells to maintain hematocrit during bypass and uncontrolled use of crystalloid, albumin, or red cells as needed postoperatively. There was a statistically significant but clinically insignificant drop in COP in the LR-primed group. This was accompanied by a pulmonary shunt fraction that was also higher. No differences in outcome were reported.

Given an appreciation of Starling's forces, these patients are not at risk for clinically significant edema secondary to crystalloid priming of their cardiopulmonary bypass pump during the first operative procedure. However, if these patients return to surgery because of ongoing postoperative hemorrhage and blood loss is replaced with packed cells and crystalloid, it would be wise to obtain a total protein level and administer colloid if the value is less than 5.2 g/dL. COP should be maintained at or above 20 mm Hg and the PCWP kept below 12 mm Hg while maintaining an adequate urine output.

Albumin in Patients With Thermal Injury

The papers recommending a formula to resuscitate volume loss in burn patients also neglect to use preinjury, intrainjury, or postresuscitation values relevant to Starling's equation to guide therapy.[48, 49] Goodwin et al.[49] took 79 patients and assigned them to receive either LR or 2.5% albumin in LR in the initial 24 hours following burn injury to maintain urine output. This resuscitation was followed by 5% dextrose in water (D_5W) to restore preburn weight. On day 2, all patients received colloid to restore plasma volume. Both groups received colloid, so we would not expect a clinically significant difference in hemodynamic parameters. In fact, the administration of colloid to patients who do not need it can be dangerous. Thermal injury directly produces a leaky membrane at the site of injury and circulating free radicals. There would be no harm in withholding albumin during the initial resuscitation until the total serum protein level drops to 5.2 g/dL, provided that the CVP is kept at 12 cm H_2O or below.

Albumin in Patients With Cirrhosis

Published reports regarding albumin use in cirrhotic patients[50-61] are characterized by formula administration of albumin whether the patient needed it or not. Patients who suffer from cirrhosis secondary to chronic alcohol consumption generally have adequate total protein levels. In fact, total protein levels are usually above average. On the other hand, albumin levels are consistently low. Since it is total protein and not albumin that produces COP, there is no reason to administer albumin to patients who are not hypo-oncotic. In the one study that recorded colloid pressures,[57] no difference was found between the study and control groups. The albumin-treated group was given 25 to 100 g daily and the dosage then titrated to keep COP between 35 and 40 cm H_2O. Recall that a normal COP is 32 to 38 cm H_2O. The CVPs were not recorded. Thus, gradients cannot be determined. No difference in outcome was noted, thus reinforcing the fact that this group of patients may not have needed albumin supplementation. One report[61] did cite the fact that albumin was necessary to maintain sodium in the circulation.

ALBUMIN AND NUTRITION

Albumin Administration and Enteral Feeding Tolerance

The movement of intestinal intraluminal fluid into the circulation is COP dependent. There is no active pump to draw water into the circulating volume. Thus, if a patient is profoundly hypoproteinemic and has hypo-oncotic interstitial edema, there may be a problem with loose bowel movements if tube feeding is

started.[62-70] The papers that dispute the correlation of low albumin concentrations with absorption[67-69] do not, however, record the patients' total protein level. Further, CVPs (P_c) are not given.

Maintenance of tissue tensile strength at the site of anastomosis is another reason to maintain a COP/CVP gradient in patients facing bowel surgery. Recall that tissue pressures are normally about -7 mm Hg. Thus, cells are packed together. If these pressures are significantly disturbed, structural integrity is lessened. Surgeons anecdotally report that the construction of an anastomosis in a profoundly hypoproteinemic patient with bowel edema is "like sewing two wet ice cream cones together." There is a recent report that documents the decrease in the ability of the hypo-oncotic edematous bowel to hold suture.[15]

Albumin Administration in Patients Receiving Total Parenteral Nutrition

There are two conflicting papers in the literature regarding albumin supplementation in patients receiving TPN. One paper[71] reports that patients receiving albumin did better. However, none of the patients in either the treated or nontreated groups had albumin levels that would be expected to be associated with clinically significant hypoproteinemia. This study did not look at edematous patients. It is the edema associated with hypoproteinemia that appears to be the most significant factor in altering outcome. A second study reporting no benefit from the administration of albumin by protocol to patients receiving TPN gave albumin to achieve a level of 2.5 g/dL.[72] This study looked at patients on the low end of the scale, that is, albumin levels between 1.9 and 2.1 g/dL. They may have administered insufficient amounts of albumin to correct hypo-oncotic edema. Nevertheless, colloid pressures, total proteins, the presence of edema, and other correlates to allow us to evaluate their data by Starling's law were not provided.

To reiterate, albumin should not be given to raise serum albumin levels alone. Albumin should be given to correct clinically significant hypo-oncotic edema by raising the total protein content. In a review of the use of albumin in TPN,[73] eight patients who had original diagnoses of ARDS and generalized anasarca because of "leaky membranes" were successfully resuscitated by adding albumin to the TPN solution. As the π_c increases above P_c, there will be a recapture by the circulating volume of interstitial edema that may necessitate diuresis with furosemide to avoid rebound hydrostatic pulmonary edema.

It is widely held that adding albumin to a TPN solution in moderate amounts (12.5 to 25 g/L) and administering it at a constant rate is more effective than giving the same amount of albumin via intravenous "piggyback" over shorter periods of time. This has not been documented. The half-life of albumin, often reported to be 20 days, has not been measured during TPN infusions. It appears that albumin administered along with TPN behaves differently.

Since inflammatory mediators suppress endogenous albumin synthesis, it will be more difficult to elevate colloid pressures to effective levels in septic patients. Under these circumstances, the old dictum of "drain the pus" remains the superseding principle of therapy. When inflammatory mediators are no longer a factor, exogenous albumin may not be necessary since the patient will be able to synthesize albumin in the uncompromised repair of malnutrition by TPN.

The most significant form of hypoproteinemia is pseudo-ARDS. The sheep animal model has been used in a plasmapheresis study to demonstrate two important observations. Lowering the π_c has twice the effect on moving fluid from the circulating volume and across the interstitial space than does elevating the PCWP.[74] In addition, replacement of

plasmapheresed colloid restores homeostasis in the pulmonary interstitial fluid flow model (Fig 8–2).[75] The observed "leak" is therefore not related to a change in σ. Hypo-oncotic edema produces a pseudoleak that is reparable.

The infusion of albumin in the clinical setting of edema has been unjustly criticized. The critiques describe albumin as leaking through the membrane and resulting in an increase in interstitial albumin and, therefore, an increase in interstitial water. This is true if σ is altered as with trauma or a chronic septic state. If this is not the case, however, profound hypoproteinemia should be viewed as a total-body albumin deficit. Under these circumstances, when albumin is administered, it will and should translocate into the interstitial space and repair the π_{if} deficit as well as the π_c deficit. This will restore the gel in the gel-sol matrix and recover series resistance to interstitial fluid flow. It complements the unaltered σ, raises π_c, and results in the mobilization of interstitial edema of the lung and intestine. The extremities, however, also need to be physically moved in order to promote lymph flow and evacuate residual dependent hypo-oncotic edema. The residual edema in muscle is mobilized by muscular contraction. Edema in the dependent skin is mobilized by a change in position or by external pressure (increase P_{if}) as generated by intermittent compression boots.

Many patients populating the intensive care unit today are different from those focused upon in the literature. Our patients now tend to be chronically malnourished and hypoproteinemic. They are different from well-nourished patients who were traumatized or underwent elective surgery and received whole blood. Hypoproteinemic patients with a total protein value of 5.2 g/dL are near the break point of edema vs. nonedema. If these patients experience increased hydrostatic pressure, decreased oncotic pressure, or decreased lymphatic flow, frank edema is likely to

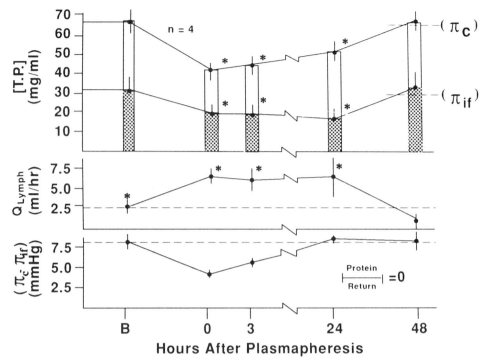

FIG 8–2.
Time courses of plasma (π_c) and lymph protein concentrations (π_{if}) and the plasma-to-lymph oncotic gradient ($\pi_c - \pi_{if}$) in four sheep. Plasmapheresis ended at B. Protein was reinfused at zero. All variables are means ± SE. * $P < 0.05$, paired Student's t-test. (From Kramer G, Harms B, Bodai B, et al: *Am J Physiol* 1982; 243:803–809. Used by permission.)

develop. Our new appreciation for total-body protein deficits, resulting in an alteration of Kf, places the clinician in the intensive care unit in a different arena than the investigators involved in many of the studies reviewed. Whole blood is simply no longer available.

Before a course of therapy is set, it is imperative to evaluate three parameters: total protein, central pressures, and the presence or absence of edema. If the total protein is 5.2 g/dL, the patient is generating a COP of approximately 17 mm Hg. A normal CVP usually produces an end-capillary hydrostatic pressure (P_c) of approximately 17 mm Hg. If a CVP determination is not available with direct monitoring, the tone of the external jugular vein can be evaluated. It is also important to check for the presence or absence of dependent pitting edema in the posterior of the thigh or calf. If the patient has no jugular venous distension, a total protein content below 5.0 g/dL, and dependent edema, then the edema

is probably secondary to a hypo-oncotic state. The obvious solution for resuscitation, whether acute or chronic, would include something to repair colloid pressure. An understanding of Starling's forces coupled with these three observations can effectively guide therapy.

Acknowledgment

The authors wish to thank J. Clarke and O. Fistrovic for their hours of library research and assistance.

REFERENCES

1. Bergstrom N, Braden B: Nutritional status during the development and resolution of pressure sores, in Funk SG, Tornquist IM, Champagne MT, et al (eds): *Key Aspects of Recovery: Improving Nutrition, Rest and Mobility in Infants, Adults and the Elderly.* New York, 1990, Springer-Verlag, pp 183–187.

2. Buzby G, Mullen J, Matthews D, et al: Prognostic nutritional index in gastrointestinal surgery. *Am J Surg* 1980; 139:160.

3. Kaminski M, Lowrie E, Rosenblatt S, et al: Malnutrition is lethal, diagnosable, and treatable in ESRD patients. *Transplat Proc* 1991; 13:1810–1817.

4. Pinchcofsky-Devin G, Kaminski M: Correlation of pressure sores and nutritional status. *J Am Geriatr Soc* 1986; 34:435–440.

5. Elwyn D, Kinney J, Gump F, et al: Metabolism and endocrine effects of fasting followed by infusion of five percent glucose. *Surgery* 1981; 90:810–816.

6. Gray C, Kaminski M: Protein-calorie malnutrition, in Kaminski M Jr (ed): *Hyperalimentation, a Guide for Clinicians.* New York, 1985, BC Dekker, pp 23–46.

7. Brenner D, Buck M, Feitelberg SP, et al: Tumor necrosis factor-α inhibits albumin gene expression in a murine model of cachexia. *J Clin Invest* 1990; 85:248.

8. Ramadore G, Van Damme J, Rieder H, et al: Interleukin 6, the third mediator of acute-phase reaction, modulates hepatic protein synthesis in human and mouse. Comparison with interleukin 1β and tumor necrosis factor-α. *Eur J Immunol* 1988; 18:1259.

9. Breslow R: Nutritional status and dietary intake of patients with pressure ulcers: Review of research literature 1943 to 1989. *Decubitus* 1991; 4:16–21.

10. Rackow E, Fein A, Siegel J: The relationship of colloid osmotic pressure gradient to pulmonary edema and mortality in critically ill patients. *Chest* 1982; 82:4.

11. Guyton AC: Capillary dynamics and exchange of fluid between the blood and the interstitial fluid, in Guyton A (ed): *Text Book of Medical Physiology,* ed 7. Philadelphia, 1986, Saunders, p 348.

12. Kaminski M, Williams S: Review of the rapid normalization of serum albumin with modified total parenteral nutrition solutions. *Crit Care Med* 1990; 18:327.

13. Mullholland J, Tui C, Wright A, et al: Protein metabolism and bedsores. *Ann Surg* 1943; 188:1015–1023.

14. Nijsten M, Hack C, Helle M, et al: Interleukin-6 and its relation to the humoral immune response and clinical parameters in burned patients. *Surgery* 1991; 109:761–767.

15. Rosas M, Kaminski M, Ninos N, et al: Intestinal edema and decreased tensile strength during hypoproteinemia (abstract). *JPEN* 1991; 15(suppl):28.

16. Kramer G, Harms B, Gunther R: The effects of hypoproteinemia on blood-to-lymph fluid transport in sheep lung. *Circ Res* 1981; 49:1173–1180.

17. Guyton A: The lymphatic system, interstitial fluid dynamics, edema and pulmonary fluid, in Guyton A (ed): *Textbook of Medical Physiology,* ed 7. Philadelphia, 1986, Saunders, p 361.

18. Civetta J: A new look at the Starling equation. *Crit Care Med* 1979; 7:84–91.

19. Kaminski M, Haase T: Use of albumin in total parenteral nutrition solutions: Understanding Starling's law and the resolution of hypo-oncotic edema, in Van Way C (ed): *Handbook of Surgical Nutrition.* Philadelphia, 1992, Lippincott, pp 272–282.

20. Kaminski M, Haase T: Albumin and colloid pressure: Implications for fluid resuscitation, in Kaufman B (ed): *Critical Care Clinics: Fluid Resuscitation of the Critically Ill.* Philadelphia, 1992, Saunders, pp 311–322.

21. Kaminski M, Haase T: Role of albumin in total parenteral solutions, in Robin A (ed): *Problems in General Surgery,* vol 8. Philadelphia, 1991, Lippincott, pp 49–56.

22. Erstad B, Gales B, Rappaport W: The use of albumin in clinical practice. *Arch Intern Med* 1991; 151:901–911.

23. Lucas C, Ledgerwood A, Higgans R, et al: Impaired pulmonary function after albumin resuscitation from shock. *J Trauma* 1980; 20:446–451.

24. Grootendorst A, van Wilhengurg M, de Laat P, et al: Albumin abuse in intensive care medicine. *Intensive Care Med* 1988; 14:554–557.

25. Zadrobilek E, Hackl W, Sporn P, et al: Effect of large volume replacement with balanced electrolyte solutions on extravascular lung water in surgical patients with sepsis syndrome. *Intensive Care Med* 1989; 15:505–510.

26. Skillman J, Restall S, Salzman E: Randomized trial of albumin vs electrolyte solutions during abdominal aortic operations. *Surgery* 1975; 78:291–303.

27. Boutros A, Ruess R, Olson L, et al: Comparison of hemodynamic, pulmonary, and renal effects of use of three types of fluids after major surgical procedures on the abdominal aorta. *Crit Care Med* 1979; 7:9–13.

28. Hauser C, Shoemaker W, Turpin I, et al: Oxygen transport responses to colloids and crystalloids in critically ill surgical patients. *Surg Gynecol Obstet* 1980; 150:811–816.

29. Zetterstrom H, Hedstrand U: Albumin treatment following major surgery, 1: Effects on plasma oncotic pressure, renal function and peripheral edema. *Acta Anaesthesiol Scand* 1981; 25:125–132.

30. Nielsen O, Engell H: Extracellular fluid volume and distribution in relation to changes in plasma colloid osmotic pressure after major surgery. *Acta Chir Scand* 1985; 151:221–225.

31. Stein L, Beraud J, Morissette M, et al: Pulmonary edema during volume infusion. *Circulation* 1975; 52:483–489.

32. Lowe R, Moss G, Jilek J, et al: Crystalloid vs colloid in the etiology of pulmonary failure after trauma: A randomized trial in man. *Surgery* 1977; 81:676–683.

33. Virgilio R, Rice C, Smith D, et al: Crystalloid vs colloid resuscitation: Is one better? *Surgery* 1981; 85:129–139.

34. Moss G, Lowe R, Jilek J, et al: Colloid or crystalloid in the resuscitation of hemorrhagic shock: A controlled clinical trial. *Surgery* 1981; 89:434–438.

35. Zetterstrom H: Albumin treatment following major surgery, II: Effects of postoperative lung function and circulatory adaptation. *Acta Anaesthesiol Scand* 1981; 25:133–141.

36. Shires T, Peitzman A, Albert S, et al: Response of extravascular lung water to intraoperative fluids. *Ann Surg* 1983; 197:515–519.

37. Rackow E, Falk J, Fein A, et al: Fluid resuscitation in circulatory shock: A comparison of the cardiorespiratory effects of albumin, hetastarch, and saline solutions in patients with hypovolemia and septic shock. *Crit Care Med* 1983; 11:839–850.

38. Skillman J, Parikh B, Tanenbaum B: Pulmonary arteriovenous admixture: Improvement with albumin and diuresis. *Am J Surg* 1970; 119:440–447.

39. Vinocur B, Artz J, Sampliner J, et al: The effect of albumin and diuretics on the alveolar-arterial oxygen gradient in patients with pulmonary insufficiency (abstract). *Chest* 1975; 68:429.

40. Appel P, Shoemaker W: Evaluation of fluid therapy in adult respiratory failure. *Crit Care Med* 1981; 9:862–869.

41. Baudendistel L, Dahms T, Kaminski D: The effect of albumin on extravascular lung water in animals and patients with low-pressure pulmonary edema. *J Surg Res* 1982; 33:285–293.

42. Metildi L, Shackford S, Virgilio R, et al: Crystalloid versus colloid in fluid resuscitation of patients with severe pulmonary insufficiency. *Surg Gynecol Obstet* 1984; 158:207–212.

43. Hallowell P, Bland J, Dalton B, et al: The effect of hemodilution with albumin or Ringer's lactate on water balance and blood use in open-heart surgery. *Ann Thorac Surg* 1978; 25:22–29.

44. Sade R, Stroud M, Crawford F, et al: A prospective randomized study of hydroxyethyl starch, albumin, and lactated Ringer's solution as priming fluid for cardiopulmonary bypass. *J Thorac Cardiovasc Surg* 1985; 89:713–722.

45. Ohqvist G, Settergren G, Bergstrom K, et al: Plasma colloid osmotic pressure during open-heart surgery using non-colloid or colloid priming solution in the extracorporeal circuit. *Scand J Thorac Cardiovasc Surg* 1981; 15:251–255.

46. Marelli D, Samson R, Edgell D, et al: Does the addition of albumin to the prime solution in cardiopulmonary bypass affect clinical outcome? *J Thorac Cardiovasc Surg* 1989; 98:751–756.

47. Bodenhamer R, Johnson R, Randolph J, et al: The effect of adding mannitol or albumin to a crystalloid cardioplegic solution: A prospective, randomized clinical study. *Ann Thorac Surg* 1985; 40:374–379.

48. Demling R: Fluid replacement in burned patients. *Surg Clin North Am* 1987; 67:15–30.

49. Goodwin C, Dorethy J, Lam V, et al: Randomized trial of efficacy of crystal-

loid and colloid resuscitation on hemo-dynamic response and lung water following thermal injury. *Ann Surg* 1983; 197:520–531.

50. Janeway C, Gibson S, Woodruff L, et al: Chemical, clinical, and immunological studies on the products of human plasma fractionation, VII: Concentrated human serum albumin. *J Clin Invest* 1944; 23:465–490.

51. Patek A Jr, Mankin H, Colcher H, et al: The effects of intravenous injection of concentrated human serum albumin upon blood plasma, ascites and renal functions in three patients with cirrhosis of the liver. *J Clin Invest* 1948; 27:135–144.

52. Faloon W, Eckhardt R, Murphy T, et al: An evaluation of human serum albumin in the treatment of cirrhosis of the liver. *J Clin Invest* 1949; 28:583–594.

53. Thorn G, Armstrong S Jr, Davenport V: Chemical, clinical, and immunological studies on the products of human plasma fractionation, XXXI: The use of salt-poor concentrated human serum albumin solution in the treatment of hepatic cirrhosis. *J Clin Invest* 1946; 25:304–323.

54. Kunkel H, Labby D, Ahrens E Jr, et al: The use of concentrated human serum albumin in the treatment of cirrhosis of the liver. *J Clin Invest* 1948; 27:305–319.

55. Wilkinson P, Sherlock S: The effect of repeated albumin infusions in patients with cirrhosis. *Lancet* 1962; 2:1125–1129.

56. McCormick P, Mistry P, Kaye G, et al: Intravenous albumin infusion is an effective therapy for hyponatremia in cirrhotic patients with ascites. *Gut* 1990; 31:204–207.

57. Gines P, Arroyo V, Quintero E, et al: Comparison of paracentesis and diuretics in the treatment of cirrhotics with tense ascites. *Gastroenterology* 1987; 93:234–241.

58. Gines P, Tito L, Arroyo V, et al: Randomized comparative study of therapeutic paracentesis with and without intravenous albumin in cirrhosis. *Gastroenterology* 1988; 94:1493–1520.

59. Tito L, Gines P, Arroyo V, et al: Total paracentesis associated with intravenous albumin management of patients with cirrhosis and ascites. *Gastroenterology* 1990; 98:146–151.

60. Spanish Group for the Study and Treatment of Ascites: Multicenter randomized comparative study of therapeutic paracentesis (TP) plus intravenous albumin and peritoneovenous shunt (PV-S) in cirrhotics with refractory ascites. *J Hepatol* 1989; 9(suppl 1):86.

61. Nelson W, Rosenbaum J, Strauss M: Hyponatremia in hepatic cirrhosis following paracentesis. *J Clin Invest* 1951; 30:738–744.

62. Brinson R, Kolts B: Hypoalbuminemia as an indicator of diarrheal incidence in critically ill patients. *Crit Cart Med* 1987; 15:506–509.

63. Brinson R, Kolts B: Diarrhea associated with severe hypoalbuminemia: A comparison of a peptide-based chemically defined diet and standard enteral alimentation. *Crit Care Med* 1988; 16:130–136.

64. Cobb L, Cartmill A, Gilsdorf R: Early postoperative nutritional support using the serosal tunnel jejunostomy. *JPEN* 1981; 5:397–401.

65. Ford E, Jennings M, Andrassy R: Serum albumin (oncotic pressure) correlates with enteral feeding tolerance in the pediatric surgical patient. *J Pediatr Surg* 1987; 22:597–599.

66. Moss G: Malabsorption associated with extreme malnutrition: Importance of replacing plasma albumin *J Am Coll Nutr* 1982; 1:89–92.

67. Benya R, Damle P, Mobarhan S: Diarrhea complicating enteral feeding after liver transplant. *Nutr Rev* 1990; 48:148–152.

68. Norton J, Ott L, McClain C, et al: Intolerance to enteral feeding in the brain-injured patient. *J Neurosurg* 1988; 68:62–66.

69. Pesola G, Hogg J, Yonnios T, et al: Isotonic vasogastric tube feedings: Do they cause diarrhea? *Crit Care Med* 1989; 17:1151–1155.

70. Edes T, Walk B, Austin J: Diarrhea in tube-fed patients: Feeding formula not necessarily the cause. *Am J Med* 1990; 88:91–93.

71. Brown R, Bradley J, Bekemeyer W, et al: Effect of albumin supplementation during parenteral nutrition on hospital morbidity. *Crit Care Med* 1988; 16:1177–1182.

72. Foley E, Borlase B, Dzik W, et al: Albumin supplementation in the critically ill. *Arch Surg* 1990; 125:739–742.

73. Kaminski M Jr, Haase T: Hypo-oncotic edema misdiagnosed as a leaky membrane can be resolved by adding albumin to TPN solutions. (abstract). *J Am Coll Nutr* 1991; 10:551.

74. Kramer G, Harms B, Bodai E, et al: The effects of hypoproteinemia and increased vascular pressure on lung fluid balance in sheep. *J Appl Physiol* 1983; 55:1514–1522.

75. Kramer G, Harms B, Bodai B, et al: Mechanisms for redistribution of plasma protein following acute protein depletion. *Am J Physiol* 1982; 243:803–809.

9

Amino Acids and Respiratory Function

Pierre Singer, M.D.

David P. Katz, Ph.D.

Jeffrey Askanazi, M.D.

Effects of protein malnutrition on the respiratory system

Quantitative and qualitative effects of amino acids on the central nervous system

Serotonin theory

Aspartate theory

Effects of amino acids on respiratory muscles

Effects of amino acids on metabolism

Amino acid effects on sleep and respiration in normal subjects

Clinical applications

Protein intake and weaning from the ventilator

Apnea in renal failure and prematurity

The interrelations between nutrition and respiratory function are well known. Calorie restriction has been associated with a decreased metabolic rate and decreased ventilatory response to hypoxemia and hypercapnia in normal subjects.[1, 2] On the contrary, nutrients that induce hypermetabolism also serve as stimuli to ventilation.[3] Patients with emphysema or chronic bronchitis are often malnourished,[4] and their weight loss is associated with an increased resting energy expenditure (REE) and a higher mortality rate.[5, 6] Carbohydrate and lipid administration is known to affect the respiratory system.[7, 8] Less appreciated are the affects of protein intake on respiratory function. Our aims in this chapter are to review the mechanisms of action of amino acids on the respiratory centers, muscle function, and the respiratory muscles. We discuss the clinical applications of amino acids as pharmacologic agents in the treatment of diseases such as sleep apnea, apnea of prematurity, muscular fatigue, and weaning from mechanical ventilation.

EFFECTS OF PROTEIN MALNUTRITION ON THE RESPIRATORY SYSTEM

Acute fasting of 1, 2, or 3 days in animals results in a reduction in body weight, diaphragm strength and endurance, and blood glucose levels.[9] However, diaphragm weight, thickness, and glycogen content are unchanged. The authors suggest that hypoglycemia may induce the reduction in diaphragmatic contractility observed in short-term fasting.

Prolonged starvation (3 weeks) has been demonstrated to decrease tissue elasticity as well as increase surface forces in rats.[10] Nutritional depletion is common in lung disease and occurs in 50% of patients with acute respiratory diseases.[11] Moreover, Rogers et al.[12] showed that 70% of patients with chronic obstructive pulmonary disease (COPD) admitted to the hospital had weight loss. Weight loss may be beneficial in overweight patients with COPD[13] because the reduced metabolic demands lead to lower respiratory requirements, lower $Paco_2$, and improved muscle strength. On the other hand, normal-weight patients with COPD who sustain weight loss may show a deterioration in their respiratory parameters. Our group suggests that the increased REE observed in malnourished patients with COPD induces the weight loss. This increase in REE may be due to an increase in the work of breathing.[14]

Arora and Rochester[15] demonstrated that the respiratory muscles were not preserved during prolonged starvation or stress catabolism. Decreased diaphragmatic muscle mass paralleled skeletal muscle loss. However, the impairment in respiratory muscle function exceeded the muscle loss. This impairment may result from decreased glycogen or bichemical alterations in the muscle cells (decreased adenosine triphosphate [ATP] levels or hypophosphatemia). Refeeding of malnourished patients with COPD improves respiratory muscle function before peripheral muscle function.[16] Undernourished patients without lung disease have reduced inspiratory and expiratory muscle strength and endurance.[17] This reduction is directly proportional to the degree of weight loss and results in a reduction in maximal voluntary ventilation.

Mechanical ventilation adversely affects respiratory muscles and leads to muscular atrophy when controlled mechanical ventilation is used. On the other hand, mechanical ventilation of patients with acute respiratory failure decreases respiratory muscle work, which compensates for the reduced efficacy of gas exchange. As soon as objective indices of adequate lung and respiratory function reappear, weaning from the ventilator should be started. Nutritional support is important to ensure adequate respiratory muscle strength and endurance for maintenance of spontaneous ventilation.[18, 19] A positive nitrogen balance and regeneration of lost lean tissue, including respiratory muscles, are important goals. The optimal weaning diet remains to be determined.

QUANTITATIVE AND QUALITATIVE EFFECTS OF AMINO ACIDS ON THE CENTRAL NERVOUS SYSTEM

Protein and amino acids have been shown to alter respiratory patterns by modifying the ventilatory drive. One thousand kilocalories of egg albumin ingested orally is followed in 2 to 3 hours by an increase in minute ventilation and oxygen consumption and a higher ventilatory response to hypoxemia and hypercapnia.[3] Eight semi-starved subjects who received 400 kcal/day for 7 days demonstrated an increase in minute volume and oxygen consumption 4 hours after receiving a 20-kcal/hr amino acid mixture. This increase persisted during the 24 hours of infusion and resulted in a leftward shift of the minute volume–$Paco_2$ relationship toward enhanced ventilatory sensitivity.[20] When nitrogen intake was modified from 7.5 mg of nitrogen per kilocalorie of REE (11 g/day) to 15 mg of nitrogen per kilocalorie of REE (21 g/day), a significant reduction in $Paco_2$ was observed, and a marked leftward shift of the relationship between minute volume and $Paco_2$ was noted. These results indicated an increased ventilatory sensitivity to CO_2 during increased protein intake.[21]

Examination of plasma amino acids during amino acid administration indicated a significant increase in the ratio of the large neutral amino acids (valine, isoleucine, leucine, tyrosine, and phenylalanine) as compared with tryptophan.[22] Takala et al. compared the effects of a standard amino acid solution (23% branched-chain amino acids [BCAAs] with a BCAA-enriched solution (85%)[23] in 6 healthy volunteers. The high-BCAA solution appeared to magnify the respiratory stimulation observed with the standard solution. The central respiratory drive was increased as shown by increased minute volume and V_T/T_I (mean inspiratory flow) and decreased $Paco_2$ with carbon dioxide production unchanged.

Serotonin Theory

Neurotransmitters are important for the transmission of electrical potentials. There are more than 40 neurotransmitters, including the amino acids glutamate, aspartate, taurine, glycine, and 5-hydroxytryptamine (5-HT) or serotonin.[24] Tryptophan is actively transported across the cell membrane to the presynaptic nerve terminal. There, it is hydroxylated to 5-HT, or serotonin. 5-HT is degraded to hydroxyindole acetic acid (5-HIAA). Transport of large neutral amino acids across the blood-brain barrier depends upon the plasma amino acid concentration. There is also competition between amino acids for a common transporter. For tryptophan, penetration into the brain depends upon the levels of other large neutral

amino acids, including BCAAs.[25]

An increase in the plasma tryptophan concentration may lead to higher levels of brain tryptophan. This increases the synthesis of 5-HT, and its concentration rises in the brain. The net result is an increase in the release of neurotransmitter into the synapse. 5-HT can induce changes in behavior[26] such as increased sleep duration, fatigue, increased pain tolerance, or altered food intake. These aspects have been discussed extensively elsewhere.[25]

The response of the ventilatory drive to amino acid infusion exceeds the observed increase in metabolic rate.[20] These ventilatory drive responses parallel the change in the ratio of tryptophan to other amino acids that compete with tryptophan for transport across the blood-brain barrier (valine, leucine, isoleucine, tyrosine, phenylalanine).[22] These findings, together with the fact that 5-HT inhibits respiration,[27, 28] led to the hypothesis that the increased respiratory sensitivity noted with amino acid infusion was mediated through inhibition of central 5-HT synthesis secondary to excess levels of amino acids that oppose tryptophan uptake through the blood-brain barrier. This phenomenon is supported by the study of Takala et al.[23] They observed that increases in the plasma ratio of large neutral amino acids to tryptophan lead to increases in respiratory drive.

Aspartate Theory

Important structures in respiratory control are located near the ventrolateral medullary surface.[29] Glutamate applied to this region increases ventilation by binding to N-methyl-D-aspartate receptors. This effect is dose dependent and additive to the CO_2 drive effect.[30]

EFFECTS OF AMINO ACIDS ON RESPIRATORY MUSCLES

It is well established that sepsis, trauma, and surgery result in a negative nitrogen balance largely because of an increase in skeletal muscle breakdown.[31] The amino acids provided by this breakdown are used for repair processes, immune system integrity, and gluconeogenesis. Muscle breakdown also provides BCAAs, which are oxidized by muscles.

Respiratory muscle fatigue is common during critical illness,[32] and there is a rationale for direct therapeutic efforts at maximizing muscle capacity and decreasing fatigue. In isolated rat diaphragm,[33] leucine (a BCAA) stimulates muscle protein synthesis and decreases protein degradation. However, valine and isoleucine have little effect on this muscle preparation. Our group investigated the direct effects of BCAAs on isometric force production, fatigue, and recovery in isolated rat hemidiaphragms in the absence of systematic and neurohumoral interactions.[34] Fatigue was induced by 10-minute stimulation with 30 trains per minute of 5 Hz at a 50% duty cycle. The effects of Krebs'-Ringer's buffer solution was compared with balanced mixtures of amino acids and a mixture of valine, leucine, and isoleucine. This last mixture had an ameliorative effect on fatigue when expressed as isometric tension elicited by single and tetanic stimuli. We next evaluated the contribution of the individual BCAA.[35] A reduction in fatigue was obtained with leucine and the BCAA mixture but not with valine or isoleucine alone.

Respiratory muscle mass and function are compromised during malnutrition and stress. Experimental data suggest that leucine may improve protein synthesis, decrease proteolysis, and decrease diaphragm fatigue. However, clinical studies confirming these findings are lacking.

EFFECTS OF AMINO ACIDS ON METABOLISM

The caloric value of protein is 4.3 kcal/g. For each gram oxidized, 965 mL of O_2 is consumed along with the production of 781 mL of CO_2, 0.41 g of water, and 0.16 g of urinary nitrogen. The result is a respiratory quotient (RQ) of 0.81. Under normal conditions, the specific dynamic action (thermic effect) of food increases energy expenditure by about 10%. This effect is almost entirely due to the protein component.[36] The protein content of the diet averages 20% of the caloric intake. Therefore, the thermic effect of protein is equal to 50% of its available energy (2 kcal/g). Most of the thermic effect of protein is due to increased protein synthesis since four to five high-energy phosphate bonds are cleared for each amino acid incorporated.[37] If 300 g of protein is synthesized in a day, the caloric cost is 225 kcal (12% of the basal metabolism).

Three hours after the administration of 1000 kcal of egg albumin solution through a nasogastric tube[3] to normal subjects, there is an increase in minute ventilation from 7.8 ± 0.3 to 9.2 ± 0.2 L/min in V_{O_2} from 241 ± 6.7 to 270 ± 5.4 mL/min, and in V_{CO_2} from 183 ± 10.6 to 213 ± 8 mL/min. The hypoxemic ventilatory response increases from 105 ± 14.5 to 219 ± 17.3 without the occurrence of systemic acidosis. Similar to carbohydrate administration, protein load is associated with an increase in REE.

This metabolic effect of amino acids was confirmed when amino acids were infused into subjects following 7 days of semistarvation.[20] Four hundred kilocalories of amino acids infused in 24 hours resulted in an increase in tidal volume, minute ventilation, oxygen consumption, and metabolic rate (by 8%).

The effects of total parenteral nutrition (TPN) (1.5 g/kg of amino acid and nonprotein energy corresponding to the pre-TPN energy expenditure with 40% as lipids) on V_{O_2}, V_{CO_2}, RQ, and REE were studied in ventilated patients with multiple trauma ($n = 10$) and sepsis ($n = 17$).[38] V_{O_2}, V_{CO_2}, and REE increased significantly. TPN also altered the CO_2 set point. In these septic patients, V_D/V_T was not modified. Therefore, an increase in alveolar ventilation was required to maintain the $Paco_2$ at stable levels. When the effect of amino acids alone (1.5 g/kg) was studied, an increase in REE to 26% above predicted levels was noted. The increase in Vo_2 was smaller (only 3%), but Vco_2 was increased to the same magnitude as REE. These data are difficult to interpret since the metabolic response to TPN has a relatively small effect on ventilatory demand during controlled mechanical ventilation. The effects of different substrates on spontaneous breathing in acutely ill patients are currently under investigation.

AMINO ACID EFFECTS ON SLEEP AND RESPIRATION IN NORMAL SUBJECTS

Over the last 25 years, many controlled studies have suggested that tryptophan increases sleep duration.[39] Sleep patterns, oxygen saturation, and end-tidal CO_2 were studied in five healthy volunteers by polysomnography, pulse oxymetry, and capnography.[40] The subjects were studied at night while receiving a normal saline infusion, no infusion (control), or a BCAA infusion. End-tidal CO_2 levels during the BCAA infusion were lower (P < .01) when compared with controls (44 ± 5 mm Hg vs. 52 ± 1 mm Hg). The BCAAs seemed to act as ventilatory stimulators during sleep.

CLINICAL APPLICATIONS

Protein Intake and Weaning From the Ventilator

Since protein increases the ventilatory drive (probably by decreasing serotonin synthesis in the brain), van den Berg et al.[41] studied the effect of different protein contents on metabolic and ventilatory variables during weaning from mechanical ventilation in patients receiving enteral feeding. Ten patients who had pulmonary, cardiac, or neuro-

logic disease and were ventilated at least 13 days and in whom weaning had failed at least once were included in the study. They received 30 hours of a diet composed of 480 kcal of carbohydrate, 360 kcal of fat, and 160 kcal of protein (moderate-protein intake) or 210 kcal of protein (high-protein intake) per 1000 mL. The study was performed as a crossover trial and revealed significant increases in Vco_2 and RQ for both regimens (as compared with baseline). During weaning, the high-protein diet was associated with a higher minute ventilation, $Paco_2$, and Vco_2 when compared with the moderate-protein diet. These data suggest an increase in ventilatory sensitivity to CO_2 secondary to high-protein intake. The authors concluded that high-protein intake may be beneficial during weaning in ventilated patients. However, the increase in Vco_2 observed in these patients may be deleterious if the increase in minute ventilation induced by the diet increases the work of breathing. Others have failed to find any differences in ventilatory parameters when using standard- or high-protein regimens and moderate or high BCAA concentrations. They reported no differences in minute ventilation, Vco_2, $Paco_2$, and the ventilatory response to CO_2 inhalation in postoperative patients ventilated with pressure support.[42]

Failure to wean is a major complication of mechanical ventilation. It probably relates to the increased oxygen cost of the work of breathing. Disconnecting intensive care patients from the ventilator can increase their Vo_2 by 24%.[43, 44] In addition to lung disease, bronchospasm, pulmonary secretions, obesity, abdominal distension, and nutrition (carbohydrate overfeeding, malnutrition) play a key role in the generation of increased work of breathing. When muscular fatigue occurs, weaning fails.

Nutrition support seems to improve muscle strength and endurance[18] and has been found to significantly improve the success of weaning[18, 19] when compared with 5% dextrose in water (D_5W).

However, overfeeding of calories may be deleterious. High glucose infusion rates are well known to elevate the metabolic rate and may induce respiratory failure in patients with COPD or respiratory compromise. High-protein intake has also be associated with increased minute ventilation and respiratory effort.[45] Therefore, recommendations regarding the exact amount of protein to administer to a patient during the weaning process remain to be determined.

BCAAs stimulate the ventilatory drive by lowering the $Paco_2$ set point in normal subjects. However, their effects during the weaning process remain unclear. Takala et al.[46] studied 30 open heart surgery patients on the first postoperative day after weaning from mechanical ventilation. They received 400 kcal of BCAAs, conventional amino acids, or dextrose over a period of 18 hours. Breathing frequency and alveolar ventilation were increased and $Paco_2$ was decreased in the BCAA-fed group. No changes were noticed in tidal volume or dead space. This study suggests a higher efficiency of CO_2 removal when BCAAs are used despite an increase in Vco_2. On the other hand, Delafosse et al. failed to observe increases in ventilatory drive while using BCAAs (lower amount than Takala et al.) in postoperative patients receiving inspiratory pressure support ventilation.[42]

Apnea in Renal Failure and Prematurity

In chronic renal failure, both obstructive and central apnea may occur.[47] Soreide et al.[48] studied seven patients receiving hemodialysis (three times per week) who had reduced sleep quality and decreased rapid eye movement (REM) sleep. They randomly received 4% BCAAs (60 mg/kg/hr) or saline for 7 hours on 2 nights of the study. The BCAA infusion was associated with a significant decrease in end-tidal CO_2 during both REM and non-REM sleep ($P < 0.05$). These findings suggest that BCAAs stimulate respiration and im-

prove sleep quality in patients with sleep disturbances.

Periodic breathing is common in premature infants. Apnea of prematurity is defined as cessation of breathing for a period of 20 seconds or more or respiratory cessation accompanied by cyanosis, bradycardia, hypotonia, metabolic acidosis, or pallor.[49] In 433 episodes of apnea of prematurity occurring in 76 premature infants, 55% were of central origin, 12% were obstructive, and the remainder was mixed. Durand et al.[50] demonstrated a decrease in minute ventilation in preterm infants with apnea that was associated with an elevation in end-tidal CO_2. There was also a significant depression in CO_2 sensitivity.[51] Others[52] have documented alterations in serotonin concentrations in selected respiratory nuclei during acute hypoxemia. Our group[53] supplemented ten newborns with TPN containing 30% BCAAs on the first day, enhanced BCAAs (53%) on the second day, and 30% BCAAs again on the third day. Computerized pulmonary function, apnea frequency, and amino acid patterns were analyzed. Following enhanced BCAA infusion, there was an increase in plasma levels of valine, leucine, and isoleucine. Dynamic compliance was increased significantly ($P < 0.05$) when day 2 data were compared with day 1 or 3 results. The peak-to-peak pressure decreased from 5.96 ± 0.93 to 4.09 ± 2.34 cm H_2O ($P < 0.05$) during the BCAA-enriched infusions and returned to baseline on day 3. Four of the ten premature infants had significant apneic spells. During the increased BCAA infusions, the number of apnea spells was decreased from 58 per 12 hours to 11 per 12 hours ($P < 0.01$). Multiple regression analysis demonstrated that the increase in dynamic compliance, the decrease in expiratory resistance, and the decrease in peak-to-peak pressure were directly related to the plasma total BCAA level. BCAAs may improve respiratory muscle function by increasing the power of diaphragmatic contractility and decreasing muscular fatigue.[34, 35]

Newborn and premature infants have low total muscle mass and a low amount of high-twitch oxidative (type I) fibers. The diaphragm of the neonate contains approximately 10% of these fibers vs. 25% in babies and 50% in adults.[54] The decrease in apneic spells may be due to the central effect of BCAAs. Moreover, apneic episodes may be of diaphragmatic origin.[55] The effect of BCAAs on the diaphragm may decrease the apnea phenomenon.

Poor nutritional status affects pulmonary function by compromising respiratory muscle strength and function, decreasing the ventilatory drive, and altering lung defense against infections. Nutritional support is mandatory in patients with respiratory disease and nutritional failure. Amino acids have physiologic and pharmacologic actions aside from the provision of nitrogen. They enhance the ventilatory drive, and this effect is related to the amino acid profile. BCAAs have a greater effect on minute volume—arterial Pco_2 relationships than do regular amino acid solutions. BCAAs, mainly leucine, alter ventilatory responses and reduce diaphragmatic fatigue. Finally, amino acids increase energy expenditure, oxygen consumption, and CO_2 production. These effects depend upon the nutritional status and the amount of protein administered. BCAA-enriched solutions may be clinically of benefit in patients with sleep apnea or hypoventilation and in neonates suffering from apnea of prematurity. However, excess amino acids may induce hyperventilation in patients with borderline COPD and may lead to respiratory decompensation. Further study of the pharmacologic effects of amino acids on the respiratory system is required to better define their clinical utility.

REFERENCES

1. Doeckel RC, Zwillich CW, Scoggin CH, et al: Clinical semi-starvation. Depression of hypoxic ventilatory response. N Engl J Med 1976; 295:358.
2. Keys A, Brozek J, Henshel A, et al: Biology of Human Starvation. Minneapolis, University of Minnesota Press, 1950.
3. Zwillich CW, Sahn SA, Weil JA: Effects of hypermetabolism on ventilation and chemosensitivity. J Clin Invest 1977; 60:900.
4. Openbrier DR, Irwin MM, Dauber JH, et al: Factors affecting nutritional status and the impact of nutritional support in patients with emphysema. Chest 1984; 85(suppl):67.
5. Goldstein S, Thomashow B, Kvetan V, et al: Nitrogen and energy relationship in malnourished patients with emphysema. Am Rev Respir Dis 1988; 138:636.
6. Vandenbergh E, Van de Woestijne KP, Gyselen A: Weight changes in the terminal stages of chronic obstructive pulmonary disease: Relation to respiratory function and prognosis. Am Rev Respir Dis 1967; 95:556.
7. Heymsfield SB, Head CA, McManus CB III, et al: Respiratory, cardiovascular and metabolic effects of enteral hyperalimentation: Influence of formula dose and composition. Am J Clin Nutr 1984; 40:116.
8. Askanazi J, Nordenstrom J, Rosenbaum SH, et al: Nutrition for the patient with respiratory failure: Glucose versus fat. Anesthesiology 1981; 54:373.
9. Shindoh C, Dimarco A, Lust W, et al: Effect of acute fasting on diaphragm strength and endurance. Am Rev Respir Dis 1991; 144:488.
10. D'Amours R, Clerch L, Massaro D: Food deprivation and surfactant in adult rats. J Appl Physiol 1983; 565:1413.
11. Pingleton SK, Eulberg M: Nutritional analysis of acute respiratory failure patients (abstract). Chest 1983; 84:1343.
12. Rogers RM, Dauber JH, Saunder MH, et al: Nutrition and COPD: State of the art. Chest 1984; 85:635.
13. Openbrier DR, Irwin MM, Rogers RM, et al: Nutritional status and lung function in patients with emphysema and chronic bronchitis. Chest 1983; 88:17.
14. See reference 5.
15. Arora NS, Rochester DF: Effect of body weight and muscularity on human diaphragm muscle mass, thickness and area. J Appl Physiol 1982; 52:63.

164   Specific Nutrients: Proteins

16. Whittaker JS, Ryan CF, Buckley PA, et al: The effects of refeeding on peripheral and respiratory muscle function in malnourished chronic obstructive pulmonary disease patients. *Am Rev Respir Dis* 1990; 142:283.

17. Arora NS, Rochester DF: Respiratory muscle strength and maximal voluntary ventilation in undernourished patients. *Am Rev Respir Dis* 1982; 126:5.

18. Mattar JA, Velasco IT, Esgaib AS: Parenteral nutrition as a useful method for weaning patients from mechanical ventilation. *JPEN* 1978; 2(suppl):50.

19. Bassili HR, Deitel M: Effect of nutritional support on weaning patients off mechanical ventilation. *JPEN* 1981; 5:161.

20. Weissman C, Askanazi J, Rosenbaum SH, et al: Amino acids and respiration. *Ann Intern Med* 1983; 98:41.

21. Askanazi J, Weissman C, Lasala PA, et al: Effect of protein intake on ventilatory drive. *Anesthesiology* 1984; 60:106.

22. Askanazi J, Weissman C, Lasala PA, et al: Nutrients and ventilation. *Adv Shock Res* 1983; 9:69.

23. Takala J, Askanazi J, Weissman C, et al: Changes in respiratory control induced by amino acids infusions. *Crit Care Med* 1988; 16:465.

24. Iversen LL: Neurotransmitters and CNS disease. *Lancet* 1982; 2:914.

25. Skeie B, Kvetan V, Gil KM, et al: Branch-chain amino acids: Their metabolism and clinical utility. *Crit Care Med* 1990; 18:549.

26. Anderson GH: Diet, neurotransmitters and brain function. *Br Med Bull* 1981; 37:95.

27. Armijo JA, Florez J: The influence of increased brain 5-hydroxytryptamine upon the respiratory activity of cats. *Neuropharmacology* 1974; 13:977.

28. Lundberg DB, Mueller RA, Breese GR: An evaluation of the mechanism by which serotoninergic activation depresses respiration. *J Pharmacol Exp Ther* 1980; 212:397.

29. Millhorn DE, Eldridge F: Role of ventrolateral medullary surface in regulation of respiratory and cardiovascular systems. *J Appl Physiol* 1986; 61:1249.

30. Mitra J, Prabhakar NR, Overholt JL, et al: Respiratory effects of N-methyl-D-aspartate on the ventrolateral medul-

31. lary surface. *J Appl Physiol* 1989; 67:1814.

31. Kinney JM, Duke JH Jr, Long CL, et al: Tissue fuel and weight loss after injury. *J Clin Pathol* 1970; 23(suppl):65.

32. Macklem PT, et al: Respiratory muscle fatigue. *Am Rev Respir Dis* 1992; 142:474.

33. Fulks RM, Li JB, Goldberg AL: Effects of insulin, glucose, and amino acids on protein turnover in rat diaphragm. *J Biol Chem* 1975; 250:290.

34. Yamada H, Ohta Y, Chaudhry I, et al: Effects of branched chain amino acids (BCAA) on diaphragm fatigue in vitro (abstract). *Anesthesiology* 1990; 73:1150.

35. Yamada H, Kvetan V, Ohta Y, et al: Effect of individual branched chain amino acids on contractility and fatigue of diaphragm (abstract). *Anesthesiology* 1990; 73:258.

36. Elwyn DH, Kinney JM, Askanazi J: Energy expenditure in surgical patients. *Surg Clin North Am* 1981; 61:545.

37. Elwyn DH: Protein metabolism and requirements in the critically ill patient. *Crit Care Clin* 1987; 3:57.

38. Takala J: Parenteral nutrition in respiratory failure, in *The Role of Nutrition in Pulmonary Disease.* Chicago, Abbott, 1990, pp 69–72.

39. Spinweber CL, Ursin R, Hilbert L, et al: L-Tryptophan: Effects on daytime sleep latency and the waking EEG. *Electroencephalogr Clin Neurophysiol* 1983; 55:652.

40. Kirvela O, Thorpy M, Takala J, et al: Respiratory and sleep patterns during nocturnal infusions of branched chain amino acids. *Acta Anaesthesiol Scand* 1990; 34:645.

41. Van den Berg B, Stam H, Hop WCJ: Effects of dietary protein content on weaning from the ventilator. *Clin Nutr* 1989; 8:207.

42. Delafosse B, Bouffard Y, Bertrand O, et al: Effects of protein intake on pulmonary gas exchange and ventilatory drive in postoperative patients. *Anesthesiology* 1989; 70:404.

43. Bursztein S, Taitelman U, De Myttenaere S, et al: Reduced oxygen consumption in catabolic states with mechanical ventilation. *Crit Care Med* 1978; 6:162.

44. Field S, Kelly SM, Macklem PT: The ox-

ygen cost of breathing in patients with cardiorespiratory disease. *Am Rev Respir Dis* 1982; 126:9.

45. Askanazi J, Weissman C, Rosenbaum SH, et al: Nutrition and the respiratory system. *Crit Care Med* 1982; 10:163.

46. Takala J, Kiiski R, Kari A: Ventilatory stimulation by branched chain amino acids after weaning from mechanical ventilation. *Clin Nutr* 1989; 8(suppl):3663.

47. Kimmel PL, Miller G, Mendelsohn WB: Sleep apnea syndrome in chronic renal disease. *Am J Med* 1989; 86:308.

48. Soreide E, Kirvela O, Ginsberg N, et al: Respiratory effects of nocturnal infusion of 4% branched chain amino acids (BCAA) solution in patients with chronic renal failure. *Clin Nutr* 1990; 9(suppl):23.

49. Klesh WK, Brozanski BS, Guthrie RD: Apnea of prematurity; current theories of pathogenesis and treatment, in Guthrie RD (ed): *Neonatal Intensive Care*. New York, Churchill Livingstone, 1988, pp 91–122.

50. Durand M, Georgie S, Barberis C, et al: Ventilatory response to CO_2 in preterm infants with idiopathic apnea, in Jones CT, Nathanielsz PN (eds): *The Physiological Development of the Fetus and Newborn*. London, Academic Press, 1985, p 211.

51. Gerhardt T, Bancalari E: Apnea of prematurity: Lung function and regulation of breathing. *Pediatrics* 1984; 74:58.

52. Lawson EE, Long WA, Gingras-Leatherman J, et al: Hypoxemia and endogenous neurotransmittors in newborns, in Bianchi AL, Denairt-Saubie B (eds): *Neurogenesis of Central Respiratory Rhythm*. Lanchester, England, MTP Press, 1985, p 422.

53. Blazer S, Reinersman GT, Askanazi J, et al: The effect of branched chain amino acid supplementation on respiratory pattern and function in the neonate (abstract). *Anesthesiology* 1991; 73:231.

54. Keens TG, Bryan AC, Levinson H, et al: Developmental pattern of muscle types in human ventilatory muscles. *J Appl Physiol* 1978; 44:909.

55. Martin RJ, Miller MJ, Carlo WA: Pathogenesis of apnea in preterm infants. *J Pediatr* 1986; 109:733.

B: Carbohydrates, Lipids, Nucleic Acids

10

Glucose vs. Lipid Calories

Fredric J. Cohen, M.D.

Carbohydrate and lipid metabolic pathways

Review of clinical trials comparing glucose with lipid calories with respect to protein metabolism

Potential adverse consequences of carbo-

hydrate feeding

Potential adverse consequences of lipid feeding

Recommendations for therapy

Controversies in the optimal delivery of any type of medical therapy usually arise as a result of insufficient or undiscovered data comparing available treatment options. This is certainly one of the reasons for the continuing controversies surrounding nutritional therapy in critically ill patients. In this diverse group of patients, experts have failed to reach consensus on the answers to questions regarding optimal nutrient balance. They have also failed to agree on just what questions need to be answered before such a consensus can be reached. Will the ideal nonprotein nutritional constituent be one that best benefits protein metabolism regardless of other possible adverse effects (i.e., impaired lung function or immune suppression)? For that matter, what constitutes the most favorable effect on protein metabolism? Most experts agree that sparing muscle protein is a major goal of nutritional therapy. However, proof that reversal of muscle protein ca-

tabolism with nutritional therapy improves patient outcome is lacking.

When critically reviewing the literature comparing glucose with lipid calories in the management of critically ill patients, one must remember that conclusions and recommendations for therapy frequently are based on individual perceptions of the principal goals of nutritional therapy. It is not surprising that no consensus on the optimal ratio of glucose to lipid calories in the nutritional management of critically ill patients has been reached since no consensus exists on the optimal goals of nutritional therapy itself. Despite this lack of consensus, there is a wealth of data comparing glucose with lipid as the primary calorie source.

In this chapter, I will attempt to reach specific conclusions regarding glucose and lipid calorie sources by comparing and contrasting their effects on protein metabolism and amino acid distribution, organ function (especially lung and liver function), and immunity. I will then try to bridge an existent gap between scientific study and clinical practice by proposing several general guidelines for therapy.

CARBOHYDRATE AND LIPID METABOLIC PATHWAYS

It is important when designing nutritional regimens to understand the body's responses to infused or enterally fed nutrients so as to optimize fuel utilization efficiency. The term "stress state" or "critical illness" refers to that condition characterized by hypermetabolism, hyperglycemia, insulin resistance, and negative nitrogen balance and is analogous to the "flow phase" of stress as described by Cuthbertson.[1] The following discussion will concentrate on the body's metabolic responses during stress.

Basal glucose production is elevated in critically ill patients and is not fully suppressed by exogenously administered glucose, as occurs in normal patients.[2-5] The increased glucose appearance in the blood results from the accelerated rate of endogenous production of glucose from gluconeogenesis and hepatic glycogenolysis and contributes to the observed "insulin resistance" seen during stress.[6] In later stages of illness and even after recovery, persistent insulin resistance may result more from defective insulin-stimulated glucose utilization than from increased glucose production.[7] Substrates for glucose production include lactate (via the Cori cycle)[4] and, to a lesser extent, glycerol, alanine, and other amino acids.[8] Hormonal stimulation of glucose production is mediated by glucagon, cortisol, and catecholamines, the levels of all of which are usually elevated in critical illness[9-11]; glucagon, however, appears to be the principal mediator of increased glucose production.[10]

Peripheral glucose clearance is mediated by insulin, except in those tissues not dependent on insulin for glucose uptake, i.e., brain, erythrocytes, wound tissue, skin, and lung. Normally, the glucose concentration is determined by the rate of glucose production and is not greatly influenced by changing rates of glucose clearance resulting from insulin release and peripheral insulin action.[12] However, in burns, trauma, and sepsis, glucose clearance is markedly enhanced because of increased insulin-independent clearance of glucose (i.e., in wound tissue).[8, 13, 14] When the rate of appearance of glucose is sufficiently high, however, the ability of insulin-independent tissues to clear glucose may be overwhelmed, and insulin, whose effectiveness for glucose clearance is diminished in critical illness, may be unable to maintain euglycemia.[10] Interestingly, glucose oxidation, previously thought to be impaired in critical illness, seems to be normal in burned and septic patients and is primarily limited only by glucose uptake.[15]

Following trauma, sepsis, and burn injury, free fatty acid (FFA) release, as reflected by FFA or glycerol turnover, is increased.[2, 16, 17] The majority (60% to 70%) of FFA released in the basal state is reesterified in the liver. Liver uptake of FFAs is determined by the rate of FFA delivery to the liver and is not under hormonal control.[2, 17] Increased esterification can result in a fatty liver if very low density lipoprotein (VLDL) production and triglyceride release are not proportionately increased. While FFA recycling rates are increased in critically ill patients, basal fat oxidation rates are also markedly increased, with fat oxidation accounting for 70% to 90% of the resting energy expenditure (REE).[2, 16-18] FFA oxidation rates are higher than expected based on FFA blood concentrations, which are usually only mildly elevated. Fat oxidation is not inhibited to a significant degree by the relatively high basal levels of glucose and insulin,[19] although fat oxidation rates are suppressible with exogenous hypertonic glucose.[20] Thus, it appears that fat is the body's preferred calorie source during critical illness, both in the fasted state and during glucose feeding.[20-22] On the other hand, during sepsis, the body does not adjust its pattern of fuel oxidation when exogenous fat is supplied over a wide range of lipid-to-glucose calorie ratios.[21] This suggests that patterns of fuel oxidation may be fixed in sepsis, thus offering no metabolic advantage to lipid administration.

REVIEW OF CLINICAL TRIALS COMPARING GLUCOSE WITH LIPID CALORIES WITH RESPECT TO PROTEIN METABOLISM

Since the widespread availability of intravenous lipid emulsions in the 1950s, researchers have sought the ideal balance of metabolic fuels for treating ill patients. Many studies have centered on protein metabolic effects.[23] Unfortunately, study designs vary widely; even studies with closely matched goals often differ markedly in their methods. In some studies, various experimental conditions are altered simultaneously, e.g., the glucose infusion rate and the amino acid infusion rate. Another area for concern and for potential misinterpretation of results lies in the measurements used to assess protein metabolic effects. Traditionally, nitrogen balance and body weight changes have been used for assessing these effects. Nitrogen balance is often considered a "gold standard" in this regard. However, nitrogen balance may not be an acceptable gold standard.[24] For many critically ill, immobile or paralyzed, ventilated, or neurologically injured patients, nitrogen loss may be the teleologically appropriate clinical response. Indeed, there may be a metabolic advantage to protein atrophy of "nonessential" tissues. Factitious nitrogen retention can also occur, especially during high nitrogen intake.[24, 25] This may result in a false or inaccurate assessment of body nitrogen. Additionally, achieving an improvement

in nitrogen balance does not necessarily indicate an improvement in clinical condition or a reversal of altered amino acid fluxes seen during sepsis and other stress states.[26] To overcome these deficiencies, other techniques such as amino acid radiolabeling and isotopic dilution have increasingly been employed to assess the rates of whole-body protein synthesis and catabolism. Unfortunately, these techniques also suffer from methodologic difficulties and make use of assumptions that may not be valid under abnormal physiologic conditions such as severe stress.[24, 25] Variable study lengths and inhomogeneous patient populations additionally complicate comparisons between experiments. Finally, most of the published studies use parenteral forms of glucose and fat. It is not clear that parenteral and enteral nutrition is equivalent. There is a growing body of literature suggesting that enteral diets are superior in many respects to parenteral feedings, and enteral diets are fast becoming the standard in intensive care nutrition.[27-29]

In catabolic patients, low-dose (150 to 200 g/day) dextrose infusion alone has little or no nitrogen-sparing effect and does not suppress gluconeogenesis or ureagenesis to a significant degree.[8, 30, 31] However, when low-dose dextrose infusion is added to hypocaloric amino acid solutions, nitrogen balance is improved progressively as dextrose infusion rates increase.[32-35] There appears to be a plateau to this phenomenon, as first suggested by Iapichino et al.[36] In their study of moderately to severely catabolic trauma patients, they found that a plateau in nitrogen balance was reached when dextrose was infused at a rate equivalent to about 120% of the daily energy requirement (determined by indirect calorimetry). Amino acids were provided at amounts equal to about 20% of the energy output (range, 230 to 280 mg/kg/day). Of note, these investigators used exogenous insulin to maintain blood glucose levels in the near-normal range

(100 to 150 mg/dL). It has since been established that supplemental insulin improves nitrogen balance in highly catabolic patients. The improved nitrogen balance noted with high rates (600 to 750 mg/day) of dextrose infusion may likely relate to the stimulation of endogenous insulin and its suppressive effects on skeletal muscle protein efflux and gluconeogenesis from alanine.[36–38] Some nutritional regimens provide large quantities of glucose in combination with insulin. However, the absolute and net rates of protein breakdown remain increased above normal during hyperinsulinemic euglycemic clamps, even when hepatic gluconeogenesis is totally suppressed and glucose uptake maximally stimulated.[38] Thus, the clinical utility of high-dose insulin infusions is questionable. These studies do suggest, however, that insulin infused at a rate sufficient to maintain normal blood glucose levels during moderate rates of dextrose infusion (at or near energy expenditure) can provide a significant improvement in nitrogen balance in catabolic patients.

There have been few published reports examining the role of fat alone as a fuel source.[39–42] These studies appear to suggest a response to fat emulsions analogous to that observed with dextrose given alone (i.e., minimal to no protein-sparing effect). The small protein-sparing effect seen with higher doses of fat alone may result from the glycerol component of the emulsion rather than the esterified triglyceride component.[41] Similar to glucose, the protein-sparing effect of intravenous fat is markedly enhanced by the addition of hypocaloric amino acids, although the relative protein-sparing efficiency of lipids is not as great as that of dextrose.[41, 43, 44]

Most of the available data concerning the appropriate selection of a fuel source comes from studies using combinations of lipid, carbohydrate, and amino acids. Bark et al. studied mildly catabolic postoperative patients.[45] Patients were given crystalline amino acids at a rate of 0.3 g N/kg/day and isocaloric quantities of fat plus fructose or hypertonic glucose plus fructose (nonprotein energy equal to 50 kcal/kg/day). Nitrogen equilibrium was similarly attained in both groups.[45] Nordenström et al. studied 18 mildly traumatized and/or septic patients and 5 nutritionally depleted patients by using dietary regimens of amino acids (0.28 to 0.40 g N/kg/day) and either glucose alone or an equicaloric mixture of lipid and glucose (energy intake of approximately 143% of REE in acutely ill patients).[46] They found no significant differences in nitrogen balance improvement between dietary regimens. Baker et al. studied 20 critically ill patients (overall mortality rate of 30%) a mean of 7.4 days after their admission to the intensive care unit (ICU).[47] The patients received calorically equivalent regimens providing 100%, 75%, or 25% of nonprotein calories as dextrose and the remainder as lipid. All patients received about 1 g of protein/kg/day and exogenous insulin to keep blood glucose levels below 250 mg/dL. No significant differences in whole-body protein synthesis or breakdown were detected. Near-zero protein balance was achieved on all regimens. High vs. low insulin infusion offered no additional improvements.[47]

In their study of 81 septic, traumatized, or cancer-affected patients, Shaw and Holdaway[48] used radioisotopically derived kinetic measurements to determine the effects of short-term infusions of either glucose (at 4 mg/kg/min) or an isocaloric amount of lipid emulsion on protein metabolism, glucose turnover, and glucose oxidation. They found that net protein catabolism was similarly suppressed by both fuel sources (by about 15%). Additionally, they discovered that the lipid emulsion did not change the rate of endogenous glucose production or the rate of glucose oxidation to any great degree, thus suggesting that "the protein-sparing effect of substrate infusion in severely ill patients occurs independent of both glucose and alanine availability."[48] They also speculated that lipid effects on protein metabolism are mediated by lipid-induced decreases in plasma cortisol concentrations.[48] Shaw and Wolfe published the results of metabolic analyses performed on 43 severely ill trauma patients fed with total parenteral nutrition (TPN) consisting of 1.7 g protein/kg/day and 2,000 to 2,500 kcal/day in equicaloric proportions of glucose and fat.[2] As before, they noted a decrease in (although not an amelioration of) net protein catabolism, due primarily to an increase in whole-body protein synthesis.[2] Finally, in a recently published report, de Chalain et al.[49] studied 50 patients in a surgical ICU who required mechanical ventilatory support for at least 4 days. Patients were fed either 100% glucose or a mixture of glucose and fat and then after 4 days were crossed over to the alternate fuel source. All patients received 1.5 g protein/kg/day. Kinetic amino acid tracer studies were conducted after 4 days of each feeding regimen. They reported that the selection of fuel source did not influence whole-body protein dynamics, with both regimens achieving greatly improved whole-body protein kinetics.[49] These patients likely had a lower catabolic stress than found in other studies[2, 48, 50] since net protein synthesis was achieved in over half the patients and positive nitrogen balance in nearly all cases. In addition, 32 of the patients meeting inclusion criteria did not complete the study for many reasons, including 13 patients who died prior to completing 4 days of study.

In summary, studies addressing the "protein-sparing" effects of glucose vs. lipid calories in mild to moderately catabolic patients indicate no benefit of one fuel source over the other. The protein-sparing effects in moderately to severely catabolic patients remain unclear. There is a disturbing paucity of data derived from severely catabolic patients, but what few data are available suggest that these fuel sources are equivalent in their protein-sparing effects. Unfortunately, the ideal study has not been published. Such a study would investigate a homogeneous group of critically ill patients at the peak of their catabolic phase over a reasonable study time duration (somewhere between 2 hours[48] and 4 days[49]), compare the effects of glucose plus amino acids vs. lipid plus amino acids vs. glucose-lipid mixtures plus amino acids, and employ a crossover design with patients serving as their own controls.

POTENTIAL ADVERSE CONSEQUENCES OF CARBOHYDRATE FEEDING

Potential undesirable effects of carbohydrate feeding include excessive production of carbon dioxide (Vco_2), hepatic steatosis, hyperglycemia, and effects related to hypertonicity, including venous sclerosis from parenteral forms of carbohydrate and osmotic diarrhea from enteral forms.

In normal subjects, carbohydrate, when administered in amounts isocaloric or hypercaloric to REE, increases minute ventilation and the work of breathing in an amount proportional to the increase in Vco_2 caused by oxidation of glucose (respiratory quotient [RQ] = 1.0) or lipogenesis (RQ = 8.0).[51–53] Askanazi and associates[54] found similar results in septic patients overfed with dextrose at 1.5 to 2.0 times REE; these patients manifested a 30% increase in oxygen consumption (Vo_2), a 57% increase in Vco_2, and an increase in minute ventilation of 71%.[54] In anecdotal reports, carbohydrate-induced increases in Vco_2 have been reported to precipitate respiratory distress in both spontaneously breathing patients[55] and mechanically ventilated patients.[56] The common factor related to the development of respiratory failure in these patients appears to be underlying lung disease with pre-existent ventilation-perfusion mismatches and/or hypercapnia. Increases in minute ventilation are required to excrete increased CO_2 resulting from carbohydrate metabolism. Patients with marginal respiratory reserve may be incapable of increasing ventilation, and hypercapnia may result. In addition, increased respiratory work may result in respiratory muscle fatigue and subsequent respiratory failure.[57]

To avoid the hypercapnia, respiratory acidosis, and muscle fatigue associated with aggressive carbohydrate feeding, lipid has been substituted for glucose or carbohydrate as a calorie source. Lipid/glucose combinations cause less CO_2 production and lower minute ventilation when compared with glucose alone.[58–60] Thus, many advocate this type of mixed–fuel source regimen for all patients at risk of ventilatory failure or patients undergoing active weaning from mechanical ventilation.[61, 62] However, few studies have addressed the clinical significance of these findings. Previous studies reporting significant increases in V_{CO_2} with carbohydrate alone vs. carbohydrate/lipid calorie sources overfed patients. When carbohydrate or carbohydrate/lipid calories are administered at rates that match energy expenditure (isocaloric), there are few if any significant differences in V_{CO_2} between groups.[63] Thus, the clinical benefit of mixed fuel diets (especially diets very high in fat) for treating patients with pulmonary disease (including weaning from the ventilator) remain unproven. Moderate caloric intake appears to be more important than the fuel source in this regard.

Hepatic complications associated with TPN have been reported since the early 1970s.[64] These complications range from hepatic steatosis to liver failure and death. Hepatic steatosis is the earliest and most frequently noted complication.[65] Steatosis becomes clinically significant in the critically ill patient when it leads to the development of intrahepatic cholestasis, detected by elevated serum alkaline phosphatase levels

and later by hyperbilirubinemia.[66] The pathogenesis of hepatic steatosis is still incompletely understood. Recent evidence suggests that enhanced hepatic uptake of fatty acids and reduced triglyceride secretion (in the form of VLDL particles) are important. These effects are closely related to the portal venous hormonal milieu,[65, 67] as reflected by the portal insulin-to-glucagon molar ratio. According to this theory, hepatic steatosis occurs not as a direct result of the fuel source per se but instead as a result of the effect of the fuel source(s) on the insulin/glucagon ratio. Nussbaum et al.[68] reported that hepatic steatosis, in the rat, is associated with high-dextrose–based TPN (25% dextrose) but not with TPN containing 17% or 25% dextrose plus 2.5% lipid. Rats that developed histologic abnormalities had significantly increased portal insulin/glucagon ratios as a result of increased portal insulin production.[68] This same group had previously shown a reversal of existent hepatic steatosis and prevention of the development of hepatic steatosis in rats by the addition of glucagon to hypertonic dextrose TPN.[67, 69]

Caution should be used when applying these data clinically since studies testing this hypothesis in humans remain to be performed. In fact, the addition of lipid to TPN in human patients does not always prevent or reverse hepatic steatosis.[66, 70] Furthermore, although the rat model is a good one for the development of steatosis, the model is not analogous to the human situation in that the progressive liver disease does not develop in rats, even with prolonged steatosis-inducing TPN.[71] Thus, although definitive recommendations await further research, it seems reasonable to conclude from available data that hypercaloric all-dextrose TPN regimens would more often be associated with hepatic abnormalities than would mixed-fuel regimens and that conservative therapy for steatosis once it has developed should include the addition of some lipid calories. The optimal concentration of lipids and/or the use of additional nutrients (such as L-glutamine) in this regard remains to be determined.

Carbohydrate administration can also result in hyperglycemia, especially when given at rates at or near maximal glucose uptake (about 6 mg/kg/min). Hyperglycemia can often be prevented by supplying insulin concomitantly and by monitoring blood glucose levels at regular intervals. If glucose levels are allowed to rise unchecked, serious complications such as nonketotic hyperosmolar syndrome and diabetic ketoacidosis (DKA) can result. Even at low to moderate glucose infusion rates (≤ 4 mg/kg/min), hyperosmolarity, osmolar diuresis, and aggravation of central nervous system (CNS) injury can occur. The ICU clinician should be aware of these potential complications and use proper precautions to prevent them.

POTENTIAL ADVERSE CONSEQUENCES OF LIPID FEEDING

Like carbohydrates, exogenously delivered lipids have been associated with organ dysfunction and unwanted side effects of variable clinical significance. Most of the published data concern lipid effects on cardiopulmonary and immune function, although there are also some reports of negative effects on microcirculation/platelet function.[72-74]

Indirect evidence that intravenous fat emulsions (IVFEs) impair lung function derives from reports of patients suffering from fat embolism syndrome who develop significant hypoxemia following the release of fat from bone marrow after trauma.[75] Clinical studies in critically ill patients reveal a somewhat discrepant picture. Van Deyk and associates[76] noted no changes in pulmonary artery pressure (PAP), right ventricular stroke work index, or the alveolar-arterial O_2 difference (A-aDO_2) before, during, or after the administration of

intravenous lipid (Lipofundin S, 20%) (0.24 g/kg/hr) over a period of 16 hours in 16 patients with multiple trauma. Venus et al.[77] also noted no significant changes associated with infusion of 20% IVFE over a period of 10 hours in adults with acute respiratory illnesses not associated with adult respiratory distress syndrome (ARDS). However, they did find higher pulmonary pressures and shunt fraction (Q_S/Q_T) in patients with ARDS.[77] In a later study, this same group confirmed these findings in patients with ARDS, and further extended their data to show a significantly worse hemodynamic response to IVFE in those patients with both ARDS and sepsis, as manifested by higher pulmonary wedge pressures, Q_S/Q_T, and peripheral vascular resistance.[78]

The mechanism(s) of impaired lung function and altered cardiopulmonary hemodynamics from infused lipid remains incompletely understood. Early studies attributed the changes to a decrease in diffusing capacity caused by hyperlipidemia.[79] More recent data from experimental models suggest an indirect role of Intralipid mediated by alterations in intrapulmonary prostaglandin (PG) production. McKeen and associates[80] demonstrated a decrease in PaO_2 and an increase in mean pulmonary artery pressures (MPAPs) in sheep with infusion of 10% Intralipid at 0.25 g/kg/hr. Indomethacin (blocks PG synthesis) but not heparin (enhances triglyceride clearance) prevented the IVFE-induced pulmonary changes, thus suggesting a role for arachidonic acid metabolites.[80] Similar results have been obtained in a rabbit model.[81, 82] In those studies, IVFE appeared to induce pulmonary changes via an increase in vasodilatory PGs, which theoretically caused increased perfusion to areas of relatively low ventilation and thus increased V/Q mismatching in injured lungs.[81, 82]

However, PG measurements performed in humans with ARDS and sepsis during Intralipid infusion have failed to demonstrate a cause-and-effect relationship between plasma PG levels and the observed pulmonary hemodynamic response to slow (increased Q_S/Q_T and no change in MPAP) or fast (increased MPAP and no change in Q_S/Q_T) Intralipid infusion.[83] Thus, while the exact mechanisms remain to be elucidated, it does seem clear that IVFEs induce pulmonary hemodynamic changes in nearly all models of injured lung, including humans with ARDS. These changes are small, however, and their clinical consequences, if any, have not been determined. These changes are not seen with enteral nutrient formulations.

The effects of IVFEs on the immune system are less clear than their pulmonary hemodynamic effects, but the clinical significance of the former may be greater. In both animals and humans, in vivo reticuloendothelial system (RES) dysfunction has been documented repeatedly during prolonged infusions of IVFEs composed primarily of long-chain triglycerides (LCTs).[84-87] In adult humans, RES clearance rates were reduced by more than 40% after just 3 days of intermittent (10-hour) lipid infusions at normally administered rates.[87] Variable effects of IVFEs on neutrophil locomotory function have been reported in both animals and humans, with some studies[88, 89] but not all[90] demonstrating decreased neutrophil chemotaxis and random migration. Similarly, studies examining the effects of IVFEs on neutrophil cytotoxicity have yielded conflicting results.[91-93] Recent evidence also suggests that metabolic products (especially PGE_2) produced from high rates of administration of linoleic acid (found in intravenous fat preparations and some enteral products) can impair immune cell function. While the immune-suppressing effects of IVFEs and linoleic acid are clear in experimental models, it is still unclear whether they have clinically significant adverse effects on immunity, infection rate, and outcome. Early data in burn patients suggest that they may have adverse clinical effects.[94] It is also unclear whether immune sup-

pression is necessarily bad. Immune suppression is a normal response to injury and may prevent the organism from instituting an immune response against damaged tissues early after injury. However, prolonged immune suppression predisposes to secondary infections. Further study concentrating on the phase of injury, the duration of immune suppression, infectious complications, and outcome are needed before the clinical relevance of the available data can be fully assessed. Furthermore, the use of lipid-induced immune suppression in transplant recipients remains an intriguing possibility.

Finally, it should be mentioned that an absence of lipid from the diets of critically ill hyperinsulinemic patients can lead to essential fatty acid deficiency (EFAD). EFAD can be prevented or corrected by the administration of parenteral or enteral lipid.[95, 96] Approximately 100 mL of a 10% LCT emulsion prevented EFAD in one study of stressed patients fed with TPN.[96] More recent work indicates that mild EFAD can occur in stressed patients receiving TPN and that a safflower-based lipid emulsion only partially corrects the condition.[97] The clinical significance of this persistent mild EFAD remains to be determined.

RECOMMENDATIONS FOR THERAPY

The ideal calorie source is efficiently delivered to and utilized by tissues during the catabolic phase of stress. It effectively causes a reduction in net protein catabolism by providing the body with the needed substrates for energy production. It does not cause large, potentially deleterious increases in oxygen consumption, nor does it cause carbon dioxide production. It does not adversely affect liver or lung function and does not interfere with the immune system. Obviously the ideal calorie source does not exist. Although alternative energy sources are being investigated, current practice is limited by the commercial availability of lipid and carbohydrate sources. Fat emulsion and dextrose (glucose) are acceptable forms of nonprotein calories for parenteral nutrition. Fat and carbohydrate sources are more variable in enteral nutritional products.

While the available data are not definitive because of limitations in the clinical studies of critically ill patients, several conclusions can be drawn and guidelines for the rational use of fuel sources made:

1. While the stressed body does use lipid preferentially as a fuel source, glucose oxidation is not impaired, and lipid infusion probably does not change patterns of fuel oxidation. Thus, there is no theoretical metabolic reason to choose one fuel over the other.

2. Glucose and lipid "spare" protein equally well, as determined by nitrogen balance and kinetic tracer measurements, in mildly to moderately hypermetabolic patients as long as a "sufficient" quantity of protein is administered simultaneously. The protein-sparing effects of glucose and lipids in severely hypercatabolic patients are not so well studied, but the available data suggest that there is no benefit of one fuel over another.

3. If glucose is used, exogenous insulin should be provided to maintain euglycemia in order to maximize glucose's protein-sparing actions.

4. Glucose infusions that meet energy expenditure do not increase Vco_2 significantly. Caution should be exercised when using hypercaloric glucose in patients with compromised lung function, especially with pre-existent hypercapnia.

5. Hepatic steatosis results from high parenteral carbohydrate administration. Its clinical consequences in adults are not usually serious. Conservative management, including the use of mixed lipid-glucose sources, can limit steatosis. Enteral feeding is rarely associated with carbohydrate-induced steatosis.

6. Intravenous lipids, even during slow administration, may cause pulmonary hemodynamic changes in injured lungs, possibly by affecting PG metabolism. These changes are small, however, and may not be of clinical significance.

7. Lipids, especially LCTs, can impair RES clearance functions, even when hypertriglyceridemia is absent. Their effects on other arms of the immune system are not as well defined, but some data suggest that lipids can impair both neutrophil and lymphocyte function.

8. Preliminary data also suggest that these effects could have an impact on the rates of infection and survival. Further study is needed on this subject.

When initiating nutritional therapy in the critically ill patient, the clinician should take into consideration all factors that could potentially have an impact on the patient's response to the infused (or enterally fed) nutrients. For example, the patient with intra-abdominal sepsis and ARDS might benefit from the short-term administration of an isocaloric glucose/protein mixture rather than one containing equal parts of glucose and fat as the nonprotein fuel since the fat could potentially impair the patient's lung function and immune response to the septic source. Alternatively, one may choose a mixed fuel that is low in long-chain triglycerides (i.e., linoleic acid) but rich in medium-chain triglycerides. A patient with severe chronic obstructive pulmonary disease (COPD) and liver damage may not tolerate an all-glucose regimen as well as a mixed-fuel regimen because of excess CO_2 production and steatosis. Until more research focusing on these types of morbidities is completed, the clinician will need to consider all potential adverse effects of the fuel source when choosing a feeding regimen. In general, we prefer to use a mixture of carbohydrate and lipid as the fuel source. These are administered at rates to meet the energy expenditure. We usually administer approximately 35% to 45% of nonprotein calories as lipid and 55% to 65% as carbohydrate. We prefer to use a lipid mixture containing both long- and medium-chain triglycerides.

REFERENCES

1. Cuthbertson DP: Post-shock metabolic response. *Lancet* 1942; 1:433–436.
2. Shaw JHF, Wolfe RR: An integrated analysis of glucose, fat, and protein metabolism in severely traumatized patients. Studies in the basal state and the response to total parenteral nutrition. *Ann Surg* 1989; 209:63–72.
3. Wolfe RR, Durkot J, Allsop JR, et al: Glucose metabolism in severely burned patients. *Metabolism* 1979; 28:1031–1039.
4. Elwyn DH, Kinney JM, Jeevanandam M, et al: Influence of increasing carbohydrate intake on glucose kinetics in injured patients. *Ann Surg* 1979; 190:117–127.
5. Long CL, Kinney JM, Geiger JW: Nonsuppressability of gluconeogenesis by glucose in septic patients. *Metabolism* 1976; 25:193–201.
6. Wilmore DW, Goodwin CW, Aulick LH, et al: Effect of injury and infection on visceral metabolism and circulation. *Ann Surg* 1980; 192:491–504.
7. Yki-Järvinen H, Sammalkorpi K, Koivisto VA, et al: Severity, duration, and mechanisms of insulin resistance during acute infections. *J Clin Endocrinol Metab* 1989; 69:317–323.
8. Shaw JHF, Klein S, Wolfe RR: Assessment of alanine, urea and glucose interrelationships in normal subjects and in patients with sepsis with stable isotopic tracers. *Surgery* 1985; 97:557–568.
9. Bessey PQ, Watters JM, Aoki TT, et al: Combined hormonal infusion simulates the metabolic response to injury. *Ann Surg* 1984; 200:264–281.
10. Jahoor F, Herndon DN, Wolfe RR: Role of insulin and glucagon in the response of glucose and alanine kinetics in burn-injured patients. *J Clin Invest* 1986; 78:807–814.
11. Gelfand RA, Matthews DE, Bier DM, et al: Role of counterregulatory hormones in the catabolic response to stress. *J Clin Invest* 1984; 74:2238–2248.
12. Wolfe RR, Allsop JR, Burke JF, et al: Glucose metabolism in man: Response to intravenous glucose infusion. *Metabolism* 1979; 28:210–220.
13. Wolfe RR, Durkot MJ, Allsop JR, et al: Glucose metabolism in severely burned patients. *Metabolism* 1979; 28:1031–1039.
14. Wilmore DW, Aulick LH, Mason AD, et al: Influence of the burn wound on local and systemic response to injury. *Ann Surg* 1977; 186:444–458.
15. Wolfe RR, Jahoor F, Herndon DN, et al: Isotopic evaluation of the metabolism of pyruvate and related substrates in normal adult volunteers and severely burned children: Effect of dichloroacetate and glucose infusion. *Surgery* 1991; 110:54–67.
16. Goodenough RD, Wolfe RR: Effect of total parenteral nutrition on free fatty acid metabolism in burned patients. *JPEN* 1984; 8:357–360.
17. Shaw JHF, Wolfe RR: Fatty acid and glycerol kinetics in septic patients and in patients with gastrointestinal cancer. The response to glucose infusion and parenteral feeding. *Ann Surg* 1987; 205:368–376.
18. Askanazi J, Carpentier YA, Elwyn DH, et al: Influence of total parenteral nutrition on fuel utilization in injury and sepsis. *Ann Surg* 1980; 191:40–46.
19. Jeevanandam M, Grote-Holman AE, Chikenji T, et al: Effects of glucose on fuel utilization and glycerol turnover in normal and injured man. *Crit Care Med* 1990; 18:125–135.
20. Nordenström J, Carpentier YA, Askanazi J, et al: Free fatty acid mobilization and oxidation during total parenteral nutrition in trauma and infection. *Ann Surg* 1983; 198:725–735.
21. Nanni G, Siegel JH, Coleman B, et al: Increased lipid fuel dependence in the critically ill septic patient. *J Trauma* 1984; 24:14–30.
22. Levinson MR, Groeger JS, Jeevanandam M, et al: Free fatty acid turnover and lipolysis in septic mechanically ventilated cancer-bearing humans. *Metabolism* 1988; 37:618–625.
23. Abbott WE, Krieger H, Holden WD, et al: Effect of intravenously administered

fat on body weight and nitrogen balance in surgical patients. *Metabolism* 1957; 6:691–702.

24. Schlichtig R, Ayres SM: Nutrient requirements of critically ill patients: Protein and nonprotein fuel, in *Nutritional Support of the Critically Ill*. St Louis, Mosby–Year Book, 1988, pp 97–127.

25. Hegsted DM: Assessment of nitrogen requirements. *Am J Clin Nutr* 1978; 31:1669–1677.

26. Cerra FB, Siegel JH, Coleman B, et al: Septic autocannibalism. A failure of exogenous nutritional support. *Ann Surg* 1980; 192:570–580.

27. Chiarelli A, Enzi G, Casadei A, et al: Very early nutrition supplementation in burned patients. *Am J Clin Nutr* 1990; 5:1035–1039.

28. Saito H, Trocki O, Alexander JW, et al: The effect of route of nutrient administration on the nutritional state, catabolic hormone secretion, and gut mucosal integrity after burn injury. *JPEN* 1987; 11:1–7.

29. Zaloga GP, Bortenschlager L, Black KW, et al: Immediate postoperative enteral feeding decreases weight loss and improves wound healing after abdominal surgery in rats. *Crit Care Med* 1992; 20:115–118.

30. Blackburn GL, Flatt JP, Clowes GHA Jr, et al: Protein sparing therapy during periods of starvation with sepsis or trauma. *Ann Surg* 1973; 177:588–594.

31. Wolfe BM, Culebras JM, Sim AJW, et al: Substrate interaction in intravenous feeding: Comparative effects of carbohydrate and fat on amino acid utilization in fasting man. *Ann Surg* 1977; 186:518–540.

32. Elwyn DH, Gump FE, Iles M, et al: Protein and energy sparing of glucose added in hypocaloric amounts to peripheral infusions of amino acids. *Metabolism* 1978; 27:325–331.

33. Askanazi J, Carpentier YA, Jeevanandam J, et al: Energy expenditure, nitrogen balance, and norepinephrine excretion after injury. *Surgery* 1981; 89:478–484.

34. Skillman JJ, Rosenoer VM, Pallotta JA, et al: Effect of isocaloric fat or glucose on albumin synthesis and nitrogen balance in patients receiving amino acid infusion. *Surgery* 1981; 89: 168–174.

35. McDougal WS, Wilmore DW, Pruitt BA Jr: Effect of intravenous near isosmotic nutrient infusions on nitrogen balance in critically ill injured patients. *Surg Gynecol Obstet* 1977; 145:408–414.

36. Iapichino G, Gattinoni L, Solca M, et al: Protein sparing and protein replacement in acutely injured patients during TPN with and without amino acid supply. *Intensive Care Med* 1982; 8:25–31.

37. Brooks DC, Bessey PQ, Black PR, et al: Insulin stimulates branched chain amino acid uptake and diminishes nitrogen flux from skeletal muscle of injured patients. *J Surg Res* 1986; 40:395–405.

38. Jahoor F, Shangraw RE, Miyoshi H, et al: Role of insulin and glucose oxidation in mediating the protein catabolism of burns and sepsis. *Am J Physiol* 1989; 257:E323–E331.

39. Van Itallie TB, Moore FD, Geyer RP, et al: Will fat emulsions given intravenously promote protein synthesis? Metabolic studies on normal subjects and surgical patients. *Surgery* 1954; 36:720–731.

40. Munro HN: Carbohydrate and fat as factors in protein utilization and metabolism. *Physiol Rev* 1951; 31:449–488.

41. Brennan MF, Fitzpatrick GF, Cohen KH, et al: Glycerol: Major contributor to the short-term protein sparing effect of fat emulsions in normal man. *Ann Surg* 1975; 182:386–394.

42. Wilmore DW, Moylan JA, Helmkamp GM, et al: Clinical evaluation of a 10% intravenous fat emulsion for parenteral nutrition in thermally injured patients. *Ann Surg* 1973; 178:503–513.

43. Munro HN, Naismith DJ: The influence of energy intake on protein metabolism. *Biochem J* 1953; 54:191–197.

44. Yamazaki K, Maiz A, Sobrado J, et al: Hypocaloric lipid emulsions and amino acid metabolism in injured rats. *JPEN* 1984; 8:360–366.

45. Bark S, Holm I, Hakansson I, et al: Nitrogen-sparing effect of fat emulsion compared with glucose in the postoperative period. *Acta Chir Scand* 1976; 142:423–427.

46. Nordenström J, Askanazi J, Elwyn DH,

et al: Nitrogen balance during total parenteral nutrition glucose vs. fat. *Ann Surg* 1983; 197:27–33.

47. Baker JP, Detsky AS, Stewart S, et al: Randomized trial of total parenteral nutrition in critically ill patients: Metabolic effects of varying glucose-lipid ratios as the energy source. *Gastroenterology* 1984; 87:53–59.

48. Shaw JHF, Holdaway CM: Protein-sparing effect of substrate infusion in surgical patients is governed by the clinical state, and not by the individual substrate infused. *JPEN* 1988; 12:433–440.

49. de Chalain TMB, Michell WL, O'Keefe SJ, et al: The effect of fuel source on amino acid metabolism in critically ill patients. *J Surg Res* 1992; 52:167–176.

50. Streat SJ, Beddoe AH, Hill GL: Aggressive nutritional support does not prevent protein loss despite fat gain in septic intensive care patients. *J Trauma* 1987; 27:262–266.

51. Rodriguez JL, Askanazi J, Weissman C, et al: Ventilatory and metabolic effects of glucose infusion. *Chest* 1985; 88:512–518.

52. Weissman C, Askanazi J: Respiratory complications of nutritional support. *Clin Anaesthesiol* 1983; 1:707–720.

53. Zwillich CW, Sahn SA, Weil JV: Effects of hypermetabolism on ventilation and chemosensitivity. *J Clin Invest* 1977; 60:900–906.

54. Askanazi J, Rosenbaum SH, Hyman AI, et al: Respiratory changes induced by the large glucose loads of total parenteral nutrition. *JAMA* 1980; 243:1444–1447.

55. Askanazi J, Elwyn DH, Silverberg PA, et al: Respiratory distress secondary to a high carbohydrate load: A case report. *Surgery* 1980; 87:596–598.

56. Covelli HD, Black JW, Olsen MS, et al: Respiratory failure precipitated by high carbohydrate loads. *Ann Intern Med* 1981; 95:579–581.

57. West JB: *Respiratory Physiology: The Essentials*, ed 3. Baltimore, Williams & Wilkins, 1985.

58. Askanazi J, Nordenström J, Rosenbaum SH, et al: Nutrition for the patient with respiratory failure: Glucose vs. fat. *Anesthesiology* 1981; 54:373–377.

59. Herve P, Simmonneau G, Girard P, et al: Hypercapnic acidosis induced by nutrition in mechanically ventilated patients: Glucose vs. fat. *Crit Care Med* 1985; 13:537–540.

60. Heymsfield SB, Head CA, McManus CB III, et al: Respiratory, cardiovascular, and metabolic effects of enteral hyperalimentation: Influence of formula dose and composition. *Am J Clin Nutr* 1984; 40:116–130.

61. Weissman C, Hyman AI: Nutritional care of the critically ill patient with respiratory failure. *Crit Care Clin* 1987; 3:185–203.

62. Schlichtig R, Sargent SC: Nutritional support of the mechanically ventilated patient. *Crit Care Clin* 1990; 6:767–784.

63. Talpers SS, Romberger DJ, Bunce SB, et al: Nutritionally associated increased carbon dioxide production. Excess total calories vs high proportion of carbohydrate calories. *Chest* 1992; 102:551–555.

64. Peden VH, Witzleben CL, Skelton MA: Total parenteral nutrition. *J Pediatr* 1971; 78:180–181.

65. Hall RI, Grant JP, Ross LH, et al: Pathogenesis of hepatic steatosis in the parenterally fed rat. *J Clin Invest* 1984; 74:1658–1668.

66. Sheldon GF, Peterson SR, Sanders R: Hepatic dysfunction during hyperalimentation. *Arch Surg* 1978; 113:504–508.

67. Li SJ, Nussbaum MS, McFadden DW, et al: Addition of glucagon to total parenteral nutrition (TPN) prevents hepatic steatosis in rats. *Surgery* 1988; 104:350–357.

68. Nussbaum MS, Li S, Bower RH, et al: Addition of lipid to total parenteral nutrition prevents hepatic steatosis in rats by lowering the portal venous insulin/glucagon ratio. *JPEN* 1992; 16:106–109.

69. Li SJ, Nussbaum MS, McFadden DW, et al: Reversal of hepatic steatosis in rats by addition of glucagon to total parenteral nutrition (TPN). *J Surg Res* 1989; 46:557–566.

70. Boelhouwer RU, King WW, Kingsnorth AN, et al: Fat-based (Intralipid 20%)

versus carbohydrate-based total parenteral nutrition: Effects on hepatic
structure and function in rats. *JPEN*
1983; 7:530–533.

71. Nussbaum MS, Fischer JE: Pathogenesis of hepatic steatosis during total
parenteral nutrition. *Surg Annu* 1991;
23:1–11.

72. Brockner J, Amris CJ, Larsen V: Fat
infusions and blood coagulation: Effect
of various fat emulsions on blood coagulability. *Acta Chir Scand Suppl* 1965;
343:48–55.

73. Jarnvig IL, Naesh O, Hindberg I, et al:
Platelet responses to intravenous infu-
sion of Intralipid in healthy volunteers.
Am J Clin Nutr 1990; 52:628–631.

74. Hageman JR, Hunt CE: Fat emulsions
and lung function. *Clin Chest Med*
1986; 7:69–77.

75. Nixon JR, Brock-Utne JG: Free fatty
acid and arterial oxygen changes following major injury: A correlation between hypoxemia and increased free
fatty acid levels. *J Trauma* 1978;
18:23–26.

76. van Deyk K, Hempel V, Münch F, et al:
Influence of parenteral fat administration on the pulmonary vascular system
in man. *Intensive Care Med* 1983;
9:73–77.

77. Venus B, Patel CB, Mathru M, et al:
Pulmonary effects of lipid infusion in
patients with acute respiratory failure
(abstract). *Crit Care Med* 1984;
12:293.

78. Venus B, Smith RA, Patel C, et al: Hemodynamic and gas exchange alterations during Intralipid infusion in patients with adult respiratory distress
syndrome. *Chest* 1989; 95:1278–1281.

79. Greene HL, Hazlett D, Demaree R: Relationship between Intralipid-induced
hyperlipemia and pulmonary function.
Am J Clin Nutr 1976; 29:127–135.

80. McKeen CR, Brigham KL, Bowers RE,
et al: Pulmonary vascular effects of fat
emulsion infusion in unanesthetized
sheep. Prevention by indomethacin. *J
Clin Invest* 1978; 61:1291–1297.

81. Inwood RJ, Gora P, Hunt CE: Indomethacin inhibition of Intralipid-
induced lung dysfunction. *Prostaglandins Med* 1981; 6:503–514.

82. Hageman JR, McCulloch K, Gora P, et
al: Intralipid alterations in pulmonary

prostaglandin metabolism and gas exchange. *Crit Care Med* 1983; 11:794–
798.

83. Mathru M, Dries DJ, Zecca A, et al: Effect of fast vs. slow Intralipid infusion
on gas exchange, pulmonary hemodynamics, and prostaglandin metabolism. *Chest* 1991; 99:426–429.

84. Park W, Paust H, Schroder H: Lipid infusion in premature infants suffering
from sepsis. *JPEN* 1984; 8:290–292.

85. Sobrado J, Moldawer LL, Pomposelli
JJ, et al: Lipid emulsions and reticuloendothelial system function in healthy
and burned guinea pigs. *Am J Clin
Nutr* 1985; 42:855–863.

86. Hamawy KJ, Moldawer LL, Georgieff M,
et al: The Henry M. Vars Award. The
effect of lipid emulsions on reticuloendothelial system function in the
injured animal. *JPEN* 1985; 9:559–
565.

87. Seidner DL, Mascioli EA, Istfan NW, et
al: Effects of long-chain triglyceride
emulsions on reticuloendothelial system function in humans. *JPEN* 1989;
13:614–619.

88. Nordenström J, Jarstrand C, Wiernik
A: Decreased chemotactic and random
migration of leukocytes during Intralipid infusion. *Am J Clin Nutr* 1979;
32:2416–2422.

89. Fischer GW, Hunter KW, Wilson SR, et
al: Diminished bacterial defenses with
Intralipid. *Lancet* 1980; 2:819–820.

90. Escudier EF, Escudier BJ, Henry-Amar
MC, et al: Effects of infused Intralipids
on neutrophil chemotaxis during total
parenteral nutrition. *JPEN* 1986;
10:596–598.

91. Loo LS, Tang JP, Kohl S: Inhibition of
cellular cytotoxicity of leukocytes for
herpes simplex virus–infected cells in
vitro and in vivo by Intralipid. *J Infect
Dis* 1982; 146:64–70.

92. Palmblad J, Brostrom O, Lahnborg G,
et al: Neutrophil functions during total
parenteral nutrition and Intralipid infusion. *Am J Clin Nutr* 1982; 35:1430–
1436.

93. Robin AP, Arain I, Phuangsab A, et al:
Intravenous fat emulsion acutely sup-
presses neutrophil chemiluminescence.
JPEN 1989; 13:608–613.

94. Alexander JW, Saito H, Trocki O, et al:
The importance of lipid type in the diet

after burn injury. *Ann Surg* 1986; 204:1–8.

95. O'Neill JA Jr, Caldwell MD, Meng HC: Essential fatty acid deficiency in surgical patients. *Ann Surg* 1977; 185:535–542.

96. Barr LH, Dunn GD, Brennan MF: Essential fatty acid deficiency during total parenteral nutrition. *Ann Surg* 1981; 193:304–311.

97. Alden PB, Svingen BA, Johnson SB, et al: Partial correction by exogenous lipid of abnormal patterns of polyunsaturated fatty acids in plasma phospholipids of stressed and septic surgical patients. *Surgery* 1986. 100:671–678.

11

Fiber

Gary Levine, M.D.

Fiber—What is it?
   Definition
   Composition of fiber
   Metabolism of fiber
Basic research

Clinical data
Use of fiber in the critical care setting
Adverse effects of fiber
Recommendations

It may seem curious that a chapter on fiber is included in a book discussing nutritional support of critically ill patients. During the past two decades our approach to feeding patients has evolved from relying on total parenteral nutrition (TPN) to recognizing the benefits of enteral feeding. Renewed interest in the benefits of enteral diets has produced a change in our diet preferences. Twenty years ago physicians were keen on using chemically defined diets that were purported to be easily absorbed across the gastrointestinal tract. Currently, nutritionists advocate widespread use of specialized, complete diets. As part of this trend, formula manufacturers have produced a large number of fiber-containing liquid diets that further expand our therapeutic choices for enteral nutritional support. This chapter will review our current knowledge concerning the role of fiber-containing enteral nutritional support in critically ill patients.

FIBER—WHAT IS IT?

Definition

Although the word "fiber" is bandied about in both the medical and popular literature, considerable confusion exists as to a precise definition. Terms such as "crude fiber," "unavailable carbohydrate," "indigestible residue," "bulk," and "roughage" have been used. Trowell's[1] definition of fiber is now the most widely accepted. Fiber is a mixture of fibrous and/or viscous undigested plant cell wall polysaccharides.

Many analytic methods have been used to measure the fiber content of food. Initially, "crude fiber" was defined as the residue remaining after treating foodstuffs with strong acid and alkali. However, this method underestimates cell wall polysaccharides such as hemicellulose. The American Organization of Analytical Chemists defined total dietary fiber as the residue remaining after enzyme digestion. However, this laboratory measurement has been criticized because it includes as fiber any "resistant starch" formed during the processing and cooking of foods. In my mind, the most logical method is Cummings and Englyst's,[2] who defined fiber as the nonstarch polymers remaining after enzyme digestion followed by chromatographic measurement of residual sugars. A determination of fiber content by this method measures both soluble and insoluble fractions but excludes lignin, which is a very minor dietary constituent.

Composition of Fiber

Outlined in Table 11–1 are the characteristics of the most common types of dietary fiber. Fiber includes the structural carbohydrates of the cell wall.[3, 4] These compounds include cellulose (a fibrillar polysaccharide), hemicellulose (a branched polysaccharide), and lignin (a polyphenolic polymer). Lignin, a noncarbohydrate, encrusts cellulose and hemicellulose during the latter stages of plant growth to provide tensile strength. Although lignin makes up only a small percentage of dietary fiber, its crystalline structure surrounds other cell wall constituents and interferes with their digestion and solubility. Among the other noncellulosic fibers present in the cell wall are the pectins (hexose-pentose uronic acid polymers), the

gums (methloxylated and acetylated polysaccharides), and the mucilages (highly branched polysaccharides).

The nonstructural polysaccharide fibers, the pectins, gums, and mucilages, are used extensively in food preparation and the compounding of medicinal products. These fibers are extremely hydrophilic and viscous. In addition, these components are most readily metabolized by hydrolases present on the exterior surface of bacterial cell walls. Soluble fibers such as the pectins, psyllium, and ispaghula are 90% to 99% digested, whereas an insoluble fiber such as cellulose is only 10% to 15% digested.

Solubility and digestibility are dependent on the chemical composition as well as the particle size of fiber preparations.[5] The smaller the particle size, the greater the solubility and digestibility. In addition to holding water, dietary fiber possesses the ability to act as a cation exchanger/binder, particularly of calcium and magnesium. In addition, the insoluble fiber lignin is an excellent adsorbent of bile acids and drugs.

Currently, soy polysaccharide is the most commonly used fiber additive in enteral products. Its constituents are mainly cellulose (20%) and hemicellulose (80%). Depending on intestinal transit time, soy polysaccharide is 70% to 90% fermented.[6] However, the administration of antibiotics may interfere with bacterial metabolism of fiber.

TABLE 11–1.

Types of Dietary Fiber*

Name	Chemical Structure	Water Solubility	Common Source
Cellulose	Glucose polymers β (1–4) units	Insoluble	Ubiquitous in all plant products
Lignins	Aromatic alcohol polymers (phenols)	Insoluble	Wood
Hemicellulose	Pentose, hexose, uronic acid polymers	Soluble	Ubiquitous in fruits, vegetables
Pectins	Galactouronic acid polymers, α (1,4) linkage; methylated side groups	Soluble	Fruits (citrus, apples, etc.)
Gums	Polysaccharides, often methoxylated and acetylated	Soluble	Seeds, (carob, karaya, guar)
Mucilages	Highly branched polysaccharides (i.e., arabinoxylans)	Soluble	Seeds (ispaghula and psyllium) seaweed

*Data from Selvendran RR: Am J Clin Nutr 1984; 39:320, and Eastwood MA, Pasmore R: Lancet 322:202, 1983.

Metabolism of Fiber

Dietary fiber, as well as unabsorbed dietary carbohydrate, undergoes fermentation predominantly in the colon by anaerobic bacteria.[2, 6] The content and composition of bacterial cell wall amylases with specificity for hydrolysis of $\alpha 1,4$ and $\beta 1-4$ linkages are variable among the bowel flora. These enzymes are inducible after exposure to different types of fiber. The bacterial population of the human intestine is unique to each individual and tends to be stable over time. The relative size of these populations can be influenced by fasting, a change in diet, and most importantly, the administration of antibiotics in critically ill patients.

The major end products of fiber metabolism are the short-chain fatty acids (SCFA) acetate, propionate, and butyrate as well as the gases hydrogen, carbon dioxide, and methane.[2-4] It has been estimated that normally 30 to 80 g of unabsorbed carbohydrate and fiber substrate enters the colon each day and results in the production of 300 to 800 mmol of SCFA. SCFAs are the predominant anions in the colon and are absorbed by both active and passive diffusive transport systems.[7] The ability to convert carbohydrates into SCFAs in the colon is a major driving force for colonic salvage of electrolytes and water. In addition, SCFA absorption represents the retention of an additional 100 to 250 kcal daily.[6] SCFAs are the preferential metabolic fuel for colonic epithelial cells and provide energy by β-oxidation. This phenomenon may account for the profound trophic effects of SCFAs on the large intestine.

Fiber metabolism also may affect nitrogen balance. The acidic milieu resulting from SCFA production and countertransport of hydrogen into the intestinal lumen traps ammonia in the gut in the form of ammonium ions. Therefore, acidification of the stool increases fecal nitrogen excretion. In addition, luminal ammonia provides a nitrogen source for bacterial growth, further facilitating fiber metabolism. Individuals receiving a high fiber diet may have enhanced excretion of nitrogenous products. This phenomenon may be effacious in the treatment of liver and kidney failure.

BASIC RESEARCH

Twenty years ago, investigators became interested in examining the effects of liquid diets on the gastrointestinal tract. Chemically defined diets maintained gastric and small intestinal structure and function but caused atrophy of the pancreas, distal part of the ileum, and entire colon.[8] These results stimulated investigation into the effects of fiber in controlling intestinal proliferation and function. In the rat, soluble, metabolizable fibers such as pectin, guar, and to a lesser extent bran stimulated mitotic activity and the cell renewal rate when compared with controls fed fiber-free diets.[9] The direct administration of SCFA into the rat colon has also been shown to be trophic.[10] Most recently, the effects of fiber and SCFA on colonic absorption were determined. Both pectin and soy polysaccharide stimulated colonic water and electrolyte absorption when compared with fiber-free control diets.[11]

Rolandelli and colleagues have extensively investigated the role of fiber in adaptation after intestinal resection or injury. Pectin as well as the direct infusion of SCFA enhanced adaptation and improved wound healing.[12] The effects of pectin and cellulose on fat absorption in the rat demonstrated that while pectin had no effect on fat absorption, cellulose appeared to decrease fat absorption.[13] Experiments carried out in my laboratory have demonstrated that metabolizable fiber and SCFAs improve colonic absorption after cecectomy in the rat.[14]

CLINICAL DATA

Unfortunately, the number and quality of animal studies surpass clinical studies in the field of fiber research. Among the many variables that confound confident interpretation of the clinical literature are the heterogeneity of the patient population studied (normal controls vs. hospitalized patients) and the type and dosage of fiber administered. The type of study design (prospective vs. retrospective, randomized vs. nonrandomized, longitudinal vs. crossover) may interfere with the interpretation of the clinical data. The end points studied (the presence or absence of constipation or diarrhea) also vary. In managing critically ill patients, the most important considerations are fiber's effects on the incidence of diarrhea, gut integrity, and improved survival. Unfortunately, no studies on the latter topics have been published.

In general, research performed on normal controls or healthy patients has documented that the addition of various types of fiber influences stool weight with a variable effect on stool frequency. In a study examining the effects of 30 and 60 g of soy fiber added to a flavored isotonic feeding (Ensure), the two doses of fiber increased fecal weight by 50% and more than 100%, respectively, without a change in stool frequency.[15] In this study, the fiber-free liquid diet increased transit time and water absorption and resulted in the passage of smaller and firmer stools as compared with periods when the subjects received the fiber-containing diet. Diarrhea rather than constipation was reported in another study where an isotonic tube feeding (Osmolite HN) was given *orally* to healthy volunteers.[16] When 15 to 30 g/day of pectin was added to the liquid diet, the experimental subjects did not experience diarrhea.

Several studies have been performed on institutionalized severely disabled patients receiving chronic tube feeding. Shankardass and colleagues compared fiber-free Ensure with Enrich (containing soy polysaccharide) in adult patients who had sustained various forms of neurologic injury. Although the fiber-containing diet did not influence stool frequency or weight, fiber did reduce the number of episodes of diarrhea in patients prone to this problem as well as reduced the laxative needs of constipated patients.[17] In another study using the same formulas, chronically institutionalized, profoundly retarded children and adolescents were studied. When these subjects received the control diet, all were chronically constipated. However, the addition of soy polysaccharide improved spontaneous stool frequency from every other day to daily and led to a doubling of stool weight.[18]

In addition to the effects previously mentioned, soluble fiber such as pectin and guar slow gastric emptying and small intestinal absorption of sugars and amino acids.[15] Delayed absorption probably results from two phenomena: slowed transit and retention of nutrients within the hydrophilic fiber gel.

USE OF FIBER IN THE CRITICAL CARE SETTING

There is a paucity of definitive, well-designed, randomized studies exploring the effects of fiber feeding in critically ill patients. Extrapolating data from normal controls and healthy, chronically institutionalized patients to the intensive care unit (ICU) setting may be inappropriate since diarrhea rather than constipation is the most frequent gastrointestinal complaint. The incidence of diarrhea in ICU patients ranges from 25% to over 50%.[19] This problem has led physicians to pay close attention to the effects of dietary modification. Gut-derived sepsis is another troublesome problem seen in the ICU that may be amenable to dietary treatment. Among the limited number of studies comparing the effects of fiber with fiber-free diets in ICU patients, none has demonstrated an improvement in the incidence of diarrhea or sepsis. Most importantly, it has not been demonstrated that dietary modification improves survival. These studies are outlined in Table 11–2.

The earliest published study of fiber treatment in ICU patients came from a burn unit.[20] In this study, psyllium (approximately 7 g/day) was added to the fiber-free feedings of patients in whom diarrhea developed. It was reported that the incidence of diarrhea fell dramatically. However, this study was uncontrolled and lacking in detail. The improvement noted may have been related to other factors such as improvement in their patients' overall medical condition and nutritional status. Hart and Dobb performed a randomized study in which 7 g/day of ispaghula was administered to half the patients receiving an isotonic tube feeding (Osmolite).[21] Thirty-five patients received fiber supplementation and 33, placebo. No difference in the incidence of diarrhea was detected. These authors did find that there was a weak statistical correlation between the incidence of diarrhea and the administration of antibiotics. There are several criticisms of this study, including the low dose of fiber used and the higher (almost double) incidence of administration of magnesium-containing antacids to the treatment group.

Another randomized, double-blind trial was reported by Frankenfield and Beyer, who studied 9 patients in a crossover trial.[22] The two products used were a fiber-free tube feeding (Ensure) and a soy polysaccharide–containing diet of similar nutrient composition (Enrich). A careful statistical analysis was performed and demonstrated that the major reduction in diarrhea observed was due to the effects of time rather than dietary treatment. In this study, a relatively high dose of fiber was administered (35 g/day), but the study periods were of relatively short duration, and no washout period was included between treatments. Interestingly, every subject in this study in whom diarrhea developed was receiving the antibiotics clindamycin and gentamicin as well as the H_2 antagonist ranitidine. Whether these drugs were the direct cause of diarrhea or a marker for more seriously ill patients prone to the development of diarrhea is unclear.

The same diets also were compared in the study performed by Dobb and Towler.[23] In this double-blind, randomized, controlled trial, 45 patients received the fiber-supplemented diet and 46, the fiber-free diet. There was no difference in the incidence of diarrhea (approximately 30% to 35% in each group). There were numerically fewer patients in whom constipation developed with the fiber-containing diet, but this finding was not statistically significant.

Guenter et al. studied 100 acutely ill patients.[24] Half received the fiber-free formula Osmolite, while the other half received Jevity, which contains soy

TABLE 11–2.

Clinical Studies in Critically Ill Patients

Study	Setting	Fiber	Study Design	End Point
Frank & Green[20]	Burn unit	Psyllium, 7 g/day	Uncontrolled	Decreased incidence of diarrhea
Hart & Dobb[21]	ICU	Ispaghula, 7 g/day	Double blind, randomized, crossover	No significant differences
Frankenfield & Beyer[22]	ICU	Soy polysaccharide, 33 g/day	Double blind, randomized, crossover	No significant differences
Dobb & Towler[23]	ICU	Soy polysaccharide, 20–40 g/day	Randomized	No significant differences
Guenter et al.[24]	ICU	Soy polysaccharide, dose not reported	Prospective	No significant differences

polysaccharide. Diarrhea developed in 34% of the patients receiving the fiber-free formula vs. 26% of the patients receiving the fiber-containing diet, a nonsignificant difference. However, the administration of antibiotics was most relevant to the presence or absence of diarrhea since 41% of the patients receiving antibiotics experienced diarrhea whereas diarrhea developed in only 3% of those not receiving antibiotics. This study suggests that any potential benefit of metabolizable fiber such as soy polysaccharide may be obviated by the concomitant administration of antibiotics.

In sum, there are no compelling, human experimental data supporting the use of fiber-containing diets in critically ill patients. However, before one abandons the use of these products, we must realize that each of these studies has serious design or analytic flaws. Large randomized studies need to look at other end points in addition to diarrhea. For example, does fiber feeding reduce the incidence of sepsis or anastomotic leaks after bowel surgery? Will fiber diets improve survival?

ADVERSE EFFECTS OF FIBER

The role of fiber in nutritional support of the critically ill remains uncertain. Experimental data from animal studies strongly support a role for fiber in maintenance of colonic integrity, wound healing, and adaptation after injury or resection. However, clinical studies in humans are equivocal at best. Are there any risks or side effects related to using fiber? Bowen et al. compared the effects of adding 40 g of soy polysaccharide per day with a conventional enteral diet on mineral absorption.[25] Although there was a significant decrease in the absorption of iron and copper, the absorption of other elements was not statistically different. Taper et al.[26] also discovered that high fiber intake (40 g/day of soy polysaccharide) caused a net loss of copper and iron. However, conventional doses of fiber (<20 g/day) had no deleterious effects. Heymsfield et al., in a study of chronically ill medical patients, compared two different soy-containing formulas, Susta II and Enrich, with Ensure.[27] In this study, the fiber-supplemented formulas led to greater fecal excretion of nitrogen and fat but did not impair mineral absorption.

RECOMMENDATIONS

Given our present state of knowledge, it appears that the currently available formulas that contain soy polysaccharide are an appropriate choice for feeding. Soy polysaccharide is highly soluble, contains mostly hemicellulose, and is present in sufficient concentration in the commercially available products to deliver at least 20 to 30 g/day to the patient (Table 11–3).[28] Since no comparative studies comparing soy polysaccharide with other fibers exist, there is no compelling reason to add exogenous fibers such as psyllium or ispaghula to non–fiber-containing feedings. Exogenous fiber often clogs feeding tubes and increases the number of tubes that need be replaced. Another rationale exists for the use of fiber in critically ill patients.

TABLE 11–3.

Fiber-Containing Enteral Diets*

Name	Manufacturer	Total Dietary Fiber/L†
Compleat	Sandoz Nutrition	4
Enrich	Ross Laboratories	16–20‡
Fibersource	Sandoz Nutrition	9–12‡
Glucerna	Ross Laboratories	18
Jevity	Ross Laboratories	18
Newtrition/Fiber	Knight Medical	16
Nutren/Fiber	Clintec	14
Profiber	Sherwood Medical	15
Sustacal/Fiber	Mead Johnson	7
Vitaneed	Sherwood Medical	11
Ultracal	Mead Johnson	14

*Adapted from Fredstrom SB, Baglien KS, Lampe JW, et al: *JPEN* 1991; 15:450.
†Including carrageenan added as an emulsifier.
‡Depends on the flavor and nutrient density.

Patients with diabetes or those in whom glucose intolerance develops during acute illness may benefit from fiber feedings. In sum, given our present state of knowledge, the best rationale for using fiber-supplemented feedings may be that fiber, at worst, is harmless and, at best, may be beneficial.

REFERENCES

1. Trowell H: Definition of dietary fiber and hypotheses that it is a protective factor in certain diseases. *Am J Clin Nutr* 1976; 29:417.
2. Cummings JA, Englyst HN: Fermentation in the human large intestine and the available substrates. *Am J Clin Nutr* 1987; 45:1243.
3. Selvendran RR: The plant cell wall as a source of dietary fiber: Chemistry and structure. *Am J Clin Nutr* 1984; 39:320.
4. Eastwood MA, Passmore R: Dietary fiber. *Lancet* 322:202, 1983.
5. Heller SN, Hackler LR, Rivers JM, et al: Dietary fibre: The effect of particle size of wheat bran on colonic function in young men. *Am J Clin Nutr* 1989; 33:117.
6. Roediger WEW: Role of anerobic bacteria in the metabolic welfare of the colonic mucosa in man. *Gut* 1980; 21:793.
7. Ruppin H, Bar-Meir S, Soergel KH, et al: Absorption of short-chain fatty acids by the colon. *Gastroenterology* 1980; 78:1500.
8. Morin CL, Ling V, Bourasso D: Small intestine and colonic changes induced by a liquid elemental diet in rats. *Dig Dis Sci* 1980; 22:808.
9. Jacobs LR, Lupton JR: Effect of dietary fibers on rat large bowel mucosal growth and cell proliferation. *Am J Physiol* 1984; 246:378.
10. Kripke SA, Fox AD, Berman JH, et al: Stimulation of intestinal mucosal growth with intracolonic infusion of short chain fatty acids. *JPEN* 1989; 13:109.
11. Levine GM, Rosenthal J: Effects of fiber containing diets on colonic structure and function. *JPEN* 1991; 15:526.
12. Rolandelli RH, Koruda MJ, Settle RG, et al: The effect of postoperative pectin supplemental enteral feedings on healing of colonic anastomosis in the rat. *Surgery* 1986; 99:703.
13. Toki A, Todani T, Watanabe Y, et al: Effects of pectin and cellulose on fat absorption after massive small bowel resection in weanling rats. *JPEN* 1992; 16:255.
14. Kelberman I, Cheetham B, Levine G, et al: Dietary fiber promotes colonic adaptation (abstract). *Gastroenterology* 1991; 100:527.
15. Slavin JL, Nelson NL, McNamara EA, et al: Bowel function of healthy men consuming liquid diets with and without dietary fiber. *JPEN* 1985; 9:317.
16. Zimmaro DM, Rolandelli RH, Koruda MJ, et al: Isotonic tube feeding formula induces liquid stool in normal subjects: Reversal by pectin. *JPEN* 1989; 13:117.
17. Shankardass K, Chuchmach S, Chelswick K, et al: Bowel function of long term tube fed patients consuming formulae with and without dietary fiber. *JPEN* 1990; 14:508.
18. Liebl BH, Fischer MH, Van Calcar SC, et al: Dietary fiber and long-term large bowel response in enterally nourished nonambulatory profoundly retarded youth. *JPEN* 1990; 14:371.
19. Cheng RWS, Jacobs S, Lee B: Gastrointestinal dysfunction among intensive care unit patients. *Crit Care Med* 1987; 15:909.
20. Frank HA, Green LC: Successful use of a bulk laxative to control diarrhea in tube feeding. *Scand J Plast Reconstr Surg* 1979; 13:193.
21. Hart GK, Dobb GJ: Effect of a fecal bulking agent on diarrhea during enteral feeding of the critically ill. *JPEN* 1988; 12:465.
22. Frankenfield DC, Beyer PL: Soy polysaccharide fiber: Effect on diarrhea in tube-fed, head injured patients. *Am J Clin Nutr* 1989; 50:533.
23. Dobb GJ, Towler SC: Diarrhea during enteral feeding in the critically ill: Comparison of feeds with and without fibre. *Intensive Care Med* 1990; 16:252.
24. Guenter PA, Settle G, Perlmutter S, et al: Tube feeding–related diarrhea in acutely ill patients. *JPEN* 1991; 15:277.

25. Bowen PE, Taper LJ, Milam R: Mineral absorption using fiber augmented liquid formula diets. *JPEN* 1982; 6:575.
26. Taper LJ, Milam RS, McCallister MS, et al: Mineral retention in young men consuming soy-fiber–augmented liquid-formula diets. *Am J Clin Nutr* 1988; 48:305.
27. Heymsfield SB, Roongspisuthipong C, Evert M, et al: Fiber supplementation of enteral formulas: Effects on the bioavailability of major nutrients and gastrointestinal tolerance. *JPEN* 1988; 12:265.
28. Fredstrom SB, Baglien KS, Lampe JW, et al: Determination of fiber content of enteral feedings. *JPEN* 1991; 15: 450.

12

Lipids

Timothy J. Babineau, M.D.

James Pomposelli, M.D.

R. Armour Forse, M.D., Ph.D.

George L. Blackburn, M.D., Ph.D.

Fat metabolism	**Long-chain fatty acids**
Short-chain fatty acids	Vegetable (ω-6) vs. fish oil (ω-3)
Medium-chain fatty acids	**Structured lipids**

The importance of diet in both health and disease has long been recognized. Recently, diets are being designed in an attempt to promote health and modify different diseases. Nutrients are being considered for their ability to improve health and not just avoid deficiencies. Our understanding of the interaction between nutrition and our immune system is unfolding, thus prompting many investigators to examine the effect of dietary manipulation on the inflammatory response to injury. The importance of lipid type in diets after a variety of stresses, including burns and sepsis, has been extensively studied.[1-3] For example, lipids may play a unique role as both a caloric source and an immunomodulator by altering the composition of cell membranes and the kinetics of prostaglandin synthesis. Today, nutritionists and physicians seeking to modify the state of inflammation in a partic-

ular disease process are looking to a variety of different nutrients. This chapter will focus on one class of nutrients, lipids (Table 12–1).

Dietary supplementation with fat serves a number of useful functions. First, fat provides a source of non-glucose/non−amino acid calories, theoretically minimizing the catabolism of endogenous protein supplies. Second, fat supplementation with polyunsaturated fatty acids (PUFAs) prevents essential fatty acid deficiency. Third, newer types of manufactured "structured" lipids are being developed and may have a favorable impact on the immune system in stressed, septic patients. Although body cells are held together via structural proteins, the cell walls themselves are held together by lipid membranes. The structure of cell membranes and receptors can be altered by the composition of dietary lipids.[4]

TABLE 12-1.

Fatty Acid Composition of Selected Oils*

	Oils			
Fatty Acids	Soybean	Safflower	MCT†	Fish Oil
6:0			<2‡	
8:0			70	
10:0			30	
12:0			<2	
14:0	0.1	0.1		7.0
16:0	10.5	6.7		17.3
16:1ω7				8.6
18:0	3.2	2.7		2.7
18:1ω9	22.3	12.9		12.9
18:2ω6	54.5	77.5		2.1
18:3ω3	8.5			0.9
20:5ω3				12.8
22:6ω3				8.7

*From Bell SJ, Mascioli EA, Bistrian BR, et al: J Am Diet Assoc 1991; 91:1. Used by permission.
†MCT = medium-chain triglyceride.
‡Values are percentages of total fatty acids.

Intravenous lipid emulsions have been in use clinically for over 25 years. Initially developed (in part) as an alternative energy source to glucose to avoid hyperglycemia during stress-induced insulin resistance, the utility, benefits, and risks of intravenous lipids have improved over the years and have expanded their role in nutrition support. An increasing body of knowledge is developing on the specific functions that lipids play in nutrition support and critical illness.[5, 6] In addition, a variety of "new" structured lipids are being developed in an effort not only to provide caloric support to the patient but also to modify a patient's metabolic response to illness and disease (Fig 12-1).

In overfed, overweight individuals, diets high in lipids have been known for some time to have an adverse effect. Adverse effects in patients' cellular and hormonal immune response have also been noted with intravenous lipid emulsions. Within the past decade, the type and quantity of lipid within a diet have been shown to influence immunologic responses. In particular, linoleic acid (a key precursor to the synthesis of prostaglandin E_2 [PGE_2]), has been shown to be immunosuppressive when given to

animals. Indeed, some studies have demonstrated that animals fed fatty acid-deficient intravenous diets are more resistant to bacterial challenge. This chapter will focus on the role of lipids as "medical foods" in the nutritional support of critically ill patients. Fat metabolism will be briefly reviewed, followed by a discussion of the three lipid types: short-, medium-, and long-chain fats. Finally, the highly *un*saturated ω-3 fish oils and structured lipids will be reviewed.

FAT METABOLISM

During illness or injury (and particularly during sepsis) the major source of energy is body fat. However, our understanding of fat metabolism during critical illness is poor. Wiener et al. point out that "many of our observations can be described but not necessarily explained."[7] It has become increasingly clear that the clinical state of the patient has an important bearing on fat metabolism. For example, observations made on patients in septic shock may not hold true in hemorrhagic shock or multisystem organ failure. Nevertheless, certain aspects of fat metabolism merit consideration in an effort to correctly feed the critically ill.

During the early phase of the physiologic response to injury there is an increase in fat mobilization (lipolysis), a rise in serum levels of free fatty acids (FFAs), and an increase in fat oxidation. Little and coworkers, using trauma patients, described a postabsorptive, fasting respiratory quotient (RQ) (ratio of carbon dioxide produced to oxygen consumed) of 0.78, i.e., the predominant fuel (>50% of the total nonprotein caloric expenditure) was fat.[8] As the patient enters the "flow" phase of injury response (as described by Cuthbertson[8a]), FFA levels and fat oxidation may increase or decrease with exogenous glucose administration and influence this energy balance. The reason for this phe-

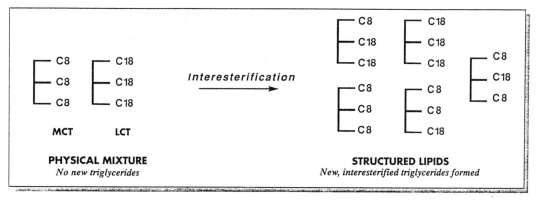

FIG 12–1.
Physical mixture vs. structured lipids. (From Stephan: *A New Frontier in Fat Nutrition.* Stepan PVO Department, 1992. Used by permission.)

nomenon is not entirely clear but most likely represents a complex balance between increased lipolysis, increased lipogenesis from reesterification (with high-dextrose total parenteral nutrition [TPN]), and substrate cycling.[9]

Although fat metabolism is incompletely understood, problems resulting from overfeeding with dextrose-alone solutions have prompted the use of intravenous lipids and the creation of mixed-fuel parenteral systems. Up until recently, 100% vegetable oil ω-6 polyunsaturated long-chain triglycerides (LCTs) derived from soybean or safflower oil were the sole source of parenteral lipid (Table 12–2). They are classified as *long*-chain triglycerides because the fatty acids that make up these triglycerides are 16 or 18 carbons long. Linoleic acid (18:2ω6) is the predominant fatty acid in these triglyceride formulas, unlike "ordinary" oral diets where it is only 10% to 15% of the dietary fat content. Linoleic acid has two double bonds in its chemical makeup and is therefore referred to as polyunsatured (Table 12–3). Concern over the possible adverse side effects that LCTs may have in critically ill patients has prompted investigators to look for "newer" forms of fats. These newer forms will be discussed in detail later.

Administering nutritional support to the critically ill patient (in the form of TPN) requires a "mixed-fuel/3-in-1" system to mimic routine macronutrient diets and to avoid the complications of glucose overfeeding. The mixed glucose/amino acid/lipid system has avoided some of the glucose-based, "overfeeding" complications of TPN while still providing adequate nutrition. However, complications with the use of boluses of exogenous vegetable fat emulsions have been observed, including impaired clotting, impaired phagocytosis, and depressed function of the reticuloendothelial system (RES).[10] These clinical problems may be related to the excessive production of prostaglandins and leukotrienes from the LCTs, which contain a high level of ω-6 PUFAs. Under these circumstances, an imbalance of eicosanoids can enhance vasoconstriction, platelet aggregation, neutrophil migration, immunosuppression, cytokine depression, and free-radical formation, all of which may predispose to secondary inflammation and sepsis. Such potential "overworking" of the immune system with TPN-based LCT lipid infusions has prompted a search for alternative lipid sources.

SHORT-CHAIN FATTY ACIDS

Fatty acids consisting of one to six carbons (C1–6) are designated short-chain fatty acids (SCFAs). Also known as "volatile" fatty acids, they are pri-

TABLE 12–2.

Components of Typical Long-Chain Triglyceride Oils*

Oil	Lauric	Myristic	Palmitic	Palmitoleic	Margaric	Stearic	Oleic	Linoleic	Linolenic	Arachidic	Gadoleic	Eicosadienoic	Behenic	Lignoceric
						Acid								
Corn			12.2	0.1		2.2	27.5	57.0	0.9	0.1				
Peanut		0.1	11.6	0.2	0.1	3.1	46.5	31.4		1.5	1.4	0.1	3.0	1.0
Safflower		0.1	6.5			2.4	13.1	77.7		0.2				
Soybean		0.1	11.0	0.1		4.0	23.4	53.2	7.8	0.3			0.1	
Sunflower seed	0.5	0.2	6.8	0.1		4.7	18.6	68.2	0.5	0.4				

*From Babayan VK: Nutr Support Serv 1986; 6:7. Used by permission.

TABLE 12–3.

Major Families of Polyunsaturated Fatty Acids*

ω9	ω6	ω3
C1–8:1ω9†	C18:2ω6	C18:3ω3
Oleic acid	Linoleic acid	α-Linolenic acid
↓	↓	↓
C18:2ω9	C18:3ω6	C18:4ω3
↓	γ-Linoleic acid	↓
C20:2ω9	↓	C20:4ω3
↓	C20:3ω6	↓
C20:3ω9	Di-homo-γ-linoleic acid	C20:5ω3
Eicosatrienoic acid	↓	Eicosapentaenoic acid
	C20:4ω6	↓
	Arachodonic acid	C22:5ω3
		Docosapentaenoic acid
		↓
		C22:6ω3
		Docosahexaenoic acid

*From Mascioli EA: Nutrition, in Walkins WD (ed): *Prostaglandins in Clinical Practice.* New York, Raven Press, 1989. Used by permission.
†The respective 18-carbon fatty acids are acted on alternately by desaturases and elongases to produce the other fatty acids of that family. Humans cannot interconvert fatty acids between families.

marily the product of microbial carbohydrate fermentation in mammalian gastrointestinal tracts.[11] The three principal SCFAs produced in mammals are acetate, propionate, and butyrate. Carbohydrate, often as dietary fiber and starch that has not been absorbed proximally, reaches the bacteria-containing portion of the distal part of the gut and is metabolized via the Embden-Meyerhof pathway into SCFAs.[12] Starvation of the gut and alteration of the microbial environment of the colon often lead to an alteration in SCFA metabolism.

The absorption of SCFAs takes place throughout the gastrointestinal tract but is highest in those areas with the greatest concentration of SCFA, namely the colon. Absorption appears to be passive and linearly related to the concentration gradient.[13] Once absorbed, SCFAs are easily metabolized in man.[14] The majority of SCFA metabolism takes place within the colonocyte. Those SCFAs not metabolized by colonocytes are transported to the liver in the portal blood, where they are rapidly metabolized. Depending on the amount of fiber in the diet, it is estimated that SCFAs

may supply up to 5% to 10% of the daily energy requirements in man. In addition to their caloric role, SCFAs also benefit the host through stimulation of increased colonic blood flow, promotion of salt and water absorption, and stimulation of mucosal proliferation.[15, 16]

The potential clinical applications for SCFAs are only beginning to be recognized. Conditions such as short-bowel syndrome, colitis, and disuse atrophy may benefit from the stimulatory effects of SCFAs.[17] Kripke and coworkers have studied the effects of a continuous colonic infusion of SCFA on intestinal mucosal growth in rats. Rats that received a continuous colonic infusion of SCFA following cecectomy and ileocolic anastomosis exhibited increased colonic mucosal growth and ileal mucosal DNA concentration.[18] In addition, animals fed a fiber-free enteral diet demonstrated enhanced healing of a colonic anastomosis following the intracolonic infusion of SCFA.[19] Finally, rats that were fed parenteral TPN supplemented with SCFAs demonstrated a reduction in the mucosal atrophy associated with TPN and enhanced adaption to small-bowel resection.[20]

Studies in man are only beginning to emerge. Harig and Soergel found that SCFAs significantly reduced colonic inflammation in patients with diversion colitis.[21] Moreover, Breur et al. found that rectal irrigation with SCFAs improved disease activity in nine of 10 patients with ulcerative colitis.[22] The role of SCFA during critical illness in man (supplied either enterally or parenterally) is just now being studied. Further investigation is warranted to elucidate the potential benefits of SCFAs on gut mucosal atrophy, which often accompanies severe critical illness. The role of enteral and parenteral SCFA needs to be investigated in man before any recommendations can be made.

MEDIUM-CHAIN FATTY ACIDS

Medium-chain fatty acids (MCFAs) have chain lengths between 6 and 12 carbons (C6–12). Commercial medium-chain triglycerides (MCTs) are principally 8 to 10 carbons in chain length. The current sources for the MCTs, palm kernel and coconut oils, have chain lengths of 8 to 10 carbons (Table 12–4). Like SCFAs, MCFAs cannot be elongated

and stored, so they act as instant oxidative fuels. Triglycerides composed mainly of LCTs are absorbed into the enterocyte as FFAs, reesterified into triglycerides, processed into chylomicrons, and transported via the lymphatic system. MCFAs are minimally reesterified and travel primarily via the portal circulation (bound to albumin) to the liver where they are metabolized. Studies in man have shown that the MCFA content of chylomicrons can be altered by changing the amount and rate at which MCFAs are consumed.[23–25] MCFA may be beneficial in patients with types I and IV hyperlipidemia who are prone to atherosclerosis secondary to LCTs.

MCTs are currently thought to be an ideal substrate for the stressed and septic state.[26] Studies in animals and man have shown that MCFAs are more rapidly and efficiently oxidized than LCTs and very little is stored as excess body fat.[27] This increased rate of oxidation is most likely due to the ability of MCFA to enter mitochondria directly, without the need for the carnitine shuttle.[28, 29] LCTs require carnitine (and conversion to carnitine transport forms) to be oxidized, which leads to a slower rate of metabolism. It is felt that rapid oxidation

TABLE 12–4.

Medium-Chain Triglycerides*

Saturates†		Monounsaturates ω-9 High Oleic	Polyunsaturates		
			ω-6		ω-3 High Linolenic
Medium chain	Long chain		High Linoleic	GLA‡ Oils	
C6–C12	C14–C24	Olive	Corn	Black current	Linseed
Kernel oils	Cocoa butter	Canola	Cotton	Borage	Fish oils
Babassu	Dairy fats	Safflower (hybrid)	Saya	Primrose	Menhaden
Coconut	Lard	Sunflower (hybrid)	Safflower (regular)		Salmon
Cohune	Tallow		Sunflower (regular)		Mackeral
Palm kernel	Palm				Tuna
Tucum	Stearine				Anchovy
MCT‡ oil					

Hydrogenation

←————————————————————→

Stearines Shortenings Margarine Salad oils

*From Babayan VK, Rosenau JR: *Food Technol*, Feb 1991. Used by permission.
†Lipids include long-chain saturates, monounsaturates, and polyunsaturates.
‡GLA = γ-linolenic acid; MCT = medium-chain triglycerides.

of MCFAs makes them less prone to fat deposition. In particular, RES shows minimal MCFA uptake as compared with LCTs.[30] Therefore, MCFA may lead to less impairment of RES function when supplied intravenously (Table 12–5).

If used as the sole fuel source, MCFA can produce toxic side effects in animals; however, these effects are limited by the use of mixtures of MCT and LCT as well as the provision of carbohydrate.[31–33] Studies employing protein kinetics and nitrogen balance have indicated that MCT/LCT solutions are associated with improved protein sparing in both animals and humans. When administered as a 75% MCT/25% LCT mixture, the improved protein sparing is associated with increased lipid oxidation and an increase in thermogenesis.[34] Improved protein sparing results in improved host defenses and evidence of improved cellular immune function.[35] Currently, MCTs are widely used in most pediatric feeding formulas and most medical enteral formulas and are approved for intravenous use in Germany.

LONG-CHAIN FATTY ACIDS

PUFAs are nutrients essential to life. They serve as important sources of fuel for metabolic work, provide substrate for inflammatory mediators and second messengers, and are building blocks for all cell membranes. Lipids are a heterogeneous group of substances that share

TABLE 12–5.

Rationale for the Use of Medium-Chain Triglycerides (Tentative Formulations)*

Physicochemical Characteristics	Physiologic Considerations	Potential Therapeutic Applications
MCTs† present more interfacial surface for enzyme action/unit time	Intraluminal enzymatic hydrolysis of MCT is more rapid and more complete than LCT†	Decreased intraluminal concentrations of pancreatic lipase (pancreatic insufficiency, cystic fibrosis) Decreased small-bowel absorptive surface (intestinal resection)
Greater water solubility of MCT hydrolysis products	Bile salts are not required for dispersion in water	Decreased intraluminal concentrations of bile salts (intrahepatic and extrahepatic biliary tract obstruction, chronic parenchymal liver disease)
Smaller molecular size of MCT vs. LCT	Small amounts of MCT may enter intestinal cell without prior hydrolysis	Pancreatic insufficiency
Shorter chain length of fatty acids derived from MCT	More efficient penetration of diseased mucosal surface	Nontropical sprue, tropical sprue
Small molecular size and lower pK of fatty acids derived from MCT	Intramucosal metabolism of MCFA† different from LCFA† Decreased affinity for esterifying enzymes Decreased affinity for activating enzymes Minimal reesterification of MCFA to MCT No chylomicron formation	Abetalipoproteinemia Hypobetalipoproteinemia
Greater water solubility of MCFA	Different routes of transport of MCT vs. LCT Portal transport of MCT (as MCFA) Lymphatic transport of LCT(as chylomicrons)	Lymphatic obstruction (lymphomas) Intestinal lymphangiectasia

*From Babayan VK: *Nutr Support Serv* 1986; 6:7. Used by permission.
†MCT = medium-chain triglycerides; LCT = long-chain triglycerides; MCFA = medium-chain fatty acid; LCFA = long-chain fatty acid.

the property of being insoluble in water. Each type of fatty acid substrate has its own unique effects on intermediary metabolism. This provides a novel nutrient-metabolic interaction with potential therapeutic implications for the critically ill patient.

In the past, nutritionists and lipid biochemists classified dietary fats into three broad categories: saturated, monounsaturated, and polyunsaturated fatty acids. Generally, it was believed that saturated fats were deleterious and were to be avoided in the diet, whereas polyunsaturated lipids were considered to be beneficial. With improvements in chromatography and fatty acid separation techniques, we now recognize that not only is the level of desaturation important but also the chain length and the position of double bonds. Saturated SCFAs and MCFAs (chains less than 12 carbons) have completely different metabolic effects when compared with their long-chain counterparts. Similarly, within the subgrouping of unsaturated long-chain fatty acids, the position of the terminal double bond also greatly influences the metabolic fate and physiologic effect of the fatty acid.

There are basically three series, or "families," of naturally occurring unsaturated fatty acids that, when introduced into the host, can be converted into higher derivatives through the process of elongation and desaturation. These are oleic acid ($18:1\omega9$), linoleic acid ($18:2\omega6$), and α-linolenic acid ($18:3\omega3$). In each case, the numerical expression reveals the number of carbon atoms followed by the number of double bonds. The ω characterizes the position of the terminal double bond (or "omega" double bond) in the fatty acid chain counting from the methyl end. Since all oxidation and reduction reactions occur on the carboxyl end of fatty acids, it is impossible to interconvert between families of fatty acids (Table 12–4).

Desaturation cannot occur in animals at positions ω-6 and ω-3 in fatty acids. As a result, linoleic acid and α-linolenic acids have to be ingested in the diet and are considered "essential." Polyunsatured essential fatty acids affect biomembrane function by influencing fluidity and permeability and form precursors for the inflammatory mediators prostaglandins and leukotrienes. There is substantial evidence that these mediators play a significant role in the pathogenesis of sepsis and the systemic inflammatory response in the critically ill patient. Through dietary engineering of designer/structured lipids, we may be able to significantly downregulate certain hyperimmune "allogeneic" aspects of the inflammatory response while maintaining desired host defenses and wound healing processes.

Following injury, infection, or trauma, numerous endogenous mediators are released such as interleukin-1 (IL-1), tumor necrosis factor (TNF), interleukin-6 (IL-6), eicosanoids, complement, procoagulants, stress hormones, and other cytokines that combine to activate and regulate the immune response. In a septic host, endogenous cytokines (i.e., IL-1, TNF and IL-6) appear particularly important since they are released into the general circulation after endotoxin administration and reproduce many features of septic shock. Although cytokines have direct activity on cell metabolism, many of their physiologic effects are mediated through second messengers such as arachidonic acid. Fever is one example. In addition, a complex regulatory feedback mechanism is hypothesized to exist between prostanoids and cytokines.

Substantial evidence has accumulated to suggest that arachidonic acid metabolites (i.e., leukotrienes, thromboxane, prostaglandins) may be a common efferent signal in the pathogenesis of septic shock. Plasma levels of prostaglandins, thromboxanes, and leukotrienes are increased during endotoxemia and after cytokine administration. Thromboxane may be a particularly critical mediator since thromboxane antagonism prevents ischemia-induced neutrophil oxidative burst in rats and improves oxygen delivery and consumption in burned sheep. In further support of this postulate, rats made essential fatty acid deficient (leading to a decreased arachidonic acid content of tissue phospholipids) demonstrate improved survival during endotoxemia and fail to have significant endotoxin-induced elevations in thromboxane A_2 levels.

The administration of antiprostaglandin agents such as aspirin or indomethacin could favorably alter the course of sepsis. Indeed, several investigators have demonstrated the benefit of pharmacologic inhibition of prostaglandin metabolites in the amelioration of septic shock. However, results to date have not been uniform. Cyclooxygenase and thromboxane synthetase inhibitors can redirect the metabolism of arachidonic acid toward the production of other intermediary eicosanoids such as the endoperoxides and leukotrienes. Unfortunately, the endoperoxides PGG_2 and PGH_2 share many of the physiologic effects of thromboxane. In addition, shunting of arachidonic acid toward the formation of leukotrienes can also result in significant inflammatory activity. This may in part explain the conflicting reports regarding the efficacy on nonsteroidal anti-inflammatory agents in septic shock.

Vegetable (ω-6) vs. Fish Oil (ω-3)

Recent studies attempting to elucidate the physiologic effects of diets enriched with ω-3 fatty acids have centered on the altered formation and metabolism of prostanoids.[38] Eicosapentaenoic acid (EPA, 20:5ω3) has been shown to be the metabolically active fatty acid in fish oil because of its structural similarity to the usual prostaglandin precursor arachidonic acid (20:4ω6). Arachidonic acid is derived from the ω-6 family of fatty acids and gives rise to the dienoic or "2" series of prostaglandins and the "4" series of leukotrienes. EPAs are de-rived from the ω-3 family of fatty acids and form the trienoic or "3" series of prostaglandins and the "5" series of leukotrienes.

The biological activities of these two families of prostaglandins differ significantly. Thromboxane A_2 synthesized by platelets from arachidonic acid, is a very potent platelet aggregator and vasoconstrictor. Thromboxane A_3, formed from EPA, is a moderate vasoconstrictor but will not aggregate platelets. Leukotriene B_4 made from arachidonic acid, is a potent chemotactic and aggregatory agent for neutrophils. Leukotriene B_5, derived from EPA, is only 12% as chemotactic and 5% as active as an aggregating agent relative to leukotriene B_4. However, prostacyclin I_2, synthesized in endothelial cells from arachidonic acid, and prostacyclin I_3 derived from EPA, are both potent vasodilators and platelet antiaggregators.

EPA competes with arachidonic acid as a substrate for the enzymes cyclooxygenase and 5-lipoxygenase, further reducing the formation of proinflammatory eicosanoids. Thus, controlled intake of select fats rich in EPA and ω-3 fatty acids can alter eicosanoid metabolism and lead to a more vasodilatory, platelet and neutrophil antiaggregatory state relative to diets enriched with ω-6 fatty acids (found in high concentrations in various vegetable oils). This altered state of vasoconstriction and neutrophil downregulation may offer a survival advantage to the patient suffering from an overly aggressive systemic inflammatory response to injury and infection.

Several studies performed in our laboratory have demonstrated that both long-term enteral (i.e., 6 weeks) and short-term parenteral (i.e., 3 days) administration of diets enriched with ω-3 fatty acids significantly alters the metabolic response to endotoxin infusion. Mascioli et al.[37] performed a series of survival studies in which guinea pigs were fed diets enriched with either vegetable or fish oil for 6 weeks or infused with lipid emulsion made from vegetable or fish oil for 3 days. In both experiments, animals given the fish oil preparations had improved survival when compared with vegetable oil–fed animals after endotoxin infusion.

In a similar set of experiments, Pomposelli et al.[51] challenged guinea pigs with endotoxin after pretreatment with diets enriched with either safflower oil or fish oil. Animals fed fish oil–containing diets demonstrated significant elevation in long-chain ω-3 fatty acid levels when compared with vegetable oil–fed animals. Significant lactic acidosis developed in animals fed safflower oil and infused with endotoxin when compared with animals fed fish oil. Safflower oil–fed animals given endotoxin and pretreated with either indomethacin or thromboxane receptor blocker had improved blood pH and lower lactate levels. However, these agents had no effect in animals fed fish oil, which consistently had the lowest lactate levels. This suggests that ω-3 fatty acids influence other systems that contribute to the pathogenesis of endotoxin-induced lactic acidosis.[36] In addition to improved lactate levels, mixed venous oxygen tension measured in endotoxin-treated animals given TPN containing fish oil was significantly higher when compared with animals given TPN containing Intralipid. Tissue oxygen delivery may have improved in the fish oil–fed animals.[46]

Endres et al.[52] demonstrated that monocytes obtained from human volunteers previously fed fish oil supplements had a reduced ability to secrete IL-1 and TNF in response to endotoxin infusion. Thus, fish oil feedings significantly reduced the systemic inflammatory response. The anti-inflammatory effects of ω-3 fatty acids have also been demonstrated histologically. Animals fed fish oil exhibit relatively normal lung morphology, whereas safflower-fed animals demonstrated bilateral interstitial infiltrates in response to endotoxin infusion. These effects may prove to be of benefit in altering the pathogenesis of adult respiratory distress syndrome (ARDS). This is supported by the work of Lee et al.,[53] who demonstrated reduced neutrophil chemotaxis and aggregation after fish oil feeding. However, it is still unclear whether the biochemical effects of fish oil feeding observed in vitro and in vivo will necessarily translate into improved clinical outcome.

In general, significant lactic acidosis develops in animals fed diets enriched with safflower oil and infused with endotoxin despite an adequate systemic arterial po_2, cardiac output, and blood pressure. The moderate decrease in blood pressure observed initially after endotoxin infusion is consistent with the hyperdynamic phase of sepsis. In a state of vasodilation, as observed acutely after endotoxin infusion, an increase in cardiac output would be expected to contribute to normalization of the blood pressure. Therefore, the observed "normal" cardiac output may represent the transition from hyperdynamic to hypodynamic sepsis because preliminary studies show that most animals exhibit rapid deterioration and death within a few hours of endotoxin infusion.

Supplementation with ω-3 fatty acids may be a useful adjunct to current therapy by reducing the development and consequences of septic shock syndromes. Indeed, several recent studies have demonstrated benefit of ω-3 fatty acid feeding in improving the outcome from experimental peritonitis, reducing myocardial reperfusion injury in animals, and having a favorable impact on the natural history of ulcerative colitis in humans.[45,48] Other fatty acids that may have use in sepsis syndromes are also under study. These include γ-linolenic acid (GLA), which is an intermediate metabolite of linoleic acid. GLA given in high doses can be metabolized to PGE_1, which demonstrates some of the same desirable actions on blood vessels and platelet antiaggregation observed with ω-3 fatty acids. Since GLA is an ω-6 fatty acid, there is the possibility that its beneficial effects may be offset by metabolism to arachidonic acid. Given the complicated network of efferent signals involved in the critically ill patient (i.e., monokines, eicosanoids, etc.), future studies should more precisely define the impact of various families of fatty acids on cellular metabolism.

STRUCTURED LIPIDS

Recently, lipid emulsions have been developed that include triglycerides containing a variety of fatty acids, so-called structured lipids or "structured triglycerides" (see Fig 12–1). These lipid emulsions are biochemically created by mixing together a variety of fatty acids (i.e., MCTs, ω-3 LCTs, and ω-6 LCTs).[39] The triglycerides are subjected to hydrolysis and subsequent reesterification after random mixing of the different fatty acid forms. This produces various triglycerides that contain one or two long-chain fatty acids, one or two MCFAs and one or two ω-3 fatty acids. The new "structured triglyceride" varies depending on the particular fatty acid complement. Presently, in the United States intravenous structured lipids are still in the experimental phase. However, they are available in the enteral form.

Lipids are important components of the host response to injury and sepsis. In addition to serving as preferred fuel substrates, they also act as modulators of cellular function. The search for the optimal lipid composition for use as both fuel and modulator has led to the development of structured lipids.

Jandacek et al. demonstrated that MCTs and LCTs are efficiently absorbed from the intestine when they are in the form of a structured lipid.[40] Structured lipids with MCTs on the 1 and 3 positions and an LCT on the 2 position are most effectively absorbed. These findings are supported by the work of others.[41]

MCT/LCT structured lipids, in stressed animal models, demonstrate improved nitrogen balance, higher serum albumin concentrations, and increased protein synthesis in liver and muscle.[42–44] These results are particularly evident with a mixture of 60% to 75% MCT and 40% to 25% LCT. When the mixture of MCT/LCT is on a 50:50 molar basis, there is no improvement in the protein-sparing effect. In addition, animal studies indicate that structured lipids improve RES function (Table 12–6).

Polyunsaturated ω-3 fatty acids have also been incorporated into structured lipids. In a burn model, animals fed a structured lipid of 60% MCT and 40% ω-3 demonstrate improved nitrogen balance, increased protein synthesis, decreased protein oxidation, and a reduced energy expenditure as compared with animals fed LCTs alone.[45] These results are explained by the improved protein-sparing effect of the MCT-based structured lipid and the decreased en-

TABLE 12–6.

Advantages and Disadvantages of Triglycerides

Long chain (LCT)
  Disadvantages
    Inhibition of neutrophil function
    Inhibition of macrophage phagocytosis
    Impairment of reticuloendothelial system
    Decreased clearance by lipoprotein lipase in sepsis
    Dependent on carnitine oxidation, which is decreased in sepsis
Medium chain (MCT)
  Advantages
    Hydrolyzed at the intestinal brush border and transported by the portal circulation
    Efficiently oxidized to acetate, ketones, and CO_2
    Decreased adipose tissue storage
    Oxidized by a carnitine-independent pathway
    Decreased blockage of the reticuloendothelial system
MCT/LCT structure lipids
  Advantages
    Advantages of MCT
    Reduced toxicity of MCT alone
    Improved LCT absorption from the intestine
    Improved LCT clearance from the blood
    Improved protein sparing in injured animals
    Decreased protein oxidation by leucine kinetics
    Increased protein synthesis in the liver and muscle
    Improved hepatic reticuloendothelial bacterial clearance
    Decreased bacterial sequestration in the lung

ergy expenditure resulting from the ω-3 lipid. Animals infused with a structured lipid of MCT/ω-3 PUFA demonstrate an improved cardiovascular response to endotoxemia as compared with LCT-fed animals.[46, 47] Finally, animals fed a structured lipid of MCT/ω-3 PUFA and then starved for 48 hours demonstrate an improved metabolic response to thermal injury,[48] thus indicating a lasting effect on cell membrane composition.

There is evidence that structured lipids can improve host defense against tumors. The structured lipid most studied is a MCT/ω-3 structured lipid. Although tumor protein turnover in tumor-bearing animals is increased in the structured lipid group, tumor growth is reduced.[49] Other experiments show that sarcoma-bearing rats infused with both TNF and structured lipid have a greater reduction in tumor volume (while maintaining carcass weight and nitrogen balance) than rats infused with TNF alone.[50]

Presently, evidence exists to suggest that structured lipids may play a role in the nutritional support of critically ill patients and improve host defenses. Structured lipid diminishes the depression of host defenses associated with LCT and takes advantage of the efficient MCT substrate and the biological activity of specific LCTs such as ω-3. Enterally, structured lipid results in a more efficient absorption of LCT, while parenterally there is evidence of improved LCT clearance. Structured lipid reduces stress-induced protein catabolism and improves net protein synthesis in the liver. Specifically, structured lipid results in improved RES function and decreased bacterial sequestration in the lungs. The RES is an important host defense against endotoxin and loss of gastrointestinal barrier function. Currently, there are a variety of enteral products being studied that contain structural lipids. The efficacy of one product over another has yet to be elucidated.

There is good evidence that lipid mixtures of triglycerides designed for special medical purposes play an important role in the nutritional support of critically ill patients. Experiments to date demonstrate that by altering the composition of lipid emulsions, the depression of host defenses often seen with traditional LCT formulas is less common. Structured lipids may provide the opportunity to take advantage of efficient MCT substrates and the biological activity of specific LCTs such as ω-3 triglycerides. Enterally, structured lipid results in more efficient absorption of LCTs, while parenterally there is increasing evidence of improved LCT clearance. Lipid research needs to determine the effect of these designer molecules during sepsis and injury, particularly with regard to specific host defenses. It is hoped that lipid modulation will improve patient outcome.

REFERENCES

1. Alexander JW, Saito H, Ogle CK, et al: The importance of lipid type in the diet after burn injury. *Ann Surg* 1986; 204:1–8.
2. Jensen GL, Mascioli EA, Meyer LP, et al: Dietary modification of chyle composition in chylothorax. *Gastroenterology* 1989; 97:761–765.
3. Gottschlich MM, Alexander JW: Fat kinetics and recommended dietary intake in burns. *JPEN* 1987; 11:80–85.
4. Stein TP, Blackburn GL: Problems and perspectives with lipids: Where next? *JPEN* 1988; 12(suppl):136–138.
5. Babineau TJ, Borlase BC, Blackburn GL: Applied total parenteral nutrition in the critically ill, in Rippe JM, et al (eds): *Intensive Care Medicine.* Boston, Little, Brown, 1991.
6. Borlase BC, Babineau TJ, Forse RA, et al: Enteral nutritional support, in Rippe JM, et al (eds): *Intensive Care Medicine.* Boston, Little, Brown, 1991.
7. Wiener M, Rothkopf MM, Rothkopf G, et al: Fat metabolism in injury and stress. *Crit Care Clin* 1987; 3:1–25.

8. Little RA, Stoner HB, Frayn KN: Substrate oxidation shortly after accidental injury in man. *Clin Sci* 1981; 61:789–791.

8a. Cuthbertson DP: Post-shock metabolic response. *Lancet* 1:433, 1942.

9. Forse RA: Fat metabolism in sepsis. Personal communication, 1993.

10. Wan JMF, Haw MP, Blackburn GL: Symposium of the interaction between nutrition and inflammation. *Proc Nutr Soc* 1989; 48:315–335.

11. Cummings JH, Branch WJ: Fermentation and the production of short chain fatty acids in the human large intestine, in Vahouny GB, Kritchevsky D (eds): *Dietary Fiber: Basic and Clinical Aspects.* New York, Plenum Publishing Corp, 1986, 131–152.

12. Demigne C, Remesy C: Stimulation of absorption of volatile fatty acids and minerals in the cecum of rats adapted to a very high fiber diet. *J Nutr* 1985; 115:53–60.

13. Ruppin H, Bar-Meir S, Soergel KH, et al: Absorption of short chain fatty acids by the colon. *Gastroenterology* 1980; 78:1500–1507.

14. Hoverstad T: Studies of short chain fatty acid absorption in man. *Scand J Gastroenterol* 1986; 21:257–260.

15. Kvietys PR, Granger ND: Effect of volatile fatty acids on blood flow and oxygen uptake by the dog colon. *Gastroenterology* 1981; 80:962–969.

16. Kripke SA, Fox AD, Berman JM, et al: Stimulation of intestinal mucosal growth with intracolonic infusion of short chain fatty acids. *JPEN* 1989; 13:117–123.

17. Koruda MJ, Rolandelli RH, Settle RG, et al: Effect of parenteral nutrition supplemented with short chain fatty acids on adaption to massive small bowel resection. *Gastroenterology* 1988; 95:715–720.

18. Kripke SA, Fox AD, Berman JM, et al: Stimulation of intestinal mucosal growth with intracolonic infusion of short-chain fatty acids. *JPEN* 1989; 13:109–115.

19. Rolandelli RH, Koruda MJ, Settle RG, et al: Effects of intraluminal infusion of short chain fatty acids on the healing of colonic anastomosis in the rat. *Surgery* 1986; 100:198–203.

20. Koruda MJ, Rolandelli RH, Settle RG, et al: The effect of short chain fatty acids on the small bowel mucosa (abstract). *JPEN* 1987; 8(suppl).

21. Harig JM, Soergel KH: Treatment of diversion colitis with short chain fatty acid (SCFA) irrigation. *N Engl J Med* 1989; 320:23–28.

22. Breur RI, Buto SK, Christ MD, et al: Rectal irrigation with short chain fatty acids for distal ulcerative colitis. *Dig Dis Sci* 1991; 36:185–187.

23. Isselbacher KJ: Mechanisms of absorption of long and medium chain triglycerides, in Senior JR (ed): *Medium Chain Triglycerides.* Philadelphia, University of Pennsylvania, 1968, pp 21–33.

24. Hill JO, Peters JC, Swift LL, et al: Changes in blood lipids during six days of overfeeding with medium chain or long chain triglycerides. *J Lipid Res* 1990; 31:407–416.

25. Swift LL, Hill JO, Peters JC, et al: Medium chain fatty acids: Evidence for incorporation into chylomicron triglyceride in humans. *Am J Clin Nutr* 1990; 52:834–836.

26. Forse RA, Blackburn GL, Bistrian BR: The role of structured lipids in host defense interactions. Submitted for publication.

27. Mascioli EA, Lopes S, Randall S, et al: Serum fatty acid profile after intravenous medium chain triglyceride administration. *Lipids* 1989; 24:793–798.

28. Johnson RC, Young SK, Cotter R, et al: Medium chain triglyceride lipid emulsion: Metabolism and tissue distribution. *Am J Clin Nutr* 1990; 52:502–528.

29. Otto DA: Relationship of the ATP/ADP ratio to the site of octanoate activation. *J Biol Chem* 1984; 259:5490–5494.

30. Sneidner DL, Mascioli EA, Istfan NW, et al: Effects of long-chain triglyceride emulsions on therapy in humans. *JPEN* 1989; 13:614–619.

31. Bach A, Guisard D, Debry G, et al: Metabolic effects following a medium chain triglyceride load in dogs. V. Influence of the perfusion rate. *Arch Int Physiol Biochim* 1974; 82:705–719.

32. Cotter R, D'Alleinne C: Medium-chain triglycerides. A preclinical perspective, in Kinney JM, Borm PR (eds): *Perspec-*

tives in Clinical Nutrition. Baltimore, Urban Scwarzenberg, 1989.

33. Mascioli EA, Porter KA, Randall S, et al: Metabolic response to intravenous medium-chain triglyerices, in Kinney JM, Borum PR (eds): *Perspectives in Clinical Nutrition.* Baltimore, Urban Schwarzenberg, 1989.

34. Mascioli EA, Randall S, Porter KA, et al: Thermogenesis from intravenous medium-chain triglycerides. *JPEN* 1991; 15:27–31.

35. Redmond HP, Shou J, Kelly CJ, et al: Immune response in mild and severe protein-calorie malnutrition. *JPEN* 1991; 15(suppl):21.

36. Pscheidl EM, Wan JM, Blackburn GL, et al: Influence of omega-3 fatty acids on splanchnic blood flow and lactate metabolism in an endotoxemic rat model. *Metabolism* 1992; 41:698–705.

37. Mascioli EA, Iwasa Y, Trimbo S, et al: Endotoxin challenge after menhaden oil diet: Effects on survival of guinea pigs. *Am J Clin Nutr* 1989; 49:277–282.

38. Pomposelli JJ, Mascioli EA, Bistrian BR, et al: Attenuation of the febrile response in guinea pigs by fish oil enriched diets. *JPEN* 1989; 13:136–140.

39. Babayan VK: Medium chain triglycerides and structured lipids. *Lipids* 1987; 22:417–420.

40. Jandacek RJ, Whiteside JA, Holcombe BN, et al: The rapid hydrolysis and efficient absorption of triglycerides with octanoic acid in the 1 and 3 positions and long-chain fatty acid in the 2 position. *Am J Clin Nutr* 1987; 45:940–945.

41. Hubbard VS, McKenna MC: Absorption of safflower oil and structured lipid preparations in patients with cystic fibrosis. *Lipids* 1987; 22:424–428.

42. Mok KT, Maiz A, Yamazaki K, et al: Structured medium-chain and long-chain triglyceride emulsions are superior to physical mixtures in sparing body protein in the burned rat. *Metabolism* 1984; 33:910–915.

43. DeMichelle SJ, Karlstad MD, Babayan VK, et al: Enhanced skeletal muscle and liver protein synthesis with structured lipid in enterally fed burned rats.

44. DeMichele SJ, Karlstad MD, Bistrian BR, et al: Enteral nutrition with structured lipid: Effect on protein metabolism in thermal injury. *Am J Clin Nutr* 1989; 50:1295–1302.

45. Teo TC, DeMichele SJ, Selleck KM, et al: Administration of structured lipid composed of MCT and fish oil reduces net protein catabolism in enterally fed burned rats. *Ann Surg* 1989; 210:100–107.

46. Pomposelli JJ, Flores E, Hirschberg Y, et al: Short-term TPN containing n-3 fatty acids ameliorate lactic acidosis induced by endotoxin in guinea pigs. *Am J Clin Nutr* 1990; 52:548–552.

47. Teo TC, Selleck KM, Wan JMF, et al: Long-term feeding with structured lipid composed of medium chain and n-3 fatty acids ameliorates endotoxic shock in guinea pigs. Submitted for publication.

48. Swenson ES, Selleck KM, Babayan VK, et al: Persistence of metabolic effects after long term oral feeding of a structured triglyceride derived from medium chain triglyceride and fish oil in burned and normal rats. Submitted for publication.

49. Ling P, Istfan N, Babayan V, et al: Effect of fish oil medium chain triglyceride structured lipid (FMS) on tumor growth and protein metabolism in Yoshida sarcoma-bearing rats. *JPEN* 1989; 13(suppl):5.

50. Mendez B, Crosby L, Babayan V, et al: Metabolic effects of structured lipid (SL) composed of MCT and fish oil (MCT/FO)d in sarcoma-bearing rats. *JPEN* 1989; 13(suppl):21.

51. Pomposelli JJ, Flores EA, Blackburn GL, et al. Diets enriched with n-3 fatty acid ameliorate lactic acidosis by improving endotoxin-induced tissue, hypoperfusion in guinea pigs. *Ann Surg* 1991; 213:166–176.

52. Endres S, Ghorbani R, Nelley VE, et al: Dietary n-3 polyunsaturated fatty acids suppress synthesis of IL-1 and tumor necrosis factor. *N Engl J Med* 1987; 317:397–403.

53. Lee TH, Mecia-Huerta JM, Shih C, et al: Characterization and biologic properties 5,12-dehydroxy derivatives of eicosapentaenoic acid including leukotriene B5 and the double lipoxygenase product. *J Biol Chem* 1984;259:2383–2389.

13

Nucleotides

Charles Van Buren, M.D.

Nucleotides are those elements in cells that direct much of the metabolic activity of the cells, tissues, and organs of living organisms. They consist of nucleobases, both purines and pyrimidines, as well as the carbohydrate ribose-phosphate. In polymeric form nucleotides are present as DNA and RNA. In these forms, nucleotides make up the genetic material that guides protein synthesis and controls much of the cell's activity. In monomeric form, such as nucleoside phosphates, these compounds serve as energy stores or as intracellular messengers responding to hormonal or external stimuli. Nucleotides are ubiquitous throughout most cells and participate in the regulation of cellular function.

cules can be synthesized de novo from other substrates. The purines adenine and guanine are synthesized from the amino acids carbamylphosphate and *N*-formyltetrahydrofolate. The pyrimidines cytosine, thymine, and uracil are synthesized de novo from asparate and carbamoylphosphate. Synthesis of phosphoribosylpyrophosphate (PRRP) is a high-energy–requiring process that occurs via the pentose shunt. PRPP is required to synthesize nucleotides, compounds combining nucleobases along with ribose-phosphate. Thus, with adequate provision of carbohydrate, protein, folate, phosphate, and other vitamins, nucleotide synthesis can take place adequately to meet the needs of an unstressed organism.

DE NOVO SYNTHESIS

As can be surmised for such an elemental part of living cells, these mole-

EXOGENOUS SOURCES

The fate of orally ingested purines has been well studied. Studies using radioactively labeled adenine showed that 90% of the label appeared either in the intestinal mucosa or in the liver.[1] Approximately 5% of labeled adenine could be found in splenic and lymphatic tissue. Other purines are degraded to uric acid or allaction, depending on the species. Intestinal epithelial cells are especially dependent on exogenous purines since these rapidly replicating cells appear to be unable to synthesize purines de novo.

Uric acid represents the major end product of purine catabolism. The catabolic products of pyrimidines are β-alanine and β-aminoisobutyric acid, which are nontoxic and easily catabolized or eliminated. A negative feedback for de novo pyrimidine synthesis is exhibited by both dietary pyrimidines and purines.[2] Thus, dietary sources of purines or pyrimidines can have an influence on the rate of de novo synthesis of these compounds and can be incorporated directly into rapidly dividing cell populations.

CONDITIONS OR TISSUES NEEDING EXOGENOUS SOURCES

Rapidly Proliferating Cells

Although dietary sources of nucleotides do have an influence on de novo synthesis rates for purines and pyrimidines in the body and can be directly found in various organs in the body, it had been assumed that body needs for these compounds could be met by de novo synthesis.[3] However, some tissues appear to have a greater need for nucleotides than can be met by de novo synthesis. A casein-based nucleotide-free diet (NFD) in rats resulted in a decrease in rat small intestinal and colonic RNA content.[4] Messenger RNA levels decreased for purine salvage enzymes in the small intestine but not in the liver. No corresponding decrease was observed in intestinal mucosal cells of

RNA-supplemented hosts. These findings suggest that rapidly proliferating cells do have a heretofore unrecognized need for exogenous sources of nucleotides.

Lymphocytes

Lymphocytes also appear to need exogenous sources of purines or pyrimidines for optimum responsiveness. Lymphocyte proliferation is enhanced in vitro by provision of exogenous nucleosides.[5] G_1 thymocytes or peripheral lymphocytes do not have de novo biosynthetic capability, whereas S-phase large thymocytes have this capacity.[6] Consistent with the lack of de novo synthetic ability is the enhanced capacity of G_1-phase thymocytes to salvage pyrimidines,[7] a capacity greater than that found in G_1-phase peripheral lymphocytes. These findings suggest that at an early phase in T-lymphocyte development and before initiation of T-lymphocyte division, these populations of cells are dependent on nucleoside salvage and are vulnerable to deprivation of these substrates.

Purine Metabolic Defects

Defects in purine metabolism have severe effects on normal immune responses. Adenine deaminase (ADA) deficiency is a disorder associated with depressed lymphocyte production and severe inhibition of both T-lymphocyte and B-lymphocyte responses.[8] Purine nucleoside phosphorylase deficiency, on the other hand, results in the less severe disorder of primarily defective cellular immunity, which is influenced by T-lymphocyte function.[9] Both of these enzymes are induced in peripheral lymphocytes and regional lymph nodes following immunostimulation.[10] Thus, increased purine metabolic activity is required to propagate a normal immune response.

Suppression of Allograft Rejection Response

Although in vitro requirements for exogenous nucleosides had been previously documented, the presumption had been that these substrates were not required for developing animal or man. This presumption was challenged by the observation that rejection of a heterotopic heart allograft in a murine model was significantly delayed in recipients maintained by NFDs for 4 weeks before transplantation. This diet, which was casein based, was equivalent in protein content to the chow-based normal rodent diet. Weight gain and albumin levels were comparable in animals maintained on chow or NFD. This suppression of the rejection response was eliminated if animals were maintained on NFD supplemented with 0.25% yeast RNA (NFR).[11]

This experiment was repeated, with BALB/c mice maintained on chow, NFD, or NFR before heart transplantation. Animals were randomly assigned to receive cyclosporine (10 mg/kg for 4 days) or olive oil by gavage feeding. This dose of cyclosporine did not prolong allograft survival in chow-fed or NFR-fed hosts. Only NFD-fed animals exhibited enhanced allograft survival, a prolongation that was statistically significant when compared with the enhanced survival with NFD alone.[12] This experiment confirmed that NFDs suppress rejection of a cardiac allograft. This immunosuppressive effect was synergistic with a subtherapeutic dose of a potent immunosuppressant, cyclosporine.

This evidence that exogenous nucleotides were required to maintain normal host responses to foreign antigens was confirmed by three separate delayed hypersensitivity models. In each model, mice were maintained on the assigned diets for 2 to 3 weeks before sensitization with an immunogen. The inoculating preparations were either complete Freund's adjuvant or sheep erythrocytes (SRBCs). The chemical immunogen was dinitrofluorobenzene (DNFB). The dietary groups, in addition to chow (F), NFD, and NFR, included NFD supplemented with 0.06% adenine (NFA) or 0.06% uracil (NFU). The nucleobases were readily interconvertible with other respective purine or pyrimidine bases, and the content by weight reflected the amount of either purines or pyrimidines present in the 0.25% RNA diet.

Following maintenance on these experimental diets, mice were rechallenged with the immunizing antigen (purified protein derivative [PPD] in the case of complete Freund's adjuvant). In each case the diet devoid of nucleotides was immunosuppressive. Both chow and the RNA-supplemented diets maintained normal delayed cutaneous hypersensitivity responses. NFA feedings did not maintain responsiveness; the uracil-supplemented diet supported a normal delayed cutaneous hypersensitivity response.[13]

The mechanism by which dietary nucleotide restriction appears to exert its suppressive effect on allograft rejection and development of delayed cutaneous hypersensitivity responses appears to be through the arrest of normal T-lymphocyte maturation. Terminal deoxynucleotidyl transferase (TdT) is a surface enzyme marker of cellular immaturity. In mice that are maintained on NFD, the concentrations of TdT-positive lymphocytes or thymocytes are elevated in the thymus and bone marrow as compared with chow-fed or RNA-supplemented hosts (Table 13-1).[14] The retardation of lymphocyte maturation does not appear to be uniform throughout lymphocyte populations. Following immunostimulation with complete Freund's adjuvant, NFD-fed hosts have depressed levels of phenotypic T-helper lymphocytes as compared with chow-fed or RNA-supplemented groups. In contrast, levels of T-suppressor and/or T-cytotoxic cells appear to be unaffected by diet. This sup-

TABLE 13–1.

Presence of Terminal Deoxynucleotidyl Transferase in Lymphoid Tissue From BALB/c Mice on Specific Diets*

Diet	Lymphoid Tissue—TdT-positive cells (%)		
	Thymus†(5)‡	Bone Marrow§(3)	Spleen¶(4)
F	11.4 ± 3.5	8.7 ± 1.0	5.4 ± 3.6
NFD	29.4 ± 4.4	27.2 ± 1.8	11.2 ± 5.6
NFR	16.3 ± 4.0	9.3 ± 0.3	5.1 ± 1.3
NFA	14.5 ± 1.5	14.8 ± 0.6	12.3 ± 4.3
NFU	15.5 ± 4.0	17.9 ± 2.1	7.9 ± 1.4

*Data from Rudolph FB, Fanslow WC, Kulkarni AD, et al: *Adv Exp Med Biol* 1985; 195:49. Used by permission.
†NFD vs. F, $P < .03$; NFD vs. NFR, $P < .05$; NFD vs. NFA, $P < .05$.
‡Numbers in parentheses indicate the number of animals.
§NFD vs. F, NFR, $P < .005$; NFD vs. NFA, NFU, $P < .05$; NFU, NFA vs. NFR, $P < .02$.
¶$P > .05$ for all groups.

pression of T-helper cell members is partially mediated by a suppression of interleukin-2 (IL-2) production in NFD-fed hosts.[15] RNA supplementation maintains normal IL-2 production, vital to normal maturation of cellular immunity and the production of antigen-specific T-killer lymphocytes.

In a model examining lymph nodes in animals that have received footpad injections of allogeneic spleen cells, the restriction of dietary nucleotides appears to alter the cellular metabolic and physiologic transformations vital to lymphocyte maturation. NFD-fed hosts fail to exhibit induction of ADA, the purine metabolic enzyme whose deficiency results in severe combined immunodeficiency. In both naive and immunostimulated NFD-fed hosts, purine nucleoside phosphorylase levels are depressed when compared with chow-fed groups.[16] Thus two vital enzymes in purine and pyrimidine metabolism are negatively influenced by the absence of nucleotides from the diet. NFD-fed hosts also exhibit decreased production of the IL-2 receptor on lymphocytes, vital early in the propagation of a normal T-cell response.[17] These alterations affected by dietary nucleotide restriction help to explain the suppression of cellular immunity previously observed.

Previously presented data were obtained in animals that had received adequate calories and protein throughout the study. However, the clinical setting in which nutritional support is usually prescribed is in patients who are protein and/or calorie malnourished. To address whether dietary nucleotides were required to reverse immunosuppression induced by protein deprivation, BALB/c mice were placed on a protein-free diet for 7 to 10 days. During this period the mice lost 20% to 25% of body weight. The mice were then randomly allocated to NFD, NFR, NFA, NFU, or chow or continued on a protein-free diet. At the time of assignment to the various diets, mice were inoculated in the hind footpad with allogeneic $C_{57}BL/6$ irradiated spleen cells. The contralateral footpad was injected with syngeneic (BALB/c) spleen cells to control for nonspecific immune stimulation. Mice were weighed daily and sacrificed 7 days following inoculation. Popliteal lymph nodes from both hind limbs were harvested, and the weights of allogeneically stimulated nodes were divided by the weight of the contralateral popliteal node to calculate a stimulation index of immune responsiveness.

All mice converted from a protein-free to an NFD, NFR, NFU, NFA, or chow diet regained lost weight. No difference was noted in restoration of weight between these groups. In contrast, mice continued on a protein-free diet continued to lose weight and had an average 30% weight loss at the time of sacrifice.

TABLE 13-2.

Effect of Various Diets on In Vivo Popliteal Lymph Node Response Following Protein Starvation*

Diet Group†	Lymph Node Weight (mg)		
	Allogenic Node	Syngeneic Node	Delta‡
PF→PF	3.1 ± 0.6§	1.2 ± 0.2	1.2 ± 0.6
PF→NFD	2.9 ± 0.2	1.4 ± 0.1	1.5 ± 0.1
PF→NFR (0.025%)	7.4 ± 0.6	1.7 ± 0.2	5.7 ± 0.5¶
PF→NFR (2.5%)	7.0 ± 0.8	1.4 ± 0.2	5.6 ± 0.9¶
PF→NFU (0.6%)	9.8 ± 1.0	1.7 ± 0.3	7.9 ± 1.0¶
F→F	8.6 ± 1.2	1.5 ± 0.3	7.1 ± 1.2¶

*Data from Kulkarni AD, et al: Used by permission.
†All animals except the F→F group were on a protein-free diet (Purina 5755) (PF) for 7 to 10 days and then randomly placed on the indicated diets and the popliteal lymph node response determined after 7 days. There were five mice per diet group.
‡The delta value is the mean of the difference between the allogeneic mode weight and the syngeneic mode weight.
§Results are expressed as the mean weight in milligrams plus or minus SEM.
¶PF, NFD vs. NFR (0.025%), NFR (2.5%), NFU (0.6%), F: $P < .05$.

Immune restoration was dependent on the presence of either RNA or uracil in the diet. The mice maintained NFD, even though they regained lost weight, had an immune response that was not better than the mice continued on protein starvation (Table 13-2). Thus, provision of calories and protein alone is inadequate to reverse the immunosuppression induced by protein starvation. Dietary nucleotides or dietary pyrimidines are necessary to restore lost immune function.[18] These findings, if extended to man, may help to explain the lack of association in previous clinical studies between improved nitrogen balance after nutritional support and changes in infection and/or mortality rates.

Infection

The above-mentioned studies focused on the influence of dietary nucleotides on lymphocyte function and cellular immunity. To test the hypothesis that these findings altered the host response to infective organisms, BALB/c mice maintained on NFD, NFU, NFR, NFA, or chow were inoculated intravenously with either fungal (Candida albicans) or bacterial (Staphylococcus aureus) pathogens. All mice were maintained on the assigned diets 3 weeks before inoc-

ulation. In the mice inoculated with Candida, survival was significantly prolonged ($P < .02$) in NFR- or NFU-fed hosts.[19] NFD- or NFA-fed mice died more rapidly. This decreased resistance to fungal infection was reflected in the ability to culture viable organisms from the spleens. NFD- and NFA-fed hosts had higher numbers of viable fungal organisms recovered from their spleens as compared with the NFR or NFU groups. These findings were expected since cellular immunity appears to play an important role in resistance to fungal infections.

Unexpectedly, a median infective dose (LD_{60}) of S. aureus in chow-fed hosts resulted in a 100% mortality rate in NFD-fed mice. RNA or uracil supplementation resulted in improved survival following bacterial inoculation, whereas adenine supplementation had no beneficial effect.[20] Since cellular immunity is not known to have an important role in defenses against gram-positive bacterial infections, macrophage responses were examined. The phagocytic capacity of macrophages could not explain the difference in survival. Although the NFR-fed group exhibited enhanced ability of de novo isolated macrophages to engulf radiolabeled bacteria, no difference was observed in the phagocytic capacity of macrophages from the NFD and chow groups. Instead, the bactericidal capacity of splenic macrophages appeared to correlate with resistance to *S. aureus*. NFR-, NFU-, and chow-fed groups exhibited a better capacity to kill phagocytosed bacteria than either NFD- or NFA-fed animals. Further studies revealed a decreased production of superoxide in macrophages of animals maintained on NFD as compared with NFR or chow.[21] Thus, the requirement for dietary nucleotides appeared to be important for nonspecific as well as specific host defenses.

Bone Marrow Engraftment

The revelation that macrophage as well as T-lymphocyte function appeared to depend on exogenous nucleotides suggested a more basic role for these substrates. To test for acute graft-vs.-host disease (GVHD) in a bone marrow transplant model, syngeneic radiation chimera bone marrow donors were maintained on NFD; it was found that the incidence of GVHD was decreased in H_2-incompatible irradiated hosts, as compared with chow-fed donors.[22] The influence was not permanent; donors that had been fed NFD for 6 to 8 weeks following bone marrow infusion had suppressed capacity to cause GVHD, whereas donors maintained for 15 weeks had a normal alloreactive capability. These findings are most consistent with a delay in maturation of T lymphocytes or their precursors. To support these conclusions, bone marrow harvested from NFD-fed mice had a decreased responsiveness to IL-3, an important cytokine for lymphocyte maturation. RNA-supplemented hosts had a normal response to IL-3.[23] Bone marrow cells, when transfused into NFD-fed hosts, had a diminished capacity to engraft as splenic colonies when compared with marrow from chow-fed or RNA-supplemented hosts. Uracil-fed hosts support normal marrow engraftment, whereas adenine-supplemented hosts have a suppressed capacity to enhance engraftment. Thus, the influence of dietary nucleotides on elements of the immune system may be much broader and affect a less-differentiated population of immunopotent cells than initially suspected.

These findings suggest that dietary nucleotides are required to support the normal growth and development of T-lymphocytes; dietary restriction of this substrate retards the development of cellular immunity and specific T-lymphocyte—mediated host responses. The mechanism appears to be based on maturation arrest in T-lymphocyte development, focused primarily on T-helper cells. This results in defective production of IL-2 and resultant clonal expansion. These diet-induced changes in T-helper lymphocyte activity result in diminished allograft rejection and increased susceptibility to fungal infection.

Nonspecific Host Defense Mechanisms

Nonspecific host defense mechanisms also appear to require dietary nucleotides for optimal function. Macrophage bactericidal activity is suppressed in NFD-fed animals. A result of this suppression of phagocytic cell function is enhanced mortality from bacterial challenge in NFD-fed hosts. Dietary RNA prevents this compromise of host defenses. In both these studies and studies of lymphoproliferative responses, pyrimidines mimic the action of RNA, whereas purines are usually ineffective in maintaining immune responsiveness.

In examining the ability to restore lost immune function following protein starvation, calories and protein alone are inadequate to restore cellular immunity. Dietary nucleotides are required to restore lost immune responsiveness. Pyrimidines in the diet exert a similar effect.

CLINICAL STUDIES

To extend these findings to clinical studies, dietary nucleotides have been incorporated in an enteral feeding formula with two other immunopotent substrates (i.e., fish oil and arginine). Fish oil, which is rich in ω-3 fatty acids, has been demonstrated to enhance lymphoproliferative responses to lectins.[24] The suggested mechanism for this effect is the enhanced production of prostaglandin E_3 (PGE_3) rather than PGE_2, the latter of which is synthesized from arachidonic acid. PGE_2 appears to suppress lymphoproliferative responses.[25] Arginine is a dibasic amino acid that enhances thymic development and increases lymphocyte numbers and responses. The mechanism by which this amino acid exerts these effects remains to be elucidated.

In single-substrate comparisons of immune-enhancing effects, fish oil and dietary RNA appeared to be equivalent in maintaining lymphoproliferative responses. Arginine appeared less effective (Fig. 13–1). Moreover, when RNA and fish oil were combined with arginine, there appeared to be an additive benefit on immune function. These observations were also documented in the staphylococcal inoculation model (Fig. 13–2). This was the basis for the development of an enteral formula combining nucleotides, fish oil, and arginine.

In two clinical studies, an enteral formula containing fish oil, nucleotides, and arginine (Impact) was compared with an isocaloric casein-based enteral formula (Osmolite). In Cerra and colleagues' study of intensive care unit patients, patients who were septic or critically ill were randomly assigned to receive one of the enteral formulas.[26] Patients were studied before nutritional intervention and throughout the study for lymphoproliferative responses to phytohemagglutinin (PHA), concanavalin A (Con A), or tetanus toxoid protein. The study was double blinded and controlled for nitrogen delivery. Since the formula containing arginine contained nearly 12 g/l more of amino acids and/or protein than Osmolite, the Impact-fed patients received fewer calories per day. Randomization was successful, with 11 Impact-fed patients and 9 Osmolite-fed patients having similar

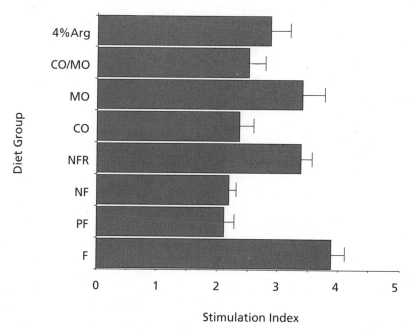

FIG 13–1.

Popliteal lymph node (PLN) assay in various dietary groups: BALB/c mice challenged with C57Bl/6 and BALB/c splenocytes after 4 weeks on various diets. The stimulation index is calculated as the ratio of weight of PLN by allostimulation and synstimulation. Only chow (F), RNA-supplemented diet (NFR), or fish oil–supplemented diets (MO) enhanced immune responsiveness. CO = corn oil–supplemented basal diet; NF = nucleotide-free casein-based diet; PF = protein-free diet.

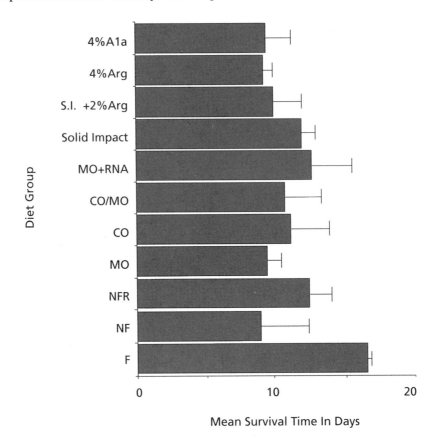

FIG 13–2.
Mean survival time of dietary groups of BALB.c mice following inoculation with 1×10^8 S. *aureus* organisms. Results are represented as the average survival time in days ± SEM. RNA-fed hosts survived longer than mice fed a casein-based diet supplemented with either fish oil or arginine. *CO* = corn oil–supplemented basal diet; *MO* = fish oil–supplemented basal diet; *NF* = nucleotide-free casein-based diet; *NFR* = NF supplemented with 0.25% RNA; *PF* = protein-free diet; *F* = chow; *Solid Impact* = Impact containing RNA, MO, and arginine.

demographics, prestudy nutritional assessments, and severity of illness. Both groups of patients remained on study for an average of 9 days. The Impact-fed patients remained in the hospital for an average of 37 days, whereas Osmolite-fed patients remained in the hospital for 55 days. The differences were not statistically significant because of the small number of patients involved; however the trend is worth noting in light of subsequent observations. What did prove to be statistically significant was the difference in immune response. Osmolite-fed patients demonstrated no difference in immune response throughout the study, with end-of-study lymphocyte proliferative responses practically identical to those observed before feeding. In contrast, Impact-fed patients demon-

strated a statistically significant and steady improvement in lymphoproliferative responses to PHA, Con A, and tetanus, with the highest responses noted at the conclusion of the study. Standard tube feeding failed to improve the initial immune suppression noted in the critically ill patients, while the solution containing nucleotides, fish oil, and arginine significantly improved immune responses. This improvement in the Impact-fed group was present despite no difference in nitrogen balance between the two groups.

In the second study, in postoperative cancer patients, Daly et al. studied the same two enteral solutions in 85 patients with gastrointestinal cancer.[27] Daly and associates controlled for caloric intake, which resulted in the

Impact-fed group receiving significantly more nitrogen despite similar calories as the Osmolite-fed patients. Nitrogen balance, as expected, was better in the Impact-fed group. However, no matter how positive the nitrogen balance in the Osmolite-fed group, no improvement was noted in the immune response of these patients. In contrast, the Impact-fed patients demonstrated a statistically significant improvement in immune function. The clinical outcome associated with this improved immune response was a 70% reduction in infectious and wound complications in the Impact-fed group as compared with the Osmolite-fed group (37% incidence of complications in Osmolite-fed patients as compared with an 11% incidence in Impact-fed patients). This reduced complication rate resulted in a 22% reduction in the length of hospital stay. These are the first two controlled clinical studies to suggest that specially formulated enteral solutions containing nucleotides have a favorable influence on the outcome of hospitalized patients.

Dietary nucleotides appear to be a conditionally essential substrate to support normal nonspecific and specific immune defenses. Investigations in the animal laboratory and the emerging clinical literature suggest that future nutritional therapy should provide patients with dietary nucleotides to minimize the risk of infectious complications, provide cost-effective therapy, and improve outcome.

REFERENCES

1. Sonoda T, Tatibana M: Metabolic fate of pyrimidines and purines in dietary nucleic acids ingested by mice. *Biochim Biophys Acta* 1978; 521:55–66.
2. Zöllner N, Grobner W: In Elliot K, Fitzsimmons DW (eds): *Purine and Pyrimidine Metabolism* Amsterdam, Elsevier, 1977;165–179.
3. Zöllner N: Purine and pyrimidine metabolism. *Prod Nutr Soc* 1982;41:329-342.
4. LeLeiko NS, Martin BA, Walsh M, et al: Regulation of types I, II, III, and IV procollagen mRNA synthesis in glucocorticoid-mediated intestinal development. *Gastroenterology* 1987; 93:1014.
5. Strauss PR, Henderson JF, Goodman MG: Nucleosides and lymphocytes: an overview. *Proc Soc Exp Biol Med* 1985; 179:413–418.
6. Cohen A, Barankiewicz J, Lederman HM, et al: Purine and pyrimidine metabolism in human T lymphocytes: regulation of deoxyribonucleotide metabolism. *Can J Biochem* 1984; 62:577–583.
7. Cohen A, Barankiewicz J, Gelfand EW: Roles of alternative synthetic and catabolic purine pathways in T lymphocyte differentiation. *Ann NY Acad Sci* 1985; 451:26–33.
8. Giblett ER, Anderson JE, Cohen F, et al: Adenosine-deaminase deficiency in two patients with severely impaired cellular immunity. *Lancet* 1972; 2:1067–1069.
9. Giblett ER, Ammann AJ, Sanderman R, et al: *Lancet* 1985; 1:1010.
10. Murray JL, Reuben JM, Munn CG, et al: Decreased 5'-nucleotase activity in lymphocytes from asymptomatic sexually active homosexual men and patients with the acquired immune deficiency syndrome. *Int J Immunopharmacol* 1985; 7:661–669.
11. Van Buren CT, Kulkarni A, Schandle VB, et al: The influence of dietary nucleotides on cell-mediated immunity. *Transplantation* 1983; 36:350-352.
12. Van Buren CT, Kulkarni A, Rudolph FB: *Transplant Proc* 1983; 15:2967–2968.
13. Kulkarni AD, Fanslow WC, Rudolph FB, et al: Nucleotide-free diet and suppression of immune response. *Transplantation* 1987; 44:847–849.
14. Rudolph FB, Fanslow WC, Kulkarni AD, et al: Effect of dietary nucleotides on lymphocyte maturation. *Adv Exp Med Biol* 1986; 195:497–501.
15. Van Buren CT, Kulkarni A, Fanslow WC: *Transplantation* 1985; 40:694–697.
16. Kulkarni AD, Fanslow WC, Rudolph FB, et al: Dietary nucleotides, a requirement for helper/inducer T lymphocytes. *Transplantation* 1992; 53:467–472.

17. Kulkarni A, Fanslow W, Higley H, et al: Expression of immune cell surface markers in vivo and immune competence in mice by dietary nucleotides. *Transplant Proc* 1989; 21:121.

18. Pizzini R, Kumar S, Kulkarni A, et al: Dietary nucleotides reverse malnutrition and starvation-induced immunosuppression. *Arch Surg* 1990; 124:86–90.

19. Fanslow WC, Kulkarni AD, Van Buren CT: Effect of nucleotide restriction and supplementation on resistance to experimental murine candidiasis. *JPEN* 1988; 12:49–52.

20. Kulkarni AD, Fanslow WC, Van Buren CT, et al: Influence of dietary nucleotide restriction on bacterial sepsis and phagocytic cell function in mice. *Arch Surg* 1986; 121:169–172.

21. Kulkarni AD, Rudolph FB, Van Buren CT: In Kabbash L (ed): *CRC Handbook on Nutrition and Immunity.* Boca Raton, Fla, CRC Press, in press.

22. Kulkarni SS, Bhateley DC, Zander AP, et al: Functional impairment of T-lymphocytes in mouse radiation chimeras by a nucleotide-free diet. *Exp Hematol* 1984; 12:694–699.

23. Kulkarni AD, Fanslow WC, Rudolph FB, et al: *Transplantation* 1992; 53:467–472.

24. Kinsella JE, Lokesh B, Broughton S, et al: *Nutrition* 1990; 6:24–44.

25. Goodwin JS: In *Prostaglandins and Immunity.* Boston, Martinus Nijhoff, 1985.

26. Cerra FB, Lehman S, Konstantinides N, et al: *Nutrition* 1990; 6:84–87.

27. Daly JM, Lieberman MD, Goldfine J, et al: *Surgery* 1992; 112:56–67.

Vitamins and Minerals

14

Vitamins

Gary P. Zaloga, M.D.

Lawrence Bortenschlager, M.D.

Fat-soluble vitamins

Vitamin A

Chemistry

Metabolism

Sources

Requirements

Deficiency states

Therapy

Preparations and adverse effects

Vitamin D

Chemistry

Metabolism/function

Sources

Requirements

Deficiency states

Therapy

Preparations and adverse effects

Vitamin E

Chemistry

Metabolism

Sources

Requirements

Deficiency states

Therapy

Preparations and adverse effects

Vitamin K

Chemistry

Metabolism

Sources

Requirements

Deficiency states

Therapy

Preparations and adverse effects

Water-soluble vitamins

Thiamine (vitamin B_1)

Chemistry

Metabolism

Sources

Requirements

Deficiency states

Therapy

Preparations and adverse effects

Riboflavin (vitamin B_2)

Chemistry

Metabolism

Sources

Requirements

Deficiency states

Therapy

Preparations and adverse effects

The word "vitamin" means life. Vitamins are substances essential for the maintenance of normal metabolic functions. They are required for the metabolism of carbohydrates, fats, and protein. Most vitamins are not synthesized in the body. Some are produced by microorganisms in the gut and absorbed via the intestine. Therefore, the body is primarily dependent upon an exogenous supply of these compounds. Healthy individuals consuming normal diets receive adequate quantities of vitamins. However, during states of abnormal body metabolism (i.e., critical illness) and malnutrition, multiple vitamin deficiencies may develop. Little is known of changes in vitamin requirements associated with critical illness, trauma, and surgery. Vitamin deficiencies impair cellular and organ function and recovery from illness. A knowledge of their properties is important when these agents are administered to patients.

The biological half-life of fat-soluble vitamins (i.e., A, D, E, K) in healthy humans is usually long. The biological half-life of vitamin A is 600 days. Thus, significant deficiencies of fat-soluble vitamnins are infrequent. The administration of adequate calories and protein with total parenteral nutrition (TPN) reduces mobilization of body fat and minimizes the release of fat-soluble vitamins. These patients are at risk for fat-soluble vitamin deficiencies if supplementation during TPN is inadequate. Tissue stores of water-soluble vitamins are small, and deficiencies occur early following the onset of malnutrition. Supplementation during TPN is mandatory. Supplements may also be required during enteral feeding in critically ill patients because of inadequate intake and/or increased requirements. In this chapter, we briefly review both the fat-soluble (i.e., A, D, E, K) and the water-soluble vitamins (Table 14−1). We discuss their basic chemistry, metabolism, sources, requirements, manifestations of deficiency, and therapeutic administration.

FAT-SOLUBLE VITAMINS

Vitamin A

Chemistry

Vitamin A is a fat-soluble vitamin found in animal tissues as retinol.[1−15] It exists in several isomeric forms. Naturally occurring vitamin A is found in animal tissues and saltwater fish but not vegetables. However, many vegetables (green leaves of plants and yellow tubers, fruit) contain carotenoid pigments that have a similar chemical structure to that of vitamin A and hence act as provitamins for conversion to vitamin A in the liver. The most important

of these carotenoids with provitamin A activity is β-carotene. In nature, the esterified form of vitamin A is often found as the acetate or the palmitate ester.

Metabolism

Foods containing retinol or carotenoids are digested by gastric and intestinal enzymes, and both forms are absorbed by the intestinal mucosa (primarily the upper tract). Eighty percent to 90% of dietary vitamin A is actively absorbed as retinol esters, while 40% to 60% of β-carotene is absorbed. Following absorption, β-carotene is cleaved to two molecules of retinal (retinaldehyde), which is then reduced to retinol. Most of the retinol is esterified with saturated fatty acids and incorporated into lymph chylomicrons, which enter the bloodstream. Chylomicrons are metabolized and taken up by the liver together with their content of retinol. Retinol is stored as retinol esters in the parenchymal cells of the liver, which contains about 90% of the total body reserves. The liver stores approximately 600,000 IU (enough for 3 to 12 months). These esters are subsequently hydrolyzed and release free alcohol (i.e., retinol). Retinol is transported to peripheral tissues by a specific transport protein, retinol-binding protein. Normal serum concentrations of retinol in the adult are 163 ± 53 IU/dL. Serum levels are maintained until stores are depleted. Thus, serum levels are unreliable indicators of body stores of vitamin A. More accurate estimates can be obtained from measuring the vitamin A content in tissues (especially liver), where 100 to 300 µg/g of tissue is normal. Vitamin A is important for epithelial integrity and is a component of photoreceptors in the retina. It is required for normal growth, vision, and bone maintenance.

Sources

Animal tissues (i.e., dairy products, margarine, liver, fish) are responsible for the daily intake of preformed vitamin A. Vegetable sources supply carotenoid provitamins. Carotenoid compounds, mainly β-carotenes, form part of the yellow and orange pigments of most fruit and vegetables (i.e., carrots, leafy green vegetables, cantaloupes, and papaya).

Requirements

Daily intake of vitamin A is expressed as micrograms of retinol equivalents (RE), where one RE is defined as 1 μg of retinol or 6 μg of β-carotene (making the overall utilization of β-carotene one

TABLE 14–1.

Vitamin Functions, Deficiencies, and Dosage

Vitamin	Functions	Deficiency	Usual Therapeutic Dosage
A	Epithelial integrity Photoreceptors	Night blindness Perifollicular hyperkeratosis Xerophthalmia Keratomalacia Panophthalmitis Blindness	10,000–20,000 μg or 30,000–60,000 IU/day
D	Maintenance of calcium homeostasis, bone mineralization	Rickets Osteomalacia Hypocalcemia	Ergocalciferol, 20–125 μg/day
E	Antioxidant, integrity of membranes	Hemolysis Neural abnormalities	30–100 mg/day
K	Blood coagulation	Hemorrhage Bruising	Phytonadione, 2.5–20 mg/day PO, SC, or IM
C (ascorbic acid)	Reducing agent, collagen and catecholamine synthesis, iron absorption, wound healing, immune function, vascular integrity	Scurvy (loose teeth, gingivitis, hemorrhages, anemia, poor healing)	50–1000 mg/day
B_{12} (cyanocobalamin)	DNA synthesis, maturation of RBCs, neural function, folate metabolism	Pernicious anemia, glossitis, diarrhea, peripheral neuropathy, posterior column disease (CNS), dementia	50 μg/day IM first 2 wk, 100 μg twice weekly for next 2 mo, then 100 μg/mo
Folic acid	Synthesis of DNA, RBC maturation, growth	Pancytopenia, stomatitis, diarrhea	1 mg/day
Riboflavin (B_2)	Energy and protein metabolism, integrity of mucous membranes	Cheilosis, stomatitis, corneal vascularization, dermatitis	5–25 mg/day
Thiamine (B_1)	Carbohydrate metabolism Myocardial function Central and peripheral nerve function	Beriberi, peripheral neuropathy, cardiac failure, Wernicke-Korsakoff syndrome	30–90 mg/day
Pyridoxine (B_6)	Nitrogen metabolism, transamination, porphyrin and heme synthesis, tryptophan conversion to niacin, linoleic acid metabolism	Seizures in infancy, anemia, neuropathy, skin lesions	25–100 mg/day
Niacin	Oxidation-reduction reactions Carbohydrate metabolism	Pellagra (dermatosis, glossitis, GI and CNS dysfunction)	Nicotinic acid, 50–500 mg/day
Biotin	Carboxylation, amino acid and fatty acid metabolism	Dermatitis Glossitis	100–300 μg/day
Pantothenic acid	Component of CoA, carbohydrate and fatty acid metabolism	Burning "feet" syndrome	10 mg/day

sixth that of retinol). The recommended dietary allowance (RDA) for vitamin A is 1000 μg (1.0 mg) of RE for adult males and 800 μg (0.8 mg) for adult females (pregnancy, 1000 μg; lactation, 1200 μg). Vitamin A allowances may also be expressed as international units. One RE (micrograms) is equivalent to 3.33 IU of retinol and 10 IU of β-carotene. Thus, the RDA expressed in international units for vitamin A is 5000 for adult males and 4000 for adult females.

Deficiency States

Vitamin A deficiency, a common problem worldwide (especially in developing countries), may account for the majority of blindness in the young. In the United States, vitamin A deficiency is usually due to fat malabsorption syndromes (i.e., sprue, cystic fibrosis, inflammatory bowel disease, intestinal bypass surgery, bile salt depletion, biliary tract obstruction), alcoholism, long-term parenteral nutrition, laxative abuse (mineral oil based), and prolonged use of drugs such as cholestyramine, colestipol, neomycin, or coichicine. Other causes of deficiency include inadequate dietary intake, rapid loss from the body, infections, and inadequate conversion of carotene to vitamin A (i.e., diabetes mellitus, hypothyroidism). The clinical manifestations of these deficiency states include night blindness, dryness of the conjunctivae (xerosis) and the cornea (xerophthalmia), development of small white patches on the sclera (Bitot spots), ulceration and necrosis of the cornea (keratomalacia), prolapse of the iris, and panophthalmitis leading to blindness. In such patients, keratinization of epithelial tissues of the eyes, lungs, and gastrointestinal and genitourinary tracts may occur and increase the propensity to infection. Vitamin A deficiency may also result in phrynoderma (skin eruption about the hair follicles), growth retardation, decreased resistance to infection, depressed synthesis of corticosteroids, mild leukopenia, and anemia (impaired hemoglobin synthesis). Except for keratomalacia, most of the manifestations of vitamin A deficiency are reversible with adequate replacement therapy. Vitamin A stores have been assessed by measuring changes in serum retinol levels following a load of retinyl palmitate and evaluation of dark adaptation (95% sensitive, 91% specific).

Therapy

When vitamin A is used for therapy, it is provided entirely in the form of retinol, and its biological potency is given in international units. Night blindness and other signs of early deficiency can be effectively treated with 30,000 IU of vitamin A daily for 1 week. Clinical features of advanced disease (i.e., corneal damage) are best treated by the administration of 20,000 IU/kg for at least 5 days followed by a maintenance dose of 10,000 to 20,000 IU (3000 to 6000 μg)/day orally in three divided doses. Vitamin A is available in a liquid form containing an emulsifier that solubilizes the vitamin. However, these forms require bile acids for absorption. When bile acids are deficient, the water-soluble forms may be of greater benefit (i.e., better absorbed).

When supplementation is administered intravenously, as much as 50% may bind to glass/plastic containers or infusion tubing. In addition, vitamin A is susceptible to oxidation and is unstable in parenteral nutrition solutions. Little if any breakdown or binding occurs in the presence of lipid emulsions (3-in-1 mixture). It is recommended that vitamin A be administered at a dose of 2500 to 8000 IU/day during TPN.

Preparations and Adverse Effects

Vitamin A capsules (oil preparation) are available in 10,000-, 25,000-, and 50,000-IU doses. Aquasol A (water-miscible form; may be used parenterally) is supplied in 25,000-IU (7.5 mg of retinol per milliliter) and 50,000-IU (15 mg of retinol per milliliter) doses; Del-Vi-A is supplied in 50,000-IU doses. Adverse effects include anaphylaxis (after intravenous administration), increased intracranial pressure, cutaneous desquamation, liver damage, hypercalcemia, bone pain, arthralgias, nausea, vomiting, anorexia, malaise, headache, diplopia, irritability, alopecia, leukopenia, polyuria, and polydipsia.

Vitamin D

Chemistry

Vitamin D, a generic term for a number of distinct but closely related sterols possessing antirachitic properties, is a fat-soluble vitamin.[1-15] The two sterol forms important in nutrition and therapeutics are vitamin D_2 (ergocalciferol) and D_3 (cholecalciferol).

Vitamin D_3 is the natural form of vitamin D and is synthesized in skin under the influence of ultraviolet (UV) irradiation in sunlight. Vitamin D_2, a synthetic vitamin D compound, is manufactured by exposing the provitamin ergosterol, found in fungi and yeasts, to UV irradiation. This active ingredient is used in a number of commercial vitamin preparations. Ergocalciferol (D_2) differs from cholecalciferol (D_3) by the presence of a methyl group at C-24 and a double bond between C-22 and C-23. Vitamins D_2 and D_3 possess similar physiologic actions in man.

Metabolism/Function

Dietary vitamin D is absorbed in the small intestine. Normal absorption requires intact fat digestion and the presence of bile salts. Once absorbed, it is carried by chylomicrons to the liver. Vitamin D (of skin or dietary origin) is converted in the liver to 25-hydroxyvitamin D (calcifediol), the major circulating form of the vitamin. In the kidney, calcifediol is 1-hydroxylated by a mitochondrial 1-hydroxylase enzyme to 1,25-dihydroxyvitamin D (calcitriol). Calcitriol is the primary active form of vitamin D.

Calcitriol functions as a hormone and along with parathyroid hormone and calcitonin regulates calcium and phosphate metabolism. In the upper portion of the small intestine and kidney, calcitriol promotes calcium absorption. In bone, calcitriol stimulates reabsorption of calcium and phosphorus (along with parathyroid hormone). These processes are important for the maintenance of normal calcium and phosphorus concentrations in plasma. Normal ion concentrations are essential for normal cardiovascular function, neuromuscular activity, mineralization of bone, and other calcium-dependent processes. Vitamin D deficiency results in hypocalcemia, osteomalacia, or rickets. Vitamin D excess causes hypercalcemia, bone loss, renal stones, and tissue calcinosis. Recent evidence also suggests a role for vitamin D metabolites in cell differentiation and immune function. The primary route of excretion of vitamin D is the bile, with small amounts found in the urine.

Sources

Endogenous production of vitamin D is the most important source of the vitamin. Over 90% of circulating 25-hydroxycholecalciferol is derived from skin synthesis in normal healthy individuals. The rate of synthesis in the skin is determined by the degree of exposure to UV light and by the amount of skin pigment.

The major dietary sources supplying vitamin D_3 (cholecalciferol) are liver, oils, egg yolk, and butter. Fortified milk and other foods with vitamin D_2 (ergocalciferol) are another major dietary source.

Requirements

The recommended daily allowance of vitamin D in adults is 200 to 400 IU (5 to 10 μg). One milligram of vitamin D is equivalent to 40,000 IU. Estimated intravenous requirements are 200 to 420 IU/day. Intakes above the recommended levels are potentially dangerous and should be avoided. Many chronically ill patients lack sunlight exposure and may require higher dietary amounts of the vitamin (i.e., especially patients with fat malabsorption, liver disease, and renal disease).

Deficiency States

Primary nutritional deficiency of vitamin D in the United States is rare. However, vitamin D deficiency may develop in ill patients with inadequate exposure to sunlight and inadequate dietary intake. An absolute or relative deficiency may occur secondary to malabsorption syndromes, liver and/or cholestatic diseases, prolonged anticonvulsant usage (phenytoin, phenobarbital), rare metabolic disorders (i.e., vitamin D–dependent rickets), hypoparathyroidism, renal diseases (i.e., chronic renal disease, Fanconi syndrome, renal tubular acidosis), and chronic corticosteroid use. Vitamin D status may be assessed by measuring calcifediol (normal, 25 to 50 ng/mL) and calcitriol (normal 20 to 45 pg/mL) serum levels. Calcifediol levels primarily reflect dietary intake and skin synthesis of vitamin D; calcitriol levels reflect renal 1-hydroxylase activity. Vitamin D status can also be indirectly assessed by measuring serum calcium (ionized form) and phosphorus, 24-hour urine calcium, alkaline phosphatase levels, and radiographic bone density.

Vitamin D deficiency may be manifested clinically as poor bone mineralization in children (rickets) or adults (osteomalacia). Bone disease (i.e., renal osteodystrophy) may also develop in patients with chronic renal disease. These patients fail to produce adequate quantities of calcitriol. This effect results in decreased calcium absorption, lowered serum calcium levels, and secondary hyperparathyroidism. The net result is bone loss. In severe deficiency states, hypocalcemia may occur. Muscle cramps, tetany, and seizures may result from hypocalcemia.

Therapy

Adequate calcium and phosphorus intake must accompany vitamin D replacement therapy. Vitamin D is available in various forms (Table 14–2) that differ in their metabolism, dose, half-lives, and cost. Ergocalciferol is the vitamin D form most commonly used to treat dietary deficiency, malabsorption syndromes, and hypoparathyroidism. Dietary vitamin D deficiency states are treated with 25 to 125 μg/day orally, malabsorption syndromes with 2.5 to 7.5 mg/day orally or 250 μg/day intramuscularly, and hypoparathyroidism with 0.625 to 2.5 mg/day orally. Calcifediol may be useful in patients whose vitamin D deficiency results from severe liver disease or chronic renal failure. Calcifediol is usually started at a dose of 50 μg/day or 100 μg on alternate days orally. The dose is increased every 4 weeks until the desired effect is achieved.

Calcitriol is used primarily in patients with chronic renal failure or other renal disease states. It is also useful in the treatment of hypoparathyroidism and is the preferred treatment for vitamin D–dependent rickets. Calcitriol is initiated at a dose of 0.25 μg/day orally. The dose is increased by 0.25 μg/day every 2 to 4 weeks until the desired effect is achieved. An injectable form of calcitriol is also available.

Preparations and Adverse Effects

Ergocalciferol (calciferol, vitamin D capsules, Deltalin Gelseals, Drisdol) is available in capsule (0.625 mg [25,000 IU], 1.25 mg [50,000 IU]), liquid (8,000 IU/mL), and injectable forms (12.5 mg [500,000 IU]/mL). Calcifediol (25-hydroxyvitamin D, Calderol) is available as capsules (20 and 50 μg). Calcitriol (1,25-dihydroxyvitamin D, Rocaltrol, Calcijex) is available in capsule (0.25 and 0.5 μg) and injectable forms (1 and 2 μg/mL). The major toxicities from vitamin D administration are hypercalcemia, hypercalciuria, renal stones, bone loss, and tissue calcium deposition. Clinical features of hypercalcemia include headache, ataxia, irritability, somnolence, convulsions, hypertension, dysrhythmias, bradycardia, dry mouth, conjunctivitis, pruritis, anorexia, nausea, vomiting, constipation, polyuria, renal insufficiency, and weakness.

Vitamin E

Chemistry

Vitamin E is an alcohol derived from phytol and trimethylhydroquinone, soluble in fat solvents, readily oxidized, and most stable in the acetate form.[1-15] Eight tocopherols and tocotrienols with vitamin E activity have been identified; they differ from each other in the number and position of methyl groups around the phenol ring of the molecule. α-Tocopherol is the most widely distributed and most active of the tocopherols. Although its exact function and mechanisms of action are somewhat unclear, the most widely accepted function of vitamin E is as an antioxidant protecting membranes and other cellular structures from attack by free radicals. The term α-tocopherol is derived from *tokos* (Gr. "childbirth") and *pherein* (Gr. "to bear"). It was named because of its fertility effects in animals.

Metabolism

The absorption of vitamin E, like that of all fat-soluble vitamins, is linked to fat absorption and requires biliary (bile salt micelles) and pancreatic (esterase) secretions. Twenty percent to 50% of dietary tocopherols are normally absorbed. This amount is decreased by excess fat in the intestinal lumen. Most ingested vitamin E is d-α-tocopherol acetate. It is hydrolyzed in the intestine, enters the blood via the lymph, and is bound to lipoproteins. There is no specific carrier protein for vitamin E. Plasma levels correlate with plasma lipid levels. Vitamin E is stored in all tissues; however, adipose tissue, liver, and muscle are the most important sites of stor-

TABLE 14-2.

Vitamin D Preparations

	Ergocalciferol (Vitamin D$_2$)	Calcifediol (25-Hydroxycholecalciferol)	Dihydrotachysterol (1-Hydroxyvitamin D)	Calcitriol (1,25-Dihydroxycholecalciferol)
Concentration in serum (ng/mL)	10	30		0.03
Physiologic dose (μg/day)	10	5	20	0.5
Pharmacologic dose (μg/day)	1200	50	200–800	0.25–1
Onset of maximal effect (days)	30	15	15	3
Dosage forms	Tablets 625 μg 1250 μg Solution 8000 units/mL Oil for injection 500,000 units/mL	Capsules 20 μg 50 μg	Tablets 125 μg 200 μg 400 μg Solution 200 μg/mL	Capsules 0.25 μg 0.50 μg
Commercial products	Calciferol	Calderol	Hytakerol	Rocaltrol
Serum half-life (days)	30	15		0.2
Time for reversal of effect (days)	17–60	7–30	3–14	2–10
Advantages	Low cost, prolonged action, parent compound	Liver disease	Renal disease, hypoparathyroidism	Renal disease, liver disease, hypoparathyroidism, rapid onset, rapid offset
Disadvantages	Instability, long toxicity	Expense	Expense	Expense

age. The major excretory route is through the feces (about 75% is excreted in bile), with the remainder excreted as glucuronides in the urine. Vitamin E functions as an antioxidant in the body. It inhibits the oxidation of unsaturated fatty acids and other substrates and stabilizes cell membranes. Vitamin E and selenium both prevent peroxidation of polyunsaturated fats in lipid membranes. Selenium is a cofactor for glutathione peroxidase (destroys peroxides) and reduces the need for vitamin E.

Vitamin E metabolism is linked to prostaglandin metabolism in animals. Vitamin E deficiency results in decreased prostacyclin synthesis in blood vessels. Therapy with vitamin E has been shown to decrease tissue levels of prostaglandins E_1, E_2, and F_2. The significance of these findings for human disease is unclear.

Sources

The richest sources of vitamin E are vegetable oils (i.e., wheat germ, sunflower seed, cotton seed, safflower, palm, and other oils). Shortening and margarine are major sources in the diet. Eggs, butter, whole-meal cereals, and broccoli are moderately good sources, while meats, fruits, and vegetables provide small amounts of vitamin E. Breast milk contains four times as much vitamin E as cow's milk. The total daily ingestion varies from 2.6 to 15.4 mg of tocopherol.

Requirements

Vitamin E requirements must take into account the intake of natural oxidants such as polyunsaturated fatty acids (which increase the requirement) and diets containing antioxidants (which decrease the requirement). In general, approximately 1 mg of vitamin E is needed for each 600 mg of polyunsaturated fatty acid. It should be remembered, however, that the food sources highest in vitamin E content

are also high in polyunsaturated fatty acids.

The RDA for vitamin E is expressed in terms of milligrams of α-tocopherol equivalents and is 10 mg/day (15 IU) for adult males and 8 mg/day (12 IU) for adult females. Women who are pregnant require between 10 and 12 mg/day of vitamin E. Normal serum concentrations in adults are greater than 0.5 mg/dL. Low serum concentrations may not indicate tissue depletion unless the duration of depletion is long (i.e., 1 year). The antioxidant protection provided by vitamin E (i.e., measure of tissue stores) can be assessed by quantitating the in vitro formation of malondialdehyde from erythrocyte membranes exposed to peroxidant stress.

Deficiency States

In view of vitamin E's wide distribution in foods, primary dietary deficiency of the vitamin is unlikely. However, in the setting of severe malabsorption (i.e., celiac sprue, Crohn's disease, etc), clinical deficiency may appear. Severe deficiency occurs in patients with abetalipoproteinemia, where both intestinal absorption and serum transport of the vitamin are defective. Vitamin E deficiency may also accompany chronic cholestatic liver disease, biliary atresia, cystic fibrosis, and the use of infant formulas that contain large amounts of polyunsaturated fats and iron. The diagnosis of vitamin E deficiency is made by measuring plasma levels of the vitamin (normal, greater than 0.5 to 0.7 mg/dL). The concentration of vitamin E correlates with plasma lipid levels. Approximately 1 μg of α-tocopherol is present per milligram of total lipid.

Vitamin E deficiency diseases are well described in experimental animals, poultry, and livestock. Deficiency diseases are less common in humans. Clinical features of Vitamin E deficiency (seen with malabsorption) include peripheral neuropathy, areflexia, reduced proprioception and vibratory sense, ataxia, ophthalmoplegia, hemolysis, anemia, and increased platelet aggregation. Vitamin E may prevent hemolysis by protecting membrane lipids from peroxidation. In premature infants, deficiency of the vitamin has been associated with retrolental fibroplasia, hemolytic anemia, intraventricular hemorrhage, edema, and thrombocytosis. Iron supplementation (a free-radical generator) may increase hemolysis in the presence of vitamin E deficiency. Vitamin E deficiency may develop in premature and full-term newborn infants due to its poor transport across the placenta.

Therapy

Vitamin E supplementation is indicated in patients with serum vitamin E levels less than 0.5 mg/dL or when a clinical deficiency state has been diagnosed. In those individuals in whom severe malabsorption is the cause of the deficiency, vitamin E (30 to 100 mg/day) should be given intramuscularly as dl-α-tocopherol acetate (1 mg = 1 IU). Deficiency manifested as neuropathy may be corrected with oral administration of high doses of vitamin E (50 to 200 IU/kg/day). If oral therapy fails, intramuscular administration of dl-α-tocopherol acetate (1 to 2 mg/kg/day) should be tried. Retrolental fibroplasia in premature infants may be prevented with the prophylactic use of oral vitamin E (100 mg/kg/day). The recommended dosage for intravenous support is 10 mg/day.

Preparations and Adverse Effects

Vitamin E may be obtained in the d or the d/l isomers of α-tocopherol, α-tocopherol acetate, or α-tocopherol succinate. Oral preparations of the fat-soluble form of tablets or capsules range from 50 to 1000 IU. The water-miscible preparation Aquasol E comes in 100- and 400-IU capsules. Parenteral forms of vitamin E are also available (200 IU/mL). Adverse effects include fatigue, nausea, vomiting, weakness, headache, blurred vision, and diarrhea. Large doses of vitamin E have been reported to lengthen clotting times in patients taking warfarin.

Vitamin K

Chemistry

Vitamin K is a fat-soluble naphthaquinone.[1-15] It occurs naturally in two forms differing from one another only in their side chains. The most active form, vitamin K_1 (phytonadione), is the only form found in plants and is the only natural vitamin K available for therapeutic use. Vitamin K_2 (menaquinone) is synthesized by the normal intestinal flora and is also found in some animal tissues. Vitamin K_3 (menadione) is the water-soluble parent compound of the vitamin K series. It is not found naturally but rather represents an artificial provitamin that can be alkylated in vivo to menaquinone.

Metabolism

The naturally occurring vitamin K derivatives are absorbed only in the presence of bile salts (like other lipids) and are distributed in the bloodstream via the lymphatics (i.e., chylomicrons). Menadione is absorbed in the absence of bile salts and enters directly into the bloodstream. The absorption of phytonadione occurs in an energy-dependent, saturable process in the proximal portion of the small bowel, whereas menaquinone and menadione are absorbed via a diffusional process in the distal part of the small bowel and colon. Once absorbed, vitamin K is stored in the liver and other tissues; however, its storage is limited. Vitamin K is metabolized in the liver and excreted in the urine and bile after conjugation with glucuronate and sulfate.

Vitamin K is required for normal blood clotting. It acts as a cofactor for a liver carboxylase that activates factors II (prothrombin), VII (proconvertin), IX (plasma thromboplastin component), and X (Stuart factor). The carboxylase converts glutamate residues to α-carboxyglutamate. This amino acid assists in binding calcium. Carboxyglutamate is also found in other proteins such as bone osteocalcin, protein S, and protein C.

Sources

The best dietary sources of vitamin K are green leafy vegetables (i.e., broccoli, lettuce, cabbage, and spinach). Beef liver is a good source, but most other animal foods, cereals, and fruits are poor sources unless they have undergone extensive bacterial putrefaction. The average diet in the United States contains approximately 300 to 500 μg/day of vitamin K. It should be noted that approximately half of the vitamin K in the body is derived from gut bacteria while the other half comes from the diet. Breast milk contains lower quantities of vitamin K as compared with formula or cow's milk (i.e., breast milk contains 1 to 2 μg/L of vitamin K_1; cow's milk contains 5 to 17 μg/L).

Requirements

The RDA for vitamin K in normal adult males is 70 to 80 μg/day, and in normal adult females it is 60 to 65 μg/day, assuming that half of the vitamin made by bacteria is absorbed and the rest supplied by the diet. The RDA would double (i.e., 140 μg/day) in cases in which bacterial vitamin is not synthesized or absorbed (i.e., patients receiving broad-spectrum antibiotics). Recommended oral supplementation during TPN is 10 mg/wk. One may also administer 5 mg intramuscularly each week.

Deficiency States

Vitamin K deficiency has not been produced in the normal human by the administration of a vitamin K–deficient diet alone. The intestinal synthesis of vitamin K_2 (by gut organisms) can supply the needs of the normal adult. Primary deficiency states occur in newborn babies as a result of poor placental transport of lipids, sterile intestines, and breast feeding (a poor source of vitamin K). Deficiency states also result from fat malabsorption (i.e., biliary obstruction, malabsorption syndromes), the use of broad-spectrum antibiotics with little enteral nutrition, severe liver disease, the use of oral anticoagulants such as warfarin, the administration of cholestyramine, and long-term total parenteral nutritional support. Prolonged antibiotic therapy suppresses the gut flora and may result in vitamin K deficiency (especially if intake is poor).

Clinically, vitamin K deficiency results in delayed blood clotting and is manifested by easy bruising and/or an increased tendency to bleeding. A diagnosis of vitamin K deficiency is suggested by finding a prolonged prothrombin time. A specific diagnosis is made by radioimmunoassay measurement of one or more of the four vitamin K–dependent clotting factors.

Therapy

Phytonadione (vitamin K_1) is the preparation of choice for treating vitamin K deficiency, but it must be remembered that vitamin K deficiency will respond rapidly to the administration of vitamin K only if liver function is normal. For prophylaxis against hemorrhagic disease of the newborn, a single intramuscular dose of phytonadione, 0.5 to 1 mg, should be administered immediately after birth. One to 2 mg/day intramuscularly or subcutaneously is administered for treating hemorrhagic disease of the newborn.

Anticoagulant-induced hypoprothrombinemic states should be treated with phytonadione, 2.5 to 20 mg orally, subcutaneously, or intramuscularly (titrated to effect). Menadiol is ineffective in reversing anticoagulant-induced hypoprothrombinemic states. In more severe hemorrhagic states secondary to anticoagulant overdose, 10 to 50 mg of phytonadione dissolved in 5% dextrose or 0.9% sodium chloride may be given intravenously at a rate not to exceed 1 mg/min. Additional doses may be given at 6- to 8-hour intervals and therapy monitored by following the prothrombin times. In such situations, the transfusion of plasma may also be indicated. Vitamin K deficiency secondary to other causes may be adequately treated with menadiol or phytonadione preparations. Oral, subcutaneous, or intramuscular doses of 5 to 10 mg/day or twice daily are usually sufficient. Whenever possible, phytonadione should be given subcutaneously or intramuscularly. If oral phytonadione is used in patients with biliary insufficiency, a bile salt preparation must be administered concomitantly. Finally, for patients receiving long-term total parenteral nutrition, phytonadione, 5 to 10 mg/wk subcutaneously or intramuscularly, is sufficient to prevent deficiency. Alternatively, 0.5 to 1.0 mg/day of Aquamephyton may be administered intravenously.

Preparations and Adverse Effects

Phytonadione (vitamin K_1, Aquamephyton, Konakion, Mephyton) is a lipid-soluble synthetic preparation. It is available in 5-mg tablets (Mephyton), 2-mg/mL injection, and 10-mg/mL injection (Aquamephyton for intravenous use, Konakion for intramuscular use). Aquamephyton is the form usually added to parenteral nutrition solutions. It is unstable when exposed to light, so the storage time after mixing should be no longer than 24 hours. Menadiol sodium diphosphate (vitamin K_4) is a water-soluble derivative. It is available as an oral preparation (Synkayvite, 5-mg tablets) and injectable form (Synkayvite solution, 5, 10, and 37.5 mg/mL). Menadiol may be administered intravenously (slow push) in doses of 5 to 20 mg. Adverse effects following oral administration are rare. Hypersensitivity reactions may occur following intravenous administration. Hemolysis has been reported in individuals with glucose-6-phosphate dehydrogenase (G6PD) deficiency. Anemia, hyperbilirubinemia, and kernicterus may occur with large doses in the newborn.

WATER-SOLUBLE VITAMINS

Thiamine (Vitamin B_1)

Chemistry

Thiamine is a water-soluble organic molecule consisting of a pyrimidine ring joined to a sulfur-containing thiazole ring by a methylene bridge.[1-15]

Metabolism

Thiamine is rapidly absorbed from the upper portion of the small intestine by an Na^+-dependent active transport system (low concentrations) and by passive diffusion (high concentrations). Oral absorption ranges from 8 to 15 mg/day. During absorption, the vitamin is phosphorylated to thiamine pyrophosphate (TPP) within the mucosal cells of the intestine. This phosphorylated form is found in all cells and constitutes the majority (80%) of stored vitamin. Other forms, stored in lesser amounts, are thiamine triphosphate, thiamine monophosphate, and free vitamin. The major site of thiamine storage is skeletal muscle, with the heart, liver, kidneys, and brain serving as secondary storage sites. Tissue stores are saturated by approximately 1 mg of thiamine per day. As the intake exceeds this minimal requirement, excess appears in the urine (either as metabolite or unchanged vitamin). Thiamine is an important precursor for TPP, the coenzyme responsible for the decarboxylation of α-keto acids, transketolase activity (hexose monophosphate shunt), and carbohydrate metabolism (i.e., pyruvate to acetylcoenzyme A). It is important for biochemical pathways that generate reduced nicotinamide adenine dinucleotide phosphate (NADPH). Additionally, thiamine modulates neuromuscular transmission. It is an important structural component of nervous system membranes.

Sources

Humans are almost entirely dependent on dietary sources for thiamine. The best dietary sources are beef, pork, whole grains, enriched cereal grains, peas, potatoes, beans, nuts, and yeast. The refining of sugar, rice (polishing), and many cereal products may lead to removal of the vitamin. Some foods such as raw fish, coffee, and tea contain thiaminases that can destroy the dietary supply of thiamine. Thiamine is rapidly destroyed at alkaline pH and is heat sensitive. Because of its water-soluble properties, much of the vitamin is extracted from dry foods when cooked in liquids.

Requirements

The RDA for thiamine in adult males is 1.4 mg/day, and in adult women it is 1.1 mg/day. Given that thiamine is essential for energy metabolism, especially of carbohydrates, the RDA may be related to caloric intake (0.5 mg/1000 kcal). This requirement increases when carbohydrates form the major dietary component, in the elderly who utilize thiamine less efficiently, in states of increased metabolism (i.e., hyperthyroidism, fever, increased activity), and during pregnancy and lactation. Needs frequently increase 50% in these situations. Intravenous requirements during TPN range from 3 to 21 mg/day.

Deficiency States

The biological half-life of thiamine is 9 to 18 days. Deficiency has been detected biochemically as early as 7 days and clinical symptoms observed as early as 9 days after dietary thiamine elimination. Deficiency of the vitamin results from decreased intake, increased tissue utilization, or both. In the United States, chronic alcoholism and advanced age are the most common causes of thiamine deficiency. Other important causes include malabsorption syndromes, diuretic therapy, prolonged antacid therapy (thiamine is destroyed in the alkaline bowel lumen), dialysis, increased metabolic rate, diarrhea, chronic malnutrition, folate deficiency, diets in which refined grains make up the major caloric source (i.e., polished rice, unenriched white flour), administration of intravenous dextrose solutions, and chronic ingestion of food high in thiaminases. Patients receiving TPN are prone to the development of thiamine deficiency because of stress, insufficient thiamine intake, and the use of high-carbohydrate diets.

Early manifestations of thiamine deficiency include weight loss, muscle cramps, anorexia, irritability, and paresthesias. Advanced deficiency affects the cardiovascular system (wet beriberi) and/or the nervous system (dry beriberi). Wet beriberi is characterized by reduced systemic vascular resistance and augmented venous return resulting in high-output cardiac failure characterized by dyspnea, tachycardia, biventricular failure, QT prolongation, pulmonary and peripheral edema, wide pulse pressure, sweating, and warm extremities. A rare low-output state (Shoshin disease) may occur and is characterized by hypotension, tachycardia, the absence of edema, and lactic acidosis.

Nervous system involvement includes both the peripheral and central nervous systems. Typically, peripheral nerve involvement is manifested by symmetrical motor and sensory neuropathy with pain, paresthesias, weakness, and loss of reflexes. Lower-extremity distal segments are commonly involved. However, arm involvement may occur after the leg signs are well established. Involvement of the central nervous system results in Wernicke-Korsakoff syndrome. Wernicke's encephalopathy consists of horizontal nystagmus, unilateral or bilateral ophthalmoplegia, fever, ataxia, confusion, and coma. Korsakoff's syndrome is characterized by retrograde amnesia, confabulation, psychosis, and an impaired ability to learn. Thiamine deficiency is best diagnosed by assessing erythrocyte or leukocyte transketolase activity (normal, <15%; mild deficiency, 15% to 25%; severe deficiency,

>25%). Hemolyzed cells are incubated with and without TPP. The increase in activity with TPP is a measure of the degree of thiamine deficiency. Other indicators of deficiency include increased blood pyruvate and lactate levels and diminished urinary thiamine excretion (<50 µg/day). Thiamine deficiency results in a decrease in the activity of the citric acid cycle and stimulation of the glycolytic pathway. The greater flux through this pathway and inhibition of pyruvate dehydrogenase results in elevated concentrations of pyruvate and lactate. In most instances, however, the clinical response to empirical thiamine therapy is used to support a diagnosis.

Therapy

Thiamine deficiency may be treated with thiamine, 10 to 20 mg intramuscularly every 8 hours for 1 to 2 weeks followed by an oral daily maintenance dose (usually in the form of a multivitamin containing 5 to 10 mg thiamine). Severe deficiency, in the form of beriberi heart disease ("wet beriberi"), is a medical emergency. Thiamine, 10 to 30 mg intravenously every 8 hours for 1 to 2 weeks followed by 25 mg orally per day, may lead to dramatic improvement. Wernicke's encephalopathy may require up to 1 g of thiamine intravenously for acute control, followed by 25 to 100 mg every 12 hours orally for maintenance. Thiamine deficiency may be prevented by the administration of 1 to 2 mg of thiamine per day.

There are a number of thiamine-responsive inborn errors of metabolism. These include pyruvic acidemia, subacute necrotizing encephalomyelopathy (SNE), maple syrup urine disease, and thiamine-responsive megaloblastic anemia.

Preparations and Adverse Effects

Thiamine hydrochloride is available in tablets (5, 10, 25, 50, 100, 250, and 500 mg), elixir (2.25 mg/5 mL), and injectable forms (100 and 200 mg/mL). It is relatively stable in parenteral nutrition solutions. Adverse effects include restlessness, allergic reactions (especially following rapid intravenous administration), nausea, vomiting, hemorrhage, and diarrhea.

Riboflavin (Vitamin B$_2$)

Chemistry

Riboflavin consists of a heterocyclic isoalloxazine ring attached to a sugar alcohol side chain, ribitol.[1-15] It is water soluble, heat stable, but unstable in alkali solution or when exposed to light.

Metabolism

Riboflavin is rapidly absorbed from the upper portion of the gastrointestinal tract by a site-specific and saturable transport process. During absorption it is phosphorylated in the intestinal mucosa to the coenzyme flavin mononucleotide (FMN). Phosphorylation also takes place in the liver and other tissues. The vitamin is stored in small concentrations in all tissues, with varying amounts being bound to serum proteins. Riboflavin is excreted in the urine. As ingestion increases, a larger proportion is excreted unchanged. Small quantities of the vitamin are found in sweat. Riboflavin is important for normal energy metabolism. It is a component of the tissue coenzymes riboflavin-5'-phosphate, FMN, and flavin adenine dinucleotide (FAD). FMN and FAD also serve as the prosthetic groups for several enzyme systems concerned with electron and hydrogen transport (oxidation) and metabolism of amino acids. Riboflavin is required for the conversion of pyridoxine to pyridoxal phosphate. Thyroid hormone enhances the conversion of riboflavin to FMN and FAD (via stimulation of flavokinase and FAD pyrophosphorylase). Adrenocorticotropic hormone (ACTH) and aldosterone also increase the synthesis of FMN and FAD. Aldosterone antagonists (i.e., spironolactone) and phenothiazines inhibit the synthesis of flavin coenzymes.

Sources

Riboflavin is widely distributed in leafy vegetables, milk, cheese, meat, fish, egg whites, kidney, liver, and whole-grain and enriched cereals. In the United States, milk and dairy products account for nearly half of the daily intake. Its biological activity can be lost by exposing it to light while being cooked. Small quantities of riboflavin are also synthesized by colonic bacteria.

Requirements

The RDA for riboflavin is 1.4 to 1.7 mg/day in adult males and 1.2 mg/day in adult females. The RDA is increased to 1.6 to 1.8 mg/day during pregnancy and lactation. Riboflavin requirements vary with caloric intake (0.6 mg/1000 calories) and increase during strenuous exercise (i.e., energy expenditure). Needs may be increased during hypermetabolic illness. The requirement for riboflavin relates more to nitrogen balance than to caloric intake. Suggested intravenous requirements during TPN range from 3.5 to 7.5 mg/day.

Deficiency States

Symptoms of riboflavin deficiency can develop within 7 days of institution of a riboflavin-deficient diet. Riboflavin deficiency usually results from chronic malnutrition or the use of parenteral nutrition solutions containing inadequate vitamin. Other factors such as drugs (i.e., phenothiazines, tricyclic antidepressants) and disease states such as hypothyroidism, chronic alcoholism, trauma, burns, dialysis, and malignancy may also lead to deficiency.

Early symptoms of riboflavin deficiency are manifested as soreness of the mouth, burning and itching of the eyes, photophobia, and personality alteration. With progression of the deficiency, cheilosis, angular stomatitis, seborrheic dermatitis, glossitis, vascularizing keratitis, corneal vascularization, anemia, and retarded intellectual development can occur. In addition to the above, the metabolism of a number of drugs can be altered by a deficiency of this vitamin.

Laboratory evaluation of riboflavin status may be assessed by measuring urinary excretion of riboflavin or erythrocyte activity of glutathione reductase (a riboflavin-dependent enzyme). Excretion of less than 50 μg of riboflavin per day is indicative of deficiency. Glutathione reductase activity is expressed as an activity coefficient (i.e., the ratio of enzyme activity after incubation with FAD in vitro to that before incubation). A value greater than 1.3 is considered to be indicative of deficiency.

Therapy

For the treatment of deficiency states, 5 to 25 mg/day of oral riboflavin should be given until clinical findings resolve. A prophylactic dose of 3 mg/day is useful when malabsorption is present. Since riboflavin deficiency usually coexists with other vitamin B deficiencies, many recommend replacement therapy in the form of B-complex vitamins.

Preparations and Adverse Effects

Riboflavin is available in oral tablet (5, 10, 25, 50, and 100 mg) and injectable forms (35 mg/mL). Riboflavin is relatively unstable in glucose–amino acid solutions but is stabilized with the addition of lipid (3-in-1 mixture). Riboflavin can result in bright yellow urine. Clinical toxicity has not been reported.

Pyridoxine (Vitamin B₆)

Chemistry

The term "vitamin B_6" or "pyridoxine" is used to refer to three closely interrelated compounds: pyridoxine (alcohol), pyridoxal (aldehyde), and pyridoxamine (amine) and their corresponding phosphates.[1–15] Pyridoxal-5'-phosphate is the major coenzyme and active form of the vitamin. All are soluble in water and alcohol. They are resistant to normal heat but degradable by alkali and UV light.

Metabolism

Vitamin B_6 is rapidly absorbed in the small intestine by passive transport following hydrolysis of its phosphorylated derivatives. It is distributed throughout the tissues as the coenzyme pyridoxal phosphate. In addition, this form makes up about 60% of the circulating vitamin. The various forms of pyridoxine are readily interconverted in the liver and by erythrocytes. Excretion of pyridoxine occurs in the urine mainly as the metabolite 4-pyridoxic acid. Vitamin B_6 as the coenzyme pyridoxal phosphate, functions in many chemical reactions related to amino acid and protein metabolism. Its most important roles are as coenzymes for transamination and decarboxylation of amino acids. Many neurotransmitters or inhibitors of neurotransmitters are formed by decarboxylation of amino acids. Pyridoxal phosphate is also involved in the metabolism of several vitamins and in the biosynthesis of heme and sphingosine. It aids in the conversion of tryptophan to nicotinamide and enhances the transport of amino acids and potassium into cells. Pyridoxal phosphate is essential for the function of phosphorylase, the enzyme that catalyzes the breakdown of glycogen to form glucose-1-phosphate. Pyridoxine is also a cofactor for dehydratases, racemases, transferases, hydroxylases, synthetases, and other enzymes.

Sources

Low concentrations of vitamin B_6 are widespread in the food supply (both plants and animals). Liver, meat, fish, egg yolk, whole-grain cereals, legumes, fruit, and vegetables are good sources. Substantial losses of the vitamin occur during prolonged cooking.

Requirements

Vitamin B_6 requirements are estimated by using a ratio of 0.016 mg of the vitamin per gram of protein ingested. The RDA is 2.0 mg/day for adult males and 1.6 mg/day for adult females, which provides a reasonable margin of safety and allows for daily intakes of more than 100 g of protein per day. During pregnancy and lactation, a 0.5-mg/day increase is recommended. The use of estrogens and diets high in protein may also necessitate an increased allowance of vitamin B_6. Recommended intravenous doses for TPN are 4 to 6 mg/day.

Deficiency States

Deficiency of pyridoxine rarely results from dietary restrictions since it is found in many foods. The major causes of vitamin B_6 deficiency are related to malabsorption syndromes, alcoholism, pregnancy, and medications such as isoniazid, L-dopa, estrogens, cycloserine, and penicillamine.

The biological half-life of pyridoxine ranges from 22 to 38 days. Clinical symptoms have developed in less than 3 weeks of starting a vitamin B_6–deficient diet. Initially, personality changes, irritability, and depression develop. Deficiency may manifest itself as seborrhea-like lesions about the eyes, nose, and mouth, acneiform papular rashes, stomatitis, glossitis, nausea, vomiting, seizures, peripheral neuritis, and hypochromic anemia. Laboratory diagnosis of pyridoxine deficiency may be accomplished by measuring urinary levels of metabolites (i.e., after a tryptophan load) or by direct assay of pyridoxal phosphate in the blood (normal is greater than 50 ng/mL). Urinary excretion of less than 1.0 mg/day of 4-pyridoxic acid is suggestive of deficiency. One may also measure the activity of erythrocyte transaminases. An activity coefficient greater than 1.5 for aspartate aminotransferase and greater than 1.25 for alanine aminotransferase is indicative of pyridoxine deficiency.

Therapy

Pyridoxine deficiency is treated with 25 to 100 mg of pyridoxine daily for 3 weeks followed by a maintenance dose of 2.0 to 2.5 mg daily in a multivitamin preparation. Prophylaxis in patients receiving isoniazid consists of 25 to 50 mg of pyridoxine daily. Pyridoxine deficiency in patients receiving isoniazid (i.e., peripheral neuritis) is best treated with 50 to 200 mg of pyridoxine daily. Isoniazid poisoning (i.e., >10 g) is treated with an equal quantity of pyridoxine (i.e., 4 g intravenously followed by 1 g intramuscularly every 30 minutes for six doses).

Preparations and Adverse Effects

Pyridoxine hydrochloride is available in oral (10, 25, 50, 100, 200, 250, and 500 mg) and injectable forms (100 mg/mL). Adverse effects include paresthesias, somnolence, headache, decreased sensation (to touch, temperature, and vibration), unstable gait, seizures, nausea, burning or stinging at injection sites, allergic reactions, and decreased serum folate levels.

Vitamin B_{12} (Cobalamin, Cyanocobalamin)

Chemistry

Vitamin B_{12} is composed of a central cobalt ion within a porphyrin-like ring (corrin ring) linked to a nucleotide base, ribose, and phosphoric acid.[1-15] In nature the vitamin usually occurs in combination with protein. Vitamin B_{12} exists in several forms. Cyanocobalamin, hydroxocobalamin, 5'-deoxyadenosylcobalamin, and methylcobalamin serve as coenzymes and are essential for cell growth and replication. Cyanocobalamin and hydroxocobalamin are both available commercially for therapeutic use, in part due to their stable structure. Vitamin B_{12} is produced commercially as a byproduct of the cultivation of *Streptomyces griseus* used in the preparation of the antibiotic streptomycin. Vitamin B_{12} is freely soluble in water and somewhat resistant to boiling in neutral solution but is unstable in alkali.

Metabolism

After ingestion, Vitamin B_{12} (released from protein by pancreatic enzymes) is bound to intrinsic factor, a protein secreted by gastric parietal cells. This intrinsic factor–cobalamin complex transits the intestine and attaches to a specific receptor in the ileal mucosa where it is absorbed. Following absorption, the vitamin is bound by a plasma protein, transcobalamin II, for transport to the tissues. Normal serum concentrations range from 200 to 900 pg/mL. The liver is the major storage site for vitamin B_{12} and contains approximately 2 mg. Normal individuals eating a standard American diet excrete about 1.3 μg/day of vitamin B_{12}. Small quantities of the vitamin are secreted in bile. However, most of this vitamin B_{12} is reabsorbed with intrinsic factor via an enterohepatic cycle. Since daily losses of vitamin B_{12} are 1 to 2 μg/day, the body has sufficient stores to last more than 3 years after vitamin B_{12} absorption ceases. Thus, Vitamin B_{12} deficiency states are unusual unless gut absorption is diminished for long periods of time.

Vitamin B_{12} serves as a transmethylating agent and functions in the synthesis of thiamine, methionine, and tetrahydrofolic acid. It is also involved in a number of other enzymatic reactions. Vitamin B_{12} is required for normal hematopoiesis and for maintenance of the integrity of the nervous system (especially myelin formation). Both folate and vitamin B_{12} are required for DNA synthesis.

Sources

The average U.S. diet supplies 5 to 15 μg/day of vitamin B_{12}. The vitamin B_{12} content of vegetables is low, and the usual dietary sources are meat and meat products, fish, oysters, clams, eggs, and to a lesser extent, milk and milk products. Vitamin B_{12} is present in several forms in food. The main forms are deoxyadenosylcobalamin and hydroxocobalamin, of which one third to one half is absorbed. Methylcobalamin is found in egg yolk and cheese, while little or no cyanocobalamin occurs in foods. Enteric microorganisms (i.e., *Actinomyces*) synthesize cyanocobalamin and supplement the dietary intake. Since it is absorbed in the small intestine, colonic production of vitamin B_{12} is not bioavailable.

Requirements

The RDA of vitamin B_{12} for adults is 3 μg/day. The minimum daily requirement is 2 μg/day. Pregnant females have a slightly higher RDA of 4 μg/day. Vitamin B_{12} requirements are higher in patients with diminished intrinsic factor production and altered ileal absorption. Suggested intravenous requirements range from 5 to 15 μg/day.

Deficiency States

There is a relatively large storage of vitamin B_{12} and an efficient enterohepatic circulation. Thus, dietary vitamin B_{12} deficiency is rare and requires years to develop. Strict vegetarians who avoid all dairy products as well as meat and fish are at risk. Pernicious anemia (i.e., lack of intrinsic factor) is a common secondary cause of vitamin B_{12} deficiency. Other causes include malabsorption syndromes (i.e., celiac disease, sprue, drugs, malignancy, pancreatic dysfunction), gastrectomy, blind loop syndrome, tapeworms, surgical resection of the ileum, Crohn's disease, transcobalamin II deficiency (rare), and liver and kidney disease.

The manifestations of vitamin B_{12} deficiency are usually insidious. The hallmark of the deficiency is megaloblastic anemia. Weakness, fatigue, and dyspnea are usually related to anemia. Other signs and symptoms include glossitis, anorexia, diarrhea, and loss of taste. Vitamin B_{12} deficiency also leads to the development of a complex neurologic syndrome. Vitamin B_{12} is essential for myelin synthesis. Peripheral nerves are affected first in the lower extremities, which is manifested as numbness and tingling. The posterior columns are affected next, with patients complaining of difficulty in balance during walking and loss of vibratory and positional sense. Dementia and psychoses may also become evident with progressive deficiency.

Assessment of the vitamin B_{12} status is usually accomplished by measuring serum levels of the vitamin (normal, 150 to 900 pg/mL) by radioimmunoassay and clinical assessment of red blood cell indices (especially mean cell volume), peripheral blood smear, and bone marrow aspirate. Findings of a macrocytic anemia, hypersegmented leukocytes, megaloblastic bone marrow, and a serum vitamin B_{12} level less than 100 pg/mL are indicative of vitamin B_{12} deficiency. Vitamin B_{12} absorption may be assessed with the Schilling test (normal, >30%).

Therapy

Vitamin B_{12} deficiency secondary to pernicious anemia is treated with 50 to 100 μg of vitamin B_{12} intramuscularly daily for 14 days or 1000 μg every 7 days for 3 weeks. This is followed by 100 μg intramuscularly twice per week for 2 months and then monthly maintenance injections of 100 μg for life.

Patients with vitamin B_{12} deficiency who have neurologic symptoms are treated with 100 μg of vitamin B_{12} intramuscularly daily for 14 days followed by 100 μg of vitamin B_{12} intramuscularly every 2 weeks for 6 months. This is followed by 100 μg intramuscularly per month for life in patients with impaired absorption. Neurologic signs and symptoms may be reversible if they are of relatively short duration (i.e., less than 6 months). For megaloblastic anemia, both vitamin B_{12} and folate should be administered until the results of folate/B_{12} levels have returned. Vitamin B_{12} may be administered orally, intramuscularly, or subcutaneously. Intramuscular or subcutaneous routes are preferred during initial therapy. Doses are 30 μg/day for 5 to 10 days followed by a monthly maintenance dose of 100 to

200 μg. Normal vitamin B_{12} absorption must be documented before relying on oral administration. Higher doses may be required in critically ill patients or those with hyperthyroidism or disease states of increased metabolic activity.

Preparations and Adverse Effects

Vitamin B_{12}, as cyanocobalamin crystalline, is available in oral (25- to 1000-μg tablets) and injectable forms (for intramuscular injection 30, 100, and 1000 μg/mL). Vitamin B_{12}, as hydroxocobalamin crystalline, is available in an injectable form (for intramuscular injection, 1000 μg/mL). Vitamin B_{12} liver preparations are available in oral (0.5 units of vitamin B_{12} with intrinsic factor concentrate and 25 μg of cobalamin) and parenteral forms (intramuscular only—2, 10, and 20 μg B_{12}/mL). The intravenous route of administration should be avoided due to the occurrence of hypersensitivity reactions. However, if intravenous vitamin B_{12} is required, multivitamin preparations containing vitamin B_{12} are available. Adverse effects from vitamin B_{12} administration include hypersensitivity reactions (i.e., anaphylaxis, urticaria, pruritis), pulmonary edema, congestive heart failure, vascular thrombosis, diarrhea, hypokalemia, polycythemia vera, and local pain at the injection site.

Vitamin C (Ascorbic Acid)

Chemistry

Ascorbic acid is a simple carbohydrate (L-ascorbic acid) that is soluble in water, stable in acid, and destroyed by alkali and oxygen.[1-15] In the body, L-ascorbic acid is reversibly oxidized to dehydroascorbic acid, a form possessing full biological activity. Further metabolism of dehydroascorbic acid yields derivatives that are void of vitamin C activity.

Metabolism

Ascorbic acid is readily absorbed in the small intestine by facilitated diffu-sion and active transport. Absorption of ascorbic acid occurs in both intestinal cells and renal tubular cells. In the intestine, dehydroascorbic acid can be reduced to ascorbic acid and subsequently absorbed. Ascorbic acid is excreted in the urine as ascorbic acid, dehydroascorbic acid, or one of several metabolites. Small amounts appear in feces and sweat. The efficiency of intestinal absorption decreases with large daily intakes (i.e., over 180 mg). Renal tubular reabsorption also varies with intake. Complete tubular reabsorption occurs when the plasma concentration is less than 15 mg/L. Consequently, large quantities of ascorbic acid in the intestine and kidney tubule result in poor absorption and tubular reabsorption, respectively, and in significant fecal and renal losses. Following absorption, all organs and tissues take up ascorbic acid. Concentrations are highest in glandular tissues (i.e., adrenals, liver) and average up to 50 times higher than the plasma concentration. The body pool of ascorbic acid averages 1500 mg in normal individuals (i.e., receiving about 80 mg of the vitamin per day). Approximately 3% is catabolized daily. Plasma concentrations reflect dietary intake and are variable. White blood cell ascorbic acid levels are used as an indicator of cellular and tissue levels. Ascorbic acid is a reducing agent involved in numerous oxidation-reduction reactions and the transfer of protons. It plays a part in the electron transport chain with cytochrome C. It is important in the synthesis of collagen, catecholamines, and corticosterone, and in the metabolism of tyrosine. It helps to maintain the integrity of connective tissue, osteoid tissue of bone, and dentin of teeth. Vitamin C enhances iron absorption and is needed for the conversion of folic acid to tetrahydrofolic acid (it protects folic acid reductase). Wound healing, vascular integrity, and immune function are also under the influence of ascorbic acid. Ascorbic acid is important in the synthesis of neurotransmitters (i.e., norepinephrine, 5-hydroxytryptophan). With the exception of collagen synthesis (hydroxylation of proline and lysine), the mechanism of action for most of these activities is poorly understood.

Sources

Vitamin C is widely distributed in foods. The best dietary sources are citrus fruits and green vegetables, especially broccoli, green peppers, tomatoes, cabbage, oranges, grapefruits, and lemons. Variation in content depends upon the degree of ripeness, storage conditions, and food preparation.

Requirements

The RDA for ascorbic acid is 40 mg/day for adults. Patients who smoke, are febrile, are undergoing surgery, have been subjected to trauma or burns, are receiving TPN, are pregnant or lactating, or have thyrotoxicosis may require increased amounts of daily vitamin C intake. Vitamin C requirements are increased in patients with malabsorption, inflammatory diseases, and achlorhydria. The RDA for pregnant females is increased to 70 mg/day, while lactating females should receive 95 mg/day of ascorbic acid. Suggested intravenous supplementation during TPN ranges from 100 to 500 mg/day.

Deficiency States

Clinical vitamin C deficiency (scurvy) is uncommon in the Western world, but when seen, it is usually due to dietary inadequacy in the chronically ill, the poor, the elderly, or chronic alcoholics. Symptoms of deficiency develop in 29 days in normal volunteers receiving an ascorbic acid–free diet. However, following a major burn (requirements may increase 100-fold), deficiency may develop in 24 to 48 hours. The manifestations of scurvy are initially nonspecific and include malaise and weakness. Progression of the deficiency state is evidenced by perifollicular hemorrhages, petechiae, bruising, follicular hyperkerato-

sis and purpura, bleeding and swollen gums, loosened teeth, joint hemorrhage, subperiosteal hemorrhage, bleeding from mucous membranes, and bone fractures. Pallor and anemia are common, and wound healing is markedly impaired. As the disease advances, edema, oliguria, and neuropathy are common. Intracerebral hemorrhage is usually followed by death.

Assessment of the vitamin C status may be accomplished by measuring plasma ascorbic acid levels (normal, greater than 1.30 mg/dL) and leukocyte ascorbic acid concentrations (normal, greater than 15 mg/dL). Vitamin C deficiency usually occurs when plasma ascorbic acid levels are less than 0.20 mg/dL and leukocyte ascorbic acid levels are less than 7 mg/dL. The diagnosis of scurvy is usually made on the basis of clinical manifestations in conjunction with low plasma and leukocyte ascorbic acid levels.

Therapy

For prophylaxis against scurvy or correction of deficiency, 40 to 60 mg of vitamin C is administered daily. The oral route is preferred. However, vitamin C may also be given parenterally (i.e., intravenously or intramuscularly). For the treatment of scurvy 300 mg to 1.0 g should be administered daily parenterally for 1 week followed by 100 mg daily for several weeks until tissue stores are replenished. For disease states requiring increased intake (i.e., surgery, trauma, febrile state), 150 mg of vitamin C should be administered daily. For severe burns, 500 mg to 2.0 g is administered daily parenterally until healing has occurred.

Preparations and Adverse Effects

Vitamin C is available in tablet, capsule, and parenteral forms. It is also a component of most multivitamin preparations. Large doses may cause diarrhea or renal stones (i.e., cystine, oxalate, or urate). Renal stones are more likely when the urine is acidic. Lightheadedness and dizziness may occur following rapid intravenous administration. Vitamin C interferes with the anticoagulant effects of heparin, with 2 mg of ascorbic acid neutralizing 1 unit of heparin.

Folic Acid (Pteroylglutamic Acid, Folate, Folacin)

Chemistry

Folic acid (i.e., folate) is composed of a pteridine ring attached to *p*-aminobenzoic acid and conjugated to one molecule of glutamic acid.[1-15] Pteroylglutamic acid is the pharmaceutical form of folic acid but not the active coenzyme or the primary form found in food. Replacement of the glutamic acid residue renders the vitamin inactive. This water-soluble vitamin is unstable when heated in a neutral or alkaline media. It is also unstable upon exposure to sunlight.

Metabolism

Three quarters of the folate in foods is in the reduced polyglutamyl form, which is normally hydrolyzed to free folate in the small intestinal epithelium. Free folate is actively absorbed from the upper portion of the small intestine, during which time it is reduced and methylated to dihydrofolate and tetrahydrofolate, the active forms of folate that are delivered to all tissues. Some vitamin remains unreduced and is metabolized by the liver. After conversion in the liver to 5-methyltetrahydrofolate the vitamin enters the plasma, is stored in tissue, or is excreted in bile. Folate stores are maintained by the diet. Folate excreted in bile is reabsorbed via the enterohepatic circulation. Total-body folate stores are approximately 70 mg, with 20 to 25 mg found in the liver. Normal serum folate concentrations range from 5 to 16 ng/mL. The serum folate concentration does not accurately reflect tissue stores. However, when serum levels are below 2 ng/mL, tissue depletion is usually present. About one fifth of ingested folate is excreted in the urine. An additional 60 to 90 μg/day is excreted in bile and lost into the stool (i.e., not reabsorbed). Folic acid is essential for growth and is required for carbon transfer, purine and pyrimidine biosynthesis, amino acid conversions, and maturation of blood cells.

Sources

Dietary folic acid exists largely as reduced polyglutamates. The average U.S. diet contains 30 to 1000 μg of folic acid per day. Foods rich in folate are green leafy vegetables, organ meats, yeast, and some fruits. Boiling, steaming, or frying of foods can destroy 80% to 95% of the folate content.

Requirements

The RDA for folic acid in adults is 400 μg/day. The RDA for pregnant and lactating females is 600 to 800 μg/day. Suggested intravenous doses for TPN range from 0.4 to 1.0 mg/day.

Deficiency States

Causes of folate deficiency include chronic alcoholism, TPN, poor dietary intake, malabsorption syndromes (i.e., sprue), drugs that cause inadequate absorption (i.e., phenytoin, barbiturates, cycloserine, ethanol), increased utilization of folate (i.e., hemolytic anemia, leukemia, chronic exfoliative dermatitis, sepsis, chronic myelofibrosis, malignancy, hyperthyroidism), folic acid antagonists (i.e., methotrexate, triamterene, trimethoprim, pyrimethamine), and pregnancy. Vitamin B_{12} deficiency may also result in folate deficiency. Vitamin B_{12} participates in the formation of tetrahydrofolic acid.

Symptoms of deficiency may occur earlier in chronic alcoholics, during severe stress, following trauma, after sepsis, and in patients receiving nasogastric suction (high levels of folate are found in bile). A deficiency of folate is manifested as anorexia, nausea, diarrhea, stomatitis, alopecia, glossitis, megaloblastic anemia, thrombocytopenia, leukopenia, hypersegmentation of polymorphonuclear leukocytes, and fatigue.

Assessment of the folate status and a diagnosis of deficiency may be accomplished by measuring folate levels in plasma and red blood cells. Plasma folate is a poor predictor of tissue folate levels but reflects dietary intake. Red blood cell folate levels correlate better with tissue levels. Normal plasma levels of folate are 6 to 20 ng/mL, and normal red blood cell levels of folate are greater than 160 to 600 ng/mL. Folate deficiency is usually present when plasma folate levels are less than 3 to 4 ng/mL. A more definitive diagnosis is made when both plasma and red blood cell levels of folate are decreased (i.e., plasma folate less than 3 to 4 ng/mL and red blood cell folate levels less than 140 ng/mL).

Therapy

Unreduced pteroylglutamic acid is the form of folic acid used therapeutically. For deficiency states, 1 to 2 mg folic acid is given orally per day. Once the symptoms have subsided, a maintenance dose of 0.4 mg/day in adults and 0.8 mg/day in pregnant and lactating females is advised. Parenteral administration is advisable for the treatment of patients with malabsorption.

For treating overdosage of folic acid antagonists (i.e., methotrexate), leucovorin calcium, 10 mg/m^2, is administered orally or parenterally every 6 hours for 72 hours (i.e., leucovorin "rescue"). If the 24-hour postmethotrexate serum creatinine level is 50% greater than premethotrexate creatinine levels, the dose of leucovorin is increased to 100 mg/m^2 every 3 hours until serum methotrexate levels are below 5×10^{-8}M. For hematologic toxicity from folic acid antagonists, leucovorin calcium, 5 to 15 mg, is administered orally daily. Adequate hydration and urinary alkalization with sodium bicarbonates should be employed to increase urinary elimination of the antagonists.

Preparations and Adverse Effects

Folic acid is available in oral (0.1-, 0.4-, 0.8-, and 1-mg tablets) and injectable forms (1, 5, and 10 mg/mL). Leucovorin calcium (folinic acid) is available in oral (5, 10, 15, and 25 mg) and injectable forms (1, 3, and 10 mg/mL). Folic acid is stable in intravenous nutritional solutions (as long as the pH is above 5). Adverse effects of both folic acid and leucovorin calcium preparations are infrequent, but hypersensitivity reactions have been reported.

Nicotinic Acid (Niacin)

Chemistry

Niacin is the generic name for nicotinic acid and nicotinamide, either of which may act as a source of the vitamin in the diet.[1–15] Nicotinic acid is a monocarboxylic acid derivative of pyridine, and nicotinamide is the corresponding amide. They are both water soluble and heat stable but labile in air, alkali, or light.

Metabolism

Both forms of niacin are nearly completely absorbed from the intestinal tract by facilitated and passive diffusion. After absorption, coenzymes are formed and distributed to all tissues. Little vitamin is stored. A small quantity of niacin is also formed from dietary tryptophan. The major metabolites are N-methylnicotinamide and 2-pyridine. Metabolites and unchanged vitamin are excreted in the urine. Nicotinic acid functions as a precursor for the coenzymes nicotinamide adenine dinucleotide (NAD) and nicotinamide adenine dinucleotide phosphate (NADP). These coenzymes are essential for a variety of oxidation-reduction reactions (i.e., carbohydrate, protein, and fat metabolism). They participate in the transfer of hydrogen. In addition, nicotinic acid has therapeutic functions because of its ability to lower serum cholesterol and triglyceride levels.

Sources

Niacin is present in whole-grain cereals, meats, liver, fish, eggs, legumes, and many vegetables. Tryptophan from protein sources is also an important precursor for endogenous niacin production.

Requirements

The RDA for niacin is 15 to 19 mg in adult males and 13 to 15 mg daily in adult females. Allowances are dependent upon the protein intake (i.e., it takes 60 mg of dietary tryptophan to form 1 mg of niacin). Niacin requirements depend upon calorie intake (6.6 mg of niacin per 1000 kcal). An additional 5 mg of niacin per day may be required in pregnant and lactating females. Suggested intravenous requirements for patients receiving TPN range from 40 to 150 mg of niacin per day.

Deficiency States

Niacin deficiency occurs when the diet is poor in both niacin and tryptophan. Historically, niacin deficiency occurred when corn, a poor source of both niacin and tryptophan, was the major source of calories. Today, niacin deficiency is more commonly due to secondary causes such as alcoholism, drugs (i.e., isoniazid and 6-mercaptopurine), rare inborn errors of metabolism (Hartnup's disease), and malnourished patients with malignant carcinoid syndrome.

The manifestations of nicotinic acid deficiency are collectively known as "pellagra." Early manifestations are vague and nondescript. They include weakness, lassitude, anorexia, and indigestion. However, with advanced deficiency, the classic triad of pellagra (dermatitis, diarrhea, and dementia) may be present. The characteristic dermatitis is symmetrical and involves the sun-exposed areas. Skin lesions are dark, dry, and scaling. The diarrhea can be severe, recurrent, and bloody. It may result in malabsorption due to atrophy of the intestinal villi. Dementia may begin as headache, dizziness, irritability, and insomnia that progress to confusion, memory loss, hallucinations, seizures, and psychosis. Death ultimately follows in an untreated patient.

A diagnosis of pellagra, especially in early cases, requires a high index of suspicion. Measurement of the niacin metabolite N-methylnicotinamide in the urine may be helpful. Low levels suggest deficiency. Blood concentrations of NAD and NADP are reduced. However, these are variable and nonspecific indicators of deficiency.

Therapy

Niacin deficiency may be prevented by administering 5 to 20 mg of nicotinic acid daily as a dietary supplement. Niacin deficiency is treated with 50 to 100 mg of oral nicotinic acid daily. Pellagra is treated with 300 to 500 mg of oral nicotinic acid daily in divided doses or 25 to 100 mg of nicotinic acid intravenously every 2 to 3 hours (maximum, 1 g/day). It should be given very slowly and diluted in 0.9% sodium chloride to run at a rate of 2 mg/min. Nicotinic acid may also be given intramuscularly (50 to 100 mg) in divided doses. For the treatment of hyperlipidemia, 1 to 2 g of nicotinic acid is administered in three divided oral daily doses.

Preparations and Adverse Effects

Nicotinic acid is available in oral prolonged-release capsules (125 to 500 mg), tablets (25 to 50 mg), and injectable forms (100 mg/mL). Nicotinamide is manufactured as oral tablets (50 to 500 mg), as timed-release capsules (1000 mg), or as an injectable (100 mg/mL). Adverse effects include headache, dizziness, syncope, flushing, burning, tingling, tachycardia, hypotension, nausea, vomiting, diarrhea, flatulence, peptic ulcers, hepatotoxicity, hyperglycemia, hyperuricemia. and blurred vision.

Biotin

Chemistry

Biotin is an imidazole derivative consisting of eight isomers, of which only d-biotin is found naturally and has vitamin activity.[1-15] This vitamin is soluble in water and alcohol, stable to heat, and unaffected by acid or alkali.

Metabolism

Ingested biotin is rapidly absorbed from the small intestine and widely distributed in all tissues. It is also synthesized by intestinal bacteria and absorbed from the colon. The intact vitamin is the major form excreted in the urine, with the metabolites biotin sulfoxide and bis-norbiotin appearing in smaller amounts. Biotin acts as a cofactor for carboxylating enzymes essential to the metabolism of both fat and carbohydrates.

Sources

Biotin is found in low concentrations in most animal and vegetable foodstuffs. Good sources are organ meats, yeast extracts, egg yolks, dairy products, grains, fruits, and vegetables.

Requirements

The RDA for biotin is 30 to 100 μg in adults. The average American diet provides 100 to 300 μg of biotin per day. Bacterial synthesis in the large intestine provides additional quantities of the vitamin. The recommendation for biotin supplementation during TPN is 60 μg/day.

Deficiency States

Causes of biotin deficiency include severe malnutrition, consumption of large quantities of raw egg whites (egg white contains avidin, a biotin antagonist), disruption of normal intestinal flora by broad-spectrum antibiotics, and long-term TPN. Only a few reports of biotin deficiency during TPN have been published. Biotin deficiency manifests itself as a maculopapular dermatitis, glossitis, lingual atrophy, muscle pain, lassitude, alopecia, paresthesia, ataxia, nausea, anorexia, anemia, and hypercholesterolemia. Cutaneous eruptions develop in cutaneomucosal areas such as the corners of the eyelids, mouth, and perineal region. Ophthalmologic manifestations include blurred vision, keratoconjunctivitis, and photophobia. The biotin status is assessed by measuring the vitamin in plasma (normal, 1.47 mg/mL; range, 0.82 to 2.7) or urine (24-hour urinary excretion: normal, 42.4 mg; range, 24 to 81).

Therapy

Most of the symptoms of deficiency are reversible with large doses of biotin (100 to 300 μg/day). Deficiency may be prevented by administering a multivitamin preparation containing biotin.

Preparation and Adverse Effects

Biotin is available as oral tablets (1, 5, and 10 mg). It is also available in various multivitamin preparations. No significant adverse effects are reported.

Pantothenic Acid

Chemistry

Pantothenic acid is a dimethyl derivative of butyric acid (pontic acid) joined by a peptide linkage to the amino acid β-alanine.[1-15] This is a water-soluble vitamin that is unstable in acid, alkali, or heat.

Metabolism

Pantothenic acid is readily absorbed from the intestinal tract and subsequently transformed to 4'-phosphopantetheine. In the tissues, this derivative forms the prosthetic group for both coenzyme A and acyl carrier protein. The vitamin does not appear to be degraded in the body, with 70% of absorbed vitamin being excreted in the urine unchanged. Pantothenic acid is an essential component of coenzyme A, which participates in enzymatic reactions important in the metabolism of carbohydrates, gluconeogenesis, fatty acid oxidation, and the synthesis of sterols, steroid hormones, and porphyrins. Its contribution to acyl carrier protein is important for fatty acid synthesis.

Sources

Pantothenic acid is widely distributed in foods. Good sources include organ meats, beef, liver, yeast, egg yolk, whole-grain cereals, and legumes.

Requirements

A recommended daily intake of 4 to 7 mg is considered adequate intake for adults. There is no RDA established for pantothenic acid. A well-balanced 2500-kcal diet contains about 10 mg of the vitamin. During pregnancy and lactation, daily intake of the vitamin should be increased.

Deficiency States

The occurrence of pantothenic acid deficiency is rare because of its wide distribution in foods. Spontaneous clinical deficiency has not been described but may occur as a constellation of symptoms in association with other B-vitamin deficiencies. Experimental deficiency has produced the following symptoms and signs: heel and foot pain, fatigue, paresthesias, weakness, leg cramps, and the so-called burning foot syndrome. In clinical practice, these symptoms rarely respond to vitamin supplementation. Assessment of pantothenic acid status is accomplished by measuring blood levels (normal, 100 to 180 µg/dL).

Therapy

For deficiency manifested as the "burning foot syndrome," 10 mg of pantothenic acid is administered orally per day.

Preparations and Adverse Effects

Pantothenic acid is available as a calcium salt preparation (oral, 10 to 500 mg). It is also present in many of the multivitamin and B-complex prepara-

tions. Adverse effects have not been reported.

Choline

Chemistry

Choline (trimethylethanolamine or trimethyl-β-hydroxyethylammonium hydroxide), is a lipotropic quaternary amine that is water soluble, strongly alkaline, and hygroscopic.[1-15] It is classified as being "vitamin-like" since this substance is synthesized within the body. The endogenous synthesis of choline, however, requires adequate amounts of the amino acids serine and methionine, along with adequate amounts of folic acid and vitamins B_{12} and B_6.

Metabolism

Choline is absorbed from the intestinal tract. Most of the free choline is metabolized by intestinal bacteria to trimethylamine, whereas dietary choline derived from lecithin is absorbed and extracted by the liver and peripheral tissues. Choline is excreted in urine and feces. The functions of choline are many: it is an important component of membrane phospholipids (i.e., lecithin and sphingomyelin), essential for the synthesis of the neurotransmitter acetylcholine, it is an integral component for normal lung development (i.e., as a component of surfactant), and it functions as a methyl donor for the synthesis of compounds such as methionine.

Sources

Choline is found in most foods. Egg yolk, liver, soybean, and fish provide a rich source. Foods high in fat contain more choline than those low in fat (i.e., vegetables and fruits).

Requirements

No deficiency state attributable to choline has been identified in humans. Given that the average American diet contains 300 to 900 mg/day of choline and that it is readily available endogenously, no RDA has been established.

CONCLUSION

Vitamins are essential compounds for the maintenance of normal metabolic functions. Requirements must be met to ensure optimal nutritional support and recovery from illness. Further research is needed to define optimal quantities during critical illness. Deficiency syndromes are not uncommon in critically ill patients. Unfortunately, many go unrecognized. Enteral nutritional formulas contain adequate quantities to meet RDAs if adequate calories and protein are administered. However, these quantities will not meet the increased needs found in many critically ill patients as a result of increased requirements or body loss. Supplementation may be required. Vitamin solutions are available for use during TPN. MVI-12 provides recommended intravenous amounts. It does not contain vitamin K.

REFERENCES

1. Marks J: The individual vitamins, in Marks J (ed): *The Vitamins—Their Role in Medical Practice.* Boston, MTP Press, 1985, pp 111–193.
2. Feldman EB: *Essentials of Clinical Nutrition.* Philadelphia, FA Davis, 1988, pp 24–42, 333–361.
3. Suter PM, Russel RM: Vitamin nutriture and requirements of the elderly, in Munro HN, Danford DE (eds): *Human Nutrition. A Comprehensive Treatise— Nutrition, Aging, and the Elderly,* vol 6. New York, Plenum Publishing Corp, 1989, pp 245–291.
4. Gibson RS: *Principles of Nutritional Assessment.* New York, Oxford University Press, 1990, pp 377–486.
5. Herbert V: Vitamins and minerals, in Herbert V, Subak-Sharpe GJ (eds): *The Mount Sinai School of Medicine Complete Book of Nutrition.* New York, St Martin's Press, 1990, pp 89–105.
6. Suter PM: Vitamin requirements, in Chernoff R (ed): *Geriatric Nutrition. The Health Professional's Handbook.* Gaithersburg, Md, Aspen Publications, 1991, pp 25–51.
7. Chaney SG: Principles of nutrition II: Micronutrients, in Devlin TM (ed): *Textbook of Biochemistry with Clinical Correlations,* ed 2. New York, John Wiley & Sons, 1986, pp 962–983.
8. Kissane JM: *Anderson's Pathology,* ed 9. St Louis, Mosby–Year Book, 1990, pp 550–561, 1377–1378.
9. Gilman AG, Rall TW, Nies AS, et al: *Goodman and Gilman's The Pharmacological Basis of Therapeutics,* ed 8. New York, Pergamon Press, 1990, pp 1510–1522, 1530–1571.
10. Wyngaarden JB, Smith LH Jr, Bennett JC: *Cecil Textbook of Medicine,* ed 19. Philadelphia, WB Saunders, 1992, pp 1170–1183, 1404–1406.
11. Bennett DR: In *Annual Drug Evaluations.* Chicago, American Medical Association, 1992, pp 368, 2017–2032.
12. Olin BR, Hebel SK, Dombek CE, et al: *Drug Facts and Comparisons,* ed 46. St Louis, Facts and Comparisons, 1992, pp 4–28, 169, 223–233.
13. Viteri FE: Vitamin deficiencies, in Paige DM (ed): *Clinical Nutrition,* ed 2. St Louis, Mosby–Year Book, 1988, pp 547–578.
14. Grant JP (ed): *Handbook of Total Parenteral Nutrition,* ed 2. Philadelphia, WB Saunders, 1992, pp 291–309.
15. Caldwell MD, Kennedy-Caldwell C, Winkler MF: Micronutrients and enteral nutrition, in Rombeau JL, Caldwell MD (eds): *Clinical Nutrition—Enteral and Tube Feeding,* ed 2. Philadelphia, WB Saunders, 1990, pp 73–117.

15

Minerals

Robert D. Lindeman, M.D.

Richard J. Roche, M.D.

Maintenance of sodium and extracellular fluid volume

Disturbances in sodium and water balance

Hyponatremia with contracted extracellular fluid volume (primary salt depletion)

Hyponatremia with normal extracellular fluid volume

    Displacement syndromes (pseudohyponatremia)

    Redistribution hyponatremia

    Syndrome of inappropriate antidiuretic hormone

    Water intoxication

Hyponatremia with expanded extracellular fluid volume (dilutional hyponatremia)

Hyponatremia in the elderly

Hypernatremia

Maintenance of potassium balance

    Hypokalemia

    Hyperkalemia

Maintenance of calcium balance

    Osteoporosis

    Hypocalcemia

    Hypercalcemia

Maintenance of magnesium balance

    Hypomagnesemia

    Hypermagnesemia

Maintenance of phosphorus balance

    Hypophosphatemia

    Hyperphosphatemia

Maintenance of body fluids and minerals (electrolytes) is essential to man's survival. With highly variable intake of fluids and minerals, preservation of the internal environment requires variable but essentially continuous urinary excretion in amounts that precisely balance the quantities acquired through ingestion or other sources. Although losses through the gastrointestinal tract and other portals, e.g., skin (sweat) and the respiratory tract, may contribute to this excretory capacity, the greatest responsibility for water and mineral conservation and excretion is borne by the kidney. Although most of the regulatory mechanisms are geared toward maintaining the integrity of the extracellular fluid volume (ECFV), the continuous exchange of water and minerals across cell membranes ensures that the kidney also regulates the volume and mineral composition of intracellular fluids.

Despite the presence of effective homeostatic mechanisms for conserving water and minerals, a minimal intake of water and minerals is necessary to maintain health. Sodium conservation is extremely efficient. Unless an abnormality in this system develops such as abnormal gastrointestinal or insensible water loss or abnormal loss in urine, it is difficult to restrict sodium intake to levels that will produce a body deficit of sodium. Potassium is conserved less well. However, unless pathology is present or rigid dietary restriction is imposed, simple dietary restriction of potassium also does not produce a body deficit. In contrast, recommended daily allowances (RDAs) for dietary intakes of calcium, magnesium, and phosphorus have been identified as necessary to maintain health.[1] These requirements are 800 mg/day for calcium, 350 mg/day for magnesium, and 800 mg/day for phosphorus. Deficient intakes as well as excessive losses can result in body deficits of these minerals.

This chapter deals with the major minerals or electrolytes: sodium, potassium, calcium, magnesium, and phosphorus, along with the water that keeps them in solution. Distribution within the body, normal physiologic and biochemical functions, normal homeostatic mechanisms, the pathophysiology of deficits and excesses, and the treatment of body fluid and electrolyte imbalances are covered. Specific attention is paid to these problems in the elderly, partly because the ability to maintain homeostasis is much more limited in the elderly and partly because that is our area of special interest.

MAINTENANCE OF SODIUM AND EXTRACELLULAR FLUID VOLUME

Sodium ions and their associated anions are the primary regulators of ECFV. The control of extracellular fluid osmolality is a function of body water balance and is under the combined control of fluid intake and renal excretion of water moderated largely by antidiuretic hormone (ADH). An active sodium-potassium transport mechanism moves sodium from inside the cell to the extracellular space in exchange for potassium so that the extracellular sodium concentration is maintained at 140 mEq/L and the intracellular sodium approximates 10 mEq/L. The sodium ion and its associated anions of chloride and bicarbonate account for more than 90% of the osmotically active solute in the ECFV. The control of the ECFV is therefore largely dependent upon the regulation of sodium balance, which in turn is dependent upon the relationship between sodium intake and renal and extrarenal sodium losses. Normal kidneys are able to excrete virtually sodium-free urine or large sodium loads depending upon the body's needs. The control of osmotic pressure of body fluids is more rapid and precise than is control of volume. If one compares the administration of isotonic saline, which expands volume, with water, which lowers osmolality, the kidneys respond to the latter with a much prompter elimination of excess fluid.

DISTURBANCES IN SODIUM AND WATER BALANCE

The serum sodium concentration alone fails to reflect total-body sodium stores; the clinical assessment of ECFV is equally important and generally much more difficult. While the presence of edema is indicative of an excess of ECFV, determination of a deficit can be more difficult. Postural hypotension, if the patient is able to stand or at least sit, is a good indicator of ECFV deficit, but it can be present in older patients with autonomic dysfunction (i.e., diabetes, Shy-Drager syndrome). Loss of skin turgor can be hard to evaluate in older per-

SERUM SODIUM CONCENTRATION		LOW	NORMAL	HIGH
	LOW	DEHYDRATION (Primary Salt Loss) Na$^+$Loss > H$_2$0 Loss	REDISTRIBUTION Hyperglycemia DISPLACEMENT Hyperlipemia Hyperproteinemia SYNDROME OF INAPPROPRIATE ADH WATER INTOXICATION	DILUTIONAL HYPONATREMIA H$_2$0 Retention > Na$^+$Retention
	NORMAL	DEHYDRATION Na$^+$Loss = H$_2$0 Loss	NORMAL	UNCOMPLICATED EDEMA H$_2$0 Retention = Na$^+$ Retention
	HIGH	DEHYDRATION (Primary Water Loss) H$_2$0 Loss > Na$^+$ Loss	HYPERALDOSTERONISM HYPERCORTISONISM	STERIOD EXCESS SALT INTOXICATION Na$^+$ Retention > H$_2$0 Retention
		LOW	NORMAL	HIGH
		EXTRACELLULAR FLUID VOLUME		

FIG 15–1.

Causes of salt and water abnormalities with relationships between serum sodium concentrations and extracellular fluid volumes.

sons with loss of subcutaneous tissue because of chronic illness and aging. Loss of sweating and decreased intraocular tension can also be hard to evaluate. The total-body sodium content approximates the product of the plasma sodium concentration and the ECFV ($T_BNa = P_{Na} \times ECFV$). Various disturbances in salt and water balance are demonstrated in Figure 15–1.

HYPONATREMIA WITH CONTRACTED EXTRACELLULAR FLUID VOLUME (PRIMARY SALT DEPLETION)

Dehydration by definition is a decrease in body water. It can result from excessive water loss with inadequate replacement (hypernatremic dehydration) or from a primary salt loss (hyponatremic dehydration). Early in primary salt loss dehydration, water is lost with sodium so that serum sodium concentrations remain normal; once sufficient volume is lost to stimulate ADH release, salt continues to be lost, but water is retained, thus creating hyponatremia.

As shown in Table 15–1, causes of hyponatremia with a contracted volume can be separated into those where the urinary sodium excretion is less than 10 mEq/L and those where it exceeds that amount. Etiologies of the former include inadequate sodium intake, excessive sweating, and gastrointestinal fluid and salt loss (diarrhea, bowel and biliary fistulas). Normal kidneys can lower urinary sodium levels to the range of 2 mEq/L during sodium depletion. In addition, during volume depletion sweat decreases its salt content. Thus, salt depletion rarely results from either inadequate salt intake or sweating alone. If urinary sodium excretion exceeds 10 mEq/L, in the face of hyponatremia and dehydration, inappropriate renal losses of sodium and water because of adrenal insufficiency, underlying renal disease, or diuretics should be suspected. Severe vomiting with metabolic alkalosis and bicarbonaturia also can result in excessive sodium losses.

Treatment of hyponatremia resulting from primary salt depletion should be with isotonic or hypertonic saline. Generally, the former is safer. Once the volume is repleted, excess water is excreted, and some salt continues to be retained, thereby raising the serum sodium concentration toward normal. If

TABLE 15–1.

Hyponatremic Syndromes

Hyponatremia with contracted ECFV*
  Urinary sodium < 10 mmol/L
    Inadequate intake
    Excessive sweating
    Excessive gastrointestinal losses
      Diarrhea
      Fistulous tracts (bowel, biliary)
  Urinary sodium > 10 mmol/L
    Severe metabolic alkalosis (bicarbonaturia)
    Excessive urinary losses
      Adrenal insufficiency
      (Addison's disease, hypoaldosteronism)
      Renal salt wasting (renal tubular acidosis, interstitial
        nephritis, acute tubular necrosis, end-stage renal
        disease)
      Diuretic induced
Hyponatremia with normal ECFV
  Redistribution
    Hyperglycemia
    Mannitol infusion
  Displacement syndromes
    Hyperlipidemia
    Hyperproteinemia
  Syndrome of inappropriate ADH*
    Malignancies, most notably lung
    Pulmonary disease, including pneumonia and
      treatment with positive-pressure breathing
    Cerebral conditions (trauma, infection, tumor,
      vascular accidents)
    Drugs (sulfonylureas, thiazides, antitumor agents)
    Myxedema
    Porphyria
    Idiopathic
  Water intoxication
Hyponatremia with expanded ECFV
  Dilutional hyponatremia
    Congestive heart failure
    Cirrhosis
    Nephrotic syndrome
    Renal insufficiency
    Hypoalbuminemia

*ECFV = extracellular fluid volume; ADH = antidiuretic hormone.

it is unclear in the differential diagnosis whether primary salt depletion or the syndrome of inappropriate antidiuretic hormone (SIADH) exists, it is wise to insert a central venous pressure (CVP) catheter to monitor right heart pressures. One can then give normal (or hypertonic, e.g., 3%) saline until the CVP rises above 4 mm Hg. If the patient is suspected of having left heart failure, a Swan-Ganz catheter would provide added safety. If one wishes to estimate the amount of salt necessary to replete a volume-contracted individual with hyponatremia, it is important to remember that even though sodium is largely an extracellular cation, as the serum sodium concentration is increased, water shifts from inside the cell to the ECFV to dilute and again lower the serum sodium concentration. Therefore, estimates of sodium deficit must be made on the basis of total-body water (60% of body weight) rather than ECFV (20% of body weight). It is best to replace deficits slowly to allow time for fluid shifts. The rise in serum sodium levels should not exceed 2.5 mEq/hr or 20 to 25 mEq/48 hr.

HYPONATREMIA WITH NORMAL EXTRACELLULAR FLUID VOLUME

Displacement Syndromes (Pseudohyponatremia)

A decrease in the serum sodium concentration does not always indicate a decrease in the osmolality of body fluids. Normally about 93% of serum is water, with the other 7% being solute. If one raises the percentage of solute, as seen in hyperproteinemia or hyperlipidemia, there is a proportionate drop in the serum sodium concentration even though the actual sodium concentration in plasma water is unchanged. This is because a small serum sample is diluted multiple times to create the solution used by the flame photometer.

Redistribution Hyponatremia

Hyperglycemia produces an increase in osmolality in the extracellular fluid followed by a movement of water from the intracellular to extracellular fluid compartments. Subsequently, the excessive extracellular fluid creates a natriuresis, through renal mechanisms, that persists until the ECFV returns to normal. Although theoretically every 100-mg/dL increase in the serum glucose concentration above the normal

100 mg/dL results in a 2.8-mEq/L decrease in the serum sodium concentration, the actual experience is a 1.6-mEq/L decrease. For example, if a patient has a serum glucose concentration of 800 mg/dL, the serum sodium content would be expected to decrease to 129 mEq/L (140 − [1.6 × 7]). Any variance from this would suggest superimposed dehydration or salt loss. Mannitol infusions produce similar effects.

Syndrome of Inappropriate Antidiuretic Hormone

A persistently high level of circulating ADH is considered inappropriate when neither hyperosmolality of the serum nor volume depletion, the usual stimuli to ADH release, are present. An inability to excrete the free water ingested (or infused) leads to volume expansion, dilutional hyponatremia, and increased urinary salt loss. SIADH is typically seen in patients with pulmonary neoplasms but may be associated with a number of other conditions (see Table 15−1). Since volume (stretch) receptors controlling ADH release are located in the left atrium and aortic arch, any pulmonary condition (e.g., positive-pressure breathing or pneumonia) that impedes the flow of blood through the lungs into the left atrium will be interpreted as volume depletion and result in the stimulation of ADH release.

The problem of differentiating salt depletion hyponatremia from SIADH frequently arises in nonedematous patients. Patients with the former diagnosis tend to raise their blood urea nitrogen (BUN) out of proportion to the serum creatinine concentration; patients with the latter diagnosis have a normal or subnormal BUN value unless underlying renal impairment is present. If urinary sodium excretion is very low, this favors the former diagnosis; a high urinary sodium excretion can be seen in either salt depletion hyponatremia (associated with diuretic use, adrenal or renal disorder) or SIADH. If one remains clinically unsure which entity is responsible, monitoring the CVP as outlined earlier may be necessary.

The first step in treating SIADH is fluid restriction. It may be necessary to restrict water to as little as 500 mL/day to prevent symptomatic hyponatremia. If symptomatic hyponatremia develops (confusion, somnolence, seizures), one can use a loop diuretic, e.g., furosemide, to cause the kidney to excrete hypotonic (dilute) urine. To prevent volume depletion, urine losses can be replaced by isotonic or hypertonic saline.[2] Since raising the serum osmolality also results in a shift of water from inside the cell to the ECFV, fluid volume replacement needs to be less than urinary volume.

One can calculate the excess water that needs to be excreted in order to fully correct the hyponatremia as follows (assuming a 70-kg man whose total-body water content is 60% of his body weight and his serum sodium concentration is 120 mEq/L):

$$70 \text{ kg} \times 0.6 = 42 \text{ L of total-body water}$$

$$\frac{120 \text{ mEq/L (patient)}}{140 \text{ mEq/L (normal)}} \times 42 \text{ L} = 36 \text{ L}$$

$$42 \text{ L} - 36 \text{ L} = 6 \text{ L excess fluid}$$

This means that correction of hyponatremia with either isotonic or hypertonic saline and a diuretic, e.g., furosemide requires that the urine volume exceed fluid input by 6 L. Again, this should be accomplished slowly.

Other agents used to treat SIADH include lithium carbonate and demeclocycline (Declomycin), which produce nephrogenic diabetes insipidus. The latter is generally preferred because it is less toxic. The recommended dosage of demeclocycline is 150 to 300 mg four times daily. A diuresis usually occurs within 5 days after initiation of therapy and reverses within 2 to 6 days after discontinuation of treatment with the drug. Rapid correction or overcorrection (>25-mEq/L change in the plasma sodium concentration in 48 hours) carries with it the risk of central pontine myelinolysis, a devastating condition with severe neurologic damage (pseudobulbar palsy or cranial nerve abnormalities).[3]

Water Intoxication

It is difficult if not impossible for a normal person to drink sufficient water (without vomiting) to cause symptomatic hyponatremia. Patients with schizophrenia, however, do appear to be capable of drinking sufficient water to become symptomatic. Treatment is merely restriction of water.

HYPONATREMIA WITH EXPANDED EXTRACELLULAR FLUID VOLUME (DILUTIONAL HYPONATREMIA)

Edematous patients with advanced cardiac, hepatic, and renal disease and with hypoalbuminemia (nephrotic syndrome) can be severely limited in their ability to eliminate both salt and water in the urine. The usual practice in such patients of restricting salt intake (but not water intake) is appropriate until hyponatremia begins to develop. At that time, it may also become necessary to place restrictions on water intake. Although the total blood volume is increased in such patients, the blood volume reaching the atria and arterial vascular system is decreased, often with a decrease in cardiac output. Low cardiac output is interpreted by the baroreceptors as a decreased effective blood volume, thereby stimulating salt and water retention. A decrease in the glomerular filtration rate concurrent with increased sodium reabsorption in the proximal tubule limits water excretion by sharply decreasing the delivery of tubular salt and fluid to the distal diluting segment of the nephron. If little salt and water reach the distal nephron, the patient is unable to dilute urine below isotonic levels. The result is hyponatremia

since the usual mix of salt and water intake consists of a hypotonic solution. Since a decrease in the effective intravascular volume is a potent stimulus to ADH release, high levels of circulating ADH also play a role in the pathogenesis of fluid retention and hyponatremia in these patients. One would expect patients with cardiac and hepatic failure, unless receiving diuretics, to have low urinary sodium concentrations (<10 mEq/L). Treatment consists of diuretics, e.g., furosemide, which decrease the concentrating ability, and fluid (as well as sodium) restriction. Treatment of the underlying disease is also necessary.

HYPONATREMIA IN THE ELDERLY

Surveys of older persons in both acute and chronic care facilities show a much higher prevalence of hyponatremia when compared with younger subjects. Kleinfeld et al.[4] for example, reported that 36 of 160 chronically ill patients (23%) had serum sodium concentrations below 132 mEq/L (mean, 120 mEq/L). In most, the low serum sodium value was not readily explainable except by the presence of debilitating disease and old age.

Anderson et al.[5] evaluated the prevalence, cause, and outcome of hyponatremia in an acute facility. The prevalence was 2.5%, with one third being hospital acquired. Furthermore, normovolemic hyponatremia (SIADH) developed in one third of the patients. Hypovolemia, hypervolemia, and hyperglycemia accounted for another one sixth each and the remaining sixth was attributed to renal failure or laboratory error. The authors demonstrated that nonosmotic (baroreceptor) stimulation of vasopressin (ADH) release was a major factor in the development of hyponatremia regardless of the cause since there were increases in serum arginine vasopressin (AVP) in the face of low serum osmolalities.

Other evidence suggests that elderly persons may be more susceptible to the development of hyponatremia because of increased ADH release from osmoreceptor stimulation. Postoperative hyponatremia and hyponatremia induced by diuretics and sulfonylureas are entities occurring almost exclusively in older patients. Helderman et al.[6] showed that older subjects increased serum AVP concentrations much more after a standardized hypertonic saline infusion (designed to raise the serum osmolality to 306 mOsm/L) than did younger subjects. In contrast, ethanol, which inhibits ADH secretion, produced a depression in serum AVP concentrations that lasted much longer in young than in older subjects. These two observations together suggest an increasing osmoreceptor sensitivity with age. Older subjects, after quiet standing, however, often failed to increase serum AVP levels as did younger subjects.[7] This observation suggests that the vasopressin response to volume-pressure stimuli might be the primary defect in the elderly and the osmotic hyperresponsiveness might in some way be a compensatory response.

HYPERNATREMIA

An increase in the serum sodium concentration usually results from a loss of body water in excess of salt (dehydration), although it also can result from the ingestion or administration of sodium without sufficient water. Among elderly patients, hypernatremia is most common in those who are bedfast or restricted and not provided adequate quantities of fluids and in those whose sensation of thirst is impaired.

Again, older patients appear to be predisposed to the development of hypernatremia (dehydration). Snyder et al.[8] reported that over 1% of their hospital admissions were for patients over the age of 60 years in whom hypernatremia developed (serum sodium concentration greater than 148 mEq/L). One half had hypernatremia on admission, and hypernatremia developed in the other half while in the hospital. Surgery, febrile illness, infirmity, and diabetes mellitus accounted for two thirds of their cases.

Older subjects have a relative inability to conserve both salt[9] and water[10] when the intake of each is eliminated or sharply restricted. The inability to conserve salt may be related to the lower renin and aldosterone levels observed in the elderly under all conditions.[11] Undoubtedly, this contributes to the development of hypernatremia, but more importantly, older subjects develop an impaired thirst response. Phillips et al.[12] studied alterations in thirst perception in healthy old vs. young subjects. After 24 hours of water deprivation, all were given free access to water. Older individuals exhibited less thirst and drank less water even though they lost more fluid during the period of water deprivation. They ended up with higher plasma sodium concentrations and osmolalities.

The earliest manifestation of hypernatremia, at least in younger individuals, is thirst, followed by confusion and lethargy. Ultimately, delirium, stupor, and coma develop. Because the intravascular volume is preserved at the expense of cell water, changes in blood pressure, pulse rate, and skin turgor are not prominent features of hypernatremia.

Factors that enhance the development of dehydration include increased insensible water loss related to fever and sweating, vomiting and diarrhea, diabetes insipidus, and an osmotic diuresis (as seen in hyperosmolar, nonketotic hyperglycemia). Insensible water losses may be an important component of dehydration, normally contributing approximately 750 mL/day. These losses are dependent on the respiratory rate, humidity, and temperature.

Once significant hypernatremia develops, parenteral restoration of fluid balance is usually necessary. The amount of water (or dextrose and water) needed can be determined by multiplying the percent increase in serum sodium concentration above normal (140 mEq/L) by the total-body water (60% of body weight in kilograms). For example, a person with a serum sodium concentration of 154 mEq/L (10% increase) and a body weight of 70 kg (42 kg or L of total-body water) would require 4.2 L to replace the water deficit (assuming that there was no salt deficit present). To prevent a recurrence, a fluid prescription (quantity of fluid to be ingested daily) may be an important component of treatment.

MAINTENANCE OF POTASSIUM BALANCE

Potassium is the primary intracellular cation. Less than 2% of the total-body potassium content is in the extracellular fluid compartment. Thus, the serum potassium concentration may not accurately reflect total-body potassium stores. A flux of potassium into cells occurs with cell growth, with intracellular nitrogen and glycogen deposition, and with increases in extracellular pH. Potassium leaves the cell with cell destruction, with intracellular glucose utilization, and with decreases in extracellular pH. Because a steep concentration gradient is normally maintained between the intracellular and extracellular compartments, factors affecting this gradient must be kept in mind when assessing any serum potassium concentration. For example, a diabetic patient with metabolic ketoacidosis is admitted with a high-normal serum potassium concentration despite a total-body potassium deficit. Treatment with rehydration (dilution), correction of the acidosis with bicarbonate, and treatment of the hyperglycemia with insulin cause the potassium to move intracellularly, and the serum potassium concentration falls dramatically. Certain clinical conditions (e.g., metabolic and respiratory ac-

idosis, congestive heart failure, cirrhosis, and renal failure) are accompanied by a decrease in the intracellular-to-extracellular potassium gradient so that the total-body potassium concentration is decreased.

Hypokalemia

The causes of hypokalemia are listed in Table 15−2.[13] Often multiple mechanisms can be implicated in the pathophysiology of hypokalemia. For example, vomiting reduces potassium intake and causes the loss of small amounts of potassium in gastric contents. More importantly, there is a loss of hydrogen ions, which creates a metabolic alkalosis that causes a shift of potassium intracellularly and increases urinary potassium losses. The contracted intravascular volume increases proximal tubular sodium and bicarbonate reabsorption, further enhancing the metabolic alkalosis and producing secondary hyperaldosteronism, which also increases urinary potassium losses.

Although the normal kidney is not as effective in conserving potassium as it is sodium, excretion should be reduced to below 20 mEq/day when the serum potassium concentration falls below 3.5 mEq/L, even in the presence of an acidosis or alkalosis. Since little potassium is normally lost through the gastrointestinal tract, it takes 2 to 3 weeks of a potassium-free diet for hypokalemia to develop, provided that other organ systems, specifically the gastrointestinal tract and kidney, are functioning normally.

The causes of excessive urinary potassium loss can be divided into four categories (see Table 15−2): (1) pituitary-adrenal excess, (2) renal pathology, (3) drug induced, and (4) idiopathic and miscellaneous. One important cause in category 4 is hypomagnesemia. In a patient with low serum calcium, phosphorus, and potassium concentrations, one should suspect magnesium depletion.

TABLE 15–2.

Causes of Hypokalemia

Inadequate intake
Excessive sweating
Dilution of extracellular fluid volume
Shift of potassium intracellularly
   Increase in blood pH (alkalosis)
   Glucose + insulin
   Familial hypokalemic periodic paralysis
Excessive gastrointestinal losses
   Vomiting
   Biliary, pancreatic, and intestinal drainage from fistulas
     and ostomies
   Diarrhea
     Chronic infections and inflammatory lesions
     Malabsorption
     Villous adenomas of the colon and rectum
     Catechol-secreting neural tumors
     Abdominal lymphomas
     Non-α, non-β islet cell tumors of the pancreas
     Excessive use of enemas and purgatives
   Ureterosigmoidostomy
Increased urinary losses
   Pituitary-adrenal disturbances
     Primary aldosteronism
     Secondary aldosteronism (renal artery stenosis)
     Cushing's syndrome (adrenal adenomas, carcinomas,
       hyperplasia, pituitary adenoma causing
       corticotropin hypersecretion)
   Renal disorders
     Proximal and distal renal tubular acidosis
     Renin-secreting renal tumor
     Salt-losing nephritis
     Diuretic phase of acute tubular necrosis
     Postobstructive diuresis
   Drug induced
     Diuretics
     Licorice extracts (glycyrrhizic acid)
     Large, nonreabsorbable anions (carbenicillin)
     Acetylsalicylic acid (respiratory alkalosis)
   Idiopathic and other pathologies
     Bartter's syndrome
     Hypomagnesemia
     Thyrotoxicosis
     Idiopathic or familial

Unless this underlying problem is first corrected, it may be difficult to correct the potassium deficit because of continued urinary wasting of potassium.

Clinical features associated with potassium deficiency include involvement of the kidney (concentrating defect), myocardium, (depressed ST segment, inversion of T waves, accentuated U waves), muscle (weakness to paralysis, tenderness, rhabdomyolysis),

gastrointestinal tract (decreased motility, paralytic ileus), and endocrine-metabolic system (carbohydrate intolerance, growth failure). Depressive reactions (weakness, lethargy, apathy, fatigue) and acute brain syndromes have also been reported.

Since alkalosis (chloride depletion) usually accompanies hypokalemia, replacement therapy should be with potassium chloride rather than with the alkaline salts of potassium. The exception to this is a patient with renal tubular acidosis. For the treatment of marginally low serum potassium levels (3.3 to 3.7 mEq/L), ingestion of foods high in potassium content (bananas, orange juice, tomato juice) is recommended. One has to be cautious about the use of commercial tomato juice because it usually has large quantities of salt. Other foods high in potassium content include squash, green vegetables, beans, and potatoes. Most commercial oral preparations for potassium replacement contain 20 mEq/15 cc, so this amount can be given without risk two to four times daily in a glass of water or juice, provided that renal function is not severely impaired. Since these liquid forms are not very palatable, even though they insure the best absorption, alternative forms (tablet, capsule, slow-release tablet) are available.

Intravenous potassium replacement may be necessary but can be hazardous, especially if infusion rates exceed 20 mEq/hr or concentrations of infusate exceed 40 mEq/L. Adequate urine output should be present and electrocardiographic monitoring initiated before potassium infusions are pushed above these levels.

A great deal of concern has been generated over the possibility that hypokalemia may precipitate life-threatening arrhythmias or sudden death in patients receiving diuretics, especially in those taking digitalis or those with acute myocardial infarction. The evidence does not support this concern.[14] In fact, more concern should be focused on the routine use of potassium supplements because there is a significant incidence of life-threatening hyperkalemia in supplemented patients. Age and azotemia are the two most significant risk factors identified in the Boston Collaborative Drug Surveillance Program for the development of hyperkalemia associated with potassium supplementation.[15] Older subjects have lower plasma renin activity and urinary aldosterone excretion, which probably explains their inability to excrete excessive potassium in the urine.[11]

Hyperkalemia

Hyperkalemia is seen most commonly in patients with impaired renal function. However, most patients with chronic renal failure are able to maintain good urine flow rates, and significant hyperkalemia does not develop until after they require some form of maintenance dialysis. Because the distal nephron has a sizable capacity for secreting potassium, hyperkalemia develops only when some contributing factor is superimposed on chronic renal failure. These include oliguria (acute renal failure), excessive potassium load (tissue catabolism, exogenous supplements), severe acidosis, administration of a diuretic that blocks sodium-potassium exchange (triamterene, spironolactone, amiloride), administration of a drug that impairs potassium excretion (angiotensin-converting enzyme [ACE] inhibitor, nonsteroidal anti-inflammatory agent), or a deficiency of endogenous steroid (cortisol, aldosterone). In older persons, especially diabetics and patients with interstitial nephritis, failure of the renin-angiotensin-aldosterone system may develop and cause type IV renal tubular acidosis.

The clinical manifestations of hyperkalemia can be very nonspecific and subtle (anxiety, restlessness, apprehension, weakness). These features may precede death from cardiac arrythmia by minutes to hours. Characteristic electrocardiographic changes are peaking of the T waves followed by widening and then loss of P waves and widening of the QRS complex.

Therapy should be started when the serum potassium concentration exceeds 5.5 mEq/L; a true medical emergency exists when it exceeds 7.0 mEq/L. Acute treatment is with glucose, insulin, and sodium bicarbonate to shift potassium intracellularly and with calcium and sodium salts, which act as physiologic antagonists. For example, 15 units of regular insulin can be added to 1 L of 5% glucose and water (50 g of glucose) along with two ampules of 7.5% sodium bicarbonate (44.6 mEq per 50-mL ampule). Calcium should not be added with bicarbonate because it will precipitate out. It is important to continue this infusion until potassium is removed from the body. Otherwise, potassium will move back into the extracellular fluid as soon as the infusion is stopped. Sodium polystyrene sulfonate (Kayexalate) resins are used to remove excess potassium from the body and can be given orally or in enema form. Orally, 15g (4 level tsp) of the powder can be given four times a day. To avoid constipation and fecal impaction with oral administration of these resins, 15 to 30 cc of a 70% sorbitol solution in one-half glass of water can be taken with the Kayexalate and this dosage titrated to maintain a mild osmotic diarrhea. Rectally, 50 g is given in 200 mL of water. Often a portion of the water (50 cc) is given as a 70% sorbitol solution to reduce water absorption. This can be repeated every hour or two until the serum potassium concentration is lowered to a safe level. When the hyperkalemia is due to a mineralocorticoid deficiency as in hyporeninemic hypoaldosteronism (type IV renal tubular acidosis), fludrocortisone acetate (Florinef) can be given in doses starting with 0.1 mg/day and increased or decreased as the need dictates. Since sodium is reabsorbed in exchange for potassium, one must be cautious not to overhydrate the patient and precipitate pulmonary edema.

MAINTENANCE OF CALCIUM BALANCE

A finely tuned endocrine system exists to maintain serum ionized calcium concentrations within a narrow normal range by controlling intestinal absorption, bone exchange, and renal excretion of calcium. Whenever serum ionized calcium concentrations decrease, parathyroid hormone (PTH) secretion increases and results in mobilization of calcium from bone, decreased renal tubular phosphate resorption with a resultant decreased serum phosphate concentration (this facilitates bone resorption of calcium), increased renal tubular calcium resorption, and increased intestinal calcium resorption, either directly or by enhancing the effect of vitamin D. Vitamin D is converted by the liver to the carrier metabolite 25-hydroxycholecalciferol (25-OHD$_3$) and by the kidney to the active metabolite 1,25-dihydroxycholecalciferol (1,25-(OH)$_2$D$_3$). The active metabolite acts primarily to increase calcium absorption in the intestine, but it also increases bone resorption of calcium and decreases urinary calcium and phosphate excretion. PTH appears to produce its effects on the intestine by accelerating renal conversion of 25-OHD$_3$ to 1,25-(OH)$_2$D$_3$. When serum calcium concentrations increase, serum thyrocalcitonin concentrations increase and produce effects generally counter to those of PTH.

Serum calcium exists in both the ionized and bound states, but only ionized calcium is physiologically active. The bound calcium either binds to serum proteins, primarily albumin, or is complexed with such anions as citrate. The binding is dependent on the concentration of serum protein (albumin) and the blood pH, with calcium binding increasing as the pH increases. The total serum calcium level declines by approximately 0.4 mmol/L (0.8 mg/dL) for each 1-g/dL decrease in serum albumin concentration. Since most laboratories report only total serum calcium concentrations,

these factors must be considered when evaluating a specific serum calcium concentration. Direct measurement of ionized calcium is the most reliable method for assessing the circulating calcium status.

Osteoporosis

Riggs and Melton[16] have postulated that at least two distinct clinical types of osteoporosis exist. Type I is referred to as postmenopausal, is caused by a deficiency of estrogen, and is characterized by loss of mineralization and fractures in trabecular bone (spine, distal thirds of the ulna and radius). Following menopause, whether natural or surgically induced, there is a rapid increase in bone mineral loss that lasts 10 to 15 years before returning to premenopausal levels. Estrogen replacement therapy greatly retards this bone loss and is associated with a much reduced risk of fracture.

Senile osteoporosis (type II) occurs later in life, is related to deficient intakes of calcium and vitamin D, and affects both trabecular and cortical (femur) bone. Because vitamin D is a major regulator of calcium absorption, the cumulative effect of a deficit of calcium intake and an inadequate intake of vitamin D is a negative calcium balance, which stimulates PTH secretion. PTH, in turn, increases bone calcium resorption and the risk of fractures with its subsequent morbidity and mortality.

The intensivist is often called on to deal with long-standing negative calcium balance (osteoporosis) with its resultant fractures of hips, compression fractures of the spine, and other difficult-to-treat fractures. Although initiation of calcium and vitamin D supplements has little immediate effect on bone mineralization, they should be started. Calcium supplements should be administered in amounts ranging from 1000 to 1500 mg/day. Oral calcium supplements come in several forms (e.g., carbonate, citrate, lactate, and phosphate). OsCal (calcium carbonate), for example, provides 500 mg of calcium in each tablet. Most vitamin D supplements (or analogues) come in dosages intended to treat vitamin D—resistant conditions (vitamin D—resistant rickets, hypoparathyroidism, renal osteodystrophy, etc.) and are sufficiently large that they may cause toxicity (hypercalcemia, renal failure) and actually increase bone resorption of calcium by stimulating osteoclast activity. Furthermore, clinical trials of vitamin D supplements, including calcitriol, have shown that vitamin D alone is ineffective in preventing calcium loss from bone.[17] For example, calciferol (ergocalciferol) is available in 50,000-unit (1.25 mg) capsules and tablets. This dose is 100-fold more than the 400 IU (10 μg) listed as the RDA.[1] Calciferol is also available in a solution with 8000 IU (200 μg)/mL, which is still a high dose. Other forms of vitamin D include calcifediol (25-OH-cholecalciferol), which comes in 20- and 50-μg capsules, calcitriol (1,25-(OH)$_2$-cholecalciferol), which comes in 0.25- and 0.5-μg capsules, and dihydrotachysterol, which comes in 0.125-mg capsules or tablets. All are used to treat vitamin D—resistant conditions in these dosages. If used for other purposes (e.g., osteoporosis), the serum calcium concentrations must be monitored closely to prevent the development of hypercalcemia and resultant renal damage. It is probably better to give one vitamin-mineral supplement daily that contains 400 IU of vitamin D until it can be shown that this dose fails to normalize the serum calcium concentration.

Calcitonin may be effective in treating acute compression fractures of the spine. Not only does it reinstitute bone mineralization, but it is often also effective in providing pain relief. It must be given by subcutaneous injection and generally cannot be used for more than 2 years because of an escape phenomenon (loss of effect). Injections of 50 or 100 units are given three times a week. Higher doses are administered initially and lower doses after pain relief is

achieved. Fluoride also has been used to increase bone mineralization in doses of 40 to 60 mg/day, along with calcium and vitamin D supplementation. Finally, the diphosphonates (bisphosphonates) show promise in treating osteoporosis. Cyclical etidronate (Didronel) has been shown to be effective at doses of 400 mg/day in improving bone mineralization and decreasing fracture rates.[18 19] Some of the newer diphosphonates appear even more promising but have yet to be released on the U.S. markets for anything but investigational use.

Hypocalcemia

The causes of hypocalcemia are listed in Table 15—3. Renal insufficiency is the most common cause of hypocalcemia and is usually associated with hyperphosphatemia. In patients with unexplained hypocalcemia, hypokalemia, or hypophosphatemia, clinicians should be aware that hypomagnesemia could be the underlying etiology. Hypomagnesemia causes a peripheral resistance to the effects of PTH, thereby inhibiting re-

TABLE 15–3.

Causes of Hypocalcemia

Renal insufficiency
Malignancies, especially with osteoblastic metastases
  (prostate)
Hypoparathyroidism; pseudohypoparathyroidism
  (resistance to PTH* action)
Disorders of vitamin D metabolism
  Dietary deficiency
  Malabsorption
  Nephrotic syndrome (urinary loss)
  Liver disease
  Vitamin D—resistant rickets
    1α-Hydroxylase deficiency (type 1)
    Resistance to 1,25-dihydroxyvitamin D action (type
    2)
Acute pancreatitis
Calcitonin-producing tumors (medullary carcinoma of the
  thyroid)
Electrolyte imbalances
  Hypomagnesemia
  Hyperphosphatemia (rhabdomyolysis, tumor lysis)

*PTH = parathyroid hormone.

lease of calcium from bone and decreasing the release of PTH.

The symptomatology associated with hypocalcemia is primarily related to increased neuromuscular excitability, as manifested by tetany and positive Chvostec and Trousseau signs. Long-term manifestations include cataracts, abnormalities of the nails, skin, and teeth, and mental and growth retardation. Urgent therapy may be required for acute hypocalcemic crises as manifested by severe tetany, laryngospasm, convulsions, or cardiovascular collapse.

Acute correction of symptomatic hypocalcemia can be accomplished with parenteral calcium salts (e.g., calcium gluconate; 10 mL of a 10% solution contains 1 g of calcium gluconate or nearly 100 mg of calcium). Intravenous administration should not exceed 200 mg (2 cc) of calcium gluconate per minute or a total of 2 g without rechecking the serum calcium concentration. Patients receiving cardiac glycosides are at increased risk for toxicity. Subcutaneous and intramuscular administration produces tissue irritation and necrosis, especially with calcium chloride. Oral calcium salts, (carbonate, citrate, lactate, phosphate) can be used to treat mild or latent hypocalcemia. Vitamin D, especially its 1,25-$(OH)_2$-cholecalciferol metabolite [calcitriol], increases the serum calcium concentration by increasing intestinal absorption and bone resorption of calcium.

Hypercalcemia

The causes of hypercalcemia are listed in Table 15–4. The most frequent cause in hospitalized patients is malignant disease. A number of mechanisms, both with and without bony metastases, are operable in causing hypercalcemia.[20, 21]

Early symptoms are vague and nonspecific and include anorexia, nausea, vomiting, constipation, fatigue, somnolence, muscle weakness, pruritus, confusion (delirium), and psychiatric dis-

TABLE 15–4.

Causes of Hypercalcemia Classified by Major Pathogenetic Mechanisms

Increased bone resorption
  Primary (and tertiary) hyperparathyroidism
  Malignancy
    Local osteolytic lesions, e.g. breast, multiple myeloma
    Humoral hypercalcemia (PTH*-like secretion), e.g.
      ovary, kidney, head and neck, colon, cervix, lung
  Thyrotoxicosis
  Immobilization, e.g., Paget's disease
Increased gastrointestinal absorption
  Vitamin D intoxication
  Malignancy due to excessive conversion of
    25-hydroxyvitamin D to 1,25-dihydroxyvitamin D,
    e.g., histiocytic lymphoma
  Sarcoidosis
  Other granulomatous disease (tuberculosis,
    coccidioidomycosis, histoplasmosis, berylliosis,
    candidiasis, eosinophilic granuloma)
  Milk-alkali syndrome
Mechanism unclear
  Vitamin A intoxication
  Addison's disease
  Acute rhabdomyolysis
  Familial hypocalciuric hypercalcemia
  Thiazide diuretics (decreases renal clearance of calcium)

*PTH = parathyroid hormone.

turbances (hallucinations, depression). Ultimately, polyuria with dehydration, azotemia, and cardiac arrhythmias are likely to occur. Nephrolithiasis, nephrocalcinosis, and extrarenal calcifications are manifestations of long-standing hypercalcemia. When serum calcium concentrations exceed 15 mg/dL, one is faced with a life-threatening emergency with the potential for serious cardiac arrhythmias. The electrocardiogram may reveal shortening of the QT interval and prolongation of the PR interval.

The initial therapy for patients with hypercalcemia is rehydration with normal saline. This decreases the serum calcium concentration by hemodilution and increases urinary calcium excretion by volume expansion. If renal function is reasonable and a good urine output is established, 300 to 500 mL/hr of saline is a reasonable infusion rate. Loop diuretics (furosemide) greatly increase urinary calcium excretion, whereas thiazide diuretics decrease urinary calcium excretion and may potentiate hypercalcemia. Twenty milligrams of furosemide intravenously every 6 to 8 hours can establish a brisk diuresis.

Oral phosphate and diphosphonate salts such as etidronate (Didronel) are effective in lowering calcium levels. They are well tolerated except for gastrointestinal disturbances (e.g., diarrhea). Etidronate is initially given as an intravenous infusion (7.5 mg/kg body weight over at least a 2-hour period) for 3 to 5 days followed by an oral intake not to exceed 20 mg/kg/day. Renal failure is the major contraindication. A number of additional, more effective diphosphonates (bisphosphonates) are available for investigational use but are not yet available in this country for general use. Two grams of oral sodium or potassium phosphate daily represents another form of management for patients with chronic hypercalcemia. Commercial preparations that provide this amount are available in liquid (Phospho-soda, 3 tsp daily), powder (Neutra-phos, 2 tsp daily), capsule (Neutra-phos, 8 capsules daily), and tablet (Phos-tabs, 12 tablets daily) forms. The major concern with the use of intravenous phosphates is the development of tissue calcification and its consequences. Prednisone in high doses (40 to 60 mg/day) is effective in lowering calcium concentrations when the mechanism of the hypercalcemia is increased vitamin D—mediated calcium absorption from the intestine (sarcoid, multiple myeloma, vitamin D intoxication). It is less effective in most malignancies, especially with metastatic bone disease, and in hyperparathyroidism.

Injections of calcitonin (50 to 100 IU/day three times a week) decreases the skeletal release of calcium, phosphorus, and hydroxyproline. The most impressive results are seen in conditions in which a high rate of bone turnover occurs (e.g., immobilization, thyrotoxicosis, and vitamin D intoxication). Nonsteroidal anti-inflammatory agents or indomethacin may be helpful in reducing the hypercalcemia in some malignancies (e.g., renal cell carcinoma in which prostaglandin E appears to be the mediator of excessive bone breakdown). Plicamycin (mithramycin) can be used in the treatment of hypercalcemia associated with malignancy unresponsive to other therapies. This antitumor agent acts by inhibiting bone resorption and blocking vitamin D action. Its application is limited by the necessity of intravenous administration. Transient nausea and vomiting, bone marrow suppression, bleeding diathesis, and hepatotoxicity are the major side effects. Bone marrow suppression usually limits the dosage. Therapy is initiated with 25 μg/g body weight per day. A fall in serum calcium concentration occurs within 48 hours. The number of doses per week is adjusted to maintain serum calcium concentrations in the normal range. If all else fails, hemodialysis is effective in acutely lowering serum calcium concentrations in life-threatening situations. Finally, gallium nitrate holds promise as an investigational drug in the treatment of hypercalcemia of malignancy.[22]

MAINTENANCE OF MAGNESIUM BALANCE

Magnesium is the second most abundant intracellular cation, with about 60% of body magnesium located in bone, 40% intracellularly, and 1% extracellularly. The normal serum magnesium concentration ranges from 0.7 to 1.1 mmol/L (1.4 to 2.2 mEq/L) and correlates poorly with intracellular magnesium. About 30% of serum magnesium is protein bound, with most of the remainder in ionized form, which makes it ultrafilterable through the kidney. Most of the intracellular magnesium is bound to protein and energy-rich phosphates. Magnesium is important in over 300 different enzyme systems. Magnesium is indispensable to the metabolism of adenosine triphosphate (ATP), thereby affecting glucose utilization. It is important in the synthesis of fat, protein, and nucleic acids, in muscle contraction, and in several membrane transport systems.

Hypomagnesemia

The most commonly encountered cause of hypomagnesemia is alcoholism. Other causes of magnesium deficiency are listed in Table 15–5. Hypomagnesemia produces neuromuscular hyperirritability (tetany, hyperacusis, seizures, muscle weakness, vertigo, tremors) and psychiatric disturbances (irritability, aggressiveness). It is often recognized because of the presence of other electrolyte disorders (hypocalcemia, hypokalemia, hypophosphatemia). Significant depletion of intracellular magnesium can occur before the serum magnesium concentration falls below the normal range.[23]

Oral magnesium repletion is limited by the development of diarrhea. Approximately 15% to 30% of orally administered magnesium-containing antacids and laxatives are absorbed. Magnesium hydroxide is the most commonly used form of oral magnesium, with each 5 mL of milk of magnesia containing 14 mEq. Generally doses in excess of 80 mEq/day produce diarrhea. Magnesium citrate

TABLE 15–5.

Causes of Hypomagnesemia

Gastrointestinal disorders with malabsorption
Chronic alcoholism
Endocrine disorders
Hyperaldosteronism
Hyperparathyroidism
Diabetic ketoacidosis
Acute pancreatitis
Renal magnesium loss
Diuretic therapy
Syndrome of inappropriate antidiuretic hormone
Magnesium wasting
Idiopathic
Gentamicin
Cisplatin
Renal tubular acidosis
Protein-calorie malnutrition

and sulfate also are available as oral salts. Symptomatic magnesium deficiencies can be treated with intravenous or intramuscular magnesium salts; the latter tend to be painful. Magnesium sulfate is available in 10% (20-mL ampule) or 50% (2-mL ampule) solutions. The rate of intravenous infusion should not exceed 150 mg/min (1.5 mL/min of a 10% solution).

Hypermagnesemia

Hypermagnesemia sufficient to produce symptoms (lethargy, respiratory depression) primarily develops in patients with renal failure treated with magnesium-containing antacids and cathartics (e.g., milk of magnesia). Although no treatment is usually needed other than stopping the exogenous magnesium, calcium gluconate or gluceptate can be administered intravenously as a physiologic antagonist in treating respiratory depression.

MAINTENANCE OF PHOSPHORUS BALANCE

Hypophosphatemia

Selective phosphorus deficiency induced in normal subjects by an inadequate diet and/or ingestion of large quantities of phosphate-binding antacids leads to a distinctive clinical syndrome characterized by anorexia, weakness, and bone pain. Symptoms appear primarily when the serum phosphorus concentration falls below 0.3 mmol/L (< 1.0 mg/dL), and clinical improvement occurs rapidly when the serum phosphorus concentration is restored by intravenous or dietary phosphorus.

Severe hypophosphatemia has been documented in association with alcohol withdrawal, diabetes mellitus, excessive antacid ingestion (e.g., phosphate-binding aluminum hydroxide), recovery from burns, unsupplemented hyperalimentation, nutritional recovery syndrome, and severe respiratory alkalosis.[24] It is important to recognize that a severely malnourished patient may have a precipitous drop in serum phosphorus concentration during refeeding unless adequate supplies of phosphorus are provided. Hypophosphatemia results from a combination of total-body phosphorus depletion, catabolic starvation, and increased cellular influx during carbohydrate refeeding with infusions of glucose and water. Respiratory insufficiency, metabolic encephalopathy, irritability, muscular weakness, hypoesthesias and paresthesias, dysarthria, confusion, seizures, coma, rhabdomyolysis, hemolysis, and leukocyte (abnormal phagocytic, chemotactic, and bacteriocidal activities of granulocytes) and platelet dysfunction may develop in patients with severe hypophosphatemia.

Dairy products are the best dietary sources of phosphorus. The phosphorus salts (mentioned earlier under hypercalcemia) can be given orally or infused intravenously. Inorganic phosphates can be buffered to a pH of 7.4 by mixing four parts of the disodium salt with one part of the monopotassium salt (4 Na_2HPO_4 : 1 KH_2PO_4). This formulation is unfortunately not commercially available.

Hyperphosphatemia

Significant hyperphosphatemia is seen primarily in patients with renal failure, but mild elevations can also be seen in patients with hypoparathyroidism, pseudohypoparathyroidism, hyperthyroidism, and acromegaly. Hyperphosphatemia does not produce symptoms directly, but high levels result in precipitation of calcium phosphate salts in arteries, muscle, periarticular spaces, kidney, and other soft tissues, and this results in symptomatology. It also can produce hypocalcemia with consequent tetany and secondary hyperparathyoidism. Magnesium- and/or aluminum-containing antacids can be used to bind phosphate in the intestine,

thereby inhibiting phosphorus absorption and lowering the serum phosphorus concentration.

REFERENCES

1. National Research Council: *Recommended Dietary Allowances,* ed 10. Washington, DC, National Academy Press, 1989.
2. Hantman D, Rossier B, Zohlman R, et al: Rapid correction of hyponatremia in the syndrome of inappropriate antidiuretic hormone. An alternative treatment of hypertonic saline. *Ann Intern Med* 1973; 78:870–875.
3. Berl T: Treating hyponatremia: What is all the controversy about? *Ann Intern Med* 1990; 113:417–419.
4. Kleinfeld M, Casimir M, Borra S: Hyponatremia as observed in a chronic disease facility. *J Am Geriatr Soc* 1979; 27:156–161.
5. Anderson PJ, Chung HM, Kluge R, et al: Hyponatremia: A prospective analysis of its epidemiology and the pathogenetic role of vasopressin. *Ann Intern Med* 1985; 102:164–168.
6. Helderman JH, Vestal RE, Rowe JW, et al: The response of arginine vasopressin to intravenous ethanol in man: The impact of aging. *J Gerontol* 1978; 33:39–47.
7. Rowe JW, Minaker KL, Sparrow D, et al: Age related failure of volume-pressure mediated vasopressin release. *J Clin Endocrinol Metab* 1982; 54:661–664.
8. Snyder NA, Feigal DW, Arieff AI: Hypernatremia in elderly patients: A heterogeneous, morbid, and iatrogenic entity. *Ann Intern Med* 1987; 107:308–319.
9. Epstein M, Hollenberg N: Age as a determinant of renal sodium conservation in normal man. *J Lab Clin Med* 1976; 87:411–417.
10. Rowe JW, Shock NW, DeFronzo RA: The influence of age on the renal response to water deprivation in man. *Nephron* 1976; 17:270–278.
11. Weideman P, DeMyttenaeu-Bursztein S, Maxwell MH, et al: Effect of aging on plasma renin and aldosterone in normal man. *Kidney Int* 1975; 8:325–333.

12. Phillips PA, Rolls BJ, Ledingham JJG, et al: Reduced thirst after water deprivation in healthy elderly men. *N Engl J Med* 1984; 311:753–759.

13. Lindeman RD: Hypokalemia: Causes, consequences, and correction. *Am J Med Sci* 1976; 272:5–17.

14. Fries ED: Diuretic induced hypokalemia: The debate over its relationship to cardiac arrhythmias. *Postgrad Med* 1987; 81:123–129.

15. Lawson DH: Adverse reactions to potassium chloride. *Q J Med* 1974; 171:433–440.

16. Riggs BL, Melton LJ III: Involutional osteoporosis. *N Engl J Med* 1986; 314:1676–1686.

17. Parfitt A: Calciferol and metabolites in osteoporosis. *Drugs* 1988; 36:513–520.

18. Storm T, Thamsborg G, Steiniche T, et al: Effect of intermittent cyclical etidronate therapy on bone mass and fracture rate in women with post menopausal osteoporosis. *N Engl J Med* 1990; 322:1265–1271.

19. Watts NB, Harris ST, Genant HK, et al: Intermittent cyclical etidronate treatment of post menopausal osteoporosis. *N Engl J Med* 1990; 323:23–79.

20. Sherwood LM: The multiple causes of hypercalcemia in malignant disease. *N Engl J Med* 1980; 303:1412–1413.

21. Fetchick DA, Mundy GR: Hypercalcemia of malignancy: Diagnosis and therapy. *Compr Ther* 1986; 12:27–32.

22. Burns Schaiff RA, Hall TG, Bar RS: Medical treatment of hypercalcemia. *Clin Pharm* 1989; 8:108–121.

23. Reinhart RA: Magnesium metabolism: A review with special reference to the relationship between intracellular content and serum levels. *Arch Intern Med* 1988; 148:2415–2420.

24. Knochel JP: The pathophysiology and clinical characteristics of severe hypophosphatemia. *Arch Intern Med* 1977; 137:203–220.

16

Trace Elements

Daniel L. Herr, M.D.

Micronutrients are required for the utilization of macronutrients (i.e., protein, carbohydrates, fats). Micronutrients belong to two main groups: vitamins and trace elements. In this chapter we discuss trace elements, inorganic elements that regulate numerous metabolic processes in the body. Many function as constituents of enzyme complexes. Depletion of these substances causes functional, biochemical, or structural abnormalities in tissues. Seven trace elements are essential for health in humans: chromium, copper, cobalt, iodine, iron, selenium, and zinc. Recommended allowances for healthy individuals have been defined; however, it is unclear how these values should be applied to critically ill patients.

CHROMIUM

Chromium is an essential trace mineral that functions primarily to potentiate the action of insulin. Chromium can assume many oxidation states, the most stable and biologically active state being trivalent chromium. Trivalent chromium is not associated with enzymes but instead acts as a coordinating compound in the control of glucose metabolism. It is associated with a low-molecular-weight organic complex termed glucose tolerance factor that acts with insulin in promoting normal glucose utilization.

In 1985, it was reported that normal subjects consumed an average of 28 μg/day of chromium in their diet. This is 50% of the recommended dietary allowance (RDA). Researchers argue that the intake of chromium in the diet of the average American is not optimal and point to an improvement in glucose tolerance with diets that are supplemented with chromium. Further, with stressful events such as trauma, strenuous exercise, and high glucose intake, chromium losses are increased; therefore a knowledge of chromium metabolism is important in the management of critically ill patients.

Metabolism

As with many of the trace minerals, the absorption and metabolism of chromium have not been fully clarified. Chromium is most likely absorbed via a nonsaturable diffusion process and, like iron, is carried on transferrin. It is primarily excreted in urine. The most studied aspect of chromium is its capacity to prevent glucose intolerance. It is well known that brewer's yeast contains a significant amount of chromium in the form of a biologically active organic co-ordination compound, chromium dinicotinatoglutathione. When highly purified, brewer's yeast exhibits glucose tolerance activity, which potentiates the action of insulin by facilitating the interaction of insulin with its all surface receptors. In humans with impaired glucose tolerance, however, increases in serum insulin are not usually accompanied by increased secretion of chromium in the urine, and chromium usually fails to reverse glucose intolerance. Besides improving glucose control, glucose tolerance factor may lower serum cholesterol and triglyceride levels. The variable response of glucose homeostasis to chromium supplementation may result from the rarity of a true cellular deficiency state. Chromium most likely improves glucose intolerance in patients with chromium deficiency but has little benefit in those without deficiency. Thus, in patients with protein-calorie malnutrition and glucose intolerance, chromium frequently improves glucose control.

Deficiency States

Rare chromium deficiency syndromes are reported in the literature, although this may reflect an inability to measure the actual biological activity of this mineral. There have been rare case reports of chromium deficiency in patients receiving long-term total parenteral nutrition (TPN) (Table 16−1) that has reversed with the addition of chromium to the TPN solution. Absorbed chromium is excreted almost completely in the

TABLE 16−1.

Signs of Marginal Chromium Deficiency in Humans

Impaired glucose intolerance
Elevated fasting insulin
Glycosuria
Elevated circulating insulin
Decreased insulin binding
Decreased insulin receptor number
Elevated cholesterol and triglycerides
Decreased high-density lipoprotein (HDL) cholesterol
Hypoglycemic symptoms

urine, but it is unclear whether excessive diuresis causes a deficiency state. Chromium supplementation in glucose-intolerant patients requires 1 to 6 months of therapy for maximum response. The recommended dietary chromium allowance in adults is 50 to 200 μg/day. It is based on the absence of signs of chromium deficiency among U.S. residents who consume an average of 50 μg/day. Although most TPN solutions have added chromium, the exact amount of chromium in the solution is difficult to assess because amino acids and lipids also contain this mineral. In a study that examined chromium content in TPN solutions, the amount of chromium ranged from 2.4 to 8.1 μg for a high-glucose formula and 2.6 to 10.5 μg for a high-lipid formula. Even when additional chromium is added to TPN, most patients still receive less than the standard chromium requirements for healthy adults. Further, the addition of extra chromium to TPN solutions has been associated with a significant reduction in blood glucose levels (without any other changes to the TPN regimen). The maximum dose of intravenous chromium is not well known, although 250 μg has been given to patients with chromium deficiency and malnutrition without side effects.

Assessment

A determination of chromium deficiency states cannot be based on the level of chromium in the bloodstream because this level is not in equilibrium with body stores. Assessment is further complicated by the fact that all needles, syringes, and containers must be free of contaminating trace metals when the sample is drawn. Since no definitive test for chromium deficiency is available, a therapeutic trial is usually undertaken when deficiency is suspected. We recommend administering 100 to 200 μg/day for 1 to 2 months. If glucose tolerance improves, chronic supplementation may be indicated. One

must be cautious since glucose control may improve over this time period because of improvement in disease activity.

Treatment

Patients should receive 50 to 200 mg/day of dietary chromium; 10 to 15 mg/day is recommended for intravenous supplementation.

COPPER

The normal adult body contains 100 to 150 mg of copper, 90% of which is found in muscle, bone, and liver. In the blood, more than 90% is found associated with ceruloplasmin, with the remainder bound to albumin and in erythrocytes. Copper is important for the function of numerous oxidative enzyme systems. These oxidative enzymes are known as cuproenzymes (Table 16–2). Clinical manifestations of copper deficiency, such as Menkes' hair syndrome, result from altered metabolic pathways that are controlled by cuproenzymes. These enzymes are integral to metabolic functions such as erythropoiesis and leukopoiesis, oxidative phosphorylation, catecholamine metabolism, antioxidant protection, and the maintenance of immunocompetence. These processes are important for the body's reaction to tissue injury and stress. Cuproenzymes are essential for consumption of molecular oxygen–related species such as superoxide radicals. Copper overload may result from Wilson's disease, a hereditary disorder of

TABLE 16–2.

"Common" Cuproenzymes

Monoamine oxidase
Diamine oxidase
Lysyl oxidase
Cytochrome c oxidase
Dopamine β-hydroxylase
Tyrosinase
Zn-Cu superoxide dismutase

copper metabolism. This autosomal recessive disease results from progressive accumulation of copper within body tissues (i.e., erythrocytes, kidney, liver, brain) and causes progressive organ failure (i.e., hepatic failure, anemia, central nervous system [CNS] damage renal tubular disease). Defective synthesis of the copper transport protein ceruloplasmin is an associated defect. Copper homeostasis, like that of many other trace elements in critically ill patients, has not been adequately studied.

Metabolism

Copper can be absorbed in the stomach, but most is absorbed in the distal end of the duodenum. The RDA for copper is 2 to 3 mg/day in adults, and the copper content of a normal diet is 2 to 5 mg/day. Copper absorption increases during deficiency states; however, absorption is not under known hormonal control but is inhibited by contact with bile, a potentially important consideration during enteral nutrition in critically ill patients. Like zinc, copper is absorbed by phytates and ascorbic acid (vitamin C) in the diet. Antacids and zinc at high doses also diminish copper absorption. Metallothionein (MT), whose synthesis is stimulated by zinc, binds copper in circulation. This binding process becomes a concern when supplementing zinc in a zinc-to-copper ratio greater than 500:1. Once copper is absorbed into the circulation, it is bound to albumin and transported to the liver. In the liver, copper is incorporated into ceruloplasmin. This transport protein provides copper to the bone marrow for red and white blood cell production and/or donates copper for incorporation into the various types of cuproenzymes. An important consideration with regard to copper metabolism and nutrition in the critically ill patient is that ceruloplasm is considered an acute-phase reaction protein. It has been dem-

onstrated that in patients with infectious diseases, ceruloplasm levels can increase up to threefold in the circulation. In the presence of bile, however, copper is primarily excreted in the feces without evidence of an enterohepatic circulation. Smaller amounts of copper may also be excreted in the urine.

Deficiency States

The most common clinical manifestations of copper deficiency are hypochromic microcytic anemia and neutropenia, although neither state specifically indicates copper deficiency. In patients with hypochromic microcytic anemia, however, failure of a reticulocyte response to iron administration is suggestive of copper deficiency. Neutropenia in the context of copper deficiency is relative since copper-deficient patients can mount a normal leukocyte response to infection. A list of documented clinical manifestations of copper deficiency can be found in Table 16–3. Menkes' kinky-hair syndrome is a sex-linked genetic abnormality caused by a defect in intestinal copper absorption. Affected infants have low levels of copper and ceruloplasmin, and progressive cerebral degeneration, retarded growth, sparse brittle hair, arterial lesions, and "scurvy-like" bone changes develop. Copper (intravenous) prevents the syndrome.

Copper restriction studies in animals and a few experiments in humans have

TABLE 16–3.

Clinical Manifestations of Copper Deficiency in Critically Ill Patients

Hypochromic microcytic anemia
Neutropenia
Skeletal demineralization*
Depigmentation of hair
Skin pallor
Vascular aneurysms*
Cerebral and cerebellar degeneration*
Hypotonia*
Hypothermia*
Subperiosteal hemorrhages

*Only demonstrated in children.

revealed numerous biochemical and laboratory abnormalities associated with copper deficiency. Knowledge of the physiologic role of cuproenzymes is based on these copper restriction studies. Normal individuals excrete only minimal amounts of copper in the urine, but injured patients excrete large amounts. Urinary excretion can rise to a mean of 256 μg/day. In the general population, copper deficiency is a rare occurrence, except in severely malnourished children. As with other trace elements, the most common cause of inadequate copper nutriture is chronic TPN therapy, but even this cause is now considered rare. It is well documented that circulating copper levels diminish rapidly in patients receiving unsupplemented TPN formulations. The American Medical Association's suggested daily intravenous copper intake for adult TPN patients is 0.5 to 1.5 mg daily. Most authorities agree that 0.3 mg of daily intravenous copper is sufficient for copper replacement in TPN patients. Patients with diarrhea have increased intravenous requirements that approach 0.5 mg/day. Copper replacement requirements can decrease to 0.1 mg/day in patients with liver disease and in patients with diseases that are susceptible to copper overload. Copper requirements of 0.5 mg/day have been recommended for critically ill patients.

Assessment

Accurate noninvasive assessment of copper concentrations in the body is difficult because there is no standardized laboratory test and because levels are highly influenced by sex, age, and hormonal state. Further, more than 90% of the body's copper is bound to ceruloplasmin—an acute-phase reactant—which makes assessment of copper status in critically ill patients even more difficult. The measurement of urinary copper excretion is not a reliable index during TPN because of aminoaciduria.

Levels of copper in hair are greatly affected by the environment. The most common method for assessing copper status is via circulating plasma or serum levels, although when dealing with a critically ill patient, a more useful method of assessing copper nutriture would be the measurement of cuproenzymes. Unfortunately, this method is not readily available. Plasma copper concentrations are elevated during pregnancy and estrogen therapy because of a rise in ceruloplasmin levels.

Adverse Effects (Copper Excess)

Although copper deficiency is usually the more important consideration when dealing with the nutritional mandates of trace elements, the effects of copper overload must also be considered. Copper excess may result from excessive copper intake, long-term exposure to hemodialysis solutions containing copper, or hereditary disorders of copper metabolism (i.e., Wilson's disease). Manifestations of acute copper intoxication include nausea, vomiting, abdominal pain, diarrhea, and diffuse myalgias. CNS damage progressing to coma and death, necrotizing pancreatitis, and hemolytic anemia also occur. Wilson's disease is a hereditary disorder associated with accelerated copper absorption and tissue copper overload. Untreated, there is progressive accumulation of copper within erythrocytes, kidney, liver, and brain. Copper accumulation results in hemolytic anemia, hepatic failure, CNS damage (tremor, choreoathetoid movements, rigidity of skeletal muscles, dysarthria, personality changes, dementia, coma, death), cirrhosis, renal dysfunction, and osteomalacia. The diagnosis is made by findings of hypocupremia, decreased ceruloplasmin levels, and compatible clinical findings. Liver biopsy findings demonstrating hepatic copper overload are confirmatory. Treatment consists of a low-copper diet and oral copper binder (i.e., penicillamine).

Treatment

Patients should be supplemented with 2 to 3 mg/day of dietary copper or 0.5 to 1.5 mg/day of intravenous copper.

ZINC

The body contains 1 to 2.5 g of zinc, which is found primarily in bones, teeth, hair, skin, liver, muscle, and testes. In plasma, 33% is bound to albumin and 66% to globulins. Zinc is known for its ability to promote wound healing and form many types of metalloenzymes that are vital to protein synthesis and maintenance of cell membrane stability. Unlike copper, the pathophysiology of zinc deficiency cannot be attributed to one particular metalloenzyme. Also unlike copper, zinc overload is not an issue, although recent evidence suggests that overfeeding of zinc may inhibit certain immunologic functions (see the assessment section). Since the discovery of the disease acrodermatitis enteropathica, an inherited skin/gastrointestinal tract disorder resulting in zinc chelation and malabsorption of zinc, the clinical signs of zinc deficiency have been well known. These signs are hallmarked by palmar bullae, scaly hyperpigmented lesions over acral surfaces and around the mouth, and other clinical manifestations that subsequently resolve with dietary zinc supplementation.

Metabolism

In humans, the distal segment of the jejunum is largely responsible for the absorption of zinc. The average diet contains 10 to 15 mg of zinc per day (1 to 2 mg absorbed). The RDA for zinc is 15 mg/day. The absorptive capacity of the jejunum is 1.5 times greater than that of the duodenum and 4 times greater than that of the ileum. It appears that intestinal pH does not affect zinc uptake. Rather, zinc is absorbed by facilitated diffusion. Chelation of dietary zinc by foods high in fiber and phytate, geophagia, and parasitism reduce absorption. A large amount of absorbed zinc is retained in the intestinal cells and bound to the intracellular protein metallo thionein (MT). The zinc then moves with MT from the intestinal cell to the blood and is bound to albumin for transport. MT also is synthesized in the liver, where it can extract zinc from albumin and thereby increase hepatic zinc concentrations. As the level of zinc decreases, the amount of absorption increases, as does the production of MT. Zinc is excreted in feces, sweat, and urine. A precise understanding of the clinical significance of zinc is lacking, except in clinical zinc deficiency syndromes. We do know, however, that one of the more important functions of zinc is to act as an essential cofactor for a variety of metalloenzymes. In order for an enzyme to be considered a metalloenzyme, the enzyme must satisfy three requirements: (1) the metal must be tightly bound to the protein, (2) there must be a stoichiometric relationship between the metal and the protein, and (3) removal of the metal must impair catalytic function of the enzyme. With this definition in mind and having an understanding of the function of the different zinc metalloenzymes, we see that zinc is important for gene expression, protein synthesis, membrane structure and function, and second messenger acute-phase response.

The role of free radicals and antioxidants is becoming increasingly important in the etiology of diseases of the critically ill such as multiorgan system failure (MOSF), adult respiratory distress syndrome (ARDS), and reperfusion injury. The role of zinc as an antioxidant is the subject of intense scientific investigation. Zinc is important for the activity of carbonic anhydrase. (For further information the reader is directed to an excellent review by Bray and Bettger.) In addition, it has recently been suggested that long-term (3 months) zinc supplementation improves the recovery rate and visceral protein synthesis in patients with severe head injury.

Deficiency States

Most cases of zinc deficiency in the United States are associated with diarrhea, gastrointestinal fluid loss, malabsorptive diseases such as inflammatory bowel disease, high-phytate diets, and insufficient zinc in TPN. Diarrhea depletes the body's stores of zinc by reducing dietary intake, impairing intestinal absorption, and increasing intestinal losses.

Zinc deficiency is associated with certain patient subpopulations such as infants, adolescents, women of reproductive age, and the elderly. Diseases commonly associated with zinc deficiency are sickle cell anemia, chronic renal failure (especially in patients with nephrotic disease and uremia), and severe hepatitis or cirrhosis.

Zinc deficiency is associated with a variety of clinical signs and symptoms (Table 16–4). These include decreased appetite, poor growth, impaired wound healing, decreased taste, hair loss, diarrhea, dermatitis, hypogonadism, depression, hyperammonemia, and impaired immune function. Diminished antioxidant defenses may also contribute to organ injury. The body willingly sacrifices growth to maintain normal plasma zinc levels and levels of metalloenzymes such as alkaline phosphatase.

Maintenance of tissue zinc levels is integral to normal physiologic function.

TABLE 16–4.

Common Manifestations of Zinc Deficiency

Growth retardation
Delayed sexual manifestation
Hypogonadism and hypospermia
Alopecia
Skin lesions
Immune deficiency
Behavioral disturbances (i.e., depression)
Night blindness
Impaired taste, decreased appetite
Impaired wound healing
Diarrhea

Zinc plays a primary role as a cofactor for antioxidant enzyme activities. In zinc-deficient animals, growth is sacrificed in order to maintain tissue zinc concentrations and other components of the antioxidant defense system. During severe zinc deficiency, zinc is mobilized from the exchangeable zinc pools found in liver and bone to organs such as skin and muscle.

The role and importance of glutamine during hypermetabolic illness, commonly found in critically ill patients, is discussed elsewhere in this book. Zinc acts as a coenzyme for the enzyme glutamine synthetase. Diminished activity of glutamine synthetase results in increased ammonia levels in the blood. Thus, zinc deficiency may contribute to the hyperammonia often found in critically ill patients.

Zinc deficiency has been implicated in the pathogenesis of night blindness in alcoholics with liver disease, presumably because of its role as a cofactor for vitamin A dehydrogenase, which is needed for the conversion of retinol to retinal. This may be important when considering zinc replacement in acutely ill patients with liver disease.

Many of the clinical abnormalities such as abnormal testicular function, peroneal nerve dysfunction, and hyperammonia that are seen in patients with renal failure and uremia are the same as those found in patients with zinc deficiency. While these clinical abnormalities are not reversed with hemodialysis, zinc supplementation has been shown to improve or normalize these conditions. Zinc deficiency in uremic patients is not related to excess urinary losses of zinc, except in nephrotic patients with proteinuria, but instead is related to poor intestinal absorption. In the care of critically ill and injured patients, knowledge of immune function has become paramount. The study of zinc and its effect on immune function adds to our knowledge of the importance of maintaining sufficient levels of zinc in the critically ill. Zinc deficiency impairs three components of immune function: antigen-mediated immunity, phagocytosis, and mucosal and barrier immunity.

Interleukin-1 (IL-1), an essential cytokine in the activation of antigen-mediated immunity, appears to have direct effects upon zinc nutriture. IL-1 decreases both plasma zinc levels and the uptake of zinc in organs such as the liver, bone marrow, and thymus. This cytokine influence on zinc uptake by immunologic tissues such as the thymus and bone marrow suggests that zinc supplementation may improve T- and B-cell production during immunologic stress. There is also evidence that zinc may be needed for the production and/or membrane binding of cytokines such as IL-1, IL-2, and interferon. Several clinical syndromes in humans reveal adverse affect of zinc deficiency on the immune system. The disease acrodermatitis enteropathica (an inherited disorder of zinc malabsorption) causes certain immunologic problems such as increased rates of infection, thymic atrophy, and impaired cell-mediated immunity. Thymic atrophy and impaired delayed hypersensitivity response develop in children with severe protein malnutrition. In both of these conditions, the immunologic deficiencies are correctable with zinc replacement therapy. Further, zinc deficiency is associated with aging, and there is some evidence that the loss of immunologic responsivity associated with aging may be related to zinc deficiency. Finally, thymulin levels are known to be decreased in sickle cell disease, nephrosis, other diseases associated with zinc deficiency, and "healthy patients" with decreased zinc levels. Most important to the nutritional care of the critically ill patient is the knowledge that the serum zinc concentration falls to 50% of premorbid levels during hypercatabolic stress. Further, trauma patients can excrete up to 2000 to 4000 mg/day of zinc in urine as compared with the normal 400 to 600 mg/day. Zinc is known to be essential for stress-induced biosynthesis of acute-phase proteins in the liver, and zinc uptake in the liver is increased during stress.

Zinc losses may be increased in the urine in patients receiving angiotensin-converting enzyme (ACE) inhibitors. As yet, the loss of zinc in the urine secondary to the use of captopril has not been proved to be clinically important, but when combined with other causes of clinically significant zinc deficiency, this loss of zinc may become clinically relevant.

Assessment

As is the case with most trace minerals, assessment of whole-body zinc requirements is difficult because of the different pools of zinc within the body. The process of collecting specimens is inherently flawed in that it can introduce contamination and thereby provide inaccurate measurements of zinc levels. Most zinc assay systems measure either serum or plasma zinc levels. Serum levels measure both exchangeable and nonexchangeable zinc pools. Plasma zinc levels are part of the exchangeable zinc pool, so when levels are low, plasma zinc is a good indicator of the size of the exchangeable pool of zinc. Neither serum zinc nor plasma zinc levels, however, are good indicators of deficiencies in dietary zinc or changes in whole-body zinc levels. Assaults to the body such as shock, trauma, infection, and burns cause zinc to be redistributed to other body sites in response to the increase in metabolic demand. This redistribution leads to an acute fall in plasma zinc levels but may not represent zinc deficiency.

Because of the problems in trying to differentiate between true zinc deficiency and low plasma zinc levels secondary to severe acute illness or injury, it has been suggested that the levels of other substances such as MT or C-reactive protein be measured in conjunction with plasma zinc concentrations. MT binds both zinc and copper and is important as a transporter of zinc to the tissues. MT production, like zinc production, is induced by stress. Plasma MT levels reflect changes in hepatic MT concentrations. These facts lead us to conclude that measurement of both plasma zinc and plasma MT levels may allow for better interpretation of zinc nutriture. A low level of plasma zinc accompanied by a high level of plasma MT suggests that zinc is being redistributed in response to stress. In this situation, zinc nutriture would *not* be compromised. In contrast, a low level of plasma zinc accompanied by a low level of MT suggests zinc *deficiency* during stress because MT is not synthesized during stress in zinc-deficient patients.

Levels of C-reactive protein have been measured in an attempt to improve assessment of zinc nutriture in elderly hospitalized patients. C-reactive protein is an α_2 acute-phase reactant that is an excellent indicator of the hepatic acute-phase response to stress. IL-2 is known to increase the hepatic uptake of zinc and stimulate hepatic synthesis of C-reactive protein. According to research, a low serum zinc level accompanied by a high level of C-reactive protein indicates severe infection (i.e., stress) in elderly patients, whereas a low serum zinc level and a normal C-reactive protein level are indicative of true zinc deficiency.

Although a variety of laboratory and diagnostic options are available for assessing zinc status, many require further experience and validation in humans. The method of assessing zinc status by using a substance closely related to zinc metabolism gives weight to the idea that measuring certain zinc-dependent metalloenzymes will be helpful in assessing zinc status. For example, at least one case report in the literature associates low levels of alkaline phosphatase with low zinc levels. Although methods vary, the most important aspect in the assessment of zinc deficiency is to recognize diseases, treatments, and clinical manifestations in patients predisposed to hypozincemia.

Such patients include those with critical illness accompanied by diarrhea, those receiving TPN, and patients with characteristic skin lesions.

Treatment

Patients should be supplemented with 15 mg/day of zinc; intravenous maintenance doses are 2 mg/day. Patients with diarrhea or excess gastrointestinal losses should receive additional zinc.

SELENIUM

Selenium deficiency states were first described in animals; in 1969 selenium was found to be essential in animals, and in 1973 selenium's function as a cofactor for erythrocyte glutathione peroxidase in humans was reported. The biochemical role of this enzyme, similar to that of the fat-soluble antioxidant vitamin E, is to reduce intracellular inorganic and organic peroxides and thus protect cells from oxidative damage. As we learn more about the destructive potential of oxygen free radicals in critically ill and injured patients, selenium may begin to play a more important nutritional role in their care.

Metabolism

Selenium is absorbed readily via the gut (primary duodenum) and transported in the blood on albumin and low- and very low-density lipoproteins (LDL and VLDL). A large portion of the selenium in the human body is in the form of selenium amino acids, which provide the selenium needed to produce glutathione peroxidase. Glutathione peroxidase functions as a major intracellular antioxidant that allows glutathione to catalyze the reduction of hydrogen peroxide and other organic hydroperoxides to nontoxic products. Removal of these oxidants prevents the initiation of membrane lipid peroxidation. Reperfusion injury and subsequent formulation of toxic oxidants that cause secondary reperfusion injury have been well studied in critically injured patients. There are a large number of enzymes that generate superoxide and hydroxyl free radicals in the cell and only a small number that remove them. The protective enzymes include selenium glutathione peroxidase, superoxide dismutase, peroxidases, and vitamins C and E. Selenium is also involved in prostaglandin metabolism; selenium deficiency reduces prostacyclin synthesis. There is no homeostatic control known to selenium, and following its metabolism, this mineral is lost via the urine, bile, sweat, and skin. Further, catabolic states are associated with increased selenium loss via the kidneys. Because of the detrimental effects of selenium deficiency, its metabolism should be studied in critically ill patients.

Assessment

In critically ill patients it is better to measure plasma selenium levels than whole blood concentrations because plasma responds more rapidly to changes in intake and disease state alterations and is less affected by blood transfusions. In the context of caring for the critically ill, the measurement of red blood cell glutathione peroxidase activity may be a more important measure of selenium nutriture. Evaluation of this enzyme activity relates well to biologically active selenium because plasma glutathione peroxidase levels increase within 1 to 2 days after initiating selenium supplementation. Breath analysis of exhaled pentane and ethane has been used to measure in vivo lipid peroxidation of endogenous fatty acids. The problem with using either of these functional indices is that neither glutathione peroxidase activity nor the breath test can differentiate between deficiencies of selenium or vitamin E. However, they do reflect antioxidant status and are useful for guiding therapy.

Deficiency States

In the general population, selenium deficiency is most clearly manifested as Keshan disease, which occurs in hyposeleniferous regions of China. It is characterized by a seasonal acute cardiomyopathy, which may be prevented via selenium supplementation. As mentioned above, critical illness that results in hypermetabolism causes excessive selenium loss. Patients with burns, severe trauma, and cancer are therefore at high risk of becoming selenium deficient. Further, these patient populations often require TPN, which over prolonged intervals causes a gradual decline in circulating levels of selenium (and other trace minerals) because the crystalline amino acid solutions utilized in TPN have a low selenium content. Its effects on the myocardium make selenium deficiency, along with that of chromium and molybdenum, a critical factor for assessment in TPN patients. Review of the literature yields two case reports in which patients chronically receiving TPN demonstrated muscle weakness and one case of cardiomyopathy responding to treatment with selenium supplementation.

Requirements/Therapy

As with many of the trace elements, the requirements for selenium in critically ill patients have not been well studied. Selenium deficiency, except for the rare manifestation of cardiomyopathy in patients from selenium-deficient areas, cannot be diagnosed on clinical findings. As with all the trace metals, there are no case reports of acute selenium deficiency. One study of trace elements in eight critically ill patients demonstrated selenium balance to be zero or negative. The American Medical Association Expert Panel did not include selenium in its recommendations for daily trace minerals requirements, but the National Research Council established adequate selenium intake for adults at 50 to 200 μg/day. In consideration of the rapid metabolism of selenium, it is prudent to assume that the selenium requirement in critically ill patients is higher than the recommended daily requirement for the general population. Therefore the minimum selenium supplementation for patients receiving TPN should be 40 to 60 μg/L to achieve a desired level of 80 to 150 μg/day. Unsupplemented TPN solutions will supply no more than 10 μg/day of selenium.

Adverse Effects

In the event of selenium toxicity in a critically ill patient, the diagnosis can be made when the characteristic "garlicky breath" (the result of the production of dimethyl selenite secondary to selenium toxicity) is encountered.

Sources/Preparations

Selenomethionine is the best supplement for selenium in parenteral solutions. Unfortunately, this source of parenteral selenium is not used; instead, selenous acid, which provides 40 μg of selenium per milliliter, is the common dosage form of selenium.

IRON

The body contains 3 to 5 g of iron. Fifty percent to 60% is in hemoglobin, and 10% is in myoglobin. Most of the remainder is found in storage pools.

Metabolism

Iron is a component of enzymes and proteins necessary for energy transfer and oxygen transport/utilization. It is a component of porphyrin-based compounds such as hemoglobin, myoglobin, flavoproteins, and cytochromes. Iron also forms an important component of enzymes such as catalase, peroxidase, xanthine oxidase, hydroxylases, and oxidases. Iron is required for synthesis of red blood cells (i.e., hemoglobin), functions as an antioxidant (i.e., catalase, peroxidase), is essential for oxidative phosphorylation (i.e., cytochromes, flavoproteins), and is involved in bacterial killing.

Iron is found in two forms in food: organic or inorganic iron in the Fe^{+2} or Fe^{+3} forms. Iron is absorbed in the small intestine (primarily duodenum) as Fe^{+2}. Much of dietary iron must be reduced from Fe^{+3} to Fe^{+2} by reducing agents such as vitamin C before absorption. Fe^{+2} enters the small intestinal cells of the mucosa and is reoxidized to Fe^{+3}. It is then bound to the storage protein ferritin in the small intestine. Ferritin releases iron (Fe^{+3}) to transferrin for transport to the liver and other tissues. The normal level of transferrin in plasma is 200 to 350 mg/dL, and normally 20% to 50% is saturated with iron. Iron bound to transferrin is transferred to ferritin for storage in tissues (i.e., liver, spleen, bone marrow). A small amount of ferritin is present in the serum (30 to 300 ng/mL) and reflects body iron storage. On average, 10% to 15% of inorganic and food iron is absorbed. Heme iron (i.e., meat) is absorbed directly (iron in hemoglobin is Fe^{+2}); nonheme iron (i.e., vegetable) requires gastric acid and digestion for absorption. Normal gastric secretion is required to release protein-bound iron in food. Ascorbic acid and organic acids enhance absorption. Large doses of trace elements, tannins, phosphates, fatty acids, and antacids bind iron and decrease its absorption. Copper deficiency also diminishes absorption. Iron absorption is increased during iron deficiency states, chronic hypoxia, and anemia.

Iron circulates in the blood bound to its transport protein transferrin. It is stored in tissues bound to ferritin or hemosiderin. Approximately 0.2 to 0.5 mg/day of iron is excreted in feces, 0.2 mg/day in urine, and small amounts in sweat. Normal men and postmenopausal women lose approximately 0.6 to

1.0 mg/day. Menstruating women lose additional iron during menses (i.e., 0.5 to 0.8 mg/day), and daily requirements are 1 to 2 mg. The RDA for iron is 10 mg in adults. This amount is increased during infancy, pregnancy, and lactation.

Deficiency States

Iron deficiency results from abnormal iron losses or diminished iron intake. Excess loss of iron may result from blood loss through the gastrointestinal tract and inflamed surfaces (i.e., peptic ulcers, ulcerative colitis, neoplasms) and from bile/small-bowel drainage. Blood loss from surgery or trauma and blood for laboratory testing may also lead to deficiency. Malabsorption of iron (i.e., sprue, celiac disease, gastrectomy, diarrhea, achlorhydria) is another cause of deficiency. Copper deficiency decreases iron mobilization and may cause anemia even in the presence of adequate iron stores.

Iron deficiency is manifested as hypochromic microcytic anemia, depressed cellular immunity, and decreased bactericidal activity of leukocytes. The activity of iron-dependent enzymes is also impaired. In addition to signs and symptoms of anemia (i.e., fatigue, shortness of breath, tachycardia), iron deficiency may result in glossitis, cheilosis, and koilonychia.

Iron Overload

Excess iron intake or absorption can result in tissue deposition of the element (i.e., hemochromatosis). The net result may be organ injury (i.e., liver, heart, kidneys, pancreas). Iron ions stimulate lipid peroxidation in cellular membranes, free radical formation, and damage to cellular processes.

Assessment

The best means of assessing body iron stores is via bone marrow examina-

tion. Ferritin levels in the plasma (normal, 30 to 300 ng/mL) reflect iron levels in the marrow and may be useful for assessing iron stores. Levels below 12 ng/mL suggest iron deficiency. However, ferritin levels may be elevated in some patients with inflammation (acute-phase reactant), with liver disease, and following iron-dextran injection.

As storage iron levels decrease, there is a compensatory increase in absorption of iron and the serum transferrin concentration (represented by a rise in iron binding capacity). When iron stores are depleted, plasma iron decreases while transferrin levels increase. Serum transferrin saturation (normal, 20% to 50%) represents iron flow to the tissues. When saturation is less than 16%, iron supply is suboptimal, and anemia develops. Levels of serum transferrin (200 to 360 mg/dL) and iron (male, 75 to 150 μg/dL; female, 65 to 165 μg/dL) may be decreased during infection and malnutrition. Thus, these tests may be unreliable as an index of iron status.

Treatment

The RDA for intravenous iron is 1 to 2 mg/day. Patients should receive at least 10 mg/day of enteral iron during nutritional support (10% to 15% absorbed). Extra iron may be required because of excess losses (i.e., blood loss). Iron may be administered intravenously (as iron dextran) or orally. The dose of intravenous iron depends upon the hemoglobin level (see the manufacturer's instructions for administration). Oral iron may be provided as ferrous sulfate or ferrous gluconate (300 mg three times per day). A reticulocyte response should occur within 7 to 10 days after initiating iron repletion. Therapy should continue for at least 6 months to replenish tissue stores. Blood is also an excellent source of iron when hemoglobin is required to support tissue oxygen delivery.

IODINE

Iodine is a component of thyroid hormones (i.e., thyroxine, triiodothyronine). More than 75% of the 10 to 20 mg of iodine in the body is found in the thyroid gland. Smaller quantities of iodine are found in the ovaries, mammary and parotid glands, gastric mucosa, and placenta.

The iodide content of foods depends upon the iodide level in soil and the amount of fertilizer used. Many soils are low or depleted of iodide, but marine foods are rich sources of iodide. Iodide is also supplemented in salts; iodized salt contains 50 μg of iodide per 5 g of NaCl. Today, iodine deficiency is rare in western countries.

Iodine is absorbed from the intestine into the circulation and cleared by the thyroid gland and kidneys. Iodine is transported in serum bound to proteins (level, 4 to 11 μg/dL). Most iodine in the blood circulates as thyroxine (4 to 10 μg/dL), with smaller amounts as triiodothyronine (90 to 200 ng/dL). The amount of inorganic iodine in serum is 0.2 to 1.0 μg/dL. Iodine is trapped by the follicular cells of the thyroid and bound to tyrosine in thyroglobulin. It is later used to synthesize thyroid hormones. However, if the level of circulating inorganic iodide exceeds 30 μg/dL, it blocks the uptake of inorganic iodide by thyroid cells, blocks iodination of tyrosine, and reduces synthesis of thyroid hormones. Iodine is excreted principally in the urine; smaller amounts are excreted through the gastrointestinal tract, sweat, and milk (mammary glands). The salivary glands and gastric glands concentrate iodide from plasma and excrete it.

The RDA for iodine is 0.15 mg for adults. Deficiency of iodine results in hypertrophy of the thyroid (goiter) and/or hypothyroidism. On the other hand, excess iodine inhibits thyroidal synthesis of thyroid hormones and can also cause hypothyroidism (especially in patients with Hashimoto's thyroiditis). Iodine metabolism has not been well studied in critically ill patients.

COBALT

Cobalt is a component of vitamin B_{12} (see the chapter on vitamins). It has no other known metabolic function.

MANGANESE

The human body contains 12 to 20 mg of manganese, which is found primarily in the mitochondria. The liver, kidney, lymph nodes, and pancreas contain the highest levels. Manganese is important for the action of vitamin K (synthesis of prothrombin) and glycosyltransferases. Manganese is a component of mitochondrial superoxide dismutase. It influences the synthesis of mucopolysaccharides, stimulates hepatic synthesis of cholesterol and fatty acids, and is a cofactor for many enzymes (i.e., arginase, alkaline phosphatase, chondroitin sulfate synthesis, RNA and DNA polymerase, malic enzyme, pyruvate decarboxylase, acetylcholine esterase, CDP-diacylglycerolinositol transferase, farnesyl pyrophosphate synthetase).

Only 3% to 4% of dietary manganese is absorbed. Absorption is inhibited by high levels of calcium and phosphate. It is transported in the blood bound to β-globulins (i.e., transferrin). Excretion occurs in bile, with smaller amounts in pancreatic juice and intestinal secretions; negligible quantities are excreted in urine.

The normal dietary intake is 2 to 20 mg/day; the recommended dietary intake for adults is 2.5 to 5.0 mg/day. Clinical deficiency of manganese has not been reported in humans. In animals, manganese deficiency causes impaired growth, defective connective tissue synthesis, skeletal abnormalities, ataxia, and defective reproduction. Manganese should be supplemented during nutritional support (especially long-term TPN); intravenous requirements are 0.15 to 0.8 mg/day.

MOLYBDENUM

Molybdenum is an essential component of xanthine oxidase, sulfite oxidase, and aldehyde oxidase. Deficiency causes hyperoxypurinemia, hypouricemia, and low sulfate excretion.

Legumes, organ meats, and yeast are relatively good sources of this element. Liver and kidney have the highest concentrations. Molybdenum is absorbed from the small intestine, transported in blood bound to serum proteins, and excreted in the urine. Absorption is inhibited by inorganic sulfates, and large losses have been reported in the stools of patients with Crohn's disease.

No clinical deficiency state has been established in humans. However, there is a genetic inborn error of metabolism resulting from the absence of liver and kidney sulfite oxidase; neurologic abnormalities, mental retardation, and early death develop. The recommended dietary intake of molybdenum is 0.15 to 0.5 mg/day.

FLUORIDE

Fluoride is absorbed from the intestine, and approximately 96% of CaF_2 is absorbed. Fluoride is concentrated in teeth and bones and has been shown to prevent dental caries when added to water (0.7 to 1.0 mg/L). On the other hand, high levels of fluoride in water (>1.5 mg/L) can cause mottled teeth. Fluoride supplementation has also been shown to prevent bone fractures from osteoporosis.

The main source of fluoride in humans is water. The RDA is 1 to 2 mg/day. A water supply containing 1 ppm of fluoride will supply 1 to 2 mg/day provided that water intake is normal.

ENTERAL FORMULAS

The trace element content of enteral nutritional formulas are listed in Appendix 16–1. These formulas meet recommended requirements for health when given in sufficient amounts to meet the energy needs of the patient. Needs in critically ill patients may exceed the recommended nutritional intakes because of diminished absorption, hypermetabolism, and excess losses.

SUGGESTED READING

Aggett PJ: Physiology and metabolism of essential trace elements: An outline. *Clin Endocrinol Metab* 1985; 14:513–543.

Anderson RA: Selenium, chromium, and manganese, in Shils ME, Young VR, (ed): *Modern Nutrition in Health and Disease,* ed. 7, Philadelphia, 1988, Lea & Febiger.

Anderson RA: Essentiality of chromium in humans. *Sci Total Environ* 1989; 86:75–81.

Anderson RA, Bryden NA, Polansky MM, et al: Urinary chromium excretion and insulinogenic properties of carbohydrates. *Am J Clin Nutr* 1987; 51:864–868.

Bray TM, Bettger WJ: The physiological role of zinc as an antioxidant. *Free Radic Biol Med* 1990; 8:281–291.

Borel JS, Majerus MM, Polansky PB, et al: Chromium intake and urinary chromium excretion of trauma patients. *Biol Trace Elem Res* 1984; 6:317–326.

Brown MR, Cohen HJ, Lyons JM, et al: Proximal muscle weakness and selenium deficiency associated with long term parenteral nutrition. *Am J Clin Nutr* 1986;43:549–554.

Cassack ZT, Prasad AS: Hyperammonia zinc deficiency activities or urea cycle related enzymes. *Nutr Res* 1987; 7:1161–1167.

Cohen HJ, Brown MR, Hamilton D, et al: Glutathione peroxidase and selenium deficiency in patients receiving home parenteral nutrition: Time course for development of deficiency and repletion of enzyme activity in plasma and red blood cells. *Am J Clin Nutr* 1989; 49:132–139.

Cornatzer WE: Trace elements, in Cornatzer WE (ed): *Role of Nutrition in Health and Disease.* Springfield, Mo, Charles C. Thomas, 1989.

Cousins RJ: Tissue specific regulation of zinc metabolism and metallothionein and cerulloplasmin. *Physiol Rev* 1985; 65:238–309.

Cousins RJ, Leinart AS: Tissue-specific regulation of zinc metabolism and metallothionein genes by interleukin-1. *FASEB J* 1988; 2:2884–2890.

Craig GM, Evan SJ, Brayshaw BJ: An inverse ratio between serum zinc and creatine protein levels in acutely ill elderly hospital patients. *Postgrad Med J* 1990; 66:1025–1028.

Dowd PS, Kelleher J, Fraker PJ: T-lymphocyte subsets and interleukin-2 production in zinc deficient rats. *Br J Nutr* 1986; 55:59–69.

King JC: Assessment of zinc status. *J Nutr* 1990; 120:1474–1479.

Fleming CR, Hodges RE, Hurley LS: A prospective study of serum copper and zinc levels in patients receiving TPN. *Am J Clin Nutr* 1976; 29(1):70–77.

Flemming CR, McCall JT, O'Brien JF, et al: Selenium status in patients receiving home parenteral nutrition. *JPEN* 1988; 8:258–262.

Giugliano R, Millward DJ: Growth and zinc homeostasis in severely zinc deficient rat. *Br J Nutr* 1984; 52:545–560.

Golden MHN, Golden BE: Effects of zinc on the thymus of recently malnourished children. *Lancet* 1977; 2:1057–1059.

Golick A, Averbukh Z, Cohn M, et al: Effect of diuretic on captopril-induced urinary zinc excretion. *Eur J Clin Pharmacol* 1990; 38:359–361.

Graham GC, Cordano A: Copper deficiency in human subjects, in Prasad AS (ed): *Trace elements of human health and disease,* vol. 1, Zinc and Copper, New York, 1976, Academic Press.

Hawker F, Stewart PM, Snitch PJ: Effects of acute illness on selenium homeostasis. *Crit Care Med* 1990; 18:442–446.

Jacobson S, Wester PO: Balance studies of twenty trace elements during total parenteral nutrition in man. *Br J Nutr* 1977; 37:107–126.

Johnson RA, Baker JT, Fallon EP, at al: An accidental case of cardiomyopathy and selenium deficiency. *N Engl J Med* 1981; 304:1210–1212.

Kararskis EJ, Shuna A: Serum alkaline phosphatase after treatment of zinc deficiency in humans. *Am J Clin Nutr* 1980; 33:2609–2612.

Keen CL, Gershwin ME: Zinc deficiency and immune function. *Annu Rev Nutr* 1990; 10:415–431.

Keshan Disease Research Group: *Chin Clin Med J* 1979; 92:471–476.

Kien CL, Ganther HE: Manifestations of chronic selenium deficiency in a child receiving total parenteral nutrition. *Am J Clin Nutr* 1983; 37:329–338.

King JC: Assessment of zinc status. *J Nutr* 1990; 120:1474–1479.

Mahajam SK: Zinc in kidney disease. *J Am Coll Nutr* 1989; 8:296–304.

Mertz W: Chromium occurence and function in biological systems. *Physiol Rev* 1969; 49:185–239.

National Research Council: *Recommended Dietary Allowance,* ed 9, Washington, DC, National Academy of Sciences, 1980.

O'Dell BL: Biochemical basis of the clinical effects of copper deficiency, in Prasad AS (ed): *Clinical Biochemical and Nutritional Aspects of Trace Elements,* New York, 1982, Alan R. Liss.

Parr RM: Recommended dietary intakes of trace elements: Some observations on their definition and interpretation in comparison with actual levels of dietary intake, in Hiroshi T (ed): *Trace Elements in Clinical Medicine,* Tokyo, Springer-Verlag, 1980.

Phillips GD, Garnys VP: Parenteral administration of trace elements to critically ill patients, *Anaesth Intensive Care* 1991; 9:221–225.

Prasad AS, Rabbani P, Abbas A, et al: Experimental zinc deficiency in humans. *Ann Intern Med* 1978; 89:483–490.

Rotnick JT, Pope AL, Ganther ME, at al: Selenium biochemical role as a component of glutathione peroxidase. *Science* 1973; 179:588–590.

Salas M, Kirchner H: Induction of interferon-gamma in human leukocyte cultures stimulated by Zn^{+2}. *Clin Immunol Immunopathol* 1987; 45:139–142.

Senapati A, Jenner J, Thompson R: Zinc in the elderly. *Q J Med* 1990; 261:81–87.

Shike E, Roulet M, Kurian R: Copper metabolism and requirements in TPN. *Gastroenterology* 1981; 81(2):290–297.

Solomons NW: Minerals, zinc and copper, in Shils (ed): *Modern Nutrition in Health and Disease*, ed. 7, Philadelphia, 1988, Lea & Febiger.

Stern J, Ross DA: Zinc supplementation improves recovery rate and visceral protein levels in patients with severe closed head injury. Presented at the 42nd Meeting of the Congress of Neurological Surgeons, Washington, D.C., October, 1992.

Subcommittee on the Tenth Edition of the RDAs, Food and Nutrition Board, Commission on Life Sciences, National Research Council: Trace elements, chromium, in *Recommended Dietary Allowances*, ed. 10, Washington DC, 1989, National Academy Press.

Tappel AL, Dillard CJ: In vitro lipid peroxidation measurement via exhaled pentane and protection by vitamin E. *Fed Proc* 1981; 40:174–178.

VanRij AM, Thompson CD, McKenzie JM, et al: Selenium deficiency in TPN. *Am J Clin Nutr* 1979; 32:2076–2085.

Wade S, Parent G, Bleiberg-Daniel F: Thymulin (Zn-FTS) activity in protein energy malnutrition: New evidence for interaction between malnutrition and infection on thymic function. *Am J Nutr* 1988; 47:305–311.

Wagner PA, Jernign JA, Bailey LB: Zinc nutriture and cell mediated immunity in the aged. *Int J Vitam Nutr Rev* 1983; 53:94–109.

Yasushito MB, Alcock NW, Shils ME: Chromium content of total parenteral nutrition solutions. *J Parenteral Enteral Nutr* 1990; 14(6):610–614.

APPENDIX 16–1.

Trace Mineral Content of Enteral Feedings*

Diets	Magnesium (mg)	Iron (mg)	Iodine (μg)	Copper (mg)	Zinc (mg)	Manganese (mg)	Selenium (μg)	Molybdenum (μg)	Chromium (μg)
Elemental diets									
Peptamen Diet	400	12	100	1.4	14	2.7	40	120	40
Peptamen—Oral Diet	400	12	100	1.4	14	2.7	40	120	40
Reabilan	251	10	74.7	1.6	10	2	50.7	N/A	82.5
Reabilan HN	248	10	76.2	0.95	10	2	50.1	N/A	62.2
Criticare HN	200	9	75	1	10	2.5	N/A	N/A	N/A
AlitraQ	267	15	100	1.3	20	3.4	50	110	75
Vital HN	267	12	100	1.4	15	3.4	47	100	67
Tolerex	220	10	83	1.1	8.3	1.6	83	83	28
Vivonex TEN	200	9	75	1	10	0.9	50	50	17
Accupep HPF	250	11.3	100	1.5	15	2.5	N/A	N/A	N/A
Disease-specific diets									
Renal									
Aminess Essential	N/A	N/A	N/A	N/A	N/A	N/A	N/A	N/A	N/A
Amino Acid Tablets									
Travasorb Renal Diet	N/A	N/A	N/A	N/A	N/A	N/A	N/A	N/A	N/A
Amin-Aid	N/A	N/A	N/A	N/A	N/A	N/A	N/A	N/A	N/A
Alterna	N/A	N/A	N/A	N/A	N/A	N/A	N/A	N/A	N/A
Nepro	105	9.5	78.9	1.1	11.8	2.63	51.1	N/A	N/A
Suplena	105	9.5	78.9	1.05	11.8	2.63	38	N/A	N/A
Hepatic									
Travasorb Hepatic Diet	179	8	66.8	0.9	6.7	1.2	N/A	N/A	N/A
Hepatic-Aid II	N/A	N/A	N/A	N/A	N/A	N/A	N/A	N/A	N/A
Pulmonary									
NutriVent Diet	400	12	100	1.4	14	2.7	40	120	40
Pulmocare†	282	12.7	106	1.4	15.9	3.5	50	106	71
Critical Care									
Replete Diet	400	18	160	2	24	4	100	220	140
Replete with Fiber Diet	400	18	160	2	24	4	100	220	140
Immun-Aid‡	200	9	75	2	25	2.5	100	75	75
TraumaCal	133	5.9	50	1	9.9	1.7	N/A	N/A	N/A
Perative	267	12	100	1.34	15	3.34	47	100	67

(Continued.)

APPENDIX 16–1 (cont.).

Diets	Magnesium (mg)	Iron (mg)	Iodine 9(µg)	Copper (mg)	Zinc (mg)	Manganese (mg)	Selenium (µg)	Molybdenum (µg)	Chromium (µg)
Impact	270	12	100	1.7	15	2	100	200	100
Impact with Fiber	270	12	100	1.7	15	2	100	200	100
Stresstein	170	7.5	63	0.8	6.3	1.7	50	130	50
Protain XL	320	21.6	120	2.4	36	6	10	150	100
Glucose intolerance									
Glucerna	282	12.7	106	1.5	15.9	3.6	50	106	71
Intact protein diets									
Nutren 1.0 Diet	340	12	100	1.4	14	2.7	40	120	40
Nutren 1.5 Diet	333	12	100	1.3	13.3	2.7	40	120	40
Nutren 2.0 Diet	340	12	100	1.4	14	2.6	40	120	40
Entrition 0.5 Diet	200	9	75	1	7.5	2	N/A	N/A	N/A
Entrition HN Diet	308	13.9	116	1.54	11.6	1.54	N/A	N/A	N/A
Isolan	302	13.5	113	1.5	11.3	1.9	113	226	113
Nutrilan	239	10.8	119	1.2	9	1.9	N/A	N/A	N/A
Ultralan	267	12	100	1.3	10	1.7	80	160	80
Isocal	200	9	75	1	10	2.5	N/A	N/A	N/A
Isocal HN	320	14	120	1.6	12	4.3	80	200	80
Isocal HCN	200	9	75	1.5	15	1.7	N/A	N/A	N/A
Lipisorb	200	9.2	75.1	1	10	1.5	N/A	N/A	N/A
Sustacal 8.8	1.52	9.2	75.2	1.1	10	200	50	124	50
Sustacal HC	227	10	86.7	1	8.7	1.7	N/A	N/A	N/A
Ensure	200	9	75	1	11.25	2.5	N/A	50	75
Ensure HN	286	12.86	107.2	1.43	16.08	3.57	50	108	72
Ensure Plus	189	8.5	70	0.96	10.6	2.34	33	71	47
Ensure Plus HN	282	12.7	106	1.42	15.9	3.52	50	106	71
Osmolite	200	9	75	1	11.5	2.5	35	75	50
Osmolite HN	286	12.86	107.2	1.43	16.08	3.57	50	108	72
TwoCal HN	211	9.5	78.9	1.05	11.85	2.63	37	79	53
Isosource	220	10	83	1.1	14	2.8	83	170	83
Isosource HN	220	10	83	1.1	14	2.8	83	170	83
Resource Liquid	200	9	75	1.1	15	2	N/A	N/A	N/A
Resource Plus	210	9.6	70	1.1	16	1.4	N/A	N/A	N/A
Attain	320	14.4	120	1.6	24	4	100	150	100
Comply	267	12	100	1.3	20	3	N/A	N/A	N/A
Magnacal	200	9	75	1	15	2.5	N/A	N/A	N/A

Product									
High protein									
Replete—Oral	400	12	100	1.4	14	2.7	N/A	N/A	N/A
Nitrolan	258	11.6	96.8	1.3	9.7	1.6	96.8	194	96.8
Sustacal	380	16.9	140	2	14.1	2.9	N/A	N/A	N/A
Promote	320	14.4	120	1.6	18	4	56	120	80
Isotein HN	190	8.6	71	0.95	7.1	1.9	71	140	71
Citrotein	629	56	235	3.1	24	7.6	N/A	N/A	N/A
Intact protein with fiber									
Nutren 1.0 with Fiber Diet	340	12	100	1.4	14	2.7	40	120	40
Fiberlan	267	12	100	1.3	10	1.7	100	200	100
Sustacal with Fiber	265	12	100	1.3	13.1	1.7	N/A	N/A	N/A
Ultracal	320	14.1	120	1.6	16	2.4	80	200	80
Ensure with Fiber	262	11.77	98.1	1.31	14.73	3.27	N/A	N/A	N/A
Jevity	286	12.9	107	1.44	16.1	3.56	50	108	72
Fibersource	220	10	83	1.1	14	2.8	83	170	83
Fibersource HN	220	10	83	1.1	14	2.8	83	170	83
Profiber	267	12	100	1.5	20	3	80	200	80
Milk-based supplements									
Carnation Instant Breakfast	400	18	180	2	15	N/A	N/A	N/A	N/A
Carnation Diet Instant Breakfast	632	23.7	237	2.63	19.7	N/A	N/A	N/A	N/A
Sustacal Powder mixed with milk	375	16.7	139	1.9	13.9	2.8	N/A	N/A	N/A
Forta Shake mixed with milk	345	15.5	129.3	1.72	18.1	2.07	N/A	N/A	N/A
Delmark Instant Breakfast	483	21.7	183	2.4	18.3	0.03	N/A	N/A	N/A

*From Clintec Nutrition Company: Enteral Product Reference Guide. 1992. Used by permission.
†Contains 1.4 mg fluoride.
‡Contains 0.76 mg fluoride.

PART III

Feeding

17

Feeding Controversies

Ronald L. Koretz, M.D.

Who gets fed?

How should Who get fed?

Who will find out who "Who" is?

Thy food shall be thy remedy.
Hippocrates (approximately 400 B.C.)

In 1936, Hiram Studley described his experience in operating on patients with peptic ulcer disease. He noted that the patients who died in the immediate postoperative period had "regularly lost preoperatively a considerable proportion of their weight."[1] In fact, the surgical mortality rate in patients who lost at least 20% of their weight prior to surgery was 33% (6/18), a figure dramatically higher than those with lesser weight loss (1/28, 4%).

Studley concluded that "there is reason to believe that more patients will be saved provided efforts are concentrated on the preoperative preparation of those who have lost a good deal of weight, regardless of other appearances in the individual." Indeed, over the next 30 years a number of investigators, perhaps best exemplified by Jonathan Rhoads, attempted to develop techniques to provide nutrition to individuals who could not or would not eat and who had lost weight.[2]

These early efforts used intravenous fluids, and the limiting factors were the volume and osmolality that could be employed. These obstacles were overcome with the use of central vein catheters and superior vena caval infusions. In 1968, Dudrick et al. described a controlled trial in beagle puppies in which the animals given parenteral feedings grew at least as well as those given oral puppy chow.[3] In this same paper, these authors also described an uncontrolled experience in patients with various complicated intestinal diseases who were maintained for 10 to 200 days.

Over the next 20 to 25 years, nutritional support (NS) has grown in popularity, and it is now a multibillion dollar-a-year industry.[4] This growth was spurred by the assumption that such an intervention would improve patient outcome. Therapeutic enthusiasts have made very optimistic claims; in 1971, Dudrick and Ruberg wrote: "the provision of adequate calories and nutrients given intravenously can significantly decrease the morbidity and mortality associated with a wide variety of disease processes."[5] Included in their list of "indications for parenteral nutrition" were hypermetabolic states, complicated trauma or surgery, burns, pancreatitis, idiopathic inflammatory bowel disease, malignant disease (as adjunctive therapy), nonterminal coma, and acute renal failure.

The basis for this wide acceptance of NS (parenteral NS [PNS] originally but subsequently enteral NS [ENS] as well) rests on five lines of "reasoning":

1. Any living organism, when deprived of nutrient intake for a long enough period, will die.
2. An individual with a given disease who is also malnourished has a poorer prognosis than does one with the same disease but who is not malnourished (Studley's observation).
3. NS improves measured parameters of malnutrition (especially such things as body weight or nitrogen balance).
4. Retrospective or prospective (with or without nonrandomized control groups) reports allegedly demonstrate therapeutic efficacy.
5. Doing something is better than doing nothing.

These lines of reasoning, as intuitively appealing as they may be, should be considered in more detail. It is certainly true that, given a long enough period of time, any living organism that is starved will die. This has been amply demonstrated with famines or prisoner-of-war experiences. These people, who may even have been in reasonable health initially (i.e., no underlying disease) did die, although the mortality statistics did not start to climb until the weight loss exceeded 40%.[6] While patients with underlying diseases may tolerate less weight loss, it may also be that they become metabolically adapted and can even tolerate greater weight loss.[7] (Remember that the body's usual response to illness is to reduce food intake!)

We do not know how much or for how long nutrient deprivation can occur before a patient is in danger of malnutrition-*caused* morbidity or mortality (in contrast to malnourished patients who become sicker from or even die of a particular disease state). In all likelihood any patient can probably tolerate a few days of "not eating"; it is equally likely that many months of starvation will carry with it its own morbidity and mortality.

The second line of reasoning is related to this point. It is important to recognize the difference between association and causation. It has been amply demonstrated (beginning with Studley) that there is an association between malnutrition and morbidity/mortality. However, it does not logically follow that the malnutrition causes the bad outcome. If the malnutrition is only a marker designating the presence of severe disease, there is no reason to believe that fixing that marker will fix the disease. For example, consider two groups of patients with colon cancer. One has disease limited to only 2 cm of the transverse colon, and the other has metastases to the liver, peritoneum, lungs, bones, and brain. It is very likely that the second group will have suffered much more weight loss than the first. It is also very likely that the life expectancies in the second group are much shorter than those in the first. However, the poorer survival is due to the increased severity of the underlying disease, not the weight loss per se. The weight loss is a message telling us that bad disease is present. The Greeks (who gave us Hippocrates) and other civilizations of past times learned that killing the messenger did not alter the content of the message.

The provision of NS has been shown to make certain nutritional parameters (tests) better. Again, if our ultimate goal is to make a test better, then these observations are quite important. However, for most health care practitioners, the objective is to make the quality and quantity of the patient's life better. What has not been shown is that improving these tests necessarily improves clinical outcome.[8]

In order to *prove* that a particular intervention alters a specific outcome, it is necessary to create a situation where only that one intervention is altered and then see whether the outcome changes. In clinical medicine, this usually requires the performance of a prospective randomized controlled trial (PRCT). Uncontrolled experiences do not allow any comparison at all with the outcome that would have occurred had no intervention been made. Nonrandomized control groups allow a comparison, but in such a case, at least two variables have been changed. The first variable is whether or not the intervention occurred; the second one is the reason for the intervention to have taken place or not. In nonrandomized control groups, the reason for an intervention not to have happened is *not* to test the efficacy of the intervention. If that had been the reason, the investigator would have performed a PRCT. While data from nonrandomized controlled trials do allow for the creation of a hypothesis, these data cannot prove the hypothesis.

The last line of reasoning relates to the perception that something good is happening. The health care workers feel good because they are delivering a service that requires their special abilities. The patient sees something being done and, since he assumes that the health care system would not do something bad, also feels good about the activity. The health care facility receives financial support for this intervention and thus also has reason to encourage its performance.

The only rational reason to provide NS to a patient is because it does improve some aspect of disease morbidity or mortality. Since both PNS and ENS have associated costs (both medical [complications] and financial), it is important to seek information establishing efficacy. As we have just noted, for almost all of the clinical conditions for which NS has been proposed, we need

data from well-designed and well-executed PRCTs.

There have been a large number of PRCTs evaluating PNS[9] and ENS.[10] Unfortunately, most of them have not been able to demonstrate a favorable impact of NS on clinical outcome. (Also, unfortunately, at least for the purposes of this chapter, there are no placebo-controlled trials of NS in adult general intensive care unit [ICU] patients.) It should be noted that many of these PRCTs are not "well designed and executed," the principal problem usually being small numbers of patients. In such studies, one cannot exclude the possibility of a "type II error," namely, a study in which inadequate numbers of subjects were enrolled to demonstrate a difference that really existed. (Of course, if NS had an extraordinarily dramatic impact on clinical outcome, even small trials would demonstrate it; it is probably true that NS will, at best, have a less-than-dramatic effect.)

With this background perspective, this chapter will look at two controversies regarding NS in the ICU. The first is a consideration of whether (and if so, when) or not NS should even be used (who gets fed). The second will look at the question of how, if a patient is to be fed, should the patient receive the feeding (ENS or PNS).

WHO GETS FED?

Journal articles emphasizing the role and encouraging the use of NS in critically ill surgical patients have been appearing since the 1970s.[11, 12] For the past decade, a similar appeal has been taken up by pulmonologists, who deal with patients on respirators in the ICU.[13] Such articles continue to appear in the 1990s.[7, 14, 15] The rationales for employing NS in burn patients, surgical or trauma patients (often with sepsis), and respirator-bound patients are summarized in Table 17–1[14–33]; for purposes of historical comparison, I have also included the arguments that were

TABLE 17–1.

Rationales for Employing Nutritional Support*

Disease State	Patient at Risk of Starvation	Malnutrition Associated With Poor Prognosis	Nutritional Support Improves Parameter	Uncontrolled/ Nonrandomized Controlled Report
Burns	High caloric needs in burn patients[16, 17]	Higher metabolic rate in worse burns[17]	Better nitrogen balance and visceral protein levels[18, 19]	"High survival rate" in uncontrolled series[16]
Critical trauma/surgical (± sepsis)	High catabolic rate in critically ill surgical patient[14, 15]	Malnourished head-injured patients and women with hip fractures had higher mortality rates[20, 21]; malnutrition correlated with poorer surgical outcome[22]	Better nitrogen balance,[23] experimental wound healing[24]	Improved morbidity and mortality in retrospective, controlled series[25]
Respiratory failure†	Pre-existent weight loss common in patients with chronic lung disease	Emphysematous patients who lost weight had a poor prognosis[27]	Reduced muscle protein degradation[28]	Better respirator weaning in retrospective controlled series[24]
Cancer (radiation or chemotherapy)	Cachexia common in patients with metastatic cancer[30]	Patients with weight loss had poorer survival[31]	Improved delayed hypersensitivity[32]	Fewer side effects of therapy in uncontrolled series[33]

*The references cited are not necessarily the only applicable references but are representative.
†This is usually an exacerbation of pre-existing chronic obstructive pulmonary disease.

put forth by oncologists advocating NS as adjunctive therapy for patients receiving radiation therapy or chemotherapy.

Although the specifics of the rationales in each disease state differ, the general thought processes are the same and encompass the first four lines of reasoning we just discussed. The cancer group was included because unlike the other disease states, a number of PRCTs are available. In fact, 24 trials have evaluated the role of PNS[34–41]; with the exception of 1 trial in bone marrow transplant recipients,[36] the results have been very disappointing. There was no apparent favorable impact of PNS on survival, tumor response, or gastrointestinal or hematologic toxicity to anticancer agents. Similar conclusions were also reached by a meta-analysis evaluating many of these reports.[42]

Ten of the PRCTs reported infection rates in both the patients who received PNS and the control groups; these data are summarized in Table 17–2. It is to be noted that in all 10 trials the recipients of PNS had higher infection rates,

TABLE 17–2.

Parenteral Nutritional Support and Cancer Chemotherapy—Infection Rates

Study	Frequency of Infection	
	PNS*	Control
Hays[35]	2/5 (40%)	0/5 (0%)
Weisdorf[36]	45/71 (63%)	33/66 (50%)
Szeluga[37]†	26/29 (90%)‡	18/28 (64%)
Clamon[40]	20/57 (35%)§	3/62 (5%)
Ghavimi[43]	7/11 (64%)‡	1/14 (7%)
Samuels[44]	7/41 (17%)‡	2/48 (4%)
Shambarger[45]	5/12 (42%)	5/15 (33%)
Van Eys[46¶]	0.71§	0.01
Jordan[47]	6/19 (32%)	2/24 (8%)
Valdivieso[48]	22/82 (27%)	17/97 (18%)

*PNS = parenteral nutritional support.
†The control group received enteral nutritional support.
‡$P < .05$ vs. control.
§$P < .01$ vs. control.
¶Data reported as the sepsis rate per patient per 100 protocol days.

a phenomenon that could not be explained simply by the presence of the central line. Did the PNS predispose these patients to infection in some manner, perhaps as a consequence of bowel rest[49, 50] or from some unfavorable immunomodulation by a component of the PNS formulation?[51] Whatever the reason, these data led the American College of Physicians to state that "parenteral nutritional support was associated with net harm" and to recommend that "the routine use of parenteral nutrition for patients undergoing chemotherapy should be strongly discouraged."[52]

George Santayana noted that "those who cannot remember the past are condemned to repeat it." With the oncology lesson in mind, especially with regard to the fact that PNS may even be harmful, what data are available from PRCTs regarding the efficacy of NS in critically ill patients?

For purposes of this section, we will only consider those PRCTs that attempted to assess the value of NS per se. In other words, unless otherwise noted, the control group did not receive any other nutrition except that available in

food brought on a tray or in 5% dextrose given intravenously. A series of other studies that compared PNS with ENS will be discussed in the next section.

Only three pertinent reports are available,[53–55] two of which were performed in the 1970s.[53, 54] The data are summarized in Table 17–3. All three trials evaluated PNS.

In the cardiac surgery study,[53] the patients randomized to receive PNS appeared to have had more complications (especially acute renal failure and pneumonia) and had higher hospital bills. However, it should be noted that the patients truly received "hyperalimentation" and were given as much fluid and nutrients as they could tolerate. The adverse consequences of overfeeding (especially CO_2 production)[51] were not recognized at the time the study was performed.

The trial by Gunn et al.[54] could raise the question of a type II error (see Table 17–3). The absolute mortality rate in the treated group was half (15%) that in the control group (30%). Is this a real difference (which would be important to know) or only a statistical variation? It

TABLE 17–3.

Prospective Randomized Controlled Trials of Nutritional Support in Critically Ill Patients

Study	Patient Population	Outcome Parameter	Treatment Group*		
			Standard NS	BCAA-NS	Control
Abel[53]	Malnourished† cardiac surgery (valve disease) patients	Survival	16/20 (80%)		21/24 (88%)
		Complications‡	16		7
		Days on respirator	5.3		3.5
		Days in hospital	31		27
		Postoperative hospital cost	$9,630§		$6,275
Gunn[54]	Neonates with respiratory distress¶	Survival	17/20 (85%)		14/20 (70%)
		Sepsis	1/20 (5%)		1/20 (5%)
		Cardiac arrests	2/20 (10%)		0/20 (0%)
		Days on respirator	5.2		4.7
Reilly[55]	Liver transplant recipients	Survival	8/8 (100%)	9/10 (90%)	8/10 (80%)
		Days on respirator	2.3	2.6	3.6
		Days in ICU	3.8§	3.6§	6
		Days in hospital	67	44	47
		Hospital cost	$158,000	$158,000	$178,000

*NS = nutritional support; BCAA = branched-chain amino acid based.
†Patients randomized to receive or not receive 5 days postoperative NS.
‡Total number of complications (if one complication per patient, differences statistically significant; the authors noted "more complications" in recipients of NS).
§$P <.05$ vs. control.
¶The control group received 10% dextrose.

should be noted, on the other hand, that two of the survivors in the treated group had major neurologic deficiencies.

The third trial[55] evaluated two PNS regimens (standard amino acid–containing solutions vs.branched-chain amino acid [BCAA] solutions) vs. no PNS. It was the only one of the three trials to show a benefit from NS, a shorter ICU stay.

All three trials did evaluate the number of days the patients were on the respirator. It is somewhat disheartening to note, in all three, that earlier weaning could not be achieved.

Some other PRCTs should be noted in passing. Moore and Jones randomized patients with abdominal trauma to have or not have a needle catheter jejunostomy placed at the time of exploratory surgery; the treated group then received elemental diet feedings through the jejunostomy beginning 12 to 18 hours postoperatively.[56] This study was not included in Table 17–3 because the control group was allowed to receive PNS if they were not eating by the fifth postoperative day; 9 of the 31 control patients (29%) were so treated.

Moore and Jones found no difference between the two groups with regard to the total postoperative complication rate, mortality from sepsis-induced multiple organ failure, or the duration or cost of hospitalization. The authors claimed that there was a statistically significant difference in postoperative infections (9/31 [29%] vs. 3/32 [9%], "$P < .025$"), although if the chi-square test is corrected for the small numbers (Yates correction), the P value is .10. Furthermore, if PNS predisposes to infection, this difference may be due to the PNS the control group received rather than any effect from early ENS.

Grahm et al. reported a trial evaluating jejunal feedings in head-injured patients.[57] However, at least 8 of the 32 patients were purposely put into the group to which they had not been assigned, and the control patients received various forms of ENS via gastric feedings. It is impossible to assess the specific impact of ENS with such a study design.

Several groups evaluated the role of essential amino acids in acute renal failure; these data were the subject of a meta-analysis.[58] None of these trials, unfortunately, are adequate to answer the question of whether NS per se is of benefit because all of the investigators gave hypertonic glucose to the control groups. This was done in an effort to balance the caloric load and thus isolate the role of the amino acid solution. Unfortunately, providing hypertonic glucose to patients who are in renal failure is probably not optimal therapy. This may have been the case for the subgroup in whom a difference may have emerged, those who required dialysis. The hypertonic glucose could have caused hyperglycemia and consequent fluid overload; if the amino acids stimulated insulin release (and leucine in particular is known to do this[59]), these experiments may have shown nothing more than the fact that hypertonic glucose is better tolerated in anuric patients if one also provides insulin!

A similar problem exists when one examines the data evaluating the role of BCAA solutions in PNS formulations given to patients with liver disease. Naylor et al., in a meta-analysis, found a potential survival benefit in studies that did not employ lipid as a calorie source.[60] Unfortunately, those were the very studies where the control group received large quantities of dextrose! BCAA solutions did appear to be effective in treating hepatic encephalopathy. However, one cannot determine from these data whether the NS was an important factor; it may be that BCAAs alone are active pharmacologic agents in treating this process.[61]

Pancreatitis is a disease that can result in a patient being admitted to the ICU. Unfortunately, the only PRCT evaluating NS in this disease was one that randomized patients with more mild disease.[62] In this trial, the recipients of the PNS had significantly longer hospitalizations (16 days vs. 10 days, $P <.05$; personal communication, H. Sax) in spite of being in better nitrogen balance. There was an arithmetic but statistically insignificant increase in the infection rate in the treated group (3/29 [10%] vs. 1/26 [4%]).

Surgery may be viewed as a model of the stressed patient, and a large number of PRCTs have evaluated preoperative as well as postoperative PNS and ENS in surgery patients. Two meta-analyses of the PNS data have suggested that there may be a trend for PNS to reduce the rate of major complications [42,63] (personal communication, S. Klein). However, the cost to prevent one such complication may be prohibitive. (If 7 to 10 days of preoperative PNS reduces the absolute rate by 5% and if the daily cost of PNS is $800,[64] the cost to prevent one complication is $112,000 to $160,000.)

Neither published meta-analysis included the data from the largest PRCT reported to date in the NS literature, the Veterans Affairs cooperative trial.[65] This study, in which almost 400 patients were randomized to preoperative PNS or immediate surgery, found that the treated group had an arithmetically (not statistically significant) higher mortality rate (13.4% vs. 10.5% in the controls) and arithmetically lower postoperative noninfectious complication rate (16.7% vs. 22.2% in the controls). Of most note and reiterating what has become a trou-

blesome theme, the treated group had a significantly higher postoperative infectious complication rate (14.1% vs. 6.4% in the controls).

Another surgical trial of PNS was stopped because an early analysis showed a trend for an increased complication rate in the treated group.[66] Again, these problems were largely infectious.

Preoperative and/or postoperative ENS has also been subjected to evaluations by PRCTs. Although the data for postoperative needle catheter jejunostomy (or nasojejunal tube) feeding could not attribute any particular gain to this form of therapy,[67] the story for preoperative ENS may be more optimistic. Four such trials have been published, and those data are summarized in Table 17–4[68–72] (S. Klein, personal communication). All of the studies evaluated patients who mostly[68] or entirely[69–72] had cancer. Although there were no differences in any of the trials regarding survival, in all four trials the postoperative complication rates were lower (significantly so in two) in the treated groups.

It should be noted, however, that there were potentially major methodologic problems in the two trials showing the greatest differences.[68, 69] In one,[68] there were significantly more patients with benign disease in the treated group than in the control group (37% vs. 16%, $P <.05$), which suggests a randomiza-

TABLE 17–4.

Preoperative Enteral Nutritional Support

Reference	ENS* (Days)	Mortality		Postoperative Complications		Duration of Hospitalization (Days)	
		ENS	Control	ENS	Control	ENS	Control
68	10	4/67 (6%)	5/43 (12%)	7/67 (10%)†	16/43 (37%)	10‡	13
69	≥1	1/28 (4%)	4/32 (13%)	5/28 (18%)†	15/32 (47%)	No data	
70	10–21§	No data		6/19 (32%)	10/17 (59%)	19	21
71,¶ 72	10	4/50 (8%)	2/50 (4%)	6/50 (12%)	8/50 (16%)	No data	

*ENS = enteral nutritional support.
†$P <.05$ vs. controls.
‡These patients also had 10 days of preoperative hospitalization.
§Outpatient treatment.
¶Personal communication, S. Klein, 1992.

tion breakdown. In the other,[69] four patients were removed from the treatment group because surgery revealed metastatic disease and/or there were preoperative biliary drainage complications. Since these patients were probably more likely to have postoperative complications, the differences between the two groups may actually be less impressive. The outcomes in these four patients were not available; if all 4 were to have had postoperative complications, the complication rates (28% vs. 47%) would no longer have been statistically different.

Almost 10 years ago I received a request from the editors of *Chest* to write a review article regarding the use of NS in the ICU. At that time I declined the offer because there did not seem to be adequate data upon which to make any conclusions. Instead I submitted an editorial[73] and subsequently two others[74, 75] pointing out the need for one (or more) properly executed PRCT to evaluate the efficacy of NS in ICU patients. Although I have subsequently heard rumors that such studies are in progress, none have yet (July 1992) become available. At this time, I can only observe that NS has not been proved to be as effective as was initially claimed in other disease states and that the arguments for using NS in the ICU bear remarkable resemblance to those used to support its use in other disorders.

So, who gets fed? From the above data, it is difficult to support the widespread application of NS to most patients, even if they are, for a short period, critically ill. It is even possible that PNS will make the situation worse. From my perspective, the time to use NS is when the patient is truly in danger of dying (or becoming sicker) *because* of starvation. Unfortunately, we have no data as to when that line is crossed. Since many of the PRCTs have not been able to show an impact of NS provided for 10 to 14 days, I suspect that most patients can tolerate 2 weeks of very limited nutrient intake without further adverse effects. My personal recommendation (based on all of these considerations) is that NS should be undertaken when the patient has not begun (or when it becomes clear that he cannot be expected to begin) regular feeding for 3 weeks.

Should allowances be made for hypermetabolism? In general, this state usually does not last for weeks, only days. For example, patients who have "uncontrolled sepsis" usually expire well before the 3-week mark unless the infection can be controlled. As such, a correction factor will probably not prove to be necessary in most cases. It should also be appreciated that NS is only being provided to prevent morbidity or mortality from the effects of long-term starvation; the fate-determining factor is whether the underlying disease can be successfully treated.

HOW SHOULD WHO GET FED?

This section will deal with a comparison of enteral and parenteral feeding. While a number of PRCTs have made such comparisons, it should be recognized that such studies are comparing two types of treatment. If differences are found, it cannot be assumed that one treatment is efficacious; since we do not know in most of these situations that NS is of benefit, it may be that the study has only shown that the other treatment is worse! We have already touched on this subject with the concern that PNS predisposes to infection.

Perhaps because there is a preconceived bias that NS is efficacious, there have been a few more trials that have compared PNS with ENS in critically ill patients. These trials are summarized in Table 17−5.[76−84]

The two burn studies[76, 77] were sequential trials from the same unit. The patients randomized to receive PNS in both studies actually received ENS with PNS supplementation. The ENS was apparently administered orally. In both tri-

TABLE 17–5.

Parenteral vs. Enteral Nutritional Support in Critically Ill Patients

Patient Population	Reference	Mortality		Infections		Cost Considerations	
		PNS*	ENS*	PNS	ENS	PNS	ENS
Burns	76†	8/13 (52%)	8/15 (53%)				
	77†	10/16 (63%)‡	6/23 (26%)				
Abdominal trauma	78			11/30 (37%)	5/29 (17%)		
	79	3/23 (13%)	1/23 (4%)	No differences§		$3,729¶	$1,346
						Dur'n Hosp Same	
	80			20/45 (44%)‡	12/51 (24%)		
Sepsis	81‖	8/35 (23%)	7/32 (22%)			$330/day‡	$228/day
Head injury	82	3/20 (15%)‡	9/18 (50%)			Dur'n Hosp Same	
	83	7/23 (30%)	9/28 (32%)	No difference			
	84**	2/10 (20%)	4/10 (40%)				

*PNS = parenteral nutritional support; ENS = enteral nutritional support; Dur'n Hosp = duration of hospitalization.
†Patients in the PNS group actually received a combination of PNS and ENS.
‡$P < .05$ vs. ENS.
§All postoperative complications.
¶No statistical analysis (total per-patient costs of nutritional support).
‖Ten patients randomized to ENS received 4 to 6 days of PNS prior to the study.
**Patients in ENS group actually received a combination of ENS and PNS.

als, the PNS recipients received about 1,000 kcal/day more energy than those given ENS alone. PNS did not appear to provide any additional benefit, and there was an increase in mortality associated with PNS in one of the studies.[77]

Although the three abdominal trauma trials[78–80] were conducted in different centers, they had similar designs. Patients were randomized to receive ENS through a jejunostomy or to receive postoperative PNS. Two of the PRCTs found at least arithmetic differences in infection rates between the two groups.[78, 80] The authors attributed this to a "benefit" of ENS, but the alternate possibility, a bad effect of PNS, is an equally tenable explanation.

One trial evaluated patients with "persistent hypermetabolism" after sepsis.[81] The patients receiving ENS had either nasoduodenal tubes or surgical jejunostomies; 10 of them had also received PNS for 4 to 6 days before the ENS was begun. The patients given ENS had more diarrhea than did those in the PNS group. The PNS cost more than the ENS, although "both forms of support represented considerable daily resources." The study was designed to see whether either form of NS was more ef-

fective at preventing the multiple organ failure syndrome or death; both forms of NS were equally effective or ineffective in this regard.

Two of the head injury trials[82, 83] were from the same center and represented consecutive studies. The protocols are very similar, although the authors claimed that the techniques for delivering ENS in the second trial[83] were more effective than in the first study (small-diameter nasogastric tube, pump, calorie-dense feeding, etc.).

The most remarkable finding was the dramatic difference in mortality in the first study (a finding that could not be duplicated in the second). The authors attributed this to the better nutrient delivery by PNS, but again, one must worry that it was a matter of the ENS doing harm. These ENS recipients[82] all had large-bore nasogastric tubes in place and had varying degrees of mental obtundation; they were certainly at risk for aspiration. In fact, if one compares the outcomes with the authors' previously reported experiences, it appeared that it was a matter of the ENS recipients doing worse rather than the PNS recipients doing better.[85]

The last head injury study[84] compared PNS with a combined program of PNS and ENS. ENS was delivered by bolus feeding through a nasogastric tube, probably a system analogous to that employed in the first head injury study.[82] Was the arithmetic difference in mortality a reflection of the same problem? One cannot really tell from the available data.

Are there any conclusions that can be drawn from these trials? No consistent patterns were seen with regard to either ENS or PNS being associated with better survival, although large-bore nasogastric tubes may be less preferable than thin-bore or jejunostomy tubes for ENS. PNS is more expensive; ENS, especially if delivered beyond the pylorus, may cause more diarrhea.[79-81] The question has been raised whether ENS, when provided through surgically created jejunostomies, may cause fewer postoperative infectious complications than PNS. This was observed in two of these trials[78, 80] and also in a meta-analysis of mostly unpublished data.[86] Even if this is true, it cannot be known whether this is a benefit attributable to ENS through surgical jejunostomies or a detriment of PNS. The time has come to perform a PRCT comparing ENS with no NS at all, i.e., to redo the trial described by Moore and Jones[56] but deleting the PNS fallback after 5 days.

Another potential benefit of NS is the prevention of stress-related upper gastrointestinal bleeding. While retrospective controlled reports have suggested that NS, especially ENS, may be associated with decreased bleeding,[87, 88] no PRCT has proved this to be the case. This issue will not be easily answered with assurance because the background incidence of major bleeding in the ICU is not high.[89]

On the basis of animal studies and some of the above information, emphasis is being placed on providing ENS to critically ill patients. It is even being speculated that ENS improves the metabolic response to injury.[90] When one is given the choice between PNS and ENS, it would seem almost obvious to opt for the enteral route, especially if one can avoid large-bore nasogastric tube feedings. However, my reason for supporting this decision is pragmatic rather than based on the possibility that the feeding is having a positive impact on the underlying disease. From the above data, there is no particular reason to think that ENS is inferior to PNS, and it is cheaper.

My perspective is that NS should only be provided to prevent primary starvation. Since that event will generally not be an issue for a few weeks, most patients will be eating on their own by then. Those who are not are likely to have nonfunctional gastrointestinal tracts, and will not be candidates for ENS.

WHO WILL FIND OUT WHO "WHO" IS?

I have been an observer of the explosion of NS as a clinical activity for 2 decades. During this time, there has been a paucity of supportive scientific data that can justify its expense. In fact, if NS had been proposed as a drug rather than a food, it is doubtful that it could have satisfied the Food and Drug Administration. Recently, challenges have been raised to the use of PNS as adjunctive therapy in cancer treatment; its effect in the perioperative state appears to be marginal at best. ENS may be more promising, but there are still very few studies that have shown it to be superior to no NS at all in improving the morbidity and mortality of a wide variety of disease process.

Curiously, I find myself writing a chapter in a book devoted entirely to NS in critical illness. As the author of the "controversy" chapter, I must conclude with an appeal that I trust my coauthors and readers will find noncontroversial. We need appropriate PRCTs to evaluate the role of NS in the ICU. These studies need to be large enough to avoid type II errors, and they must include non-treated controls. The argument that it is unethical not to provide NS to such patients assumes data not in existence, namely, that NS has established benefit. As we have already noted, some NS (i.e., PNS) may actually have established harm. Hippocrates may have been wrong.

It is what we think we know already that often prevents us from learning.
Claude Bernard

Acknowledgment

My appreciation is extended to Sylvia Anguiano for her tireless repreparation of manuscripts. My gratitude is also extended to Bud Abbott and Lou Costello for introducing me to their first baseman. Who would have been a great ballplayer if he had been able to stay away from alcohol and subsequent ICU hospitalizations.

REFERENCES

1. Studley H: Percentage of weight loss. *JAMA* 1936; 106:458–460.
2. Dudrick SJ, Rhoads JE: New horizons for intravenous feeding. *JAMA* 1971; 215:939–949.
3. Dudrick SJ, Wilmore DW, Vars HM, et al: Long-term parenteral nutrition with growth, development, and positive nitrogen balance. *Surgery* 1968; 64:134–142.
4. Howard L, Heaphey L, Fleming CR, et al: Four years of North American registry home parenteral nutrition outcome data and their implications for patient management. *JPEN* 1991; 15:384–393.
5. Dudrick SJ, Ruberg RL: Principles and practices of parenteral nutrition. *Gastroenterology* 1971; 61:901–910.
6. Keys A: Caloric deficiency and starvation, in Jolliffe N (ed): *Clinical Nutrition,* ed 2. New York, Harper & Brothers, 1962.
7. Schlichtig R, Sargent SG: Nutritional support of the mechanically ventilated patient. *Crit Care Clin* 1990; 6:767–784.
8. Koretz RL: Nutritional support: Are we shooting the messenger? (abstract). *Gastroenterology* 1980; 96:269.
9. Koretz RL: What supports nutritional support? *Dig Dis Sci* 1984; 29:577–588.
10. Koretz RL, Meyer JH: Elemental diets—facts and fantasies. *Gastroenterology* 1980; 78:393–410.
11. Liljedahl SO, Birke G: The nutrition of patients with extensive burns. *Nutr Metabol* 1972; 14(suppl):110–113.
12. Blackburn GL, Bistrian BR: Nutritional care of the injured and/or septic patient. *Surg Clin North Am* 1976; 56:1195–1224.
13. Barrocas A, Tretola R, Alonso A: Nutrition and the critically ill pulmonary patient. *Respir Care* 1983; 28:50–61.
14. Burzstein S, Elwyn DH, Kvetan V: Nutritional and metabolic support. *Crit Care Clin* 1991; 7:451–461.
15. McCarthy MC: Nutritional support in the critically ill surgical patient. *Surg Clin North Am* 1991; 71:831–841.
16. Bartlett RH, Allyn PA, Medley T, et al: Nutritional therapy based on positive caloric balance in burn patients. *Arch Surg* 1977; 112:974–980.
17. Love RT: Nutrition in the burned patient. *J Miss State Med Assoc* 1972; 13:391–392.
18. Liljedahl SO, Larsson J, Schildt B, et al: Metabolic studies in severe burns. *Acta Chir Scand* 1982; 148:393–400.
19. Alexander JW, MacMillan BG, Stinnett JD, et al: Beneficial effects of aggressive protein feeding in severely burned children. *Ann Surg* 1980; 192:505–517.
20. Savitz MH, Bryan-Brown CW, Elwyn DH, et al: Postoperative nutritional failure and chronic cerebral edema in neurosurgical patients. *Mt Sinai J Med* 1978; 45:394–401.
21. Bastow MD, Rawlings J, Allison SP: Undernutrition, hypothermia, and injury in elderly women with fractured femur: An injury response to altered metabolism? *Lancet* 1983; 1:143–146.
22. Buzby GP, Mullen JL, Matthews DC, et al: Prognostic nutritional index in gastrointestinal surgery. *Am J Surg* 1980; 139:160–167.
23. Wernerman J, von der Decken A, Vinnars E: Protein synthesis in skeletal muscle in relation to nitrogen balance

after abdominal surgery: The effect of total parenteral nutrition. *JPEN* 1986; 10:578–582.

24. Steiger E, Daly JM, Allen TR, et al: Postoperative intravenous nutrition: Effects on body weight, protein regeneration, wound healing, and liver morphology. *Surgery* 1973; 73:686–691.

25. Mullen JL, Buzby GP, Matthews DC, et al: Reduction of operative morbidity and mortality by combined preoperative and postoperative nutritional support. *Ann Surg* 1980; 192:604–613.

26. Braun SR, Keim NL, Dixon RM, et al: The prevalence and determinants of nutritional changes in chronic obstructive pulmonary disease. *Chest* 1984; 86:558–563.

27. Boushy SF, Adhikari PK, Sakamoto A, et al: Factors affecting prognosis in emphysema. *Dis Chest* 1964; 45:402–411.

28. Aguilaniu B, Goldstein-Shapses S, Pajon A, et al: Muscle protein degradation in severely malnourished patients with chronic obstructive pulmonary disease subject to short-term total parenteral nutrition. *JPEN* 1992; 16:248–254.

29. Bassili HR, Deitel M: Effect of nutritional support on weaning patients off mechanical ventilators. *JPEN* 1981; 5:161–163.

30. Anonymous: Cancer cachexia (editorial). *Lancet* 1984; 1:833–834.

31. Dewys WD, Begg C, Lavin PT, et al: Prognostic effect of weight loss prior to chemotherapy in cancer patients. *Am J Med* 1980; 69:491–497.

32. Daly JM, Dudrick SJ, Copeland EM: Intravenous hyperalimentation. *Ann Surg* 1980; 192:587–592.

33. Copeland EM, MacFadyen BV, Lanzotti VJ, et al: Intravenous hyperalimenation as an adjunct to cancer chemotherapy. *Am J Surg* 1975; 129:167–172.

34. Koretz RL: Parenteral nutrition—is it oncologically logical? *J Clin Oncol* 1984; 2:534–538.

35. Hays DM, Merritt RJ, White L, et al: Effect of total parenteral nutrition on marrow recovery during induction therapy for acute nonlymphocytic leukemia in childhood. *Med Pediatr Oncol* 1983; 11:134–140.

36. Weisdorf SA, Lysne J, Wind D, et al: Positive effect of prophylactic total par-enteral nutrition on long-term outcome of bone marrow transplantation. *Transplantation* 1987; 43:833–838.

37. Szeluga DJ, Stuart RK, Brookmeyer R, et al: Nutritional support of bone marrow transplant recipients: A prospective, randomized clinical trial comparing total parenteral nutrition to an enteral feeding program, *Cancer Res* 1987; 47:3309–3316.

38. Serrou B, Cupissol D, Favier F, et al: Opposite results in two randomized trials evaluating the adjunct value of peripheral intravenous nutrition in lung cancer patients, in Salmon SE, Jones SE (eds): *Adjunctive Therapy of Cancer III*, New York, Grune & Stratton, 1981.

39. Moghissi K, Teasdale P: Supplementary parenteral nutrition in disseminated cancer of the lung treated by surgery (abstract). *JPEN* 1979; 3:292.

40. Clamon GH, Feld R, Evans WK, et al: Effects of adjuvant central IV hyperalimentation in the survival and response to treatment of patients with small cell lung cancer: A randomized trial. *Cancer Treat Rep* 1985; 69:167–176.

41. Drott C, Unsgaard B, Schersten T, et al: Total parenteral nutrition as an adjuvant to patients undergoing chemotherapy for testicular carcinoma: Protection of body composition—a randomized, prospective study. *Surgery* 1988; 103:499–506.

42. Klein S, Simes J, Blackburn GL: Total parenteral nutrition and cancer clinical trials. *Cancer* 1986; 58:1378–1386.

43. Ghavimi F, Shils ME, Scott BF, et al: Comparison of morbidity in children requiring abdominal radiation and chemotherapy, with and without total parenteral nutrition. *J Pediatr* 1982; 101:530–537.

44. Samuels ML, Selig DE, Ogden S, et al: IV hyperalimentation and chemotherapy for stage III testicular cancer: A randomized study. *Cancer Treat Rep* 1981; 65:615–627.

45. Shambarger RC, Brennan MF, Goodgame JT, et al: A prospective, randomized study of adjuvant parenteral nutrition in the treatment of sarcomas: Results of metabolic and survival studies. *Surgery* 1984; 96:1–12.

46. Van Eys J, Copeland EM, Cangir A, et

al: A clinical trial of hyperalimentation in children with metastatic malignancies. *Med Pediatr Oncol* 1980; 8:63–73.

47. Jordan WM, Valdivieso M, Frankmann C, et al: Treatment of advanced adenocarcinoma of the lung with Ftorafur, doxorubicin, cyclophosphamide, and cisplatin (FACP) and intensive IV hyperalimentation. *Cancer Treat Rep* 1981; 65:197–205.

48. Valdivieso M, Frankmann C, Murphy WK, et al: Long-term effects of intravenous hyperalimentation administered during intensive chemotherapy for small cell bronchogenic carcinoma. *Cancer* 1987; 59:362–369.

49. Fong Y, Marano MA, Barber A, et al: Total parenteral nutrition and bowel rest modify the metabolic response to endotoxin in humans. *Ann Surg* 1989; 210:449–457.

50. Zaloga GP, Knowles R, Black KW, et al: Total parenteral nutrition increases mortality after hemorrhage. *Crit Care Med* 1991; 19:54–59.

51. Phelps SJ, Brown RO, Helms RA, et al: Toxicities of parenteral nutrition in the critically ill patient. *Crit Care Clin* 1991; 7:225–253.

52. American College of Physicians: Parenteral nutrition in patients receiving cancer chemotherapy. *Ann Intern Med* 1989; 110:734–736.

53. Abel RM, Fischer JE, Buckley MJ, et al: Malnutrition in cardiac surgical patients. *Arch Surg* 1976; 111:45–50.

54. Gunn T, Reaman G, Outerbridge EW, et al: Peripheral total parenteral nutrition for premature infants with the respiratory distress syndrome: A controlled study. *J Pediatr* 1978; 92:608–613.

55. Reilly J, Mehta R, Teperman L, et al: Nutritional support after liver transplantation: A randomized prospective study, *JPEN* 1990; 14:386–391.

56. Moore EE, Jones TN: Benefits of immediate jejunostomy feeding after major abdominal trauma—a prospective, randomized study. *J Trauma* 1986; 26:874–881.

57. Grahm TW, Zadrozny DB, Harrington T: The benefits of early jejunal hyperalimentation in the head-injured patient. *Neurosurgery* 1989; 25:729–735.

58. Naylor CD, Detsky AS, O'Rourke K, et al: Does treatment with essential amino acids and hypertonic glucose improve survival in acute renal failure? A meta-analysis. *Renal Failure* 1987; 10:141–152.

59. Adibi SA: Roles of branched-chain amino acids in metabolic regulation. *J Lab Clin Med* 1980; 95:475–484.

60. Naylor CD, O'Rourke K, Detsky AS, et al: Parenteral nutrition with branched-chain amino acids in hepatic encephalopathy. *Gastroenterology* 1989; 97:1033–1042.

61. Koretz RL: Nutritional support: How much for how much? *Gut* 1986; 27(suppl 1):85–95.

62. Sax HC, Warner BW, Talamini MA, et al: Early total parenteral nutrition in acute pancreatitis: Lack of beneficial effects, *Am J Surg* 1987; 153:117–124.

63. Detsky AS, Baker JP, O'Rourke K, et al: Perioperative parenteral nutrition: A meta-analysis. *Ann Intern Med* 1987; 107:195–203.

64. Twomey PL, Patching SC: Cost-effectiveness of nutritional support. *JPEN* 1985; 9:3–10.

65. The Veterans Affairs Total Parenteral Nutrition Cooperative Study Group: Perioperative total parenteral nutrition in surgical patients. *N Engl J Med* 1991; 325:525–532.

66. Ellis LM, Copeland EM, Souba WW: Perioperative nutritional support. *Surg Clin North Am* 1991; 71:493–507.

67. Koretz RL: Predigested diets: Should we mash the meat when we mash the potatoes? *Nutr Clin Pract* 1990; 5:241–246.

68. Shukla HS, Rao RR, Banu N, et al: Enteral hyperalimentation in malnourished surgical patients. *Indian J Med Res* 1984; 80:339–346.

69. Foschi D, Lavagna G, Callioni F, et al: Hyperalimentation in malnourished surgical patients. *Br J Surg* 1986; 73:716–719.

70. Flynn MB, Leightly FF: Preoperative outpatient nutritional support of patients with squamous cancer of the upper aerodigestive tract. *Am J Surg* 1987; 154:359–362.

71. von Meyenfeldt MF, Meyerink WJHJ, Soeters PB, et al: Perioperative nutri-

tional support results in a reduction of major postoperative complications especially in high risk patients (abstract). *Gastroenterology* 1991; 100:553.

72. Meijerink WJHJ, von Meyenfeldt MF, Rouflart MMJ, et al: Efficacy of perioperative nutritional support (letter). *Lancet* 1992; 340:188–189.

73. Koretz RL: Breathing and feeding—can you have one without the other? (editorial). *Chest* 1984; 85:288–289.

74. Koretz RL: Nutritional support— whether or not some is good, more is not better (editorial). *Chest* 1985; 88:2–3.

75. Koretz RL: Things that go around come around, even in the intensive care unit (editorial). *Chest* 1990; 98:524–526.

76. Herndon DH, Stein MD, Rutan TC, et al: Failure of TPN supplementation to improve liver function, immunity, and mortality in thermally injured patients. *J Trauma* 1987; 27:195–204.

77. Herndon DH, Barrow RE, Stein M, et al: Increased mortality with intravenous supplemental feeding in severely burned patients. *J Burn Care Rehabil* 1989; 10:309–313.

78. Moore FA, Moore EE, Jones TN, et al: TEN vs TPN following major abdominal trauma—reduced septic morbidity. *J Trauma* 1989; 29:916–923.

79. Adams S, Dellinger EP, Wertz MJ, et al: Enteral versus parenteral nutritional support following laparotomy for trauma: A randomized prospective trial. *J Trauma* 1986; 26:882–891.

80. Kudsk KA, Croce MA, Fabian TC, et al: Enteral vs. parenteral feeding. *Ann Surg* 1992; 215:503–513.

81. Cerra FB, McPherson JP, Konstantinides FN, et al: Enteral nutrition does not prevent multiple organ failure syndrome (MOFS) after sepsis. *Surgery* 1988; 104:727–733.

82. Rapp RP, Young B, Twyman D, et al: The favorable effect of early parenteral feeding on survival in head-injured patients. *J Neurosurg* 1983; 58:906–912.

83. Young B, Ott L, Twyman D, et al: The effect of nutritional support on outcome from severe head injury. *J Neurosurg* 1987; 67:668–676.

84. Hausmann D, Mosebach KO, Caspari R, et al: Combined enteral-parenteral nutrition versus total parenteral nutrition in brain-injured patients. *Intensive Care Med* 1985; 11:80–84.

85. Koretz RL: Nutritional support in acute head injuries (letter). *J Neurosurg* 1984; 60:1334–1335.

86. Anderson JD, Moore FA, Moore EE: Enteral feeding in the critically injured patient. *Nutr Clin Pract* 1992; 7:117–122.

87. Pingleton SK, Hadzima SK: Enteral alimentation and gastrointestinal bleeding in mechanically ventilated patients. *Crit Care Med* 1983; 11:13–16.

88. Kuric J, Lucas CE, Ledgerwood AM, et al: Nutritional support: A prophylaxis against stress bleeding after spinal cord injury. *Paraplegia* 1989; 27:140–145.

89. Koretz RL: Should patients in the intensive care unit be provided routinely with antacids, sucralfate, or H_2 blocker prophylaxis to prevent stress bleeding?—Negative, in Gitnick G, Barnes HV, Lewis RP, et al (eds): *Debates in Medicine,* vol 4. St Louis, Mosby–Year Book, 1991.

90. Lowry SF: The route of feeding influences injury responses. *J Trauma* 1990; 12(suppl):S10–S15.

18

Timing and Route of Nutritional Support

Gary P. Zaloga, M.D.

Timing of nutrition support

    Malnutrition

    Gut integrity

    Wound healing

    Infection/sepsis

    Hypermetabolism

    Outcome

Route of nutrition support

    Nutrient availability

    Studies of enteral vs. parenteral nutrition

        Animal studies

        Human Studies

            Trauma/burn

    Neuroinjury

    Perioperative nutritional support

    Cancer

    Bone marrow transplantation

    Inflammatory bowel disease

    Intestinal fistulas

    Pancreatitis

Metabolic effects of parenteral and enteral nutrition

    Gastrointestinal tract and liver

    Bacterial translocation

    Immunity

    Miscellaneous

The optimal quantity, quality, route, and timing of nutritional support in the critically ill patient remain poorly defined. In this chapter, we address the timing and route of nutritional support in the postinjury period. Clearly, preinjury prevention of malnutrition is also extremely important. Prevention of malnutrition is more effective in reducing complications and cost and in improving outcome than is posttreatment. Other chapters in this text address the quality of nutrient administration.

TIMING OF NUTRITION SUPPORT

Many patients "tolerate" a short period of starvation. On the other hand, prolonged starvation results in loss of organ function, increased morbidity, prolonged hospital stay, and increased mortality. Early institution of nutritional support may provide essential nutrients for maintenance of gut integrity, prevention of bacterial translocation, preservation of organ function (i.e., cardiovascular, respiratory, renal, liver, intestine), wound healing, and immune function. The net result from early nutritional support may be improved organ function, decreased infections, reduced morbidity and mortality, and decreased hospital stay and cost.

The optimal timing of nutritional support is patient and disease specific. Malnourished patients with burn injury or multitrauma may benefit from immediate nutritional support, while others (i.e., elective surgery for hernia repair) may tolerate a few days of starvation without adverse consequences.

Our concept of nutritional support goes beyond the delivery of calories and protein. It includes the use of specific nutrients that are capable of protecting and improving organ function (i.e., metabolic resuscitation). Current research indicates that the delivery of specific nutrients can support gut integrity, improve gut and liver blood flow, minimize liver injury from shock, improve liver function, speed wound healing, modulate cardiovascular function, improve the immune status, decrease infection rates, and improve outcome. It is true that some patients "tolerate" short periods of starvation. However, their recovery may be improved with nutritional support. In this section, we discuss animal and human studies addressing the timing of nutritional support.

Malnutrition

Protein-energy malnutrition (PEM) becomes important clinically when it is severe enough to impair physiologic function sufficiently to prolong recovery from illness, increase morbidity, or increase mortality. Physiologic impairments are associated with loss of body protein.[1] When more than 20% of body protein is lost, most physiologic functions are diminished. Physiologic impairments include maximum voluntary grip strength, ulnar nerve-muscle stimulation, maximum inspiratory and expiratory pressures, maximum minute ventilation, the ventilatory response to

hypoxia and hypercapnia, and wound healing.

Patients with PEM have more postoperative complications and longer hospital stays than do well-nourished patients.[1-3] Hill[1] evaluated the outcome of 101 patients after major gastrointestinal surgery. Protein-depleted patients had significantly more complications (50% vs. 23%), pneumonia (23% vs. 8%), and wound infection (19% vs. 9%) and a longer hospital stay (19.2 days vs. 14.6 days). However, the amount of protein loss required to alter physiologic function during critical illness (i.e., major surgery, trauma, sepsis) is unknown. Recent studies suggest that immune and gut function are more susceptible to PEM than muscle wasting is.

The degree of wasting of various organs that accompanies weight loss has been evaluated in necropsy studies. Most organs have a percent mass loss roughly similar to total-body weight, the exception being the brain.[1] Protein losses are large but nutritional therapy may be unable to achieve net protein anabolism in many critically ill patients. However, protein losses can be reduced with early nutritional support.[1, 4, 5]

Widespread defects in cellular chemistry and physiologic function occur in patients with PEM[1] and may result in organ dysfunction. Both parenteral and enteral nutrition can improve these abnormalities. A few days of nutritional repletion can replenish muscle adenosine triphosphate (ATP) and adenosine diphosphate (ADP) stores.[1] Three to 4 days of parenteral feeding improves respiratory (i.e., muscle strength, peak expiratory flow) and skeletal muscle strength (i.e., grip strength) in patients with inflammatory bowel disease (IBD).[6]

The patient groups most at risk for complications and prolonged hospital stay are those with moderate to severe PEM and physiologic impairments (i.e., organ dysfunction).[1] These patients have more sepsis, pneumonia, wound infections, and other complications and may be the patients who most benefit from early nutritional support (before organ failure sets in).

Gut Integrity

Gut integrity (i.e., function and mass) is maintained via stimulation from enteral nutrients, trophic hormones, adequate blood flow, and neurologic input. Gut function begins to deteriorate when nutrients are lacking (i.e., starvation). Thus, it would seem logical that the gut would benefit from early nutritional support (see the section on the route of nutrition support).

Experimental studies of gut integrity in guinea pigs following thermal injury indicate that the bowel becomes edematous, loses mucosal integrity, and allows for bacterial translocation within 24 to 72 hours of the burn. Initiation of enteral nutrition immediately following a burn injury protects the gut from atrophy and injury.[7-9] Early enteral feeding also improves blood flow to the gastrointestinal tract and liver, diminishes free radical production, reduces the hypermetabolic response to burn injury, prevents bacterial translocation, and improves survival.

Early enteral feeding protects the liver from damage following experimental hemorrhage.[10] Food digestion products are known to produce a hyperemic response in the gut.[11, 12] We believe that enteral nutrients improve gut and liver blood flow by dilating mesenteric blood vessels and prevent gut/hepatic ischemia. In support of this hypothesis, Inoue et al.[13] studied cardiac output and intestinal blood flow responses to experimental burn injury. Regional blood flow to the gut was compared in animals fed an electrolyte solution and diet formula. Despite similar cardiac outputs, the diet group had significantly higher blood flow to the jejunum and cecum (common sites of bacterial translocation). Vasoconstrictors and other toxins released following burn injury are believed to be responsible for gut hypoperfusion. Enteral nutrients appear to antagonize the vasoconstrictor effects of these mediators. We routinely administer enteral nutrition to patients receiving vasopressors and inotropic agents, and have had excellent success, with no increase in bowel ischemia/infarction. We are careful to volume-resuscitate the patient first.

Wound Healing

Wound healing is impaired in malnourished animals and humans.[14] Early nutritional support improves wound healing rates. We reported a doubling of wound strength (at 1 week) in animals following abdominal surgery with early vs. 3-day enteral feeding.[15] The early fed group also maintained better body weight. Moss et al.[16] measured the strength of colorectal healing following anastomoses in dogs. Animals fed enterally immediately after surgery had twice the wound strength (at 1 week) and improved wound collagen synthesis when compared with animals not receiving early feeding. Luminal nutrients improve gut healing via direct trophic effects and by stimulating the production of gut trophic hormones.

Windsor et al.[17] reported improved wound healing following surgery in patients with adequate food intake prior to surgery vs. patients with decreased food intake. Schroeder et al.[18] reported improved wound healing in patients receiving immediate postoperative enteral nutrition. Early institution of parenteral nutrition also improves wound healing.[19-21] Haydock and Hill[19] compared wound healing in malnourished patients receiving total parenteral nutrition (TPN) and well-nourished patients. Wound healing was diminished in malnourished patients and improved significantly (above controls) with TPN. Wound healing following a period of preoperative nutrition was better than what occurred with only postoperative nutrition. From these data, Hill[1] concluded that an improvement in the wound healing response occurs after only 1 week of TPN and before there is a measurable improvement in nutritional status. In surgery patients, the improvement in wound healing response is more marked when TPN is given before rather than after the surgical procedure.[1, 19] Collins et al.[21] reported improved wound healing following a 2-week postoperative course of TPN (after rectal excision for ulcerative colitis). Early institution of parenteral nutrition also decreased the hospital stay following surgery.[21]

Malnutrition may decrease healing following fracture of a bone. In a prospective, randomized controlled study,[22] the administration of an oral protein-containing supplement was associated with fewer complications and deaths and shorter hospital stays in elderly patients with femoral neck fractures. Others[23, 24] also reported improved outcome after hip fractures with protein-containing supplements given parenterally or enterally. The primary nutrient improving healing was protein.[25] Protein supplementation improved osteocalcin levels, a marker of osteoblast activity.[25]

Infection/Sepsis

Chiarelli et al.[26] randomized 20 patients to early (average, 4 hours) vs. delayed (average, 57 hours) enteral nutrition following burn injuries (average, 38% total-body burn). The early-fed patients had reduced infections, improved nitrogen balance, and decreased hospital stay. Jenkins et al.[27] reported fewer infections in burned patients with early vs. delayed feeding. Recently, Jenkins and colleagues[28] extended these observations to include intraoperative enteral nutrition. Burn injury patients were randomized to two early feeding regimens (40 patients per group). One group was fed following burn injury and throughout hospitalization (including surgery). The second group was fed following burn injury but had enteral feed-

ing stopped for operative procedures. The first group, receiving continuous enteral feeding, had lower wound infection rates and a significantly decreased hospital stay.

Moore and Jones[29] randomized trauma patients to early or delayed (day 5) postoperative enteral nutrition. The early-fed group had fewer infections during their hospital stay (10% vs. 28%). Grahm et al.[30] randomized 32 head-injured patients to nasojejunal ($n = 17$) or gastric ($n = 15$) feedings. Nasojejunal nutrition was initiated within 36 hours of admission (early group). Gastric feedings were initiated after 72 hours or when gastric function returned (late group). The early-fed group had fewer infections (18% vs. 88%).

Ryan and coworkers[31] reported a reduction in septic complications with early postoperative feeding. Sagar et al.[32] randomized patients to early postoperative nutrition. Early-fed patients demonstrated decreased infections, less weight loss, and decreased hospital stay when compared with delayed (day 3) nutritional support. Daly et al.[33] randomized 85 gastrointestinal surgery patients to a low-nitrogen enteral formula and a formula supplemented with arginine, RNA, and ω-3 fatty acids. The patients in the supplemented formula group received significantly more nitrogen (0.22 vs. 0.12 g/kg/day) and calories (20 vs. 16.7 kcal/kg/day). The supplemented patients had fewer infections and shorter hospital stays.

Peck et al.[34, 35] studied the effect of protein malnutrition on the response to infection in mice. Mice received normal or low-protein diets for 3 and 6 weeks and were injected intraperitoneally with *Salmonella typhimurium*. Protein malnutrition was associated with greater weight loss and increased mortality. Protein malnutrition is known to suppress cell-mediated immunity and may have been the cause of the poorer outcome. Others have also reported impairment of immune function[36–39] and increased susceptibility to infection in malnourished animals.[40-43] Interestingly, calorie restriction (3 weeks) but not protein restriction was associated with a lower mortality rate following infection.[35]

Failure of gut barrier function is implicated in the pathogenesis of sepsis and multiple organ failure. Nutrition depletion is associated with a loss of gut mass and function and impaired immune responses. Thus, malnutrition may predispose to gut bacterial invasion (i.e., translocation) and dissemination.

To study the influence of early enteral feeding on gut bacterial translocation, Alexander et al.[44] evaluated the effect of food deprivation in mice following burn injury. Starvation increased the amount of translocation to mesenteric lymph nodes following a 20% total-body burn. In a second experiment, animals were randomized to receive enteral lactated Ringer's solution or an enteral diet immediately following a 40% total-body burn. Translocation was tenfold higher in the group receiving lactated Ringer's solution. These studies indicate that early enteral feeding decreases bacterial translocation following experimental burn injury. Alexander[44] also evaluated the effect of nutrient quantity on bacterial translocation. Guinea pigs received 40% total-body burns and were fed with isovolumetric quantities of feedings at full strength, 75% strength, 50% strength, and 25% strength and with lactated Ringer's solution. Bacterial translocation was minimized in animals receiving 50% or greater quantities of nutrients.

Complement activation is implicated in the inflammatory response occurring in the adult respiratory distress syndrome and multiple organ failure. Deitch et al.[45] examined the effect of zymosan-activated complement on bacterial translocation in mice. Zymosan promotes bacterial translocation to mesenteric lymph nodes primarily by injuring the intestinal mucosa. A protein-free diet did not promote bacterial translocation in otherwise normal mice. However,

protein-malnourished mice were more susceptible to zymosan-induced bacterial translocation when compared with normally nourished mice. In addition, protein malnutrition allowed translocating bacteria to spread past the mesenteric lymph nodes to invade the liver, spleen, and blood. Although the exact number of days of protein malnutrition required to predispose to infection is uncertain, 7 days of protein malnutrition resulted in bacterial translocation to mesenteric lymph nodes (100%), liver/spleen (70%), and blood (60%). Well-nourished mice translocated bacteria to mesenteric lymph nodes (80%) and the liver/spleen (10%). Protein malnutrition also increased mortality and zymosan-induced gut mucosal damage.[45]

Deitch and coworkers[46] have also reported that protein malnutrition increases susceptibility to the lethal effects of endotoxin in mice. The increased mortality is due to a failure of protein-malnourished mice to control the systemic spread of bacteria translocating from the gastrointestinal tract. These results suggest that protein-malnourished mice are more susceptible to inflammatory-induced gut origin sepsis than are normally nourished mice.

Hypermetabolism

Early enteral nutrition diminishes the hypermetabolic hypercatabolic response to burn injury.[8, 9, 47, 48] Early enteral feeding is associated with decreased secretion of counterregulatory hormones such as catecholamines and cortisol.[9] Early enteral feeding may prevent gut bacterial translocation, cytokine release, and the subsequent increase in stress hormones. The net result would be a decrease in hypercatabolism.

Outcome

In a nonrandomized retrospective review, Rapp et al.[49] reported a higher mortality rate in neurosurgical patients when nutrition support was delayed. It is unclear whether the patients who had nutrition support delayed were sicker. Grahm et al.[30] randomized patients with head injuries to early enteral feeding (nasojejunal tubes) or delayed enteral feeding (gastric tubes). The early-fed patients had significantly fewer infections (18% vs. 88%) and decreased length of intensive care unit (ICU) hospitalization (7 vs. 10 days).

Sagar et al.[32] randomized postoperative patients (gastrointestinal surgery) to early enteral nutrition (first postoperative day; feeding tube) vs. conventional postoperative oral feeding. The early-fed patients had significantly decreased hospital stays (median stay, 14 vs. 19 days). However, other studies (employing needle catheter jejunostomies) failed to confirm shortened hospital stays in early-fed postoperative patients.[24, 50] For example, Yeung et al.[50] compared 20 postoperative (gastrointestinal surgery) patients fed by jejunostomy with 20 control patients (retrospective, nonrandomized). Feedings were initiated 3 ± 1.8 days after surgery and slowly increased over a period of 24 to 48 hours. All patients had access to food. There were no differences in complication rates or hospital stay between groups. However, the patients fed by jejunostomy maintained better weight, lean body mass, and prealbumin levels.

In a study of ten matched pairs of patients undergoing proctocolectomy, Collins et al.[21] reported more rapid healing and a shorter hospital stay in the group receiving early postoperative (day 2) nutritional support with TPN (when compared with a group receiving no added nutrition). There were no differences in infections. All patients had free access to food. Oral food intake usually occurred 4 to 6 days after surgery. In a follow-up report,[51] the early fed patients maintained better body weight, total-body nitrogen, prealbumin, transferrin, and retinol-binding protein levels.

Abel et al.[52] randomized malnour-ished patients undergoing cardiac surgery to immediate postoperative TPN ($n = 24$) vs. an oral diet ($n = 20$). Oral intake was allowed as soon as the endotracheal tube was removed. TPN was administered for 5 to 6 days and delivered 1000 kcal and 5 g of nitrogen per day. When compared with well-nourished patients, malnourished patients had more complications. However, more postoperative complications developed in the malnourished TPN group (early-fed group) than in the malnourished oral diet group (late-fed group).

In a nonrandomized study, Mullen et al.[53] noted that patients receiving adequate preoperative nutrition (with TPN) had reduced postoperative complications, less sepsis, and lower mortality when compared with patients receiving no preoperative TPN. Subsequently, numerous prospective randomized studies have evaluated early postoperative parenteral nutrition vs. standard postoperative hospital diets or tube fed diets. In general, these studies have failed to demonstrate an outcome advantage for early parenteral feeding over early enteral nutrition or oral diets.[54–60] Of special note, the Veterans Affairs Total Parenteral Nutrition Study Group randomized 395 malnourished patients who required laparotomy or noncardiac thoracotomy to TPN or an oral diet.[56] The TPN patients received both preoperative (7 to 15 days) and postoperative intravenous nutrition. The rates of major complications and mortality were similar between groups. However, there were significantly more infections in the TPN group (14.1% vs. 6.4%). These studies did not compare early aggressive enteral feeding with standard oral postoperative feeding. They indicate that routine preoperative intravenous nutritional support is of little benefit when compared with enteral feeding (primarily oral).

Malnutrition is often observed in patients with hip fractures (many are elderly) and may contribute to morbidity. Voluntary nutritional intake is frequently depressed in these patients. In prospective randomized trials,[22, 23] enteral supplementation with a protein-containing formula decreased the hospital stay, complications, and mortality rates following hip fracture. Tkatch et al.[25] randomized hip fracture patients to receive a protein-containing or a non-protein-containing oral nutritional supplement. These formulas were matched for vitamins and minerals. The clinical course was improved in the protein-supplemented group. The rate of complications and deaths was significantly lower (52% vs. 80%) and the length of hospital stay decreased (69 vs. 102 days) in the protein-supplemented group. Gallagher et al.[61] randomized 97 malnourished patients with hip fractures to receive an oral diet (control) or diet plus tube feedings (tube). Tube feedings were started on the first postoperative day and continued until the patient could eat 75% of his caloric needs for 3 consecutive days. The tube-fed group demonstrated more rapid rises in visceral protein levels, a decrease in rehabilitation length of stay, and fewer surgical or gastrointestinal complications. These data suggest that early enteral supplementation with protein-containing formulas improves the outcome following hip fracture.

Alexander et al.[62] randomized 18 burned children to "control" or "high-protein" diets. Control patients were encouraged to voluntarily take as much of a normal diet as possible. They were supplemented with a standard intact protein formula (orally or by tube) or TPN. The high-protein group consumed the normal diet supplemented with protein. Parenteral nutrition was used when the gastrointestinal tract was intolerant of nutrients. The control group required more TPN than the high-protein group did. Despite lower caloric consumption (but higher protein intake), the high-protein group had significantly better survival rates (100% vs. 56%). These data suggest that early aggressive enteral supplementation also improves survival following thermal injury.

Parenteral nutrition has been compared with oral diets in patients receiving chemotherapy and radiotherapy for cancer (see the section on the route of nutrition support).[63, 64] Parenteral nutrition improves calorie/protein intake. However, it is associated with a higher rate of infection, poorer tumor response, and higher mortality. Few studies have evaluated early aggressive enteral nutrition vs. standard oral intake in cancer patients receiving chemotherapy. Infection rates, tumor response, and outcome are similar in these groups.

Nutrition debility is common in patients undergoing bone marrow transplantation. Cytoreduction therapy (i.e., chemotherapy, radiotherapy) produces toxic effects upon the gastrointestinal tract. The debilitated condition of these patients predisposes to infection and other complications. Institution of early nutritional support with parenteral nutrition results in a more rapid return of bone marrow function.[65, 66] In a prospective randomized trial, Weisdorf et al.[67] reported that early institution of supplemental parenteral nutrition (vs. diet alone) improved overall survival (2 year survival rates, 50% vs. 35%), the time to relapse, and disease-free survival in patients receiving bone marrow transplants. Engraftment, the duration of hospitalization, and the incidence of graft-vs.-host disease and bacteremia were not different.

Reilly et al.[68] randomized 28 hypoalbuminemic cirrhotic patients undergoing liver transplantation to receive an oral diet or TPN immediately posttransplant. The TPN group (early nutritional support) achieved earlier respiratory independence (2.3 vs. 3.6 days) and had a shorter ICU stay (3.8 vs. 6 days). There were no differences between groups in renal function, hepatic function, or encephalopathy. Serum 3-methyhistidine levels (a marker of muscle catabolism) were lower in the early-fed group.

Kalfarentzos et al.[69] administered TPN to patients with acute pancreatitis. Patients whose TPN was started within 72 hours of the disease had a 23.6% complication rate and a 13% mortality rate. Patients whose TPN was started later in the course of the disease had a 95.6% complication rate and a 38% mortality rate. It is unclear whether the group receiving delayed nutritional support was sicker.

Prospective randomized controlled clinical trials of adequate size are needed to further delineate the clinically important benefits of early nutritional support. These studies should evaluate the cost-effectiveness of early nutritional support and which patients are most likely to benefit from this therapy.

At the present time, the available data suggest that early nutritional support may improve the clinical outcome of selected patients. It may decrease gut atrophy, bacterial translocation, and infection rates and improve host defenses and survival. The enteral route is preferred over the parenteral route (see the section on the route of nutrition support). It is clear that many patients do not require early enteral nutritional support. They do fine with standard oral nutrition until such time that depletion occurs. On the other hand, certain high-risk patients (i.e., critically ill, malnourished, burn, or trauma patients) may benefit from early nutrient administration. Patients most likely to benefit are those with protein depletion, weight loss, and physiologic impairments. The data indicate that early nutritional support does not harm patients or worsen the outcome. Thus, if one is undecided on whether a patient would benefit from early nutrient support, we favor early feeding.

ROUTE OF NUTRITION SUPPORT

The supply of adequate cellular nutrients is important for optimal recovery from illness. Nutrients may be supplied via the parenteral or enteral routes. Although techniques are available for delivery of both enteral and parenteral nutrients, the composition and types of nutrients that can be delivered via each route are different. Accumulating data also indicate that nutrients have different physiologic actions when delivered via different routes. In this section, we review and summarize studies comparing both the physiologic actions and clinical effects of parenteral and enteral nutrition.

Nutrient Availability

The major classes of nutrients include proteins, carbohydrates, lipids, nucleic acids, minerals, vitamins, and trace elements (Table 18–1). Parenteral and enteral nutrition delivers minerals, vitamins, and trace elements in similar amounts. However, they differ considerably in their ability to deliver proteins, carbohydrates, lipids, and nucleic acids.

Protein is available as intact protein, hydrolyzed protein (i.e., peptides), and amino acids.[70] Parenteral nutrition uses only amino acids as its nitrogen source. Glutamate and aspartate are not administered intravenously (in most formulas) because these "excitatory" amino acids have a variety of toxic ef-

TABLE 18–1.

Nutrients Found in Enteral and Parenteral Formulas

Component	Parenteral Nutrition	Enteral Nutrition
Protein		
Intact	No	Yes
Peptides	No	Yes
Amino acids	Yes	Yes
Glutamine	No	Yes
Arginine	Yes	Yes
Cysteine	No	Yes
Carbohydrate		
Simple	Yes	Yes
Complex (i.e., fiber)	No	Yes
Lipids		
Long chain ω-6	Yes	Yes
Long chain ω-3	No	Yes
Medium chain	No	Yes
Nucleotides	No	Yes

fects upon cells (especially the central nervous system).[71, 72] Glutamine and asparagine are not delivered in parenteral nutrition formulas because these amino acids break down in solution and liberate ammonia and "excitatory" amino acids. However, recent evidence indicates that glutamine is a major fuel for the gastrointestinal tract and plays a major role in maintenance of the immune system.[73-75] Body demands for this amino acid exceed endogenous supply during stress and critical illness. Thus, glutamine is now considered to be "semiessential." Arginine, present in low concentrations in parenteral nutritional formulas, is important for wound healing, nitrogen balance, and immune function.[76-78] Similar to glutamine, arginine demands exceed endogenous supply during severe illness and stress. Parenteral nutritional formulas also lack cysteine, an important amino acid in the synthesis of glutathione (γ-glutamylcysteinylglycine).

Recent studies suggest that intact protein and peptides are better nitrogen sources for the body than are amino acids.[70] Peptides possess biological activities that are important for normal physiologic activity. Studies have demonstrated a role for peptides in maintenance of the gastrointestinal tract, support of liver function, stimulation of hormonal responses, nitrogen utilization, growth, and wound repair.[70] Intact protein (which is digested to peptides) and peptides are only available for use in enteral nutritional support.

Complex carbohydrate in the form of fiber produces unique effects upon gastrointestinal tract structure and function.[79-81] Certain fibers are metabolized to short-chain fatty acids, which are preferential fuels for the colon.[80, 81] In addition, bulk fiber is important for stimulating gut motility (ensuring distal nutrient flow) and maintenance. Complex carbohydrate is only available with enteral nutrition.

Long-chain ω-6 polyunsaturated fatty acids (i.e., linoleic acid) are precursors

to arachidonic acid, which upon subsequent metabolism produces prostaglandins and leukotrienes (of the 2 series). These lipids have profound affects upon cardiovascular and immune function.[82, 83] Reducing the quantity of ω-6 long-chain fatty acids in the diet may be associated with improved immune function and reduced infections.[82-85] Lipids used during parenteral nutritional support are high in linoleic acid (50% to 66%). On the other hand, lipid formulations used for enteral nutrition are lower in linoleic acid content. Improved immune function and reduced infection rates during enteral nutrition may partially relate to the lipid content.

Nucleotides may play a beneficial role in stimulation of the immune system.[86] Nucleotides are absent from parenteral nutrition formulas. Although absent from most enteral formulas, nucleotides are present in some enteral diets.

In summary, parenteral nutritional formulas lack many important nutrients, whereas enteral nutrition provides many of these nutrients.

Studies of Enteral vs. Parenteral Nutrition

Animal Studies

Kudsk et al. randomized rats to receive dextrose—amino acid solutions via the parenteral or enteral route[87, 88] (Table 18−2). Following 12 to 14 days of feeding, animals were subjected to *Escherichia coli*—hemoglobin peritonitis. Survival was significantly higher in enterally fed malnourished[87] and well-nourished[88] rats. The mortality rate (2 day) in malnourished animals was 60% for intravenous feeding and 40% for enteral feeding.[87] Similarly, the mortality rate (2 day) in well-nourished animals was 80% with intravenous nutrition and 40% with enteral feeding.[88] Petersen and coworkers[89] studied normal and protein-depleted rats. Survival following *E. coli*—hemoglobin peritonitis was 66% in normal animals as opposed to 15% in protein-depleted rats. Protein-

TABLE 18–2.

Animal Studies Comparing Enteral and Parenteral Nutrition

Reference	Animal	Model	Mortality Rate
87	Rat	E. coli peritonitis	60% TPN; 40% enteral
88	Rat	E. coli peritonitis	80% TPN; 40% enteral
89	Rat	E. coli peritonitis	95%–100% TPN; 47% enteral
91	Rat	Hemorrhagic shock	63% TPN; 0% enteral
92	Rat	Methotrexate	100% TPN; 25%–50% enteral

depleted rats refed with regular diets had a 53% survival rate, while rats repleted with intravenous hyperalimentation had survival rates of 0% to 5%.

Kudsk et al.[90] studied the effect of enteral and parenteral feeding on body composition in malnourished rats. Following protein depletion, animals were fed dextrose–amino acid solutions for 14 days via the enteral or parenteral routes. Parenterally fed animals gained more weight (with greater fat formation) than did the enteral group but had lower intestinal mass and nitrogen.

Zaloga et al.[91] evaluated the effect of parenteral and enteral feeding on survival in rats following hemorrhagic hypotension. The mortality rate (24 hours) was significantly increased in animals receiving parenteral nutrition (63%) as compared with peptide-based enteral diets (0%). Interestingly, the mortality rate was 0% in animals receiving enteral and intravenous saline.

Zaloga and coworkers[92] administered high-dose methotrexate to rats receiving parenteral and enteral nutrition. The mortality rate was 100% in parenterally fed animals as compared with 50% in animals fed a defined-formula enteral diet and 25% in animals receiving chow. All tissues (i.e., mesenteric lymph nodes, liver, spleen, lung) in the parenterally fed animals contained large quantities of bacteria, while most tissues in chow-fed animals were free of bacteria. Tissue bacterial counts were intermediate in animals fed the defined-formula diet.

These data indicate that intravenous feeding is associated with higher mortality rates in animals following peritonitis, hemorrhage, and high-dose methotrexate treatment. Parenteral nutrition is associated with increased bacterial translocation and tissue dissemination following methotrexate administration. In addition, intravenous feeding does not improve survival in protein-depleted animals with peritonitis. On the other hand, enteral feeding does improve the outcome following peritonitis in protein-depleted animals.

Human Studies

Trauma/Burn.—Adams and coworkers[93] compared the efficacy of enteral and parenteral nutrition in 46 trauma patients (Table 18–3). Patients were randomized during admission laparotomy to receive central venous parenteral nutrition ($n = 23$) or enteral nutrition via jejunostomy ($n = 23$; intact protein formulas). Nutritional support began on the first postoperative day, and the study continued for a maximum of 14 days. There were no significant differences between groups for injury severity, hours to full nutritional support, the number of days receiving nutritional support, average daily caloric intakes, nitrogen balance, or complication rates. TPN patients had more hyperglycemia while enterally fed patients had more diarrhea (48% vs. 26%). The cost of delivering enteral nutrition was less than that for parenteral nutrition. The cost difference for delivering nutritional support between groups (accounting for line and tube placement) was $2,383.00 per patient. The authors concluded that early postoperative jejunostomy feeding

TABLE 18–3.

Human Studies Comparing Enteral Nutrition and Parenteral Nutrition

Reference	No.	Result
Trauma/burn		
93	46	EN* and PN* equally effective, PN more expensive
94	46	Better visceral proteins with EN, more sepsis with PN
95	59	Better visceral proteins with EN, more sepsis with PN
96	98	Sepsis higher with TPN
97	Meta-analysis of 8 trials	Sepsis higher with TPN
98	39	Survival better with EN
Neuroinjury		
100	45	No differences in outcome between EN and PN
101	41	No differences in outcome between EN and PN
Perioperative		
102	Meta-analysis of 18 trials	Routine use of TPN not justified
103	34	Preoperative TPN vs. no Preoperative TPN, no differences
104	24	PN vs. EN, PN had higher cost
105	15	PN vs. EN, no differences noted
106	28	PN vs. EN, no differences noted
107	20	PN vs. EN, no differences except that TPN had higher cost
108	395	PN vs. oral, more infections with TPN
109	66	PN vs. EN, no differences noted
Cancer chemotherapy and radiotherapy		
110	17 trials	PN vs. oral, sepsis higher with PN
111	28 trials	PN vs. oral, sepsis higher with PN
112	Meta-analysis of 12 trials	PN vs. oral, PN associated with decreased survival, lower tumor response, higher infection rate
Bone marrow		
113	137	PN vs. fluids, better survival with PN
114	57	PN vs. EN, no differences except that PN cost more

*EN = enteral nutrition; PN = parenteral nutrition.

was safe and efficacious for multiple-trauma patients.

Peterson et al.[94] investigated isocaloric, isonitrogenous total enteral nutrition (TEN; amino acid–based diet) vs. TPN in 46 trauma patients. Patients with an abdominal trauma index (ATI) between 15 and 40 were randomized to receive TEN or TPN. Acute-phase proteins increased more in TPN patients. Visceral protein levels (albumin, transferrin, retinol-binding protein) increased to a greater extent in TEN patients. Clinical outcomes analyzed by the route of nutritional support were comparable for ICU and hospital stay. Septic complications were more common in TPN patients (2/21 vs. 8/25; $P = .08$). The authors concluded that postinjury TEN attenuated reprioritization of hepatic protein synthesis in patients sustaining major trauma. In a follow-up study, Moore et al.[95] reported on 59 patients randomized to TEN or TPN. Visceral protein levels improved more in the TEN than the TPN group. The overall septic morbidity was 17% in the TEN group and 37% in the TPN group. Pneumonia occurred in 6 of 30 (20%) in the TPN group and in 0 of 29 (0%) in the TEN group. The authors concluded that TEN was well tolerated in severely injured patients and that early feeding via the gut reduced septic complications in stressed patients.

Kudsk et al.[96] randomized 98 patients with an ATI of at least 15 to enteral (peptide-based formula) or parenteral feeding within 24 hours of injury. Groups were matched for the severity of injury, age, and the mechanism of injury. The length of hospital stay was comparable between groups. One patient died in each group. Septic morbidity was defined as pneumonia, intraabdominal abscess, empyema, line sepsis, or fasciitis occurring during the first 15 days of hospitalization. Septic morbidity was significantly lower in the enteral group (24% vs. 76%). The enteral group had fewer pneumonias (11.8% vs. 31%), intra-abdominal abscesses (1.9% vs. 13.3%), and line sepsis (1.9% vs. 13.3%).

Moore and coworkers[97] reported the results from eight prospective randomized trials comparing the efficacy of early enteral (amino acid–based diet) vs. early parenteral nutrition in high-risk surgery patients. Two of these trials were published previously.[95, 107] The data were analyzed by meta-analysis. The TEN and TPN groups were comparable. Septic complications were lower in TEN patients (18% vs. 35%; P = .01), and TEN patients had a lower incidence of pneumonia, intra-abdominal abscesses, and catheter sepsis.

Herndon et al.[98] randomized 39 patients with burns (>50% of their body surface area) to receive intravenous nutrient supplementation of enteral calories (n = 16) or enteral nutrients alone (n = 23). The mortality rate was significantly higher in the intravenously supplemented group (63%) when compared with the group receiving enteral nutrients alone (26%). The authors recommended that "the use of intravenous supplemental nutrition in the early postburn period should be discouraged and its use limited only to nutritional support of patients whose enteral function has failed totally."

Neuroinjury.—Rapp and colleagues[99] compared the effects of early parenteral nutrition with delayed enteral nutrition on outcome in patients following head injury. Thirty-eight head-injured patients were randomly assigned to receive TPN or standard enteral nutrition. Eight of 18 (44%) patients with delayed enteral nutrition died within 18 days of injury, whereas none of the TPN patients died within this period. TPN patients had improved nitrogen balance and higher serum albumin levels. The authors concluded that early nutrition could improve survival following head injury. This study primarily compares early with delayed feeding. It is difficult to draw conclusions regarding the route of nutrient delivery since the parenteral and enteral groups were not comparable for nutritional support.

Hadley et al.[100] randomized 45 patients with acute head injury to receive TPN or enteral nutrition (intact protein formula). TPN patients had a significantly higher mean daily nitrogen intake. However, there were no differences between groups for maintenance of serum albumin levels, weight loss, incidence of infection, nitrogen balance, and outcome.

Young et al.[101] studied 41 brain-injured patients randomized to receive TPN or enteral nutrition (intact protein formulas). The TPN group received significantly more protein (1.35 vs. 0.91 g/kg/day) and calories (76% vs. 59% of requirements) than the enteral group did. Nitrogen balance was significantly better in the TPN patients. The incidence of infection and sepsis was not significantly different between groups. Early (<18 days after injury) and late (>18 days after injury) deaths were not statistically different between groups. Ten of 23 (43%) of the TPN patients and 10 of 28 (36%) of the enterally fed patients died. The authors concluded that more patients in the TPN group had favorable outcomes (43.5% vs. 32.1% at 6 months). However, the definition of favorable neurologic outcome was arbitrary and based upon the Glasgow Coma Scale (GCS). Five patients (22%) in the TPN group had peak admission GCS scores of 5 or less while 10 patients in the enteral group (36%) had admission GCS scores of 5 or less. One would not have expected the enteral group to have done as well neurologically. Thus, despite lower calorie and protein intake, there was no difference in outcome between patients receiving enteral or parenteral nutrition.

Perioperative Nutritional Support.— Detsky et al.[102] used meta-analysis to evaluate the results of 18 controlled trials (1966 to 1986) that measured the effectiveness of perioperative TPN. Many of the trials suffered from poor methodologies. In 4 studies, TPN was administered only during the postoperative period; in 5, only during the preoperative period; and in 10, during both the preoperative and postoperative periods. In 15 studies, patients with gastrointestinal malignancies were involved; in 1, head and neck cancers; and in 1, bladder cancer. Most studies compared TPN with oral diets (not tube feeding). The evidence suggested that the "routine use of perioperative total parenteral nutrition in unselected patients having major surgery was not justified." There was no significant reduction in complication rates or mortality. The health and public policy committee of the American College of Physicians[115] published a position paper on perioperative parenteral nutrition in 1987. The committee agreed that "routine use of perioperative parenteral nutrition for unselected patients having major surgery was not justified." The committee called for further trials in subgroups of high-risk patients (i.e., severely malnourished patients having major surgery, postoperative patients with complications that result in prolonged periods of inadequate nutritional intake). The committee also suggested that some of these patients may be able to receive their nutrients through enteral feeding tubes.

We will review selected studies from the meta-analysis. Moghissi et al.[116] studied patients with carcinoma of the esophagus (with dysphagia) who were randomized to receive preoperative TPN (n = 10; 34 to 36 kcal/kg/day and 0.18 to 0.20 g nitrogen/kg/day) or no TPN (6

kcal/kg/day and no nitrogen). The TPN group had better nitrogen balance and weight gain. No significant differences in complications or mortality were reported. Holter and Fischer[117] randomized patients with gastrointestinal malignancies to receive perioperative TPN or no preoperative TPN. There were no differences in complications or mortality. Heatley et al.[118] randomized patients with cancer of the esophagus and stomach to receive a hospital diet or a hospital diet plus parenteral nutrition (amino acids, ethanol, sorbitol). There was no difference in mortality. However, the complication rate (primarily wound infections) was lower in the patients receiving supplemental parenteral nutrition. Thompson et al.[119] randomized 21 patients with gastrointestinal cancers and weight loss (>10%) to receive TPN (n = 12; starting an average of 8 days before surgery) or no TPN (n = 9). There were no differences between groups for postoperative complications or mortality. Muller and associates[120] randomized 125 patients with cancer of the gastrointestinal tract to receive preoperative TPN (n = 66) or a hospital diet (n = 59). The diet group had more malnourished patients (62% vs. 41%). The overall major complication rate was 30% in the control group and 20% in the TPN group. The mortality rates were 18.6% in the control group and 4.5% in the TPN group. Lim et al.[121] randomized 24 patients with esophageal carcinoma to receive TPN (n = 12) or gastrostomy feedings (n = 12; blenderized diet). The TPN group attained earlier positive nitrogen balance. The percent increase in serum albumin concentration was similar between groups. Catheter sepsis developed in 2 patients (17%) in the TPN group and thrombosis of the subclavian vein in 1 patient. One gastrostomy patient had a mild wound infection. One patient died in the TPN group, and 2 died in the gastrostomy group. There were no significant differences in complications between groups. TPN was significantly more expensive than enteral feeding. Abel et al.[122] randomized malnourished patients undergoing cardiac surgery to receive postoperative TPN (n = 24) or diet (n = 20). A separate group of well-nourished patients undergoing cardiac surgery were also studied. TPN was continued for 5 to 6 days postoperatively (average daily intake, 1000 kcal, 5 g nitrogen). Oral intake was allowed as soon as the patients were extubated. The malnourished patients had more complications than the well-nourished patients. In addition, the TPN malnourished patients had more complications than the non-TPN malnourished patients. Collins et al.[123] studied 30 patients undergoing abdominal perineal resections. Patients were divided into three matched groups: intravenous fluids, postoperative intravenous amino acids, and postoperative TPN. There were no significant differences between groups for septic morbidity or mortality. The TPN group had better wound healing and decreased hospital stays.

The retrospective study by Mullen et al.[124] was also included in the meta-analysis.[102] They studied patients referred to the nutritional support service who underwent major intra-abdominal or intrathoracic surgery. The study was not randomized. The decision to use TPN was made by the primary surgeon. Patients not receiving preoperative TPN served as the control group. Patients were retrospectively stratified by Prognostic Nutritional Index (PNI). Data were reported on 145 patients (50 TPN patients, 95 controls). Complications in 9 patients developed (18%), and 2 died (4%) in the TPN group. Complications developed in 37 patients (38.9%), and 27 died (29.4%) in the control group. Significant differences between groups was demonstrated only for those patients identified as high risk by a PNI of 50% or greater. Preoperative nutritional support was associated with a reduction in complications, sepsis, and mortality. Daly et al.[125] also retrospectively as-

sessed the effect of preoperative TPN in malnourished patients with esophageal cancer. Patients receiving preoperative TPN had lower wound infection rates as compared with patients not receiving preoperative TPN.

Smith and Hartemink[103] randomized 34 surgery patients with a PNI greater than 30% to receive preoperative parenteral nutrition (10 days) or surgery without preoperative nutritional support (controls). This study was not part of the meta-analysis.[102] Patients underwent major gastrointestinal surgery. Preoperative nutritional support in these malnourished patients was associated with weight gain, increased triceps skin fold, improved delayed skin hypersensitivity responses, and improved PNI (5.5%). There were 3 major complications and 1 death in the preoperative nutrition group and 6 major complications and 3 deaths in the control group (not significant). The average hospital stay was 38 days in the control group and 44 days in the treatment group. This study did not compare TPN with enteral nutrition but rather preoperative intravenous nutritional support with no preoperative intravenous nutritional support.

McArdle et al.[104] studied 24 surgical patients (i.e., burns, trauma, cancer, head injury, respiratory failure) with greater than 15% weight loss in a prospective randomized study. Patients were randomized to receive a parenteral nutrition solution (amino acids and dextrose) via the intravenous or enteral routes. Both groups achieved nitrogen balance by the third day of nutritional support. Serum insulin levels were higher and free fatty acid levels lower (decreased fat mobilization) in the parenterally fed patients. The cost of delivering the enteral solution was 50% less than the cost of the parenteral solution. Complications and outcome were not reported.

Muggia-Sullam et al.[105] studied 15 patients undergoing abdominal surgery. Patients received an elemental diet via needle catheter jejunostomy or

TPN (nonrandomized). Both nutritional groups were similar for nitrogen balance, body weight preservation, and visceral protein levels. No data were presented for complications.

Fletcher et al.[106] randomized 28 patients undergoing aortic grafting for aneurysms or occlusive disease to receive standard intravenous fluids, parenteral nutrition, or early postoperative enteral feeding. Nitrogen balance was similar in the parenteral and enteral groups. As expected, both nutritional groups had better nitrogen balance than the intravenous fluid group did. There were no deaths and no significant differences between groups for complications or length of stay.

Bower et al.[107] randomized 20 patients undergoing major upper gastrointestinal or pancreaticobiliary surgery to receive postoperative nutritional support by TPN or enteral nutrition (amino acid–based formula; needle catheter jejunostomy). Both routes of nutritional support provided adequate nutrition, although nitrogen balance was better in the TPN group. Serum albumin and transferrin levels decreased more in the TPN group. Prealbumin decreased more in the enteral group. Serum glutamate oxaloacetate transaminase (SGOT) and serum glutamate pyruvate transaminase (SGPT) levels increased to a greater extent in the TPN group. There was no difference in complications between groups, and the enteral nutrition was cheaper.

The Veterans Affairs Total Parenteral Nutrition Cooperative Study Group evaluated perioperative TPN in 395 malnourished surgery patients.[108] Patients who required laparotomy or noncardiac thoracotomy were randomly assigned to receive either TPN for 7 to 15 days before surgery and 3 days afterward or no perioperative TPN (diet alone). Patients were monitored for complications for 90 days after surgery. The rates of complications during the first 30 days after surgery were similar between groups (25.5% with TPN, 24.6% in the control group). Mortality rates (90 day) were similar between groups (13.4% for TPN, 10.5% for the control group). However, there were more infectious complications in the TPN group than the controls (14.1% vs. 6.4%; $P = .01$). Severely malnourished patients who received TPN had fewer complications than controls (5% vs. 43%). The TPN group averaged 2944 kcal/day in the preoperative period, while the control group received 1280 kcal/day. Some have argued that the increased infectious complications in the TPN group may have resulted from overfeeding. However, it must also be pointed out that this study did not compare isocaloric isonitrogenous enteral with parenteral nutrition. Many would also argue that enteral nutrition (via feeding tube) could be used for nutritional support in all the malnourished patients and there was little if any need for TPN in these patients.

Cerra et al.[109] randomized 66 surgery patients with sepsis and persistent hypermetabolism to receive TPN or enteral nutrition. They reported no reduction in the incidence of multiple organ failure or mortality between groups. The authors concluded that the route of nutrient delivery had little effect on outcome after organ failure developed.

In summary, the routine use of preoperative TPN appears unjustified in unselected patients. In addition, routine perioperative use of TPN does not decrease surgical complications or infections or improve outcome. However, it is more costly than perioperative enteral nutrition.

Cancer.—Retrospective and uncontrolled trials have reported a benefit from TPN in patients with cancer. However, therapeutic efficacy can only be established by careful prospective, randomized, controlled trials. In 1984, Koretz[110] evaluated survival data, tumor response, and therapeutic toxicity from 17 randomized controlled trials using parenteral nutrition as an adjunct to chemotherapy and radiation therapy.

Most of the control groups received oral nutrition (diet). Parenteral nutrition did not improve survival, tumor response, or toxicity. Sepsis was more common in patients receiving parenteral nutrition. Klein et al.[111] evaluated 28 prospective randomized controlled clinical trials of TPN in cancer patients in 1986. Control patients were treated with diet in most trials. The authors concluded that TPN may be useful (reduces surgical complications and mortality) when used preoperatively in patients with gastrointestinal tract cancer. No significant benefit from TPN could be demonstrated for survival, treatment tolerance, treatment toxicity, or tumor response in patients receiving chemotherapy or radiotherapy. There was a significant increase in infections ($P < .0001$) in TPN patients receiving chemotherapy.

A position paper from the American College of Physicians evaluated parenteral nutrition in patients receiving cancer chemotherapy in 1989.[112] Meta-analysis was used to pool the results from 12 randomized controlled trials. Patients receiving parenteral nutritional support were 81% as likely to survive as control patients ($P = .05$), 68% as likely to achieve a complete or partial tumor response ($P = .12$), and 400% more likely for significant infection to develop ($P < .0001$). The report concluded that "parenteral nutritional support was associated with net harm, and no conditions could be defined in which such treatment appeared to be of benefit." The full meta-analysis was published in a separate report.[126] The increased risk of infection persisted when catheter-related septicemia was excluded. The use of TPN also prolonged the hospital stay by a median of 14 days.

Bone Marrow Transplantation.— Weisdorf et al.[113] studied the impact of TPN ($n = 71$) vs. intravenous fluids ($n = 66$) on the clinical outcome of well-nourished patients receiving bone marrow transplants for malignant disease. The study period began 1 week prior to

marrow transplantation and continued for 4 weeks posttransplant. All patients were encouraged to maintain enteral intake during the study. Calorie and protein intake was significantly higher in the TPN-treated patients. In addition, 61% of the control patients were eventually treated with intravenous nutrition (average start, 21 days posttransplant). Survival was significantly longer in the patients receiving TPN than in control patients (2-year survival rate for TPN, 50%, and for controls, 35%). The time to relapse and disease-free survival were significantly longer in the TPN patients. There was no difference between groups for engraftment, graft vs. host disease, or hospital days. Time to bacteremia was not significantly different for the two groups when all patients were included. However, in patients receiving allogeneic transplants, the incidence of bacteremia was higher in TPN patients (72% vs. 48%, $P = .001$). This study evaluated the role of TPN supplementation to an enteral diet. It was not a comparison of isocaloric isonitrogenous parenteral vs. enteral diets. The study suggested that improved nutrient intake could improve survival after bone marrow transplantation.

Szeluga et al.[114] compared TPN ($n = 27$) with enteral nutrition ($n = 30$) in a prospective randomized trial of patients receiving bone marrow transplants. Enteral nutrition was provided by oral supplements and/or tube feeding. TPN was associated with more days of diuretic use, more frequent hyperglycemia, and more frequent catheter removal (prompted by catheter-related complications) but less frequent hypomagnesemia. There were no significant differences in the rate of hematopoietic recovery, length of hospitalization, or survival, but nutrition-related costs were 2.3 times greater in the TPN group. The authors concluded that TPN was not superior to enteral feeding and recommended that TPN be reserved for bone marrow transplant recipients who demonstrate intolerance to enteral feeding.

Inflammatory Bowel Disease.—TPN is frequently employed as primary therapy for patients with severe IBD. Recent attention has also focused on the use of enteral nutrition as primary therapy for patients with IBD (primarily Crohn's disease). Few studies of nutritional support of IBD compare isocaloric isonitrogenous parenteral and enteral nutrition. Most studies are retrospective and uncontrolled. They are difficult to interpret because of small size and the fact that many patients received different medications (i.e., corticosteroids). In most of the controlled studies, the control group received corticosteroids, while the nutrition therapy group did not. Some studies attempted to evaluate nutritional therapy as an adjunct to medical or surgical therapy. Others evaluated the nutritional therapy as primary therapy for the disease.

To compare the benefits of TPN vs. enteral nutrition for induction of remission in Crohn's disease, we tabulated known studies of TPN and enteral nutrition (with elemental diets) in patients with Crohn's disease. TPN (Table 18–4) was associated with a 65% early (in-hospital) remission rate and a 41% long-term (3 to 64 month) remission rate. Elemental enteral diets were associated with a 68% early remission rate and 47% long-term remission rate (Table 18–5). These results were not statistically different from each other. To further evaluate the route of nutritional support in the treatment of Crohn's disease, we evaluated only prospective controlled studies (Table 18–6). Seven studies compared TPN with control diets.[127–133] Both short- (74% and 76%) and long-term (40% and 41%) remission

TABLE 18–4.

Parenteral Nutrition in the Treatment of Crohn's Disease

Series	No.	Short-Term Remission	Long-Term Remission	Type
Anderson (1973)	8	7 (88%)	1 (13%)	R
Fischer (1973)	7	3 (43%)	—	R
Vogel (1974)	8	8 (100%)	4 (50%)	R
Reilly (1976)	23	14 (61%)	—	R
Dean (1976)	11	4 (36%)	—	R
Harford (1978)	30	23 (77%)	4/21 (19%)	R
Mullen (1978)	50	19 (38%)	—	R
Milewski (1980)	7	2 (29%)	—	R
Bos (1980)	86	24 (28%)	7 (8%)	R
Houcke (1980)	36	27 (75%)	22 (61%)	R
Holm (1981)	8	7 (88%)	7 (88%)	R
Shiloni (1983)	9	9 (100%)	6 (67%)	R
Ostro (1985)	100	77 (77%)	50/93 (54%)	R
Elson (1980)	20	13 (65%)	8 (40%)	P
Greenberg (1981)	43	33 (77%)	29 (67%)	P
Muller (1983)	30	25 (83%)	17 (57%)	P
Lerebours (1986)	20	19 (95%)	3 (15%)	P
Dickinson (1980)	6	4 (67%)	1 (17%)	PC
Lochs (1983)	10	6 (60%)	5 (50%)	PC
Greenberg (1985)	17	12 (71%)	8 (47%)	PC
McIntyre (1986)	9	9 (100%)	3 (33%)	PC
Greenberg (1988)	17	12 (71%)	5 (29%)	PR
Jones (1987)	16	14 (88%)	—	PR
Cravo (1991)	24	18 (75%)	12/23 (52%)	PR
Totals		389/595 (65%)	192/464 (41%)	

R = retrospective; P = prospective; PC = prospective controlled; PR=prospective randomized.

TABLE 18–5.

Elemental Diets in the Treatment of Crohn's Disease

Series	No.	Short-Term Remission	Long-Term Remission	Type
Voitk (1973)	7	3 (43%)	—	R
Rocchio (1974)	25	10 (40%)	—	R
Axelsson (1977)	11	8 (73%)	4 (36%)	R
O'Morain (1980)	27	24 (89%)	18 (67%)	P
Lochs (1978)	25	15 (60%)	12 (48%)	P
O'Morain (1984)	11	9 (82%)	8 (73%)	PC
Saverymutti (1985)	21	15 (71%)	—	PC
Greenberg (1985)	19	11 (58%)	2 (11%)	PC
Jones (1987)	16	14 (88%)	—	PR
Giaffer (1990)	16	12 (75%)	—	PC
Totals		121/178 (68%)	44/93 (47%)	

R = retrospective; P = prospective; PC = prospective controlled; PR=prospective randomized.

TABLE 18–6.

Parenteral vs. Enteral Nutrition in the Treatment of Crohn's Disease (Prospective, Controlled Studies)

Reference	Series	Group	Short-Term Remission	Long-Term Remission
Parenteral				
127	Dickinson (1980)	Control	3/3	0/3
		PN	4/6	1/6
128	Lochs (1983)	Control	6/10	6/10
		PN	6/10	5/10
129	Greenberg (1985)	Control	9/15	6/15
		PN	12/17	8/17
130	McIntyre (1986)	Control	5/7	2/7
		PN	9/9	3/9
131	Jones (1987)	Enteral	14/16	—
		PN	14/16	—
132	Greenberg (1988)	DFD	11/19	6/19
		PN	12/17	5/17
		PN + food	9/15	5/15
133	Cravo (1991)	Control	35/42	18/38
		DFD	11/15	4/13
		PN	18/24	12/23
Totals		Control	83/112 (74%)	38/96 (40%)
		PN	75/99 (76%)	34/83 (41%)
Enteral				
	O'Morain (1984)	Control	8/10	7/10
		Elemental	9/11	8/11
	Saverymutti (1985)	Control	16/16	—
		Elemental	15/21	—
	Greenberg (1985)	Control	9/15	6/15
		Elemental	11/19	2/19
	Malchow (1990)	Control	32/44	—
		Pep-Diet	21/51	—
	Giaffer (1990)	Control	5/14	—
		Elemental	12/16	—
Ttotals		Control	70/99 (71%)	13/25 (52%)
		Enteral	68/118 (58%)	10/30 (33%)

PN = parenteral nutrition; DFD = defined-formula diet; Pep-Diet = peptide-based diet.

rates were similar with both nutritional regimens (see Table 18–6). In addition, elemental diets were no better than control diets for inducing remission in Crohn's disease (see Tables 18–5 and 18–6). Abad-Lacruz et al.[134] evaluated liver function in 29 patients with IBD who were randomized to receive TEN or TPN. Patients receiving enteral nutrition had better liver function (measured by serum bilirubin and albualbumin levels) and less hepatic damage (measured by alkaline phosphatase, γ-glutamyltransferase (GGT), aspartate aminotransferase (AST), and alanine aminotransferase (ALT).

Patients with active ulcerative colitis respond poorly to TPN. The majority of patients continue to have active disease. Only 4 of 22 (18%) patients treated with TPN by Sitzmann et al.[135] had acceptable responses to therapy. In a prospective controlled trial, Dickinson et al.[127] reported no difference in clinical response between conventional medical therapy (with diet) and TPN. In-hospital remission rates were 57% for controls vs. 46% for TPN patients. One-year follow-up revealed 36% of the controls and 31% of the TPN patients to be in remission. McIntyre et al.[130] reported a 58% in-hospital remission rate in control diet patients and 40% in TPN patients. Long-term remission rates were 25% and 13%, respectively.

Malnutrition is a risk factor for patients undergoing operative procedures. Although there is a lack of controlled trials evaluating preoperative nutritional support in patients with IBD, preoperative nutritional support may benefit many of these patients. Patients with significant underlying malnutrition are those most likely to benefit from preoperative nutritional support. The best route to deliver nutrients remains undefined.

These studies support the conclusion that nutritional therapy can reverse the nutritional deficits caused by IBD and aid in the healing process. However, these studies do not support a role for nutritional therapy as primary therapy for IBD. In addition, TPN may result in bowel starvation rather than bowel rest.[136]

On the basis of these clinical studies, it appears that TPN offers little advantage over enteral nutrition plus medical therapy (i.e., corticosteroids, sulfasalazine) for the treatment of IBD in most patients. Enteral nutrition is preferable to parenteral nutrition as initial therapy for IBD. TPN should be reserved for patients who do not tolerate enteral nutrition, patients with short guts, patients with bowel obstruction, and patients with high-output fistulas.

Intestinal Fistulas.—Gastrointestinal fistulas may develop as a result of abdominal surgery, IBD, cancer, pancreatitis, radiation, trauma, and other etiologies. The reported mortality rate of patients with gastrointestinal fistulas is 6% to 67%.[137] Most patients with fistulas are malnourished or become malnourished secondary to anorexia, infection and sepsis, protein losses, or an inability to tolerate enteral diets. Adequate nutritional support is an integral part of the management of these patients. Mortality is higher in malnourished patients vs. well-nourished patients with enterocutaneous fistulas.[137]

Many clinicians routinely treat patients with gastrointestinal fistulas with TPN. TPN is believed to improve nutritional status, close the fistulas, and improve outcome. TPN decreases fluid losses from fistulas. Hamilton et al.[138] reported that TPN decreased fistula output by 80% to 85% within 2 to 3 days. Wolfe et al.[139] studied enterocutaneous fistulas in the dog. Fistula output decreased by 81% with an elemental diet and 93% with TPN. On the other hand, Fischer[140] noted only a 31.5% decrease in fistula output with TPN.

Fistula closure rates average around 50% to 59% when using enteral feeding.[141–143] Fistula closure rates have been reported to be as high as 73% to 89% with TPN.[144, 145] However, prospective controlled randomized studies evaluating the effect of TPN vs. enteral nutrition on the closure rate and mortality in patients with gastrointestinal fistuals have not been performed. Reber et al.[146] compared 82 patients with fistulas treated between 1968 and 1971 (35% receiving intravenous nutrition) with 104 patients treated between 1972 and 1977 (71% receiving intravenous nutrition). Spontaneous fistula closure rates were 26% (1968 to 1971) and 35% (1972 to 1977). Mortality rates were 22% and 29%, respectively. These differences were not significant. Soeters et al.[147] reviewed 404 patients with gastrointestinal fistulas. The mortality rate was 15.1% from 1960 to 1970 (before TPN) and 25.6% from 1970 to 1975 (after the introduction of TPN). The major cause of death was uncontrolled sepsis. Spontaneous closure rates increased from 10% to 23.3%. Similarly, Deitel et al.[148] compared the outcome in patients with fistuals before and after TPN. The mortality rate decreased from 40% to 9.3%, and the closure rate increased from 34.4% to 81%. Many studies indicate that increased spontaneous closure rates of fistulas can be achieved with TPN. Although some reports have shown decreased mortality with TPN, mortality figures in several large series range from 6.5% to 22% with TPN and 15% to 28% without TPN.[137]

The anatomic location of a fistula and the volume of drainage should determine the optimal means of nutritional support. Patients with high-output fistulas and high small-bowel fistulas (i.e., upper part of the jejunum) are difficult to replete with enteral nutrition. These patients may better be repleted with parenteral nutrition. Enteral nutrition (perhaps with elemental diets) should be tried in most of the remaining patients. Distal or colonic fistulas can usually be supported with enteral feedings. Patients with high upper gastrointestinal fistulas (i.e., stomach, duodenum) can be fed by placing a feeding tube 30 to 40 cm beyond the fistula. Radiation-induced fistulas and fistulas in patients with Crohn's disease are less likely to close and are associated with high mortality rates. These patients frequently require surgery.

Pancreatitis.—The pancreas possesses both exocrine and endocrine functions. It secretes bicarbonate, electrolytes, digestive enzymes (i.e., amylase, lipase, phospholipase, trypsin, chymotrypsin), and hormones (i.e., insulin, glucagon, somatostatin). Because it is the major source of digestive enzymes and insulin, malfunction of the pancreas has important nutritional implications. Pancreatic secretion is stimulated by vagal efferents from the brain in response to the sight, smell, or taste of food (cephalic phase), stimulation of the pancreas because of food in the stomach (gastric phase), and the presence of acid or food in the intestine (intestinal phase). Undigested proteins have little or no stimulatory effect upon pancreatic secretion. On the other hand, peptides and amino acids have a strong stimulatory effect. Pancreatic secretion is inhibited by the consumption of hypertonic glucose solutions and gastrointestinal hormones (i.e., glucagon, somatostatin, pancreatic polypeptide). Infusion of trypsin and chymotrypsin into the duodenum inhibits pancreatic secretion.[149, 150]

Elemental (amino acid, low fat) diets cause less stimulation of pancreatic exocrine secretion than do complex diets. Oral consumption of nutrients stimulates more pancreatic secretion than does intragastric administration. The administration of nutrients into the stomach stimulates more pancreatic secretion than does infusion into the duodenum; duodenal infusion stimulates more secretion than jejunal administration does. Jejunal administration results in pancreatic juice that is "enzyme poor." In addition, acidic diets stimulate more pancreatic secretion than basic diets do. It is clear that use of the gastrointestinal tract for nutritional support induces some pancreatic secretion. Stimulation can be minimized by infusion of elemental, neutral pH diets into the proximal portion of the jejunum. Elemental enteral diets also have a smaller trophic effect upon the pancreas and gastrointestinal tract than do complex diets.

Intravenous glucose (i.e., 25% to 40%) inhibits secretin- and cholecystokinin-induced pancreatic secretory output (i.e., fluid, protein, amylase, lipase). Intravenous infusion of glucose, amino acids, and fat stimulates little if any pancreatic secretion.[151-153] The secretory response to intravenous nutrition is less than that to the intraduodenal administration of elemental diets.[141-153] Bodoky et al.[154] compared pancreatic secretion in patients receiving pancreatoduodenectomy for chronic pancreatitis. Patients were randomized to receive enteral feeding by needle catheter jejunostomy (n = 7) or TPN (n = 5). No difference in exocrine secretion was observed between groups.

Chronic pancreatitis results in a loss of exocrine function, and patients with this are usually managed with enteral nutrition. Limitation of dietary fat intake can help prevent steatorrhea. Vitamin and mineral deficiencies can usually be treated with oral supplements. Malabsorption frequently results from insufficient pancreatic enzyme secretion. Enzyme supplementation aids in nutrient digestion and absorption; it can also help reduce pain.[155, 156]

Acute pancreatitis is manifested as a systemic illness characterized by pain, fluid and electrolyte imbalance, shock, organ failure, and even death. This systemic response is felt to result from the release of pancreatic enzymes, bioactive digestion products, and cytokines. During recovery from an attack of acute pancreatitis, the patient is at risk for nutritional depletion, immune compromise, and infection/sepsis. Many of these patients have been traditionally fed with TPN. TPN provides nutritional support and can "rest" the pancreas.

If continued production of pancreatic enzymes during acute pancreatitis is responsible for systemic manifestations and complications, then suppression of these enzymes may ameliorate the severity of the attack. Some evidence suggests that pancreatic enzyme production is already low as a result of pancreatitis. Few studies have compared TPN with enteral feeding in patients with acute pancreatitis. Goodgame and Fischer[157] reported data from a retrospective study of 46 cases of acute pancreatitis treated with parenteral nutrition (mortality rate, 20%). Results were compared with complications and mortality rates (23%) found in the medical literature. They concluded that parenteral nutrition had little effect on disease pathophysiology as judged by mortality and morbidity. TPN was associated with a higher incidence of catheter-related sepsis. Similar conclusions were drawn from a retrospective analysis by Grant et al.[158] In a more recent uncontrolled retrospective analysis of 67 patients with acute pancreatitis, Kalfarentzos et al.[159] reported an overall complication rate of 55.2% and a mortality rate of 24% in patients treated with TPN. An increased incidence of catheter-related sepsis was also reported. Sax and associates[160] performed a randomized, prospective trial of early TPN in acute pancreatitis. Patients were randomized to receive conventional therapy (i.e., intravenous fluids, analgesics, antacids, nasogastric suction) or conventional therapy plus TPN (dextrose plus amino acids initially, 10% lipid added when the triglyceride levels were normal). Patients not eating in 7 days were crossed over to parenteral nutrition. TPN patients maintained better nitrogen balance. However, early institution of TPN had no advantage over conventional therapy. Catheter-related sepsis was higher in the TPN group (10.5% vs. 1.5%). Days to full oral intake ($P < .06$) and the length of hospitalization ($P < 0.04$) were longer in the TPN group. Total hospital charges were greater in the TPN patients.

Overall, at the present time there are no data to indicate that TPN alters the course of acute pancreatitis. Enteral nutrition is the preferred method for initial nutritional support of patients with pancreatitis. Acute pancreatitis has also been successfully managed with enteral nutrition.[161, 162]

Metabolic Effects of Parenteral and Enteral Nutrition

Gastrointestinal Tract and Liver

Luminal nutrients are important for the maintenance of normal gastrointestinal tract structure and function. Luminal nutrients directly stimulate the gut. They also produce indirect effects via stimulation of gut trophic hormones. Intravenous feeding is associated with a loss of gut weight, mucosal protein and DNA content, villous height, glucose absorption, and mucosal enzyme activities.[163-171] TPN is also associated with atrophy of the pancreas.[164, 172] Thompson et al.[166] measured diamine oxidase (DAO) activity, an intestinal mucosal enzyme that serves as a marker of gut cellular maturity and integrity, in animals given TPN or enteral diets. DAO activity decreased with TPN and correlated with a decrease in gut mass.

Intestinal growth and development may be delayed in premature neonates given intravenous nutrition. Immature sucking rats given TPN during weaning demonstrate delayed intestinal growth, decreased mucosal mass, and reduced enzyme activity.[173-175] These effects are reversed by enteral nutrition.[174]

Guedon et al.[165] performed duodenal endoscopic biopsies in seven adults with IBD who were placed on a regimen of TPN and corticosteroids. The patients had moderate weight loss at the time of study. Following 21 days of TPN, there were significant decreases in disaccharidase (72% to 83%) and peptidase (23% to 78%) enzyme activities. These activities increased after oral refeeding. There

were also significant decreases in microvillus height (13%) in comparison with pre-TPN values. No data were presented from normal controls for comparison. Biasco et al.[176] followed an adult patient with serial jejunal biopsies after intestinal resection for superior mesenteric artery thrombosis. Intestinal hypoplasia was found after 30 days of TPN; cell proliferation and intestinal hyperplasia occurred within 14 days of oral refeeding.

Greene et al.[177] studied 16 infants with protracted diarrhea and malnutrition who were allocated to receive TPN or parenteral nutrition plus enteral feedings. The enterally fed group had earlier recovery of intestinal sucrase and maltase activities and shorter hospital stays (34 vs. 46 days). Orenstein[178] prospectively randomized infants with intractable diarrhea to receive parenteral or enteral nutrition. Parenteral and enteral nutrition produced similar weight gain; however, enteral feeding was associated with faster resolution of malabsorption and diarrhea, fewer complications, and less expensive hospitalization.

Gut trophic hormones are also important for maintaining the integrity of the gastrointestinal tract. Adams et al.[179] constructed isolated bowel loops in rats. Structural hypoplasia occurred in intact and isolated intestines in animals fed with parenteral nutrition. However, intestinal integrity was maintained in both intact and isolated gut of enterally fed animals. These findings indicated that some systemic (i.e., hormonal) factor(s) affected gut mass. Intravenous feeding results in lower levels of gut trophic hormones as compared with enteral feeding. These hormones include gastrin,[164, 180, 181] cholecystokinin and secretin,[182] insulin,[183] enteroglucagon,[181, 183, 184] motilin,[181] neurotensin,[181] and epidermal growth factor.[185, 186] The administration of gastrin,[180] cholecystokinin and secretin,[182] and epidermal growth factor[185, 186] has been shown to improve gut mass and/or function during TPN. Saito et al.[187] have also shown that enteral nutrition, when compared with parenteral feeding, diminishes the secretion of catabolic hormones (i.e., vanillylmandelic acid [VMA], cortisol, glucagon) following burn injury in animals.

Elevations in the levels of serum aminotransferase, bilirubin, and bile salts are frequently seen in patients receiving TPN. These findings suggest that TPN may have deleterious effects on hepatic function. Knodell et al.[188, 189] evaluated the effect of enteral and parenteral nutrition on liver function in rats. Hepatic microsomal cytochrome P-450 oxidase activity and the capacity for demethylation of meperidine and hydroxylation of pentobarbital were significantly reduced in TPN-fed animals. Katayama et al.[190] randomized rats to receive parenteral or enteral nutrition (using the same formula) and measured hepatic energy charge and mitochondrial phosphorylation rates. The TPN group showed a deterioration of the hepatic phosphorylation rate and energy charge. Charland et al.[191] also randomized rats to receive parenteral or enteral feeding and found that parenteral nutrition was associated with a decrease in hepatic cytochrome P-450 activity. Zamir et al.[192] randomized rats to receive oral chow, TPN, and TPN plus chow diets for 7 days. TPN was associated with hepatic steatosis, but the addition of enteral feeding to TPN reduced hepatic steatosis. These data suggest that the route of delivery of nutrients may have a significant impact upon liver function.

Bacterial Translocation

The intestinal mucosa and immune system function as major defense barriers preventing bacteria and endotoxin contained within the gut from invading distant organs. Bacterial translocation is reported to occur in animals following endotoxin,[193] hemorrhage,[194] trauma,[195] burn injury,[196] and methotrexate administration.[92]

Alverdy et al.[197] randomized animals to receive food, oral TPN fluid, or intravenous TPN. Animals were fed for 2 weeks. Two thirds of the TPN animals had culture-positive mesenteric lymph nodes as compared with one third of oral TPN animals and none of the food group. Spaeth et al.[198] divided rats into three groups: food, oral TPN, and intravenous TPN. Bacterial translocation occurred in 60% of the intravenous and oral TPN-fed animals. Translocation did not occur in animals receiving food. The addition of oral cellulose powder to the oral and intravenous TPN groups reduced bacterial translocation to 8% and 0%. Thus, oral administration of fiber appeared to maintain the intestinal barrier and reduced bacterial translocation. We[92] randomized methotrexate-treated animals to receive TPN or enteral diets. Bacterial translocation and mortality were significantly greater in TPN animals. These data suggest that TPN promotes bacterial translocation in animals. Illig et al.[199] fed rats with TPN plus 0%, 6%, 12%, or 25% of calories supplied as an intact protein oral diet (diets were isocaloric and isonitrogenous). Translocation of bacteria to the mesenteric lymph nodes decreased (67% to 10%) as oral nutrition increased.

Many have questioned the role of bacterial translocation in human disease. However, recent studies suggest that bacterial/toxin translocation occurs in humans following injury.[200–202] Reed et al.[200] harvested mesenteric lymph nodes from 25 patients undergoing exploratory celiotomy for abdominal injury. Six patients (25%) had bacteria in their lymph nodes by culture. However, all patients received preoperative antibiotics. Brathwaite et al.[201] sampled portal venous blood and mesenteric lymph nodes from 10 patients with trauma. Portal venous blood was culture-positive in 2 (20%), and mesenteric lymph nodes were culture-positive in 1 patient (10%). However, when mesenteric lymph nodes were reacted with monoclonal antibody to *E. coli* β-galactosidases, all the mesenteric lymph nodes were positive. Reed et al.[202] confirmed these findings. They harvested mesenteric lymph nodes from 16 patients with abdominal trauma. All received preoperative antibiotics. One patient had bacteria in the mesenteric lymph nodes by culture, 9 by electron microscopy, and 3 by both techniques. Overall, bacteria were identified in the mesenteric lymph nodes in 13 of 16 (81%) patients. These studies indicate that bacteria/toxins may be present in mesenteric lymph nodes (indicating translocation) even though cultures are negative. Clearly, preoperative antibiotics may interfere with culture results. Together, these data indicate that bacterial translocation is common in humans after abdominal trauma.

Immunity

Immune responsiveness was assessed in animals fed orally or intravenously for 7 days.[203] Lymphocyte reactivity to concanavalin A remained unchanged over a period of 7 days in orally fed rats. On the other hand, lymphocyte reactivity was depressed by 60% in TPN-fed animals. Renk et al.[204] measured the lymphocyte response to concanavalin A and phytohemagglutinin in traumatized rats (bilateral femoral fracture) randomized to receive TPN or enteral nutrition. Lymphocyte responses were depressed in both groups 1 day after injury but returned to normal by 7 days postinjury in the enteral group but not the TPN group. Meyer et al.[205] studied endotoxin-induced neutrophil activation in enterally vs. parenterally fed volunteers. Neutrophil chemotaxis in response to leukotriene B$_4$ was significantly lower in TPN-fed individuals. Neutrophil chemotaxis induced by zymosan and N-formyl-methionyl-leucyl-phenylalanine were similar in the parenteral and enteral groups. Shou et al.[206] evaluated the effect of TPN on pulmonary alveolar macrophage antimicrobial function in rats. Animals were randomized to receive a chow diet or isocaloric/isonitrogenous TPN for 7 days. TPN administration impaired pulmonary mac-

rophage function (killing of *Candida albicans,* superoxide production, tumor necrosis factor production), decreased pulmonary *E. coli* clearance, and was associated with greater translocation of bacteria to mesenteric lymph nodes. Alverdy and coworkers[207] measured secretory IgA in animals fed intravenously or enterally. Secretory IgA levels were significantly higher in enterally fed animals.

The immune response of patients receiving TPN vs. enteral nutrition has not been evaluated in prospective randomized trials. However, there is worry that the lipid composition (i.e., high in long-chain ω-6 fatty acids) and protein composition (i.e., amino acids, no glutamine, low arginine) of TPN may result in suppression of immune responses.

Miscellaneous

A number of studies (human and animal) have evaluated the effect of TPN and enteral nutrition on nitrogen balance during stress. Overall, studies indicate that protein and calories administered via the enteral route result in the same or better nitrogen balance than when administered via the parenteral route.[208, 209]

Delany et al.[210] evaluated wound healing in rats fed for 6 days via the parenteral and enteral routes. There were no significant differences between groups for weight change, nitrogen balance, colonic bursting strength, or skin incision bursting strength. Similar results were obtained by Zaloga et al.[211]

Differences in the response to infection may exist between enterally and parenterally fed individuals. Mortality from infection is higher in animals[87–92] and humans[112] fed with parenteral vs. enteral nutrition. The acute-phase protein response to infection[94] and catabolic hormone secretion[187] are higher in animals fed parenterally vs. enterally. Endotoxin triggers many of the hemodynamic, metabolic, and immune responses associated with injury and infection. To determine whether parenteral nutrition altered the host response to infection, Fong et al.[212] administered endotoxin to human volunteers (prospective, randomized) maintained on 1 week of enteral or parenteral nutrition. In response to endotoxin, higher body temperature, higher heart rates, and lower blood pressures developed in parenterally fed patients. Individuals receiving TPN had higher stress hormone responses (i.e., epinephrine, glucagon, C-reactive protein), hepatic venous tumor necrosis factor levels, and lactate levels and greater peripheral amino acid mobilization. These data indicate that TPN produces alterations in the host response to "infection" independent of nutritional status.

We have reviewed a large quantity of data comparing enteral and parenteral nutrition. Results have been grouped into three major categories: nutrient availability, studies of enteral vs. parenteral nutrition (animal and human), and the metabolic effects of enteral vs. parenteral nutrition. The following conclusions are based upon the data presented:

1. Parenteral and enteral nutrition differ in the ability to deliver proteins, carbohydrates, and fats. Parenteral nutritional formulas lack many important nutrients (i.e., glutamine, peptides, complex carbohydrates such as fiber, medium- and short-chain fatty acids, ω-3 long-chain fatty acids, and nucleotides).

2. Prospective randomized studies of infection in animals demonstrate higher mortality rates in animals fed with parenteral vs. enteral nutrition.

3. Parenteral nutrition (vs. enteral nutrition) is associated with a higher rate of sepsis in humans following trauma.

4. Enteral and parenteral nutrition is associated with similar outcomes following head injury.

5. Routine use of perioperative TPN in unselected patients having major surgery is not justified.

6. Enteral nutrition is as good or better than parenteral nutrition in patients following surgery. Enteral nutrition is safe, is cheaper than parenteral nutrition, and may be associated with a lower infection rate.

7. Parenteral nutrition is associated with lower survival, poorer tumor response, and more infections in unselected patients receiving chemotherapy or radiotherapy for cancer.

8. Parenteral nutrition has no beneficial effects on the course of IBD or pancreatitis. Enteral nutrition should be the primary mode of nutritional support in these patients.

9. Parenteral and enteral nutrition is of equal efficacy in most patients with gastrointestinal fistulas. However, some patients with fistulas (i.e., high output, high jejunal, pancreatic) may benefit from TPN.

10. When compared with enteral nutrition, parenteral nutrition induces gut atrophy, liver dysfunction, gut bacterial translocation (animals), and immune dysfunction.

In summary, enteral nutrition is superior to parenteral nutrition as a means of nutritional support in most patients. The primary indication for the use of parenteral nutrition is a failure of enteral nutrition.

REFERENCES

1. Hill GL: Body composition research—Implications for the practice of clinical nutrition. *JPEN* 1992; 16:197–218.
2. Windsor JA, Hill GL: Weight loss with physiologic impairment—a basic indicator of surgical risk. *Ann Surg* 1988; 207:290–296.
3. Windsor JA, Hill GL: Risk factors for postoperative pneumonia: The importance of protein depletion. *Ann Surg* 1988; 208:209–214.
4. Shaw JHF, Wildbore M, Wolfe RR: Whole body protein kinetics in severely septic patients. *Ann Surg* 1987; 205:288–294.

5. Shaw JHF, Wolfe RR: An integrated analysis of glucose, fat, and protein metabolism in severely traumatised patients. *Ann Surg* 1989; 209:63–72.

6. Christie PM, Hill GL: Effect of intravenous nutrition on nutrition and function in acute attacks of inflammatory bowel disease. *Gastroenterology* 1990; 99:730–736.

7. Saito H, Trocki O, Alexander JW, et al: The effect of route of nutrient administration on the nutritional state, catabolic hormone secretion, and gut mucosal integrity after burn injury. *JPEN* 1987; 11:1–7.

8. Dominioni L, Trocki O, Mochizuki H, et al: Prevention of severe postburn hypermetabolism and catabolism by immediate intragastric feeding. *J Burn Care Rehabil* 1984; 5:106–112.

9. Mochizuki H, Trocki O, Dominioni L, et al: Mechanism of prevention of postburn hypermetabolism and catabolism by early enteral feeding. *Ann Surg* 1984; 200:297–310.

10. Zaloga GP, Black KW, Prielipp R: Enteral feeding minimizes liver damage following hemorrhage. *Chest* 1991; 100(suppl):135.

11. Gallavan RH, Chou CC, Kvietys PR, et al: Regional blood flow during digestion in the conscious dog. *Am J Physiol* 1980; 238:220–225.

12. Hernandez LA, Kvietys PR, Granger DN: Postprandial hemodynamics in the conscious rat. *Am J Physiol* 1986; 251:117–123.

13. Inoue S, Lukes S, Alexander JW, et al: Increased gut blood flow with early enteral feeding in burned guinea pigs. *J Burn Care Rehabil* 1989; 10:300–308.

14. Haydock DA, Hill GL: Impaired wound healing in surgical patients with varying degrees of malnutrition. *JPEN* 1986; 10:550–554.

15. Zaloga GP, Bortenschlager L, Black KW, et al: Immediate postoperative enteral feeding decreases weight loss and improves wound healing after abdominal surgery in rats. *Crit Care Med* 1992; 20:115–118.

16. Moss G, Greenstein A, Levy S, et al: Maintenance of GI function after bowel surgery and immediate enteral full nutrition. I. Doubling of canine colorectal anastomotic bursting pressure and intestinal wound mature collagen content. *JPEN* 1980; 4:535–538.

17. Windsor JA, Knight GS, Hill GL: Wound healing response in surgical patients: Recent food intake is more important than nutritional status. *Br J Surg* 1988; 75:135–137.

18. Schroeder D, Gillanders L, Mahr K, et al: Effects of immediate postoperative enteral nutrition on body composition, muscle function, and wound healing. *JPEN* 1991; 15:376–383.

19. Haydock DA, Hill GL: Improved wound healing response in surgical patients receiving intravenous nutrition. *Br J Surg* 1987; 74:320–323.

20. Law NW, Ellis H: The effect of parenteral nutrition on the healing of abdominal wall wounds and colonic anastomoses in protein-malnourished rats. *Surgery* 1990; 107:449–454.

21. Collins JP, Oxby CB, Hill GL: Intravenous amino acids and intravenous hyperalimentation as protein-sparing therapy after major surgery. A controlled trial. *Lancet* 1978; 1:788–791.

22. Delmi M, Rapin CH, Bengoa JM, et al: Dietary supplementation in elderly patients with fractured neck of the femur. *Lancet* 1990; 1:1013–1016.

23. Bastow MD, Rawlings J, Allison SP: Benefits of supplementary tube feeding after fractured neck of femur: A randomized controlled trial. *BMJ* 1983; 287:1589–1592.

24. Smith RC, Hartemink RJ, Hollinshead JW, et al: Fine-bore jejunostomy feeding following major abdominal surgery: A controlled randomized clinical trial. *Br J Surg* 1985; 72:458–461.

25. Tkatch L, Rapin CH, Rizzoli R, et al: Benefits of oral protein supplementation in elderly patients with fracture of the proximal femur. *J Am Coll Nutr* 1992; 11:519–525.

26. Chiarelli A, Enzi G, Casadei A, et al: Very early nutrition supplementation in burned patients. *Am J Clin Nutr* 1990; 51:1035–1039.

27. Jenkins M, Gottschlich M, Alexander JW, et al: Effect of immediate enteral feeding on the hypermetabolic response following severe burn injury. *JPEN* 1989; 13(suppl):12.

28. Jenkins M, Gottschlich M, Baumer T,

et al: Enteral feeding during operative procedures. *JPEN* 1991; 15(suppl):22.

29. Moore EE, Jones TN: Benefits of immediate jejunostomy feeding after major abdominal trauma—a prospective randomized study. *J Trauma* 1986; 26:874–881.

30. Grahm TW, Zadrozny DB, Harrington T: The benefits of early jejunal hyperalimentation in the head-injured patient. *Neurosurgery* 1989; 25:729–735.

31. Ryan JA, Page CP, Babcock L: Early postoperative jejunal feeding of an elemental diet in gastrointestinal surgery. *Am Surg* 1981; 47:393–403.

32. Sagar S, Harland P, Shields R: Early postoperative feeding with elemental diet. *BMJ* 1979; 1:293–295.

33. Daly JM, Lieberman MD, Goldfine J, et al: Enteral nutrition with supplemental arginine, RNA, and omega-3 fatty acids in patients after operation: Immunologic, metabolic, and clinical outcome. *Surgery* 1992; 112:56–67.

34. Peck MD, Alexander JW: Interaction of protein and zinc malnutrition with the murine response to infection. *JPEN* 1992; 16:232–235.

35. Peck MD, Babcock GF, Alexander JW: The role of protein and calorie restriction in outcome from *Salmonella* infection in mice. *JPEN* 1992; 16:561–565.

36. McMurray DN, Yetley EA, Burch T: Effect of malnutrition and BCG vaccination on macrophage activation in guinea pigs. *Nutr Res* 1981; 1:373–384.

37. Christadoss P, Talal N, Lindstrom J, et al: Suppression of cellular and humoral immunity to T-dependent antigens by calorie restriction. *Cell Immunol* 1984; 88:1–8.

38. Heresi G, Chandra RK: Effects of severe calorie restriction on thymic factor activity and lymphocyte stimulation response in rats. *J Nutr* 1980; 110:1888–1893.

39. Chandra RK: Nutrition, infection and immunity: Present knowledge and future directions. *Lancet* 1983; 1:688–691.

40. Petersen SR, Kudsk KA, Carpenter G, et al: Malnutrition and immunocompetence: Increased mortality following an infectious challenge during hyper-alimentation. *J Trauma* 1981; 21:528–533.

41. Cooper WC, Good RA, Mariani T: Effects of protein insufficiency on immune responsiveness. *Am J Clin Nutr* 1974; 27:647–664.

42. Price P, Bell RG: The toxicity of inactivated bacteria and endotoxin in mice suffering from protein malnutrition. *J R E Soc* 1975; 18:230–243.

43. Sobrado J, Maiz A, Kawamura I, et al: Effect of dietary protein depletion on nonspecific immune responses and survival in the guinea pig. *Am J Clin Nutr* 1983; 37:795–801.

44. Alexander JW: Early enteral feeding—Animal studies. Presented at the 17th Clinical Congress, American Society for Parenteral and Enteral Nutrition, San Diego, Calif, 1993, pp 58–60.

45. Deitch EA, Ma WJ, Ma L, et al: Protein malnutrition predisposes to inflammatory-induced gut-origin septic states. *Ann Surg* 1990; 211:560–568.

46. Deitch EA, Winterton J, Li M, et al: The gut as a portal of entry for bacteremia: Role of protein malnutrition. *Ann Surg* 1987; 205:681–692.

47. McArdle AH, Palmason C, Brown RA, et al: Early enteral feeding of patients with major burns: Prevention of catabolism. *Ann Plast Surg* 1984; 13:396–401.

48. Jenkins M, Gottschlich M, Alexander JW, et al: Effect of immediate enteral feeding on the hypermetabolic response following severe burn injury. *JPEN* 1989; 13(suppl):12.

49. Rapp RP, Young B, Twyman D, et al: The favorable effect of early parenteral feeding on survival in head-injured patients. *J Neurosurg* 1983; 58:906–912.

50. Yeung CK, Young GA, Hackett AF, et al: Fine-needle catheter jejunostomy—an assessment of a new method of nutritional support after major gastrointestinal surgery. *Br J Surg* 1979; 66:727–732.

51. Young GA, Hill GL: A controlled study of protein-sparing therapy after excision of the rectum: Effects of intravenous amino acids and hyperalimentation on body composition and plasma amino acids. *Ann Surg* 1980; 192:183–191.

52. Abel RM, Fischer JE, Buckley MJ, et al: Malnutrition in cardiac surgery patients: Results of a prospective randomized evaluation of early postoperative parenteral nutrition. *Arch Surg* 1976; 111:45–50.

53. Mullen JL, Buzby GP, Matthews DC, et al: Reduction of operative morbidity and mortality by combined preoperative and postoperative nutritional support. *Ann Surg* 1980; 192:604–613.

54. Detsky AS, Baker JP, O'Rourke K, et al: Perioperative parenteral nutrition: A meta-analysis. *Ann Intern Med* 1987; 107:195–203.

55. American College of Physicians: Perioperative parenteral nutrition. *Ann Intern Med* 1987; 107:252–253.

56. Veterans Affairs Total Parenteral Nutrition Cooperative Study Group: Perioperative total parenteral nutrition in surgical patients. *N Engl J Med* 1991; 325:525–532.

57. Allison SP: Nutritional Support—Efficacy versus cost. *Nutr Int* 1987; 3:19–24.

58. Bower RH, Talamini MA, Sax HC, et al: Postoperative enteral versus parenteral nutrition: A randomized controlled trial. *Arch Surg* 1986; 121:1040–1045.

59. Sako K, Lore J, Kaufman S, et al: Parenteral hyperalimentation in surgical patients with head and neck cancer—a randomized study. *J Surg Oncol* 1981;16:390–402.

60. Fletcher JP, Little JM: A comparison of parenteral nutrition and early postoperative enteral feeding on the nitrogen balance after major surgery. *Surgery* 1986; 100:21–24.

61. Gallagher J, Schermbeck J, Dixon L, et al: Aggressive early management of malnutrition in hip fracture patients. *JPEN* 1992; 16(suppl):19.

62. Alexander JW, MacMillan BG, Stinnett JD, et al: Beneficial effects of aggressive protein feeding in severely burned children. *Ann Surg* 1980; 192:505–517.

63. Klein S, Simes J, Blackburn GL: Total parenteral nutrition and cancer clinical trials. *Cancer* 1986; 58:1378–1386.

64. American College of Physicians: Parenteral nutrition in patients receiving cancer chemotherapy. *Ann Intern Med* 1989; 110:734–736.

65. Hays DM, Merritt RJ, White L, et al: Effect of total parenteral nutrition on marrow recovery during induction therapy for acute nonlymphocytic leukemia in childhood. *Med Pediatr Oncol* 1983; 11:134–140.

66. Weisdorf S, Hofland C, Sharp HL, et al: Total parenteral nutrition in bone marrow transplantation: A clinical evaluation. *J Pediatr Gastroenterol Nutr* 1984; 3:95–100.

67. Weisdorf SA, Lysne J, Wind D, et al: Positive effect of prophylactic total parenteral nutrition on long-term outcome of bone-marrow transplantation. *Transplantation* 1987; 43:833–838.

68. Reilly J, Mehta R, Teperman L, et al: Nutritional support after liver transplantation: A randomized prospective study. *JPEN* 1990; 14:386–391.

69. Kalfarentzos FE, Karavias DD, Karatzas TM, et al: Total parenteral nutrition in severe acute pancreatitis. *J Am Coll Nutr* 1991; 10:156–162.

70. Zaloga GP: Studies comparing intact protein, peptide, and amino acid formulas, in Bounous G (ed): *Uses of Elemental Diets in Clinical Situations.* Boca Raton, Fla, CRC Press, 1993, pp 201–217.

71. Buchan AM: Do NMDA antagonists protect against cerebral ischemia: Are clinical trials warranted? *Cerebrovasc Brain Metab Rev* 1990; 2:1–26.

72. Weiss JH, Hartley DM, Koh J, et al: The calcium channel blocker nifedipine attenuates slow excitatory amino acid neurotoxicity. *Science* 1990; 247:1474–1477.

73. Proceedings of an international glutamine symposium: Glutamine metabolism in health and disease—Basic science and clinical aspects. *JPEN* 1990; 14(suppl):39–146.

74. Hwang TL, O'Dwyer ST, Smith RJ, et al: Preservation of small bowel mucosa using glutamine enriched parenteral nutrition. *Surg Forum* 1986; 37:56–58.

75. Souba WW, Smith RJ, Wilmore DW: Glutamine metabolism by the intestinal tract. *JPEN* 1985; 9:608–617.

76. Barbul A: Arginine—Biochemistry, physiology, and therapeutic implications. *JPEN* 1986; 10:227–238.

77. Barbul A: Arginine and immune function. *Nutrition* 1990; 6(suppl):53–58.

78. Barbul A, Fishel RS, Shimazu S, et al: Intravenous hyperalimentation with high arginine levels improves wound healing and immune function. *J Surg Res* 1985; 31:328–334.

79. Palacio JC, Rombeau JL: Dietary fiber—A brief review and potential application to enteral nutrition. *Nutr Clin Pract* 1990; 5:99–106.

80. Settle RG: Short-chain fatty acids and their potential role in nutritional support. *JPEN* 1988; 12(suppl):104–107.

81. Rombeau JL: Colonic infusions of short-chain fatty acids. *JPEN* 1988; 12(suppl):102–103.

82. Zaloga G: Nutrition and prevention of systemic infection. *Crit Care State Art* 1991; 12:31–79.

83. Kinsella JE, Lokish B: Dietary lipids, eicosanoids, and the immune system. *Crit Care Med* 1990; 18:(suppl):94–113.

84. Meydani SN, Nicolosi RJ, Hayes KC: Effect of long term feeding of corn oil or coconut oil on immune response and prostaglandin E_2 synthesis on squirrel and cebus monkeys. *Nutr Res* 1985; 5:993–1002.

85. Wan JMF, Teo TC, Babayan VK, et al: Lipids and the development of immune dysfunction and infection. *JPEN* 1988; 12(suppl):43.

86. Van Buren CT, Rudolph FB, Kulkarni A, et al: Reversal of immunosuppression induced by a protein-free diet. Comparison of nucleotides, fish oil, and arginine. *Crit Care Med* 1990; 18(suppl):114–117.

87. Kudsk KA, Carpenter G, Petersen S, et al: Effect of enteral and parenteral feeding in malnourished rats with *E. coli*–hemoglobin peritonitis. *J Surg Res* 1981; 31:105–110.

88. Kudsk KA, Stone JM, Carpenter G, et al: Enteral and parenteral feeding influences mortality after hemoglobin–*E. coli* peritonitis in normal rats. *J Trauma* 1983; 23:605–609.

89. Petersen SR, Kudsk KA, Carpenter G, et al: Malnutrition and immunocompetence: Increased mortality following an infectious challenge during hyperalimentation. *J Trauma* 1981; 21:528–533.

90. Kudsk KA, Stone JM, Carpenter G, et al: Effects of enteral and parenteral feeding of malnourished rats on body composition. *J Trauma* 1982; 22:904–906.

91. Zaloga GP, Knowles R, Black KW, et al: Total parenteral nutrition increases mortality after hemorrhage. *Crit Care Med* 1991; 19:54–59.

92. Zaloga GP, Roberts P, Black KW, et al: Gut bacterial translocation/dissemination explains the increased mortality produced by parenteral nutrition following methotrexate. *Circ Shock* 1993; 39:263–268.

93. Adams S, Dellinger EP, Wertz MJ, et al: Enteral versus parenteral nutritional support following laparotomy for trauma: A randomized prospective trial. *J Trauma* 1986; 26:882–891.

94. Peterson VM, Moore EE, Jones TN, et al: Total enteral nutrition versus total parenteral nutrition after major torso injury: Attenuation of hepatic protein reprioritization. *Surgery* 1988; 104:199–207.

95. Moore FA, Moore EE, Jones TN, et al: TEN versus TPN following major abdominal trauma—Reduced septic morbidity. *J Trauma* 1989; 29:916–923.

96. Kudsk KA, Croce MA, Fabian TC, et al: Enteral versus parenteral feeding. Effects on septic morbidity after blunt and penetrating abdominal trauma. *Ann Surg* 1992; 215:503–513.

97. Moore FA, Feliciano DV, Andrassy RJ, et al: Early enteral feeding, compared with parenteral, reduces postoperative septic complications. The results of a meta-analysis. *Ann Surg* 1992; 216:172–183.

98. Herndon DN, Barrow RE, Stein M, et al: Increased mortality with intravenous supplemental feeding in severely burned patients. *J Burn Care Rehabil* 1989; 10:309–313.

99. Rapp RP, Young B, Twyman D, et al: The favorable effect of early parenteral feeding on survival in head-injured patients. *J Neurosurg* 1983; 58:906–912.

100. Hadley MN, Grahm TW, Harrington T, et al: Nutritional support and neurotrauma: A critical review of early nutrition in forty-five acute head injury patients. *Neurosurgery* 1986; 19:367–372.

101. Young B, Ott L, Twyman D, et al: The effect of nutritional support on outcome from severe head injury. *J Neurosurg* 1987; 67:668–676.

102. Detsky AS, Baker JP, O'Rourke K, et al: Perioperative parenteral nutrition: A meta-analysis. *Ann Intern Med* 1987; 107:195–203.

103. Smith RC, Hartemink R: Improvement of nutritional measures during preoperative parenteral nutrition in patients selected by the prognostic nutritional index: A randomized controlled trial. *JPEN* 1988; 12:587–591.

104. McArdle AH, Palmason C, Morency I, et al: A rationale for enteral feeding as the preferable route for hyperalimentation. *Surgery* 1981; 90:616–623.

105. Muggia-Sullam M, Bower RH, Murphy RF, et al: Postoperative enteral versus parenteral nutritional support in gastrointestinal surgery. *Am J Surg* 1985; 149:106–111.

106. Fletcher JP, Little JM: A comparison of parenteral nutrition and early postoperative enteral feeding on the nitrogen balance after major surgery. *Surgery* 1986; 100:21–24.

107. Bower RH, Talamini MA, Sax H, et al: Postoperative enteral vs parenteral nutrition. *Arch Surg* 1986; 121:1040–1045.

108. The Veterans Affairs Total Parenteral Nutrition Cooperative Study Group: Perioperative total parenteral nutrition in surgical patients. *N Engl J Med* 1991; 325:525–532.

109. Cerra FB, McPherson JP, Konstantinides FN, et al: Enteral nutrition does not prevent multiple organ failure syndrome (MOFS) after sepsis. *Surgery* 1988; 104:727–733.

110. Koretz RL: Parenteral nutrition: Is it oncologically logical? *J Clin Oncol* 1984; 2:534–538.

111. Klein S, Simes J, Blackburn GL: Total parenteral nutrition and cancer clinical trials. *Cancer* 1986; 58:1378–1386.

112. Position paper: Parenteral nutrition in patients receiving cancer chemotherapy. *Ann Intern Med* 1989; 110:734–736.

113. Weisdorf SA, Lysne J, Wind D, et al: Positive effect of prophylactic total parenteral nutrition on long-term outcome of bone marrow transplantation. *Transplantation* 1987; 43:833–838.

114. Szeluga DJ, Stuart RK, Brookmeyer R, et al: Nutritional support of bone marrow transplant recipients: A prospective randomized clinical trial comparing total parenteral nutrition to an enteral feeding program. *Cancer Res* 1987; 47:3309–3316.

115. Health and public policy committee: Perioperative parenteral nutrition. *Ann Intern Med* 1987; 107:252–253.

116. Moghissi K, Hornshaw J, Teasdale PR, et al: Parenteral nutrition in carcinoma of the esophagus treated with surgery: Nitrogen balance and clinical studies. *Br J Surg* 1977; 64:125–128.

117. Holter AR, Fischer JE: The effects of hyperalimentation on complications in patients with carcinoma and weight loss. *J Surg Res* 1977; 23:31–34.

118. Heatley RV, Lewis MH, Williams RHP: Pre-operative intravenous feeding—a controlled trial. *Postgrad Med J* 1979; 55:541–545.

119. Thompson BR, Julian TB, Stremple JT: Peri-operative total parenteral nutrition in patients with gastrointestinal cancer. *J Surg Res* 1981; 30:497–500.

120. Muller JM, Dienst C, Brenner U, et al: Preoperative parenteral feeding in patients with gastrointestinal carcinoma. *Lancet* 1982; 1:68–71.

121. Lim STK, Choa RG, Lam KH, et al: Total parenteral nutrition versus gastrostomy in the preoperative preparation of patients with carcinoma of the oesophagus. *Br J Surg* 1981; 68:69–72.

122. Abel RM, Fischer JE, Buckley MJ, et al: Malnutrition in cardiac surgical patients: Results of a prospective randomized evaluation of early postoperative parenteral nutrition. *Arch Surg* 1976; 111:45–50.

123. Collins JP, Oxby CB, Hill GL: Intravenous amino acids and intravenous hyperalimentation as protein sparing therapy after major surgery. A controlled clinical study. *Lancet* 1978; 1:788–791.

124. Mullen JL, Buzby GP, Matthews DC, et al: Reduction of operative morbidity

and mortality by combined preoperative and postoperative nutritional support. *Ann Surg* 1980; 192:604–613.

125. Daly JM, Massar E, Giacco G, et al: Parenteral nutrition in esophageal cancer patients. *Ann Surg* 1982; 196:203–208.

126. McGeer AJ, Detsky AS, O'Rourke K: Parenteral nutrition in cancer patients undergoing chemotherapy: A meta-analysis. *Nutrition* 1990; 6:233–240.

127. Dickinson RJ, Ashton MG, Axon ATR, et al: Controlled trial of intravenous hyperalimentation and total bowel rest as an adjunct to the routine therapy of acute colitis. *Gastroenterology* 1980; 79:1199–1204.

128. Lochs H, Meryn S, Marosi L, et al: Has total bowel rest a beneficial effect in the treatment of Crohn's disease? *Clin Nutr* 1983; 21:61–64.

129. Greenberg GR, Fleming CR, Jeejeebhoy KN, et al: Controlled trial of bowel rest and nutritional support in the management of Crohn's disease. *Gut* 1988; 29:1309–1315.

130. McIntyre PB, Powell-Tuck J, Wood SR, et al: Controlled trial of bowel rest in the treatment of severe acute colitis. *Gut* 1986; 27:481–485.

131. Jones VA: Comparison of total parenteral nutrition and elemental diet in induction of remission of Crohn's disease. *Dig Dis Sci* 1987; 32(suppl):100–107.

132. Greenberg GR, Fleming CR, Jeejeebhoy KN, et al: Controlled trial of bowel rest and nutritional support in the management of Crohn's disease. *Gut* 1988; 29:1309–1315.

133. Cravo M, Camilo ME, Correia JP: Nutritional support in Crohn's disease: Which route? *Am J Gastroenterol* 1991; 86:317–321.

134. Abad-Lacruz A, Gonzalez-Huis F, Esteve M, et al: Liver function tests abnormalities in patients with inflammatory bowel disease receiving artificial nutrition: A prospective randomized study of total enteral nutrition vs total parenteral nutrition. *JPEN* 1990; 14:618–621.

135. Sitzmann JV, Converse RL, Bayless TM: Favorable response to parenteral nutrition and medical therapy in Crohn's colitis. *Gastroenterology* 1990; 99:1647–1652.

136. Culpepper-Morgan JA, Floch MH: Bowel rest or bowel starvation: Defining the role of nutritional support in the treatment of inflammatory bowel diseases. *Am J Gastroenterol* 1991; 86:269–271.

137. Tarazi R, Steiger E: Enterocutaneous fistulas, in Kinney JM, Jeejeebhoy KN, Hill GL, et al (eds): *Nutrition and Metabolism in Patient Care.* Philadelphia, WB Saunders, 1988, pp 243–257.

138. Hamilton RF, Davis WC, Stephenson DV, et al: Effects of hyperalimentation on upper gastrointestinal tract secretions. *Arch Surg* 1971; 102:340–352.

139. Wolfe BM, Keltner RM, Willman VL: Intestinal fistula output in regular, elemental, and intravenous alimentation. *Am J Surg* 1972; 124:803–806.

140. Fischer JF: The management of high-output intestinal fistulas. *Adv Surg* 1975; 9:139–176.

141. Voitk AJ, Echave V, Brown RA, et al: Elemental diet in the treatment of fistulas of the alimentary tract. *Surg Gynecol Obstet* 1973; 137:68–72.

142. Rocchio MA, Cha C, Haas KF, et al: Use of chemically defined diets in the management of patients with high output gastrointestinal cutaneous fistulas. *Am J Surg* 1974; 127:148–156.

143. Bury KD, Stephens RV, Randall HT: Use of a chemically defined liquid elemental diet. *Am J Surg* 1971; 121:174–183.

144. Graham JA: Conservative treatment of gastrointestinal fistulas. *Surg Gynecol Obstet* 1977; 144:512–514.

145. Silberman H, Granson M, Fong G, et al: Management of external gastrointestinal fistulas with glucose and lipids. *Surg Gynecol Obstet* 1980; 150:856–858.

146. Reber HA, Roberts C, Way LW, et al: Management of external gastrointestinal fistulas. *Ann Surg* 1978; 188:460–467.

147. Soeters PB, Ebeid AM, Fischer JE: Review of 404 patients with gastrointestinal fistulas: Impact of parenteral

nutrition. *Ann Surg* 1979; 190:189–202.

148. Deitel M: Nutritional management of external gastrointestinal fistulas. *Can J Surg* 1976; 19:505–511.

149. Slaff J, Jacobson D, Tillman CR, et al: Protease-specific suppression of pancreatic exocrine secretion. *Gastroenterology* 1984; 87:44–52.

150. Green GM, Lyman RL: Feedback regulation of pancreatic enzyme secretion as a mechanism for trypsin inhibitor–induced hypersecretion in rats. *Proc Exp Biol Med* 1972; 140:6–12.

151. Kelly GA, Nahrwold DL: Pancreatic secretion in response to an elemental diet and intravenous hyperalimentation. *Surg Gynecol Obstet* 1976; 143:87–91.

152. Stabile BE, Debas HT: Intravenous versus intraduodenal amino acids, fats, and glucose as stimulants of pancreatic secretion. *Surg Forum* 1981; 32:224–226.

153. Stabile BE, Borzatta M, Stubbs RS: Pancreatic secretory responses to intravenous hyperalimentation and intraduodenal elemental and full liquid diets. *JPEN* 1984; 8:377–380.

154. Bodoky G, Harsanyi L, Pap A, et al: Effect of enteral nutrition on exocrine pancreatic function. *Am J Surg* 1991; 161:144–148.

155. Sarles H, Sahel J, Staub JL, et al: Chronic pancreatitis, in Howat HT, Sarles H (eds): *The Exocrine Pancreas*. London, WB Saunders, 1979, pp 402–439.

156. Isaksson G, Ihse I: Pain reduction by oral pancreatic enzyme preparation in chronic pancreatitis. *Dig Dis Sci* 1983; 28:97–102.

157. Goodgame JT, Fischer JE: Parenteral nutrition in the treatment of acute pancreatitis: Effect on complications and mortality. *Ann Surg* 1977; 186:651–658.

158. Grant JP, James S, Grabowski V, et al: Total parenteral nutrition in pancreatic disease. *Ann Surg* 1984; 200:627–631.

159. Kalfarentzos FE, Karavias DD, Karatzas TM, et al: Total parenteral nutrition in severe acute pancreatitis. *J Am Coll Nutr* 1991; 10:156–162.

160. Sax HC, Warner BW, Talamini MA, et al: Early total parenteral nutrition in acute pancreatitis: Lack of beneficial effects. *Am J Surg* 1987; 153:117–124.

161. McArdle AH, Echave W, Brown RA, et al: Effect of elemental diet on pancreatic secretion. *Am J Surg* 1974; 128:690–692.

162. Voitk A, Brown RA, Echave V, et al: Use of an elemental diet in the treatment of uncomplicated pancreatitis. *Am J Surg* 1973; 125:223–227.

163. Levine GM, Deren JJ, Steiger E, et al: Role of oral intake in maintenance of gut mass and disaccharide activity. *Gastroenterology* 1974; 67:975–982.

164. Johnson LR, Copeland EM, Dudrick SJ, et al: Structural and hormonal alterations in the gastrointestinal tract of parenterally fed rats. *Gastroenterology* 1975; 68:1177–1183.

165. Guedon C, Schmitz J, Lerebours E, et al: Decreased brush border hydrolase activities without gross morphologic changes in human intestinal mucosa after prolonged total parenteral nutrition of adults. *Gastroenterology* 1986; 90:373–378.

166. Thompson JS, Vaughan WP, Forst CF, et al: The effect of the route of nutrient delivery on gut structure and diamine oxidase levels. *JPEN* 1987; 11:28–32.

167. Hughes CA, Dowling RH: Speed of onset of adaptive mucosal hypoplasia and hypofunction in the intestine of parenterally fed rats. *Clin Sci* 1980; 59:317–327.

168. Kotler DP, Levine GM, Shiau YF: Effects of luminal nutrition and metabolic status on in-vivo glucose absorption. *Am J Physiol* 1981; 240:432–436.

169. Hosoda N, Nishi M, Nakagawa M, et al: Structural and functional alterations in the gut of parenterally or enterally fed rats. *J Surg Res* 1989; 47:129–133.

170. Czernichow B, Galluser M, Hasselmann M, et al: Effects of amino acids in mixtures given by enteral or parenteral route on intestinal morphology and hydrolases in rats. *JPEN* 1992; 16:259–263.

171. Morin CL, Ling V, Bourassa D: Small intestinal and colonic changes in-

duced by a chemically defined diet. *Dig Dis Sci* 1980; 25:123–128.

172. Hughes CA, Prince A, Dowling RH: Speed of change in pancreatic mass and in intestinal bacteriology of parenterally fed rats. *Clin Sci* 1980; 59:329–336.

173. Castillo RO, Pittler A, Costa F: Intestinal maturation in the rat: The role of enteral nutrients. *JPEN* 1988; 12:490–495.

174. Ford WD, Boelhouwer RU, King WW, et al: Total parenteral nutrition inhibits intestinal adaptive hyperplasia in young rats: Reversal by feeding. *Surgery* 1984; 96:527–534.

175. Morgan W, Yardley J, Luk G, et al: Total parenteral nutrition and intestinal development: A neonatal model. *J Pediatr Surg* 1987; 22:541–545.

176. Biasco G, Callegari C, Lami F, et al: Intestinal morphologic changes during oral refeeding in a patient previously treated with total parenteral nutrition for short bowel resection. *Am J Gastroenterol* 1984; 79:585–588.

177. Greene HL, McCabe DR, Merenstein GB: Protracted diarrhea and malnutrition in infancy; changes in intestinal morphology and disaccharidase activities during treatment with total intravenous nutrition or oral elemental diets. *J Pediatr* 1975; 87:695–704.

178. Orenstein SR: Enteral versus parenteral therapy for intractable diarrhea of infancy: A prospective randomized trial. *J Pediatr* 1986; 109:277–286.

179. Adams PR, Copeland EM, Dudrick SJ, et al: Maintenance of gut mass in bypassed bowel of orally vs parenterally nourished rats. *J Surg Res* 1978; 24:421–427.

180. Johnson LR, Lichtenberger LM, Copeland EM, et al: Action of gastrin on gastrointestinal structure and function. *Gastroenterology* 1975; 68:1184–1192.

181. Aynsley-Green A, Lucas A, Lawson GR, et al: Gut hormones and regulatory peptides in relation to enteral feeding, gastroenteritis, and necrotizing enterocolitis in infancy. *J Pediatr* 1990; 117(suppl):24–32.

182. Hughes CA, Bates T, Dowling RH: Cholecystokinin and secretin prevent the intestinal mucosal hypoplasia of total parenteral nutrition in the dog. *Gastroenterology* 1978; 75:34–41.

183. Lickley HLA, Track NS, Vranic M, et al: Metabolic responses to enteral and parenteral nutrition. *Am J Surg* 1978; 135:172–175.

184. Sagor GR, Ghatei MA, Al-Mukhtar MYT, et al: Evidence for a humoral mechanism after small intestinal resection. *Gastroenterology* 1983; 84:902–906.

185. Jacobs DO, Evans DA, Mealy K, et al: Combined effects of glutamine and epidermal growth factor on the rat intestine. *Surgery* 1988; 104:358–364.

186. Bragg LE, Hollingsed TC, Thompson JS: Urogastrone reduces gut atrophy during parenteral alimentation. *JPEN* 1990; 14:283–286.

187. Saito H, Trocki O, Alexander JW, et al: The effect of route of nutrient administration on the nutritional state, catabolic hormone secretion, and gut mucosal integrity after burn injury. *JPEN* 1987; 11:1–7.

188. Knodell RG, Steele NM, Cerra FB, et al: Effects of parenteral and enteral hyperalimentation on hepatic drug metabolism in the rat. *J Pharmacol Exp Ther* 1984; 229:589–597.

189. Knodell RG, Spector MH, Brooks DA, et al: Alterations in pentobarbital pharmacokinetics in response to parenteral and enteral alimentation in the rat. *Gastroenterology* 1980; 79:1211–1216.

190. Katayama T, Tanaka M, Tanaka K, et al: Alterations in hepatic mitochondrial function during total parenteral nutrition in immature rats. *JPEN* 1990; 14:640–645.

191. Charland SL, Dickerson RN, Rajter JJ, et al: The effect of sepsis on hepatic cytochrome P-450 activity in parenterally fed rats (abstract). *Clin Res* 1991; 39:682.

192. Zamir O, Nussbaum MS, Bhadra S, et al: The effect of enteral feeding on hepatic steatosis induced by total parenteral nutrition (TPN). *JPEN* 1993; 17(suppl):30.

193. Deitch EA, Specian RD, Berg RD: Endotoxin-induced bacterial translocation and mucosal permeability: Role

of xanthine oxidase, complement activation, and macrophage products. *Crit Care Med* 1991; 19:785–791.

194. Baker JW, Deitch EA, Li M, et al: Hemorrhagic shock induces bacterial translocation from the gut. *J Trauma* 1988; 28:896–906.

195. Deitch EA, Bridges RM: Effect of stress and trauma on bacterial translocation from the gut. *J Surg Res* 1987; 42:536–542.

196. Maejima K, Deitch E, Berg R: Promotion by burn stress of the translocation of bacteria from the gastrointestinal tracts of mice. *Arch Surg* 1984; 119:166–172.

197. Alverdy JC, Aoys E, Moss GS: Total parenteral nutrition promotes bacterial translocation from the gut. *Surgery* 1988; 104:185–190.

198. Spaeth G, Berg RD, Specian RD, et al: Food without fiber promotes bacterial translocation from the gut. *Surgery* 1990; 108:240–247.

199. Illig KA, Ryan C, Hardy DJ, et al: Differential effects of partial enteral nutrition (PEN) on gut function. *JPEN* 1993; 17(suppl):25.

200. Reed L, Martin M, Kocka F, et al: Bacterial translocation following abdominal injury. *Circ Shock* 1992; 37:57.

201. Brathwaite CEM, Ross S, Nagele R, et al: Significance of bacterial translocation after multiple trauma with hemorrhagic shock. (abstract). *Circ Shock* 1992; 37:50.

202. Reed L, Martin M, Manglano R, et al: Bacterial translocation following abdominal trauma in humans. *Crit Care Med* 1991; 19(suppl):95.

203. Birkhahn RH, Renk CM: Immune response and leucine oxidation in oral and intravenous fed rats. *Am J Clin Nutr* 1984; 39:45–53.

204. Renk CM, Owens DR, Birkhahn RH, et al: Effect of intravenous or oral feeding on immunocompetence in traumatized rats (abstract). *JPEN* 1980; 4:587.

205. Meyer J, Yurt RW, Duhaney R, et al: Differential neutrophil activation before and after endotoxin infusion in enterally versus parenterally fed volunteers. *Surg Gynecol Obstet* 1988; 167:501–509.

206. Shou J, Lappin J, Minnard E, et al: Impairment of pulmonary macrophage function using total parenteral nutrition (TPN). *JPEN* 1993; 17(suppl):29.

207. Alverdy J, Chi HS, Sheldon GF: The effect of parenteral nutrition on gastrointestinal immunity: The importance of enteral stimulation. *Ann Surg* 1985; 202:681–684.

208. Rowlands BJ, Giddings AEB, Johnston AOB, et al: Nitrogen-sparing effect of different feeding regimens in patients after operation. *Br J Anaesth* 1977; 49:781–787.

209. Hulten L, Andersson H, Bosaeus I, et al: Enteral alimentation in the early postoperative course. *JPEN* 1980; 4:455–459.

210. Delany HM, Teh E, Dwarka B, et al: Infusion of enteral vs parenteral nutrients using high-concentration branch-chain amino acids: Effect on wound healing in the postoperative rat. *JPEN* 1991; 15:464–468.

211. Zaloga GP, Bortenschlager L, Black K: Early postoperative administration of enteral or parenteral nutrients improves wound healing. *JPEN* 1992; 16(suppl):28.

212. Fong Y, Marano MA, Barber A, et al: Total parenteral nutrition and bowel rest modify the metabolic response to endotoxin in humans. *Ann Surg* 1989; 210:449–457.

19

Enteral Nutrition

Kenneth A. Kudsk, M.D.

Gayle Minard, M.D.

Over the past 25 years, significant amounts of clinical and experimental research have been devoted to determining the impact of specialized nutritional support on the outcome of critically ill patients. Although nutritional support professionals have always agreed that "when the gut works, use it," patients were often given total parenteral nutrition (TPN) because it was easier and more reliable than enterally administered nutrients. This "traditional" approach to feeding of patients in our intensive care units (ICUs) has recently been questioned since TPN in general and specialized amino acid solutions in particular have failed to demonstrate significant effects upon the morbidity and mortality of critically ill patients. Certainly, there is a definite ICU population that will not tolerate enteral feeding because of difficulty with access, major dysfunction or loss of the gastrointestinal tract, or uncontrollable sepsis with multiple-system organ dysfunction and intolerance of feeding. With recent

interest in the use of the gastrointestinal tract and a commitment to enteral
delivery of nutrients, new techniques for
access and specialized formulas have
made enteral feeding feasible in the majority of critically ill patients. The commitment by health care professionals to
deliver nutrients enterally remains the
most important factor in successful enteral nutritional support.

RATIONALE FOR ENTERAL FEEDING

Sepsis remains the most important
clinical complication occurring in ICUs,
with a nosocomial infection rate of at
least 60% in patients requiring ICU admission for 6 days or longer. Sepsis
stimulates a hyperdynamic, hypermetabolic state that generates rapid mobilization of lean tissues from the somatic
muscle compartment, reprioritizes hepatic protein synthesis, and stimulates
various immunologic alterations.[1-3]
This "sepsis syndrome" is not always associated with intra-abdominal abscess,
pneumonia, or bacteremia, and a syndrome of "nonbacteremic clinical sepsis"
is not infrequently found in patients receiving potent antibiotics, multiple intravascular cannulas, ventilator support, and intravenous nutrition. In this
setting, multiple-organ dysfunction involving the pulmonary, renal, and hepatic systems has been well documented, but recently attention has been paid
to the gastrointestinal tract as a major
organ in this syndrome.[4-6] The gastrointestinal tract is not spared the edema,
increased vascular permeability, and
clinical dysfunction seen in other organs. Although gastrointestinal hemorrhage from diffuse gastritis has almost
been eliminated in the ICU population,
changes in motility, perme ability, and
normal architecture of the intestine
have, nevertheless, been well documented experimentally and clinically.

Acute starvation produces dramatic
histologic changes in the intestinal mucosa of animals with loss of villus
height, cellular proliferation, mucosal
protein, and overall mucosal mass.[7]
Most of these changes occur in the proximal portion of the small intestine in association with atrophy of the pancreas
and the proximal part of the stomach.
As the body diminishes the mass of
these metabolically expensive tissues
and functions, brush border disaccharidases simultaneously decrease. The mucosa increases its permeability to macromolecular proteins as the gastrointestinal tract of animals atrophies.[8] By
using models of fluorescein isothiocyanate–dextran as well as lactulose and mannitol,[9] starvation of the gut
with its attendant atrophy has been
shown to increase permeability to these
markers. Similar changes in permeability to lactulose and mannitol have been
noted in acute and chronically burned
patients and, more recently, trauma patients.[10] As patients recover from their
injuries, however, permeability returns
to normal.

Although still hypothetical, there has
been recent concern that the increase in
mucosal permeability may allow bacteria to translocate into the bloodstream
or lymphatics from the gastrointestinal
tract.[10] Mucosal permeability to macromolecular proteins increases with starvation alone[11]; however, there appears
to be no simultaneous breakdown of the
barrier to bacteria. Gut malnutrition in
the presence of endotoxin, hemorrhagic
shock, or burns is associated with a
much higher incidence of bacterial
translocation to systemic organs than
that produced by these insults in animal
models with normal gastrointestinal
tracts.[12] Changes in humoral and cellular immunity associated with the lack of
enteral nutrition have been implicated
as potential mechanisms in gut failure.[12, 13] Weakened barriers, changes in
bacterial populations and concentrations associated with increased gastrointestinal pH, decreased intestinal motility, and multiple antibiotics favor the
overgrowth of resistant, pathogenic or-

ganisms, including yeast, enterococci, and streptococci, as well as gram-negative organisms. Unfortunately, intravenous delivery of nutrients fails to maintain these barriers and increases susceptibility to infection in animals.[14, 15]

The results of these animal studies have been confirmed clinically. Alexander et al.[6] first noted that pediatric burn patients randomized to a high-protein enteral diet had a higher survival rate and fewer septic complications than did patients given a standard enteral diet. More recently, Herndon et al.[16] randomized 30 patients with burns covering more than 50% of their body to either intravenous supplementation with enteral feeding or enteral feeding alone. They noted that intravenous feeding reduced the amount of enteral calories consumed by patients. While both groups showed significant decreases in natural killer cell activity and T-helper/suppressor ratios vs. controls at 7 and 14 days following burns, the survival rate was 37% in the intravenously supplemented group vs. 74% in the enteral-fed group. Similar findings were noted in patients with closed head injuries. Rapp et al.[17] prospectively studied 38 patients randomized to receive TPN or standard enteral nutrition administered via nasogastric tube. Because of the gastric atony that occurs following severe closed head injury, many of the enterally fed patients were not able to tolerate early feeding. As a result, this study should be interpreted as comparing early TPN with late enteral feeding. Sepsis complicated the postinjury course of 6 of the 8 patients with delayed enteral feeding and a significant number of patients in the TPN group. A high sepsis rate of approximately 30% was noted in a follow-up study[18] by the same authors when 51 patients with severe closed head injury were randomized to receive early TPN vs. delayed enteral feeding. Both of these studies demonstrated no protective effect of delayed enteral feeding in patients with closed head inju-

ries. Subsequently, Grahm et al.[19] studied patients with severe closed head injury who were randomized to receive either early enteral feeding via a nasojejunal tube placed fluoroscopically within 36 hours of injury vs. delayed feeding into the stomach after gastric atony was resolved. Although there were no significant differences in age, Glasgow Coma Scale scores, or the type of neurologic injuries, the incidence of bacterial infection and the number of days in the ICU were significantly lower with early enteral feeding, thus suggesting that the early delivery of nutrients via the gastrointestinal tract was beneficial. These results were consistent with the Veteran Affairs (VA) cooperative[20] study of preoperative intravenous nutrition, which documented a significant rate of infectious complications in mildly and moderately malnourished patients and the beneficial effects of TPN only in severely malnourished patients. Even in the severely malnourished population, septic complications were frequent.

Patients sustaining penetrating and blunt trauma are the most intensively studied population to date. In 1986, Moore et al.[21] randomized a select population of trauma patients to early enteral nutrition vs. delayed TPN and documented a significant reduction in intra-abdominal abscess formation in patients randomized to receive enteral feeding. Subsequently, Moore et al.[22] investigated patients randomized to receive early enteral vs. early parenteral feeding and noted a significant reduction in postinjury septic complications in the enterally fed group. Recently, our group[23] randomized 98 patients sustaining severe blunt and penetrating trauma to enteral vs. parenteral feeding. Enterally fed patients sustained significantly fewer pneumonias, intra-abdominal abscesses, and line sepsis. Additionally, they experienced fewer infections per patient and fewer infections per infected patient. The severity of injury was noted to be an important factor since significant differences in

infection rates between groups occurred only in the most severely injured
patients with an Injury Severity Score
(ISS) greater than 20 or an Abdominal
Trauma Index (ATI) score greater than
24.

Critically ill patients are at increased
risk of septic complications developing
due to modern supportive therapies (antibiotics, intubation, vascular cannulation, and surgical intervention); there is
also a potential risk from themselves.
There is strong clinical evidence that the
route of nutrient support affects the
morbidity and potentially the mortality
of the critically ill patient. It appears
that delayed enteral feeding (>5 days)
fails to provide this protection but early
enteral feeding (<48 hours) appears to
be important in maintaining resistance
to these infections. Successful delivery
of enteral nutrition requires a planned
approach to the management of these
patients to ensure access to the gastrointestinal tract. Enteral feedings must
be delivered by using good clinical judgment since serious complications ranging from significant abdominal distension to wound dehiscence and frank
gastrointestinal necrosis can occur with
the unwise administration of nutrients.
Some patients will not tolerate the calculated goal rate of nutrients, and the
clinician must approach the critically ill
patient with caution, commitment, and
patience. Whether the nature of the nutrients is more beneficial than the route
of nutrition has not been determined,
but it is clear that delivery of nutrients
via the gastrointestinal tract influences
the outcome of critically ill patients.

ALGORITHM FOR ENTERAL DELIVERY OF NUTRIENTS IN CRITICALLY ILL PATIENTS

The decision to provide specialized
nutritional support depends upon an
assessment of prior nutritional status,
the period of expected restricted or inadequate voluntary intake, the adequacy of the gastrointestinal tract for
absorption, and the potential for complications. Nutritional assessment is
discussed in further detail in Chapter 2,
but it is clear that the patient with a recent history of weight loss, evidence of
depressed visceral and somatic protein
stores, and specific nutrient deficiencies
requires early administration of specialized nutritional support. It must be recognized that nutrition is but an adjunct
to overall patient care. Resuscitation, resection of necrotic bowel, drainage of
abscesses, appropriate therapy for
pneumonia or other invasive infection,
and debridement of necrotic tissue may
provide the most important aids to nutritional support by removing the trigger for the hypermetabolic state.

Assuming that maximal surgical and
medical management is undertaken,
the clinician must evaluate the usefulness of the gastrointestinal tract as a
means for delivery of enteral nutrition.
Clearly there are contraindications to
gastrointestinal feeding, such as gastrointestinal hemorrhage, which may require repeated endoscopies, angio-
graphic procedures, or early surgical
intervention. In addition, intestinal obstruction such as esophageal carcinoma, gastric outlet obstruction from
benign or malignant disease, or small-
bowel obstruction from adhesions, malignancy, or inflammation may be clear
contraindications to enteral feeding,
and early institution of intravenous nutrition should be considered. In general,
we have not attempted gastrointestinal
feeding of patients with partial intestinal obstruction except in the case of patients with inflammatory bowel disease
who are being aggressively treated with
steroids and antibiotic therapy. Abdominal distension by itself should not be
considered a contraindication since the
important factor is gastrointestinal motility; often patients distended with ascites or pseudo-obstruction of the colon
will have relatively normal small-bowel
function.

Motility is also an important issue in

the management of patients without intestinal obstruction. Frequently, sepsis or abdominal surgery produces "ileus" of the gastrointestinal tract. Most clinical experience supports the concept that the ileus is localized to the stomach and colon. If nutrients can be delivered directly to the small intestinal mucosa, absorption can occur without significant distension, discomfort, or complications in the majority of patients.[24] The ileus associated with severe closed head injury produces a gastric atony that resolves after approximately 4 days. If bilious nasogastric output exceeds 250 mL per 8 hours after day 4 in patients with closed head injuries, we clamp the nasogastric tube and check residuals every 4 hours. Not infrequently the nasogastric tube has migrated into the duodenum, or there is considerable reflux of duodenal contents into the stomach. By clamping the nasogastric tube, the stomach often empties without significant residuals, and gastric feeding can be started. Feedings should not be instituted through a standard large-bore nasogastric tube because the tube renders the gastroesophageal junction incompetent and increases the risk of reflux and aspiration.[25] This is particularly important in children or adults with a tendency toward gastrointestinal reflux by history. It is our practice to deliver all nutrients into the stomach via a small-bore nasoenteric tube by using continuous infusion while monitoring residuals.

Gastric feeding is preferred since less expensive, more concentrated, complex nutrient formulas can be administered while taking advantage of gastric control of emptying and the elements of digestion and absorption. Gastric feedings are certainly indicated in patients with an intact gastrointestinal tract and normal motility, but are also used in patients with short-gut syndrome (to maintain maximal gastrointestinal stimulation), inflammatory bowel disease involving the small intestine and colon or distal intestinal fistulas, or in

patients with burns or closed head injury who have no problems with gastric atony. Gastric feeding should not be given to patients who have abnormal gastric emptying (high nasogastric output unresponsive to tube clamping) or patients in whom pancreatic or biliary stimulation is contraindicated such as those with pancreatitis, pancreatic ascites, or a high-output pancreatic-duodenal fistula. Delivery into the stomach stimulates the maximal hormonal response of gastrin, secretin, cholecystokinin, etc., which in turn causes maximal secretion of the liver and pancreas.[26] Feeding into the duodenum reduces this hormonal stimulation by approximately half. With direct feeding into the intestine distal to the ligament of Treitz, there may be some increase in cholecystokinin, but there is almost no stimulation of pancreatic or biliary secretions. This was shown convincingly in patients who underwent cannulation of their pancreatic duct following pancreaticoduodenectomy. Jejunal feeding produced no more pancreatic drainage than did TPN.[27]

Postpyloric feeding should be used whenever gastric atony persists or when there is a risk of aspiration due to gastroesophageal reflux. Intragastric feeding is an invitation to disaster in patients who are unable to swallow and/or protect their airway. Some authors[28, 29] have noted that recurrent aspiration may not be reduced with postpyloric jejunal feeding; however, when previous aspiration has been documented, postpyloric feeding is the standard of care.

Postpyloric feeding is also necessary in patients with gastric atony from sepsis or diabetic paresis or in the first 4 or 5 days following closed head injury.[30] Burn patients will often tolerate gastric feeding if instituted promptly after admission to the hospital; however, if the gastrointestinal tract is not stimulated early, atony will develop within 24 hours. Duodenal or proximal intestinal fistulas are also contraindications to gastric feeding and indications for feeding distal to the fistula. A feeding tube can often be placed through an established proximal small-bowel fistula and advanced into the distal part of the lumen. Enteral feeding can then be instituted and well tolerated.

Postpyloric feedings can also be instituted in patients with active pancreatitis.[31] However, it is often difficult to position a nasoenteric tube beyond the ligament of Treitz in nonoperated patients during the early stages of acute pancreatitis or if the disease is complicated by pancreatic abscess or pseudocyst formation. Clearly, intragastric feedings are unsafe because of gastric atony, outlet obstruction secondary to the inflammatory process, and the potential for aggravating the inflammatory disease process.

Finally, many trauma patients should have cannulation of the gastrointestinal tract to allow postpyloric feeding. Our data[23] suggest that only patients with significant abdominal injuries and an ATI greater than 25 or those with a high ISS benefit from early enteral feeding. We also obtain postpyloric access during celiotomy for trauma in patients with lower ATI scores who have spinal cord injury, closed head injury, flail chest, multiple fractures, or significant pulmonary contusion because of the frequency of pneumonia, sepsis, prolonged ventilator support, and gastric atony. Since these extra-abdominal injuries prolong recovery and increase subsequent complications, postpyloric feeding avoids the problems of recurrent gastric atony and inadequate enteral nutrition during the hospitalization. Postpyloric access with either direct jejunostomy or transgastric jejunostomy may be obtained at the time of initial celiotomy in patients who will require multiple orthopedic operations (e.g., multiple open fractures), patients with perineal degloving injuries in whom repeated debridements and reconstructive surgery is necessary, or patients with other massive soft-tissue injuries requiring repeated operative debridement.[32] For these procedures, intragastric feedings

are usually discontinued 8 to 10 hours prior to general anesthesia, which severely limits the amount of calories and protein administered daily to these patients. In our experience, jejunal delivery of nutrients prior to the time of transport to the operating room has not resulted in aspiration or other complications during general anesthesia. Feedings are reinstituted immediately after surgery in hemodynamically stable patients.

In general, continuous feeding is used whether delivered into the stomach or small intestine in the acute phase of patients' illnesses. Gastric residuals should be checked every 4 hours; this is not necessary with jejunostomies. To ease nursing care, patients can be converted to bolus-type feedings via gastrostomy prior to discharge from the hospital. Because of the expense of infusion pumps for continuous jejunal infusion, only patients with recurrent episodes of aspiration due to gastroesophageal reflux should remain on jejunostomy tube feedings.

OPERATIVE PATIENTS

General Approach

The ideal time to gain enteral access is just prior to closure of the abdominal cavity following the definitive surgical procedure. There are some contraindications to enteral access, however.[33-41] For two reasons, it is unwise to cannulate the gastrointestinal tract of patients who have or are expected to have massive abdominal ascites in the postoperative period. First, there is the potential for contamination of the ascites with enteric bacteria; and second, during the formation of massive ascites and abdominal distension there is a possibility of dislodgement of the jejunostomy or gastrostomy from the anterior abdominal wall. It is also unwise to cannulate through areas involved with inflammatory bowel disease because of the potential for enterocutaneous fistulas. Diffuse suppurative peritonitis is also a relative contraindication, particularly if all of the gastrointestinal tract is severely inflamed and edematous. Severe immunosuppression is a contraindication because of the noted increased incidence of necrotizing fasciitis in this patient population. Finally, an irradiated bowel with signs of radiation enteritis should not be cannulated through the irradiated area because of the potential for complications. Fortunately, most irradiated patients have pathology limited to the distal part of the small bowel and distal portion of the colon and rectum, while the stomach or the proximal part of the intestine is normal.

The surgeon is frequently faced with the decision to obtain definitive enteral access by cannulating the stomach, the jejunum, both, or neither. If a relatively well nourished patient undergoes a surgical procedure in which the risk of complications is relatively small and it is expected that the patient will resume oral intake within 3 to 4 days with resolution of the ileus, enteral access is probably not necessary.[37] In those patients in whom there is a risk of complications from proximal anastomotic dehiscence, intra-abdominal sepsis, or prolonged ventilatory dependence or in patients with moderate to severe malnutrition in whom adequate oral intake may be delayed, obtaining enteral access is a wise decision. Even if a jejunostomy or gastrostomy is used only a short period of time postoperatively, the risk of complications is low with these surgical procedures. In patients in whom sepsis, pancreatitis, or obstruction at a gastric, duodenal, or proximal jejunal site is likely, gastrostomy is an inappropriate access for providing nutrition support. In these cases, gastrostomy is suitable only for gastric decompression; access distal to the pylorus with either a formal jejunostomy or a transgastric jejunostomy is more appropriate. Despite septic complications such as pneumonia or subdiaphragmatic abscess or the development of pancreatitis or proximal gastrointestinal complications, access dis-

tal to the ligament of Treitz ensures the ability to deliver nutrients to the small intestine. Since atony is usually limited to the stomach and colon, postpyloric access into the proximal part of the small intestine provides the most reliable means for intestinal feeding. Anastomosis in the colon or small bowel is not a contraindication to small-bowel feedings, although we delay feedings 3 to 4 days following an anastomosis in the mid or proximal portions of the small bowel.

Operative Jejunal Access

Surgical Techniques

The two most common types of jejunal access are a Witzel jejunostomy with a size 14, 16, or 18 F red rubber catheter and a needle catheter jejunostomy (NCJ) with a 16-gauge polyvinyl catheter. There are several advantages of large-bore red rubber catheters. First, they provide long-term enteral access through which both medications and tube feedings can be administered. If the tubes become occluded and have been in place at least a week, the catheters can usually be removed and replaced immediately with a tube of the same diameter. This is particularly valuable in debilitated patients needing chronic enteral access in whom aspiration from gastric feedings has been a problem or in patients in whom a prolonged postoperative recovery is expected, such as with major pancreaticoduodenal injuries, pancreatic abscesses, severe closed head injury, or the elderly with severe multiple trauma. NCJs are ideal for short-term enteral access and can be expected to remain patent for 3 to 6 weeks if strict nursing care is maintained following their placement. It is absolutely imperative that no medications be given via NCJs since crushed tablets can easily obstruct the tube and the elixirs in liquified medications such as KCl, etc., cause tube feedings to precipitate and rapidly block the tube. Unfortunately, once an NCJ is occluded, it is often permanently lost. Although flushing may open these catheters for short periods of time, in our experience, once an obstruction has occurred, the life span of NCJs is very short.

Enteral access for a jejunostomy should be obtained at a sufficient distance from the ligament of Treitz so that the jejunostomy will not be pulled away from the anterior abdominal wall if the abdomen should become maximally distended. Usually this is 15 to 20 cm distal to the ligament of Treitz. The intestine of most patients will tolerate either an NCJ or a red rubber catheter; however, when the bowel is very edematous, it is not always safe to place a red rubber catheter. If the small intestine can be easily wrapped around the red rubber catheter with a Witzel technique, the tube can be safely inserted. If the bowel is so edematous that wrapping it around the catheter would be difficult, only an NCJ should be placed. If the bowel is so indurated and edematous that it would not tolerate a Witzel tunnel around an NCJ, then no jejunostomy should be placed since the potential for leakage is high. The small intestine should be fixed to the anterior abdominal wall for 2 to 3 in. with at least three sutures so that torsion can be avoided. This will prevent one of the more common complications that occurred in jejunostomies that were fixed to the anterior abdominal wall with a single stitch. Our group has placed over 450 jejunostomies, and no episodes of torsion have occurred, although there was a single episode of volvulus of the distal portion of the small intestine around a jejunostomy tube site.

Witzel Jejunostomy.—If the decision is made to use a Witzel jejunostomy with a red rubber catheter, a pursestring 2-0 silk suture is inserted in the antimesenteric surface of the bowel at the selected site. Electrocautery is used to perforate the bowel wall, and the red rubber catheter is inserted so that all but approximately 5 to 7 cm of the tube exits the jejunum. Three centimeters to 5 cm of this externalized catheter is buried with interrupted Lembert sutures, and the needles are left on the distal and proximal sutures to sew the bowel to the anterior abdominal wall. The short, 2-cm segment of red rubber catheter is brought out through a stab wound in the anterior abdominal wall, and the jejunum is fixed to the parietal peritoneum with the two sutures. Another suture is used to fix the jejunum to the anterior abdominal wall just proximal to the tube and complete the seal around the red rubber catheter. A 2-0 silk suture secures the jejunostomy to the skin. Only a short amount of jejunostomy tube should protrude from the skin to minimize chances of dislodgement. In otherwise uncomplicated cases, tube feedings are begun the morning following surgery at 25 mL/hr.

Needle Catheter Jejunostomy.—After choosing a site in the bowel wall that will ensure a tension-free jejunostomy if distension occurs, a pursestring suture is placed and a 14-gauge needle inserted along the antimesenteric surface of the bowel for a distance of approximately 3 to 4 cm prior to entry into the lumen. The polyvinyl catheter and guidewire are inserted at least 18 in. into the small intestine through this needle, with the flexible end of the guidewire used as the leading point. We create a short Witzel tunnel over the external catheter in the bowel wall, although this is not described by most authors. Needles are left on three (proximal, mid, and distal) of the five Lembert sutures used to create the Witzel tunnel. A second 14-gauge needle is used to exit the NCJ from the peritoneal cavity. The catheter should exit at a slight angle rather than being brought out perpendicular to the abdominal wall to reduce the incidence of catheter kinking. The three previously described stay stitches are used to fix the jejunum to the anterior abdominal wall distal to the jejunotomy, and an additional stitch is placed proximal to the entrance point of the catheter to complete the seal. With this technique, there is no need for x-ray confirmation of placement, and we have had no episodes of displacement into the peritoneal cavity. If a catheter is accidentally withdrawn several inches postoperatively, there is sufficient length of catheter still residing in the jejunum to safely continue feeding.

To minimize the incidence of dislodgement, the catheter should be trimmed so that only a short segment extends onto the anterior abdominal wall. A 2-0 silk suture secures the catheter at the skin exit site, and a second suture is used to fix the wings of the jejunostomy needle to the anterior abdominal wall. A clear occlusive dressing placed over the entire catheter, except at the junction with the feeding apparatus, minimizes removal since there is little to be grasped. When this technique is used, the NCJ will survive 3 to 6 weeks without problems as long as the catheter is flushed every 4 to 6 hours and no medications are administered through it. To avoid catheter occlusion, the needle catheter should be treated as an inviolate line for feedings.

The two most common causes for NCJ occlusion are kinking at its exit from the fascia and clogging by tube feedings.[42] If the NCJ stops flowing within the first 3 days, there is usually a kink where the catheter exits the fascia. By flushing with a 10-cc syringe filled with normal saline as the catheter is withdrawn 1 to 2 in., the kink will be released, and flow will resume. The catheter should be pulled out until the kink is exposed and cut. The needle can be reattached to the catheter and sutured to the anterior abdominal wall. In our experience, in the few instances where the catheter has kinked, it has not reoccurred once repaired. If the NCJ occludes at 3 to 6 weeks, flushing with saline should be attempted, but it is unlikely that the catheter will function more than another week. A technique[43] has been described for using a guidewire to exchange the NCJ with a larger tube, but we have limited experience with this.

As mentioned above, liquid medications in the form of elixirs cause the nutrient formulas to precipitate and lead to rapid catheter occlusion. We attempted to increase the protein component of our tube feedings by adding a protein supplement (Promod). While this is easily infused through a red rubber catheter, it will rapidly occlude an NCJ. We have had extensive experience with fiber-containing formulas through NCJs, and at our institution they have not obstructed the catheters (see the section on diarrhea). However, the tubes must be irrigated with saline every 4 to 6 hours religiously.

Transgastric Jejunostomy.—Several transgastric jejunostomy tubes have been developed that allow a gastric suction port and jejunal feeding port to be placed through a single enterotomy in the stomach, the first of which was made by Moss Tubes, Inc. The technique is a modification of the Stamm gastrostomy. After a laparotomy incision is made, an appropriate site on the anterior stomach wall is chosen, along with a corresponding site on the abdominal wall. An incision is made on the abdominal wall and a Kelly clamp or Vanderbilt clamp passed through it. The transgastric jejunostomy tube is then pulled through the abdominal wall. One of the prepackaged kits provides a trocar that is passed from the intraperitoneal to the extraperitoneal side of the abdominal wall (Medical Innovations Inc. [MIC]). A "stent" is placed over the trocar, again from the inside out, and the trocar is removed. The transgastric jejunostomy tube is passed through the abdominal wall via the stent and the stent removed. Two pursestring sutures are placed in an appropriate spot on the anterior gastric wall, and a gastrotomy is made between them. The Moss transgastric jejunostomy tube is fed by hand through the pylorus into the duodenum. The MIC tube utilizes a slotted introducer that facilitates passage through the gastrotomy and pylorus into the jejunum. The intragastric balloon is filled with saline, the pursestring sutures are tied, and the stomach is fixed to the anterior abdominal wall. Most of these tubes have an external retention disk that is positioned to prevent migration of the feeding tube. Care should be taken to not put too much tension between the intragastric balloon and the disk in order to prevent gastric or abdominal wall ischemia. The transgastric jejunostomy tube allows gastric decompression at the same time as feeding distal to the ligament of Treitz.

Roux-en-Y Jejunostomy.—In a small population of patients, a permanent feeding jejunostomy can be constructed by using a Roux-en-Y technique, but this is rarely indicated initially for critically ill patients. The jejunum and mesentery are divided 20 cm beyond the ligament of Treitz and the end of the proximal part of the jejunum anastomosed to the distal portion some 40 to 50 cm distal to the site of jejunal division. The free jejunal end is brought out to the skin as a stoma.

Operatively Placed Nasojejunal Feeding Tube.—One final method of gaining postpyloric access can be obtained operatively. In patients requiring nutritional support for very short periods, a long nasoenteric tube can be passed distal to the ligament of Treitz. This eliminates enterotomy and allows early feeding postoperatively. The tube is inserted nasally by the anesthesiologist until it reaches the stomach. The surgeon directs the distal end of the tube through the pylorus and into the jejunum. It has all the disadvantages of nasoenteric tubes such as dislodgement, sinusitis, aspiration, etc., which are dealt with elsewhere in this chapter.

Enteral Feeding Via the Small Bowel

After obtaining small-bowel access, feeding should be started at a slow rate, usually about 25 cc/hr, provided that there are no contraindications.[44] Early small-bowel feedings should not be administered to patients following release of a small-bowel obstruction when the intestine is still edematous and fluid filled. Also, hemodynamically unstable patients should not be fed because of the potential for mucosal and intestinal necrosis, which occurs in 0.5% to 0.75% of patients. Small-bowel intestinal feedings should be immediately stopped if there is evidence of reflux of tube feeding into the stomach. For this reason, stomach decompression via the nasogastric or gastrostomy tube is indicated for at least the first 2 to 3 days.

Although some authors have maintained that abdominal distension is a contraindication to small-bowel feeding, we have proceeded at a slow rate of 15 to 25 cc/hr unless the cause of distension is fluid-filled loops of small bowel. Frequently, gastric or colonic dilatation causes the distension, but this is not a contraindication to small-bowel feeding. In fact, we have successfully used chemically defined diets to stimulate diarrhea and decompress colonic pseudo-obstruction in two patients. If there is no significant difficulty, tube feedings are continued.

Because of the potential for small-bowel necrosis, tube feedings are not begun in patients who are hemodynamic unstable, have a tachycardia of greater than 125, or are receiving inotropic drugs or vasopressors. The sole exception is low-dose dopamine, which may actually increase splanchnic blood flow. In patients who have been recently unstable, tube feedings are begun at 15 mL/hr for the first 12 hours and then progressed to 25 mL/hr. If tolerated, feedings are cautiously advanced to the goal rate. We do not advocate immediate enteral feeding in the recovery room but would rather wait in order to assess hemodynamic stability.

Complications of Postpyloric Feeding

Approximately 1% to 2% of patients undergoing jejunostomy will have serious complications.[45][46] Diarrhea, aspiration, occlusion of the catheter, bowel necrosis, and bowel obstruction related to the procedure have all been described. Each can be minimized by attention to technique and a logical approach to complications when they develop.

Mechanical Complications.—The most common complications associated with jejunostomy are dislodgement of the catheter, intraperitoneal migration of the tube, occlusion of the tube, and volvulus.[44, 45] As described above, fixation of the tube to the anterior abdominal wall will minimize the incidence of dislodgement. Many disoriented patients pull at tubes, and by using an occlusive dressing and keeping the external catheter short, this complication can be minimized. Volvulus can occur either by the distal part of the small bowel migrating superiorly over the tube in a medial-to-lateral direction or by twisting of the bowel at the jejunostomy site. The former can be minimized by aligning the jejunostomy site along the lateral edge of the rectus sheath rather than adjacent to the midline. We have only had one episode of volvulus of the small intestine over the jejunostomy in approximately 450 patients. The location of the jejunostomy was unclear in this case. We attach the bowel wall to the abdominal wall for 3 to 4 inches and have had no problems with torsion of the jejunostomy or displacement of the catheter into the peritoneal cavity. Occlusion of the catheter can be minimized by maintaining the NCJ as an inviolate line and only administering tube feedings through the catheter. If medications are given, the catheter should be flushed with 40 to 50 cc of water in order to reduce the possibility of subsequent occlusion. At no time should crushed tablets or viscous substances be given through the NCJ. Red rubber catheters will accept liquid medications as long as they are well flushed after administration.

Diarrhea.—In a randomized prospective study of severely injured trauma patients administered tube feeding, watery diarrhea that could compromise the skin developed in approximately 22% of patients.[23] Jones et al. studied 153 patients undergoing emergency laparotomy for major trauma, half of whom had NCJs.[35] A chemically defined diet was begun approximately 12 hours postoperatively and advanced both in volume and concentration at 8-hour intervals. Fifty percent of the patients had gastrointestinal complaints, the most frequent of which were cramping and abdominal distension. Diarrhea only occurred in 2 of the 71 patients administered the enteral diet. The symptoms were usually short-lived and resolved by decreasing the rate or concentration, thus demonstrating that adherence to a feeding schedule and daily monitoring together with reassurance by medical personnel allowed the majority of patients to tolerate full-scale NCJ feedings. Approximately 13% of patients never tolerated feedings and were converted to TPN regimens. Of these 11, most had a very high ATI, and the majority had injuries to the gastrointestinal tract itself. In another study,[47] patients with the most severe organ dysfunction, including pulmonary and renal insufficiency, had the greatest rate of intolerance. This implies that the magnitude of injury and the associated shock, ischemia, and hypoxemia produced gastrointestinal failure as part of the spectrum of multiple organ system failure. Patients who failed to tolerate enteral feeding also had the highest mortality rate.

Our approach to a patient with diarrhea is to first assess whether medications such as sorbitol or elixirs could be causing the problem. Liquid medications are the most frequent culprit,[48] and aminophylline given in a sorbitol-containing elixir is a major cause of these symptoms. If necessary, these drugs should be administered in an intravenous form. A stool sample is sent for *Clostridium difficile* detection, and if the stools are heme-positive, proctoscopy and/or sigmoidoscopy are performed to rule out pseudomembranous enterocolitis. Transient diarrhea develops in the majority of patients as the rate of feeding is advanced. If diarrhea persists, the rate is decreased to the highest rate tolerated by the patient, and again attempts are made to increase the rate over subsequent days. Not infrequently, metoclopramide[49] has been administered to patients who are being fed via a nasoenteric tube in order to stimulate gastric emptying, and this should not be overlooked as a cause of diarrhea. When treatment with the drug is stopped, the diarrhea frequently resolves.

Hypoalbuminemia[50-53] has been implicated as a source of diarrhea secondary to edema within the villi. Patterson et al.[50] studied this relationship but could find no statistical difference in the frequency of diarrhea in patients with an albumin concentration less than or greater than 2.5 g/dL. Patients with an albumin content less than 2.5 g/dL received 80% of their estimated requirements 97% of the time. In a recent study from our institution,[54] an intact protein diet was compared with one of the specialty peptide formulas in patients with hypoalbuminemia. There appeared to be no increase in diarrhea with the intact protein diet and, in general, a low rate of diarrhea despite hypoalbuminemia.

Recently, attention has been given to fiber-containing diets to control diarrhea induced by tube feeding.[55, 56] If the previously described maneuvers have been unsuccessful, we manage diarrhea by switching patients to a fiber-containing diet. In our experience, the majority of patients will respond to this therapy. Soluble fiber provides the substrate for short-chain fatty acid production by gut bacteria, which serves as a specific energy fuel for the colonic enterocyte. Since the colonic enterocyte is important in water absorption, increasing its fuel supply may be part of the mechanism by which fiber administration controls diarrhea. Although the use of fiber-containing diets to control diarrhea in patients fed via gastrostomy has met with mixed success, we have successfully used fiber-containing diets in NCJs.[57] With the initial fear that tube occlusion would occur with these diets, we reviewed 57 patients fed our hospital's low-bid, fiber-containing formula to determine the incidence of catheter occlusion and diarrhea. Forty-four of 57 catheters remained patent until oral feeding resumed, and an additional 8 catheters temporarily occluded but were reopened with flushes and remained patent for an additional 6.3 ± 3.1 days until patients were taking an oral diet. This was an overall success rate of 91%. Five catheters were lost after an average of 6.2 ± 1.8 days. Four of these 5 patients tolerated gastric feedings, but 1 patient required a permanent jejunostomy for nursing home placement. Four of the 5 complete occlusions occurred in the first 10 patients, and after reinstructing the nurses in standard flushing technique, the incidence of occlusion decreased significantly. During a randomized prospective study at our institution, diarrhea occurred in six of 57 (10.5%) patients given the fiber-containing diet vs. 11 of 51 (22%) patients fed a chemically defined diet. It appears that fiber-containing diets provide a clinical benefit to patients with diarrhea and that they can be administered through NCJs without a high rate of occlusion. Because of these advantages, fiber-containing diets have become the primary feeding through NCJs at our institution.

Fewer than 5% of patients have persistent diarrhea despite all therapy.[44] Administration of *Lactobacillus* has been used in these patients with mixed success, but often the patients cannot tolerate feeding at a full rate. In our patient population, we are satisfied if we administer at least two thirds of the calculated nutritional goals via the gastrointestinal tract and only start supplemental intravenous nutrition if 60% or fewer of the goals are met by 1 week following surgery.

Pneumatosis Intestinalis/Bowel Necrosis.—A rare but devastating complication of jejunal feeding is that of pneumatosis intestinalis and/or bowel necrosis. Tube feedings are not always associated with pneumatosis. It has been reported with many disease states, such as chronic obstructive pulmonary disease, cancer and chemotherapy, pseudomembranous enterocolitis, diverticulitis, bowel strangulation, intra-abdominal sepsis, and inflammatory bowel disease among others. When tube feedings have been implicated, it is postulated that hyperosmolar feedings, the introduction of bacteria through tube feedings into the upper portion of the jejunum, a low-flow state secondary to hypovolemia, or mesenteric ischemia due to shock, trauma, and sepsis may be contributory factors.

Although pneumatosis intestinalis is frequently a benign condition when associated with tube feedings, it may be accompanied by abdominal pain and distension along with diarrhea and occasionally gastrointestinal bleeding. In exceptional cases, it may be an early marker of gastrointestinal intolerance and subsequent bowel necrosis. Experimentally, splanchnic blood flow increases in response to enteral feeding, and in the conditions of a low-flow state, metabolic demands of the gastrointestinal tract stimulated by enteral feeding may not be met by limited splanchnic flow.[58]

In most cases, pneumatosis intestinalis follows a benign course. Smith and Sarr[59] evaluated its incidence in 217 patients following placement of NCJs during bariatric surgery or complicated abdominal procedures. In two (1%) patients pneumatosis developed, but responded to discontinuation of tube feedings and administration of parenteral antibiotics. Smith-Choban and Max[60] reported 5 cases of fatal small-bowel necrosis in 143 patients with jejunostomy tubes. In addition, significant abdominal distension developed in 17 patients. All of the patients had evidence of low-flow states, which should be a major contraindication to jejunostomy tube feeding.

We have cared for three patients in whom early jejunal feedings appeared to be an important etiologic factor in subsequent bowel necrosis. Each of these patients became massively distended within a few hours of the institution of enteral feeding and had reflux of tube feeding into the stomach. One of these patients had tolerated enteral feeding and a regular diet following a gunshot wound to the abdomen, but a small-bowel obstruction subsequently developed. Tube feedings were started soon after lysis of the adhesions, the patient's abdomen promptly became distended, and necrotic bowel was found at exploration. Two patients were hemodynamically unstable when feedings were instituted. In each of the patients acute onset of tachycardia with a heart rate greater than 130, an extremely elevated or depressed white count with a left shift, metabolic acidosis, significant fluid requirements, hypotension, and/or abdominal pain developed. As a result of this experience, postoperative jejunal feedings are not started in patients until they are hemodynamically stable and fluid and blood resuscitation is complete. If in the postoperative period a patient is significantly tachycardiac (a heart rate greater than 120), has marginal urine output, requires pressors or inotropic agents for blood pressure support, or is still requiring significant volumes of resuscitation fluids, jejunostomy feedings are not instituted. No tube feedings are given to patients following release of a small-bowel obstruction until mobilization of fluid and diuresis begin. If these principles are followed, the incidence of bowel necrosis should be minimized.

Metabolic Complications.—Hypokalemic metabolic alkalosis can develop in patients with severe diarrhea, but usually the supplementation of tube feeding with potassium is adequate to treat this problem. Severe hypophosphatemia is not commonly reported following enteral nutrition, but Hayek and Eisenberg[61] noted significant decreases in serum phosphate levels within 2 to 5 days after institution of isotonic enteral feedings. It is apparent that the enteral feeding of hypermetabolic or severely malnourished patients can produce significant hypophosphatemia and hypokalemia and that occasional supplementation of formulas with potassium phosphate is appropriate. Approximately 10% of our critically ill patients require supplemental K_2PO_4.

Operative Gastric Access

General Approach

Gastrostomy tubes are often placed in order to decompress the stomach and avoid the discomfort and complications of nasogastric tubes. They may also be used as a primary route of feeding in patients in whom immediate postoperative feeding is not necessary but in whom long-term access will be required.[44, 62] The benefits of gastric feeding include the ability to take advantage of all functions of the gastrointestinal tract, including controlled gastric emptying and normal absorptive processes, the reduced cost of complex formulas, and the ability to bolus-feed.

Gastrostomy is one of the oldest and most frequent operations performed by general surgeons, and the technique has been modified considerably since the first successful human gastrostomy by Verneuil in 1876. The advantages of avoiding a nasogastric tube are appreciated by both the patient and most surgeons.

Operative Gastrostomy Techniques

Gastrostomy tubes can be inserted by several methods. With the Witzel technique, an appropriate point in the anterior abdominal wall is chosen, a gastrostomy made, and the tube inserted. The stomach wall is invaginated over the tube with nonabsorbable Lembert sutures and fixed to the anterior abdominal wall. With the Stamm technique, two pursestring sutures, usually 2-0 silk, are placed in a circumferential manner. The first is placed 1 cm from the proposed puncture site; the second suture is placed 1 cm outside the first suture. This allows invagination of the gastric wall after the tube is placed into the stomach and the pursestring sutures are tied. As in the Witzel technique, the stomach is fixed to the anterior abdominal wall, and the gastrostomy tube is brought out through a separate incision. The Dragstedt gastrostomy is performed by wrapping the omentum around the gastrostomy tube between the stomach and the abdominal wall to prevent leakage. This is particularly valuable following a partial gastric resection when the stomach will not reach the abdominal wall.

Numerous types of catheters have been used, including red rubber catheters, Malecots, Foleys, dePezzars, and specially constructed tubes made by various manufacturers, most of which have inflatable gastric balloons. Although ardent supporters of each type exist, there are probably no major differences between the tubes. The use of gastrostomies with a cross piece or retention disk on the extra-abdominal portion of the tube may be helpful in preventing migration of the feeding tubes through the pylorus. If this occurs, it can cause a gastric outlet obstruction that may be misdiagnosed as prolonged gastric atony. It is imperative to not create too much tension between the anterior gastric wall and extra-abdominal fixation device in order to avoid necrosis of the stomach or abdominal wall.

Enteral Feeding Via the Gastrostomy

Most hospitalized patients tolerate continuous enteral feeding. If the gastric output is low and there is no evidence of abdominal distension, feedings are started at approximately 25 cc/hr and residuals checked every 4 to 6 hours. If this rate is tolerated, tube feedings are aggressively advanced over another 24 to 48 hours to the goal rate. Gastrostomy offers the advantage of intermittent bolus feeding on a long-term basis in the outpatient setting without the complications of diarrhea. Feedings can be scheduled and adapted to accommodate the needs of the patient or care personnel.[63] In addition, free water can be administered easily to avoid the problem of dehydration that occasionally occurs with standard tube feedings, particularly in debilitated patients. In hospitalized patients, the head of the bed should be elevated 30 degrees when feeding into the stomach and residuals checked every 4 hours, at least initially. The acute onset of abdominal distension or high residuals should prompt discontinuation of feedings and evaluation of the cause.

Complications of Operative Gastrostomy Tube Placement

Hemorrhage.—Significant hemorrhage from the gastrotomy site occurs in fewer than 1% of cases but can pose significant problems for the operative surgeon. The use of meticulous technique at the operative table can avoid this complication. Since the blood supply to the stomach enters perpendicular to its long axis, placement of a full-thickness suture in the long axis of the stomach 1 cm from the gastrotomy will occlude most vessels. If bleeding occurs nonetheless, the advantage of gastrostomy tubes with inflatable balloons includes the ability to use the balloon to tamponade blood vessels by putting traction on the gastrotomy tube itself. This cannot be done with mushroom-type catheters for fear of dislodgement of the tube from the anterior abdominal wall. This must be done for no longer than 12 to 24 hours, however, in order to prevent gastric or abdominal wall necrosis.

Improper Placement of the Tube.—Although improper tube placement rarely occurs during operative gastrostomy, it can occur when enteral access is obtained through a limited incision in the upper portion of the abdomen. Reports of cannulation of the duodenum, colon, and small bowel have been reported. Identification of the stomach should be made by using the omentum as a marker. The pylorus should be palpated to avoid placing the tube into the antrum and causing gastric outlet obstruction.

Dislodgement of the Stomach From the Anterior Abdominal Wall.—Dislodgement occurs less than 1% of the time after an operatively placed gastrostomy if several sutures are used to secure the stomach to the anterior abdominal wall. This complication is more likely to occur when there has been some delay in replacement of a gastrostomy tube once it has been removed. Blind probing with a clamp or tube through the previous gastrotomy site after the hole has sealed is fraught with the potential to displace the stomach from the anterior abdominal wall and insert the tube into the peritoneal cavity. If there is any question about tube location, confirmation with contrast radiographic studies will ensure that the stomach has been recannulated.

Site Leakage.—Leakage around the gastrostomy tube site is a frequent and annoying complication that occurs regardless of the technique of insertion. This can lead to severe irritation of the skin, granulation tissue, and secondary infections. This problem can be compounded by the use of excessive tension when securing the tube. Enlargement of the exit site through the abdominal wall as a result of pivoting the gastrostomy tube may also lead to leakage. This complication may be increased if the gastrostomy tube is brought out through the operative incision. The initial tendency is to replace the gastrostomy tube

346 Feeding

with a larger size. This, however, will cause more erosion and increased leakage. Shortening the tube to prevent pivoting may help. Cauterization or the use of silver nitrate to decrease granulation tissue and temporary removal of the tube may be necessary to control this problem.

Wound Infection.—In addition to the problems related to the feeding tube itself, wound complications are not uncommon. As with any laparotomy incision, there is a small but significant risk of superficial or deep wound infection, dehiscence, or evisceration. In addition, dehiscence and wound infection may dispose to subsequent ventral hernias requiring repair. Wound complications occur in approximately 2% to 8% of patients undergoing operative gastrostomies.[64, 65] This is probably more related to concomitant surgical procedures and medical conditions than the type of insertion technique used.

Gastrostomy Site Infections.—Abdominal wall infection at the point of gastrostomy tube insertion occurs in 0% to 4% of all cases.[66] Infection can often be difficult to diagnose, and the gastrostomy site should be inspected for induration or swelling in patients in whom fever, leukocytosis, and signs of infection are present with no obvious source of fever. Since other infectious processes such as pneumonia are often present in these patients, an abdominal wall abscess may not be suspected. If untreated, it may lead to the development of severe fasciitis. Aspiration of the area or even incision along the tract is occasionally indicated to rule out this complication. Another cause of infection at the gastrostomy site is the use of internal and external bumpers or retention devices. Excessive compression between the two may cause abdominal and/or gastric wall necrosis. It may appear as ischemia of the skin, erosion of the bumper into the abdominal wall, perforation of the stomach with intra-

peritoneal leakage of tube feedings, or rarely necrotizing fasciitis. Strict attention to the amount of tension between the internal and external fixation devices should minimize this complication.

NONOPERATIVE PATIENTS

General Approach

Many critically ill patients, especially patients in the medical ICU or burn unit, either never undergo abdominal surgery or do not have enteral access obtained at the time of surgery. In these cases, a new set of problems faces the clinician. First, the patient must be assessed as to the estimated length of time that nutritional support will be required. If the problem precluding oral intake is expected to resolve within 6 to 8 weeks and the patient is expected to be in the hospital the entire time, nasoenteric access is probably warranted. Examples of this are patients with acute infections such as pneumonia that are expected to resolve within weeks, patients with resolving neurologic deficits whether due to trauma or embolic events, and those with multiple fractures among others. Even though these patients may remain on prolonged ventilator support, the expectation of their recovery from the acute process is high, and operative or endoscopic manipulation of the gastrointestinal tract is probably not necessary. One exception to this would be patients with severe intractable sinusitis. On the other hand, patients with irreversible problems, e.g., fixed neurologic deficits, vocal cord paralysis, aspiration, and impassable upper gastrointestinal tract obstruction such as esophageal cancer, are candidates for permanent feeding tubes. Once the decision for a permanent feeding tube is made, the operative vs. nonoperative approach must be considered. The operative enteral access techniques have been previously discussed.

Nasogastric vs. Nasoenteric Feedings

Direct gastric feeding is feasible only when there is no evidence of gastric atony and gastric emptying is adequate either with or without metoclopramide therapy. Patients without intraabdominal pathology and who have no septic complications frequently tolerate gastric feeding. If the patients have not required nasogastric decompression, a small-bore nasoenteric tube can be inserted into the stomach and the position checked by aspiration of bilious gastric contents and, if necessary, radiography.[67-69] It is not reliable to simply inject air into the tube and listen over the upper part of the abdomen since this does not eliminate the possibility of inadvertent placement into the left lower lobe of the lung. Unfortunately, many critically ill patients do not react by coughing to bronchial placement of feeding tubes.

Even when gastric atony is not a problem, a history of aspiration secondary to reflux is often a contraindication to intragastric feeding. Studies comparing postpyloric vs. gastric feeding of patients with known aspiration have produced conflicting results. Whether intragastric feeding is from a percutaneous endoscopic gastrostomy (PEG) or a nasoenteric tube appears to have little effect upon the incidence of aspiration. Fay et al.[70] investigated 80 patients undergoing PEG vs. 29 patients with nasoenteric tubes and noted aspiration pneumonia occurring within 14 days of tube placement in 6% of PEG patients and 24% of nasoenteric tube patients. Mortality was similar in both groups, and in the long term, there appeared to be minimal difference in aspiration pneumonia. Weltz et al.[34] studied 100 patients with neurologic disease, obtundation, or oral pharyngeal dysmotility who were at risk for aspiration. None of the patients with feeding-related preoperative aspiration pneumonia had recurrence of aspiration when fed by jejunostomy, although several patients aspirated prior to the institution of jejunal feeding. These authors concluded that jejunostomy can be performed with a low morbidity rate and substantially reduces the risk of subsequent aspiration. These data contradict the data by Strong et al.[28] who placed 10 F nasoenteric tubes either into the stomach or beyond the second portion of the duodenum. The authors were careful to monitor the tubes with radiographs and replace tubes that migrated out of the desired position. If liberal criteria are used, aspiration pneumonia as documented by chest radiography occurred in approximately 33% of the patients fed into the stomach and 40% of the patients fed distal to the pylorus. The authors concluded that postpyloric feeding could not ensure protection from aspiration. Although the literature is controversial, postpyloric feedings are probably safer than direct intragastric feeding.

Positioning Nasoenteric Tubes

Positioning nasoenteric tubes beyond the pylorus is difficult and spontaneous migration through the pylorus is uncommon in critically ill patients despite weighted tubes.[71] Various reports have documented spontaneous migration from the stomach into the duodenum in 5% to 80% of patients, with the lowest rate of migration occurring in the sickest patients. Often, fluoroscopic or endoscopic manipulation is necessary.[72-77] Zaloga[78] described a corkscrew technique in which the guidewire was bent and the nasoenteric tube advanced into the duodenum with a 96% success rate in 200 patients. The tube advanced into the jejunum in approximately 30% of the patients. At no time should the guidewire be forceably advanced to pass beyond an obstruction for fear of perforation.

If this technique fails and if normal motility of the stomach does not carry the tube into the duodenum, tubes can be placed using endoscopic techniques. A small suture is tied to the end of the tube and grasped by forceps through the biopsy port of an endoscope with subsequent advancement into the small intestine. Stark et al.[76] successfully placed 13 of 14 feeding tubes by using this technique. The method was used only after fluoroscopy had failed, although fluoroscopy was successful in 94% of cases in which it was attempted. Gutierrez and Balfe[72] surveyed the results of 882 fluoroscopically guided feeding tube placements in 448 patients. The authors noted success in 86.6% of attempts, with successful positioning of the tubes distal to the third portion of the duodenum. Unfortunately, the average tube life was 7.8 days, thus reflecting the difficulty in maintaining long-term nasoenteric postpyloric feeding. There were four major complications, three arrhythmias and one tracheal bronchial injury, during the fluoroscopic placement. Although fluoroscopy appears to be an ideal solution, it is difficult to transport many critically ill patients into the radiology suite for repeated attempts to place tubes. With dislodgement of tubes in as many as 40% of patients,[79] continued postpyloric placement often taxes medical personnel, and frequent trips to the radiology suite are not without risk. Although bridle techniques have been described,[80] percutaneous gastrostomy or percutaneous jejunostomy may be helpful in these cases.

Starting Feeding

The principles of direct jejunal feedings have been previously discussed. Gastric feedings, however, require special attention. Only after confirmation of placement should gastrointestinal feedings be started, and then at a slow rate of 25 cc/hr. Gastric residuals should be checked every 4 hours and tube feeding stopped if 150 to 175 cc or more is aspirated. If residuals remain high for more than 24 hours, metoclopramide therapy can be started in order to increase motility; a substantial number of patients can be expected to respond. Once tube feedings reach the goal rate, treatment with the drug should be discontinued in order to avoid the complication of diarrhea. If patients who have been tolerating gastric feeding at or near the goal rate suddenly become intolerant and high gastric residuals develop, the most common cause is the onset of sepsis secondary to pneumonia, intra-abdominal abscess, etc. Over the past 4 years at our institution, acute gastric outlet obstruction developed in six patients secondary to the development of duodenal ulcers and resulted in intolerance of feedings. If patients suddenly become intolerant of feedings and heme-positive gastric aspirates develop, sepsis should be ruled out, and upper endoscopy should be considered to look for the presence of an acute antral or duodenal ulcer. In three of the patients with this clinical history, either acute upper gastrointestinal hemorrhage or gastric perforation developed. Two of these patients subsequently died as a complication of ulcer disease.

Complications of Nasoenteric/ Nasogastric Tubes

Atelectasis, discomfort, dysphagia, gastroesophageal reflux, irritation of the nasal, pharyngeal, esophageal, or gastric regions, and dislodgement are much more common with nasogastric tubes. In chronically intubated patients, the nasogastric tubes and endotracheal or tracheostomy balloon can produce pressure necrosis and tracheoesophageal fistulas. Because of chronic irritation, sinusitis is a real possibility any time nasal passages are intubated. The risk becomes much higher if tubes are left in place for long periods since associated swelling will obstruct drainage of sinuses into the nasopharynx. The risk particularly increases if there is a history of facial fractures. In a review of 2,368 trauma patients admitted to the Maryland Institute of Emergency Medical Services,[81] 32 patients had documented sinusitis. All had indwelling nasal tubes and were on mechanical ventilation. The usual pathogens were gram-negative rods. Treatment required removal of the nasal tubes, antibiotics, and decongestants. Antrostomy with aspiration of the sinuses for diagnosis and treatment is a common practice in patients with nasal tubes in ICUs.

A relatively unappreciated complication is the "nasogastric tube syndrome." The etiology appears to be a postcricoid ulceration with variable symptoms including hoarseness, earache, and sore throat. On examination, the ulceration may be missed, although unilateral or bilateral vocal cord paralysis may be present. Although patients with nasogastric tubes will have sore throats, excessive complaints should be investigated. Vocal cord paralysis is a complication of the most severe cases. Rigid cervical esophagoscopy is required to identify these patients and obtain good visualization of the postcricoid area.[82] Treatment consists of removal of the tube, tracheostomy, and possibly antibiotics. The etiology appears to be pressure necrosis from the tube, particularly when it is lying in the midline.

Additional complications of nasoenteric tubes include ulceration at the gastroesophageal junction, as well as anywhere along the tube, and aspiration. A gastrostomy is often employed to avoid these complications in patients who will need long-term gastric decompression.

Percutaneous Placement of Tubes

General Approach

In 1980, Gauderer et al.[83] published a description of PEG, a new type of gastrostomy without laparotomy. Several modifications of this technique have been proposed along with improvements in the ready-made equipment available. The most recent development is that of the nonsurgical percutaneous gastrostomy under fluoroscopic or ultrasound control. Each of these techniques will be described, including advantages, disadvantages, and key points of management.

As stated earlier, semipermanent feeding tubes such as PEGs are usually placed in patients who have a prolonged or lifelong need for assisted nutritional support. This technique may be performed on awake patients with sedation, comatose patients on ventilators, and patients under general anesthesia. Since it is a purely elective procedure, patient conditions must be selected so as to minimize risk. Previous abdominal surgery is not a contraindication; however, extra care must be taken to prevent puncture of overlying organs. Patients who have upper aerodigestive tract obstructions, i.e., esophageal or massive head and neck cancers precluding passage of an endoscope, are not candidates for endoscopic procedures. Although mechanical ventilation is not a contraindication, severe respiratory insufficiency requiring high levels of positive end-expiratory pressure (PEEP) should be in a resolving or at least stable phase prior to endoscopic placement of feeding tubes. Hemodynamic instability requiring pressors and/or inotropes precludes feeding the gastrointestinal tract, so elective feeding tube placement can also be postponed. The choice of local anesthesia with sedation vs. general anesthesia is patient dependent and must be individualized. Sedation with diazepam or midazolam is generally safe but may predispose to aspiration since the patients cannot protect their airway as well as when fully alert. Apnea and hypotension have also been associated with the use of either drug. Monitoring by electrocardiography (ECG), blood pressure measurements, and pulse oximetry are important components of the procedure. Supplemental oxygen and a resuscitation cart should be available. The new benzodiazepine antagonist flumazenil will help reverse the sedation but, unfortunately, will not reverse the respiratory depression. If narcotic sedation is used, naloxone should be available.

The use of local anesthesia with sedation is commonly used for PEG tube placement in intubated patients. Larger doses are possible, and muscle relaxants can be added, if necessary, while ventilation can be controlled. If these drugs are to be used, it is important to switch patients to an assist control mode or at least increase the rate of ventilations to prevent hypoventilation. In general, patients should have tube feedings stopped 8 to 12 hours prior to the procedure. At our institution, we have placed PEG tubes as early as 4 hours after cessation of feedings as long as gastric residuals have been low.

Specific Techniques
Percutaneous Endoscopic Gastrostomy.—In the original description, Gauderer et al.[83] used a two-endoscopy technique that is still the most frequently used. After adequate patient sedation the endoscope is introduced and a routine esophagogastroduodenoscopy performed to rule out conditions that may preclude the procedure, such as gastric outlet obstruction, pathology of the anterior gastric wall, or other conditions requiring surgical intervention. The stomach is distended with air to oppose the gastric wall against the anterior abdominal wall. This maneuver lessens the chance of leakage and injury to adjacent organs such as the colon and liver. It is usually necessary to dim the room lights in order to see the point of maximal illumination of the abdominal wall, which is produced by directing the endoscope anteriorly. The assistant pushes on the point of maximal illumination so that the endoscopist can confirm the position. Some endoscopists assert that in patients with burns of the abdominal wall and in those who are obese this latter maneuver is all that is necessary and illumination of the anterior abdominal wall may be omitted. Most surgical endoscopists, however, are hesitant to proceed without both criteria being met. It is probably unwise to remove previously placed feeding tubes or open the sterile PEG set until this maneuver has been successfully completed.

Confirmed enteral access and sterile PEG sets are both valuable commodities and should not be wasted, if possible. Leaving nasoenteric tubes in place during the procedure also facilitates the passage of the endoscope, particularly in critically ill patients who cannot or will not swallow. The tube must be clamped, however, or it will be impossible to insufflate the stomach.

After the site on the abdominal wall has been selected, the abdomen is prepared and draped in a sterile fashion. The operative site is anesthetized with several milliliters of 1% or 2% lidocaine. During this time a snare is passed through the endoscope and positioned on the anterior gastric wall in preparation for puncture. An incision of approximately 1½ times the diameter of the gastrostomy tube is made in the anterior abdominal wall. The commercially supplied catheter or a 16-gauge intravenous catheter is inserted through this incision and the abdominal wall and into the stomach, optimally through the snare. The needle is withdrawn and the plastic catheter left. A guidewire is inserted through the catheter and grasped with the snare. During this time the assistant prevents leakage of gastric air through the catheter by placing his finger over the end. The guidewire is withdrawn through the mouth with the endoscope while the assistant feeds the wire through the abdominal wall. The catheter may then be removed. The gastrostomy tube is tied or looped around the guidewire. This end must be tapered to permit transit through the abdominal wall. The assistant withdraws the guidewire and pulls the gastrostomy tube through the anterior abdominal wall. Most currently available PEG tubes have an internal fixation device shaped somewhat like a cup. It is convenient to place the endoscope into the end of this catheter prior to withdrawal through the mouth or esophagus to facilitate the second passage of the endoscope. Previously placed nasoenteric tubes can also be used as a guide during the second insertion. Under the direct vision of the endoscopist, the assistant withdraws the gastrostomy tube until the internal retention device abuts the abdominal wall. There is rarely a need to withdraw the tube to less than the 2-cm mark on the catheter. The loop on the external end of the gastrostomy tube is cut, and the external retention device is placed over the tube, which is facilitated by the use of sterile lubricating jelly. While still under the direct visualization of the endoscopist, the catheter is fixed to the abdominal wall by using sutures or an external retention disk. The tapered end of the gastrostomy tube is removed and a connector piece attached. The tube may be placed for gravity drainage or merely clamped and is usable the next day. The previous description is applicable to most commercially available PEG tubes. The reader is referred to the original description of Gauderer et al.[83] if a manufactured tube is not available. Because the gastrostomy tube is placed through the mouth, abdominal wall infections are a problem. Prophylactic antibiotics have been found to help prevent gastrostomy site infections.[84]

The preceding description of PEG placement is also known as the Ponsky or pull method since the feeding tube is pulled through the mouth and up through the abdominal wall by using a traction guidewire. A variation of this is the push method with a Sacks-Vine gastrostomy tube. The only difference in insertion is that the specially designed gastrostomy tube is fed over the wire and pushed in an antegrade fashion up through the abdominal wall until it can be grasped by the assistant.

Modifications of Percutaneous Endoscopic Gastrostomy

T-Anchor System.—Concerns about separation of the stomach from the anterior abdominal wall have produced other variations such as that published by Wu et al.[85] After insufflation of the stomach through the gastroduodeno-

scope, the stomach is secured to the anterior abdominal wall by using "T" nylon anchoring devices similar to those used to attach price tags to clothing. The anchors are placed in a square 1½ cm apart, and each pair is tied together after insertion. This is done under direct vision via the endoscope to prevent injury to adjacent organs. A scalpel is used to make a stab wound in the center of the square, a hemostat is advanced into the stomach to widen the tract, and a 22F or 24F Foley catheter is inserted through the tract by using a metal stylet. In addition to fixing the stomach against the abdominal wall with T-anchors, this technique also eliminates dragging the feeding catheter through the mouth, which might decrease infectious complications.

Introducer Method.—Another major variation in the PEG procedure is the introducer technique, first published by Russell et al. in 1984.[86] Endoscopy is performed in the usual manner. After preparation of the abdominal wall, a 16-gauge needle is used to puncture the abdominal wall and stomach. A guidewire is inserted and the needle removed. The introducer and outer peel-away sheath, like that used for the placement of pacemakers, are then inserted over the guidewire. This may be facilitated by twisting the introducer and outer sheath. The introducer and guidewire are removed, and a 14 F Foley catheter is passed through the sheath into the abdominal wall. The balloon of the Foley catheter is inflated with saline. The peel-away sheath is removed, and the Foley catheter is pulled up against the anterior abdominal wall and sutured to the skin. This technique has the advantage of not passing the feeding tube through the mouth. It does run the risk, however, of gastric leakage because the stomach is theoretically pushed away from the abdominal wall with insertion of the introducer and peel-away sheath. Another problem with this type of insertion is that a small Foley catheter, which becomes clogged more easily, must be used. There is some evidence that the latex from which these catheters are constructed may be easily degraded by stomach acid and predispose them to early rupture. This may lead to distraction of the stomach from the intra-abdominal wall and secondary intra-abdominal gastric content leakage.

Fluoroscopically Placed Gastrostomy.—Radiologists have modified this introducer method to eliminate the use of endoscopy. Instead, it is performed under ultrasonic and/or fluoroscopic control. With these modalities, the abdomen is first checked to make sure that no organs such as the colon or liver intervene between the stomach and abdominal wall. A nasogastric tube is inserted and the stomach insufflated. Again by using fluoroscopy, an appropriate site on the anterior abdominal wall is marked, and the abdomen is prepared and draped in a sterile fashion. The area is anesthetized with a local anesthetic, and a skin incision is made on the anterior abdominal wall. The stomach is punctured with a needle through this incision, a guidewire inserted, and the needle removed. The tract is then dilated. Finally, a peel-away sheath-and-dilator assembly is inserted over the guidewire, and the guidewire and dilator are removed. A Foley or Malecot catheter is inserted through the peel-away sheath and the sheath removed. Alternatively, a catheter with a "Cope loop" can be passed over the guidewire. In one radiologic method,[87] an 8 F orogastric feeding tube is inserted and then exchanged for a Dotter intravascular sheath and retrieval basket. The needle placed through the anterior abdominal wall into the stomach is directed toward this basket and a guidewire inserted. Under fluoroscopy the guidewire is grasped with the basket and withdrawn through the mouth. By using the typical push method, a Sacks-Vine gastrostomy tube is passed over the wire until

it appears in the abdominal wall. The tube is completely withdrawn through the abdominal wall until tension is felt on the stomach. The position of all radiologically placed tubes is confirmed with fluoroscopy with or without contrast; the amount of tension generated cannot really be assessed except by feel from the outside. The tube is sutured in place, or a retention disk is applied.

Percutaneous Endoscopic Jejunostomy.—Although open methods of obtaining jejunal access are acceptable when a laparotomy is performed, a modification of the PEG procedure—percutaneous endoscopic jejunostomy (PEJ)—is another option and avoids an abdominal incision. A prepackaged PEJ is used, or one can be fashioned from a 16 or 18 F mushroom catheter and a weighted Silastic feeding tube. The weighted tube is placed through the mushroom catheter with its tip exiting through one of the holes in the mushroom. Alternatively, a separate side hole can be cut in the head of the mushroom catheter. The feeding tube is threaded through the head of the catheter and also through an incision made in the distal end. A suture is placed through the distal end of both tubes, and they are wedged into the plastic cone of a no. 16 Medicut intravenous cannula. A crossbar is placed over both tubes adjacent to the mushroom tip as in Gauderer's original description of the PEG procedure. The endoscope is passed into the stomach and routine endoscopy performed. After the light is visualized through the abdominal wall and the endoscopist perceives the indentation made by the assistant's finger on the stomach wall, the abdominal wall is prepared and anesthetized, and an incision large enough to accommodate both tubes is made. A catheter-over-needle assembly is inserted through the incision until the endoscopist sees it entering the stomach into the loop of the snare placed through the endoscope. A guidewire is placed *t*hrough the catheter, grasped by the snare, and withdrawn through the mouth. The distal end of the feeding tube combination is secured to the guidewire, and the guidewire is pulled through the abdominal wall by the assistant until the mushroom catheter approximates the gastric wall. The weighted end of the Silastic tube still remains in the mouth at this point. A suture tied to the weighted end can be grasped with a biopsy forceps placed through the channel of the endoscope and dragged down into the stomach with the second passage of the endoscope. Alternatively, the assistant can withdraw the weighted Silastic tube until the weighted end is in the stomach. In any event, the suture tied on the weighted end of the Silastic tube is grasped with biopsy forceps and dragged through the pylorus using the endoscope. The extra length of the Silastic tube is left in the stomach so that peristalsis will carry the tube further into the small bowel.

Prepackaged PEJ kits have been developed (Moss Tubes, Inc.). As in any other percutaneous feeding tube, the appropriate spot is chosen on the gastric and abdominal walls. Four (T) anchors are placed in a square approximately 1 in. apart. A "J" guidewire is placed into the stomach via an introducer. At this point the wire may be placed through the pylorus by using biopsy forceps under endoscopic visualization. Alternatively, a dilator "breakaway" introducer is placed into the stomach via the guidewire and advanced toward the pylorus. The wire may then be directed into the pylorus. Once the "J" wire has passed the pylorus, the dilator is removed and the transgastric jejunostomy tube passed through the introducer, over the guidewire, and into the duodenum. This is facilitated by grasping a traction suture on the end of the tube with biopsy forceps and advancing the tube endoscopically. The introducer is peeled away similarly to the peel-away sheath used for the placement of pacemakers.

Complications of Percutaneously Placed Feeding Tubes

Dislodgement of the Stomach From the Anterior Abdominal Wall.—Dislodgement of the stomach from the anterior abdominal wall resulting in intraperitoneal spillage of gastric contents has been reported following all types of gastrostomy insertion techniques. As stated previously, this is uncommon following operative gastrostomy. It happens most often when the tube is inadvertently dislodged prior to a fibrous tract being formed. On reinsertion of the tube, the stomach can be pushed away from the abdominal wall, or the tube may slip between the two. If this is not recognized, tube feedings may be infused into the peritoneum. This has been reported to occur approximately 1% of the time after PEG tube insertion.[88] It is slightly more frequent after radiologically guided percutaneous gastrostomies, 1.5% to 4%[87, 89] perhaps because apposition of the stomach to the anterior abdominal wall is only checked radiologically vs. visually in the operating room or through the endoscope. Dislodgement without leakage occurs in a small percentage of all tubes but, again, more frequently in radiologically guided gastrostomies. In a study of 100 cancer patients, the dislodgement rate was 11%.[90] The use of the "Cope loop" may have been a significant factor in that study.

Gastrostomy Exit Site Infection.—Infection at the exit site of the gastrostomy tube occurs more frequently after PEG than after open gastrostomy. In a study of 107 patients divided into three groups based on antibiotic prophylaxis for pain, wound infections resulting from PEG placement developed in none of the patients receiving antibiotics therapeutically for other problems. Wound problems developed in 7% of those receiving prophylactic antibiotics as compared with a 32% infection rate in the group not given any antibiotics.[84] This increased incidence over standard gastrostomy is probably due to the PEG tube being brought through the mouth. The risk may be lessened with the radiologic insertion technique.[91]

Abdominal Wall Necrosis.— One of the complications related to the use of internal and external bumpers or retention devices is abdominal and/or gastric wall necrosis, probably secondary to too much tension between the two. It may present as ischemia of the skin, erosion of one or the other bumper into the abdominal wall, perforation of the stomach with intraperitoneal leakage of tube feedings, or rarely necrotizing fasciitis. Since many critically ill patients are obtunded, perforation with intraperitoneal leakage may not be reliably diagnosed by clinical findings. Since the gastric perforation is located in the most nondependent portion of the stomach, intraperitoneal leakage of gastric contents may be relatively minimal and be manifested as fever and leukocytosis. The course of many of these patients is complicated by multiple infections such as pneumonia, line sepsis, etc., and multiple antibiotics may be instituted and mask the symptoms of intraperitoneal soilage. In patients with unexplained fever, evidence of skin ischemia, or sudden intolerance of gastrostomy feedings, the diagnosis of occult gastric perforation should be entertained. Lateral decubitus radiographs or computed tomographic (CT) scans should be obtained to document evidence of penumoperitoneum, which may not be obvious on supine abdominal films. Simple gastric studies with contrast may not diagnose an anterior perforation, and endoscopy or laparotomy may be necessary in unusual cases to diagnose the pathology. Strict attention to the amount of tension between the internal and external fixation devices should minimize this complication.

Gastrointestinal Hemorrhage.—Gastrointestinal bleeding has also been associated with all methods of insertion. Occasionally patients have pre-existing ulcer disease or ulcerogenic conditions such as sepsis and head injury that can produce this problem. When using the endoscopic method, major vessels in the gastric wall can be visualized with the scope and, it is hoped, avoided. In addition, since the site is observed after insertion of the tube, most bleeding can be identified. Unfortunately, there are no such safeguards for the radiologic percutaneous method. Most studies report the incidence of this complication following all methods as less than 1%. Some authors give higher percentages; however, most of these studies report only 1 patient with gastrointestinal bleeding in a series of fewer than 50 patients.

Pneumoperitoneum.—One complication peculiar to percutaneous insertion of feeding tubes is that of pneumoperitoneum, which has been reported as frequently as 38% in a prospective study.[92] Although free air under the diaphragm is seen almost universally after any laparotomy, it is quite disconcerting to see it in a patient who has undergone a percutaneous procedure. The air most likely comes from inside the stomach, particularly since it is routinely insufflated prior to the percutaneous approach. Obviously, the concern is that if air could have leaked out, so could gastric contents. Although this is almost always a benign condition, patients must be observed closely. The persistence or an increase in pneumoperitoneum or late manifestation may be clues that this condition is not benign. Since many patients undergoing percutaneous procedures have altered mental status, the results of abdominal examination may be totally unreliable. Particular care must be taken when following patients with severe head or spinal cord injuries. Although computed axial tomographic (CAT) scanning and/or instillation of radiopaque contrast into the catheter may be helpful, it is not 100% sensitive, particularly because the leaking site will be anterior on the stomach wall and the contrast pools posteriorly. Occasionally exploratory laparotomy will be required to assure the clinician that there is no leak from the tube.

Aspiration.—Aspiration is a common problem in all patients with chronic gastrostomy tubes. It is very difficult to determine whether insertion of the tube or concomitant medical disease is the most important contributory factor. Aspiration may occur as frequently as 8% of the time following PEG.[93] More commonly the incidence is reported at about 2%.[66] It occurs just as frequently after operative insertion and has been reported to occur from 2% to 10% of the time.[94, 95] It was thought that gastrostomy insertion may lower the pressures of the lower esophageal sphincter and thus increase the incidence of reflux and aspiration; however, several studies have not borne this out.[96, 97]

Catheter Occlusion.—Tube blockage is a frequent complication no matter what the method of insertion or route of feeding. This problem increases with decreasing size of the feeding tube used and with use of the gastrostomy or jejunostomy tubes for medications, especially crushed pills. This is not a major problem with gastrostomies that are at least 8 to 10 days old since a fibrous tract has usually been formed. Prior to this time, however, changing the tube may place the tube in the abdominal cavity and feedings may be infused into the peritoneum; therefore, any time a tube is replaced before approximately 2 weeks, it should be checked with radiopaque water-soluble contrast. This is particularly a problem when the tube has not been secured to the abdominal wall as in the standard PEG, in percutaneous insertion under radiologic control, and in the Dragstedt technique.

Inadvertent Organ Perforation.—Bowel perforations have occasionally been reported after the insertion of gastrostomies. It is extremely rare after operative insertion of the feeding tube; however, Gauderer reported a 2.2% incidence[88] following PEG. The radiologically controlled method is associated with approximately a 1% risk.[90] In addition, perforations of the duodenum, esophagus, and kidney have been described with percutaneous techniques.

Persistent Gastrocutaneous Fistula.—A late complication that may occur after removal of the gastrostomy tube is a persistent gastrocutaneous fistula. Most gastrostomy sites will close in several days; however, if the tract has been lined with epithelium, this may not occur. Simple cauterization may be enough to eliminate the epithelialization; however, persistent gastrocutaneous fistulas must be excised operatively. Difficulties in removing the catheter can also be encountered, particularly with some of the older prepackaged PEG tubes that actually required endoscopic removal. With better product development, this problem has dropped to almost zero.

Other Complications of Percutaneous Feeding Tubes.—Numerous other complications have been reported. Fortunately, they consist mainly of case reports. Without an external retention device or adequate suturing, the gastrostomy tube may migrate into the duodenum. With an intact inflated balloon, this can cause a gastric outlet obstruction. At least one report of a hernia through the PEG site exists.[98] A gastrostomy tube has been reported to migrate into the duodenum, erode into another portion of bowel, and cause an internal fistula.[99] Intussusception around the gastrostomy tube has also been reported.

In the last decade, renewed interest has evolved in the role of enteral nutrition as a primary therapy in the critically ill patient. Evidence that enteral feeding appears to augment host defenses has stimulated the search for special nutrient formulas and improved equipment for nutrient delivery. Potential pharmacologic benefits of certain nutrients such as glutamine, ω-3 fatty acids, and arginine hold significant promise for critically ill patients. As the mechanism for reduced morbidity is better defined, clinicians can expect to have tools that will enhance the recovery of critically ill patients. Clinicians must be educated in the importance of enteral nutrition and the potential techniques for obtaining enteral access to ensure the opportunity for safe delivery of enteral nutrition. Although many patients will continue to require intravenous nutrition, a larger portion of critically ill patients can be supported with enteral nutrition through a team commitment. Enteral processing of nutrients remains the first choice whenever possible.

REFERENCES

1. Carrico CJ, Meakins JL, Marshall JC, et al: Multiple-organ failure syndrome. *Arch Surg* 1986; 121:196–208.
2. Border JR, Chenier R, McMenamy R, et al: Multiple systems organ failure: Muscle fuel deficit with visceral protein malnutrition. *Surg Clin North Am* 1976; 56:1147–1169.
3. Deitch EA: Multiple organ failure: Pathophysiology and potential future therapy. *Ann Surg* 1992; 216:117–134.
4. Border JR, Hassett J, LaDuca J, et al: The gut origin septic states in blunt multiple trauma (ISS = 40) in the ICU. *Ann Surg* 1987; 206:427–448.
5. Zaloga GP, MacGregor DA: What to consider when choosing enteral or parenteral nutrition: Is the guideline still "if the gut works, use it"? *J Crit Illness* 1990; 5:1180–1200.
6. Alexander JW, Macmillan BG, Stinnett JD, et al: Beneficial effects of aggressive protein feeding in severely burned children. *Ann Surg* 1980; 182:505–517.
7. Johnson LR, Copeland EM, Dudrick SJ, et al: Structural and hormonal alterations in the gastrointestinal tract of parenterally fed rats. *Gastroenterology* 1975; 68:1177.
8. Rothman D, Latham MC, Walker WA: Transport of macromolecules in malnourished animals. *Nutr Res* 1982; 2:467.
9. Deitch EA: Intestinal permeability is increased in burn patients shortly after injury. *Surgery* 1990; 107:411–416.
10. Deitch EA: Does the gut protect or injure patients in the ICU? *Prospect Crit Care* 1988; 1:1–31.
11. Purandare S, Offenbartl K, Weseröm B, et al: Increased gut permeability to fluorescein isothiocyanate–dextran after total parenteral nutrition in the rat. *Scand J Gastroenterol* 1989; 24:678–682.
12. Alverdy JC, Chi HS, Sheldon GF: The effect of parenteral nutrition on gastrointestinal immunity: The importance of enteral stimulation. *Ann Surg* 1985; 202:681–684.
13. Birkhahn RH, Rank CM: Immune response and leucine oxidation in oral- and intravenous-fed rats. *Am J Clin Nutr* 1984; 39:45–53.
14. Kudsk KA, Carpenter G, Petersen SR, et al: Effective enteral and parenteral feeding in malnourished rats with hemoglobin–*E. coli* adjuvant peritonitis. *J Surg Res* 1981; 31:105–110.
15. Kudsk KA, Stone JM, Carpenter G, et al: Enteral and parenteral feeding influences mortality after hemoglobin–*E. coli* peritonitis in normal rats. *J Trauma* 1983; 23:605–609.
16. Herndon DN, Barrow RE, Stein M, et al: Increased mortality with intravenous supplemental feeding in severely burned patients. *J Burn Care Rehabil* 1989; 10:309–313.
17. Rapp RP, Young D, Tyman D, et al: The favorable effect of early parenteral feeding on survival in head-injured patients. *J Neurosurg* 1983; 58:906–911.
18. Young B, Ott L, Twyman D, et al: The effect of nutritional support on outcome from severe head injury. *J Neurosurg* 1987; 67:668–676.
19. Grahm TW, Zadrozny DB, Harrington T: The benefits of early jejunal hyperalimentation in the head-injured patient. *Neurosurgery* 1989; 25:729–735.

20. The Veteran Affairs Total Parenteral Nutrition Cooperative Study Group: Perioperative total parenteral nutrition in surgical patients. *N Engl J Med* 1991; 325:525–532.

21. Moore FA, Moore EE, Jones TN: Benefits of immediate jejunostomy feeding after major abdominal trauma—A prospective randomized study. *J Trauma* 1986; 26:874–881.

22. Moore FA, Moore EE, et al: TEN vs. TPN following major abdominal trauma—Reduced septic morbidity. *J Trauma* 1989; 29:916–923.

23. Kudsk KA, Croce MA, Fabian TC, et al: Enteral vs parenteral feeding: Effects on septic morbidity following blunt and penetrating trauma. *Ann Surg* 1992; 215:503–513.

24. Gottschlich M, Alexander JW, Bower RH: Enteral nutrition in patients with burns and trauma, in Rombeau J, Caldwell MD (eds): *Clinical Nutrition: Enteral and Tube Feeding,* ed 2. Philadelphia, WB Saunders, 1990.

25. Forlaw L, Guenter P: Enteral delivery systems, in Rombeau J, Caldwell MD (eds): *Clinical Nutrition: Enteral and Tube Feeding,* ed 2. Philadelphia, WB Saunders, 1990.

26. Kellum JM, Holland GF, McNeill P: Traumatic pancreatic cutaneous fistula: Comparison of enteral and parenteral feedings. *Am J Surg* 1988; 155:112–117.

27. Bodoky G, Harsanyi L, Pap A, et al: Effect of enteral nutrition on exocrine pancreatic function. *Am J Surg* 1991; 161:144–148.

28. Strong RM, Condon SC, Solinger MR, et al: Equal aspiration rates from postpylorus and intragastric-placed small-bore nasoenteric feeding tubes: A randomized, prospective study. *JPEN* 1992; 16:59–63.

29. Lazarus BA, Murphy JB, Culpepper L: Aspiration associated with long-term gastric versus jejunal feeding: A critical analysis of the literature. *Arch Phys Med Rehabil* 1990; 71:46–53.

30. Kirby DF, Clifton GL, Turner H, et al: Early enteral nutrition after brain injury by percutaneous endoscopic gastrojejunostomy. *JPEN* 1991; 15:298–302.

31. Kudsk KA, Campbell SM, O'Brien T, et al: Postoperative jejunal feedings following complicated pancreatitis. *Nutr Clin Pract* 1990; 5:14–17.

32. Kudsk KA, McQueen MA, Voeller GR, et al: Management of complex perineal soft-tissue injuries. *J Trauma* 1990; 30:1155–1160.

33. Ryan JA, Page CP: Intrajejunal feeding: Development and current status. *JPEN* 1984; 8:187–198.

34. Weltz CR, Morris JB, Mullen JL: Surgical jejunostomy in aspiration risk patients. *Ann Surg* 1992; 215:140–145.

35. Jones TN, Moore FA, Moore EE, et al: Gastrointestinal symptoms attributed to jejunostomy feeding after major abdominal trauma—a critical analysis. *Crit Care Med* 1989; 17:1146–1150.

36. McDonald WS, Sharp CW Jr, Deitch EA: Immediate enteral feeding in burn patients is safe and effective. *Ann Surg* 1991; 213:177–183.

37. Cade RJ: Feeding jejunostomy: Is its routine use in major upper gastrointestinal surgery justified? *Aust N Z J Surg* 1990; 60:621–623.

38. al-Shehri M, Makarewicz P, Freeman JB: Feeding jejunostomy: A safe adjunct to laparotomy. *Can J Surg* 1990; 33:181–184.

39. McGonigal MD, Lucas CE, Ledgerwood AM: Feeding jejunostomy in patients who are critically ill. *Surg Gynecol Obstet* 1989; 168:275–277.

40. Page CP: Edgar J. Poth lecture. The surgeon and gut maintenance. *Am J Surg* 1989; 158:485–490.

41. Feldtman RW, Archie JP: A three-year experience with needle catheter jejunostomy in a community hospital. *Surg Gynecol Obstet* 1984; 159:23–26.

42. Nicholson LJ: Declogging small-port feeding tubes. *JPEN* 1987; 11:594–597.

43. Walters AM, Bender CE, Sarr MG: Percutaneous conversion of needle catheter jejunostomy to large bore jejunostomy for long term use. *Surg Gynecol Obstet* 1991; 173:397–398.

44. Rombeau JL, Palacio JC: Feeding by tube enterostomy, in Rombeau JL, Caldwell MD (eds): *Clinical Nutrition: Enteral and Tube Feeding,* ed 2. Philadelphia, WB Saunders, 1990.

45. Cataldi-Betcher EL, Seltzer MH, Slocum BA, et al: Complications occurring during enteral nutrition support: A

prospective study. *JPEN* 1983; 7:546–552.

46. Murphy JI: Tube feeding problems and solutions. *Adv Clin Care* 1990; 5:7–11.

47. Chang RWS, Jacobs S, Lee B: Gastrointestinal dysfunction among intensive care unit patients. *Crit Care Med* 1987; 15:909–914.

48. Edes TE, Walk BE, Austin JL: Diarrhea in tube-fed patients: Feeding formula not necessarily the cause. *Am J Med* 1990; 89:697.

49. Kittinger JW, Sandler RS, Heizer WD: Efficacy of metoclopramide as an adjunct to duodenal placement of small bore feeding tubes on a randomized placebo-controlled double blind study. *JPEN* 1987; 11:33.

50. Patterson ML, Dominquez JM, Lyman B, et al: Enteral feeding in the hypoalbuminemic patient. *JPEN* 1990; 14:362–365.

51. Brinson RR, Kolts BE: Diarrhea associated with severe hypoalbuminemia: A comparison of peptide-based, chemically-defined diet and standard enteral alimentation. *Crit Care Med* 1988; 16:130–136.

52. Ford EG, et al: Serum albumin (oncotic pressure) correlates with enteral feeding tolerance in the pediatric surgical patient. *J Pediatr Surg* 1987; 22:597–599.

53. Gottschlich MM, Warden GD, Michel MA, et al: Diarrhea in tube-fed burn patients: Incidence, etiology, nutritional impact, and prevention. *JPEN* 1988; 12:338.

54. Mowatt-Larssen CA, Brown RO, Wojtysiak SL, et al: Comparison of tolerance and nutritional outcome between a peptide and a standard enteral formula in critically ill, hypoalbuminemic patients. *JPEN* 1992; 16:20–24.

55. Hart GK, Dobb GJ: Effect of a fecal bulking agent on diarrhea during enteral feeding in the critically ill. *JPEN* 1988; 12:465–468.

56. Dobb GJ, Towler SC: Diarrhoea during enteral feeding in the critically ill: A comparison of feeds with and without fibre. *Intensive Care Med* 1990; 16:252–255.

57. Collier P, Brown RO, Glezer J, et al: Compatibility of a fiber containing formula with needle catheter jejunostomies. Presented at American Society for Parenteral and Enteral Nutrition, 17th Clinical Congress, Feb 14–17, 1993, San Diego, p. 468.

58. Inoue S, Lukes S, Alexander JW, et al: Increased gut blood flow with early enteral feeding in burned guinea pigs. *J Burn Care Rehabil* 1989; 10:300–308.

59. Smith CD, Sarr MG: Clinically significant penumatosis intestinalis with postoperative enteral feedings by needle catheter jejunostomy: An unusual complication. *JPEN* 1991; 15:328–331.

60. Smith-Choban P, Max MH: Feeding jejunostomy: A small bowel stress test? *Am J Surg* 1988; 155:112.

61. Hayek ME, Eisenberg PG: Severe hypophosphatemia following the institution of enteral feedings. *Arch Surg* 1989; 124:1325–1328.

62. Gauderer MW, Stellato TA: Gastrostomies: Evolution techniques indications and complications. *Curr Prob Surg* 1986; 23:657–719.

63. Powers T, Cowan GS Jr, Deckard M, et al: Prospective randomized evaluation of two regimens for converting from continuous to intermittent feedings in patients with feeding gastrostomies. *JPEN* 1991; 15:405–407.

64. Anderson PH, Woodward ER: Gastrostomy, an evaluation of the Dragstedt method. *Am J Surg* 1972; 124:581–586.

65. Scott JS, de la Torre RA, Unger SW: Comparison of operative versus percutaneous endoscopic gastrostomy tube placement in the elderly. *Am Surg* 1991; 57:338–340.

66. Grant JP: Comparison of percutaneous endoscopic gastrostomy with Stamm gastrostomy. *Ann Surg* 1988; 207:598–603.

67. Harris MR, Huseby JS: Pulmonary complications from nasoenteral feeding tube insertion in an intensive care unit: Incidence and prevention. *Crit Care Med* 1989; 17:917.

68. Metheny NA, Spies MA, Eisenberg P: Measures to test placement of nasoenteral feeding tubes. *West J Nurs Res* 1988; 10:367–383.

69. Guenter P, Jones S, Jacobs DO, et al: Administration and delivery of enteral nutrition, in Rombeau JL, Caldwell MD

(eds): *Clinical Nutrition: Enteral and Tube Feeding*, ed 2. Philadelphia, WB Saunders, 1990.

70. Fay DE, Poplausky M, Gruber M, et al: Long-term enteral feeding: A retrospective comparison of delivery via percutaneous endoscopic gastrostomy and nasoenteric tubes. *Am J Gastroenterol* 1991; 86:1604–1609.

71. Levenson R, Turner WW Jr, Dyson A, et al: Do weighted nasoenteric feeding tubes facilitate duodenal intubations? *JPEN* 1988; 12:135–137.

72. Gutierrez ED, Balfe DM: Fluoroscopically guided nasoenteric feeding tube placement: Results of a 1-year study. *Radiology* 1991; 178:759–762.

73. Ott DJ, Mattox HE, Gelfand DW, et al: Enteral feeding tubes: Placement by using fluoroscopy and endoscopy. *AJR* 1991; 157:769–771.

74. Cardoza JD, Jeffrey RB Jr: Nasojejunal feeding tube placement in immobile patients. *Radiology* 1988; 166:893.

75. Lewis BS, Mauer K, Bush A: The rapid placement of jejunal feeding tubes: The Seldinger technique applied to the gut. *Gastrointest Endosc* 1990; 36:139–141.

76. Stark SP, Sharpe JN, Larson GM: Endoscopically placed nasoenteral feeding tubes. Indications and techniques. *Am Surg* 1991; 57:203–205.

77. Caulfield KA, Page CP, Pestana C: Technique for intraduodenal placement of transnasal enteral feeding catheters. *Nutr Clin Pract* 1991; 6:23–26.

78. Zaloga GP: Bedside method for placing small bowel feeding tubes in critically ill patients: A perspective study. *Chest* 1991; 100:1643.

79. Meer JA: Inadvertent dislodgement of nasoenteral feeding tubes: Incidence and prevention. *JPEN* 1987; 11:187–189.

80. Meer JA: A new nasal bridle for securing nasoenteral feeding tubes. *JPEN* 1989; 13:331–334.

81. Caplan ES, Hoyt NJ: Nosocomial sinusitis. *JAMA* 1982; 247:639–645.

82. Sofferman RA, Haisch CE, Kirchner JA, et al: The nasogastric tube syndrome. *Laryngoscope* 1990; 100:962–968.

83. Gauderer MWL, Ponsky JL, Izant RJ: Gastrostomy without laparotomy: a percutaneous endoscopic technique. *J Pediatri Surg* 1980; 15:872–875.

84. Jain NK, Larson DE, Schroeder KW, et al: Antibiotic prophylaxis for percutaneous endoscopic gastrostomy. A prospective, randomized, double-blind clinical trial. *Ann Intern Med* 1987; 107:824–828.

85. Wu TK, Pietrocola D, Welch HF: New method of percutaneous gastrostomy using anchoring devices. *Am J Surg* 1987; 153:230–232.

86. Russell TR, Brotman M, Norris F: Percutaneous gastrostomy. A new simplified and cost-effective technique. *Am J Surg* 1984; 148:132–137.

87. Towbin RB, Ball WS, Bissett GS III: Percutaneous gastrostomy and percutaneous gastrojejunostomy in children: Antegrade approach. *Radiology* 1988; 168:473–476.

88. Gauderer MWL: Percutaneous endoscopic gastrostomy: A 10-year experience with 220 children. *J Pediatr Surg* 1991; 26:288–294.

89. Ho HS, Yee ACN, McPherson R: Complications of surgical and percutaneous non-endoscopic gastrostomy: review of 233 patients. *Gastroenterology* 1988; 95:1206–1210.

90. O'Keeffe F, Carrasco CH, Charnsangavej C: Percutaneous drainage and feeding gastrostomies in 100 patients. *Radiology* 1989; 172:341–343.

91. Hicks ME, Surratt RS, Picus D, et al: Fluoroscopically guided percutaneous gastrostomy and gastroenterostomy: Analysis of 158 consecutive cases. *AJR* 1990; 154:725–728.

92. Stossen W, McCullough A, Marshall J, et al: Percutaneous endoscopic gastrostomy: Another cause of benign pneumoperitoneum. *Gastrointest Endosc* 1984; 30:296–297.

93. Llaneza PP, Menendez AM, Roberts R, et al: Percutaneous endoscopic gastrostomy: Clinical experience and follow-up. *South Med J* 1988; 81:321–324.

94. Shellito PC, Malt RA: Tube gastrostomy. Techniques and complications. *Ann Surg* 1984; 201:180–185.

95. Apelgren KN, Zambos J: Is percutaneous better than open gastrostomy? A clinical study in one surgical department. *Am Surg* 1989; 55:596–600.

96. Black TL, Fernandes ET, Ellis DG, et

al: The effect of tube gastrostomy on gastroesophageal reflux in patients with esophageal atresia. *J Pediatr Surg* 1991; 26:168–170.

97. Johnson DA, Hacker JF III, Benjamin SB, et al: Percutaneous endoscopic gastrostomy effects on gastroesophageal reflux and lower esophageal sphincter. *Am J Gastroenterol* 1987; 82:622–624.

98. Sangster W, Cuddington GD, Bachulis BL: Percutaneous endoscopic gastrostomy. *Am J Surg* 1988; 155: 677–679.

99. Tom W, Zachary K, Fruchter G, et al: Endoscopy corner, case report: Prolapse of gastrostomy tube resulting in enteroenteric fistula and intussusception. *Am Surg* 1988; 54:245–247.

20

The Initiation and Progression of Tube Feeding

Diana Fullen Bowers, Ph.D., R.D., L.D.

Specialized nutritional support: Enteral feeding mode

Issues concerning feeding method, rate, osmolality, and formula dilution

  Method of formula infusion: Bolus vs. continuous feeding

    Cycled continuous formula infusion

Tube feedings and circadian rhythms

Infusion rate

  Determining the goal infusion rate

Osmolality, formula dilution, and gastrointestinal tolerance

SPECIALIZED NUTRITIONAL SUPPORT: THE ENTERAL FEEDING MODE

Tube feeding is the preferred method of nutritional support for patients with functioning gastrointestinal tracts who are unable to consume adequate nutrition orally. The prevalence of enteral tube feeding has increased over the past decade as a result of significantly lower costs and the reduced incidence of complications when compared with parenteral nutrition. Concomitant with the increase in the use of tube feedings, clinicians have developed a greater appreciation of the complexities of the relationship between intraluminal foodstuff and gastrointestinal function in critical and chronic illness.

Research over the past decade has provided considerable insight into the physiologic and metabolic benefits of enteral nutrition in relation to gastrointestinal function and metabolic homeostasis. Not only does the gut have a remarkable capacity to digest, absorb, and utilize nutrients, it is also intricately involved in immune function, intraorgan substrate flux, and metabolic homeostasis. The gastrointestinal tract is the largest endocrine gland, and the secretion of gut hormones and regulatory peptides has a profound effect on digestion and metabolic homeostasis. Investigators are just beginning to explore and understand how enteral feeding has an impact on the secretion and function of gut hormones and regulatory peptides.

It has been established that the ability of the gastrointestinal tract to carry out its various functions is largely dependent upon the presence of intraluminal nutrients. Experience with parenteral nutrition as the sole source of nutrition has demonstrated that a lack of intraluminal foodstuff results in atrophy of the gut, particularly the jejunum, and a reduced capacity of the gastrointestinal tract to limit bacterial translocation. As our understanding of gastrointestinal function in critical and chronic illness has evolved, so have methods for the formulation and delivery of enteral nutrition. Clinicians now realize that methods of nutrient delivery into the gut as well as the composition of the nutrients themselves have an impact upon gut function. To ensure success, the initiation of enteral feeding must strike a balance between many factors directly and indirectly related to formula infusion.

Practices involving the issues of feeding rate, osmolality, formula dilution, and bolus vs. continuous nutrient infusion have been investigated in recent clinical studies. Early protocols for the initiation and progression of enteral feeding dictated slow progression in the volume infused followed by cautious increases in formula concentration in an effort to avoid gastrointestinal side effects. This practice resulted in significant delays in reaching optimal intakes, and many clinicians chose to use parenteral nutrition to provide optimal nutrition within 48 to 72 hours.[1] We now know, however, that the gut is capable of assimilating nutrients starting at rates approaching actual daily energy needs[2–4] and that in most cases gastrointestinal side effects are not directly related to the enteral formula infusion.[5]

Enteral feeding is recognized and appreciated as a sophisticated form of specialized nutrition support and an important part of medical treatment plans. Successful feeding regimens are those that are individualized and carefully monitored and reflect the knowledge of gastrointestinal physiology in critical and chronic illness.

ISSUES CONCERNING FEEDING METHOD, RATE, OSMOLALITY, AND FORMULA DILUTION

Method of Formula Infusion: Bolus vs. Continuous Feedings

Formula may be given through the feeding tube as a bolus feeding or via a continuous drip method. For bolus feedings a prescribed volume of formula, usually 200 to 300 mL is given via a syringe over a period of about 30 minutes every 3 to 4 hours. This method is used when the tube placement is intragastric and when patients are fully alert, thus decreasing the risk of aspiration.

The continuous drip method involves the slow, controlled delivery of formula by using a volumetric pump and is the method of choice for critically ill patients. Infusion rates usually range from 50 to 125 mL/hr, and formula is infused over the entire 24-hour period. This method is used for intraduodenally or intrajejunally placed feeding tubes. The use of volumetric pumps for continuous feeding is recommended and is reported to decrease nursing time, maintain tube patency, and avoid fluxes in feeding volume.[6]

Cycled Continuous Formula Infusion

Recently the concept of cycled continuous feedings has emerged whereby formula is administered on a controlled delivery basis for 10 to 16 hr/day, with provisions for bowel rest and a postabsorptive period during the 24-hour cycle. Research investigating this approach focuses on the issues of energy expenditure, protein metabolism, and the physiologic and metabolic impact of continuous 24-hour vs. cycled continuous feeding on circadian rhythms and the normal cascade of gut hormone release. When compared with bolus feeding, continuous 24-hour nutrient infusion is associated with increased energy efficiency.[7, 8] However, in a study comparing continuous (24-hour) enteral feeding and cycled continuous feeding at night only, Campbell et al.[9] found that patients fed on a 24-hour basis had significantly higher oxygen consumption ($P < .01$), higher catecholamine excretion ($P < .05$), and better nitrogen balance ($P < .05$) than cyclically fed patients. The improved performance in nitrogen balance in the 24-hour–fed group was in contrast to an earlier study by Campbell et al.[10] in which patients fed intermittently via bolus infusion every 2 hours with an 8-hour pause (10 P.M. to 6 A.M.) had better nitrogen balances than the 24-hour–fed group. These conflicting results may be due to the limited time of entrainment to night feedings in the 24-hour vs. cycled continuous feeding study, which resulted in poorer nitrogen utilization.

Pinchcofsky-Devin and Kaminski[11] examined the effect of a cycled vs. 24-hour continuous enteral feeding schedule on serum albumin and transferrin levels by using two groups of ten afebrile matched control patients. Both groups received continuous (24-hour) enteral feeding for 19 ± 6 days with no improvement in serum albumin or transferrin levels. This feeding schedule remained the same for ten of the patients, while the other ten were changed to an 8-hour interrupt (16-hour night feeding, 8-hour day fast) infusion schedule, with calories, protein, and total volume remaining the same. Repeat serum albumin and transferrin levels after 10 days showed a significant increase ($P < .005$) in those patients changed to an interrupted feeding schedule.

Tube Feedings and Circadian Rhythms

In an investigation of modifications in the circadian cortisol rhythm by cyclic and continuous total enteral nutrition, Saito et al.[12] assigned 18 patients who were in vegetative states and had been receiving enteral nutrition to one of three groups: 6 patients were fed on a 24-hour continuous basis, 6 patients were fed continuously during the day

from 8 A.M. to 8 P.M., and 6 patients were fed continuously during the night from 8 P.M. to 8 A.M. The results showed a clear cortisol rhythm in patients fed during the day, with a peak cortisol level at 8 A.M. This pattern is similar to the cortisol rhythm of normal subjects. Patients fed nocturnally also demonstrated a cortisol rhythm; however, the peak appeared at 4 P.M. No significant difference was found in the amplitude of the rhythm between the diurnally and nocturnally fed groups. Patients fed on a continuous 24-hour basis did not show any consistent circadian cortisol rhythm. Plasma levels of glucose, insulin, and free fatty acids also showed circadian fluctuations corresponding to the pattern of nutrient infusion in the day and night interrupted schedules but remained almost constant throughout the day in the group fed on a continuous 24-hour basis.

Gastric emptying has also been shown to occur with circadian variation. In a study to determine whether gastric emptying could explain the circadian changes in drug absorption of orally administered drugs, Goo et al.[13] measured changes in gastric emptying rates at 8 A.M. and 8 P.M. in 16 healthy male subjects synchronized with diurnal activity and nocturnal rest. The subjects received standardized test meals 8 hours prior to testing and were allowed only tap water for the following 7.5 hours. At the test time, a second standardized meal was taken, this one with added radioisotopic markers. Results indicated that the solid-phase gastric emptying of the standardized meal consumed in the morning was significantly more rapid ($P < 0.001$) than the solid-phase emptying of the evening meal. Liquid-phase emptying was also consistently more rapid in the morning than the evening, but the difference was not statistically significant. This circadian difference in gastric emptying may prove to have clinical significance in the timing of the delivery of enteral feeding.

Administering enteral feeding by using a continuous cyclic approach more closely simulates the usual pattern of fed and postabsorptive states to which man has evolved. Postabsorptive physiology is characterized by lower insulin and higher glucagon levels and results in a shift to the utilization of glycogen, fat, and amino acids as fuel molecules. This postabsorptive pattern of substrate utilization seems to allow more efficient amino acid and nitrogen metabolism and promote visceral protein synthesis.

The usual cascade of gut hormone release and feedback mechanisms may be disrupted by 24-hour continuous enteral feeding because of continuous stimulation of hormone release. This disruption may have a significant impact on homeostasis and the utilization of fuel molecules. Endocrine cells that synthesize and secrete gastrointestinal hormones are scattered throughout the stomach and small intestine. Different cell types secrete their hormones directly into the gut and the circulation in response to distension of the gut wall, the presence of intraluminal nutrients, or a low pH. Some hormones like gastrin, cholecystokinin, and secretin enhance the digestive process by influencing gastrointestinal motility and stimulating the secretion of digestive enzymes and acid. Other hormones, however, are inhibitory to the digestive process and may function to signal the end of the digestive process. Constant release of both types of hormones because of the infusion of foodstuff on a 24-hour continuous basis perpetuates a paradoxical situation. By cycling the feeding schedule and allowing a postabsorptive state, the usual pattern of hormonal release and feedback can occur.

The method of continuous cyclic feeding with day infusion and night fast may be the most desirable schedule for optimizing nursing time and patient safety. Although digestive enzyme secretion, hormone release, and perhaps gastric emptying can adjust to a circadian pattern of night feeding, it seems safer to feed patients during the day when the ratio of nurses to patients is usually higher and patients are usually alert and more likely to be in an upright position. These factors may decrease the risk of aspiration when compared with night feeding, when the nurse-to-patient ratio is generally lower and the patient is more likely to be lying flat and asleep. One drawback to daytime feeding, however, is that there may be more interruptions in the feeding schedule because of medical procedures and tests.

Infusion Rate

Issues to consider when determining the initial formula infusion rate include the position of the feeding tube and the length of time the patient has been without feeding. Patients being fed intrajejunally will require a slower initiation of formula because of the limited reservoir capacity of the jejunum. An initial feeding rate of 50 mL/hr is usually well tolerated, with increases of 25 mL/hr every 8 to 12 hours until the goal rate is reached. By using isosmotic formula via 12 F catheter feeding jejunostomies, Hinsdale et al.[14] were able to achieve optimal feeding volumes with this schedule in 91% of the patients studied by the fourth postoperative day (the second to third feeding day).

Patients who have experienced a prolonged period without intraluminal food will also require a slower administration of enteral formula initially. The lack of stimulation by enteral foodstuff results in gut atrophy and reduced concentrations of digestive enzymes. By beginning slowly, the gastrointestinal tract will have a chance to readjust to intraluminal feeding. Reports indicate[15] that the regeneration of gut mucosa in response to feeding begins as early as 4 hours after the initiation of feeding. An initial rate of 30 to 50 mL/hr of isotonic formula for the first 24 hours is reasonable, followed by increases of 25 mL/hr every 8 to 12 hours until the goal volume is reached.

Recent studies[2, 3, 16] demonstrate the capacity of the gastrointestinal tract to assimilate enteral feedings delivered at initial rates and concentrations that provide a full complement of estimated energy requirements on the first feeding day. Elimination of "starter regimens" expedites the achievement of optimal energy intake and nitrogen balance. Rees and colleagues[2] initiated hyperosmolar (630 mOsm/kg) enteral feedings via intragastric feeding tubes continuously at 87 mL/hr in 12 patients with exacerbation of inflammatory bowel disease and 2 patients with short-bowel syndrome. Five patients experienced transient gastrointestinal symptoms of nausea, abdominal bloating, and colicky pain, but it was never necessary to reduce the rate of infusion due to these symptoms. There was no significant difference in the number of stools per day, as measured 24 hours before the feeding was begun and upon completion of the feeding. It is important to note, however, that these patients were fed intragastrically, thus having the advantage of the pylorus to regulate solute loads delivered to the upper part of the small intestine.

In a study using intraduodenally fed healthy male volunteers, Zarling et al.[16] compared the effect of various formula flow rates (50, 100, and 150 kcal/hr) and osmolalities (325, 345, 650, and 690 mOsm/kg) on clinical intolerance or carbohydrate malabsorption. The group found no significant differences between the low and high infusion rates for symptoms of abdominal pain, bloating, rectal gas, and bowel movements. The authors suggest that well-nourished patients requiring maintenance enteral feeding need not be started at low flow rates or with hypoosmolar formula.

Ott et al.[17] report that enteral feeding into the stomach is poorly tolerated in the immediate posttrauma period for head-injured patients. In a prospective study of 12 patients with moderate to severe head injuries, the group found delayed and abnormal biphasic responses to gastric emptying in the first 2 weeks postinjury that prohibited the use of gastric feeding. By the third week the majority of patients demonstrated an improvement in gastric emptying, although delays and abnormal biphasic responses were still observed. By day 16 postinjury, all but 2 patients were able to tolerate full-strength, full-rate feedings. Feeding into the duodenum or the jejunum using a continuous drip method will circumvent issues related to gastric emptying in this patient population.

Data suggest that with the exception of head-injured patients, it is possible to initiate intragastric or intraduodenal feeding at rates providing up to 150 kcal/hr and concentrations up to 690 mOsm/L in patients who have not experienced a prolonged period with nothing by mouth (NPO) and are previously well fed. Although initiation in this manner provides immediate optimal nutrition, one could also argue that with patients who are well fed up to the point of injury, a more cautious approach of initiating feeding at a lower rate is prudent. Establishing early tolerance to a smaller volume of feeding and reaching optimal intakes over a period of 24 to 36 hours may provide greater benefit without adversely affecting the overall nutritional status in this population.

Determining the Goal Infusion Rate

Estimating Caloric Needs.—The goal rate of formula infusion is calculated from the total caloric needs, the caloric density of the formula, and the number of feedings or hours of daily infusion. The provision of an appropriate caloric dose is a crucial factor in achieving feeding tolerance and metabolic homeostasis in the critically ill patient. Energy needs tend to be overestimated and this results in higher infusion rates of enteral formula than necessary. Overfeeding is associated with many metabolic complications including increased CO_2 production, increased minute ventilation, fatty liver infiltration, electrolyte imbalance, excess fluid accumulation, and poor gastrointestinal tolerance. Increased CO_2 production and minute ventilation may prolong weaning from the ventilator in patients with respiratory compromise. Although many methods have been developed to estimate energy needs, experience has shown that energy needs in hospitalized patients rarely exceed 25 to 35 kcal/kg.[18] In a study of resting energy expenditure of critically ill patients, Hunter et al.[19] found that body weight alone was as predictive as the Harris-Benedict formula without a multiplication factor in predicting energy needs when compared with actual needs measured by indirect calorimetry. Although less predictive in individual cases, the group suggested that 22 times the weight in kilograms gives a good mean estimate ($P < .05$) of resting energy expenditure.

Liggett and Renfro[20] also document the adequacy of the Harris-Benedict formula, without modifications for the severity of disease or other factors, in predicting the energy expenditure in mechanically ventilated, nonsurgical, critically ill patients. Caloric requirements based on the Harris-Benedict equation were compared with actual energy expenditures derived by the Fick method, which estimates energy expenditure by utilizing the Vo_2 from the measured thermodilution cardiac output and the O_2 content differences between arterial and mixed venous blood. Results showed no significant differences in measured vs. estimated energy expenditures for patients with cardiogenic shock, cardiogenic pulmonary edema, adult respiratory distress syndrome, (ARDS), or pneumonia or those classified as "other" (pulmonary emboli, dehydration, chronic interstitial lung disease, or chronic obstructive pulmonary

disease [COPD]). The difference was significant ($P < .0001$), however, for patients with septic shock, with the measured energy expenditure (1982 ± 97 kcal/day) being greater than the estimated value (1534 ± 56). The authors conclude that in mechanically ventilated nonsurgical patients without sepsis, no modifications of the Harris-Benedict formula are necessary and, in those patients with sepsis, an increase of 20% over the predicted value is appropriate.

Regardless of the method used to calculate energy needs, care should be taken to avoid overfeeding. During critical illness, a therapeutic goal of maintaining a eucaloric state will avoid creating additional stress through oversupply of nutrients. Calculations of energy needs should be based on dry body weight; careful assessment of the patient's hydration status will prevent overdosage or underdosage of calories due to edema or dehydration. Laboratory and clinical parameters helpful in the assessment of hydration status include serum sodium, the blood urea nitrogen-to-creatinine ratio, urine specific gravity, weight, and skin turgor.

Osmolality, Formula Dilution, and Gastrointestinal Tolerance

Osmolality reflects the number of particles per kilogram of solution. At a given concentration, solutions with smaller particle sizes will have a higher osmolality because of the larger number of particles present. The osmolality of enteral formulas is primarily affected by carbohydrate, proteins, and electrolytes. Formulas containing hydrolyzed nutrients will have higher osmolalities than those with intact nutrients because more particles will exist per volume of solution. Hyperosmolar (>300 mOsm) solutions in the gastrointestinal tract cause the movement of water from surrounding areas into the lumen, thereby effecting a lowered solution concentration and osmolality.

Early protocols for tube feeding promoted the initial infusion of isotonic or hypotonic formulas to prevent the influx of water into the lumen of the gastrointestinal tract, a phenomenon presumably responsible for tube feeding diarrhea or the dumping syndrome. It is now evident, however, that many factors other than the feeding formula may be responsible for gastrointestinal intolerance to enteral feeding, including medications and *Clostridium difficile* toxin.[5] Recent studies have demonstrated[4, 16] the ability of the gastrointestinal tract to assimilate full-strength hypertonic formulas administered intragastrically or intraduodenally at rates up to 150 kcal/hr without ensuing diarrhea or abdominal cramping.

To determine the relationship between diet tonicity and gastrointestinal side effects and to evaluate the efficacy of "starter regimens" beginning with hypotonic diets, Keohane et al.[4] randomly allocated 118 patients in a double-blind fashion to receive one of three nasogastric feeding regimens administered over a period of 24 hours: 1900 mL of undiluted hypertonic (430 mmol/kg) diet (40 patients), 2625 mL of an undiluted isotonic diet (39 patients), or the hypertonic feeding (1900 mL/day) with a 3-day starter regimen in which nitrogen intake and osmolality were gradually increased from day 1 to day 4 (39 patients). The mean duration of feeding was 8.8 days for patients receiving the full-strength hypertonic and isotonic diets and 8.5 days for patients receiving hypotonic formula with the starter regimen. The results showed a significantly better ($P < .05$) nitrogen intake and balance in the group receiving 1900 mL of hypertonic formula when compared with the other two groups. Although no difference was found among the groups in the incidence of gastrointestinal side effects related to the diet, diarrhea was significantly associated ($P < .001$) with the use of antibiotics.

As previously described, Zarling et al.[16] have also shown that normal volunteers can tolerate continuous intraduo-denal feedings with osmolalities up to 690 mOsm delivered at up to 150 kcal/hr without adverse gastrointestinal side effects. This work demonstrated the capacity of the duodenum to assimilate directly infused hypertonic formula in previously well fed individuals.

Most commercially available enteral formulas are isotonic or moderately hypertonic (>700 mOsm). In comparison, the osmolality of many foods provided on clear and full liquid diets exceeds that of enteral formula.[21] Juices, fruit ice, and gelatin, in particular, tend to have osmolalities greater than 600 mOsm (Table 20–1). Patients are routinely advanced to full-strength clear liquid diets postsurgically or after extubation without suffering adverse gastrointestinal symptoms, yet if those same patients were to require tube feeding, the tendency for most clinicians would be to dilute the initial formula to isotonicity or hypotonicity.

Dilution of enteral formulas is associated with an increased risk of bacterial contamination of the feeding.[22] Sources for this contamination include the water used for dilution, mixing utensils, or microbes present on the skin of persons handling the feeding. In contrast, formulas poured directly from the can into the delivery set and used full strength or those prepackaged in ready-to-use delivery sets show a reduced incidence of

TABLE 20–1.

Osmolality of Selected Foods*

Food Item	Osmolality (mOsm/kg)
Prune juice	1076
Water ice	1064
Cranberry juice	836
Jello, cherry	735
Cola	714
Apple juice	705
Orange juice	601
Ginger ale	565
Chicken broth, low sodium, low fat	452
Chicken broth, regular	389

*Adapted from Bell SJ, Anderson FL Bistrian BR, et al: *Nutr Clin Pract* 1987; 2:241–244.

contamination as compared with those that have been manipulated in any way.

When choosing an enteral formula, priority should be placed on the mix of nutrient substrates rather than the formula osmolality or caloric density. If formula osmolality is of significant concern (e.g., the patient has had an extended NPO period), allowance should be made for gastrointestinal adaptation by beginning with a slower rate of infusion (30 to 50 mL/hr) rather than diluted formula. Likewise, jejunal feeding can also be initiated with full-strength hypertonic formula. If the diameter of the feeding tube is of sufficient size, a formula having intact nutrients may be used. However, if feeding via a needle catheter jejunostomy, a monomeric formula is necessary to maintain tube patency.

Protocols for the initiation of enteral feeding have become less restrictive over the past decade as research has demonstrated the tremendous capacity of the gastrointestinal tract to digest, absorb, and assimilate nutrients (Table 20–2). The delivery method of enteral nutrients has an impact on gastrointestinal function as well as metabolic homeostasis.

TABLE 20–2.

Suggestions for Initiating Enteral Feeding

Method of feeding: Use the continuous method of infusion via volumetric pump[6] for intraduodenal or intrajejunal feedings. Cycle the feeding when possible to allow a postabsorptive state, gut rest, and adjustment to circadian rhythms.[9, 11–13]

Rate: If prolonged NPO status, head injury, or initial jejunostomy feeding, begin with 50 mL/hr and advance by 25 mL/hr every 8 to 12 hr as tolerance allows to the optimal feeding rate.[14, 17].

If the patient is previously well fed (NPO no longer than 72 hr), with intragastric or intraduodenal tube placement, begin with the optimal feeding rate.[2, 3, 16]

Caloric intake: Use the Harris-Benedict formula without a multiplication factor.[19, 20] Begin with dry body weight. If sepsis is present, increase the result by 20%.[20] Evaluate adequacy once the full amount of formula infusion is achieved with N_2 balance and/or indirect calorimetry.

Osmolality: Do not dilute the formula,[4, 16, 22] Use isotonic formula if necessary or regulate osmolality via the rate of feeding delivery.

Evidence suggests that cycled continuous feeding may promote greater metabolic efficiency than continuous 24-hour feedings.

Optimal intakes can be achieved with enteral feeding within 24 to 36 hours after initiation. In uncomplicated cases, it is possible to initiate feedings at the goal infusion rate. An accurate estimation of the patient's energy requirement is a critical factor in promoting feeding tolerance. In patients without sepsis, the Harris-Benedict formula without a multiplication factor will provide a good estimation of energy needs. For patients with sepsis, this figure may be increased by 20%.

When tube feeding is properly managed, the osmolality of an enteral formula is not associated with an increase in gastrointestinal intolerance, and the formula should not be diluted. The occurrence of gastrointestinal intolerance is usually related to factors other than the formula, such as medication or *C. difficile* toxin. Moreover, the practice of formula dilution provides a primary route for bacterial contamination. In patients needing time for gastrointestinal adaption to enteral feeding, a slower rate of infusion rather than a hypotonic formula should be initiated.

REFERENCES

1. Bowers DF: The logistics of enteral nutrition support: Current practices for the initiation and progression of tube feeding, in *Enteral Nutrition Support for the 1990s: Innovations in Nutrition, Technology, and Techniques.* Report of the Twelfth Ross Roundtable on Medical Issues, Columbus, Ohio, Ross Laboratories, 1992, pp 30–34.
2. Rees RGP, Keohane PP, Grimble GK, et al: Elemental diet administered nasogastrically without starter regimens to patients with inflammatory bowel disease. *JPEN* 1986; 10:258–262.
3. Rees RGP, Keohane PP, Grimble GK, et al: Tolerance of elemental diet ad-

ministered without starter regimen. *BMJ* 1985; 290:1869–1870.

4. Keohane PP, Attrill H, Love M, et al: Relation between osmolality of diet and gastrointestinal side effects in enteral nutrition, *BMJ* 1984; 288:678–680.

5. Edes TE, Walk BE, Austin JL: Diarrhea in tube-fed patients: Feeding formula not necessarily the cause. *Am J Med* 1990; 88:91–93.

6. Jones BJM, Payne S, Silk DBA: Indications for pump-assisted enteral feeding. *Lancet* 1980; 1:1057–1058.

7. Grant J, Denne SC: Effect of intermittent versus continuous enteral feeding on energy expenditure in premature infants. *J Pediatr* 1991; 118:928–932.

8. Hemsfield S, Casper K, Grossman G: Bioenergetic and metabolic response to continuous v intermittent nasoenteric feeding. *Metabolism* 1987; 36:570–575.

9. Campbell IT, Morton RP, Macdonald IA, et al: Comparison of the metabolic effects of continuous postoperative enteral feeding and feeding at night only. *Am J Clin Nutr* 1990; 52:1107–1112.

10. Campbell IT, Morton RP, Cole JA, et al: A comparison of the effects of intermittent and continuous nasogastric feeding on the oxygen consumption and nitrogen balance of patients after major head and neck surgery. *Am J Clin Nutr* 1983; 38:870–878.

11. Pinchcofsky-Devin GD, Kaminski MV: Visceral protein increase associated with interrupt versus continuous enteral hyperalimentation. *JPEN* 1985; 9:474–476.

12. Saito M, Nishimura K, Kato H: Modifications of circadian cortisol rhythm by cyclic and continuous total enteral nutrition. *J Nutr Sci Vitaminol (Tokyo)* 1989; 35:639–647.

13. Goo RH, Moore JG, Greenberg E, et al: Circadian variation in gastric emptying of meals in humans. *Gastroenterology* 1987; 93:515–518.

14. Hinsdale JG, Lipkowitz GS, Pollock TW, et al: Prolonged enteral nutrition in malnourished patients with nonelemental feeding: Reappraisal of surgical technique, safety, and costs. *Am J Surg* 1985; 149:334–338.

15. Bristol JB, Williamson RCN, Chir M: Nutrition, operations, and intestinal adaptation. *JPEN* 1988; 12:299–309.

16. Zarling EJ, Parmar JR, Mobarhan S, et al: Effect of enteral formula infusion rate, osmolality, and chemical composition upon clinical tolerance and carbohydrate absorption in normal subjects. *JPEN* 1986; 10:588–590.

17. Ott L, Young B, Phillips R, et al: Altered gastric emptying in the head-injured patient: Relationship to feeding intolerance. *J Neurosurg* 1991; 74:738–742.

18. Driscoll DF, Blackburn GL: Total parenteral nutrition 1990. A review of its current status in hospitalized patients, and the need for patient-specific feeding, *Drugs* 1990; 40:346–363.

19. Hunter DC, Jaksic T, Lewis D, et al: Resting energy expenditure in the critically ill: Estimations versus measurement. *Br J Surg* 1988; 75:875–878.

20. Liggett SB, Renfro AD: Energy expenditures of mechanically ventilated nonsurgical patients. *Chest* 1990; 98:682–686.

21. Bell SJ, Anderson FL, Bistrian BR, et al: Osmolality of beverages commonly provided on clear and full liquid menu. *Nutr Clin Pract* 1987; 2:241–244.

22. Kohn CL, Keithley JK: Enteral nutrition. Potential complications and patient monitoring. *Nurs Clin North Am* 1989; 24:339–353.

21

Parenteral Nutrition

Michael S. Nussbaum, M.D.

Josef E. Fischer, M.D.

The multiple advances in the overall management of critically ill patients in recent years have improved the clinician's ability to successfully treat patients who otherwise might have died. An understanding of the nutritional and metabolic derangements and requirements have played a central role in the care of these patients. The hypermetabolic response to injury is a generalized response that is initiated by a variety of stimuli such as shock, severe inflammation, and the extensive tissue injury associated with major burns and traumatic injury. Regardless of the patient's underlying nutritional status prior to the illness or injury, this marked hypercatabolic response can rapidly lead to severe wasting of lean body mass, impairment of vital organ function, and a delayed or diminished response to inflammatory and infectious processes. Therefore, it is clear that most critically ill patients will require some nutritional intervention in order to maintain and support their metabolic needs during their illness and recovery until they are able to meet these needs on their own.

Critically ill individuals often have a multitude of complex physical and physiologic derangements that will take precedence over their metabolic needs. Emergent operative intervention and stabilization of the patient's ventilatory, hemodynamic, acid-base, and fluid/electrolyte status remain the priorities in their initial management. Nutritional intervention should only be considered once these factors have been corrected or optimized and adequate cardiopulmonary function and tissue oxygenation have been restored so as to allow for optimal delivery and utilization of the supplemental nutrients. Generally, these derangements can be addressed rapidly, and prompt initiation of nutrition support within the first 24 to 48 hours is almost always possible.

Traditionally, support by total parenteral nutrition (TPN) has been the mainstay of nutritional therapy for critically ill or injured patients. Clearly, parenteral nutrition is required in patients whose gastrointestinal tracts are nonfunctional or in whom bowel rest is desired. However, the early institution of enteral nutrition is generally safe and effective and appears to improve the overall outcome in this population of patients. Although still controversial there appears to be a significantly lower incidence of septic morbidity in patients fed enterally after severe injury.[1] Enteral nutrition is considerably less expensive than parenteral feeding and may also prevent the atrophy of gastrointestinal villi that is theoretically linked to a loss of the barrier function of the intact intestinal mucosa, a concept that has yet to be demonstrated in man in clinical circumstances. Although gastric and colonic motility is often impaired in critical illness, small intestinal motility and absorption are usually intact, and small-bore nasoenteric feeding tubes can be easily placed at the bedside in most intensive care units (ICUs). Nevertheless, it is often difficult to adequately meet the metabolic needs of these patients via the gastrointestinal tract because of complications that limit the amount of nutrients that can be delivered. Mechanical problems with the delivery system, gastrointestinal dysfunction, interruptions of feeding in preparation for operative procedures and diagnostic tests, and metabolic complications may limit the effectiveness of enteral therapy.[2, 3] Therefore, concomitant parenteral nutrition is frequently required until enteral feedings can be advanced to meet the individual's needs or in cases where the patient is intolerant of enteral nutrition.[4, 5] The advantages of enteral feeding may be unrelated to the total nutrient intake, and any amount of enteral feeding may be better than no enteral feeding at all, even when TPN provides the majority of caloric intake.[6] The exact amount of enteral feeding that may exert a beneficial effect is not known, but it may be as little as 10% to 20% of caloric needs given enterally.

The effective delivery of parenteral nutrition in the intensive care setting requires a detailed understanding of the indications for the initiation of nutrition support and the techniques for accurately determining the patient's metabolic requirements. Safe and effective techniques for gaining access to the central venous system and maintaining sterility for that access in a nosocomially hostile environment are essential in the majority of cases where parenteral nutrition is indicated. Finally, specific disease states and organ dysfunction often demand that the nutritional formulation be tailored to meet specific needs and restrictions.

INDICATIONS FOR INITIATING PARENTERAL NUTRITION

The length of time an individual can withstand inadequate nutritional intake depends upon a number of variables, including the previous state of health and nutrition, the degree of pre-existing malnutrition, age, the severity of the illness, the presence of sepsis, and the length of time expected until oral intake resumes. A patient who is malnourished prior to injury or illness will certainly benefit from early, aggressive nutrition support. Similarly, a septic or injured patient in whom a prolonged ICU course is anticipated should also benefit from early nutritional intervention. Techniques of nutrition support are generally better for preservation of lean body mass than for repletion in patients who have lost considerable lean body mass. Therefore, it is preferable to initiate nutrition support in appropriate patients as soon as the need is identified.[7] Few definitive data are available regarding specific indications for the institution of nutritional support. However, certain guidelines are helpful.

Patients who are candidates for parenteral nutrition support are those who cannot eat, patients in whom bowel rest is desired, or those who are unable to take in sufficient enteral nutrients. If gastrointestinal tract function is present, enteral nutrient administration is the preferred route. As the metabolic rate increases, one has to take into consideration the patient's prior nutritional state in determining a reasonable threshold for instituting appropriate nutrition support (Fig 21–1). As a general rule, an adult aged 60 years or less with previously normal nutrition who is moderately catabolic will usually tolerate up to 14 days of starvation without dem-

onstrating a significant nutritional deficit. We do not advocate waiting this prolonged a period of time, but it is usually tolerated. Patients who are 60 to 70 years old tolerate only about 10 days of starvation, and patients who are over 70 years of age will tolerate no more than 5 to 7 days of starvation. In critically ill patients, however, deficits generally occur after 7 to 10 days regardless of age. Therefore, nutritional intervention should be initiated well before this time to avoid compromising physiologic function in these catabolic patients.

Clinical settings where TPN should be a part of routine care include severely catabolic patients whose gastrointestinal tracts will be unusable for more than 5 to 7 days, severe malnutrition and a nonfunctional gastrointestinal tract, severe pancreatitis, massive small-bowel resection, diseases of the small intestine, radiation enteritis, intractable diarrhea, intractable vomiting, high-dose chemotherapy or radiotherapy, and bone marrow transplantation.

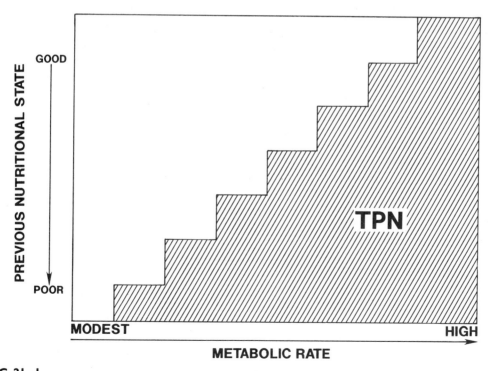

FIG 21–1.
The relationship between nutritional status and metabolic rate. As the metabolic rate increases, the threshold for initiating nutrition support is dependent upon the baseline nutritional state of the patient. (*TPN* = total parenteral nutrition.)

TPN is usually helpful in moderately malnourished patients who require intensive medical or surgical intervention, in patients in whom adequate enteral nutrition cannot be established within 7 to 10 days, and in the treatment of enterocutaneous fistulas, inflammatory bowel disease, hyperemesis gravidarum, and inflammatory adhesions with small-bowel obstruction. Parenteral nutrition is of limited value in a well-nourished patient suffering minimal stress or trauma when the gastrointestinal tract is expected to be usable within 10 days or in a proven or suspected untreatable disease state. TPN is not indicated when patients have a functional and usable gastrointestinal tract capable of absorption of adequate nutrients, when the sole dependence on TPN will be less than 5 days, when TPN therapy would delay an urgently needed operation, when aggressive nutrition support is not desired by the patient or legal guardian and when such action is in accordance with hospital policy and existing law, in patients whose prognosis does not warrant aggressive nutrition support, and when the risks of TPN are judged to exceed the benefits.[8]

A recent study by the Veterans Affairs TPN Cooperative Study Group in patients undergoing elective surgery suggested that except for severely malnourished patients, the infectious complication rate was higher when TPN was given preoperatively than in the control group.[9] These complications included both catheter-related and non−catheter-related infections, mainly pneumonia and wound infections, which suggests impairment of the immune mechanism in these patients. Similar conclusions were drawn by McGeer et al. in cancer patients with moderate malnutrition who were receiving chemotherapy. In these patients, TPN was also associated with an increased risk of infection.[10]

The goals of nutrition support in the critically ill patient include the minimization of starvation effects, attainment of nitrogen balance and reasonable visceral protein levels, prevention of specific nutrient deficiencies, and support of the acute-phase/inflammatory response until the patient heals and the hypermetabolic response resolves. It is important to recognize that as long as the source of infection or stress is present, septic/critically ill patients will not be capable of increasing or even maintaining their lean body mass. Thus, it is not enough to support these patients nutritionally, the sources of stress hypermetabolism must also be aggressively sought and treated. Because of the complex array of factors that affect these patients' nutritional needs, accurate assessment of their caloric and nutrient requirements is essential to meet the individual's needs and avoid the complications of overfeeding.

DETERMINATION OF ENERGY AND SUBSTRATE REQUIREMENTS

Energy Requirements

Critically ill patients demand very careful assessment of their caloric and nutrient needs, which generally require specific tailoring of the rate of delivery and formulation of the parenteral solutions. The goal of nutrition support in this setting is weight maintenance rather than weight gain. This approach will generally avoid complications of overfeeding while ensuring that nutrient metabolism is optimized. The basal energy expenditure (BEE) of a critically ill patient can be initially estimated by using the Harris-Benedict equations, which are based on the patient's age, sex, height, and weight (Table 21−1, A).[11] Additional adjustments for stress and activity are made by multiplying the basal values by Long's activity and stress factors, which are generally in the range of 1.2 to 2.1 (Table 21−1, B).[12] Another method for estimating energy requirements in critical illness is based upon providing 30 to 35 kcal/kg/day. These "rules of thumb" can be used to

TABLE 21–1.

Formulas for Estimating Energy Expenditure

A. Harris-Benedict equation[11]
    Males: BEE* (kcal) = 66.5 + [13.8 × weight (kg)] + [5 × height (cm)] − [6.8 × age (yr)]
    Females: BEE (kcal) = 655.1 + [9.6 × weight (kg)] + [1.9 × height (cm)] − [4.7 × age (yr)]
    Infants: BEE (kcal) = 22.1 + [31.1 × weight (kg)] + [1.2 × height (cm)]
B. Activity and stress factors[12]
    Total estimation of energy requirements = BEE × activity factor × stress factor
        Activity factor:
            Confined to bed = 1.2
            Out of bed = 1.3
        Stress factor:
            Minor operation = 1.2
            Skeletal trauma = 1.35
            Major sepsis = 1.6
            Major thermal injury = 2.1
C. Calculation of the metabolic rate (in patients with a thermodilution pulmonary artery catheter)
    Metabolic rate (kcal/hr) = V_{O_2} (mL/min) × 60 min/hr × 1 L/1,000 mL × 4.83 kcal/L
    V_{O_2} (mL/min) = Cardiac output (L/min) × [arterial oxygen content (CaO_2, mL/L) − mixed venous oxygen content (Cmv_{O_2}, mL/L)]

*BEE = basal energy expenditure.

identify approximate needs when initiating nutrition support. However, these methods are often inaccurate in complicated ICU patients. The formulas commonly underestimate the energy needs of mechanically ventilated surgical[13] patients, injured[14] patients, or patients with chronic obstructive pulmonary disease (COPD),[15] whereas the activity factors often overestimate the caloric requirements in other mechanically ventilated, sedated patients. In addition to the problems of underfeeding such catabolic patients, a major advance in recent years has been the recognition of excessive feeding as a complication. Therefore, although these formulas and stress factors are sufficient for initiating nutrition support, they will only accurately predict an individual's needs about one third of the time in the ICU setting.

The majority of critically ill patients who require nutrition support will benefit from assessment by indirect calorimetry. Actual measurement of the patient's oxygen consumption and carbon dioxide production by utilizing an automated metabolic cart is useful in the determination of energy expenditure in a resting, fed patient. This allows for an accurate prediction of the patient's actual resting energy expenditure (REE) and respiratory quotient (RQ) during the period of measurement (Fig 21–2).[16] Such measurements are most accurate and reproducible in patients who are endotracheally intubated. However, carefully conducted measurements can be performed in a cooperative, normally breathing (nonintubated) patient by utilizing canopy measurements. For many years these devices were subject to large errors that limited their clinical use, but recent improvements in equipment and technique have led to much wider use in the critical care setting.[17, 18] In general, candidates for indirect calorimetric measurement include patients with multiple risk and stress factors that may considerably skew Harris-Benedict equation results and patients who fail to respond adequately to estimated nutritional needs.

More specifically, the metabolic cart measurement should include but is not restricted to a variety of critically ill patient populations. Patients in whom multiple nutritional risk and stress factors or disease states affect their energy and nutrient requirements or otherwise make the Harris-Benedict or other en-

UNIVERSITY OF CINCINNATI MEDICAL CENTER
NUTRITION SUPPORT DIAGNOSTICS
<u>INDIRECT CALORIMETRIC MEASUREMENT</u>

Brief Diagnosis/Indication:

Nutrition Therapy During Testing: [ ] TPN Formula_____[ ] Lipids___ Rate____
                                  [ ] IVF_____ Rate_____
                                  [ ] TF Formula_____ Rate_____
                                  [ ] PO Diet_____

Activity Profile: Bed Rest_____
Ambulatory_____ PT_____
Other_____Temperature_____
Medications_____
Canopy_____Mask_____Ventilator____
Settings: FIO_2____V_E____Freq_____
V_T_____$FECO_2$_____$PaCO_2$_____

MEASUREMENT RESULTS

$\dot{V}O_2$_____mL/min

$\dot{V}O_2$_____mL/min
RQ_____
REE_____

5000 –

4000 –

3000 –

2000 –

1000 –

Estimated Energy Expenditure	Measured Energy Expenditure	Current Total qd Intake

Special considerations:_____
Interpretation:_____
_____
Recommendations:_____
_____

Date:___/___/___

Time:_____

_____
Operator

_____
Nutrition Support Attending

Transaction Code: Description:

| NSSR | CART | 1 2 9 3 4 |
| RESP | CART | 0 2 9 3 4 |

White - Medical Record   Yellow - MD   Pink - Billing   Goldenrod - Department

FIG 21–2.
Form used for reporting of indirect calorimetric measurement and assessment at the University of Cincinnati Medical Center. (*TPN* = total parenteral nutrition; *IVF* = intravenous fluids; *TF* = tube feeding; *PO* = oral; *PT* = physical therapy; *RQ* = respiratory quotient; *REE* = resting energy expenditure.) (Courtesy of the Department of Parenteral and Enteral Nutrition, University of Cincinnati Medical Center.)

ergy equations less accurate will benefit from indirect calorimetry. These include patients with neurologic trauma or major neurologic disease, amputations, paralysis, cancer with residual tumor bur-den, acute pancreatitis, COPD, and multiple trauma. Other clinical situations in which REE measurement is likely to improve the accurate determination of energy requirements include patients in whom the height and weight cannot be accurately obtained, patients who fail to respond sufficiently to estimated nutritional needs, all ICU patients who remain in critical care units for 5 days' duration or longer, severely hypermetabolic or hypercatabolic patients, all liver transplant patients and other transplant patients as deemed necessary, and morbidly obese patients. There are also certain clinical scenarios in which metabolic cart analysis will not be accurate. These include patients maintained on high-frequency ventilation, patients in whom canopy measurements are inappropriate (e.g., claustrophobics), canopy-measured patients who are at significant risk of nosocomial infection (e.g., neutropenia, acquired immunodeficiency syndrome [AIDS], reverse isolation), patients with chest tubes and a significant air leak, patients with incompetent tracheal cuffs, patients in whom the Fio_2 is greater than 60% when open circuit measurement systems are utilized, and patients in whom dialysis is in progress (defer measurement until after dialysis).[19]

Metabolic carts have become more commonplace in large ICUs and medical centers where many critically ill patients are cared for. In addition, newer methods are on the horizon for the continuous measurement of oxygen consumption by replenishment techniques or by mass spectrophotometry.[17, 18, 20–22] This will allow for more accurate determination of continuous energy expenditure as opposed to the "snapshot" that the current technology affords. These advanced technologies are not available in all settings. Another method for determining the REE is to calculate the metabolic rate from measurements of oxygen consumption (Vo_2). This requires the placement of a thermodilution pulmonary artery catheter (see Table 21–1, C).

Substrate Requirements

Once the ICU patient's energy requirements have been determined, it is important to provide these calories in a substrate formulation that can be utilized efficiently. It remains unclear what the ideal energy substrate is in critically ill patients receiving TPN. Glucose is the primary source of calories. However, the maximum rate of glucose oxidation is approximately 5 mg/kg/min (7.2 g/kg/day).[23] A portion of this glucose will be provided by ongoing gluconeogenesis, which is much higher than normal in an injured or septic patient. Much of this increase is related to an increased use of anaerobic glucose in healing and inflammatory tissue with the resulting lactate being recycled back to glucose in the liver. Gluconeogenesis decreases with increasing glucose intake. In critically ill patients it is completely suppressed at intakes of greater than 600 g/day.[24] Therefore, a reasonable starting point would be to provide approximately 5 g (20 kcal) of glucose per kilogram of body weight per day. Glucose has known protein-sparing effects.[25, 26] However, critically ill patients often tolerate large glucose loads poorly. Glucose intolerance, excess CO_2 production, and hepatic dysfunction may develop.[27, 28]

While glucose may be poorly tolerated, fat appears to be an obligatory fuel source in critical illness. Fat oxidation is increased with stress and is accompanied by increases in fat mobilization and turnover. Triglyceride hydrolysis is increased to a much greater extent than fat oxidation, thus accounting for a net increase in lipolysis in the face of injury, sepsis, or burns. In contrast, ketone synthesis is decreased with severe illness or injury.[24] Despite the increased utilization of fat, the provision of fat calories does not decrease gluconeogenesis as significantly as in the normal individual.

Protein requirements are increased in the critically ill patient. During stress both protein catabolism and protein synthesis are increased. However, there is an imbalance of protein breakdown relative to synthesis that results in a rapid decrease in lean body mass and overall nitrogen loss.[29] It has been hypothesized that there is a plasma factor that is capable of inducing muscle proteolysis in the face of trauma and sepsis.[30] Amino acids mobilized from skeletal muscle, connective tissue, and unstimulated intestine are used to support wound healing, inflammation, the acute-phase response, and gluconeogenesis. Ideally, one would prefer to provide these substrates via TPN. However, it is not certain whether the changes in protein metabolism induced by critical illness are influenced by the specific admixture of TPN.

Since part of the response to injury includes increased lipolysis and decreased glucose oxidation, TPN with a mixture of glucose, lipid, and nitrogen would be expected to reduce lipolysis and increase glucose oxidation. Furthermore, such feeding would be expected to increase protein synthesis. However, many patients remain in a state of net catabolism despite TPN.[31] While nitrogen balance can be improved, tissue catabolism may not be reversed.[32] Thus, as the degree of illness increases or when sepsis supervenes, the achievement of net protein synthesis becomes increasingly difficult and may not be attainable. The specific types of fuel sources used in parenteral feeding of the critically ill patient do not significantly alter these protein dynamics.[28, 33–36]

In hypermetabolic or septic patients, carbohydrate should constitute 60% to 70% of the nonprotein calories in order to avoid the complications of excess glucose infusion.[27, 28] In the face of a limited capacity to oxidize glucose, fat should be provided not only as a deterrent to essential fatty acid deficiency (2% to 5% of the total calories one to two times weekly) but also as a substantial portion of the nonprotein calories as well. As a general rule, lipid should be provided on a daily basis and should constitute 25% to 30% of the calories in a hypermetabolic patient. The maximum rate of lipid infusion is 1 g/kg/day in order to avoid the complications

of excess lipid infusion. The normal requirement for protein is 0.8 g/kg/day (60–70 g of protein per day), while in critical illness this requirement may increase to 1.5 to 2.0 g/kg/day. While protein catabolism is unresponsive to protein, glucose, or lipid administration, protein synthesis is responsive to amino acid infusion, and nitrogen balance can be attained through support of protein synthesis.[37–39] Nitrogen balance is an end point in metabolic support of critically ill patients. Conventional TPN formulas have a nonprotein calorie-to-nitrogen ratio of 150:1. Stressed, hypermetabolic patients with increased protein requirements and decreased calorie needs require a calorie-to-nitrogen ratio that is less (80 to 100:1) than that found in standard formulations. The administration of conventional TPN in this setting will result in excessive calorie and insufficient protein delivery. In order to determine whether an adequate quantity and composition of protein are being provided, nitrogen balance should be calculated and followed at least weekly and whenever it appears that the patient is not responding to the current parenteral regimen. In addition, the determination of short-turnover proteins such as transferrin, retinol-binding protein, and thyroxine-binding prealbumin will give some indication as to the adequacy of protein and calorie intake.

Provision of the major electrolytes (sodium, potassium, chloride, phosphorus, calcium, and magnesium) is dependent upon measured serum levels and monitoring of excessive losses resulting from fistulas, diarrhea, vomiting, etc. The major intracellular ions (potassium, phosphorus) require close monitoring during initiation of TPN and once the patient has reached a state of anabolism. The exact dosages of trace element and vitamin replacement in hypermetabolic patients are unknown. Zinc requirements are usually increased and should be supplemented in accord with serum levels. Vitamin C and B complex may also be required in increased amounts in some of these patients. Although the remainder of the vitamins and trace elements can be administered in increased amounts, there is little evidence that any benefit would be derived. Therefore, in the majority of ICU patients, the standard amounts of trace elements and multivitamins should be provided unless specific losses or deficiencies are identified.

VENOUS ACCESS FOR PARENTERAL NUTRITION DELIVERY

Establishing Venous Access[19]

The optimal method for delivering the required calories in an acceptable volume of solution is to provide the formulation in a hypertonic mixture infused into a central vein. It is preferable but not always possible to access the central venous system with a single-lumen catheter placed percutaneously via the subclavian vein. This should be a new catheter that has not been used for other infusions or monitoring before the initiation of parenteral nutrition and is used solely for its administration.

Prior to placement of the central line, the patient should be prepared physiologically. Adequate restoration of intravascular volume is of primary importance. Critically ill patients who require nutrition support can be markedly hypovolemic early in the course of their illness or injury. At least 2 to 3 L of a balanced intravenous salt solution should be administered to patients who are volume depleted prior to central venous cannulation. In addition, coagulation abnormalities as indicated by a prolonged bleeding time or thrombocytopenia (platelet count below 50,000/mm^3) in a multiply transfused and/or septic patient must be considered. When identified, they should be corrected with specific component transfusion prior to attempted line placement. Adequate explanation of the indications and risks of the procedure, sedation, and proper

positioning of the patient are of equal importance once the patient is physiologically prepared.

The nature of the procedure is explained in detail with special attention given to describing the position of the patient during the procedure and to teaching the Valsalva maneuver. The physician informs the patient of the risks of the procedure, including possible misdirection of the catheter tip (requiring replacement or redirection of the catheter under fluoroscopy) and the risk of pneumothorax or hemothorax. Adequate documentation of patient teaching, discussion of procedural risks, and a signed consent should be available in the patient's medical record. Once consent has been obtained, the patient should be sedated with small doses of an intravenous benzodiazepine administered slowly via a peripheral intravenous line. The patient should be sedated and relaxed but still able to respond to commands. A rolled blanket is placed from the base of the patient's neck to the small of the back beneath the thoracic spine. This roll allows the patient's shoulders to extend back against the mattress when the patient is in a supine position. An analogy is the position of a "soldier at attention" with his head and shoulders dropped back and his arms at his side, a position that enables a horizontal approach to the subclavian vein. The patient's bed is placed in the Trendelenburg position to distend the subclavian vein. The patient's head is turned slightly away from the side of insertion.

Central venous access for parenteral nutrition administration is best accomplished via subclavian vein cannulation with the Seldinger technique (Fig 21−3). The side of choice is a matter of personal preference and experience. The left subclavian vein is generally easier to cannulate and follows a gentler curve than the right. However, there is a small but finite risk of thoracic duct injury during cannulation on this side. If there has been extensive injury to the subcla-

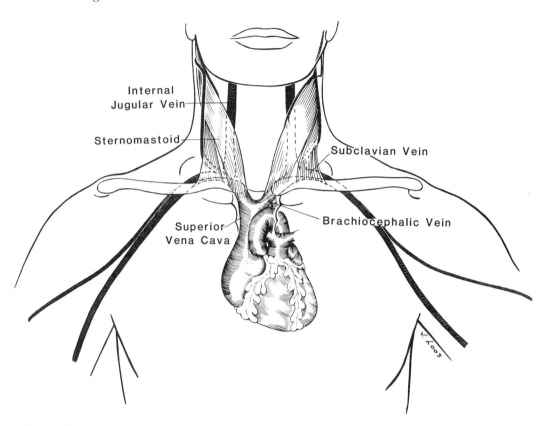

FIG 21–3.
Venous anatomy of the thoracic inlet. (From Hiyama DT (ed): *The Mont Reid Surgical Handbook,* ed 2. St Louis, Mosby–Year Book, 1990. Used by permission.)

vian region or known anatomic abnormalities on one side, the contralateral side should be used. In a situation where a tube thoracostomy is already in place and all other factors are equal, the catheter should be placed on the same side as the chest tube to protect against the development of a pneumothorax and avoid the need for contralateral tube thoracostomy.

Central line insertion is a surgical procedure and mandates the use of strict aseptic technique. Surgical caps and masks should be worn by all personnel in attendance and sterile drapes used to drape the field and shield the patient's face. The operator puts on a sterile gown and sterile gloves. Items present on the subclavian catheter insertion tray should be prepared and laid out in an orderly fashion prior to preparation of the patient's skin. Preparation of the skin is done in three steps. Initially, the

skin is cleansed with gauze sponges soaked in alcohol (the area of preparation is bounded laterally by the anterior axillary line and shoulder, superiorly by a line from the shoulder to the angle of the mandible, anteriorly along the mandible, medially by the midline, and inferiorly by a horizontal line through the nipple). Next, the area is cleansed three times with a povidone-iodine solution that should remain in contact with the skin for 2 minutes. Finally, the povidone-iodine is removed with alcohol. Three small towels or drapes should border the lateral, superior, and medial edges of the field, and a large drape should border the inferior edge of the field and extend over the lower part of the patient's chest and the abdomen to provide a work surface.

The point of insertion of the catheter is chosen at a spot near the junction of the proximal and middle thirds of the clavicle (Fig 21−4). This point is often found 1 cm inferior to and 1 cm medial to the bend of the clavicle. With a 25-gauge needle and syringe filled with lidocaine, a skin weal is made at the point of insertion by injecting 1% lidocaine. A 22-gauge needle and the lidocaine syringe are then advanced from the point of insertion toward an area below the fingertip of the operator's contralateral hand (placed in the sternal notch). The needle is passed in a horizontal position (not more than 10 degrees off the horizontal). As the needle is advanced, negative pressure is maintained by pulling on the plunger until the needle enters the subclavian vein and there is a return of blood into the syringe. The entire track is then anesthetized by injecting 1% lidocaine while slowly withdrawing the needle. A syringe with an 18-gauge

thin-walled Seldinger needle is then inserted along the same track immediately following removal of the small needle. The 18-gauge needle should be advanced slowly with negative pressure applied to the syringe barrel until a "pop" is felt as the vein is entered and the syringe fills with dark (venous) blood. When good intravascular position is attained, there will be free aspiration of blood into the syringe. In the absence of free aspiration of blood, threading of the guidewire is unlikely. The patient is then asked to perform a Valsalva maneuver, and a soft J-tipped intravascular guidewire is passed through the needle into the superior vena cava. The needle is withdrawn and the central venous catheter carefully passed over the wire into the superior vena cava. If the patient is being mechanicaly ventilated,

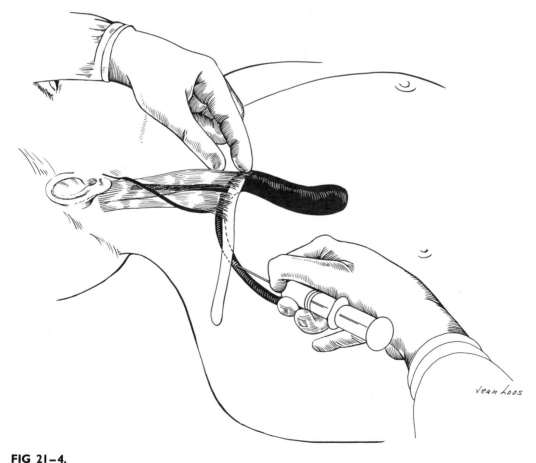

FIG 21−4.
Infraclavicular subclavian venipuncture. (From Hiyama DT (ed): *The Mont Reid Surgical Handbook*, ed 2. St Louis, Mosby−Year Book, 1990. Used by permission.)

positive-pressure ventilation should be temporarily stopped during the time of venipuncture and insertion of the guidewire. The catheter should be anchored to the skin with a single 3-0 silk suture placed at the insertion site. A 5- to 10-mm bite of skin should be taken medial to the point of catheter insertion and the knot tied loosely to avoid pressure necrosis of skin. The free ends of the suture are then passed around the catheter and tied securely.

Several points of precaution need to be mentioned. The wire should never be withdrawn through the needle because shearing may result and the wire may migrate and require fluoroscopic retrieval. Similarly, when the catheter is being threaded over the guidewire, the operator should always hold the guidewire either at the skin level or at the hub end of the catheter to prevent loss of the guidewire through the puncture site. Finally, suturing of the catheter should take place while the wire is still in the catheter lumen to avoid occluding the catheter with the suture and to prevent spillage of blood, leakage of air, or the development of a thrombus in the catheter. A single suture should be used to anchor the catheter. No additional sutures need to be placed in the catheter hub or along the catheter. The placement of multiple sutures usually results in catheter problems and provides difficulty in cleansing the entire subclavian region during subsequent dressing changes.

The catheter is now ready to be attached to the infusion system. The operator asks the patient to perform a Valsalva maneuver while the guidewire is removed, and a 500-mL bag of 5% dextrose in water is attached to the catheter via sterile intravenous tubing. Opening the roller clamp of the dextrose infusion establishes free flow through the catheter. Lowering the infusion bag below the level of the patient should result in a reflux of blood into the administration tubing to confirm intravascular tip position of the catheter. The bag is then raised to its original height to flow. The infusion should be given via an infusion device and run at a rate of 40 mL/hr until proper catheter tip position is confirmed. The rolled sheet is removed from beneath the patient, the bed is taken out of the Trendelenburg position, and a sterile occlusive dressing is applied.

Proper positioning of the catheter must be immediately confirmed by portable chest roentgenography. Acceptable positions of the catheter tip include the superior vena cava or the junction of the innominate vein and vena cava. A retrograde location of the catheter tip in the internal jugular or a location in the contralateral subclavian vein is unacceptable and can predispose the patient to thrombosis. Such misdirected catheters should be manipulated with aseptic technique under fluoroscopic guidance until they are in an acceptable position. Similarly, location of the catheter tip in the right atrium or ventricle is unacceptable because the stiffness of percutaneous catheters can cause endocardial lesions that subsequently become a nidus for bacterial or fungal infection. Erosion and perforation of the right atrium has been reported. The procedure has not been completed until the chest radiograph is seen and proper catheter position ensured.

At the conclusion of the procedure the operator should write a procedure note documenting the site of insertion, the type and dosage of sedative drug and local anesthetic, the type and size of catheter used, the number of needle passes, any complications encountered, and the position of the catheter tip on chest radiographs as well as any roentgenographic abnormalities that are seen on the postinsertion radiograph.

Occasionally the subclavian veins are not available or cannot be cannulated. In this situation central venous access for parenteral nutrition administration should be obtained via internal jugular venous cannulation (Fig 21–5). The same preparation and precautions are

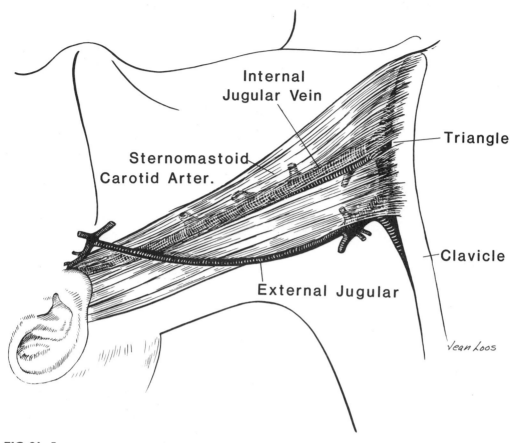

FIG 21–5.
Anatomy of the internal jugular vein. (From Hiyama DT (ed): *The Mont Reid Surgical Handbook,* ed 2. St Louis, Mosby–Year Book, 1990. Used by permission.)

necessary when accessing the internal jugular vein. However, the maintenance of a sterile occlusive dressing on the neck is more difficult than at the subclavian site, thus making these catheters more susceptible to contamination and subsequent catheter sepsis. Hence the subclavian site is preferred whenever possible.

To insert the internal jugular vein catheter, a point of insertion is selected approximately 5 cm above the clavicle along the posterior edge of the sternocleidomastoid muscle (Fig 21–6). Local anesthesia is used to infiltrate the skin, subcutaneous tissue, and the catheter insertion track from the point of insertion toward the suprasternal notch or slightly toward the ipsilateral nipple. After localization of the vein with a 22-gauge needle, an 18-gauge Seldinger

needle is used for catheter insertion over a guidewire in the same fashion as described above for the subclavian vein.

On rare occasions, the only route for central access is via the femoral veins or a peripherally inserted 24-in.-long central line. Neither of these options is very optimal, and often the risks inherrent with these methods outweigh any benefit that can be obtained. Femoral lines are associated with much higher complication rates because of the high density of skin pathogens in the region. Strict care of the entrance site along with frequent replacement of the catheter is required to decrease the incidence of complications. Peripherally inserted central lines are also associated with high infection rates and should be removed after 5 days. A much better approach to an ICU patient with limited ve-

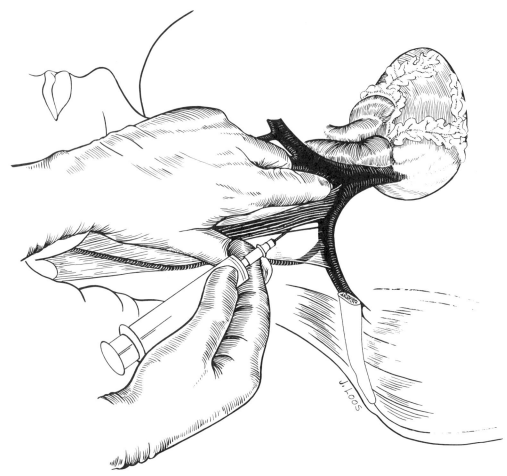

FIG 21-6.
Posterior approach for internal jugular venipuncture.

nous access is to utilize multiple-lumen catheters placed via the subclavian or internal jugular veins.[40]

Catheter Selection

Central venous access in a critically ill patient is often required for hemodynamic monitoring with pulmonary artery catheters and for infusions of a variety of intravenous solutions including TPN. In a patient with limited access, it is often necessary to infuse TPN through a multilumen catheter or through the venous infusion port of a pulmonary artery catheter. The use of these catheters allows for efficient care of the patient and management of multiple infusions while decreasing the risks of individual central line insertions. However, it is controversial as to whether infusion of TPN via these devices will increase the risk of catheter-related sepsis. It is crucial to limit the use of multilumen catheters for TPN infusion to instances where noncompatible solutions are being continuously infused in a patient with limited venous access. The least possible number of lumens should be utilized, and breaks in the continuity of the line for intermittent infusions and blood drawing should be discouraged.

Since the 7 F triple-lumen catheter was first introduced into clinical practice in 1983, there have been numerous reports and studies comparing infection rates of these vs. single-lumen catheters. The literature on this topic has yielded conflicting results. Some studies have demonstrated markedly increased catheter sepsis rates,[41, 42] while others have not been able to demonstrate a significant difference in the infection rate.[43-47] In one of the latter studies, Lee et al. hypothesize that the equivalent infection rate may be due to greater attention to skin preparation before insertion and during subsequent dressing changes.[44] The incidence of multilumen catheter–related sepsis appears to increase with the duration of catheter placement.[44] Guidewire exchange of central catheters has long been an accepted method for replacing existing lines with no increased incidence of infection[48, 49] unless the catheter and the subcutaneous tunnel have already been colonized by infectious organisms.[49-52] Routine exchange of triple-lumen catheters over a guidewire every 3 to 4 days has been shown to decrease the incidence of catheter-related sepsis to a rate equivalent to single-lumen catheters, which are not routinely exchanged.[53]

In our routine at the University of Cincinnati we require that all multilumen catheters that have TPN infusing through one of the ports be exchanged over a guidewire every 3 days. If there is suspected catheter-related sepsis, both the patient's blood and the catheter tip are cultured, and when catheter sepsis is documented or strongly suspected, the line is removed and a new line inserted at a different site. Occasionally, the only central venous access that an ICU patient has is a pulmonary artery catheter. Horowitz et al. have shown that the use of a pulmonary artery catheter for TPN infusion is a viable alternative to the use of the triple-lumen catheter, with no difference in the rate of catheter-related sepsis as long as the catheter is changed every 3 days.[47] It is the policy at our institution that the pulmonary artery catheter and introducer be exchanged over a guidewire at 3 days and removed at 6 days and be placed at a different site. By adhering to these guidelines we have been able to maintain an acceptable catheter-related sepsis rate. Between July 1989 and June

1992, 2114 central lines were placed for the administration of TPN (477 single-lumen, 1562 triple-lumen, and 75 pulmonary artery catheters) with an overall catheter-related sepsis rate of 4.5%. No difference in sepsis rates between groups was detected (Table 21–2). We define catheter-related sepsis very liberally as either culture-documented catheter infection or resolution of fever and signs of sepsis within 24 hours after removal of the line in a patient with no other identifiable source of infection. Between 1989 and 1991 the rate of colonization of the central lines, with or without positive blood cultures, was 3.6% (single lumen, 2.5%; triple lumen, 4.2%; pulmonary artery, 1.9%). While the incidence of sepsis is higher than one would like to see, the patient population has changed significantly. Many patients are severely traumatized and immunocompromised.

The role of catheter composition in the development of venous thrombus formation and subsequent development of catheter-related infection is well recognized. Rigid catheters such as those composed of polyethylene or Teflon are more often responsible for thromboses than are soft silicone or polyurethane catheters.[54, 55] In a study comparing a variety of catheter materials for thrombogenicity in an animal model, Borrow and Crowley demonstrated that polyurethane coated with hydromer was the least thrombogenic, the next least being silicone and plain polyurethane being

TABLE 21–2.

Central Venous Catheter Sepsis Rates*: University of Cincinnati Medical Center July 1989 to June 1992

Type of Catheter	Number of Catheters	Catheter Sepsis (%)†
Single lumen	477	20 (4.2)
Triple lumen	1562	69 (4.4)
Pulmonary artery	75	6 (8.0)
Total	2114	95 (4.5)

*Catheter related sepsis is defined as either culture-documented catheter infection or resolution of fever and signs of sepsis within 24 hours after removal of the line in a patient with no other identifiable source of infection.
†No significant difference between groups by analysis of variance.

the most thrombogenic.[56] Newer catheter materials containing elastomeric hydrogel become softer upon insertion and may prove to be even less thrombogenic than the materials currently available.[57]

A variety of antibiotics and antiseptic agents have been bonded to central venous catheters or catheter cuffs and have been associated with significantly lower bacterial colonization and sepsis rates.[58–60] A recent study evaluated the use of subcutaneous implantable biodegradable silver-impregnated collagen cuffs at triple-lumen catheter sites. These cuffs prolonged the time of catheter site use in nonseptic critically ill patients. However, they were of no benefit in reducing infection in septic patients and appeared to predispose these patients to fungal colonization and fungemia.[61] As new technologies develop more effective materials for the manufacture of central venous catheters along with antibiotic bonding to the catheters and catheter cuffs, catheter-related thrombosis and sepsis should continue to decline. Further studies are required to determine the long-term effectiveness and safety of antibiotic-bonded catheters and cuffs. These newer devices may allow for less frequent catheter exchanges. However, these will not replace the need for careful surveillance of all catheters and meticulous dressing care in the critically ill patient. Safe and efficient central venous access for delivery of parenteral nutrition is crucial in the nutritional support of critically ill patients. The risks of mechanical and infectious complications can be minimized by adhering to the guidelines outlined above.

PARENTERAL NUTRITION FORMULATIONS

The traditional TPN formula contains 25% dextrose, 4.25% to 5.0% amino acids, electrolytes, vitamins, and trace elements. In addition, lipid emulsions are provided as a separate infusion to prevent essential fatty acid deficiency. The population of patients considered "critically ill" represents a very heterogeneous group with varied nutritional requirements and metabolic deficits. Therefore, the provision of nutrition support in the ICU must be individualized to each unique clinical setting and the formulations modified accordingly.

A recent advance in the delivery of parenteral nutrition has been the widespread use of total nutrient admixtures (TNAs) in which all components, including lipid, are mixed in a single bag for continuous infusion. This technology allows for the daily administration of a mixed-substrate solution and avoids the transient hyperlipidemia seen with separate lipid infusion. This also allows for provision of the required calories while at the same time delivering fewer glucose calories. It is not clear what the ideal energy substrates for critically ill patients are and whether altering this fuel source might affect whole-body protein metabolism.[36] While provision of glucose calories is known to have a beneficial protein-sparing effect,[26, 62] this may be countered by various metabolic complications.[27, 28] Provision of calories in a mixed substrate of glucose and fat is as effective as pure glucose in achieving anabolism.[28, 33–36] Several studies have suggested that injured and/or septic patients may have an obligatory need for fat oxidation,[24, 31, 63] while others have not been able to conclusively demonstrate a benefit in protein sparing with the use of a combination of lipid and glucose.[64, 65] It is clear that as the degree of critical illness increases, it becomes increasingly difficult to support protein synthesis regardless of the energy source. Overall, delivery of 30% to 50% of the patient's estimated caloric needs as lipid appears to be as effective as glucose alone while decreasing the metabolic complications inherent in the use of high concentrations of glucose.[36] On the other hand, lipid may not be as effective as glucose in sparing lean body mass in severely septic or catabolic patients.[62]

As a general estimate protein requirements will be approximately 1.5 to 2.0 g of protein per kilogram of body weight per day, and caloric requirements will be around 30 to 35 kcal/kg/day. Overfeeding with excessive glucose or lipid may be detrimental and should be avoided. If administering a mixed substrate, the RQ should be in the 0.8 to 0.9 range. If this value is higher, it generally indicates overfeeding, especially with glucose, and the calories provided should be reduced. Serum glucose must be closely monitored and may be regulated over the short term by subcutaneous regular insulin administration and over the long term by insulin infusion or adding regular insulin to the TPN formulation. Serum lipid levels should also be monitored, and if consistently elevated (triglyceride levels greater than 500 mg/ dL), the amount of lipid calories provided should be reduced.

Appropriate provision of nutrition support for ICU patients should include the administration of adequate calories (especially glucose calories), utilization of moderate doses of lipid emulsions as energy substrate, and increases in the dose of nitrogen administered, provided that the blood urea nitrogen (BUN) concentration does not increase. Critically ill patients often require further modification of the standard TPN formulation because of alterations in the function of one or several vital organ systems (Table 21–3). Specific formulations can be tailored to better meet the nutritional requirements of patients with renal failure, hepatic failure, pulmonary failure, cardiac insufficiency, and severe metabolic stress (see Table 21–3). Frequently one is faced with a patient suffering from multisystem organ failure, this demands a clear understanding of the benefits of each of the specialized formulas and may require the use of a combination of specific nutrients.

Acute Renal Failure

Patients with renal failure may have a wide spectrum of metabolic abnormalities, including increased protein catabolism with an inability to excrete the products of nitrogen metabolism (urea); this leads to a rise in the BUN concen-

TABLE 21–3.

Total Parenteral Nutrition Formulations: University of Cincinnati Medical Center*

Component	Standard	High Dextrose	Renal	Hepatic	Cardiac	Stress	Peripheral
Dextrose (%)	15	20	46.6	25	35	17.5	5
Amino acids (%)	5	5	1.7†	4‡	5	5.2§	3.5
Protein (g)	50	50	17	40	50	52	35
Fat (g) (as TNA¶)	40	40	—	40	—	40	40
kcal/mL (renal and cardiac mixtures are not formulated as TNA)							
TNA	1.1	1.3	—	1.3	—	1.0	0.71
Non-TNA	0.71	0.88	1.65	1.0	1.4	0.80	—
Nonprotein calorie:N							
TNA	119	141	—	208	—	114	104
Non-TNA	67	89	794	142	156	82	—
Electrolytes (standard minimum concentrations as mEq/L and phosphate as mM/L)‖							
Potassium	18	18	0	12	0	13	10
Sodium	30	30	2	5	5	23	40
Magnesium	5	5	0	8	8	8	8
Calcium	4.5	4.5	0	4.7	0	4.7	4.7
Phosphate	10	10	0	5	5	9	5
Chloride	37	37	1	13.5	2	10	40
Acetate	55	55	14	31	45	51	52

*All values are expressed per liter of solution.
†As essential amino acids (Nephramine, McGaw,Inc.).
‡As Hepatamine, McGaw, Inc.
§As FreAmine HBC, McGaw, Inc.
¶TNA = total nutrient admixture.
‖Maximum total concentrations are K, 80; Na, 154; Mg, 12; Ca, 9.4; phosphate, 15; Cl, limited by cation; acetate, 80.

tration. Anuric and oliguric patients will also have increased fluid retention and elevated serum electrolyte levels, including potassium, magnesium, and phosphate. In addition to the catabolic effect of critical illness, renal failure alone increases the catabolic response and may further impair wound healing and resistance to infection. The goal of nutritional management in these patients is to improve the metabolic state while avoiding the accumulation of excess urea, fluid, and electrolytes. Hemodialysis is very effective in managing fluid retention and controlling azotemia and electrolyte abnormalities. However, hemodialysis itself causes increased catabolism and a negative nitrogen balance[66] because of the loss of amino acids across the dialysis membrane[67] and release of granulocyte proteinases after contact of blood with the membrane.[68]

Patients with acute renal failure who are not anuric, who are able to handle a modest fluid load, and who have no life-threatening electrolyte abnormalities may be managed with a modified renal failure TPN formulation. This solution may contain either essential amino acids[64] or a modest dose of standard amino acids[69] in a high-concentration (50% to 70%) dextrose solution. The former have been formulated to prevent the development of hyperuremia. Essential amino acids provide protein of high biological value and may allow recycling of urea for protein synthesis.[70] An increased survival rate was demonstrated in one study; however, the number of patients in this study was too small to demonstrate efficacy.[64] Therefore, despite the theoretical advantages offered by solutions high in essential amino acids, the clinical efficacy of these solutions in acute renal failure has not been conclusively proved.[71] Glucose is the primary energy source because of its protein-sparing effect in catabolic patients[62] and it can be delivered in high concentrations when fluid requirements are limited. Fat may also be utilized as an energy source in moderate

amounts (30% of the caloric requirements), particularly if the patient is consistently glucose intolerant. However, fat does not provide as much of a protein-sparing effect as carbohydrate,[62] and the lipid emulsion contains 15 mmol/L of phosphate, which may be contraindicated if the patient is already hyperphosphatemic. Serum electrolytes should be closely monitored, especially when initiating TPN, since potassium, phosphate, and magnesium levels may decline rapidly in the face of a hypertonic dextrose infusion. Caloric requirements may be administered along with essential amino acids and electrolytes in a minimal volume.

If the patient requires hemodialysis for the maintenance of fluid and electrolyte balance or for control of BUN, the TPN regimen may be liberalized to a more standard mixture of nonessential and essential amino acids, carbohydrate, and lipid. It is not necessary to reduce the nutrient or volume intake since any excess can be dialyzed off. In certain circumstances, critically ill anuric patients may not be able to tolerate the dialysis regimen because of hemodynamic instability. More recent methods of continuous fluid removal are now available and may be particularly useful in patients with hemodynamic instability. These methods include slow continuous ultrafiltration (SCUF), continuous arteriovenous hemofiltration (CAVH), and continuous arteriovenous hemodialysis (CAVHD). Each of these methods requires a different approach to the parenteral nutrition regimen.

SCUF uses hydrostatic pressure across a membrane to produce ultrafiltration rates of up to 5 mL/min.[72] No dialysis fluid is used, so there is minimal solute removal, thus necessitating intermittent hemodialysis therapy. In this regimen, a "renal formulation" containing minimal fluid, high-concentration dextrose, and essential amino acids might decrease the need for intermittent hemodialysis when control of volume excess is the primary concern. Approximately 90% of the nutrients provided are retained by the patient.[73]

CAVH also relies upon hydrostatic pressure generated by cardiac output across a membrane that is more permeable than those used for hemodialysis.[74] This allows for an increased rate of hemofiltration of 10 mL/min, which effects removal of solute by convection and may be adequate to maintain acceptable levels of BUN, creatinine, and electrolytes without supplemental hemodialysis. Because of the large volume of fluid removed by this technique, volume restriction is not a concern, and in fact, the majority of patients on CAVH will require supplemental intravenous fluids in addition to TPN. CAVH allows for the administration of a more balanced, standard TPN solution with up to 150 g/day of amino acids. There is usually good control of fluid balance and nitrogen accumulation.[75, 76]

The third method, CAVHD, is a continuous therapy that utilizes a reduced flow rate of standard dialysate fluid.[77–79] At such low flow rates, nutrients may be added to the dialysate and are taken up by the patient. This may reduce the efficiency of the dialysis but may obviate the need for separate administration of TPN. Using this technique of "nutritional hemodialysis" with a dialysate containing 5% dextrose and 0.4% amino acids and a flow rate of 27 mL/min, Feinstein et al. demonstrated that 49 g/hr of glucose and 4 g/hr of amino acids were absorbed by the patients.[77]

Hepatic Failure

Critically ill patients commonly have some degree of hepatic dysfunction when their illness is complicated by intra-abdominal sepsis. Such dysfunction does not usually warrant any protein restriction or modification in the TPN solution. In contrast, patients with acute fulminant hepatic failure secondary to acute viral or alcoholic hepatitis or patients with acute-on-chronic liver

disease may have their clinical course complicated by the development of hepatic encephalopathy. These patients have low serum levels of branched-chain amino acids (BCAAs) and elevated levels of serum aromatic amino acids.[80] In hepatic dysfunction, BCAAs may supply up to 30% of the total energy needs in contrast to the 6% to 7% of calories derived from BCAAs in normal patients. The increased aromatic amino acids are thought to contribute to encephalopathy by effectively competing with reduced BCAAs at the blood-brain barrier, thereby providing precursors for the synthesis of false neurotransmitters within the brain. A modified hepatic formulation containing 35% BCAAs and decreased amounts of the aromatic amino acids and methionine has been shown to induce a positive nitrogen balance with increased protein synthesis, improve ammonia metabolism in muscle, correct the plasma amino acid profile, and ameliorate encephalopathy.[81] Those patients with acute-on-chronic liver disease who have either mild (grade 1) or no encephalopathy may tolerate a limited amount (50 to 60 g) of protein in a standard amino acid mixture. If these patients do not tolerate a standard formula or if they have a grade 2 or greater encephalopathy, then a modified hepatic solution as described above is indicated. Meta-analysis of prospective randomized trials utilizing modified (high-BCAA, low-aromatic) formulas compared with standard mixtures reveals improvement in encephalopathy[82] and in some cases increased survival.[83]

Some patients with hepatic dysfunction and ascites may require fluid and sodium restriction in order to minimize the intra-abdominal accumulation of fluid. Cirrhotic patients frequently have folic acid and zinc deficiency. In addition to standard multivitamins and occasionally large amounts of thiamine, additional folate and zinc should be provided to these patients. Excess levels of copper in jaundiced patients may develop since this trace element is excreted primarily via the biliary system. Thus, copper replacement should be limited, and trace element solutions without copper should be used in such patients. In patients with multiple organ failure, with both hepatic and renal failure, one may have to choose between higher BUN levels and less encephalopathy (modified high-BCAA, low-aromatic formulas) or lower BUN levels and greater encephalopathy (essential amino acid formulations).

Pulmonary Failure

Acute respiratory failure requiring mechanical ventilation in a critically ill patient results in increased catabolism and hypermetabolism.[84] This is further amplified in patients with pre-existing chronic lung disease, in whom weight loss and malnutrition are common.[85] Protein-calorie malnutrition in critically ill mechanically ventilated patients leads to further derangements in pulmonary function and structure,[86] a reduction in respiratory muscle strength and contractility,[86-89] abnormal ventilatory drive,[90] decreased production of surfactant,[91, 92] and altered pulmonary defense mechanisms.[86] Early aggressive nutrition support is essential to avoid these complications of protein-calorie malnutrition in mechanically ventilated patients. Refeeding malnourished patients with respiratory failure may lead to large shifts of sodium and water from the intracellular to the extracellular compartment. This may further compromise ventilatory function because of the development of pulmonary edema. Thus, it is often necessary to restrict sodium and volume administration in these patients.

In addition to serving as substrates for nutrition, the caloric components (amino acids, carbohydrate, and lipid) in parenteral nutrition solutions have important direct effects upon pulmonary mechanics and ventilatory function that must be considered. Amino acids have been shown to increase minute ventilation, oxygen consumption, and the ventilatory response to hypoxia and hypercarbia.[90, 93, 94] Specifically, the BCAAs appear to stimulate ventilatory drive.[95] Therefore, in addition to their nutritional value, the administration of amino acids appears to also provide a beneficial effect upon ventilatory efficiency by stimulating respiratory function.

The administration of glucose in the clinical setting of respiratory failure may lead to an increased CO_2 production[96] and increased ventilatory response to hypoxia.[93] Under rare circumstances, overfeeding with large quantities of carbohydrate in a malnourished, septic patient with inadequate respiratory reserve secondary to COPD may lead to excess CO_2 production and difficulty in weaning from the ventilator.[97, 98] The administration of mixed-substrate glucose-lipid solutions should prevent the potential complications of carbohydrate overfeeding in these patients. It is emphasized that despite all the publicity that this complication has received, it occurs only rarely. It should be recalled that in the original publication, excessive CO_2 production and difficulty in weaning only occurred when depleted septic patients suddenly had large loads of glucose administered without adaptation.

Despite the concern that fat emulsions might cause further impairment of pulmonary function, intravenous administration of lipids is well tolerated in the clinical setting of pulmonary failure. Furthermore, lipid emulsions have been shown to improve pulmonary mechanical properties and surfactant production in an animal model[99] and, as previously discussed, may be a preferred fuel source for injured and septic patients.[24, 100] It is clear that in the face of respiratory failure, overall outcome is improved with careful assessment and provision of a mixed-substrate fuel formulation. Indirect calorimetry with determination of the patient's REE and RQ allows for accurate determination of patient caloric and substrate needs. Lipid calories, with their lower RQ, may be used to provide up to 50% of the energy needs while decreasing overall CO_2 production. This becomes important when one is attempting to wean such patients from mechanical ventilation. In addition to monitoring nutritional parameters, the respiratory rate, vital capacity, minute ventilation, and arterial blood gases must be continually assessed as nutrition support is instituted and advanced. Substrate manipulation should be instituted to keep the RQ less than 0.9, which reduces minute ventilation and may promote weaning. When proper initial assessment and interval follow-up are applied early in the course of the illness and appropriate amounts of mixed-substrate fuel are provided as a TNA, excessive CO_2 production and a need for major changes in the nutritional formulation during weaning should be a rare occurrence.

Cardiac Failure

For some six decades, the standing dictum that the heart is spared the ravages of starvation was unquestioned. However, over the past decade the deleterious effects of protein-calorie malnutrition on cardiac muscle have been demonstrated.[101] In addition, once depleted, normal cardiac function does not easily return.[102] In the acute setting, the myocardium is affected by starvation. Provision of adequate nutrition is essential for efficient cardiac function. In general, the myocardium utilizes fatty acids for energy under resting conditions and carbohydrate in the face of ischemia and increased energy demands. Provision of amino acids affects protein turnover in ischemic and septic cardiac muscle. In particular, BCAA-enriched solutions have been shown to improve cardiac function in isolated rat heart preparations.[102] In addition to serving as nutritional substrate, hypertonic glucose,[103] amino acids,[104] and secondarily, insulin and glucagon provide positive inotro-

pic effects in the face of cardiac dysfunction.[105–107] Thus, the nutritional needs of critically ill patients with cardiac failure can be met by utilizing a mixed-substrate solution containing glucose, balanced amino acids, and lipid emulsion.

The challenge of providing parenteral nutrition for this population of patients is to provide an adequate amount of calories in a sodium- and volume-restricted solution. By utilizing more concentrated solutions of amino acids (10%), dextrose (70%), and lipid emulsion (20%) while limiting sodium to approximately 1.5 g/day, one can generally meet the cardiac patient's needs in a limited volume of approximately 1500 mL/day. Because of the high density of carbohydrate calories utilized in this setting, blood glucose levels should be monitored closely. Insulin should be added to the formulation in amounts necessary to control hyperglycemia. Diuretic therapy is often required to maintain an optimal volume status. Vigorous diuresis may lead to substantial losses of potassium, magnesium, and zinc. These losses should be anticipated, and when indicated, additional supplementation of these elements should be provided.

Stressed/Septic Patient

The serum amino acid profile in stressed and septic patients is similar to the profile seen in hepatic failure.[108] In this setting, BCAAs are used for fuel by skeletal muscle and may become depleted. Provision of BCAAs may stimulate protein synthesis while inhibiting protein degradation. Infusion of a conventional TPN solution is also associated with intestinal atrophy. Parenteral nutrition solutions enriched with glutamine have been found to partially reverse gut atrophy,[109] although this has not been universally confirmed.[110] The potential benefit of such solutions in stressed patients is to prevent translocation of potentially pathogenic bacteria and their products across the intestinal wall and into the systemic circulation.[111] However, glutamine is excluded from conventional TPN solutions because it is unstable at room temperature. Infusion of BCAA-enriched solutions increases the synthesis and release of glutamine from skeletal muscle[112–114] and may be as effective as glutamine in limiting gut atrophy.[115]

TPN formulations containing adequate amounts of essential and nonessential amino acids and enriched with 45% BCAAs may theoretically be beneficial in stressed and septic patients by improving nitrogen retention, increasing visceral protein synthesis, preserving intestinal integrity, improving immune status, and normalizing the plasma amino acid profile.[116] Clinical studies comparing BCAA-enriched formulations with conventional solutions have shown only marginal improvement in nitrogen balance, decreased ureagenesis, and improved plasma levels of short-turnover proteins. However, despite the apparently more efficient source of protein provided by BCAA solutions, little major effect on outcome has been demonstrated.[117, 118] Because of the increased cost, this formulation should only be reserved for the rare circumstance when stressed patients fail to respond to conventional TPN solutions.

Peripheral Parenteral Nutrition

Peripheral parenteral nutrition (PPN) solutions have a low caloric density since they must be isotonic or slightly hypertonic in order to be infused via a peripheral vein. The solution contains a final concentration of 5% dextrose, and in order to provide an adequate calorie-to-nitrogen ratio, 200 mL of a 20% lipid emulsion must be administered along with the PPN. This can be compounded as a TNA with a caloric density of 0.71 K cal/mL and a calorie-to-nitrogen ratio of 104:1. On rare occasions PPN may be useful in the ICU setting when patients have no central venous access or when

central venous catheterization is contraindicated. However, large volumes of solution are required if PPN is the sole source of calories for the patient, and the volume status must be monitored closely (usually requiring central venous access for monitoring). Another use for this formulation is in a patient without central access who is unable to tolerate full enteral nutrition or is unable to take in adequate oral intake. In these instances, PPN may be used for 5 to 7 days to provide supplemental calories and protein.

REFERENCES

1. Kudsk KA, Croce MA, Fabian TC, et al: Enteral versus parenteral feeding: Effects on septic morbidity after blunt and penetrating abdominal trauma. *Ann Surg* 1992; 215:503.
2. Cataldi-Betcher EL, Seltzer MH, Slocum BA, et al: Complications occurring during enteral nutrition support: A prospective study. *JPEN* 1983; 7:546.
3. Abernathy GB, Heizer WD, Holcombe BJ, et al: Efficacy of tube feeding in supplying energy requirements of hospitalized patients. *JPEN* 1989; 13:387.
4. Kemper M, Weissman C, Hyman AI: Caloric requirements and supply in critically ill surgical patients. *Crit Care Med* 1992; 20:344.
5. Wagner DR, Elmore MF, Tate JT: Combined parenteral and enteral nutrition in severe trauma. *Nutr Clin Pract* 1992; 7:113.
6. Bower RH, Talamini MA, Sax HL, et al: Postoperative enteral vs parenteral nutrition. *Arch Surg* 1986; 121:1040.
7. Bower RH: Nutrition for critically ill patients, in Cameron J (ed): *Current Surgical Therapy*, ed 4. St Louis, Mosby–Year Book, 1992.
8. ASPEN Board of Directors: Guidelines for use of total parenteral nutrition in the hospitalized adult patient. *JPEN* 1986; 10:441.
9. VA TPN Cooperative Study Group: Perioperative total parenteral nutrition in surgical patients. *N Engl J Med* 1991; 325:525–532.

10. McGeer AJ, Detsky AS, O'Rourke K: Parenteral nutrition in cancer patients undergoing chemotherapy: A meta-analysis. *Nutrition* 1990; 6:233.

11. Harris JA, Benedict FG: *Biometric Studies of Basal Metabolism in Man.* Washington, DC, Carnegie Institute, 1979, Publication No. 279.

12. Long CL, Schaffel N, Geiger JW, et al: Metabolic response to injury and illness: Estimation of energy and protein needs from indirect calorimetry and nitrogen balance. *JPEN* 1979; 3:452.

13. Weissman C, Kemper MC, Askanzi, J, et al: Resting metabolic rate of critically ill patients: Measured vs predicted. *Anesthesiology* 1986; 64:673.

14. Hess D, Daugherty A, Large E, et al: A comparison of four methods of determining caloric requirements of mechanically ventilated patients. *Respir Care* 1986; 86:1197.

15. Branson RD, Hurst JM, Warner BW, et al: Measured versus predicted energy expenditure in mechanically ventilated patients with chronic obstructive pulmonary disease. *Respir Care* 1987; 32:748.

16. Bursztein S, Elwyn DH, Askanazi J, et al: *Energy Metabolism, Indirect Calorimetry and Nutrition.* Baltimore, Williams & Wilkins, 1989.

17. Westenskow DR, Roberts SE, Pace NL: Evaluation of a replenishment type oxygen consumption monitor. *Crit Care Med* 1989; 17:798.

18. Steinhorn DM, Rozenberg AL, Boyle MJ, et al: Modular indirect calorimeter suitable for long-term measurements in multipatient intensive care units. *Crit Care Med* 1991; 19:963.

19. Bower RH, Nussbaum MS, Orr ME, et al: *Protocol for Nutrition Support,* ed 2. Cincinnati, University of Cincinnati, 1992.

20. Nelson LD, Anderson HB, Garcia H: Clinical validation of a new metabolic monitor suitable for use in critically ill patients. *Crit Care Med* 1987; 15:951.

21. Skootsky SA, Abraham E: Continuous oxygen consumption measurement during initial emergency department resuscitation of critically ill patients. *Crit Care Med* 1988; 16:706.

22. Hankeln KB, Gronemeyer R, Held A, et al: Use of continuous noninvasive measurement of oxygen consumption in patients with adult respiratory distress syndrome following shock of various etiologies. *Crit Care Med* 1991; 19:642.

23. Wolfe RR, Allsop J, Burke JF: Glucose metabolism in man: Responses to intravenous glucose infusion. *Metabolism* 1979; 28:210.

24. Askanazi J, Carpentier YA, Elwyn DH, et al: Influence of TPN on fuel utilization in injury and sepsis. *Ann Surg* 1980; 191:40.

25. Long JM III, Wilmore DW, Mason AD, et al: Fat-carbohydrate interaction: Effects on nitrogen sparing in total intravenous feeding. *Surg Forum* 1974; 25:61.

26. Woolfson AMJ, Healey RV, Allison SP: Insulin to inhibit protein catabolism after injury. *N Engl J Med* 1979; 300:14.

27. Nanni G, Siegel JH, Coleman B: Increased lipid fuel dependence in the critically ill septic patient. *J Trauma* 1984; 24:14.

28. Meguid M, Akahoshi MP, Jeffers S, et al: Amelioration of metabolic complications of conventional TPN. *Arch Surg* 1984; 119:1294.

29. O'Keefe SJ, Sender PM, James WPT: Catabolic loss of body nitrogen in response to surgery. *Lancet* 1974; 2:1035.

30. Clowes GHA, George BC, Villee CA, et al: Muscle proteolysis induced by a circulating peptide in patients with sepsis or trauma. *N Engl J Med* 1983; 308:545.

31. Shaw JHF, Wolfe RR: An integrated analysis of glucose, fat and protein metabolism in severely traumatized patients: Studies in the basal state and the response to total parenteral nutrition. *Ann Surg* 1989; 209:63.

32. Larsson J, Lennmarken C, Martensson J, et al: Nitrogen requirements in severely injured patients. *Br J Surg* 1990; 77:413.

33. Paluzzi M, Meguid MA: A prospective, randomized study of the optimal source of nonprotein calories in TPN. *Surgery* 1987; 987:717.

34. Baker JP, Detsky AS, Stewart S, et al: Randomized trial of TPN in critically ill patients: Metabolic effects of vary-

ing glucose-lipid ratios as the energy source. *Gastroenterology* 1984; 87:53.

35. Tracey KJ, Legaspi A, Albert JD, et al: Protein and substrate metabolism during starvation and parenteral refeeding. *Clin Sci* 1988; 74:123.

36. DeChalain TMB, Michell WL, O'Keefe SJ, et al: The effect of fuel source on amino acid metabolism in critically ill patients. *J Surg Res* 1992; 52:167.

37. Cerra FB, Siegel JH, Colman B, et al: Septic autocannibalism, a failure of exogenous nutritional support. *Ann Surg* 1980; 192:570.

38. Shaw JHF, Wildbore M, Wolfe RR: Whole body protein kinetics in severely septic patients. *Ann Surg* 1987; 205:288.

39. Long CL, Jeevanaudan M, Kinney JM: Whole body protein synthesis and catabolism in septic man. *Am J Clin Nutr* 1977; 30:1340.

40. Rombeau J, Rolandelli R, Wilmore D: Nutritional support, in Wilmore D, Brennan M, Harken AH, et al (eds): *Care of the Surgical Patient*, vol 1. New York, Scientific American, 1989.

41. Pemberton LB, Lyman B, Lander V, et al: Sepsis from triple- vs. single-lumen catheters during total parenteral nutrition in surgical or critically ill patients. *Arch Surg* 1986; 121:591.

42. McCarthy MC, Shives JK, Robison RJ, et al: Prospective evaluation of single and triple lumen catheters in total parenteral nutrition. *JPEN* 1987; 11:259.

43. Kelly CS, Ligas JR, Smith CA, et al: Sepsis due to triple lumen central venous catheters. *Surg Gynecol Obstet* 1986; 163:14.

44. Lee RB, Buckner M, Sharp KW: Do multi-lumen catheters increase central venous catheter sepsis compared to single-lumen catheters? *J Trauma* 1988; 28:1472.

45. Gil RT, Kruse JA, Thill-Baharozian MC, et al: Triple vs single-lumen central venous catheters. *Arch Intern Med* 1989; 149:1139.

46. Johnson BH, Rypins EB: Single-lumen vs double-lumen catheters for total parenteral nutrition. *Arch Surg* 1990; 125:990.

47. Horowitz HW, Dworkin BM, Savino JA, et al: Central catheter-related infections: Comparison of pulmonary artery catheters and triple lumen catheters for the delivery of hyperalimentation in a critical care setting. *JPEN* 1990; 14:588.

48. Newsome HH Jr, Armstrong CW, Mayhall GC, et al: Mechanical complications from insertion of subclavian venous feeding catheters: Comparison of de novo percutaneous venipuncture to change of catheter over guidewire. *JPEN* 1984; 8:560.

49. Armstrong CW, Mayhall CG, Miller KB, et al: Prospective study of catheter replacement and other risk factors for infection of hyperalimentation catheters. *J Infect Dis* 1986; 154:808.

50. Graeve AH, Carpenter CM, Schiller WR: Management of central venous catheters using a wire introducer. *Am J Surg* 1981; 142:752.

51. Pettigrew RA, Lang SDR, Haydock DA, et al: Catheter-related sepsis in patients on intravenous nutrition: A prospective study of quantitative catheter cultures and guidewire changes for suspected sepsis. *Br J Surg* 1985; 72:52.

52. Olson ME, Lam K, Bodey G, et al: Evaluation of strategies for central catheter replacement. *Crit Care Med* 1992; 20:797.

53. Pomp A, Varella L, Caldwell MD, et al: Catheter-related sepsis: Single lumen catheters vs. triple lumen catheters (abstract). *JPEN* 1988; 12:23.

54. Linder LE, Curelaru I, Gustvsson B, et al: Material thrombogenicity in central venous catheterization: A comparison between soft, antebrachial catheters of silicone elastomer and polyurethane. *JPEN* 1984; 8:399.

55. DiConstanzo J, Sastre B, Choux R, et al: Mechanism of thrombogenesis during total parenteral nutrition: Role of catheter composition. *JPEN* 1988; 12:190.

56. Borrow M, Crowley JG: Evaluation of central venous catheter thrombogenicity. *Acta Anaesthiol Scand* 1985; 81:59.

57. Crocker KS, Devereaux GB, Ashmore DL, et al: Clinical evaluation of elastomeric hydrogel peripheral catheters during home infusion therapy. *J Intravenous Nurs* 1990; 13:89.

58. Trooskin SZ, Donetz AP, Harvey RA,

et al: Prevention of catheter sepsis by antibiotic bonding. *Surgery* 1985; 97:547.

59. Kamal GD, Pfaller MA, Rempe LE, et al: Reduced intravascular catheter infection by antibiotic bonding: A prospective, randomized, controlled trial. *JAMA* 1991; 265:2364.

60. Maki DG, Cobb L, Garman JK, et al: An attachable silver-impregnated cuff for prevention of infection with central venous catheters: A prospective randomized multicenter trial. *Am J Med* 1988; 85:307.

61. Norwood S, Hajjar G, Jenkins L: The influence of an attachable subcutaneous cuff for preventing triple lumen catheter infections in critically ill surgical and trauma patients. *Surg Gynecol Obstet* 1992; 175:33.

62. Long JM III, Wilmore DW, Mason AD Jr, et al: Effect of carbohydrate and fat intake on nitrogen excretion during total intravenous feeding. *Ann Surg* 1977; 185:417.

63. Burke JF, Wolfe RR, Mullany CJ, et al: Glucose requirements following burn injury: Parameters of optimal glucose infusion and possible hepatic and respiratory abnormalities following excessive glucose uptake. *Ann Surg* 1979; 190:274.

64. Douglas RG, Shaw JHF: Metabolic response to sepsis and trauma. *Br J Surg* 1989; 76:115.

65. Long CL: Fuel preferences in the septic patient; glucose or lipid. *JPEN* 1987; 11:333.

66. Borah MF, Schoenfeld PY, Gotch FA, et al: Nitrogen balance during intermittent dialysis therapy of uremia. *Kidney Int* 1978; 14:491.

67. Wolfson M, Jones MR, Kopple JD: Amino acid losses during hemodialysis with infusion of amino acids and glucose. *Kidney Int* 1982; 21:500.

68. Horl WH, Heidland A: Evidence for the participation of granulocyte proteinases on intradialytic catabolism. *Clin Nephrol* 1984; 21:314.

69. Abel RM, Shih VE, Abbott WM, et al: Amino acid metabolism in acute renal failure: Influence of intravenous essential *l*-amino acid hyperalimentation therapy. *Ann Surg* 1974; 180:350.

70. Abel RM, Beck CH Jr, Abbott WM, et al: Improved survival from acute renal failure after treatment with intravenous essential *l*-amino acids and glucose: Results of a prospective double-blind study. *N Engl J Med* 1973; 288:695.

71. Feinstein EI, Blumenkrantz MJ, Healy H, et al: Clinical and metabolic responses to parenteral nutrition in acute renal failure. A controlled double-blind study. *Medicine (Baltimore)* 1981; 60:124.

72. Paganini EP: Continuous replacement modalities in acute renal dysfunction, in Paganini EP (ed): *Acute Continuous Renal Replacement Therapy.* Boston, Martinus Nijhoff, 1986.

73. Paganini EP, Flaque J, Whitman G, et al: Amino acid balance in patients with oliguric acute renal failure undergoing slow continuous ultrafiltration (SCUF). *Trans Am Soc Artif Intern Organs* 1982; 28:615.

74. Kramer P, Wigger W, Rieger J, et al: Arteriovenous hemofiltration: A new simple method for treatment of overhydrated patients resistant to diuretics. *Klin Wochenschr* 1977; 55:121.

75. Kramer P, Bohler J, Kehr A, et al: Intensive potential of continuous arteriovenous hemofiltration. *Trans Am Soc Artif Intern Organs* 1982; 28:28.

76. Kaplan AA, Longnecker RE, Folkert VW: Continuous arteriovenous hemofiltration—a report of six months experience. *Ann Intern Med* 1984; 3100:358.

77. Feinstein EI, Collins JF, Blumenkrantz MJ, et al: Nutritional hemodialysis, in Atsumi K, Maekawa M, Ota K (eds): *Progress in Artificial Organs.* Cleveland, ISAO Press, 1984.

78. Geronemus R, Schneider N: Continuous arteriovenous hemodialysis: A new modality for treatment of acute renal failure. *Trans Am Soc Artif Intern Organs* 1984; 30:610.

79. Sigler M, Teehan BP: Solute transport in continuous hemodialysis: A new treatment for acute renal failure. *Kidney Int* 1987; 32:562.

80. James JH, Ziparo V, Jeppsson B, et al: Hyperammonemia, plasma amino acid imbalance, and blood-brain amino acid transport: A unified theory of portal-systemic encephalopathy. *Lancet* 1979; 2:772.

81. Fischer JE, Rosen HM, Ebeid AM, et al: The effect of normalization of plasma amino acids on hepatic encephalopathy in man. *Surgery* 1976; 80:77.

82. Naylor CD, O'Rourke K, Detsky AS, et al: Parenteral nutrition with branched-chain amino acids in hepatic encephalopathy: A meta-analysis. *Gastroenterology* 1989; 97:1033.

83. Cerra FB, Cheung NK, Fischer JE, et al: Disease-specific amino acid infusion (FO80) in hepatic encephalopathy: A prospective, randomized, double-blind, controlled trial. *JPEN* 1985; 9:288.

84. Driver AG, LeBrun M: Iatrogenic malnutrition in patients receiving ventilatory support. *JAMA* 1980; 244:2195.

85. Hunter AMB, Carey MA, Larsh HN: The nutritional status of patients with chronic obstructive pulmonary disease. *Am Rev Respir Dis* 1981; 124:376.

86. Edelman NH, Rucker RB, Peavy HH: Nutrition and the respiratory system. *Am Rev Respir Dis* 1986; 134:347.

87. Gertz I, Hedenstierna G, Hellers G, et al: Muscle metabolism in patients with chronic obstructive lung disease and acute respiratory failure. *Clin Sci Mol Med* 1977; 52:395.

88. Thurlbeck WM: Diaphragm and body weight emphysema. *Thorax* 1978; 33:483.

89. Rochester DF: Body weight and respiratory muscle function in chronic obstructive pulmonary disease. *Am Rev Respir Dis* 1986; 134:646.

90. Wilson DO, Rogers RM, Hoffman RM: Nutrition and chronic lung disease. *Am Rev Respir Dis* 1985; 132:1347.

91. Faridy EE: Effect of food and water deprivation on surface activity of lungs of rats. *J Appl Physiol* 1970; 29:493.

92. Sahebjami H, Vassallo CL, Wirman JA: Lung mechanics and ultrastructure in prolonged starvation. *Am Rev Respir Dis* 1978; 117:77.

93. Zwillich CW, Sahn SA, Weil JV: Effects of hypermetabolism upon respiratory gas exchange in normal man. *J Clin Invest* 1977; 66:900.

94. Askanazi J, Weissman C, LaSala PA, et al: Effect of protein intake on ventilatory drive. *Anesthesiology* 1984; 60:106.

95. Takala J: Branched chain amino acids and respiratory function in man, in Kinney JM, Borum PR (ed): *Perspectives in Clinical Nutrition.* Baltimore, Urban & Schwarzenberg, 1989.

96. Rodriguez JL, Askanazi J, Weissman C, et al: Ventilatory and metabolic effects of glucose infusions. *Chest* 1985; 88:512.

97. Askanazi J, Rosenbaum SH, Hyman AL, et al: Respiratory changes induced by large glucose loads of total parenteral nutrition. *JAMA* 1980; 243:1444.

98. Freund HR: Nutritional support in cardiac and pulmonary diseases, in Fischer JE (ed): *Total Parenteral Nutrition,* ed 2. Boston, Little, Brown, 1991.

99. Bahrami S, Strohmaier W, Redl H, et al: Mechanical properties of the lungs of posttraumatic rats are improved by including fat in total parenteral nutrition. *JPEN* 1987; 11:560.

100. Robin AP, Nordenstrom J, Askanazi J, et al: Influence of parenteral carbohydrate on fat oxidation in surgical patients. *Surgery* 1984; 95:608.

101. Abel RM, Grimes JB, Alonso D, et al: Adverse hemodynamic and ultrastructural changes in dog hearts subjected to protein-calorie malnutrition. *Am Heart J* 1979; 97:733.

102. Freund HR, Dann EJ, Burns F, et al: The effect of branched chain amino acids on systolic properties of the normal and septic isolated rat heart. *Arch Surg* 1985; 120:483.

103. Ko KK, Paradise RR: The effects of substrate on contractility of rat atria depressed with halothane. *Anesthesiology* 1969; 31:532.

104. Abel RM, Subramaniam VA, Gay WA Jr: Effects of an intravenous amino acid nutrient solution on left ventricular contractility in dogs. *J Surg Res* 1977; 23:201.

105. Kao RL, Christman EW, Lun SL, et al: The effect of insulin and anoxia on the metabolism of isolated mature rat cardiac myocytes. *Arch Biochem Biophys* 1980; 203:587.

106. Farah AE, Alousi AA: The actions of

insulin on cardiac contractility. *Life Sci* 1981; 29:975.

107. Markovitz LJ, Hasin Y, Freund HR: The effect of insulin and glucagon on systolic properties of the normal and septic isolated rat heart. *Basic Res Cardiol* 1985; 80:377.

108. Freund H, Ryan J, Fischer JE: Amino acid derangements in patients with sepsis. *Ann Surg* 1978; 188:423.

109. O'Dwyer ST, Smith RJ, Hwang TL, et al: Maintenance of small bowel mucosa with glutamine-enriched parenteral nutrition. *JPEN* 1989; 13:579.

110. Li S, Nussbaum MS, McFadden DW, et al: Addition of L-glutamine to total parenteral nutrition (TPN) and its effect on portal insulin and glucagon and the development of hepatic steatosis in rats. *J Surg Res* 1990; 48:421.

111. Deitch EA, Winterton J, Li M, et al: The gut as a portal of entry for bacteremia. *Ann Surg* 1987; 205:681.

112. Johnson DJ, Smith RJ, Colpoys M, et al: Branched chain amino acid uptake and muscle free amino acid concentrations predict postoperative muscle nitrogen balance. *Ann Surg* 1986; 204:513.

113. Bower RH, Kern K, Fischer JE: Use of branched chain amino acid enriched solutions in patients under metabolic stress. *Am J Surg* 1985; 149:266.

114. McCauley R, Platell C, Hall J, et al: The influence of branched chain amino acid infusions on wound healing. *Aust N Z J Surg* 1990; 60:471.

115. Platell C, McCauley R, McCulloch R, et al: Influence of glutamine and branched chain amino acids on the jejunal atrophy associated with parenteral nutrition. *J Gastroenterol Hepatol* 1991; 6:345.

116. Teasley KM, Buss RL: Do parenteral nutrition solutions enriched with high concentrations of branched chain amino acids offer significant benefits to stressed patients? *Ann Pharmacol* 1989; 23:411.

117. Bower RH, Muggia Sullam M, Vallgren S, et al: Branched chain amino acid–enriched solutions in the septic patient: A randomized, prospective trial. *Ann Surg* 1986; 203:13.

118. Cerra FB, Blackburn G, Hirsch J, et al: The effect of stress level, amino acid formula, and nitrogen dose on nitrogen retention in traumatic and septic stress. *Ann Surg* 1987; 205:282.

22

Care and Maintenance of Feeding Tubes and Central Venous Catheters

Sharon Lehmann, R.N., C.C.R.N., C.N.S.N.

Marsha Orr, R.N., C.N.S.N.

Standards for the care and maintenance of feeding tubes and central venous catheters (CVCs) have been established on the basis of tradition rather than science. Procedures within these standards have more frequently been the subject of research during the past decade as their use has expanded. Prospective, randomized, controlled studies, however, remain the exception.

Procedures related to feeding tubes include verification of placement of small-bore feeding tubes, methods used to secure nasal tubes, mucous membrane care, clearance of obstruction of feeding tubes, and medication administration via feeding tubes. Procedures related to CVCs include application of CVC dressing, irrigation of the catheter, removal and application of CVC caps, and insertion of tubing into the CVC hub.

This chapter will review procedures related to the care and maintenance of feeding tubes and CVCs. The primary goals presented within this text are to prevent complications, control costs, provide for patient comfort, and stimulate ideas within the reader for further areas of research.

NASAL FEEDING TUBES

Verifying Placement of Small-Bore Feeding Tubes

Most nasoenteral feeding tubes in use today are of the soft, small-bore (<12 F), polyurethane or silicone variety. Small-bore tubes are thought to be more comfortable for patients and less likely to cause local tissue irritation than are firm, large-bore feeding tubes.[1-8] In addition, the tips of these tubes may be positioned into the small bowel by various means (e.g., fluoroscopy, endoscopy) such that the risk of vomiting and aspiration is significantly reduced. However, the very properties that make these tubes more comfortable may cause problems with their management.

One of the most potentially dangerous problems that exists is "silent" dislodgement of the small-bore tube. The tube appears to be in the correct place externally but has moved internally. Several authors have reported that small-bore tubes became dislodged during episodes of coughing, vomiting, or nasotracheal suctioning; during extubation of endotracheal tubes; and when patients experienced a decreased level of consciousness that predisposed them to an altered swallowing and gag reflex and slowed gastric motility.[5, 8-10]

According to current standards of care in many critical care settings, feeding tube placement should be verified not only at the time of insertion but also on every shift during continuous feeding or before each intermittent feeding and appropriately documented in the health care record. It is generally accepted that radiography is the most accurate method for ensuring initial placement of small-bore nasogastric and nasointestinal feeding tubes.[1-5, 10-14] It is not common practice, however, to test tube placement by radiography regularly after tube feedings are initiated because repeated radiographs are not feasible in terms of either radiation risk or cost. Thus, the problem of how to assess continued proper positioning of the small-bore feeding tube still remains.

In a recent descriptive clinical study, 15% of small-bore nasogastric tubes, 27% of weighted, and 50% of unweighted nasointestinal tubes were found to be out of their intended position.[10] Unknown to the staff, these tubes had been spontaneously displaced. The distal tips had moved upward in the gastrointestinal tract while the external position of the tube remained intact. Therefore, no evidence of dislocation was visible until radiographic examination was performed. Two risk factors, coughing and a decreased level of consciousness, were found to occur with significantly greater frequency in patients with displaced weighted nasogastric tubes. Coughing, tracheal suctioning, and upper airway intubation predisposed to dislodgement of unweighted nasointestinal tubes.

A variety of techniques have been suggested to verify tube placement. However, none are completely reliable. These techniques include aspiration of gastrointestinal contents, pH testing of aspirates, and auscultation of insufflated air.

Aspiration of Gastrointestinal Contents

This method is recommended not only to verify tube placement but also to measure residual volumes, and should be performed whether the tube is placed in the stomach or the small intestine.[1, 3, 4, 12, 15, 16] The technique involves irrigating the tube with 5 to 10 mL of water to moisten the tube and prevent the feeding solution from sticking to it. Then, with a 35 to 60-mL syringe, aspirate to verify that gastrointestinal fluid is obtained. Several authors believe that the smaller the syringe size the greater the negative pressure created within the tube and the less likelihood of success the practitioner will have in aspirating gastrointestinal contents.[1, 3–5, 13, 16]

Metheny et al. conducted a descriptive clinical study in which nurses were asked to record the frequency with which they were able to aspirate at least 5 mL of fluid from a variety of tubes.[8] There were 34 successful attempts out of 43 (79.1%) when large-bore (primarily 14 to 18 F) nasogastric tubes were used, with a mean volume of 56.1 mL. However, only 116 out of 324 attempts (33.8%) were successful with the small-bore (8 F) pliable tube. The mean volume of fluid aspirated from small-bore pliable nasoenteral tubes was 17.4 mL in comparison to 56.1 mL from the less pliable polyvinylchloride tube. It was felt that the walls of the feeding tubes collapsed on syringe aspiration.

In a study conducted by Eisenberg and associates it was found that the volume of fluid aspirated was significantly affected by the material the tube was made of and by its diameter.[17] The mean volume aspirated per attempt was greater with polyurethane than with silicone tubes for all diameters tested. In addition, the aspirated volume was greater with 10 F ($P < .05$) tubes than with 8 F tubes.

pH Testing of Aspirates

Metheny and associates suggest that one look for recognizable secretions when checking gastric aspirates and distinguish gastric secretions from pulmonary secretions by testing the aspirate pH.[11] In most instances it has been found that gastric aspirates have a pH

of 1.0 to 4.0, intestinal aspirates have a pH of 5.0 to 8.0, and respiratory aspirates have pH values of 7.0 or greater. The practitioner must be aware that certain factors can alter the gastrointestinal pH. For example, H_2-receptor antagonists elevate the gastric pH by inhibiting the action of histamine at the receptor sites of the parietal cells, thereby decreasing gastric acid secretion.

In a recent clinical study, the mean gastric pH of 120 readings was 3.02 vs. 6.57 for 127 intestinal readings.[11] Findings indicated that pH readings were often effective in differentiating between gastric and intestinal placement ($P < .0001$). Approximately 81% of the aspirates from nasogastric tubes had pH values ranging from 1.0 to 4.0, while almost 88% of the aspirates from nasointestinal tubes had pH values of 6.0 or greater.

Auscultation of Insufflated Air

This technique consists of insufflating a small quantity of air (10 to 20 mL) through a tube while auscultating the epigastrum or left upper quadrant with a stethoscope and listening for a distinctive "whooshing or gurgling" sound.[1, 4, 8, 15, 16]

In a study using the auscultatory method, nurses reported hearing air in the epigastric region 18 times when the tubes were documented by radiography to be located in the stomach.[8] However, they also reported hearing air in the epigastric region when the tip of the tube was not in the stomach (e.g., 11 times in the duodenum, 3 times in the jejunum, and 2 times in the esophagus). In other words, the nurses were unable to predict the exact location of the tube tip in the alimentary tract by auscultating the epigastrum.

Eighty-five critically ill adults were studied to determine the extent to which sounds generated by air insufflation through a feeding tube could be used to predict tube position in the gastrointestinal tract (e.g., esophagus, stomach, or proximal portion of the small bowel).[18] Overall, the percentage of correct classification of auscultatory sounds was 34%. The stomach lies in the upper left quadrant of the abdomen. It frequently extends under the left lower ribs. Thus, ascultation of sounds generated by air insufflation cannot reliably distinguish between a feeding tube located in the stomach from one positioned in the left lower lobe of the lung.

Newer methods for checking tube placement need to be developed. Until that time a thorough abdominal assessment is essential and should include auscultation for bowel sounds at regular intervals and monitoring for signs and symptoms of nausea and vomiting, changes in stool habits, a feeling of fullness, or abdominal distension.[1, 13, 16, 19] At the time of insertion a black permanent ink pen is used to mark tube placement at the point where it exits the nose so that the position can be verified externally.[1, 9, 19] Also, the oropharynx should be checked regularly for a coiled tube.

The patient must also be observed for signs and symptoms of pulmonary aspiration: elevated temperature, tachycardia, pulmonary congestion (crackles, rhonchi, wheezing, productive cough), tachypnea, dyspnea, or cyanosis.[1, 6, 9, 13] Blue dye no. 1 can also be added to the formula, to assist in early detection of aspiration for those at risk.

Methods Used to Secure Nasal Tubes

Maintenance of nasal tubes can be a challenge for the practitioner.[1, 2, 16, 20–24] Skin irritation from tape is common, and loosening of tape with accidental removal of the tube occurs frequently. While accidental removal can occur in an oriented cooperative patient, it more often occurs in a confused patient. Inadvertent dislodgement can result in increased morbidity. There is risk of aspirating tube feeding solution should the tube only be partially displaced such that the solution is infused into the pharynx. Repeated replacements are also undesirable because of cost, interruption of nutrition support, and patient discomfort.

In a prospective study by Jeffers et al., 109 patients received various forms of enteral tube feedings. Unintentional removal of the feeding tube occurred in 38% of all the tubes placed.[20] This included 172 nasogastric tubes placed in 60 patients, 42 esophagostomies in 28 patients, 32 gastrostomies in 22 patients, and 9 jejunostomies in 8 patients. A retrospective study of 31 patients by Keohane et al. reported the inadvertent removal of feeding tubes in 52% of cases.[21] Silk et al. reported a 41% incidence of inadvertent tube removal.[22]

Meer performed a retrospective study of 78 patients and found that 40% of patients receiving nasoenteral tube feeding experienced inadvertent dislodgement of their feeding tubes.[23] There were 78 episodes of tube dislodgement; 71 of these episodes occurred while the patients were confused, disoriented, or obtunded. Barclay and Litchford prospectively observed 45 patients and reported a 39% incidence of tube removal.[24] Sixty-six percent of those tubes were pulled out by patients despite the use of wrist restraints, whereas the remaining 34% were pulled out by patients not restrained by soft wrist devices.

Most commonly the tube is taped securely to the face.[2, 4, 16] Two possible locations are the side of the face adjacent to the nare containing the tube or on the forehead. The tube should be taped so that neither traction nor pressure is applied to the nares. Activity level as well as perspiration causes problems in maintaining a securely taped tube. To ensure adhesion, it is best to cleanse the skin and thoroughly dry it before taping. Male patients should be shaved prior to taping. If adhesive or hypoallergenic tape is not desirable, a transparent moisture-vapor permeable dressing such as Op Site should be used and the dressing pinched along the side of the tube. This dressing can remain in place up to 7 days. Then, the tube can be draped over the outer part of the ear. An alternative device being used is the XOMED Naso-tube Clip, which has a self-adhesive backing. The device is taped to the patient's cheek or forehead, with the nasoenteral feeding tube being placed through a slot to hold the tube firmly in place. Problems noted with this device are that it may need to be changed as frequently as tape and the self-adherent backing may be irritating to the skin.

Another means for securing a feeding tube is with a "nasal bridle".[2, 23] This involves securing the feeding tube to a 5 F polyvinylchloride tube (the bridle) that has been secured around the nasal septum. This device discourages a patient from pulling out the tube because any traction on the bridle will cause some discomfort due to pressure on the posterior of the nasal septum. The nasal bridle, however, has several disadvantages. A physician skilled in placing bridles usually requires 5 to 20 minutes to place this device, depending on the degree of patient cooperation. In addition, patients have pulled out their feeding tubes by snaring the tube with their finger within the nose or oropharynx proximal to the site of attachment to the bridle. There is also the possibility of a patient forcefully pulling on a bridle that is too securely attached around the nasal septum and injuring the latter structure. Commercial feeding tube bridle kits are available.

Care of the Mucous Membranes

Mucosal irritation of the nasopharynx may occur anywhere along the path of the feeding tube.[1, 3, 4, 6, 7, 9, 15, 16, 19] Complications from mechanical irritation include nasopharyngeal discomfort; hoarseness; nasal, laryngeal, or esophageal erosion; necrosis or stenosis; acute sinusitis; acute otitis media; esophagitis; treacheoesophageal fistula;

and ruptured esophageal varices. Signs and symptoms may include a sore throat, difficulty in swallowing, thirst, dry mouth, pain, pressure, malodorous breath, fever and chills, and heartburn. The use of small-bore feeding tubes may decrease the risk of irritation along the path of the feeding tube.

Proper care of the nares and oral cavity will also help prevent mucous membrane breakdown. For patients with a nasoenteric feeding tube, the nare should be inspected daily for redness, sloughing, or the presence of lesions. Any suspicious lesions should be cultured. The nare should be cleansed daily with hydrogen peroxide and exposed areas lubricated with petroleum jelly. If skin breakdown is present, it may be necessary to switch the nasal tube to the other nare and alternate between them.

Basic oral care should be provided every 2 to 4 hours to alleviate dryness and maintain an intact mucosa. Patients should be allowed to rinse their mouth, chew gum, or suck on hard candy. Mouthwashes should be avoided because the alcohol content may have a drying effect on the oral mucous membranes. Lubricating the lips with petroleum jelly may also enhance patient comfort. To prevent dental and gum disease, the patient's teeth should be brushed once or twice daily even though the patient is not eating by mouth.

Occlusion of Feeding Tubes

Occlusion of feeding tubes occurs in 6% to 12% of patients.[24, 25] Most instances are a result of poorly crushed medications being instilled into the tube, intraluminal buildup of formula residue, or a failure to irrigate the tube after an intermittent feeding.[1, 6, 7, 9, 25–31] Medications that do not crush or dissolve are most likely to lead to obstruction. Some liquid medications such as antacids or syrups with a pH less than 4.0 may cause problems by adhering to the inner lumen and causing blockage. When tube occlusion occurs, the formula infusion will slow down or stop. This is especially important in critically ill patients because it can result in electrolyte imbalance, fluid volume deficit, and malnutrition.

Several studies have been conducted to determine the best agent to use to maintain tube patency or unclog a feeding tube. Cranberry juice has traditionally been used because of its acidic properties (pH 2.6 to 2.8).[4, 9, 26, 27] However, in a clinical study comparing the efficacy of cranberry juice and water as irrigants to maintain feeding tube patency, Wilson and Haynes-Johnson studied 30 subjects being fed through 12 F polyurethane nasointestinal feeding tubes.[26] The subjects were randomly assigned to receive either 30 mL of cranberry juice or 30 mL of water as irrigants every 4 hours. All subjects received their isotonic enteral formula by means of a continuous infusion pump. Tubes irrigated with water had a significantly lower incidence of occlusion and a significantly longer duration of use when compared with tubes irrigated with cranberry juice.

In a 3-day laboratory study, Metheny and associates studied 108 feeding tubes, 54 polyurethane and 54 silicone, of 8, 10, and 12 F sizes (18 of each of the six types).[27] At 4-hour intervals, flow regulators on the feeding bags were adjusted to a rate of 50 mL/hr. Fluid volumes delivered per minute were measured for each tube at 2-hour intervals. One set of tubes at each station was irrigated periodically with cranberry juice, cola, or water. On each of the 3 days, analysis revealed significant ($P < .05$) effects for tube material, cranberry juice contrasted with cola and water as irrigants, and time on tube patency. Polyurethane was consistently superior to silicone as a tube material, and cranberry juice was consistently inferior to cola and water as an irrigant.

Marcuard and Perkins studied (in vitro) the effect of luminal pH and added protein on clotting of feeding formulas. Ten different enteral feeding products were tested by applying one tenth of a milliliter of each to a series of buffer solutions with pH concentrations from 1.2 through 10.1.[28] A protein supplement was added to some of the products. Clotting was observed in premixed intact protein formulas but not in elemental products or polymeric mixtures in powder form. The addition of protein increased clotting only minimally. Luminal occlusion was primarily associated with nasogastric feeding in certain formulas, which clotted instantly when mixed with gastric acid (pH 1.5) but not with jejunal aspirate (pH 7.6).

In an in vitro study, Marcuard et al. evaluated the ability of six solutions (Adolf's Meat Tenderizer, Viokase, Sprite, Pepsi, Coca-Cola, Mountain Dew) to dissolve five different clotted enteral feedings.[25] Distilled water served as the control. The best dissolution score was obtained with Viokase (pancrelipase) in a pH solution of 7.9 ($P < .01$). The initial pH of Viokase in water was 5.9, and there was little dissolution activity. The optimum environment for chymotrypsin to work is when the pH is 7.9. Nicholson also reported successful declogging of feeding tubes by using solutions with chymotrypsin, papain, and distilled water for 4 hours.[29] Unfortunately, the pH of these solutions was not listed, and the amount of water used appeared to be small and varied for each product. Nicholson dissolved the Viokase in 1 mL of distilled water, which failed to clear the obstructed tube after 4 hours.

Currently the most effective method of unclogging feeding tubes is with the use of pancreatic enzymes (e.g., pancrelipase).[1, 4, 30, 31] Marcuard and Stegall report a 96% success rate.[30] The recommended procedure is to mix one-fourth teaspoon of pancreatic enzyme in 15 to 30 mL of warm tap water. Sodium bicarbonate (324-mg tablet) is added to increase the pH of the solution. The dissolved pancreatic enzyme solution is instilled into the feeding tube with a 6- to 12-mL syringe by using a massaging action on the feeding tube. The pancreatic enzyme solution is allowed to remain in the feeding tube for 30 minutes before irrigating the tube. This procedure may be repeated as necessary.

Enteral formulas that come in powder form need to be mixed thoroughly with water. The use of a blender can promote effective mixing and avoid clumping of the formula. Feeding tubes should be irrigated before and after checking for a residual volume, before and after an intermittent feeding, every 4 to 6 hours during continuous feeding, and anytime feedings are stopped to eliminate acid precipitation of formula in the feeding tube. Fifty to 100 mL of tap water should be used and, if fluids are restricted, 10 to 30 mL of tap water. Tap water is acceptable unless the patient is immunocompromised, in which case sterile water should be used. Marcuard and Stegall also suggest that whenever possible the patient should be fed beyond the pylorus.[30] They found that only 15% of tubes placed in the duodenum clogged whereas 49% of tubes placed in the stomach clogged.

Reinsertion of the stylet into an indwelling feeding tube should never be considered as a means of restoring the patency of a clogged tube because of the potential for bowel perforation. Researchers have had varying success unclogging tubes with such items as a Drum cartridge catheter, an Intro-Reducer (a very tiny, hollow 19-gauge catheter), or pancreatic/bicarbonate solution.[25, 30, 31]

Medication Administration via Feeding Tubes

Feeding tubes have long been used as an avenue for medication administration.[32-43] Studies supporting administration of medications via this route are minimal. The practitioner must consider drug-nutrient interactions because these interactions can involve an alteration in the dissolution and absorption of medications resulting from the "presence of food," the degradation and/

or inactivation of nutrient components, alteration of drug bioavailability, alteration in the disposition of nutrient components because of the effects of a medication or other interactions between medications and enteral nutrition.

When using the feeding tube as a means for medication administration, the practitioner needs to consider the following points. Incompatibility of enteral formulas and medications can often lead to the particle aggregation causing clumping of the formula and clogging of the feeding tube. The large number of variables involved makes effective delivery of medications difficult to define.[32-39] Gastrointestinal complications such as nausea, vomiting, abdominal cramping, and diarrhea can be caused by the underlying pathology, the formula administration technique, and the osmolality of enteral formulas and medications.[32, 37] The distal end of the feeding tube may be located in the stomach, duodenum, or jejunum, thus altering the site of delivery and absorption of medications given via a feeding tube.[40, 41]

Cutie et al. reported on the compatibility of 52 liquid medications with three polymeric, nutritionally complete enteral formulas.[38] In general, most suspensions, elixirs, and emulsions were physically compatible when placed directly into these enteral formulas. The liquid pharmaceutical preparations found to be incompatible included syrups and elixirs with a pH less than 4. These products caused clumping of the enteral formula and increased viscosity, tackiness, and particle size. Altman et al. repeated these experiments with a chemically defined formula and several high-nitrogen enteral formulas, with essentially the same results.[39]

Holtz et al. reported on the compatibility of liquid preparations of digoxin, theophylline, phenytoin, methyldopa, and furosemide added to three polymeric, nutritionally complete enteral formulas.[44] Methyldopa and phenytoin concentrations decreased substantially when added to the enteral formulas, and theophylline elixir markedly increased the osmolality of the enteral formulas. The authors recommend avoiding the addition of phenytoin suspension, theophylline elixir, and methyldopa suspension to enteral feedings. Burns et al. reported on the compatibility of 39 pharmaceutical preparations added to a fiber-enriched formula, a nutrient-dense formula, and a free amino acid formula.[41] Physical incompatibility occurred in 26% of the preparations in fiber-enriched formula, 36% of the preparations in nutrient-dense formula, and 100% of the preparations in free amino acid formula. Only 28% of clogged tubes could be unclogged easily.

A recent review by Gora et al. listed six drugs most likely to clog feeding tubes: hydrochlorothiazide/triamterene, ibuprofen, magnesium oxide, psyllium hydrophilic mucilloid, sustained-release potassium chloride capsules, and theophylline sprinkles.[40] If these drugs must be administered via a feeding tube, proper flushing of the tube before and after administration is essential.

Phenytoin

The results of studies suggest interference with phenytoin absorption by continuous tube feeding.[45-48] This interaction is of particular concern because of the narrow therapeutic range (10 to 20 mg/L) for phenytoin. Bauer reported that subtherapeutic phenytoin levels were observed in 53 neurosurgery patients receiving the drug with continuous enteral feeding.[45] In two thirds of the patients, serum phenytoin levels were almost undetectable (2.5 μg/mL). He also reported similar findings in prospective studies of patients and normal volunteers given enteral feedings and suggested that the problem might be obviated by holding the enteral feedings for 2 hours before and 2 hours after phenytoin administration. A study by Ozuna and Friel suggests that high doses of phenytoin suspension are still required to obtain therapeutic levels even with withholding of feedings.[46]

While it is still possible to administer enteral phenytoin concomitantly with enteral tube feedings, the practitioner needs to be aware that if the enteral feeding is interrupted or discontinued, the dosage of phenytoin will need to be readjusted to a lower level. Saklad et al. reported a case study in which the enteral feeding was interrupted but the patient continued to receive phenytoin and achieved toxic levels within a short period of time.[49] Intravenous administration of phenytoin is an alternative in patients receiving enteral nutrition.

Warfarin

Vitamin K is present in all enteral formulas in varying amounts. Several case studies have shown that vitamin K has contributed to warfarin resistance in the presence of enteral feedings.[32, 36, 50-52] Prothrombin times should be followed closely, especially after the enteral feedings are interrupted or discontinued, because the warfarin dose will need to be readjusted.

Theophylline

A case study was reported in which a patient was receiving continuous nasogastric tube feedings and liquid theophylline.[53] The patients' drug levels were found to be subtherapeutic, with recurrent bronchospasm developing. When the enteral feedings were interrupted for 1 hour before and after administration of the medication, drug levels rose to the therapeutic range. Close monitoring of this drug level will need to be performed, especially when enteral feedings are interrupted or discontinued, because the theophylline dose will need to be readjusted.[35, 36, 44]

Many problems with medication administration remain unsolved. As new drugs enter the market, the effect of the drug and its absorption and metabolism when administered with nutrients will need to be addressed. Table 22-1 highlights general considerations for the administration of medications via feeding tubes.[35, 40, 42, 43] Table 22-2 highlights principles to consider when administer-

TABLE 22–1.

General Considerations for Medication Administration via Feeding Tubes

Simple compressed tablets
- May always be crushed, even if they have a sugar film coating (e.g., cimetidine, digoxin).
- Designed for immediate dissolution and release.
- A mortar and pestle will be needed to crush the tablet.
- Thoroughly mix the crushed tablet in 15–30 mL of water.

Hard gelatin capsules
- Contain a powder in a gelatin envelope that separates in the middle (e.g., ampicillin, doxycline).
- The contents may be poured out and usually will not need to be crushed.
- Mix the powder thoroughly in 15–30 mL of water.

Soft gelatin capsules
- To administer the contents of these capsules, poke a pinhole into the end of the capsule and squeeze out the contents (e.g., nifedipine, chloral hydrate).
- Be aware that even careful squeezing will not remove all of the capsule contents.
- If the entire dose is needed, dissolve the contents in 15–30 mL of warm water. Although this method can be very time-consuming (up to 1 hr), it ensures that the entire dose will be administered.

Sustained action capsules
- These capsules are filled with beads or pellets that dissolve and release the medication at different rates into the small intestine (e.g., Feosol Spansule, Slo-Bid). This method of drug release results in the delivery of the equivalent of two to three doses. Therefore, if the beads or pellets are crushed, all doses of the medication would be released at one time. This would defeat the purpose of "sustained action."
- Sometimes the beads or pellets are designed to reduce gastrointestinal irritation rather than to give a sustained release action (e.g., Micro-K, Eryc). Therefore, crushing the contents of these capsules may lead to gastrointestinal upset.

Enteric coated tablets
- These tablets are formulated to allow passage from the stomach into the intestine before releasing the active form of the medication (e.g., Feosol, Azulfidine).
- The coating process is used for two basic reasons: to prevent stomach irritation and to avoid denaturation of the medication in the stomach. Therefore, crushing the tablet is likely to produce undersirable side effects or cause destruction of the active ingredient.

Sustained release tablets
- These tablets are coated with a wax matrix designed to dissolve and release medication at a slower rate.
- They contain the equivalent of two to three doses of a medication (Procan SR, Theolair SR).

ing medications via feeding tubes, timing of medications, and actual administration techniques.[32, 34, 35, 37–40, 42]

CENTRAL VENOUS CATHETERS

Catheter Infection

Infection Rates

Nosocomial infections are estimated to occur in approximately 5% of hospitalized patients and increase medical costs by 1.3 billion dollars per year.[54] Intravascular catheters are responsible for about 33% of all nosocomial infections, or about 50,000 cases per year.[55, 56] The reported incidence of CVC sepsis ranges from 3.6% to 20.4% in a general population of hospitalized patients and is estimated to be twofold to fivefold higher in critically ill patients.[55, 57–60] Patients in critical care units are at particular risk because they often have multiple intravascular catheters, have impaired host defenses, and may have multisystem organ failure. When multiple intravascular catheters are present, a patient's risk of bacteremia increases by 5% to 17%.[58]

Definition of Catheter-Related Infection and Culture Methods

Maki and Ringer's definition of CVC septicemia has emerged as a standard by which this complication is most often defined in the clinical and research setting (Table 22–3).[61] Colonization of the catheter tip via the subcutaneous insertion tract is thought to be a primary mechanism that causes subsequent septicemia. Bjornson and associates reported a significant association between colonization of CVCs and 10^3 bacterial or fungal colony-forming units

TABLE 22–2.

Administration of Medications Through an Enteral Feeding Tube

Summary of principles to consider in administration
- If the patient is able to take medications by mouth, this is the preferred route.
- The nurse must be knowledgeable of the location of the feeding tube because this will affect drug utilization. Is the tip *above* or *below* the pylorus?
- If there is a nasogastric tube in place as well as a feeding tube, use the nasogastric tube as the preferred mode for medication delivery. *Do not administer medications in a Miller Abbott Tube.*
- The administration of diluted crushed medications into a feeding tube should be avoided whenever possible. Physicians should order liquid forms when possible.
- Calculate equivalent liquid doses carefully. Many liquid dosage forms are intended for pediatric use, and the dose of the drug must be adjusted for adults or vice versa.
- Consider the use of granule formulations, effervescent tablets, and other solid dosage forms when preformulated liquid preparations appear to present a problem.
- The use of oral medications that are not meant to be crushed for enteral tube administration should be avoided.
- Reconstitute capsules with 10–15 mL of water.
- Dilute viscous liquids with 15–30 mL of water (a highly concentrated solution should be diluted with 30–60 mL of water).
- Drugs that are hypertonic or irritating to the gastrointestinal mucosa (such as potassium chloride) should be diluted in at least 15–30 mL of water before administering to avoid gastrointestinal irritation and diarrhea (sometimes 60–90 mL of water is needed).
- Drugs that are usually administered with meals to avoid gastrointestinal irritation (i.e., indomethacin) should be diluted with 15–30 mL of water prior to administration.
- Avoid mixing drugs with enteral formulas in the feeding bag whenever possible. Not only can this practice alter the therapeutic effect of the drug, it can also disrupt the emulsion of the formula and result in a formula that resembles curdled milk. If medication other than a nutrient (i.e., sodium chloride) is ordered to be added to the feeding, check with the pharmacist first. Observe the feeding after the addition for any reaction or precipitation. Shake the solution thoroughly. Label the feeding with the name and amount of the drug added.

How to time medications with tube feedings
- Intermittent gastric feeding schedules should be timed to coincide with medications that require a full or empty stomach, such as with antibiotics.
- For continuous feedings going into the stomach, stop the feeding for 15 minutes before the administration time of the medication to allow some emptying of the stomach.
- Feedings being administered beyond the pylorus are less problematic since feedings are not held in this part of the intestine. The feeding may be discontinued just prior to administration of the medication.
- Assess the patient's response to the medication to determine whether the patient is receiving the desired therapeutic effect.
- Always check for residual volume before administering the medication.

Administration of medications
- Verify tube placement by aspirating gastrointestinal contents *or* by inflating the tube with 5 mL of air (via a 35-mL or larger syringe) while listening at the epigastric area with a stethoscope for transmission of the sound of air. Record the length of the tube from the nose and note any change. Check the oropharynx area for coiled tubing.
- Flush feeding tube with 15–30 mL of water before medication administration.
- Administer each medication separately, and flush the feeding tube with at least 5 mL of water between each medication.
- Flush the feeding tube with 15–30 mL of water after medication administration

(CFUs) on the skin at the catheter insertion site.[62] Armstrong and associates found that skin site cultures with 50 or more CFUs of an organism other than coagulase-negative staphylococci carried the greatest relative risk for catheter-related infection when compared with erythema at the site, temperature elevation, hyperglycemia, or leukocytosis.[63]

Catheter-related septicemia diagnosed by positive blood cultures and positive catheter cultures can be missed if blood cultures are performed inadequately. Three blood cultures, obtained no less than 1 hour apart, are recommended to achieve a 99% chance of detecting bacteremia.[64, 65] The specificity and sensitivity of a variety of blood and catheter culture methods have been described by Curtas and Tramposch, who conclude that the semiquantitative

TABLE 22–3.

Definitions of Catheter Infection*

Infection	Definition
Local catheter-related infection	Positive semiquantitative culture with 15 or more colony-forming units
Catheter-related septicemia	Semiquantitative culture and blood culture positive for the same species. Clinical data that show no other source of septicemia
Septicemia from contaminated infusate	Isolation of the same species from the infusate and from peripheral blood cultures. Negative semiquantitative culture of the catheter

*Adapted from Maki DG, Ringer M: *JAMA* 1987; 258:2396–2403.

catheter culture method may be most practical for clinicians (Table 22–4).[66] Isolator cultures in which semiquantitative blood cultures are drawn through the CVC and through a peripheral vein have been described by several investigators.[67–69]

Catheter Insertion Site and Infection Risks

The site of insertion of CVCs can influence catheter infection rates, in part because of the ease of maintaining the catheter dressing, the propensity for catheter movement, and the likelihood of catheter dressing soilage. Collignon et

al.[70] and Gil et al.[71] reported catheter colonization rates of 34% and 47% with femorally placed catheters, and 10% and 16% with subclavian catheters. Collignon and associates found that internal jugular catheters had a 28% colonization rate. However, Gil et al. reported only a 2% colonization rate for internal jugular catheters.

Catheter Materials and Infection

The materials that are used in the composition of CVCs has been thought to influence catheter-related sepsis. A number of studies have compared the thrombogenicity of various catheter materials. In 1977, Stillman and colleagues reported that the polymers used in catheter construction influenced catheter-related infection through the propensity of the catheter to cause thrombus formation.[72] The thrombus provides a nidus for infection. Bozzetti et al. found that venous thrombosis was demonstrated by venography in 46% of the polyvinylchloride catheters and 11% of the silicone catheters after an average duration of about 12 days.[73] None of the patients experienced frank symptoms of thrombosis. Borow and Crowley compared various catheter materials for thrombogenicity when the catheters were inserted into the arteries and veins of dogs.[74] Polyurethane was found to be

TABLE 22–4.

Culture Methods to Determine Catheter Sepsis*

Method	Specificity	Sensitivity	Comments
Blood cultures			
Peripheral	Increases with the number drawn over a 24-hr period		May be false positives secondary to contamination
Catheter	++	++	Positive cultures may result from hematogenous seeding
Quantitative	+++	+++	Can determine the source of infection; high contamination rate
Device			
Qualitative	+	+++	Requires catheter removal; high degree of false positives secondary to contamination
Semiquantitative	++	++	Requires catheter removal; may only indicate colonization
Quantitative	++++	++++	Technically difficult and labor intensive

*From Curtas S, Tramposch K: *Nutr Clin Pract* 1991; 6:43–48. Used by permission.

the most thrombogenic material, followed by silicone. Hydromer-coated polyurethane was the least thrombogenic material. In a rabbit study, DiCostanzo and others found that thrombosis occurred more often with rigid catheters, such as those composed of Teflon and polyethylene, than with soft catheters composed of silicone.[75] The softer catheters, however, had a higher incidence of fibrin sleeve development.

Newer catheter materials include an elastomeric hydrogel (Aquevene) that is very rigid prior to insertion but absorbs body fluid to become 50 times softer once it is inserted.[76] In addition, a polyurethane elastomer (Vialon) has been developed for use in peripheral catheters that also becomes softer after insertion and may be less likely to damage the intima of the vein.[77] These catheter materials are currently not available for conventionally inserted percutaneous CVCs (subclavian or internal jugular approaches).

Hydromer Coating.—Damage to the intima of the vein is the first step in the development of a thrombosis. Stiffer catheters are more likely to cause this injury to the vein. The injury is followed by aggregation of platelets and, subsequently, by deposition of fibrin. Although most catheter materials appear smooth, under electron magnification their irregular surface becomes apparent. Kristinsson studied the adherence of *Staphylococcus epidermidis* and *Staphylococcus aureus* to silicone elastomer, thermoplastic polyurethane, and hydromer-coated polyurethane.[78] The hydromer-coated catheters had less bacterial adherence.

Antibiotic Bonding.—The interest in coating CVCs with agents that would reduce the adherence of bacteria has led to studies using antibiotics that are bonded to catheters. Trooskin and associates pretreated polyethylene catheters and silicone catheters with benzylpenicillin-^{14}C and a bonding agent,

tridodecylmethylammonium chloride (TDMAC).[79] The C-penicillin TDMAC-bonded catheters were compared with TDMAC-bonded catheters inserted into the jugular veins of rats. The catheter exit sites were inoculated with *S. aureus* to provide a bacteriologic challenge. The TDMAC-bonded catheters had colonization rates of up to 80%, whereas the antibiotic-bonded catheters did not become colonized.

In 1991, Kamal et al. reported a 2% catheter-related septicemia rate with cefazolin/TDMAC-bonded arterial and central venous catheters for patients in a surgical intensive care unit vs. a 14% rate for conventional polyethylene catheters.[80] Skin colonization at the insertion site did not differ between the control and bonded catheter groups.

Maki and associates reported the results of a clinical trial using a multiple-lumen CVC coated with silver-sulfadiazine and chlorhexidine, an antiseptic combination that is inhibitory to staphylococci, enterococci, and yeast.[81] Antiseptic-coated catheters were two times less frequently colonized than uncoated catheters and four times less likely to cause septicemia. Further studies of antibiotic or antiseptic catheters are needed to determine their long-term effectiveness and safety.

Antimicrobial Cuffs.—In a prospective randomized trial of a silver-impregnated cuff made of collagen that was placed on percutaneously inserted CVCs, Maki et al. reported a significantly ($P = .002$) lower catheter colonization rate (9.1%) on the cuffed catheters than on conventional catheters (28.9%).[82] The cuffed catheters were four times less likely to produce septicemia. A disadvantage of the cuff, however, is that it can be technically challenging to insert and must be placed deep enough to prevent extrusion. When correctly placed, the cuff presumably acts as an antimicrobial barrier to organisms that would migrate down to the tip of the catheter through the subcutaneous tract.

Catheter Design and Infection

The question of whether multiple-lumen CVCs increase the risk of catheter-related infection over single-lumen catheters has been the subject of debate for nearly as long as these catheters have been available for use. There is no doubt that they are widely used in critical care. Of the studies that have attempted to evaluate whether there is an increased risk of sepsis with multiple-lumen catheters, only two (Johnson and Reypins 1990, and McCarthy 1987) were prospective and randomized (Table 22–5).[83–89] Most of the studies did not report a significant difference in catheter-related septicemia between types of catheters. However, Gil et al. reported a significant increase in catheter colonization when the duration of catheterization exceeded 6 days $(P < .1)$.[71] This finding suggests that the length of time that a catheter is in place is more of a risk factor than the number of catheter lumina. The timing and method of catheter exchange has also created debate.

Duration of Catheterization and Catheter Exchange Over a Guidewire

Protocols for changing CVCs vary widely. In some centers, there is a pre-scribed duration of catheterization, whereas in others the CVCs are left in place until catheter-related sepsis is suspected. Armstrong et al. reported that the appearance of the exit site and the presence of fever, hyperglycemia, or leukocytosis are poor predictors of catheter-related infection.[63] In a French study, Richet et al. found that the use of a semipermeable transparent dressing, the use of the jugular insertion site, and the duration of catheterization were significantly associated with positive catheter tip cultures.[90] These authors recommend that central catheters be replaced every 5 days because the positive culture rate increases significantly $(P = .04)$ after this duration. Maki also recommends that the duration of CVC placement not exceed 5 days in critical care patients.[91]

Catheter Care Protocols

Skin Antisepsis

The primary goal of catheter dressing change protocols is to reduce the level of microbial growth on the skin that surrounds the CVC insertion site. Research suggests that the catheter can become colonized with skin organisms via the catheter's subcutaneous insertion tract

TABLE 22–5.

Multiple-Lumen Catheters and Catheter Sepsis

Investigators	No. of Catheters	Sepsis Rate	Comments
Kelly et al.[83] 1986	96 TLC	3.1%	TLC only
Pemberton et al.[84] 1986	59 TLC	19%, S	Prospective
	68 SLC	3%	
McCarthy et al.[85] 1987	39 TLC	12.8%, S	Prospective, randomized
	38 SLC	0%	
Lee et al,[86] 1988	307 TLC	1.3%, NS	
	68 SLC	0%	
Gil et al.[71] 1989	157 TLC	No difference	Prospective
	68 SLC		
Johnson and Rypins,[87] 1990	51 DLC	2.0%	Prospective, randomized
	48 SLC	2.1%, NS	
Horowitz et al.[88] 1990	158 PAC	2.5%	Prospective
	214 TLC	6.5%, NS	
Clark-Christoff et al.[89] 1992	78 SLC	2.6%	Randomized
	99 TLC	13.1%, S	

TLC = triple-lumen catheter; DLC = double-lumen catheter; SLC = single-lumen catheter; PAC = pulmonary artery catheter; S = significant; NS = Not significant.

and that skin colonization can approach a level that increases the risk of subsequent catheter tip colonization.[62, 63] In recent years, a number of studies have evaluated the effectiveness of various skin-cleansing agents. Skin cannot be sterilized; all skin antiseptics produce bactericidal and fungicidal effects that depend upon contact time and differ in their duration of effect. Most desirable is an antiseptic that produces a rapid (2 minutes or less) reduction of organisms, has a long duration of action, and is not irritating to the skin. Traditionally, one or more skin antiseptics have been applied during a catheter dressing procedure.

Acetone.—A defatting agent such as acetone was initially used in many catheter dressing protocols. The rationale for this practice was based on the belief that the removal of skin oils allows a more effective removal of skin organisms, and defatting was used as a "first step" in the dressing protocols. A 1987 study by Maki and McCormack showed that acetone was irritating to the skin and of no benefit as an adjunctive measure.[92]

Alcohol.—Alcohols provide antisepsis by the denaturation of proteins and are effective against most gram-positive and gram-negative organisms and the tubercle bacillus. Alcohols are also effective against many fungi and viruses.[93] Seventy percent alcohol by weight is most commonly used for catheter care protocols. Alcohols have a rapid action; washing with alcohol for 3 minutes is as effective as a 20-minute scrub.[94] Unfortunately, alcohol can be drying to the skin, and it has no residual antiseptic activity.

Iodophors.—Tincture of iodine was used as a preoperative scrub for many years. However, it cannot be left on the skin because it will cause irritation. Iodophors contain free iodine that is released during skin cleansing, and they require about 2 minutes of contact time for adequate antiseptic activity. Iodophors are effective against gram-positive and gram-negative bacteria, fungi, viruses, and some bacterial spores.[94] Iodophor can cause sensitivity and skin irritation in some patients, and the duration of antiseptic activity ends when the iodophor is dry. Povidone-iodine is the most common iodophor that is used for CVC dressing protocols.

Iodophor ointment is used over the catheter exit site in some centers. Maki and Band compared the efficacy of two antimicrobial ointments, polyantibiotic and povidone-iodine, in the prevention of vascular catheter-related infection.[95] These researchers found only a marginally protective benefit of the polymicrobial ointment. However, the study demonstrated greater benefit for catheters that remained in place for more than 4 days. The authors also stated that povidone-iodine ointment may be preferable when catheters are used for parenteral nutrition because of the increased risk of fungal and gram-negative infections.

Chlorhexidine Gluconate.—Approved for use in the United States in the 1970s, chlorhexidine is effective against gram-positive and some gram-negative bacteria, many viruses, and some fungi.[93] It has an intermediate speed of killing organisms. The most desirable aspect of chlorhexidine is its duration of activity of at least 6 hours. Maki and associates conducted a randomized prospective trial that compared the effectiveness of povidone-iodine, alcohol, and chlorhexidine in the prevention of central venous and arterial catheter sepsis.[96] Chlorhexidine was associated with a significantly lower ($P = .02$) incidence of bacteremia. Maki and associates used 2% aqueous chlorhexidine gluconate, which differs from the commonly available 2% or 4% alcoholic solution of chlorhexidine.

Skin antiseptics are a major area of focus for research dealing with prevention of related sepsis. Of particular interest are agents that have a high rate of bacterial kill, are nonirritating and nontoxic, and have a prolonged duration of action.

Catheter Dressing Materials

A variety of dressing materials have been used to cover the CVC insertion site. Sterile dressing material covers the area of the skin that is cleansed with antiseptics, thus providing an occlusive barrier to further contamination. However, the organisms that remain on the skin will eventually reach a significant level; therefore, reapplication of the dressing is necessary. Dressing adherence, comfort, propensity for irritation, bulk, absorbency, transparency, and cost are some of the factors that determine the suitability of dressing materials. In addition, certain dressing materials may effect microbial growth on the skin and thus contribute to catheter-related septicemia.

Gauze/Tape.—Gauze is the traditional type of dressing material used for CVCs. It is absorbent, nonirritating, and inexpensive. Gauze must be affixed to the skin with tape, and its average duration of adherence is between 48 and 72 hours. It is rather bulky and is completely opaque. Gauze-and-tape dressing is susceptible to contamination by liquids; thus any secretions that reach the dressing will destroy its resistance to contamination. For this reason and because of its shorter duration of adhesion, the gauze-and-tape dressing is not considered ideal. Alternative dressing materials are being used for CVCs in many critical care units.

Transparent Adherent Dressing.—Transparent, semipermeable, polyurethane dressings were first devised as dressings for wounds and for skin graft donor sites. The first reports of their use for CVCs began to appear in the early 1980s.[97-99] Transparent adherent dressings (TADs) seem ideal for CVCs; they are light, waterproof, adherent, transparent, and nonirritating and can remain adherent for up to 7 days. Cur-

rently, however, these dressings are the subject of controversy. Although early studies did not clearly demonstrate an increased risk of catheter sepsis with their use, more recent studies suggested that TADs are associated with increased rates of skin colonization near the catheter insertion site.

Conly and others reported a significantly ($P = .002$) greater colonization rate (62%) with TADs than with standard gauze-and-tape dressing (24%).[100] The increased colonization rate occurred despite dressing changes every 48 hours. In a meta-analysis of seven studies that compared infectious complications of CVCs when transparent dressings were used, Hoffman and associates reported statistically significant differences in the relative risks for catheter tip colonization.[101] The TAD groups had higher colonization rates (Conly's study was included in this meta-analysis). There was an increased relative risk for bacteremia and catheter sepsis. However, the pooled data did not reach statistical significance. The results of this meta-analysis are of concern. Catheter colonization is a well-recognized prelude to catheter sepsis. The authors of the meta-analysis commented that the covariates within the studies may have confounded the analysis; within a study, the frequency of dressing changes or the use of ointments for control and experimental groups was not always consistent. Craven and associates have commented that the moisture that accumulates under the TAD may contribute to bacterial growth.[102] TADs may also vary in their moisture permeability. Further study in this area is needed to identify factors that promote or inhibit growth under a dressing material that otherwise has very pleasing characteristics.

Catheter Hub Contamination

Procedures that involve the removal or insertion of caps or tubing into the hub of the CVC are developed to prevent inadvertent contamination at this area. Although contamination of the catheter hub is thought to occur less frequently than migration of organisms along the subcutaneous tract, its occurrence has been well documented.

Sitges-Serra and associates reported that hub colonization by coagulase-negative staphylococci led to catheter sepsis in 21 of 23 culture-positive catheters.[103] Stotter et al. reported a significant reduction in catheter infection rates by using an absolute alcohol spray at the catheter hub-tubing junction and by covering the junction with a plastic cuff lined with providone-iodine–impregnated foam.[104]

Many centers have adopted the practice of cleansing the catheter hub-tubing junction with a disinfectant such as iodophor or alcohol whenever this area is manipulated. The use of stopcocks, which can readily become colonized, is discouraged. The use of Leur-lock connections vs. the taping of connections has not been studied, nor has the frequency of catheter cap changes been investigated. The advent of "needleless" systems to protect hospital staff against needlestick injuries has brought a plethora of new intravenous devices and connectors. How these devices will affect the incidence of CVC sepsis is unknown at present.

Catheter Flushes

Heparinized saline is the traditional flush solution for CVCs. Heparin is thought to decrease the incidence of catheter occlusion. However, the dosage of heparin that is used to flush CVCs has varied widely from 1000 units/mL to 10 units/mL or less. A standard frequency of catheter flushes has not been established. In a survey of critical care nurses, 40% used 100 units/mL, 37% used 10 units/mL, and 23% used other solutions or dilutions to flush peripheral heparin locks.[105]

Smith and associates reported a randomized crossover study that compared twice-daily heparin flushes with once-per-week saline flushes for children with cancer who had indwelling CVCs.[106] Five milliliters of heparin was used twice daily or 10 mL of isotonic saline. The investigators found no significant difference between the two groups in the incidence of occlusion, sepsis, or other catheter complications.

Heparin is thought to be innocuous in dosages that are commonly used for catheter irrigation, but it has been reported to cause thrombocytopenia and thrombosis.[107, 108] In addition, heparin is incompatible with many medications, and it is more expensive than saline. Although the efficacy of saline as a flush solution for peripheral intravenous catheters has been more thoroughly studied, the best flush solution for CVCs has not been established.[105] Of particular concern is the risk of occlusion of tunneled CVCs and implanted ports with non–heparin-containing solutions.

Catheter Occlusion

CVC occlusion can result from a variety of causes that include catheter pinch-off related to the position of the patient or the catheter, thrombosis of the central vein, fibrin sleeve development on the catheter, and a blood clot or drug precipitate within the catheter lumen. Catheter pinch-off is usually resolved by changing the patient's position or having the patient cough or take a deep breath. Thrombosis or fibrin sleeve development is suspected when the catheter can be flushed but no blood can be aspirated from it.

Thrombosis of the central vein is a serious complication and may be heralded by physical symptoms such as swelling of the arm, neck, or shoulder on the side of the catheter. Thrombosis is diagnosed by venography, and fibrin sleeve development is often apparent during a fluoroscopic study. Clotted blood or drug precipitates are amenable to pharmacologic therapy.

Thrombolytic Therapy

Thrombolytic therapy began to be used to restore the patency of occluded CVCs around 1980.[109–111] Streptokinase or urokinase 5000 units/mL is instilled into the catheter in a total volume equal to the internal volume of the catheter. The thrombolytic agent is allowed to remain in the catheter for 5 to 15 minutes before attempts to withdraw blood from the catheter occur. If the initial attempt is unsuccessful, repeated attempts can occur every 5 to 15 minutes until the patency of the catheter is established or 60 minutes has passed. Investigators have reported success rates of 32% to 100% when using thrombolytic therapy.[112]

Atkinson and associates reported the use of tissue-type plasminogen activator (t-PA) in CVCs that failed to clear after initial installations of 10,000 units of urokinase.[113] The t-PA was instilled as a 2 mg/2 mL dosage and allowed to dwell for 4 hours; it was successful in five of six attempts. Further studies are required to determine whether t-PA is superior to standard thrombolytic agents in efficiacy and safety.

Hydrochloric Acid

CVCs can become occluded by drug precipitates, particularly by calcium and phosphorus salts. Thrombolytic agents are ineffective in clearing the catheter in this instance. A drug precipitate should be suspected when occlusion in conjunction with or immediately after an infusion. Occlusion by a blood clot is most often discovered at the time of the next attempt to begin an infusion or withdraw blood. In particular, infusions that contain sodium bicarbonate and acetate salts are prone to precipitation. Hydrochloric acid has been used to clear drug precipitates in CVCs. Shulman and others reported the use of 0.1N hydrochloric acid to clear CVCs that were occluded by precipitates.[114] The hydrochloric acid is instilled in the same manner as urokinase and left to dwell for up to 4 hours.

Ethanol

Catheter occlusion can result from a buildup of lipid within the catheter lumen. The use of total nutrient admixtures has increased in the last decade,

and thus the potential for catheter occlusion from lipid deposition may become more commonplace. Thrombolytic therapy and hydrochloric acid are unlikely to reestablish patency of the catheter when line occlusion results from lipid. Pennington and Pithie reported the use of 70% ethanol to clear five CVCs that were presumed to be occluded by lipid buildup.[115] The CVCs in this study had failed to open with urokinase. An instillation of 70% ethanol in a volume that approximated the internal volume of the catheter was instilled and allowed to remain in the catheter for 1 hour. Ethanol was successful in reestablishing patency in four of the five catheters.

Catheter occlusion is a significant problem that interrupts therapy and can lead to rupture of the catheter or the need to replace a catheter. Thrombolytic therapy, hydrochloric acid, and ethanol have been used to restore catheter patency. Careful assessment of the circumstances prior to and during the time that the catheter becomes occluded is important in determining which of these agents is most likely to be successful.

REFERENCES

1. Teasley-Strausburg KM, Cerra FB, Lehmann S, et al (eds): *Nutrition Support Handbook: A Compendium of Products With Guidelines for Usage.* Cincinnati, Harvey Whitney Books, 1992.
2. Forlaw L, Chernoff R, Guenter P: Enteral delivery systems, in Rombeau JL, Caldwell MD (eds): *Clinical Nutrition: Enteral and Tube Feeding,* ed 2. Philadelphia, WB Saunders, 1990.
3. Guenter P, Jones S, Jacobs DO, et al: Administration and delivery of enteral nutrition, in Rombeau JL, Caldwell MD (eds): *Clinical Nutrition: Enteral and Tube Feeding,* ed 2. Philadelphia, WB Saunders, 1990.
4. Farley JM: Current trends in enteral feeding. *Crit Care Nurs* 1988; 8:23–28.
5. Jones S: Simpler and safer tube-feeding techniques. *RN* 1984; 47:40–47.

6. Petrosino BM, Meraviglia M, Becker H: Mechanical problems with small-diameter enteral feeding tubes. *J Neurosci Nurs* 1987; 19:276–280.

7. Petrosino BM, Christian BJ, Wolf J, et al: Implications of selected problems with nasoenteral tube feedings. *Crit Care Nurs Q* 1989; 12:1–18.

8. Metheny NA, Spies MA, Eisenberg P: Measures to test placement of nasoenteral feeding tubes. *West J Nurs Res* 1988; 10:367–383.

9. Haynes-Johnson V: Tube feeding complications: Causes, prevention, and therapy. *Nutr Supp Serv* 1986; 6:17–18.

10. Metheny NA, Spies M, Eisenberg P: Frequency of nasoenteral tube displacement and associated risk factors. *Res Nurs Health* 1986; 9:241–247.

11. Metheny N, Williams P, Wersema L, et al: Effectiveness of pH measurements in predicting feeding tube placement. *Nurs Res* 1989; 38:280–285.

12. Metheny N: Measures to test placement of nasogastric and nasointestinal feeding tubes: A review. *Nurs Res* 1988; 37:324–329.

13. Bockus S: Troubleshooting your tube feedings. *Am J Nurs* 1991; 91:24–28.

14. Patterson RS: Enteral nutrition delivery systems, in Grant JA, Kennedy-Caldwell C (eds): *Nutrition Support in Nursing*. Philadelphia, Grune & Stratton, 1988.

15. Metheny NM: Twenty ways to prevent tube-feeding complications. *Nursing* 1985; 15:47–50.

16. Hatchett-Cohen L: Nasoduodenal tube feeding. *Geriatr Nurs* 1988; 9:88–91.

17. Eisenberg P, Metheny N, McSweeney M: Nasoenteral feeding-tube properties and the ability to withdraw fluid via syringe. *Appl Nurs Res* 1989; 2:168–172.

18. Metheny N, McSweeney M, Wehrle MA, et al: Effectiveness of the auscultatory method in predicting feeding tube location. *Nurs Res* 1990; 39:262–267.

19. Heitkemper MM, Williams S: Prevent problems caused by enteral feedings. *J Gerontol Nurs* 1985; 119:25–30.

20. Jeffers SL, Dorr LA, Meguid MM: Mechanical complications of enteral nutrition: Prospective study of 109 con-secutive patients (abstract). *Clin Res* 1984; 32:233.

21. Keohane PP, Attrill H, Jones BJM, et al: Limitations and drawbacks of fine-bore nasogastric feeding tubes. *Clin Nutr* 1983; 2:85.

22. Silk DBA, Rees RG, Keohane PP, et al: Clinical efficacy and design changes of "fine bore" nasogastric feeding tubes: A seven-year experience involving 809 intubations in 403 patients. *JPEN* 1987; 11:378.

23. Meer JA: Inadvertent dislodgement of nasoenteral feeding tubes: Incidence and prevention. *JPEN* 1987; 11:187–189.

24. Barclay BA, Litchford MD: Incidence of nasoduodenal tube occlusion and patient removal of tubes: A prospective study. *J Am Diet Assoc* 1991; 91:220–222.

25. Marcuard SP, Stegall, KL, Trogdon S: Clearing obstructed feeding tubes. *JPEN* 1989; 13:81–83.

26. Wilson MF, Haynes-Johnson V: Cranberry juice or water? A comparison of feeding tube irrigants. *Nutr Supp Serv* 1987; 7:23–24.

27. Metheny N, Eisenberg P, McSweeney M: Effect of feeding tube properties and three irrigants on clogging rates. *Nurs Res* 1988; 37:165–169.

28. Marcuard SP, Perkins AM: Clogging of feeding tubes. *JPEN* 1988; 12:403–405.

29. Nicholson LJ: Declogging small-bore feeding tubes. *JPEN* 1987; 11:594–597.

30. Marcuard SP, Stegall KS: Unclogging feeding tubes with pancreatic enzyme. *JPEN* 1990; 14:198–200.

31. Bommarito AA, Heinzelmann ML, Boysen DA: A new approach to the management of obstructed enteral feeding tubes. *Nutr Clin Pract* 1989; 4:111–114.

32. Melnick G, Wright K: Pharmacologic aspects of enteral nutrition, in Rombeau JL, Caldwell MD (eds): *Clinical Nutrition: Enteral and Tube Feeding*, ed 2. Philadelphia, WB Saunders, 1990.

33. Strom JG, Miller SW: Stability of drugs with enteral nutrient formulas. *Drug Intell Clin Pharm* 1990; 24:130–134.

34. Wright B, Robinson L: Enteral feeding tubes as drug delivery systems. *Nutr Supp Serv* 1986; 6:33–48.

35. Egging P: Enteral nutrition from a pharmacist's perspective, *Nutr Supp Serv* 1987; 7:17, 18, 34.

36. Fagerman KE, Ballou AE: Drug compatibilities with enteral feeding solutions coadministered by tube. *Nutr Supp Serv* 1988; 8:31–32.

37. Niemiec PW, Vanderveen TW, Morrison JL, et al: Gastrointestinal disorders caused by medications and electrolyte solution osmolality during enteral nutrition. *JPEN* 1983; 7:387–391.

38. Cutie AJ, Altman E, Lenkel L: Compatibility of enteral products with commonly employed drug additives. *JPEN* 1983; 7:186–191.

39. Altman E, Cutie AJ: Compatibility of enteral products with commonly employed drug additives. *Nutr Supp Serv* 1984; 4:8–17.

40. Gora ML, Tschampel MM, Visconti JA: Considerations of drug therapy in patients receiving enteral nutrition. *Nutr Clin Pract* 1989; 4:105–110.

41. Burns PE, McCall L, Wirsching R: Physical compatibility of enteral formulas with various common medications. *J Am Diet Assoc* 1988; 88:1094–1096.

42. Lehmann S, Barber J: Giving medications by feeding tube: How to avoid problems. *Nursing* 1991; 21:58–61.

43. Mitchell JF, Pawlicki KS: Oral dosage forms that should not be crushed: 1992 revision. *Hosp Pharm* 1992; 27:690–692, 695–699.

44. Holtz L, Milton J, Sturek J: Compatibility of medication with enteral feedings. *JPEN* 1987; 11:183–186.

45. Bauer LA: Interference of oral phenytoin absorption by continuous nasogastric feedings. *Neurology* 1982; 32:570–572.

46. Ozuna J, Friel P: Effect of enteral feeding on serum phenytoin levels. *J Neurosurg Nurs* 1984; 16:289–291.

47. Olsen KM, Hiller FC, Ackerman BH, et al: Effect of enteral feeding on oral phenytoin absorption. *Nutr Clin Pract* 1989; 4:176–178.

48. Hooks MA, Lange RL, Taylor At, et al: The recovery of phenytoin from an enteral nutrient formula. *Am J Hosp Pharm* 1986; 43:685–688.

49. Saklad JJ, Graves RH, Sharp WP: Interaction of oral phenytoin with enteral feedings. *JPEN* 1986; 10:322–323.

50. Howard PA, Hannaman KN: Warfarin resistance linked to enteral nutrition products. *J Am Diet Assoc* 1985; 85:713–714.

51. Parr MD, Record KE, Griffith GL, et al: Effect of enteral nutrition on warfarin therapy. *Clin Pharm* 1982; 1:274–278.

52. Martin JE, Lutomski DM: Warfarin resistance and enteral feedings. *JPEN* 1989; 13:206–208.

53. Gal P, Layson R: Interference with oral theophylline absorption by continuous nasogastric feedings. *Ther Drug Monit* 1986; 8:421–423.

54. Perkins CM, Dascomb HE: Intravascular device–related infections. *Probl Crit Care* 1990; 4:21–44.

55. Hampton AA, Sherertz RJ: Vascular-access infections in hospitalized patients. *Surg Clin North Am* 1988; 68:57–71.

56. Maki DG: Infection due to infusion therapy, in Bennett JV, Brachman PS (eds): *Hospital infections,* ed 2. Boston, Little, Brown, 1986.

57. Maki DG: Risk factors for nosocomial infection in intensive care. *Arch Intern Med* 1989; 149:30–35.

58. Wenzel RP, Thompson RL, Landry SM, et al: Hospital-acquired infections in intensive care unit patients: An overview with emphasis on epidemics. *Infect Control* 1983; 4:371–375.

59. Brown RB, Hosmer D, Chen HC, et al: A comparison of infections in different ICU's within the same hospital. *Crit Care Med* 1985; 13:472–476.

60. Donowitz LG: High risk of nosocomial infection in the pediatric critical care patient. *Crit Care Med* 1986; 14:26–28.

61. Maki DG, Ringer M: Evaluation of dressing regimens for prevention of infection with peripheral intravenous catheters. *JAMA* 1987; 258:2396–2403.

62. Bjornson HS, Colley R, Bower RH, et al: Association between microorganism growth at the catheter insertion

site and colonization of the catheter in patients receiving total parenteral nutrition. *Surgery* 1982; 92:4:720–726.

63. Armstrong CW, Mayhall G, Miller KB, et al: Clinical predictions of infection of central venous catheters used for total parenteral nutrition. *Infect Control Hosp Epidemiol* 1990; 11:71–78.

64. Needham C: Specimen collection, in Wentworth B (ed): *Diagnostic Procedure for Bacterial Infection*, ed 7. Washington, DC, American Public Health Association, 1987, pp 3–26.

65. Washington J: Blood cultures: Principles and techniques. *Mayo Clin Proc* 1975; 50:91–98.

66. Curtas S, Tramposch K: Culture methods to evaluate central venous catheter sepsis. *Nutr Clin Pract* 1991; 6:2:43–48.

67. Raucher HS, Hyatt AC, Barzilai A, et al: Quantitative blood cultures in the evaluation of septicemia in children with Broviac catheters. *J Pediatr* 1984; 104:29–33.

68. Mosca R, Curtas S, Forbes B, et al: The benefits of isolator cultures in the management of suspected catheter sepsis. *Surgery* 1987; 102:718–723.

69. Flynn PM, Shenep JL, Stokes DC, et al: In situ management of confirmed central venous catheter–related bacteremia. *Pediatr Infect Dis J* 1987; 6:729–734.

70. Collignon P, Soni N, Pearson I, et al: Sepsis associated with central vein catheters in critically ill patients. *Intensive Care Med* 1988; 14:227.

71. Gil RT, Kruse JA, Thill-Baharozian MC, et al: Triple vs single-lumen central venous catheters: A prospective study in a critically ill population. *Arch Intern Med* 1989; 149:1139.

72. Stillman RM, Soliman F, Garcia L, et al: Etiology of catheter-associated sepsis. *Arch Surg* 1977; 112:1497–1499.

73. Bozzetti F, Scarpa D, Terno G, et al: Subclavian thrombosis due to indwelling catheters: A prospective study on 52 patients. *JPEN* 1983; 7:560–562.

74. Borow M, Crowley JG: Evaluation of central venous catheter thrombogenicity. *Acta Anaesthesiol Scand* 1985; 815:59–64.

75. DiCostanzo J, Sastre B, Choux R, et al: Mechanism of thrombogenesis during total parenteral nutrition: Role of catheter composition. *JPEN* 1988; 12:190–194.

76. Crocker KS, Devereaux GB, Ashmore DL, et al: Clinical evaluation of elastomeric hydrogel peripheral catheters during home infusion therapy, *J Intraven Nurs* 1990; 13:89–97.

77. McKee JM, Shell JA, Warren TA, et al: Complications of intravenous therapy: A randomized prospective study—Vialon vs Teflon. *J Intraven Nurs* 1989; 12:288–295.

78. Kristinsson KG: Adherence of staphylococci to intravascular catheters. *J Med Microbiol* 1989; 28:249–257.

79. Trooskin SZ, Donetz AP, Harvey RA, et al: Prevention of catheter sepsis by antibiotic bonding. *Surgery* 1985; 97:547–551.

80. Kamal GD, Pfaller MA, Rempe LE, et al: Reduced intravascular catheter infection by antibiotic bonding. *JAMA* 1991; 265:2364–2368.

81. Maki DG, Wheeler SJ, Stoltz SM, et al: Clinical trial of a novel antiseptic-coated central venous catheter (ICAAC abstract). Washington, DC, *American Society for Microbiology*, 1991.

82. Maki DG, Cobb L, Garman JK, et al: Attachable silver-impregnated cuff for prevention of infection with central venous catheters: A prospective randomized multicenter trial. *Am J Med* 1988; 85:307–314.

83. Kelly CS, Ligas JR, Smith CA, et al: Sepsis due to triple lumen central venous catheters. *Surg Gynecol Obstet* 1986; 163:14–16.

84. Pemberton LB, Lyman B, Lander V, et al: Sepsis from triple vs single lumen catheters during total parenteral nutrition in surgical or critically ill patients. *Arch Surg* 1986; 121:591–594.

85. McCarthy MC, Shives JK, Robison RJ, et al: Prospective evaluation of single and triple lumen catheters in total parenteral nutrition. *JPEN* 1987; 11:259–262.

86. Lee RB, Buckner M, Sharp KW: Do multi-lumen catheters increase central venous catheter sepsis compared to single-lumen catheters? *J Trauma* 1988; 28:1472–1475.

87. Johnson BH, Rypins EB: Single-lumen vs double-lumen catheters for

total parenteral nutrition. *Arch Surg* 1990; 125:990–992.

88. Horowitz HW, Dworkin BM, Savino JA, et al: Central catheter-related infections: Comparison of pulmonary artery catheters and triple lumen catheters for the delivery of hyperalimentation in a critical care setting. *JPEN* 1990; 14:588–592.

89. Clark-Christoff N, Watters VA, Sparks W, et al: Use of triple-lumen subclavian catheters for administration of total parenteral nutrition. *JPEN* 1992; 16:403–407.

90. Richet H, Hubert B, Nitemberg, G, et al: Prospective multicenter study of vascular-catheter–related complications and risk factors for positive central catheter cultures in intensive care unit patients. *J Clin Microbiol* 1990; 28:2520–2525.

91. Maki DG: Pathogenesis, prevention and management of infections due to intravascular devices used for infusion therapy, in Bisno AL, Waldvogel FA (eds): *Infections Associated With Indwelling Medical Devices.* Washington, DC, American Society for Microbiology, 1986, pp 166–171.

92. Maki DG, McCormack KN: Defatting catheter insertion sites in total parenteral nutrition is of no value as an infection control measure. *Am J Med* 1987; 83:833–840.

93. Larson E: APIC guidelines for infection control practice: Guideline for use of topical antimicrobial agents. *Am J Infect Control* 1988; 16:253–266.

94. Altemeier WA: Surgical antiseptic, in Block SS (ed): *Disinfection, Sterilization and Prevention,* ed 3. Philadelphia, Lea & Febiger, 1983, pp 493–504.

95. Maki DG, Band JD: A comparative study of polyantibiotic and iodophor ointments in prevention of vascular catheter–related infection. *Am J Med* 1981; 70:739–744.

96. Maki DG, Ringer M, Alverado CJ: Prospective randomized trial of povidone-iodine, alcohol, and chlorhexidine for prevention of infection associated with central venous and arterial catheters. *Lancet* 1991; 338:339–343.

97. Jarrard M: Use of transparent polyurethane dressing (Op Site) for cen-

tral venous catheter care. Presented at the 4th Clinical Congress of the American Society for Parenteral and Enteral Nutrition, Chicago, 1980.

98. Palidar PJ, Simonowitz DA, Oreskovich MR, et al: Use of Op Site as an occlusive dressing for total parenteral nutrition catheters. *JPEN* 1982; 6:150–151.

99. Powell C, Regan C, Fabri PJ, et al: Evaluation of Op Site catheter dressing for parenteral nutrition: A prospective randomized study. *JPEN* 1982; 6:43–46.

100. Conly JM, Grieves K, Peters B: A prospective, randomized study comparing transparent and dry gauze dressings for central venous catheters. *J Infect Dis* 1989; 159:310–319.

101. Hoffman KK, Weber DJ, Samsa GP, et al: Transparent polyurethane film as an intravenous catheter dressing. *JAMA* 1992; 267:2072–2076.

102. Craven DE, Lichtenberg DA, Kunches M, et al: A randomized study comparing a transparent polyurethane dressing to a dry gauze dressing for peripheral intravenous catheter sites. *Infect Control* 1985; 6:361–366.

103. Sitges-Serra A, Puig P, Linares J, et al: Hub colonization as the initial step in an outbreak of catheter-related sepsis due to coagulase negative staphylococci during parenteral nutrition. *JPEN* 1984; 8:668–672.

104. Stotter A, Ward H, Waterfield AH: Junctional care: The key to prevention of catheter sepsis in intravenous feeding. *JPEN* 1987; 11:159–162.

105. Goode CJ, Titler M, Rakel B, et al: A meta-analysis of effects of heparin flush and saline flush: Quality and cost implications. *Nurs Res* 1991; 40:324–330.

106. Smith S, Dawson S, Hennessey R, et al: Maintenance of the patency of indwelling central venous catheters: Is heparin necessary? *Am J Pediatr Hematol Oncol* 1991; 13:141–143.

107. Rizzoni WE, Miller K, Rick M, et al: Heparin induced thrombocytopenia and thromboembolism in the postoperative period. *Surgery* 1988; 103:470–476.

108. Heeger PS, Baclestrom JT: Heparin flushes and thrombocytopenia. *Ann Intern Med* 1986; 105:143.

109. Hurtubise MR, Bottino JC, Lawson M, et al: Restoring patency of occluded central venous catheters. *Arch Surg* 1980; 115:212–213.

110. Glynn MFX, Langer B, Jeejeebhoy KN: Therapy for thrombotic occlusion of long-term intravenous alimentation catheters. *JPEN* 1980; 4:387–390.

111. Lawson M, Bottino JC, Hurtubise MR, et al: The use of urokinase to restore patency of occluded central venous catheters. *Am J Intraven Ther Clin Nutr* 1982; 9:29–32.

112. Monturo CA, Dickerson RN, Mullen JL: Efficacy of thrombolytic therapy for occlusion of long-term catheters. *JPEN* 1990; 14:312–314.

113. Atkinson JB, Bagnall HA, Gomperts E: Investigational use of tissue plasminogen activator (t-PA) for occluded central venous catheters. *JPEN* 1990; 14:310–311.

114. Shulman RJ, Reed T, Pitre D, et al: Use of hydrochloric acid to clear obstructed central venous catheters. *JPEN* 1988; 12:509–510.

115. Pennington CR, Pithie AD: Ethanol lock in the management of catheter occlusion. *JPEN* 1987; 11:507–508.

23

Nutritional Support During Peritoneal Dialysis

Robert Wolk, Pharm.D.

Patients with end-stage renal disease (ESRD) are commonly malnourished.[1-4] This is due primarily to uremia as well as the previously prescribed protein-restricted diets.[1-3]

Uremia is known to induce anorexia, nausea, and vomiting and thus result in reduced intake and malnutrition.[1, 2] Uremic metabolic disturbances can lead to carbohydrate and fat intolerance and protein catabolism with loss of lean muscle mass.[1, 3] Uremia-induced hormone imbalances such as reduced insulin and somatomedin concentrations and increased glucagon, parathyroid hormone, and interleukin-1 levels contribute to net catabolism.[2, 3] Uremia represents a catabolic state and is associated with increased nutritional requirements.[3, 4] Uremia and malnutrition together can lead to diminished immune status and increased potential for infection, which may result in further reductions in appetite and malnutrition.[2, 3]

Dietary intervention and dialysis have been used as a means to reduce the signs and symptoms of uremia.[2, 4, 5] In the long term, these interventions have been shown to reduce the morbidity and mortality of ESRD and improve the quality of life.[2, 3, 5]

The type of dialysis selected can also affect the nutritional status of the patient.[1, 3, 5] This review will examine the relationship between nutrition and peritoneal dialysis (PD) and the requirements of nutrition support.

HISTORY AND TYPES OF PERITONEAL DIALYSIS

Peritoneal fluid infusions were first used in humans by Ganter in 1923[6] when he demonstrated the ability to remove metabolites in a uremic patient.[6] In the 1940s, Fine et al. demonstrated the utility of hypertonic dialysis solutions for fluid removal.[7] The first long-term closed systems for intermittent PD were developed and used in dogs by Grollman et al. in 1951.[8]

Developments in the 1960s made possible improved access devices, commercially available solutions, and closed administration systems.[9, 10] These improvements, in conjunction with a reduced incidence of peritonitis, made PD an effective and acceptable form of maintenance therapy for ESRD.[9, 10]

In 1978 Popovich et al.[11] described the so-called equilibrium PD technique or, as it became known, continuous ambulatory peritoneal dialysis (CAPD). This method allowed for continuous toxin removal while allowing the patient greater mobility with reduced equipment load as compared with other PD methods or hemodialysis (HD).[6] The continuous removal of fluid and waste products has made CAPD the most physiologic and popular method of PD.[6, 10, 12-15]

CAPD, one of three common methods of PD,[1] consists of three to five fluid exchanges per day (typically 1 to 3 L per exchange in adults and 1200 mL/m^2 of body surface area or 40 mL/kg of body weight per exchange in children).[1, 3, 5, 6, 12] CAPD is performed 24 hours per day, 7 days per week, and is well tolerated in adult and pediatric populations including infants.[1, 3, 12, 16]

Continuous cycling peritoneal dialysis (CCPD) is similar to CAPD except that fluid exchanges are primarily at night with the use of an automated cycler.[1, 12] CCPD requires nightly hookup and therefore loss of mobility.[12] Three to four exchanges are performed at night with dwell times of 2 to 3 hours each.[1, 6, 12] A smaller volume of fluid dwells the rest of the day when the patient does not use the automated cycler.[1] CCPD is well tolerated in children and adults.[12]

Intermittent peritoneal dialysis (IPD) was the first common method of PD, and its schedule most closely resembles HD which was developed at about the same time.[3, 12] IPD is performed with 2-L exchanges every hour for 12 to 24 hours at a time, two to three times per week. IPD is not as efficient as HD or CAPD for waste clearance and is used primarily in patients in acute situations or in patients with significant residual renal function.[3]

When compared with HD, PD is not as efficient for removal of waste products on a per-hour basis.[12] However, continuous PD has several advantages over HD and IPD. Patients can remain ambulatory and provide their own care. Continuous PD provides constant urea and metabolite removal and improved fluid, acid-base, and electrolyte control and provides glucose as an energy source. Dietary restriction is minimized, so increased dietary intake may occur.[3, 12] PD is also preferred over HD because it is better tolerated in patients with unstable heart disease. It is more suitable in patients with vascular access problems or patients who live a long distance from a dialysis center or hospital.[1] In addition, infants and toddlers tolerate PD well, and access is easier to achieve and maintain.[3, 12]

PERITONEAL ANATOMY AND PHYSIOLOGY

The peritoneal cavity, while typically holding approximately 100 mL of fluid, can expand to hold several liters of fluid at a time.[13] The surface area of the peritoneal membrane is approximately 1 to 1.5 m^2 in children and 2 m^2 in adults, which makes it similar in size to skin.[7, 9, 13] This membrane provides a large surface area for absorption and exchange of fluids, electrolytes, nutrients, and medications.[1, 9, 10] Figure 23–1 shows the location of and access to the peritoneum.

The peritoneum can be divided into three regions: the visceral peritoneum, parietal peritoneum, and the lymphatics.[14] The visceral peritoneum covers the visceral organs, omentum, and mesenteric blood supply.[9, 10] The parietal peritoneum covers the abdominal wall and related blood supply.[9, 10] The relative contributions of the visceral and parietal peritoneum to solute transport are unknown.[9, 13] The lymphatics are located throughout the peritoneum but are primarily situated in the region of the diaphragm.[17]

PD entails fluid and solute exchange between the peritoneal capillary blood supply and the dialysis solution in the peritoneum.[9, 13] The exchange of solutes and fluids occurs by at least four methods. The first and probably the most important is passive diffusion, or osmosis.[8–10] Based on concentration gradients, osmosis plays a significant role in peritoneal exchange of electrolytes, small solutes, and fluids.[7, 8, 18] Three other possible methods of ex-

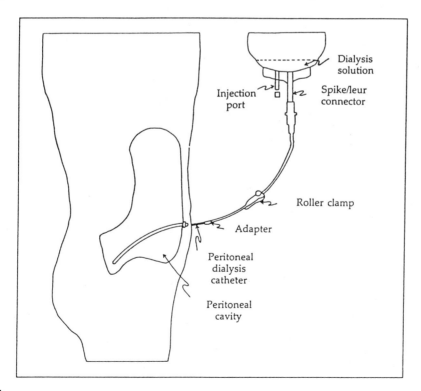

FIG 23–1.
Location and access of the peritoneum. (From Diamond S, Hernrich W: Nutrition and peritoneal dialysis, in Mitch W, Klahr S (eds): *Nutrition and the Kidney.* Boston, Little, Brown, 1988. Used by permission.)

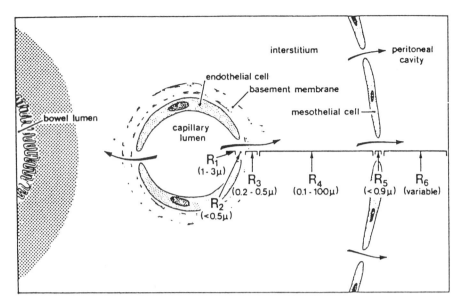

FIG 23-2.
Peritoneal membrane cross section and sites of resistance *(R)*. Exchange pathway: R_1, fluid film of the capillary; R_2, endothelium; R_3, basement membrane; R_4, peritoneal interstitium; R_5, mesothelial layer; R_6, stagnant fluid film of the peritoneal cavity. (From Nolph K, Twardowski Z: The peritoneal dialysis system, in Nolph K (ed): *Peritoneal Dialysis*, ed 3. Boston, Kluwer Academic Publishers, 1989. Used by permission.)

change are transcapillary pressure, vesicles, and intracellular gaps.[9, 13] More studies are needed to establish their relative importance.

Figure 23–2 illustrates the osmotic migration path that a solute must take to get from the capillary to the dialysis fluid or vice versa.[9] The figure identifies regions of resistance and distances, as measured in the rat.[9] There is evidence that the interstitium (R_4) and fluid film or unstirred water layers (R_1, R_6) may be the major points of resistance for the exchange of small solutes.[9] In general, molecules with a molecular weight of 20,000 or less move relatively freely across the membrane.[18] The basement membrane (R_3) is thought to be permeable to most solutes except proteins.[13] Overall, the microvascular wall provides the major resistance to larger molecules.[9]

Absorbed solutes less than 39,000 in molecular weight (e.g., electrolytes and amino acids) enter the peritoneal capillaries and then the portal circulation of the parietal peritoneum or the systemic circulation of the visceral peritoneum before reaching the central venous circulation.[10] Absorption of large molecules greater than 39,000 in molecular weight (e.g., proteins and lipids) is by convection via the peritoneal lymphatics, which are primarily located in the diaphragm.[9, 13] When the diaphragm is relaxed, fluid moves between mesothelial cells into low-pressure spaces. These are emptied during diaphragmatic contraction, which pushes fluid into the lymphatics.[9] From there the fluid moves to the thoracic duct primarily, and finally into the superior vena cava.[10, 17]

BASICS OF PERITONEAL DIALYSIS

The goal of PD is the removal of fluid and metabolic waste from the body. For small molecules, traditional principles of diffusion apply.[10] Limitations to solute osmosis in the peritoneum are based on the resistance points mentioned previously.[9] Water and metabolic products move across the membrane as well, usually in the opposite direction of the PD electrolytes in an attempt to equalize solute concentrations.[10, 13] PD solutions with an osmolarity greater than blood result in increased movement of fluid into the peritoneum to decrease the osmolarity.[4, 6, 7] A net gain or loss of fluid depends on the glucose concentration utilized (osmolarity), the dwell time, and the amount of fluid provided.[9, 8, 13, 18] A 4.25% glucose dialysis solution provides more dialysis capability in terms of glucose exchange and fluid removal than does a 1.5% solution because of these osmolarity differences.[6, 7] Many other factors may have an influence on the rate of diffusion, water loss, and solute absorption.[1, 9, 13] Warm solutions are absorbed from the peritoneum more quickly than cold ones.[10] Vasodilators such as nitroglycerin, isoproterenol, prostaglandin E_2 (PGE$_2$), and other compounds may also increase the absorption of diffusible compounds from the peritoneum by increasing permeability, although the actual amount of increased absorption has not been quantified.[1, 10, 13] Mechanical pressure caused by filling the peritoneal cavity or by abdominal binders also increases absorption.[10]

The final osmolarity is an important factor in tolerance to peritoneal dialysis solutions.[9-11] The higher the osmolarity, the greater the fluid removal, but this introduces a greater risk of peritonitis.[10, 13, 19-21] Peritonitis may result from a reduction in phagocytosis and bacterial killing.[21] Peritonitis can, in the long term, cause sclerosis of the peritoneal membrane, which results in a reduction in exchange capability and dialysis efficiency.[10, 21] PD solutions are therefore typically limited to osmolarities of 500 mOsm or less to avoid these inflammatory complications. Glucose, the primary osmotic agent currently used, provides 5 mOsm/g. Other carbohydrates have been tried (e.g., xylitol and sorbitol) but are not as effective.[20, 22, 23] The dialysate solution, because of its low pH and glucose content and osmolarity, has been implicated as a cause of increased levels of cytokines, reduced viability of leukocytes, and changes in the intercellular gaps and microvilli of the peritoneal layer, all of which may further reduce dialysis efficiency.[21]

EFFECTS OF PERITONEAL DIALYSIS ON NUTRITION

The following sections look specifically at PD and nutrient exchange.

Dextrose

The main solute used for PD is glucose, and it is available in a variety of concentrations (Table 23–1).[24] Glucose absorption from the peritoneal cavity can be extensive and can be estimated by using numerous methods[13, 17, 25-27] (Fig 23–3 and Table 23–2). High glucose concentrations, large dialysate volumes, long dwell times, and peritonitis all increase the amount of glucose ab-

TABLE 23–I.

Typical Peritoneal Dialysis Solutions*†

Component	Dianeal, 1.5% Dextrose (Travenol)	Impersol, 2.5% Dextrose (Abbott)	Dianeal 4.25% Dextrose (Travenol)
Dextrose (g/L)	15	25	42.5
Sodium (mEq/L)	141	132	141
Calcium (mEq/L)	3.5	3.5	3.5
Magnesium (mEq/L)	1.5	1.5	1.5
Chloride (mEq/L)	101	102	101
Lactate (mEq/L)	45	35	45
Osmolarity (mOsm/L)	364	398	503

*Data from Kastrup E (ed): *Facts and Comparisons.* Philadelphia, JB Lippincott, 1992, p 702.
†Typically available in 1- or 2-L sizes.

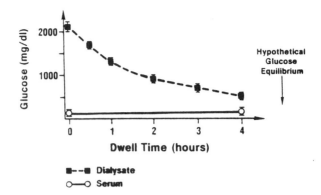

FIG 23–3.

Intraperitoneal glucose concentrations (mean ± SEM) during 4-hour exchanges in 18 CAPD patients. Twenty-two samples of a 2.5% dextrose dialysis solution were used. The percentage of glucose absorbed is based on identifying the dwell time and comparing the glucose level remaining with the starting glucose concentration. The glucose lost represents glucose absorbed. (From Mactier R, Khanna R: Peritoneal cavity lymphatics, in Nolph K (ed): *Peritoneal Dialysis*, ed 3. Boston, Kluwer Academic Publishers, 1989. Used by permission.)

sorbed.[8, 9, 13, 18] Wideroe et al.[26] looked at six patients on CAPD and found increased glucose absorption over time that ranged from 29% at 1-hour dwell times to 86% at 8-hour dwell times. They also found similar glucose absorption in diabetic patients. Insulin-dependent patients required less insulin when it was administered intraperitonealy vs. subcutaneously because of more efficient insulin absorption. Grodstein et al.[27] developed a useful formula to calculate glucose absorption that was based on four patients undergoing long-term CAPD. Mactier and Khanna[17] evaluated dialysate glucose loss (absorption) over time in 18 CAPD patients. Their findings were similar to those of Wideroe et al., with a reduction in dialysate glucose content of 50% in 2 hours and approximately 75% in 4 hours. Glucose absorption when using 2 L of a 4.25% glucose PD solution with a typical 6-hour dwell time (four exchanges per day) is approximately 60% to 80%. This quantity of glucose provides up to 270 g/day, or 900 kcal/day. Glucose absorption may represent 10% to 30% of the daily calorie intake of patients.[28, 29]

Lipids

Hyperlipidemia was first described in IPD and later CAPD.[28] It appears to be

TABLE 23–2.

Glucose Absorption Estimate

3. Dwell time data*

Dwell Time (hr)	Glucose Absorbed From Dialysate (%)
1	29 ± 4
4	74 ± 4
8	86 ± 3

Glucose concentrations and volumes are needed to determine dialysate glucose administered.

2. Glucose absorption formula†

Absorbed dextrose (g/L) = 11.3 Average dialysate dextrose (g/dL) − 10.9

Average dialysate dextrose is based on the average dextrose concentration used per day, converted to grams per deciliter

Total *absorbed dextrose* is the total number of liters per day times the absorbed dextrose.

*Data from Wideroe T-E, Smebly L, Berg K, et al: *Kidney Int* 1983; 23:22–28.
†Data from Grodstein G, Blumenkrantz M, Kopple J, et al: *Kidney Int* 1981; 19:564–567.

closely related to the hyperlipidemia of uremia but is different from HD dyslipidemias.[28]

Increased triglyceride levels develop in 50% to 70% of PD patients, while 30% have increased cholesterol levels at some time during therapy.[15, 28] The increased triglyceride and possibly cholesterol levels are believed to be due to increased glucose intake, particularly peritoneally. Hyperlipidemia results from increased triglyceride hepatic synthesis and reduced clearance, especially from lipoprotein lipase activity.[15, 25, 28] Stable hyperlipidemia develops in most patients, and levels may return to normal or close to normal over time.[15]

Protein Losses

Protein losses during PD typically range from 5 to 20 g/day.[1, 14, 25, 29] Albumin losses represent approximately 50% to 60% of the protein lost.[1, 3, 14, 23, 25, 30] IgG represents 15% to 20% of the protein lost. Many other proteins are also lost.[1, 25] Protein losses in pediatric patients can be up to 10% of their dietary intake, while it might be 20% in some elderly adults.[5, 29] Even with these losses, serum protein levels tend to remain normal or slightly below normal, usually because of increased synthesis. Protein losses increase with greater frequency of exchanges, peritonitis, and the use of various medications (especially vasodilators).[1, 3, 13] Peritonitis can increase protein losses 50% to 100%.[3, 10, 14, 25, 31]

Amino Acid Losses

Amino acid losses can also be significant, 1.7 to 3.4 g/day.[1, 3, 25, 29, 32] These amino acid losses correlate with serum levels, which suggests that diffusion is the principal method of loss.[1, 3, 29, 30, 32] The resulting plasma amino acid levels are similar to those in nondialyzed uremic patients and probably reflect metabolic and nutritional derangements.[3, 29] One study found relatively normal amino acid levels, although valine, leucine, and serine concentrations were low.[3, 32]

Electrolytes and Minerals

Electrolytes can readily cross the peritoneal membrane and are typically lost during PD.[9, 10] They are therefore included in PD solutions to reduce the osmotic gradient and ultimately to maintain normal serum levels (see Table 23–1). Potassium and phosphorus are not standard additives in any PD solution because of the elevated levels in uremic patients. PD losses of electrolytes have been reported to reach 300 mg/day for phosphorus and 31 mg/day for magnesium.[1, 11] Calcium losses vary with the ionized state, with ionized or free calcium lost most rapidly.[1, 30] The glucose concentration also appears to affect calcium clearance.[30] Along with dialysis losses, electrolyte levels can also be affected by dietary intake.[1]

Vitamins

Vitamins, especially water-soluble vitamins, can be lost in PD.[3, 30, 33] Several studies have reported low water-soluble vitamin levels in patients receiving PD, especially thiamine, pyridoxine, ascorbic acid, and folic acid.[3, 30, 33] Low levels are due in part to losses in the dialysate. It has been reported that dialysis fluid contains vitamin C levels of approximately 60% of that found in serum, thus producing a significant daily loss.[33]

Some vitamin levels such as pyridoxine and vitamin A are abnormal due in part to the underlying uremia.[34, 35] Ross et al., in a study of 11 long-term dialysis patients, found that low serum pyridoxine concentrations (as pyridoxal-5-phosphate) resulted from impaired oxidation and phosphorylation of precursors as well as enhanced hydrolysis by alkaline phosphatase. The actual dialysate losses were small.[34] Continuous

PD, however, may result in significant losses over time.

Vitamin A levels tend to increase in uremia along with retinol binding protein.[34, 35] Vitamin A toxicity in uremic patients receiving the recommended dietary allowance (RDA) for vitamin A may result from increased serum vitamin A levels and reduced retinol binding protein concentrations and result in increased free vitamin A.[35]

Several studies in patients receiving PD reported that levels of fat-soluble vitamins, especially vitamins A and E, are usually normal or slightly elevated.[3, 30, 33] Only 2% of vitamin A and E serum levels appear in the dialysate, probably because of protein binding.[33] Vitamin D losses have also been reported in PD patients.[3, 5, 16, 30]

Trace Elements

Trace element abnormalities occur in patients receiving PD and are due to several factors, including reduced intake, reduced renal clearance, dialysis input, and/or dialysis clearance.[3, 30, 36, 37] Because trace elements are protein bound, low trace element levels are believed to result from inadequate intake as well as dialysis losses.

Other factors may be involved. As an example, plasma and muscle zinc levels are reduced in uremia and during PD, but the total-body zinc level is increased.[36] These data suggest that zinc may be translocated to other organs or there is an increased need for zinc to obtain the same functional levels.[36] Low red blood cell levels for zinc and copper suggest tissue depletion and the potential need for additional supplementation.[1, 3, 30] Thomson et al.[38] investigated 31 patients receiving CAPD. A marked reduction in red cell zinc and copper levels was noted, while chromium levels were increased. The clinical significance of these findings could not be established. Additionally, dialysis solutions contain more than 40 different trace elements, with a few exceeding the

levels of dietary requirements.[39] The zinc and iron content provides 2.7 and 1.9 mg/wk respectively if fully absorbed. Aluminum is also found in small amounts in PD solutions. Little is known about other trace elements, including concerns of net accumulation and removal by dialysis.[40] More studies are required.

Carnitine

Carnitine deficiency has been reported to occur in patients undergoing dialysis, including CAPD.[41] The deficiency in carnitine has been attributed to losses in the dialysate, deficient precursors (methionine and lysine), and impaired carnitine biosynthesis.[3, 41]

NUTRITION STATUS OF PATIENTS WITH END-STAGE RENAL DISEASE

PD relieves some of the complications of uremia. However, dialysis fluids can lead to other potential problems. Reduced appetite and intake may result from abdominal filling and "bloating" and continuous glucose uptake.[11, 19] The high glucose load contributes to hyperglycemia, hypertriglyceridemia, and obesity in some PD patients.[1, 3, 10, 15, 29] Nutritional status is further compromised by protein, amino acid, vitamin, and possibly trace element losses from PD.[11, 19, 20] Nutritional needs tend to be increased in patients with ESRD who are receiving PD.[3, 4] Appropriate and adequate nutrition is important to reduce these complications, improve patient tolerance to PD, and maximize the outcome.

NUTRITIONAL REQUIREMENTS FOR ADULTS

Nutritional requirements for adults undergoing PD have been developed (Table 23–3).[1, 3, 25, 30, 42, 43] These require-

TABLE 23–3.

Recommended Nutritional Intake in Adult Patients Undergoing Peritoneal Dialysis*

Intake	Amount
Energy	35–42 kcal/kg or 1.3–1.7 times the Harris-Benedict basal metabolic rate
Protein	1.2 g/kg/day
Fluid	As tolerated by fluid balance/sodium levels
Sodium chloride	As tolerated by fluid balance/sodium levels
Potassium	60–80 mEq/day
Magnesium	200–300 mg/day
Calcium	1–1.4 g/day
Phosphate	800–1200 mg/day
Supplemental vitamins	
Ascorbic acid	100 mg/day
Pyridoxine	10 mg/day
Folic acid	1 mg/day
Vitamins A, E, K	None
Trace elements	Standard doses

*Because of variable absorption, especially for electrolytes and trace elements, lower doses may be needed intravenously.

ments represent general guidelines; there may be increased needs with malnutrition and acute illness or decreased needs secondary to obesity.[11] In addition, PD calories reduce the calories that need to be consumed.[29]

Energy

Energy requirements range from 35 to 42 kcal/kg/day, or an estimated 1.3 to 1.7 times the Harris-Benedict resting metabolic expenditure.[11, 14, 25, 42] Glucose calories from the dialysate can be as high as 20% to 30% of the calorie needs[28, 29] and may rise an additional 50% during episodes of peritonitis.[44] The PD-derived calories should be subtracted from the calculated caloric needs.[29] Dietary histories indicate that dialysis patients consume only 23 to 27 kcal/kg/day, far below the recommended amount.[3] This reduced intake does not appear to be adaptive because uremic energy expenditures are not decreased.[45] Calorie intake should be adequate to meet needs, with 35% provided as complex polysaccharide.[1, 2, 25, 30]

Ten percent to 15% of patients receiving PD actually become obese as a result of peritoneal carbohydrate absorption, and glucose control problems can occur.[1] Dietary counseling may be necessary for compliance to a low-carbohydrate diet.[1]

The remainder of nonprotein calories should be provided as fat.[1, 3] A ratio of polyunsaturated to saturated fatty acids of 1.5 to 1.0 has been recommended to reduce high triglyceride levels.[1, 3, 30] Uremic patients may have defective removal of triglycerides, and therefore fat intake must be appropriately monitored.[1, 28] An adequate energy intake must be provided to maintain a neutral or positive nitrogen balance during CAPD.

Protein

The recommended protein intake for adults receiving PD is 1.2 g/kg/day. The goal is to maintain a positive nitrogen balance.[1, 3, 15, 30, 43, 45] In one study of eight patients undergoing CAPD, as daily protein intake rose above 1.1 g/kg, no significant additional benefit on nitrogen balance was seen.[30] Figure 23–4 illustrates this plateauing of protein needs.[30] Blumenkrantz et al.[40] found similar results when nitrogen balance studies were obtained on eight patients receiving IPD and CAPD for 20 days.

Giordano et al.[46] reported that 1.2 g/kg/day of protein plus adequate calories was capable of maintaining a positive nitrogen balance in seven of eight patients. Another study of CAPD patients found positive nitrogen balance in patients consuming 0.8 to 2.1 g/kg/day of protein.[37] Protein intake correlated with weight gain.[3, 37]

Overconsumption of protein, especially the amino acids methionine and lysine, can lead to elevated blood urea nitrogen (BUN) levels, acidosis, and hyperphosphatemia.[3, 47] A protein intake exceeding 1.8 g/kg/day may require additional phosphate binders and sodium bicarbonate.[3] Protein restriction is usu-

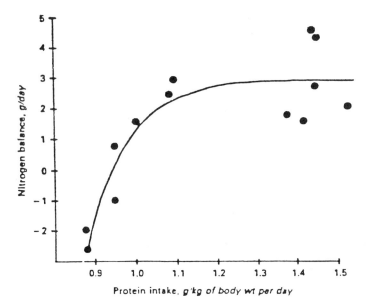

FIG 23–4.

Relation between dietary protein intake and nitrogen balance. Each *circle* represents the mean data obtained during 14 to 33 days of balance studies. The *curved line* repre-sents the calculated relationship between protein intake and nitrogen balance. (From Kopple JD, Blumenkrantz MJ: *Kidney Int* 1983; 24(suppl):295–302. Used by permission.)

ally not an issue with BUN levels below 100 mg/dL in adults.[48]

Peritonitis may further increase protein needs.[9, 29] In one study[44] peritonitis increased protein needs from 1.1 to 1.35 g/kg/day to maintain a positive nitrogen balance. This is due to increased dialysate losses.[44] Patients with peritonitis may require up to 1.6 g/kg/day because of increased protein losses.[1, 3, 9]

It is recommended that PD patients receive 1.2 g/kg/day of protein. Protein intake should be adjusted to achieve tolerance and a positive nitrogen balance. This increased requirement of protein in CAPD patients as compared with nondialyzed patients results from increased protein losses to 0.05 to 0.3 g/kg/day.[3] Adequate calories are needed since nitrogen balance has been found to be positively correlated with protein intake and total energy intake.[1, 3, 30]

Fifty percent of the oral/enteral protein should be of high biological value to provide adequate essential amino acids.[1, 2, 14, 25, 30] Enteral products with high protein and low electrolyte concentrations such as Nepho and Osmolyte

are recommended. Patients receiving total parenteral nutrition (TPN) should receive mixed amino acid solutions because of dialysate losses of proteins, peptides, and amino acids.[42, 48]

Fluid and Electrolytes

Generally speaking, the fluid and mineral status is directly affected by diet intake.[30] Therefore, attention must be paid to dietary intake or parenteral nutrition additives, as well as to the contents of the dialysate.

Sodium and water can be removed easily with CAPD, and most patients can be allowed a fairly liberal intake.[30] Some patients may tolerate 4 to 8 g/day (170 to 350 mEq/day) of sodium and 1500 to 3000 mL/day of water.[3, 30] Therefore, fluid and sodium chloride should be provided as necessary based on the patient's fluid status and serum sodium levels. More concentrated PD dextrose solutions may be needed to remove excess volume during fluid overload.[1]

Acidosis may result from the accumulation of phosphate, sulfate, and organic acids and from bicarbonate loss during dialysis.[3] The major source of these acids is dietary protein.[3] Acidosis is reported to be better controlled by CAPD than other methods of dialysis.[3, 49] Control is achieved by exchanging sodium chloride salts for sodium bicarbonate or bicarbonate precursors such as acetate, lactate, or citrate.[3]

Potassium needs remain similar to standard RDA needs.[1] In one study, a potassium intake of 67 mEq/day produced a positive potassium balance.[43] Dialysate losses account for 70% of the daily potassium losses.[3, 43] The dietary allowance is 70 to 80 mEq/day.[1]

Peritoneal losses of minerals have been discussed. CAPD provides for a more consistent balance of calcium and phosphate than IPD or HD does.[50] Additionally, PD removes parathyroid hormone, corrects acidoses better, and results in less bone disease.[50]

The minimum requirement of phosphorus is usually met by an adequate diet. Hypophosphatemia may indicate insufficient intake of energy and protein. Substantial amounts of phosphorus are also removed by CAPD.[50] Higher protein diets result in increased phosphorus intake and a more positive balance.[3, 43] Hyperphosphatemia may be due to excessive intake and may require diet adjustments with protein restriction and/or phosphate binders.[3, 50] Standard phosphorus recommendations are 800 to 1200 mg/day orally.[1]

Many uremic patients are hypocalcemic because of calcitriol deficiency, hyperphosphatemia, and reduced intestinal absorption.[50] Dialysate calcium usually corrects hypocalcemia.[50] Calcium needs remain similar to standard RDA needs,[1] although calcium balance is improved with a high protein diet.[3, 43] Calcium balance has been reported to be neutral or positive with a dietary intake of 720 mg/day or greater.[43] Calcium loss in dialysis solutions is affected negatively by the amount of serum ionized calcium available and by fluid and high dialysate glucose concentrations.[30] Oral calcium supplements, while less a necessity than in nondialyzed uremic patients, may benefit the patient by reducing intestinal phosphate absorption and correcting mild acidosis.[3]

Dietary magnesium intake and balance are greater with high-protein diets. Patients using dialysis fluids containing 1.5 mEq/L of magnesium have only minimal losses.[3, 43] Low concentrations of dialysate magnesium usually keep the magnesium levels stable.[50]

Intravenous electrolyte supplementation should be provided during TPN and adjusted according to serum levels. Reductions in potassium, phosphate, and magnesium may be required, while calcium needs may be increased. Additionally, because of variable absorption, the electrolyte requirements listed in Table 23–3 may need to be reduced for intravenous administration.

Vitamins

Specific dietary requirements for vitamins in patients receiving PD have not been established.[1] Inadequate dietary intake, altered metabolism in uremia, and vitamin loss in the dialysate may lead to vitamin deficiency.[3, 33] Several authors recommend additional supplementation with water-soluble vitamins.[1, 3, 33, 34, 51, 52]

In one of the most complete[33] vitamin studies, Blumberg and coworkers evaluated vitamin status in ten stable CAPD patients by measuring blood vitamin levels and evaluating diet histories. Even with an adequate intake of calories and protein, they discovered low blood levels of vitamins B_1, B_6, C, and folate. The low levels were felt to be due to losses in the dialysate and inadequate dietary intake. Vitamin A and E levels were frequently elevated. Seven weeks of oral supplementation normalized vitamin C, folate, and vitamin B_6 levels, while the vitamin B_1 concentration remained low.

Shah et al. raised concerns about the level of vitamin C supplementation and oxalate stone formation in renal patients.[53] In a study of seven adults undergoing CAPD, it was shown that vitamin C supplementation produced a moderate increase in serum oxalate levels.[53] Vitamin B_6, which has been associated with oxalate production in deficiency states, did not reduce oxalate levels when provided as a supplement of 10 mg/day. The authors cautioned against vitamin C supplements greater than 100 mg/day until more data are available. In addition, neuropathy has occurred with large doses of pyridoxine.[53]

Boeschoten et al.[51] evaluated the vitamin status of 31 patients who received CAPD for 0.5 to 36 months. In 24 dialysate collections, only vitamin C and folic acid levels exceeded urine losses in healthy patients. The deficiency of vitamin B_6 could not be explained. The authors concluded that patients should receive supplemental vitamin B_6, C, and folic acid. Several authors suggest that PD patients be supplemented with a water-soluble vitamin preparation or pyridoxine, 10 mg/day, folic acid, 0.5 mg/day, and vitamin C, 100 mg/day.[1, 3, 33, 34, 51] Thiamine supplementation remains controversial. Suggested doses vary widely from 0 to 40 mg/day.[1, 3, 33] Polyvitamin preparations containing vitamin A should be avoided because of concerns with vitamin A toxicity.[3] No supplemental vitamin K or E is recommended. Acutely ill patients fed by TPN should receive standard multivitamin infusion products, with supplements as above. In long-term situations, patients should receive standard vitamins and supplements but be followed closely for vitamin A toxicity. An alternative is to provide only water-soluble vitamin preparations.

Trace Elements

Specific trace element dietary requirements for patients receiving PD do not exist.[1] Trace elements are lost during dialysis,[3] but no agreement on supplementation beyond the RDA for oral or Food and Drug Administration/American Medical Association (FDA/AMA) guidelines for intravenous administration has been established.[1, 3] Fournier et al.[54] studied dialysis patients and found negative immune skin reactions along with low serum zinc levels. The authors postulated that reduced immune function was related to reduced serum zinc levels.[54] Additional research is needed to determine trace element metabolism and requirements during PD.

The single most important trace element abnormality associated with ESRD is aluminum accumulation. Restriction of aluminum-containing products is important to prevent osteodystrophy.[3, 16] Oral and intravenous products, including PD fluids, should be evaluated for their potential aluminum content.

Carnitine

Carnitine loss occurs during PD, but no supplemental dose has been established. Patients with poor oral intake may be at risk and require oral or dialysate fluid supplementation.[3] Elevated triglyceride levels may be related to carnitine deficiency and should be monitored. Carnitine supplementation has reduced elevated triglyceride levels in rats[41] and humans[55] with ESRD. Carnitine supplementation may be necessary in deficient patients.[55]

NUTRITIONAL REQUIREMENTS IN PEDIATRICS

Children with ERSD show reduced growth. There is a reduction in growth velocity, weight gain, and linear growth.[1, 5, 12, 14, 37, 56] One goal of PD is to allow these children increased intake so that they can be adequately nourished and thus obtain growth and stature increases.[4, 5, 12, 14, 16, 37] Appropriate and sufficient nutrition must be provided with PD to optimize their growth and development.[16, 37]

PD has become an effective method for managing ESRD in infants and children.[14, 16] PD is preferred over HD because it does not induce rapid volume swings and allows for better control of electrolytes and pH and for removal of waste products.[16] PD has been used both acutely and chronically in pediatric patients. Nutrient requirements in pediatric patients are usually prescribed according to body weight and age.[23] The RDAs are used as a starting point, although modifications will be needed for PD.[4, 16, 37, 57] CAPD is the dialysis of choice in children under 2 years of age.[1, 5, 12, 14, 16] Pediatric requirements are outlined in Table 23–4.[5, 12, 14, 16, 37, 57, 58]

Energy

Energy requirements in uremic children have not been defined[12] but should meet the RDAs and be adjusted for age.[16, 57] Energy requirements in infants start at 100 to 140 kcal/kg/day but may be higher depending on the severity of illness.[4, 14, 16] Calorie needs decrease with age. Adolescent males and females require 48 and 60 kcal/kg/day respectively.[13, 23] Intravenous calorie needs are similar.[58]

Peritoneal glucose absorption should be calculated and subtracted from the total calories provided. Additional calories may be needed for growth and weight gain.[12] Formulas for infants may require supplements of carbohydrates or lipids (e.g., medium-chain triglyceride [MCT] oil) to provide adequate calories and maintain stable electrolyte levels.[14, 16]

Protein

The specific protein requirements for uremic pediatric patients are not known.[12] Protein needs generally reflect the RDAs.[14, 16] Several authors suggest 2.2 g/kg/day for infants,[4, 14] while others suggest a range adjusted for age, weight, and PD losses: 3 g/kg/day for infants, 2.5 g/kg/day for 3 years to puberty, 2 g/kg/day for pubescent children, and 1.5 g/kg/day for children past puberty.[5, 12, 16] Protein intakes of 5 to 6 g/kg/day may be needed in infants to maintain growth.[14, 16] Protein intake may need to be reduced and energy intake assessed when BUN concentrations rise to 80 to 100 mg/dL.[12, 14] Salusky et al. studied 12 patients less than 10 years old and 12 patients older than 10 years of age.[5] The results showed that protein intake and losses in the dialysate were higher for the younger patients and were related to their proportionally larger peritoneal surface area.[5]

Protein losses from dialysis represent 7% to 10% of normal protein intake.[12, 48] Oral protein should contain 50% high-quality protein (high in essential amino acids).[12, 39] Standard mixed amino acid formulations should be used in patients receiving TPN[42, 48] to provide for losses of essential and nonessential amino acids.

Fluid and Electrolytes

The requirements for fluid and sodium are variable in children undergoing dialysis,[5, 12] and each child should

TABLE 23–4.

Recommended Nutritional Intakes in Pediatric Patients Undergoing Peritoneal Dialysis

Intake	Amount
Energy	
Infants	Minimum of RDA for stature and age (100–140 kcal/kg)
Children/adolescents	Minimum of RDA for height and age
Protein	
<5 yr	3 g/kg/day
5–10 yr	2.5 g/kg/day
10–12 yr	2 g/kg/day
≥12 yr	1.5 g/kg/day
Electrolytes	Meet RDA needs
Vitamins to meet RDA plus vitamin supplements	
Ascorbic acid	75–100 mg/day
Pyridoxine	5–10 mg/day
Folic acid	0.5–1 mg/day
Calcitriol (vitamin D)	As needed to keep calcium in the high normal range
Trace elements	Meet RDA needs

be managed individually.[5, 12] Generally, unrestricted sodium, potassium, calcium, magnesium, and fluid intake is used initially.[5, 12, 16] This is due to potential dialysate losses as well as low dietary intake.[5, 12, 14, 16] Neonates, in particular, are prone to hyponatremia and may require additional supplements.[12]

Renal osteodystrophy with its elevated phosphorus and alkaline phosphatase and reduced calcium levels may require electrolyte adjustment.[16] Typically, additional calcium may be needed along with phosphate binders to prevent osteodystrophy.[14, 16, 59, 60] Formulas similar to breast milk with low electrolyte levels and high calcium-phosphate ratios appear best. Similac PM 60:40, Wyeth S29, and Enfamil are such formulas.[4, 14, 16] Long-term phosphate binders include calcium carbonate or citrate.[12, 16] Aluminum-containing phosphate binders, because of their potential toxicity, should be limited to acute hyperphosphatemia.[16, 37]

In general, the RDA for electrolytes and minerals should be provided. Standard intravenous supplements are administered with TPN. Serum levels should be measured and electrolyte and mineral intake adjusted accordingly.

Vitamins

Daily vitamin requirements have not been established for children undergoing peritoneal dialysis.[12] Vitamin D is lost during dialysis and should be replaced to prevent renal osteodystrophy.[3, 5, 12, 16, 30] Supplements of folic acid (1 mg/day), vitamin B_6 (5 to 10 mg/day), and vitamin C (75 to 100 mg/day) are recommended by some authors in order to replace losses (based on data in the adult literature).[12, 33] RDA amounts for the other water-soluble vitamins are appropriate. No supplements are recommended for vitamins A, E, or K.[12, 14, 16] Warady and Kriley[52] demonstrated similar serum vitamin levels in eight dialysis and six control pediatric patients. They concluded that a standard water-soluble vitamin supplement and adequate dietary intake should prevent vitamin deficiency.[52]

Trace Elements

Trace element requirements have not been established for uremic pediatric patients,[12, 16] so standard trace element doses are recommended because of the lack of data.[4, 12, 14, 16] Aluminum, because of potential osteodystrophy and growth retardation, should be avoided.[16, 59, 60]

Carnitine

Murakami et al. identified serum carnitine deficiency after 4 months of CAPD.[55] Elevated triglyceride levels and reduced carnitine levels vs. controls developed in all 17 patients who ranged in age from 2 to 15 years.[55] It appeared that carnitine deficiency in children can be produced by inadequate intake (enteral or TPN) and accelerated by PD losses. Carnitine supplementation may be required.[55, 61]

In summary, adequate protein, calories, minerals, and vitamins should be administered to obtain a positive nitrogen balance.[3, 12, 14, 16, 30] A malnourished patient may require additional nutrients.[30] Even in stable healthy patients, a change in dialysate composition or regimen may change needs.[30] It is important to optimize nutritional intake to improve tolerance to PD and provide for adequate growth and development.[16] Finally, excess nutrients may be detrimental to the patient. Therefore, monitoring is very important.[3, 12, 14, 30]

Nutrition Assessment

Patients with ESRD typically report weight loss, and nutritional assessment reveals reductions in skin fold thickness (loss of fat), midarm muscle circumference (loss of lean muscle loss), and visceral proteins (reduced total protein, albumin).[3] Once on dialysis, the patient may feel improved with reduced uremic symptoms and a liberalized diet.[3] Regular assessment, however, is very important to ensure good nutritional status.[30]

One of the most important parameters is weight; dry weight and weight changes must be followed closely. In addition, physical examination and a dietary history are very important to assess nutritional status.[1, 2] Laboratory tests should be obtained frequently during acute illness or unstable periods and less often when the patient is stable. Short-term indicators such as prealbumin and transferrin may be useful to assess visceral protein status along with nitrogen balance if the patient is at a steady state. During long-term therapy anthropometric measurements by a skilled dietitian together with determinations of nitrogen balance are very useful.[29] Patients at increased risk for complications or intolerance such as elderly patients, those with poor appetites, and diabetics should be monitored closely.[29]

In addition to standard assessments, it is important in pediatrics to obtain height, weight, and head circumference to assess growth and development.[4, 14, 16] Most infants in renal failure fall below the 5th percentile for age. However, with appropriate nutrition they can achieve acceptable growth patterns.[14]

Assessing the nitrogen status in patients receiving PD is difficult. Typical indicators do not appear to apply.[62] Albumin, one of the most common indicators of nutritional status, is not by itself a good predictor of outcome in PD patients.[62] Albumin levels are affected by age, sex, other disease states, and diet intake, as well as the type of dialysis, the length of time on dialysis, and other dialysis factors.[62] Winchester, in his review of albumin,[62] reports that CAPD patients have a twofold higher risk of mortality when albumin levels fall below 2.5 g/dL. Fine and Cox[63] studied 19 adult patients receiving CAPD for 15 months. They found that all had a modest reduction in albumin to levels of 2.5 to 3.3 g/dL. This persisted to the end of the study. Protein catabolic rates and urea nitrogen accumulation (UNA) were stable, thus indicating adequate nutrition. The authors felt that slight decreases in albumin were common in CAPD patients and, if stable, did not indicate a poor prognosis.

Standard nitrogen balance assessments are not accurate because of abnormal nitrogen excretion.[48] Nitrogen balance should include calculations for urea nitrogen appearance,[48, 58, 64] although with stable CAPD it may be negligible. Recommendations for nutritional assessment are reviewed in several references[56, 65] and elsewhere in this book. Assessment and monitoring are the keys to achieving nutritional goals and minimizing complications.[14, 16]

Intraperitoneal Parenteral Nutrition

Intraperitoneal nutrition as a means of nutritional support has received a lot of interest since the 1970s. Using amino acids as the primary osmotic agent is believed to be advantageous by providing additional protein supplementation and reducing carbohydrate intake in CAPD while providing an equivalent osmotic force.[10, 20, 66]

Human studies have shown amino acid solutions to be safe and tolerated, but they have been too brief in time or too few in patient numbers to demonstrate significant nutritional benefit.[29, 65–69] Animal studies have shown tolerance and absorption of all nutrients and some nutritional benefits.[70–72] More studies in humans are needed, especially in severely malnourished patients undergoing CAPD, in order to determine the most appropriate solutions for the best nutritional benefit.[6, 58] Two reviews are available.[10, 73]

CONCLUSION

Malnutrition is a problem in patients with ESRD. Improved nutrition and dialysis can improve outcome while reducing the mortality and morbidity of these patients. PD-induced protein losses and glucose absorption also affect the nutritional status of patients. Nutritional requirements should reflect these factors. While calorie and protein requirements are known, more work is needed to detail the electrolyte, vitamin, and trace element requirements. The interaction of PD with the patient's nutritional needs and nutritional status is a dynamic relationship that requires ongoing monitoring.

REFERENCES

1. Diamond S, Henrich W: Nutrition and peritoneal dialysis, in Mitch W, Klahr S (eds): *Nutrition and the Kidney.* Boston, Little, Brown, 1988, pp 198–223.
2. Kratka R, Shuler C, Wolfson M: Nutrition in hemodialysis and peritoneal dialysis patients, in Nissenson AR, Fine RN, Gentile DE (eds): *Clinical Dialysis,* ed 2. Norwalk, Conn, Appleton & Lange, 1990, pp 350–365.
3. Lindholm B, Bergstrom J: Nutritional management of patients undergoing peritoneal dialysis, in Nolph K (ed): *Peritoneal Dialysis,* ed 3. Boston, Kluwer Academic Publishers, 1989, pp 230–260.
4. Wassner SJ, Abitbol C, Alexander S, et al: Nutritional requirements for infants with renal failure. *Am J Kidney Dis* 1986; 7:300–305.
5. Salusky IB, Fine RN, Nelson P, et al: Nutritional status of children undergoing continuous peritoneal dialysis. *Am J Clin Nutr* 1983; 38:599–611.
6. Boen S: History of peritoneal dialysis, in Nolph K, (ed): *Peritoneal Dialysis,* ed 3. Boston, Kluwer Academic Publishers, 1989, pp 1–12.
7. Fine J, Frank H, Seligman A: The treatment of ARF by peritoneal irrigation. *Ann Surg* 1946; 124:857–875.
8. Grollman A, Turner L, McLean J: Intermittent peritoneal lavage in nephrectomized dogs and its application to the human being. *Arch Intern Med* 1951; 87:379–390.
9. Nolph K, Twardowski Z: The peritoneal dialysis system, in Nolph K (ed): *Peritoneal Dialysis,* ed 3. Boston, Kluwer Academic Publishers, 1989, pp 13–27.
10. Sell L, Salley S, Whittlesey G, et al: Peritoneal nutrition—an emerging concept with clinical relevance. *Nutrition* 1987; 3:297–303.
11. Popovich R, Moncrief J, Nolph K, et al: Continuous ambulatory peritoneal dialysis. *Ann Intern Med* 1978; 88:449–456.
12. Salusky IB: Nutritional management of pediatric patients on chronic dialysis, in Fine RN, Gentile DE, Nissenson AR (eds): *Clinical Dialysis,* ed 2. Norwalk, Conn, Appleton & Lange, 1990, pp 676–686.
13. Korthius R, Granger D: Role of the peritoneal microcirculation, in Nolph K (ed): *Peritoneal Dialysis,* ed 3. Boston, Kluwer Academic Publishers, 1989, pp 28–47.
14. Hetrick A, Shah R: Dietary management of infants on CAPD. *Am Assoc Nephrol Nurs Techn* 1982; 9:46–48.
15. Kush RD, Hallett MD, Ota K, et al: Long term continuous ambulatory peritoneal dialysis. *Blood Purif* 1990; 8:1–13.
16. Sedman E: Dialysis in pediatrics, in Gellis SS, Kagan BM (eds): *Current Pediatric Therapy,* vol 12. Philadelphia, WB Saunders, 1986, pp 370–376.
17. Mactier R, Khanna R: Peritoneal cavity lymphatics, in Nolph K (ed): *Peritoneal Dialysis,* ed 3. Boston, Kluwer Academic Publishers, 1989, pp 48–66.
18. Putnam TJ: Living peritoneum as a dialyzing membrane. *Am J Physiol* 1923; 63:548–555.
19. Moncrief J, Popovich R: CAPD, in Nolph K (ed): *Peritoneal Dialysis,* ed 3. Boston, Kluwer Academic Publishers, 1989, pp 152–168.
20. Twardowski Z, Nolph K, Khanna R (eds): *Peritoneal dialysis: New Concepts and Applications.* New York, Churchill Livingstone, 1990, pp 29–52, 67–100.
21. Jorres A, Topley N, Gahl G: Biocompatibility of peritoneal fluids. *Int J Artif Organs* 1992; 15:79–83.
22. Hanning R, Balfe W, Zlotkin S: Effectiveness and nutritional consequences of amino acid–based versus glucose-based dialysis solutions in infants and children receiving CAPD. *Am J Clin Nutr* 1987; 46:22–30.
23. Rubin J: Comments on dialysis solution, antibiotic transport, poisonings

and novel uses of peritoneal dialysis, in Nolph K (ed): *Peritoneal Dialysis,* ed 3. Boston, Kluwer Academic Publishers, 1989, pp 199–229.

24. Kastrup E (ed): *Facts and Comparisons.* St Louis, JB Lippincott, 1992, p 702.

25. Gahl G, Hain H: Nutrition and metabolism in continuous ambulatory peritoneal dialysis in evolution and trends in peritoneal dialysis. *Contrib Nephrol* 1990; 84:36–44.

26. Wideroe T-E, Smeby L, Berg K, et al: Intraperitoneal (125 I) insulin absorption during intermittent and continuous peritoneal dialysis. *Kidney Int* 1983; 23:22–28.

27. Grodstein G, Blumenkrantz M, Kopple J, et al: Glucose absorption during CAPD. *Kidney Int* 1981; 19:564–567.

28. Thomas ME, Moorhead JF: Lipids in CAPD: A review. *Contrib Nephrol* 1990; 85:92–99.

29. Walls J, Bennett MB: Maintaining nutrition in CAPD patients. *Contrib Nephrol* 1990; 85:79–83.

30. Kopple JD, Blumenkrantz MJ: Nutritional requirements for patients undergoing continuous ambulatory peritoneal dialysis. *Kidney Int* 1983; 24(suppl):295–302.

31. Dabbagh S, Fassinger N, Clement K, et al: The effect of aggressive nutrition on infection rates in patients maintained on peritoneal dialysis. *Adv Peritoneal Dial* 1991; 7:161–164.

32. Kopple JD, Blumenkrantz MJ, Jones MR, et al: Plasma amino acid levels and amino acid losses during continuous ambulatory peritoneal dialysis. *Am J Clin Nutr* 1982; 36:395–402.

33. Blumberg A, Hanck A, Sander G: Vitamin nutrition in patients on CAPD. *Clin Nephrol* 1983; 20:244–250.

34. Ross, E, Shah G, Reynolds R, et al: Vitamin B_6 requirements of patients on chronic peritoneal dialysis. *Kidney Int* 1989; 36:702–706.

35. Gleghorn EE, Eisenberg LD, Hack S, et al: Observations of vitamin A toxicity in 3 patients with renal failure receiving parenteral nutrition. *Am J Clin Nutr* 1986; 44:107–112.

36. Smythe WR, Allen AC, Craswell PW, et al: Trace element abnormalities in chronic uremia. *Ann Intern Med* 1982; 96:302–310.

37. Kohaut EC: Growth in children treated with continuous ambulatory peritoneal dialysis. *Int J Pediatr Nephrol* 1983; 4:93–98.

38. Thomson NM, Stevens BJ, Humphrey TJ, et al: Comparison of trace elements in peritoneal dialysis, hemodialysis and uremia. *Kidney Int* 1983; 23:9–14.

39. Padovese P, Gallieni M, Brancaccio D, et al: Trace elements in dialysis fluids and assessment of the exposure of patients on regular hemodialysis, hemofiltration and continuous ambulatory peritoneal dialysis. *Nephron* 1992; 61:442–448.

40. Hosokawa S, Yoshida O: Role of trace elements on complications in patients undergoing chronic hemodialysis. *Int J Artif Organs* 1992; 15:5–9.

41. Bartel L, Hussey J, Elson C, et al: Depletion of heart and skeletal muscle carnitine in the normal rat by peritoneal dialysis. *Nutr Res* 1981; 1:261–266.

42. Wolk RA, Swartz RD: Nutrition support of patients in acute renal failure. *Nutr Suppl Serv* 1986; 6:38–41, 45–46.

43. Blumenkrantz MJ, Kopple JD, Moran JK, et al: Metabolic balance studies and dietary protein requirements in patients undergoing continuous ambulatory peritoneal dialysis. *Kidney Int* 1982; 21:849–864.

44. Robin J: Nutritional support during peritoneal dialysis–related peritonitis. *Am J Kidney Dis* 1990; 15:551–555.

45. Kopple JD, Monteon FJ, Shaib JK: Effect of energy intake on nitrogen metabolism in non-dialyzed patients with chronic renal failure. *Kidney Int* 1986; 29:734–742.

46. Giordano C, DeSanto NG, Pluvio M, et al: Protein requirement of patients on CAPD: A study on nitrogen balance. *Int J Artif Organs* 1980; 3:11–14.

47. Goodship TH, Arfeen S, Kirkwood A, et al: Amino dialysate. *Contrib Nephrol* 1990; 85:84–91.

48. Mirtallo J, Schneider P, Ruberg R, et al: Monitoring protein requirements of the patient receiving hemodialysis and total parenteral nutrition. *Am J Hosp Pharm* 1981; 38:1483–1486.

49. Nissenson AR: Acid-base homeostasis in peritoneal dialysis patients. *Int J Artif Organs* 1984; 7:175–176.

50. Hamdy NA, Brown CB, Boletis J, et al:

Mineral metabolism in CAPD. *Contrib Nephrol* 1990; 85:100–110.

51. Boeschoten EW, Schrijuer J, Krediet RT, et al: Vitamin deficiencies in CAPD patients (abstract). *Peritoneal Dial Bull* 1984; 4(suppl):7.

52. Warady BA, Kriley M: Vitamin status of pediatric patients receiving long-term peritoneal dialysis (abstract 185). Presented at the Tenth Annual International Conference on Peritoneal Dialysis, Dallas, 1990.

53. Shah GM, Ross EA, Sabo A, et al: Effect of ascorbic acid and pyridoxine supplementation on oxalate metabolism in peritoneal dialysis patients. *Am J Kidney Dis* 1992; 20:42–49.

54. Fournier AG, Corvazier M, Man W: Skin test sensitivity in zinc deficient patients in hemo and peritoneal dialysis abstract. *Artif Organs* 1989; 13:296.

55. Murakami R, Momota T, Yoshiya K, et al: Serum carnitine and nutritional status in children treated with continuous ambulatory peritoneal dialysis. *J Pediatr Gastroenterol Nutr* 1990; 11:371–374.

56. Feinstein E: Nutrition in acute renal failure, in Rombeau JL, Caldwell MD (eds): *Parenteral Nutrition,* vol 2. Philadelphia, WB Saunders, 1986, pp 586–601.

57. Food and Nutrition Board of the National Research Council: *Recommended Dietary Allowances.* Washington, DC, National Academy Press, 1989, p 285.

58. Wesley JR, Khalidi N, Faubian WC, et al: *The University of Michigan Medical Center Parenteral and Enteral Nutrition Manual,* ed 6. Ann Arbor, Mich, University Press, 1990, p 46.

59. Nebeker HG, Coburn JW: Aluminum and osteodystrophy. *Annu Rev Med* 1986; 37:79–95.

60. Sedman A: Aluminum toxicity in childhood. *Pediatr Nephrol* 1992; 6:383–393.

61. Dahlstrom KA, Ament ME, Moukarzel A, et al: Low blood and plasma carnitine levels in children receiving long term parenteral nutrition. *J Pediatr Gastroenterol Nutr* 1990; 11:375–379.

62. Winchester JF: The albumin dilemma. *Am J Kidney Dis* 1992; 20:76–77.

63. Fine A, Cox D: Modest reduction of serum albumin in continuous ambulatory peritoneal dialysis patients is common and of no apparent clinical consequences. *Am J Kidney Dis* 1992; 20:50–54.

64. Blumenkrantz MJ, Kopple JD, Moran JK, et al: Nitrogen and urea metabolism during continuous ambulatory peritoneal dialysis. *Kidney Int* 1981; 20:78–82.

65. Giordano C, Capodicisa G, DeSanto N: Artificial gut for total parenteral nutrition through the peritoneal cavity. *Int J Artif Organs* 1980; 3:326–330.

66. Williams P, Marliss E, Anderson G, et al: Amino acid absorption following intraperitoneal administration in CAPD patients. *Peritoneal Dial Bull* 1982; 2:124–130.

67. Oren A, Wu G, Anderson E: Effective use of amino acids dialysate over four weeks in CAPD patients. *Trans Am Soc Artif Intern Organs* 1983; 29:604–609.

68. Dombros N, Prutis K, Tong M: Six month overnight intraperitoneal amino acid infusion in CAPD patients. *Peritoneal Dial Int* 1990; 10:79–84.

69. Arfeen S, Goodship T, Kirkwood A, et al: The nutritional/metabolic and hormonal effects of 8 weeks of CAPD with a 1% amino acid solution. *Clin Nephrol* 1990; 33:192–199.

70. Gilsdorf R, Selby R, Schon D, et al: Total nutritional support through the peritoneal cavity. *J Am Coll Nutr* 1985; 4:461–469.

71. Klein M, Coran A, Drongowski R: The quantitative transperitoneal absorption of a fat emulsion: Implications for intraperitoneal nutrition. *J Pediatr Surg* 1983; 18:724–730.

72. Pessa M, Sitern H, Copeland E: Nutritional support by intraperitoneal dialysis in the rat: Maintenance of body weight with normal liver and plasma chemistries. *JPEN* 1988; 12:63–67.

73. Wolk RA: Intraperitoneal nutrition. *Hosp Pharm* 1992; 27:893–896, 901–905.

24

Enteral Nutrition Products

Barbara Hopkins, MMSc, RD

The enteral formula market has grown significantly over the past several years with more than 80 products available. Choices now include formulas with peptides, fiber, and β-carotene; formulas that are disease specific; and products designed to improve immune function.

Appropriate formula selection requires knowledge about the nutrient requirements of specific patient populations, awareness of the digestive and absorptive capabilities of patients, and knowledge about the potential effects of formulas on gastrointestinal, metabolic, and immunologic functions. Critical evaluation of formula composition should be undertaken to ensure the efficacy and safety of product use. Formulas developed for particular disease states or clinical conditions should be supported by well-designed clinical trials.

NUTRIENT COMPOSITION

Protein

The protein content of an enteral nutrition product is probably the most significant component.[1, 2] Protein is the source of amino acids that are essential for body cell maintenance and physiologic functions. The amount of protein in enteral formulas ranges from 4% to 32% of the total calories. With percent calories used as a reference point, formulas can be classified as low protein ($\leq$10%), standard protein (11% to 15%), intermediate protein (16% to 20%), or high protein (>20%).[2] Table 24–1 lists the currently available enteral products according to protein content. Low-protein products are usually reserved for clinical situations that warrant protein restriction, e.g., renal failure. Standard protein formulas are recommended for individuals who do not have increased

TABLE 24–1.

Enteral Product Classification According to Protein Content (Percentage of Total Calories)

Low Protein (≤10%)*	Standard Protein (11%–15%)*		Intermediate Protein (16%–20%)*		High Protein (>20%)*
Amin Aid (M)	Criticare HN (MJ)	Nepro (R)	Accupep HPF (SM)	Nitrolan (EP)	AlitraQ (R)
Suplena (R)	Ensure (R)	Nutrilan (EP)	Attain (SM)	Nutren 1.0 (C)	Immun-Aid (M)
Tolerex (S)	Ensure Plus (R)	Osmolite (R)	Compleat Modified	Nutren 1.0 with	Impact (S)
Travasorb Renal (C)	Ensure with Fiber (R)	Reabilan (EP)	(S)	Fiber (C)	Impact with Fiber (S)
	Entrition .5 (C)	Resource (S)	Compleat Regular (S)	Nutren 1.5 (C)	Isotein HN (S)
	Entrition (C)	Resource Plus (S)	Comply (SM)	Nutren 2.0 (C)	Perative (R)
	Entrition RDA (C)	Sustacal 8.8 (MJ)	Ensure HN (R)	Nutrivent (C)	Promote (R)
	Fibersource (S)	TwoCal HN (R)	Entrition HN (C)	Osmolite HN (R)	Replete (C)
	Hepatic Aid II (M)	Ultracal (MJ)	Ensure Plus HN (C)	Peptamen (C)	Replete with Fiber
	Isocal (MJ)	Ultralan (EP)	Entrition 1.5 (C)	Pre-Attain (SM)	(C)
	Deliver 2.0 (MJ)	Vital HN (R)	Entrition with Fiber	Profiber (SM)	Sustacal (MJ)
	Isolan (EP)	Vitaneed (SM)	(C)	Pulmocare (R)	Traumacal (MJ)
	Isosource (S)	Vivonex TEN (S)	Fiberlan (EP)	Reabilan HN (EP)	
	Magnacal (SM)		Fibersource HN (S)	Sustacal Plus (MJ)	
			Glucerna (R)	Sustacal with Fiber	
			Introlite (R)	(MJ)	
			Isocal HN (MJ)	Travasorb HN (C)	
			Isosource HN (S)	Travasorb MCT (C)	
			Jevity (R)	Travasorb Standard	
			Lipisorb (MJ)	(C)	

*C = Clintec Nutrition Company; EP = Elan Pharma; M = McGaw; MJ = Mead Johnson; R = Ross Laboratories; S = SANDOZNUTRITION; SM = Sherwood Medical.

protein requirements. Intermediate- and high-protein products are indicated for patients with increased nitrogen requirements, e.g., trauma, burns, etc.

There are three types of protein in commercial formulas: intact protein, protein hydrolysates, and crystalline amino acids (see the chapter on intact protein, peptide, and amino acid formulas) (Table 24–2). *Intact proteins* require digestion to smaller peptides and amino acids for absorption. Therefore, absorption is dependent on sufficient quantities of pancreatic proteases and brush border peptidases.[3] Since intact proteins have large molecular weights,

TABLE 24–2.

Sources of Protein in Enteral Nutrition Products

Intact Proteins	Peptides	Amino Acids
Beef	Hydrolyzed	L-Amino acids
Milk	Casein	
Caseinates	Whey	
Lactalbumin	Soy	
Soy protein isolate	Lactalbumin	
Whey		
Casein		

they contribute very little to the osmolality of a product. *Protein hydrolysates* are obtained from enzymatic hydrolysis of intact proteins. The end products of hydrolysis include dipeptides and tripeptides, oligopeptides, and free amino acids. Oligopeptides require further breakdown by brush border peptidases before absorption takes place. Dipeptides and tripeptides can be directly absorbed. These peptides are absorbed faster than free amino acids.[3, 4] However, the efficacy of peptide absorption in humans remains controversial.[4–8] The benefit of products with high–molecular-weight peptides has not been established. Table 24–3 provides information about the types of peptides (according to molecular weights) in current enteral products. *Crystalline amino acids* are the third type of protein found in enteral formulas. They do not require pancreatic or brush border activity for absorption. Small peptides and free amino acids greatly affect product osmolality; the smaller the molecular weight, the greater the contribution.

Another important factor is the qual-

TABLE 24–3.

Estimated Peptide Lengths of Selected Enteral Products*

Products	Free Amino Acids	Molecular Weights†				
		500	500–1000	500-5000	1000–5000	5000
Accupep HPF	15‡	40	30		15	0
AlitraQ	52	15	—	13	—	22
Criticare HN	50	—	40		10	0
Peptamen	1	3	—		50	30
Perative	0	10–15		10–18	—	67–77
Reabilan	8	—	56		30	6
Reabilan HN	8	—	56		30	6
Vital HN	20	37	—		8	30–35
Vivonex TEN	100	0	—		0	0

*Information based on published product information.
†Molecular weights less than 1000 represent small peptides.
‡All values are percentages.

ity of the protein. Quality is dependent on protein digestibility, absorption, and its amino acid composition. The two most commonly used methods for assessing protein quality are chemical score (CS) and biologic value.[9] CS is a comparison of the amino acid profile of a particular protein to that of whole egg (CS = 100) or an ideal reference pattern. Biologic value is calculated by using the following formula:

$$\text{Biologic value} = \frac{\text{Dietary nitrogen} - \left(\text{Urinary nitrogen} + \text{Fecal nitrogen}\right)}{\text{Dietary nitrogen} - \text{Fecal nitrogen}}$$

Table 24–4 lists the biologic value of proteins found in enteral products and shows a comparison to the standard reference protein, whole egg.[1, 9] The higher the biologic value, the smaller the quantity of protein needed to obtain nitrogen balance.

FIG 24–4.

Biologic Value of Proteins in Enteral Nutrition Products

Protein	Biologic Value
Whole egg	100
Cow milk	90
Lactalbumin	84
Beef	76
Soy	75
Casein	72

Nitrogen Sources of Current Interest

Glutamine has been labeled a conditionally essential amino acid during times of metabolic stress.[10–12] Glutamine is the preferred substrate of the small bowel; it is necessary for maintenance of normal gastrointestinal structure and function and may play a role in the prevention of bacterial translocation[12] (see the chapter on glutamine). Glutamine contains two nitrogen moieties and is able to shuttle nitrogen from muscle to visceral organs. Most enteral products contain glutamine as either free glutamine, glutamic acid (only one nitrogen), or protein-bound glutamine. The presence of glutamine in enteral products is of little importance when feeding unstressed patients since glutamine is synthesized endogenously. The glutamine content is more significant when nourishing critically ill patients. The amount and form of glutamine required during metabolic stress in humans is currently unknown and remains a much-debated issue. The glutamine and glutamic acid amounts in enteral formulas designed for metabolically stressed patients are found in Table 24–5.

Arginine is also considered semiessential during some stress states[13, 14] (see the chapter on arginine). Supplementation in burns and trauma may improve or preserve cellular immune

TABLE 24–5.

Glutamine, Glutamic Acid, Arginine, and Branched-Chain Amino Acid Content of Selected Enteral Products*

Component	AlitraQ	Immun-Aid	Impact	Impact with Fiber	Perative	Reabilan HN	Traumacal	Vivonex TEN
Glutamine	27.0†	15.60	21.1‡	21.1‡	18.3‡	15.9‡	24.0‡	12.85
Glutamic acid	7.0	—						—
Arginine	8.5	19.25	25	25	21.1	3.3	4.1	5.18
BCAA	18.5	36.25	17.1	17.1	18.2	21.0	23.0	33.00
Nucleotides	No	Yes	Yes	Yes	No	No	No	No

*Information based on product information.
†Values are grams per 100 g of protein.
‡Represents the total of protein/peptide-bound glutamine and glutamic acid.

function. Arginine enhances protein and wound collagen synthesis, improves cell-mediated immunity, and has secretagogue properties.[15, 16] The arginine content of selected enteral products can be found in Table 24–5.

Levels of branched-chain amino acids (BCAAs: leucine, isoleucine, and valine) are often reduced in patients with trauma or stress (see the chapter on BCAAs). Since BCAAs may be a preferred energy source during metabolic stress, supplemental BCAAs may reduce muscle-protein breakdown and stimulate protein synthesis.[17]

Nucleotides are present in three enteral products: Impact, Impact with Fiber, and Immun-Aid. Nucleotides contain a nitrogen base (purine or pyrimidine), a pentose, and one or more phosphate groups. Nucleotides are the major structural units of DNA, RNA, adenosine triphosphate (ATP), nicotinamide adenine dinucleotide (NAD), flavin adenine dinucleotide (FAD), and coenzyme A. Nucleotides are usually synthesized in adequate quantities by the liver, but exogenous sources may be necessary during critical illness secondary to impaired hepatic synthesis. The normal cellular immune response may be dependent on the supply of adequate levels of nucleotides (see the chapter on nucleotides). Improved immune function may reduce susceptibility to infection during periods of metabolic stress.[18–21]

Carnitine and taurine have been added to several enteral formulas. Carnitine is necessary for the transport of long-chain fatty acids across the mitochondrial membrane. Carnitine deficiency leads to impairment in fat metabolism. Although rare, carnitine deficiency may occur in individuals with an inadequate dietary intake of carnitine (protein malnutrition) or an impairment in the biosynthesis of carnitine.[22] Carnitine can be made endogenously from lysine and methionine. Taurine, an amino acid synthesized from cysteine, is involved in bile acid conjugation and is able to enhance insulin activity. Taurine deficiency is rare in adult humans.[23] The addition of these two nutrients to enteral formulas is not essential for most enterally fed patients.

Carbohydrate

Carbohydrate is the major fuel source in the average American diet. Approximately half of dietary carbohydrate is derived from polysaccharides (starches and dextrins), with the remainder coming from sugars.[24] Carbohydrates can be classified as either monosaccharides, oligosaccharides, or polysaccharides. Oligosaccharides contain short chains

TABLE 24–6.

Sweetness of Carbohydrates in Enteral Nutrition Products

Carbohydrate	Sweetness
Fructose	115–170
Sucrose	100
Glucose	70
Glucose syrup	30–60
Maltose	40
Lactose	20

TABLE 24–7.

Carbohydrate Sources in Enteral Nutrition Products

Polysaccharides	Oligosaccharides	Monosaccharides
Pureed vegetables	Hydrolyzed cornstarch	Fructose
Modified starch	Corn syrup	
Tapioca	Glucose polymers	
Pureed fruit	Lactose	
	Sucrose	
	Pureed fruit	

of monosaccharides (two to eight units); polysaccharides contain many (greater than eight) monosaccharide units. The form of carbohydrate greatly influences the osmolality, sweetness (Table 24–6), and digestibility of the enteral product.[1] The smaller the molecular weight, the sweeter and more hyperosmolar the product. Glucose polymers are more soluble than starch and are rapidly hydrolyzed by the small intestine. They contribute more to product osmolality than starch does. Carbohydrate sources commonly found in enteral products are listed in Table 24–7. Most carbohydrates, except lactose, are easily digested and absorbed by the small bowel. Symptoms of carbohydrate intolerance range from abdominal discomfort to flatulence and diarrhea.[25]

Fiber

Evidence to date supports the theory that fiber is necessary to maintain normal gut function[26] (see the chapter on fiber). Agreement exists that fiber is a necessary component of a healthful diet; however, the "ideal" fiber intake has not been established, particularly for critically ill and hospitalized patients. The recommended level of dietary fiber intake for healthy individuals (excluding children and the elderly) is 10 to 13 g per 1000 calories consumed.[27]

Fiber can be classified as either non-polysaccharide (lignin) or nonstarch polysaccharides (cellulose and noncellulose [hemicellulose, gums, mucilages and pectins]). Nonstarch polysaccharides undergo fermentation (Table 24–8)

by colonic bacteria, and the degree of fermentation is dependent on the type and source of fiber, the quantity consumed, and the amount of colonic flora present.[28] The end products of colonic fermentation are volatile fatty acids and gases (H_2, CH_4, CO_2). The most important short-chain fatty acids (SCFAs) include butyric, acetic, and propionic acids. SCFAs serve as energy sources for colonocytes, increase bacterial mass, enhance water and sodium absorption, and stimulate mucosal growth (butyrate).[26, 28] Pectins are the most fermentable of the nonstarch polysaccharides (Table 24–8).

Cellulose, hemicellulose, and lignin can increase fecal bulk, decrease intestinal transit time, and increase gastric emptying. Mucilages, gums, and pectins are rapidly fermented by gut flora, decrease gastric emptying, and delay absorption of glucose. Sources of fiber in enteral formulas include soy polysaccharide, oat fiber, pureed fruits and vegetables, and modified guar (Table 24–9). Fiber supplements are also available (Table 24–10). Assessment of the compatibility of the enteral formula and fi-

FIG 24–8.

Fementability of Dietary Fibers*

Fiber	Percent Fermented
Lignin	0
Cellulose	15–60
Hemicellulose	56–87
Mucilages	85–95
Pectins	90–95

*Data from Frankenfield DC, Beyer P: *J Am Diet Assoc* 1991; 91:590–599.

TABLE 24–9.

Total Dietary Fiber in Enteral Nutrition Products*

Product	Fiber Source	TDF† (g/L)	Estimated Percentage Fermented
Compleat Regular	Vegetables, fruits	4.24	60–90
Compleat Modified	Vegetables, fruits	4.24	60–90
Ensure with Fiber	Soy polysaccharide	14.4	70–93
Fiberlan	Soy polysaccharide	14.0	70–93
Fibersource	Soy polysaccharide	10.0	70–93
Fibersource HN	Soy polysaccharide	6.8	70–93
Glucerna	Soy polysaccharide	14.4	70–93
Impact with Fiber	Soy polysaccharide Modified guar	10.0	70–93 85–95
Jevity	Soy polysaccharide	14.4	70–93
Nutren 1.0 with Fiber	Soy polysaccharide	14.0	70–93
Profiber	Soy polysaccharide	12.0	70–93
Replete with Fiber	Soy polysaccharide	14.0	70–93
Sustacal with Fiber	Soy polysaccharide	5.9	70–93
Ultracal	Soy polysaccharide (60%) Oat fiber (40%)	14.4	70–93 50–55
Vitaneed	Vegetables, fruits Soy polysaccharide	8.0	60–90 70–93

*Data from Frankenfield DC, Beyer P: *J Am Diet Assoc* 1991; 91:590–599 and Jenkins DJA: Diet and colonic function, in Shils ME, Young VR (eds): *Modern Nutrition in Health and Disease*. Philadelphia, Lea & Febiger, 1988.
†TDF = total dietary fiber.

ber additive should be completed before administration to patients. Liquid pectin can solidify enteral formulas when mixed with intact proteins.[29]

The ability of fiber formulas to alleviate diarrhea in critically ill patients is questionable.[28] However, small amounts of fermentable fiber may preserve gut integrity.[26, 30, 31] An area requiring research is the effect of fiber on drug absorption.

High-fiber intake should be accompanied by increased free water intake to prevent colonic obstruction. Fiber formulas should be initiated slowly to prevent discomfort and flatulence.

Fat

Essential Fatty Acids

Fat is a source of energy and essential fatty acids. With the establishment of a second essential fatty acid (i.e., linolenic acid), many products contain fats that do not provide adequate quantities of both linoleic (ω-6) and linolenic (ω-3) acids. These two fatty acids are essential because they cannot be synthesized by humans. The amount of linoleic and linolenic acids required to prevent deficiencies are 1% to 2% and 0.2% to 0.3% of the total daily calories, respectively.[32] Linoleic acid is found in high levels in most vegetable oils; linolenic acid, on the other hand, is not. Primary sources of linolenic acid include soybean oil, canola oil (rapeseed), linseed, wheat germ, and walnuts. Linolenic acid along with its derivatives eicosapentaenoic acid (EPA) and docosahexanoic acid

TABLE 24–10.

Selected Fiber Supplements*†

Fiber Source	Amount	Characteristics
Banana flakes	100 g	2.14 g soluble fiber 5.21 g insoluble fiber 80%–90% fermented
Liquid pectin	100 mL	7.7 g soluble fiber 90%–95% fermented
Ispaghul Psyllium	100 g	85 g soluble fiber 80%–90% fermented
Purified cellulose	100 g	100% insoluble fiber 10%–20% fermented

*Data from Frankenfield DC, Beyer P: *J Am Diet Assoc* 1991; 91:590–599.
†Information also obtained from product literature and the manufacturer.

(DHA) is found in marine fish, shellfish, and fish oils.

Fat sources in enteral products include soy, corn, safflower and sunflower oils, canola oil, beef fat, refined marine fish oil, medium-chain triglycerides (MCTs), and structured lipids. The linoleic, linolenic, EPA, and DHA contents of fats used in enteral products are listed in Table 24–11.

An adequate intake of linoleic acid is important for normal immune function, but excessive amounts can be immunosuppressive[33-36] (see the chapter on lipids). Many enteral products contain high levels of linoleic acid, which may be contraindicated in conditions of metabolic stress. The ω-3 fatty acids can alter the negative effects of ω-6 fatty acids by inhibiting the formation of prostaglandins of the 2 series.[32] EPA and DHA may also be key players in the management of inflammatory diseases, where they decrease production of inflammatory cytokines.

Medium-Chain Triglycerides

MCTs (C6:0 to C12:0) are important energy sources (8.3 calories per gram) in conditions where long-chain triglyceride (LCT) digestion, absorption, or transport is impaired. MCTs require little or no pancreatic lipase activity or bile salts for absorption and are delivered directly to the liver by way of the portal vein.[37] MCTs are more water soluble than LCTs, but they do not provide the two essential fatty acids.

Since MCTs are quickly hydrolyzed intraluminally, increased levels of intake may increase the luminal osmotic concentration and cause abdominal distension and diarrhea.[1, 37] MCTs are metabolized in the liver; ingestion of high levels may be contraindicated in cirrhosis. The inability of the liver to clear C8:0 fatty acids could cause an increased amount of octanoate and induce a situation similar to hepatic encephalopathy.[37] MCTs are also ketogenic and should not be given to patients with hyperosmolar diabetic syndrome.[37]

Structural Lipids

Structured lipids are new to enteral nutrition products, and currently only two products, Impact and Impact with Fiber, contain them. Structured lipids are made by transesterification of MCTs with an oil high in polyunsaturated fatty acids.[35] The result is a triglyceride with medium- and long-chain fatty acids on the same glycerol molecule. Structured lipids may help prevent the immunosuppression associated with high levels of LCT.

Vitamins and Minerals

Most enteral products meet 100% of the U.S. recommended dietary allow-

TABLE 24–11.

Approximate Essential Fatty Acid Content of Fats Used in Enteral Nutrition Products*

Fat	Linoleic Acid (%)	Linolenic Acid (%)	EPA† (%)	DHA† (%)
Canola oil	22	11.1	0	0
Corn oil	58	0.8	0	0
Safflower oil	74	0.0	0	0
Soybean oil	51	6.8	0	0
Hydrogenated	39	2.8	0	0
Sunflower oil	66	0.3	0	0
Beef fat	—	0.6	—	—
Refined menhaden oil‡	—	—	4.7	1.6
Structured lipid‡	9	0	0	0

*Data from MacBurney MM, Russell C, Young LS: Formulas, in Rumbeau JL, Caldwell MD (eds): *Clinical Nutrition, Enteral and Tube Feeding.* Philadelphia, WB Saunders, 1990; Nettleson J: *J Am Diet Assoc* 1991; 91:331–337; and Gottschlich MM: *Nutr Clin Pract* 1992; 7:152–165.
†EPA = eicosapentaenoic acid; DHA = docosahexanoic acid.
‡Information obtained from product literature.

TABLE 24–12.

Approximate β-Carotene Content of Selected Enteral Nutrition Products*

Product	β-Carotene (IU/L)
Immun-Aid	1333
Impact	3350
Impact with Fiber	3350
Perative	4333
Replete	3332
Replete with Fiber	3332

*Information obtained from product literature.

ance (RDA) at a given volume of formula (excluding renal and hepatic formulas). The U.S. RDAs were first published in 1973 and are based on the 1968 RDAs. They are generous and are based on the greatest need of each sex-age group greater than 4 years of age. RDAs do not reflect needs during critical illness or severe hypermetabolism. With the current changes in nutritional labeling and the abandonment of the U.S. RDAs, different reference standards will be adopted

by manufacturers of enteral formulas.[38]

Of current interest is the relationship between β-carotene and immune function.[39–41] β-Carotene may increase the cytotoxicity of natural killer cells, enhance the immune response, and increase levels of T-helper cells. Presently there are six enteral products that contain β-carotene, and they are listed in Table 24–12.

PHYSICAL CHARACTERISTICS

Osmolality

Osmolality represents the number of active particles per kilogram of water. Particle size affects osmolality; high–molecular-weight proteins and carbohydrates contribute less to the osmolality of formulas than do peptides, amino acids, and simple sugars. Enteral products range in osmolality from 270 mOsm/kg to approximately 700 mOsm/kg.

TABLE 24–13.

Nutrient Composition of Modular Enteral Products per 100 g Powder or 100 mL

Product*	Source	Protein	CHO	Fat	Calories	Lactose	Ca	Na	K	P	Cl	Form
Protein modular												
Casec (MJ) (Tbs = 4.7 g)	Calcium caseinate	88	—	2	370	—	1600	120	10	800	—	Powder
ProMod (R) (Tbs = 4.0 g)	Whey	75	10	9	420	4.5	390	225	975	395	—	Powder
Propac (SM) (Tbs = 4.0 g)	Whey	75	—	8	395	6.0	350	225	500	300	50	Powder
Carbohydrate modular												
Moducal (MJ) (Tbs = 8 g)	Hydrolyzed cornstarch	—	95	—	380	—	—	70	10	—	150	Powder
Polycose (R) (Tbs = 6 g)	Hydrolyzed cornstarch	—	94	—	380	—	30	110	10	5	223	Powder
Polycose (R) (Tbs = 15 mL)	Hydrolyzed cornstarch	—	50	—	200	—	20	70	6	3	140	Liquid
Sumacal (SM) (Tbs = 5 g)	Maltodextrin	—	95	—	380	—	†	100	†	†	210	Powder
Fat modular												
MCT oil (MJ) (Tbs = 15 mL)	MCT‡	—	—	92	767	—	—	—	—	—	—	Liquid
Microlipid (SM) (Tbs = 15 mL)	Safflower oil	—	—	50	450	—	—	—	—	—	—	Liquid

*MJ = Mead Johnson; R = Ross Laboratories; SM = Sherwood Medical.
†Less than 1 mEq.
‡MCT = medium-chain triglyceride

TABLE 24–14.

Classification of Enteral Nutrition Products

Classification	Formula Characteristics	Sample Products
Intact protein		
Blenderized	Isotonic; nutritionally complete; contain fiber; lactose containing and lactose free	Compleat Regular, Vitaneed, Compleat Modified
Low-residue		
Standard protein	Isotonic; nutritionally complete; lactose free	Entrition 1.0, Isocal, Isosource, Isolan, Osmolite, Resource
Intermediate-high protein	Isotonic; nutritionally complete; lactose free	Entrition HN, Isocal HN, Osmolite HN, Isosource HN
Concentrated	Calorically dense (1.5–2.0 cal/mL); lactose free; nutritionally complete; hyperosmolar	Isocal HCN, Magnacal, TwoCal HN, Nutren 2.0
Fiber-supplemented	Isotonic; nutritionally complete; lactose free; fiber ranges from 5–14.4 g/L; standard to intermediate protein	Fibersource, Jevity, Ultracal, Fiberlan
Disease specific		
Renal	Low and standard protein; low mineral, vitamin A, and vitamin D content; lactose free; calorically dense; hyperosmolar	Nepro, Suplena
Glucose intolerant	Low CHO, high fat; lactose free; isotonic; contain fiber; nutritionally complete	Glucerna
Pulmonary	Low CHO, high fat; lactose free; nutritionally complete; hyperosmolar; calorically dense	Nutrivent, Pulmocare, Respalor
Trauma/stress	High protein; isotonic to hyperosmolar; lactose free; nutritionally complete; some contain fiber, hydrolyzed protein, supplemental amino acids (BCAA, arginine, glutamine), and β-carotene; low to high fat	AlitraQ, Impact, Impact with Fiber, Immun-Aid, Isotein HN, Replete, Replete with Fiber, Traumacal, Promote
Hydrolyzed Protein		
Very low fat	Nutritionally complete, lactose free, fewer than 10% of the calories from fat, hyperosmolar, vary in peptide length, contain amino acids	Accupep HPF, Criticare HN, Vital HN
Low fat	Nutritionally complete, lactose free, 11%–30% of the calories from fat, hyperosmolar, vary in peptide length, contain amino acids	Travasorb HN, Travasorb STD
Moderate fat	Nutritionally complete, lactose free, 30%–35% of the calories from fat (high MCT*); hyperosmolar, vary in peptide length, contain amino acids	Peptamen, Reabilan
Disease specific: trauma	Nutritionally complete, lactose free, intermediate to high protein content, 25%–35% of the calories from fat (high MCT), vary in peptide length, contain amino acids, may contain supplemental arginine and β-carotene	Perative, Reabilan HN
Crystalline amino acids	Nutritionally complete, lactose free, low fat (1%–3% of the total calories), low to standard protein content, hyperosmolar	Tolerex, Vivonex TEN
Disease specific		
Hepatic failure	High BCAA,* nutritionally incomplete, lactose free, low to moderate fat	Hepatic Aid II, Travasorb Hepatic
Renal failure	Essential amino acids plus histidine, nutritionally incomplete, lactose free, hyperosmolar, low fat	Amin-Aid
	Essential and nonessential amino acids, nutritionally incomplete but contain water-soluble vitamins, hyperosmolar, lactose free, low fat	Travasorb Renal

*MCT = medium-chain triglyceride; BCAA = branched-chain amino acid; LCT = long-chain triglyceride.

Osmolality may affect patient tolerance to a particular formula. Hypo-osmolar and hyperosmolar feedings delay gastric emptying[3]; hyperosmolar formulas may increase the intraluminal osmotic concentration and create gastrointestinal intolerance. To prevent any potential problems, hyperosmolar feedings may be initiated at a smaller volume. Data indicate that these feedings can be advanced at a fairly rapid rate without any problems.[42]

The nutrient profiles of the currently available enteral nutrition products can be found in Table 24–13 and Appendix 24–1.

CLASSIFICATION OF ENTERAL NUTRITION PRODUCTS

Several methods have been used to classify enteral products: complete vs. incomplete, polymeric vs. monomermic, and a descriptive classification based on the overall characteristics of the product. Since protein is considered to be the most significant formula component, it seems more appropriate to classify enteral formulas according to the type of protein. This system has three major categories: intact protein, hydrolyzed protein, and crystalline amino acids. Subcategories, formula characteristics, and examples of each are listed in Table 24–14. Molecular formulas are found in Table 24–3.

A product's intended use (per product literature) may not always equate with sound scientific principles. Careful evaluation of studies supporting a product should be conducted by all clinicians in nutrition support before recommending a product for patient use.

REFERENCES

1. MacBurney MM, Russell C, Young LS: Formulas, in Rombeau JL, Caldwell MD (eds): *Clinical Nutrition. Enteral and Tube Feeding.* Philadelphia, WB Saunders, 1990.
2. Heimburger DC, Weinsier RL: Guidelines for evaluating and categorizing enteral feeding formulas according to therapeutic equivalence. *JPEN* 1985; 9:61–67.
3. Johnson LR: *Gastrointestinal Physiology,* ed 2. St Louis, Mosby–Year Book, 1991.
4. Zaloga GP: Physiological effects of peptide-based enteral formulas. *Nutr Clin Pract* 1990; 5:231–237.
5. Silk DB, Fairclough PD, Clark ML, et al: Use of a peptide rather than free amino acid nitrogen source in chemically defined "elemental" diets. *JPEN* 1980; 4:548–553.
6. Grimble GK, Rees RG, Keohane PP, et al: Effect of peptide chain length on absorption of egg protein hydrolysates in the normal human jejunum. *Gastroenterology* 1987; 92:136–142.
7. Brinson RB, Pitts VL, Taylor AE: Intestinal absorption of peptide enteral formulas in hypoproteinemic (volume expanded) rats; a paired analysis. *Crit Care Med* 1989; 17:657–660.
8. Mowatt-Larssen C, Brown R, Wojtysiak S, et al: Comparison of tolerance and nutritional outcome between a peptide and a standard enteral formula in critically-ill, hypoalbuminemic patients. *JPEN* 1992; 16:20–24.
9. Munro HN, Crim MC: The proteins and amino acids, in Shils ME, Young VR (eds): *Modern Nutrition in Health and Disease.* Philadelphia, Lea & Febiger, 1988.
10. Lacy J, Wilmore D: Is glutamine a conditionally essential amino acid? *Nutr Rev* 1990; 48:297–309.
11. Souba W: Glutamine: A key substrate for the splanchnic bed. *Annu Rev Nutr* 1991; 11:285–308.
12. Souba W, Klimberg S, Plumley D, et al: The role of glutamine in maintaining a healthy gut and supporting the metabolic responses to injury and infection. *J Surg Res* 1990; 48:383–391.
13. Daly JM, Lieberman M, Goldfine J, et al: Enteral nutrition with supplemental arginine, RNA and omega-3 fatty acids in postoperative patients after operation: Immunologic, metabolic and clinical outcome. *Surgery* 1992; 112:56–67.
14. Cerra FB: Nutrient modulation of inflammatory and immune function. *Am J Surg* 1991; 161:230–234.

15. Barbul A: Arginine: biochemistry, physiology and therapeutic implications. *JPEN* 1986; 10:227–238.

16. Kirk S, Barbul A: Role of arginine in trauma, sepsis and immunity. *JPEN* 1990; 14(suppl):226–229.

17. Cerra FB, Blackburn G, Hirsch J, et al: The effect of stress level, amino acid formula and nitrogen dose on nitrogen retention in traumatic and septic stress. *Ann Surg* 1987; 205:282–287.

18. Kulkarni AD, Fanslow WC, Rudolph FB, et al: Effect of dietary nucleotides on response to bacterial infections. *JPEN* 1986; 10:169–171.

19. Carver JD, Cox WI, Barness LA: Dietary nucleotide effects upon murine natural killer cell activity and macrophage activation. *JPEN* 1990; 14:18–22.

20. Van Buren CT, Rudolph FB, Kulkarni A: Reversal of immunosuppression induced by a protein-free diet: Comparison of nucleotides, fish oil and arginine. *Crit Care Med* 1990; 18(suppl):114–117.

21. Cerra FB, Lehmann S, Konstantinides N, et al: Improvement in immune function in ICU patients by enteral nutrition supplemented with arginine, RNA and menhaden oil is independent of nitrogen balance. *Nutrition* 1991; 7:193–199.

22. Broquist HP: Carnitine, in Shils ME, Toung VR (eds): *Modern Nutrition in Health and Disease.* Philadelphia, Lea & Febiger, 1988.

23. Hyes KC: Taurine, in Shils ME, Young VR (eds): *Modern Nutrition in Health and Disease.* Philadelphia, Lea & Febiger, 1988.

24. Hunt SM, Groff JL: *Advanced Nutrition and Human Metabolism.* St Paul, Minn, West Publishing Co, 1990.

25. Granger DN, Barrowman JA, Kvietys PR: *Clinical Gastrointestinal Physiology.* Philadelphia, WB Saunders, 1985.

26. Palacio JC, Rombeau JL: Dietary fiber; a brief review and potential application to enteral nutrition. *Nutr Clin Pract* 1990; 5:99–106.

27. Ad Hoc Expert Panel on Dietary Fiber: Physiological and health consequences of dietary fiber. *FASEB* June 1987.

28. Frankenfield DC, Beyer P: Dietary fiber and bowel function in tube fed patients. *J Am Diet Assoc* 1991; 91:590–599.

29. Vargas X, Bergman G, Hopkins B: Effects of addition of liquid pectin to commercial formulas, (abstract). Presented at the Annual Meeting of the American Society for Parenteral and Enteral Nutrition, Orlando, Fla, 1992.

30. Jenkins DJA: Diet and colonic function, in Shils ME, Young VR (eds): *Modern Nutrition in Health and Disease.* Philadelphia, Lea & Febiger, 1988.

31. Scheppach W, Richter A, Bartram P, et al: Stimulation of colonic proliferation by short chain fatty acids (abstract). *Gastroenterology* 1989; 96:447.

32. Sardesai VM: The essential fatty acids. *Nutr Clin Pract* 1992; 7:179–186.

33. Nettleton J: Omega-3 fatty acids: Comparison of plant and seafood sources in human nutrition. *J Am Diet Assoc* 1991; 91:331–337.

34. Kinsella JE, Lokesh B: Dietary lipids, eicosanoids and the immune system. *Crit Care Med* 1990; 18(suppl):94–113.

35. Gottschlich MM: Selection of optimal lipids. *Nutr Clin Pract* 1992; 7:152–165.

36. Kinsella JE, Lokesh B, Broughton S, et al: Dietary PUFA and eicosanoids: Potential effects on the modulation of inflammatory and immune cells: An overview. *Nutrition* 1990; 6:24–44.

37. Bach AC, Babayan VK: Medium-chain triglycerides: An update. *Am J Clin Nutr* 1982; 36:950–962.

38. Langseth L, Vanderveen J, Frattali V: Point-counterpoint: The new reference daily intakes: For better or for worse. *Nutr Rev* 1992; 50:119–124.

39. Prabhala RH, Garewal HS, Meyskens FL, et al: Immunomodulation in humans caused by beta-carotene and vitamin A. *Nutr Res* 1990; 10:1473–1486.

40. Goodwin TW: Metabolism, nutrition and function of carotenoids. *Annu Rev Nutr* 1986; 6:273–297.

41. Watson RR, Prabhala RH, Plezia PM, et al: Effect of beta-carotene on lymphocyte subpopulations in elderly humans: Evidence for a dose-response relationship. *Am J Clin Nutr* 1991; 53:90–94.

42. Cerra FB, Shronts EP, Raup S, et al: Enteral nutrition in hypermetabolic surgical patients. *Crit Care Med* 1989; 17:619–622.

Enteral Nutrition Products: Nutrient Sources and Approximate Analysis per Liter

Product (Manufacturer*)	Protein Source	Carbohydrate Source	Fat Source
Accupep HPF (SM)	Hydrolyzed lactalbumin	Maltodextrin	MCT† oil (50%), corn oil (50%)
AlitraQ (R)	Soy hydrolysate, lactalbumin hydrolysate, whey protein, L-glutamine, L-arginine	Hydrolyzed cornstarch Sucrose, fructose	MCT (50%), safflower oil (50%)
Amin-Aid (M)	Crystalline amino acids	Maltodextrin, sucrose	Soybean oil
Attain (SM)	Sodium and calcium caseinates	Maltodextrin	MCT oil (50%), corn oil (50%)
Compleat Modified (S)	Beef, calcium caseinate	Maltodextrin, vegetables, fruits	Corn oil, beef
Compleat Regular (S)	Beef, nonfat milk	Maltodextrin, vegetables, fruits, lactose	Corn oil, beef
Comply (SM)	Sodium and calcium caseinates	Maltodextrin	Corn oil
Criticare HN (MJ)	Hydrolyzed casein (50%), amino acids (50%)	Maltodextrin, modified cornstarch	Safflower oil
Deliver 2.0	Sodium and calcium caseinates	Corn syrup	Soy oil (70%), MCT (30%)
Ensure (R)	Sodium and calcium caseinates, soy protein isolate	corn syrup, sucrose	Corn oil
Ensure HN (R)	Sodium and calcium caseinates, soy protein isolate	Corn syrup, sucrose	Corn oil
Ensure Plus (R)	Sodium and calcium caseinates, soy protein isolate	Corn syrup, sucrose	Corn oil
Ensure Plus HN (R)	Sodium and calcium caseinates, soy protein isolate	Hydrolyzed cornstarch, sucrose	Corn oil
Ensure with Fiber (R)	Sodium and calcium caseinates	Hydrolyzed cornstarch, starch, sucrose, soy polysaccharide	Corn oil
Entrition .5 (C)	Sodium and calcium caseinates	Maltodextrin	Corn oil
Entrition 1.0 (C)	Sodium and calcium caseinates	Maltodextrin	Corn oil
Entrition HN (C)	Sodium and calcium caseinates, soy protein isolate	Maltodextrin	Corn oil
Entrition RDA (C)	Sodium and calcium caseinates	Maltodextrin	Corn oil
Entrition with Fiber (C)	Sodium and calcium caseinates	Maltodextrin, soy polysaccharide	Canola oil, MCT (25%), corn oil
Entrition 1.5 (C)	Potassium and calcium caseinates	Maltodextrin	MCT (46%), corn oil, canola oil
Fiberlan (EP)	Sodium and calcium caseinates	Maltodextrin, soy polysaccharide	Corn oil (50%), MCT (50%)
Fibersource (S)	Sodium and calcium caseinates	Hydrolyzed cornstarch, soy polysaccharide	MCT (50%), canola oil (50%)
Fibersource HN (S)	Sodium and calcium caseinates	Hydrolyzed cornstarch, soy polysaccharide	MCT (50%), canola oil (50%)
Glucerna (R)	Sodium and calcium caseinates	Glucose polymers, soy polysaccharide, fructose	High-oleic safflower oil, soy oil
Hepatic Aid II (M)	Crystalline amino acids	Maltodextrin, sucrose	Soybean oil
Immun-Aid (M)	Lactalbumin, supplemental amino acids (L-arginine, L-glutamine, BCAA†), nucleic acid	Maltodextrin	MCT (50%), canola oil (50%)
Impact (S)	Sodium and calcium caseinates, L-arginine	Hydrolyzed cornstarch	Structured lipids (60%), menhaden oil (40%)

*C = Clintec Nutrition Company; EP = Elan Pharma; M = McGaw; MJ = Mead Johnson; Ross Laboratories; S = SANDOZNUTRITION; SM = Sherwood Medical.
†MCT = medium-chain triglyceride; NA = not available; BCAA = branched-chain amino acid.

Caloric Density (Calorie/mL)	Protein		Carbohydrate		Fat		Total Dietary Fiber (g)	H_2O (%)	Osmolality (mOsm/kg)
	g	Calories (%)	g	Calories (%)	g	Calories (%)			
1.0	40	16	188	75.5	10	8.5	0	84	490
1.0	52.5	21	165	66	15.5	13	0	83	480
2.0	19	4	366	75	46	21	0	70	700
1.0	40	16	135	54	35	30	0	84.6	300
1.07	43	16	140	53	37	31	4.2	83.8	300
1.07	43	16	130	48	43	36	4.2	84.3	450
1.5	60	16	180	48	60	36	0	77.5	410
1.06	38	14	220	81.5	5.3	4.5	0	83	650
2.0	75	15	200	40	102	45	0	71	640
1.06	37.2	14	145	54.5	37.2	31.5	0	85	470
1.06	44.4	16.7	141.2	53.2	35.5	30.1	0	84	470
1.5	54.9	14.7	200	53.3	53.3	32	0	77	690
1.5	62.6	16.7	199.9	53.3	50	30	0	77	650
1.1	39.7	14.5	162	55	37.2	35.5	14.4	83	480
0.5	17.5	14	68	54.5	17.5	31.5	0	92.6	120
1.0	35	14	136	54.5	35	31.5	0	84	300
1.0	44	17.6	114	45.6	41	36.8	0	84	300
1.0	36	14.4	135	54.1	35	31.5	0	84	300
1.0	40	16	127	51	38	33	14	82	300
1.5	60	16	170	45	68	39	0	76.8	420
1.2	50	17	160	53	40	30	14	78	310
1.2	43	14	170	56	41	30	10	79.6	390
1.2	53	18	160	52	41	30	6.8	80	390
1.0	41.8	16.7	93.7	33.3	55.7	50	14.4	87.3	375
1.1	44	15	169	57	36	28	0	80	560
1.0	80	32	120	48	22	20	0		460
1.0	56	22	132	53	28	25	0	78	375

Product (Manufacturer)	Vitamins								
	A (IU)	D (IU)	E (IU)	K (µg)	C (mg)	Thiamine (mg)	Riboflavin (mg)	Niacin (mg)	B₆ (mg)
Accupep HPF (SM)	3125	250	30	35	60	1.13	1.28	15	1.5
AltraQ (R)	3998	267	30	54	200	2.0	2.3	27	2.7
Amin-Aid (M)	—	—	—	—	—	—	—	—	—
Attain (SM)	4000	320	48	80	144	1.8	2.04	24	2.4
Compleat Modified (S)	3300	270	30	67	60	1.5	1.7	20	2.0
Compleat Regular (S)	3300	270	30	67	60	1.5	1.7	20	2.0
Comply (SM)	5000	400	60	50	180	2.25	2.55	30	3
Criticare HN (MJ)	2600	210	40	132	159	2	2.3	26	2.6
Deliver 2.0	5000	400	75	250	300	3.8	4.3	50	5.0
Ensure (R)	2650	212	23.9	43	159	1.6	1.9	21.2	2.2
Ensure HN (R)	3811	303	34.1	61	228	1.8	2.0	22.8	2.3
Ensure Plus (R)	3519	282	31.7	57	212	2.2	2.4	28.2	2.9
Ensure Plus HN (R)	5280	423	47.6	85	317	3.2	3.6	42.3	4.4
Ensure with Fiber (R)	3595	288	32.4	58	216	1.7	1.9	21.6	2.2
Entrition .5 (C)	1250	100	15	50	75	0.75	0.85	10	1.0
Entrition 1.0 (C)	2500	200	30	100	150	1.5	1.7	20	2.0
Entrition HN (C)	3845	308	23	54	116	1.7	2.0	23.1	2.31
Entrition RDA (C)	3333	267	30	67	100	1.5	1.7	20	2.0
Entrition with Fiber (C)	3333	267	30	67	120	1.5	1.7	20	2.0
Entrition 1.5 (C)	5000	400	45	100	180	2.25	2.55	30	3.0
Fiberlan (EP)	4000	320	24	80	144	1.2	1.36	16	1.6
Fibersource (S)	3300	270	30	48	200	2	2.3	27	2.7
Fibersource HN (S)	3300	270	30	48	200	2.0	2.3	27	2.7
Glucerna (R)	3520	282	31.7	57	212	1.6	1.8	21.2	2.2
Hepatic Aid II (M)	—	—	—	—	—	—	—	—	—
Immun-Aid (M)	2666	200	50	40	60	.76	.86	10	10
Impact (S)	6700	270	60	67	80	2.0	1.7	20	1.5

Vitamins					Minerals				
Folic Acid (µg)	Pantothenic Acid (mg)	B_{12} (µg)	Biotin (µg)	Choline (mg)	Sodium (mg)	Potassium (mg)	Chloride (mg)	Calcium (mg)	Phosphorus (mg)
300	7.5	4.5	230	200	680	1150	1064	625	625
267	14	8.0	400	400	1000	1200	1300	733	733
—	—	—	—	—	173	117	—	—	—
360	12	6.0	240	400	805	1600	1346	960	800
270	6.7	6.0	200	200	1000	1400	1100	670	870
270	6.7	6.0	200	200	1300	1400	1100	670	1200
600	15	9.0	450	450	1100	1850	1700	1000	1000
210	13.2	7.9	159	260	630	1320	1060	530	530
400	25	15	300	500	800	1700	1200	1000	1000
424	10.6	6.4	320	320	846	1564	1312	530	530
455	11.4	6.9	350	460	802	1564	1326	758	758
563	14.4	8.5	430	430	1055	1943	1904	704	704
845	21.2	12.7	640	640	1184	1818	1606	1056	1056
432	10.8	6.5	330	440	846	1693	1351	719	719
200	5	3	150	200	350	600	500	250	250
400	10	6	300	400	700	1200	1000	500	500
460	11.5	6.92	346	346	845	1529	1540	770	770
300	10	6	300	267	800	1333	1333	667	667
300	10	6	300	400	550	1250	1000	400	400
450	15	9	450	650	750	1850	1500	1000	1000
320	8	4.8	240	300	920	1560	1365	800	800
270	13	8	400	330	870	1800	1100	670	670
270	13	8	400	330	870	1800	1100	670	670
423	10.6	6.4	317	423	928	1561	1435	704	704
—	—	—	—	—	288	196	—	—	—
200	5.0	3	150	210	580	1060	888	500	500
400	6.7	8.0	200	270	1100	1300	1300	800	800

(Continued.)

APPENDIX 24–1 (cont.).

Product (Manufacturer)	Minerals							
	Magnesium (mg)	Iron (mg)	Iodine (μg)	Copper (mg)	Zinc (mg)	Manganese (mg)	Selenium (mg)	Molybdenum (μg)
Accupep HPF (SM)	250	11.3	100	1.5	15	2.5	—	—
AlitraQ (R)	267	15	100	1.4	20	3.4	50	110
Amin-Aid (M)	—	—	—	—	—	—	—	—
Attain (SM)	320	14.4	120	1.6	24	4	100	150
Compleat Modified (S)	270	12	100	1.3	15	2.7	67	200
Compleat Regular (S)	270	12	100	1.3	15	2.7	67	200
Comply (SM)	400	18	150	2.0	30	4.5	—	—
Criticare HN (MJ)	210	9.5	79	1.1	10.6	2.6	—	—
Deliver 2.0	400	18	150	2.0	20	3.0	100	250
Ensure (R)	212	9.6	80	1.1	12	2.7	38	80
Ensure HN (R)	303	13.7	114	1.6	17.1	3.8	53	76
Ensure Plus (R)	282	12.7	106	1.5	15.9	3.6	50	106
Ensure Plus HN (R)	423	19.1	159	2.2	23.8	5.3	74	159
Ensure with Fiber (R)	288	13	108	1.5	16.2	3.6	51	108
Entrition .5 (C)	100	4.5	37.5	0.5	3.75	1.0	—	—
Entrition 1.0 (C)	200	9	75	1.0	7.5	2.0	—	—
Entrition HN (C)	308	13.9	116	1.54	11.6	1.54	—	—
Entrition RDA (C)	267	12	100	1.33	11.3	2.0	100	200
Entrition with Fiber (C)	320	12	100	1.4	15	2.7	60	120
Entrition 1.5 (C)	450	18	150	2	20	4.0	60	120
Fiberlan (EP)	320	14.4	120	1.6	12	2.0	120	240
Fibersource (S)	270	12	100	1.3	17	3.3	100	200
Fibersource HN (S)	270	12	100	1.3	17	3.3	100	200
Glucerna (R)	282	12.7	106	1.5	15.9	3.6	50	106
Hepatic Aid II (M)	—	—	—	—	—	—	—	—
Immun-Aid (M)	200	9.0	76	2.0	26	2.6	100	76
Impact (S)	270	12.0	100	1.7	15	2.0	100	200

NA = not available.

Chromium (μg)	Taurine (mg)	L-Carnitine (mg)	Volume to Meet (100% US RDA)	Form
—	—	—	1600	Powder
74	200	100	1500	Powder
—	—	—	NA†	Powder
100	—	—	1250	Liquid/prefilled
100	—	—	1500	Liquid/prefilled
100	—	—	1500	Liquid/prefilled
—	—	—	1000	Liquid/prefilled
—	—	—	1890	Liquid
100	—	—	1000	Liquid
53	—	—	1887	Liquid
114	—	—	1391	Liquid
71	—	—	1420	Liquid
106	—	—	937	Liquid
72	—	—	1391	Liquid
—	—	—	4000	Prefilled
—	—	—	2000	Prefilled
—	—	—	1300	Prefilled
100	—	—	1500	Prefilled
60	—	—	1500	Prefilled
60	—	—	1000	Prefilled
120	—	—	1250	Liquid/prefilled
100	—	—	1500	Liquid/prefilled
100	—	—	1500	Liquid/prefilled
71	106	141	1422	Liquid
—	—	—	NA	Powder
76	200	100	2000	Powder
100	—	—	1500	Liquid

(Continued.)

Product (Manufacturer)	Protein Source	Carbohydrate Source	Fat Source
Impact with Fiber (S)	Sodium and calcium casinates, L-arginine	Hydrolyzed cornstarch, Soy polysaccharide, modified guar	Structured lipids (60%), menhaden oil (40%)
Introlan (EP)	Sodium and calcium caseinates	Maltodextrin	MCT (50%), corn oil (50%)
Introlite (R)	Sodium and calcium caseinates, soy protein isolate	Hydrolyzed cornstarch	MCT (50%), corn oil (50%)
Isocal (MJ)	Sodium and calcium caseinates, soy protein isolate	Maltodextrin	Soy oil (80%), MCT oil (20%)
Isocal HN (MJ)	Sodium and calcium caseinates, soy protein isolate	Maltodextrin	Soy oil (60%), MCT oil (40%)
Isolan (EP)	Sodium and calcium caseinates	Maltodextrin	Corn oil (50%), MCT (50%)
Isosource (S)	Sodium and calcium caseinates, soy protein isolate	Hydrolyzed cornstarch	MCT (50%), canola oil (50%)
Isosource HN (S)	Sodium and calcium caseinates, soy protein isolate	Hydrolyzed cornstarch	MCT (50%), canola oil (50%)
Isotein HN (S)	Delactosed lactalbumin	Hydrolyzed cornstarch, fructose	Partially hydrogenated soybean oil (80%), MCT (20%)
Jevity (R)	Sodium and calcium caseinates	Hydrolyzed cornstarch, soy polysaccharide	MCT (50%), corn oil (50%)
Lipisorb (MJ)	Sodium and calcium caseinates	Maltodextrin, sucrose	MCT oil (85%), soy oil (15%)
Magnacal (SM)	Sodium and calcium caseinates	Maltodextrin, sucrose	Soy oil
Nepro (R)	Calcium, sodium, and magnesium caseinates	Hydrolyzed cornstarch, sucrose	High-oleic safflower oil, soy oil
Nitrolan (EP)	Sodium and calcium caseinates	Maltodextrin	Corn oil (50%), MCT (50%)
Nutren 1.0 (C)	Potassium and calcium caseinates	Maltodextrin, corn syrup solids	Canola oil (52%), MCT (24%), corn oil
Nutren 1.0 with Fiber (C)	Potassium and calcium caseinates	Maltodextrin, corn syrup solids, soy polysaccharide	Canola oil (52%), MCT (24%), corn oil
Nutren 1.5 (C)	Potassium and calcium caseinates	Maltodextrin	MCT (48%), canola oil (34%), corn oil
Nutren 2.0 (C)	Potassium and calcium caseinates	Corn syrup solids, maltodextrin, sucrose	MCT (75%), canola oil (15%), corn oil (4%), lecithin
Nutrilan (EP)	Calcium and sodium caseinates	Maltodextrin, sucrose, glucose syrup	Corn oil (80%), MCT (20%)
Nutrivent (C)	Calcium and potassium caseinates	Maltodextrin, sucrose	Canola oil, MCT (40%), corn oil
Osmolite (R)	Sodium and calcium caseinates, soy protein isolate	Glucose polymers	MCT (50%), corn oil, soy oil
Osmolite HN (R)	Sodium and calcium caseinates, soy protein isolate	Glucose polymers	MCT (50%), corn oil, soy oil
Peptamen (C)	Hydrolyzed whey protein	Maltodextrin, starch, guar gum	MCT (70%), sunflower oil (17%), 8% residual milk fat
Perative (R)	Partially hydrolyzed sodium caseinate, lactalbumin hydrolysate, L-arginine	Hydrolyzed cornstarch	Canola oil (40%), MCT (40%), corn oil (20%)
Pre-Attain (SM)	Sodium caseinate	Maltodextrin	Corn oil
Profiber (SM)	Sodium caseinate	Hydrolyzed cornstarch, soy polysaccharide	Corn oil

Caloric Density (Calorie/mL)	Protein		Carbohydrate		Fat		Total Dietary Fiber (g)	H$_2$O (%)	Osmolality (mOsm/kg)
	g	Calories (%)	g	Calories (%)	g	Calories (%)			
1.0	56	22	140	53	28	25	10	86.8	375
.53	22.5	17	70	53	18	30	0	91.5	150
.53	22.2	16.7	70.5	53.3	18.4	30	0	92	200
1.06	34	13	135	56	44	37	0	84	270
1.06	44	17	123	46	45	37	0	84	270
1.06	40	15	144	54	36	31	0	81.5	300
1.2	43	14	170	56	41	30	0	80.7	360
1.2	53	18	160	52	41	30	0	80.7	330
1.2	68	23	160	52	34	25	0	85.6	300
1.06	44.4	16.7	151.7	53.3	36.8	30	14.4	83.3	310
1.35	57	17	161	48	57	35	0	80	630
2.0	70	14	250	50	80	36	0	83	590
2.0	69.9	14	215.2	43	95.6	43	0	70	635
1.24	60	19	160	52	40	29	0	77	310
1.0	40	16	127	51	38	33	0	86	300
1.0	40	16	127	51	38	33	14	86	303
1.5	60	16	170	45	68	39	0	78	410
2.0	80	16	196	39	106	45	0	70	710
1.06	38	14	143	54	37	31	0	82	320
1.5	68	18	100.8	27	94.8	55	0	78	450
1.06	37.2	14	145	54.6	38.5	31.4	0	84	300
1.06	44.4	16.7	141.2	53.3	36.8	30	0	84.1	300
1.0	40	16	127.2	51	39.2	33	0	84	270
1.3	66.6	20.5	177.2	54.5	37.4	25	0	80	425
0.5	20	16	60	48	20	36	0	93	150
1.0	40	16	132	48	40	36	12	84.5	300

(Continued.)

Product (Manufacturer)	Vitamins								
	A (IU)	D (IU)	E (IU)	K (μg)	C (mg)	Thiamine (mg)	Riboflavin (mg)	Niacin (mg)	B_6 (mg)
Impact with Fiber (S)	6700	270	60	67	80	2.0	1.7	20	1.5
Introlan (EP)	2500	200	15	50	144	0.75	0.85	10	1.0
Introlite (R)	3788	304	34.1	61	228	1.71	1.94	22.8	2.28
Isocal (M)	2700	210	40	132	159	2.0	2.3	26	2.6
Isocal HN (MJ)	4200	340	63	106	250	3.2	3.6	42	4.2
Isolan (EP)	4000	320	24	80	144	1.2	1.36	16	1.6
Isosource (S)	3300	270	48	30	200	2.0	2.3	27	2.7
Isosource HN (S)	3300	270	48	30	200	2.0	2.3	27	2.7
Isotein HN (S)	2800	230	17	56	51	1.3	1.5	11	1.7
Jevity (R)	3786	305	343	61.5	227	1.74	1.95	22.7	2.29
Lipisorb (MJ)	3750	300	22.5	60	50	1.17	1.29	15	1.5
Magnacal (SM)	5000	400	60	300	300	3.0	3.4	40	4.0
Nepro (R)	1053	84	47.6	84	105	2.53	2.9	33.7	8.7
Nitrolan (EP)	4000	320	24	80	144	1.2	1.36	16	1.6
Nutren 1.0 (C)	5000	280	28	80	140	2.0	2.4	28	4
Nutren 1.0 with Fiber (C)	5000	280	28	80	140	2	2.4	28	4
Nutren 1.5 (C)	7600	400	40	120	210	3	3.4	40	6
Nutren 2.0 (C)	10,000	560	56	160	280	4	4.8	56	8
Nutrilan (EP)	3165	253	25	38	151	1.6	1.81	21.1	2.1
Nutrivent (C)	7500	420	42	120	208	3	3.6	42	6
Osmolite (R)	2650	212	23.9	42	159	1.59	1.8	21.2	2.12
Osmolite HN (R)	3786	303	34	61.5	228	1.71	1.94	22.8	2.28
Peptamen (C)	5000	280	28	80	140	2	2.4	28	4
Perative (R)	8658	346	39	69	260	1.95	2.2	26	2.56
Pre-Attain (SM)	3125	250	30	35	60	1.13	1.28	15	1.5
Profiber (SM)	3334	267	40	50	120	1.5	1.7	20	2

	Vitamins					Minerals			
Folic Acid (μg)	Pantothenic Acid (mg)	B$_{12}$ (μg)	Biotin (μg)	Choline (mg)	Sodium (mg)	Potassium (mg)	Chloride (mg)	Calcium (mg)	Phosphorus (mg)
400	6.7	8.0	200	270	1100	1300	1300	800	800
200	5.0	3.0	150	150	345	585	624	500	500
455	11.4	6.82	341	454	930	1590	1440	758	758
210	13.2	7.9	159	260	530	1320	1060	630	530
340	21	12.7	250	420	930	1610	1440	850	850
320	8	4.8	240	300	690	1170	1085	800	800
270	13	8.0	400	330	730	1700	1100	670	670
270	13	8.0	400	330	730	1700	1100	670	670
230	5.6	3.4	170	56	620	1100	960	560	560
458	11.4	7.2	343	454	933	1567	1314	912	759
300	7.5	4.5	225	342	733	1250	1167	700	700
400	10	12	300	500	1000	1250	950	1000	1000
1053	16.8	10.1	510	640	829	1057	1011	1373	686
320	8	4.8	240	300	690	1170	1085	800	800
540	14	8	400	450	500	1250	1000	700	700
540	14	8	400	450	500	1250	1000	700	700
800	20	12	600	680	750	1880	1500	1040	1040
1080	28	16	800	900	1000	2500	2000	1400	1400
253	6.33	6.33	190	211	633	1057	728	630	630
810	21	12	600	676	750	2240	1500	1200	1200
424	10.6	6.36	318	318	636	1018	848	530	530
455	11.4	6.75	341	455	933	1567	1442	758	758
540	14	8	400	448	500	1252	1000	800	700
519	13	7.79	390	519	1039	1732	1645	866	866
300	7.5	4.5	230	200	340	575	531	313	313
400	10	6	300	300	730	1250	1200	667	667

(Continued.)

	Minerals							
Product (Manufacturer)	Magnesium (mg)	Iron (mg)	Iodine (μg)	Copper (mg)	Zinc (mg)	Manganese (mg)	Selenium (mg)	Molybdenum (μg)
Impact with Fiber (S)	270	12.0	100	1.7	15	2.0	100	200
Introlan (EP)	200	9.0	7.5	1.0	7.5	1.0	70	140
Introlite (R)	304	13.7	114	1.52	17.1	3.79	53	114
Isocal (MJ)	210	9.5	79	1.1	10.6	1.6	53	131
Isocal HN (MJ)	340	15.2	127	1.7	16.9	2.5	85	210
Isolan (EP)	320	14.4	120	1.6	12	2.0	120	240
Isosource (S)	270	12	100	1.3	17	3.3	100	200
Isosource HN (S)	270	12	100	1.3	17	3.3	100	200
Isotein HN (S)	230	10	85	1.1	8.5	2.3	85	170
Jevity (R)	303	13.7	114	1.53	17	3.77	53	114
Lipisorb (MJ)	200	9.2	75	.99	9.99	1.5	—	—
Magnacal (SM)	400	18	150	2.0	30	5	—	—
Nepro (R)	211	18.9	158	2.1	23.6	5.3	101	—
Nitrolan (EP)	320	14.4	120	1.6	12	2	120	240
Nutren 1.0 (C)	340	12	100	1.4	14	2.7	40	120
Nutren 1.0 with Fiber (C)	340	12	100	1.4	14	2.7	40	120
Nutren 1.5 (C)	500	18	152	2.0	20	4	60	180
Nutren 2.0 (C)	680	24	200	2.8	28	5.2	—	—
Nutrilan (EP)	253	11.4	126.6	1.27	9.5	2	—	—
Nutrivent (C)	600	18	150	2.1	21	4	60	180
Osmolite (R)	212	9.5	79.5	1.06	12.2	2.65	37	80
Osmolite HN (R)	303	13.5	114	1.52	17	3.78	53	114
Peptamen (C)	400	12	100	1.4	14	2.7	40	120
Perative (R)	346	15.6	130	1.7	19.5	4.3	61	130
Pre-Attain (SM)	250	11.3	100	1.5	15	2.5	—	—
Profiber (SM)	267	12	100	1.5	20	3	80	200

Chromium (μg)	Taurine (mg)	L-Carnitine (mg)	Volume to Meet (100% US RDA)	Form
100	—	—	1500	Liquid
70	—	—	2000	Prefilled
76	—	—	1321	Prefilled
53	—	—	1890	Liquid/prefilled
85	—	—	1179	Liquid/prefilled
120	—	—	1250	Liquid/prefilled
100	—	—	1500	Liquid/prefilled
100	161	263	1500	Liquid/prefilled
85	—	—	1770	Powder
76	114	114	1321	Liquid/prefilled
—	—	—	1920	Powder/liquid
—	—	—	1000	Liquid
—	—	—	NA	Liquid
120	—	—	1250	Liquid/prefilled
40	80	80	1500	Liquid
40	80	80	1500	Liquid
60	120	120	1000	Liquid
—	—	—	750	Liquid
—	—	—	1585	Liquid
60	120	120	1000	Liquid
53	79.5	79.5	1887	Liquid/prefilled
76	114	114	1321	Liquid/prefilled
40	80	80	1500	Liquid/prefilled
87	130	130	1155	Liquid
—	—	—	1600	Liquid/prefilled
80	—	—	1500	Liquid/prefilled

(Continued.)

Product (Manufacturer)	Protein Source	Carbohydrate Source	Fat Source
Promote (R)	Sodium and calcium caseinates, soy protein isolate	Hydrolyzed cornstarch, sucrose	High-oleic safflower oil (50%), canola oil (30%), MCT (20%)
Pulmocare (R)	Sodium and calcium caseinates	Sucrose, hydrolyzed cornstarch	Corn oil
Reabilan (EP)	Hydrolyzed casein and whey	Maltodextrin, tapioca	MCT (14%), soy oil, oneothera biennis oil
Reabilan HN (EP)	Hydrolyzed casein and whey	Maltodextrin, tapioca	MCT (40%), soy oil, oneothera biennis oil
Replete (C)	Calcium and potassium caseinates	Maltodextrin, corn syrup solids	Canola oil (75%), MCT (25%)
Replete—Oral (C)	Potassium and calcium caseinates	Maltodextrin, sucrose	Corn oil
Replete with Fiber (C)	Calcium and potassium caseinates	Maltodextrin, corn syrup solids, soy polysaccharide	Canola oil (75%), MCT (25%)
Resource (S)	Sodium and calcium caseinates, soy protein isolate	Hydrolyzed cornstarch, sugar	Corn oil
Resource Plus (S)	Sodium and calcium caseinates, soy protein isolate	Hydrolyzed cornstarch, sugar	Corn oil
Suplena (R)	Sodium and calcium caseinates	Hydrolyzed cornstarch, sucrose	High-oleic safflower oil, soy oil
Sustacal (MJ)	Sodium and calcium caseinates, soy protein isolate	Sugar, corn syrup	Partially hydrogenated soy oil
Sustacal 8.8 (MJ)	Casein, soy protein isolate	Corn syrup, sugar	Soy oil
Sustacal Plus (MJ)	Sodium and calcium caseinates	Corn syrup, sugar	Corn oil
Sustacal with Fiber (MJ)	Sodium and calcium caseinates, soy protein isolate	Maltodextrin, sugar, soy polysaccharide	Corn oil
Tolerex (S)	Crystalline amino acids	Glucose oligosaccharides	Safflower oil
Traumacal (MJ)	Sodium and calcium caseinates	Corn syrup, sugar	Soy oil (70%), MCT (30%)
Travasorb Hepatic (C)	Crystalline amino acids (50% BCAA)	Glucose oligosaccharides, sucrose	MCT (70%), sunflower oil (30%)
Travasorb HN (C)	Hydrolyzed lactalbumin	Glucose oligosaccharides	MCT (60%), sunflower oil (40%)
Travasorb MCT (C)	Lactalbumin, sodium and potassium caseinates	Corn syrup solids	MCT (80%), sunflower oil (20%)
Travasorb Renal (C)	Crystalline amino acids	Glucose oligosaccharides	MCT (70%), sunflower oil (30%)
Travasorb STD (C)	Hydrolyzed lactalbumin	Glucose oligosaccharides	MCT (60%), sunflower oil (40%)
TwoCal HN (R)	Sodium and calcium caseinates	Hydrolyzed cornstarch, sucrose	Corn oil (80%), MCT (20%)
Ultracal (MJ)	Sodium and calcium caseinates	Maltodextrin, oat fiber, soy fiber	Canola oil (60%), MCT (40%)
Ultralan (EP)	Sodium and calcium caseinates	Maltodextrin	MCT (50%), corn oil (50%)
Vital High Nitrogen	Partially hydrolyzed whey, meat and soy, l-amino acids	Hydrolyzed cornstarch, sucrose	Safflower oil (55%), MCT (45%)
Vitaneed (SM)	Pureed beef, sodium and calcium caseinates	Maltodextrin, soy fiber, pureed vegetables and fruit	Corn oil, beef fat
Vivonex TEN (S)	Crystalline amino acids	Maltodextrin, modified starch	Safflower oil

Caloric Density (Calorie/mL)	Protein		Carbohydrate		Fat		Total Dietary Fiber (g)	H_2O (%)	Osmolality (mOsm/kg)
	g	Calories (%)	g	Calories (%)	g	Calories (%)			
1.0	62.4	25	130	53	26	23	0	84	350
1.5	62.6	16.7	105.7	28.1	92.1	55.2	0	78.6	520
1.0	31.5	12.5	131.5	52.5	39	35	0	85	350
1.33	58	17.5	157.7	47.5	51.9	35	0	80	490
1.0	62.5	25	113	45	34	30	0	84.4	290
1.0	62.5	25	113	45	33	30	0	86	350
1.0	62.5	25	113	45	34	30	14	84	300
1.06	37	14	140	54	37	32	0	84.2	430
1.5	55	15	200	53	53	32	0	76.4	600
2.0	29.8	6	255.2	51	95.6	43	0	71	615
1.06	61	24	140	55	23	21	0	85	650
1.06	37	14	148	56	35	30	0	85	500
1.52	61	16	190	50	58	34	0	78	670
1.06	46	17	140	53	35	30	5.9	84	480
1.0	21	8	230	91		1	0	86	550
1.5	83	22	145	38	68	40	0	78	490
1.1	29.4	10.6	215.2	77.4	14.7	12	0	82	600
1.0	45	18	175	70	13.5	12	0	85.5	560
1.0	49.6	19.8	122.8	49	33	31	0	86	312
1.35	22.9	6.7	270.5	80	17.7	13.3	0	77	590
1.0	30	12	189.9	76	13.5	12	0	85.5	560
2.0	83.7	16.7	217.3	43.2	90.9	40.1	0	71.2	690
1.06	44	17	123	46	45	37	14.4	85	310
1.5	60	16	202	54	50	30	0	75.5	610
1.0	41.7	16.7	184.7	73.9	10.8	9.4	0	86.7	500
1.0	40	16	128	48	40	36	8.0	84.5	300
1.0	38	15	210	82	2.8	3	0	85	630

(Continued.)

Product (Manufacturer)	Vitamins								
	A (IU)	D (IU)	E (IU)	K (μg)	C (mg)	Thiamine (mg)	Riboflavin (mg)	Niacin (mg)	B$_6$ (mg)
Promote (R)	4000	320	36	64	240	1.8	2.1	24	2.4
Pulmocare (R)	5280	423	47.6	85	317	3.17	3.6	42.3	4.23
Reabilan (EP)	2667	200	14.9	50	100	1.49	1.49	20	1.99
Reabilan HN (EP)	3541	140	20	67	133	1.99	1.99	27	2.58
Replete (C)	7333	400	60	80	340	3	2.4	28	4
Replete—Oral (C)	5000	280	28	80	140	2	2.4	28	4
Replete with Fiber (C)	7333	400	60	80	340	3	2.4	28	4
Resource (S)	2600	210	24	38	160	1.6	1.8	21	2.1
Resource Plus (S)	3700	290	33	55	160	2.7	2.7	32	3.2
Suplena (R)	1053	84	48	84	105	2.53	2.9	33.7	8.7
Sustacal (MJ)	4700	380	28	240	56	1.4	1.7	20	2
Sustacal 8.8 (MJ)	2700	210	40	66	97	1.6	1.8	21	2.1
Sustacal Plus (MJ)	4200	340	25	210	76	1.9	2.2	25	2.5
Sustacal with Fiber (MJ)	3500	420	21	97	127	1.6	1.8	21	2.1
Tolerex (S)	2800	220	17	37	33	0.8	0.9	11	1.1
Traumacal (MJ)	2500	200	38	125	150	1.9	2.2	25	2.5
Travasorb Hepatic (C)	735	197	10	51.5	44.1	0.69	0.78	8.82	1.07
Travasorb HN (C)	2455	201	15	75	45	0.75	0.84	10	1.0
Travasorb MCT (C)	2500	200	30	75	150	1.5	1.7	20	2
Travasorb Renal (C)	—	—	—	—	42.6	0.71	0.80	9.49	4.84
Travasorb STD (C)	2499	201	15	75	45	0.75	0.84	10	1
TwoCal HN (R)	5264	422	47	86	316	252	2.86	33.6	3.36
Ultracal (MJ)	4200	340	63	106	250	3.2	3.6	42	4.2
Ultralan (EP)	5000	400	30	125	180	1.5	1.7	20	2
Vital High Nitrogen	3333	267	30	54	200	2.0	2.27	26.7	2.67
Vitaneed (SM)	3334	267	40	50	120	1.5	1.7	20	2
Vivonex TEN (S)	2500	200	15	22.3	60	1.5	1.7	20	2

	Vitamins					Minerals			
Folic Acid (μg)	Pantothenic Acid (mg)	B₁₂ (μg)	Biotin (μg)	Choline (mg)	Sodium (mg)	Potassium (mg)	Chloride (mg)	Calcium (mg)	Phosphorus (mg)
480	12	7.2	360	480	928	1980	1263	960	960
845	2.12	12.7	634	634	1311	1733	1688	1056	1056
251	4.98	1.99	99	200	699	1245	1970	499	499
333	6.66	2.98	133	266	1000	1661	2464	451	499
540	14	8	400	450	500	1560	1000	1000	1000
540	14	8	400	450	500	1560	1000	800	720
540	14	8	400	450	500	1560	1000	1000	1000
210	5.3	6.3	160	530	890	1600	1000	530	530
310	8.7	9.4	240	520	1100	2100	1600	620	620
1053	16.8	10.1	510	640	783	1116	926	1385	728
380	9.7	5.6	280	240	930	2100	1480	1010	930
420	10.6	6.3	320	320	850	1610	1440	630	530
510	12.7	7.6	380	210	850	1480	1270	850	850
420	10.6	6.3	320	—	720	1390	1390	840	700
220	5.6	3.3	170	41	470	1200	950	560	560
200	12.5	7.5	150	250	1200	1400	1600	750	750
197	5	2.94	147	197	235	892	697	491	491
201	5.1	3.0	150	144	921	1170	1365	501	501
200	5	6	150	225	350	1000	1215	500	500
47.6	2.62	—	142.5	190.1	—	—	—	—	—
201	5.1	3	150	144	921	1170	1500	501	501
674	16.8	10.2	506	632	1306	2442	1642	1052	1052
340	21	12.7	250	420	930	1610	1444	850	850
400	10	6	300	375	1035	1755	1680	1000	1000
533	13.3	8	400	400	567	1400	1033	667	667
400	10	6	300	300	680	1250	1000	667	667
400	10	6	300	73.7	460	782	819	500	500

(Continued.)

Product (Manufacturer)	Minerals							
	Magnesium (mg)	Iron (mg)	Iodine (μg)	Copper (mg)	Zinc (mg)	Manganese (mg)	Selenium (mg)	Molybdenum (μg)
Promote (R)	320	14.4	120	1.6	18	4	56	120
Pulmocare (R)	423	19.1	159	2.12	23.8	5.28	74	159
Reabilan (EP)	251	10	75	1.59	10	1.99	51	—
Reabilan HN (EP)	331	13.3	101	1.27	13.3	2.66	67	—
Replete (C)	400	18	160	2	24	4	100	220
Replete—Oral (C)	400	12	100	1.4	14	2.7	—	—
Replete with Fiber (C)	400	18	160	2	24	4	100	220
Resource (S)	210	9.5	79	1.1	16	2.1	—	—
Resource Plus (S)	310	14	110	1.6	24	2.1	—	—
Suplena (R)	211	18.9	158	2.1	23.6	5.3	76	—
Sustacal (MJ)	380	16.9	139	2	13.9	2.8	—	—
Sustacal 8.8 (MJ)	210	9.7	79	1.1	11	1.6	53	131
Sustacal Plus (MJ)	340	15.2	127	1.7	12.7	2.5	59	85
Sustacal with Fiber (MJ)	280	12.7	105	1.4	13.9	1.8	—	—
Tolerex (S)	220	10	83	1.1	8.3	1.6	83	83
Traumacal (MJ)	200	9	75	1.5	15	2.5	—	—
Travasorb Hepatic (C)	197	8.8	73.5	0.98	7.35	1.23	—	—
Travasorb HN (C)	201	9	75	0.99	7.5	1.26	—	—
Travasorb MCT (C)	200	9	75	1.0	15	2	—	—
Travasorb Renal (C)	—	—	—	—	—	—	—	—
Travasorb STD (C)	201	9	75	0.99	7.5	1.26	—	—
TwoCal HN (R)	422	19	158	2.1	23.7	5.26	74	158
Ultracal (MJ)	340	15.2	127	1.7	16.9	2.5	85	210
Ultralan (EP)	400	18	150	2	15	2.5	120	240
Vital High Nitrogen	267	12	100	1.3	15	3.33	47	100
Vitaneed (SM)	267	12	100	1.5	20	3	—	—
Vivonex TEN (S)	200	9	75	1.0	10	0.94	50	50

Chromium (μg)	Taurine (mg)	L-Carnitine (mg)	Volume to Meet (100% US RDA)	Form
80	120	120	1250	Liquid
106	—	—	947	Liquid
83	—	—	3000	Liquid
83	189	—	2857	Liquid
40	100	100	1000	Liquid
—	—	—	1500	Liquid
140	100	100	1000	Liquid
—	—	—	1890	Liquid/powder
—	—	—	1600	Liquid
—	—	—	NA	Liquid
—	—	—	1060	Liquid
53	—	—	1890	Liquid
85	—	—	1420	Liquid
—	—	—	1420	Liquid
28	—	—	3160	Powder
—	—	—	2000	Liquid
—	—	—	2060	Liquid
—	—	—	2000	Powder
—	—	—	2000	Powder
—	—	—	NA	Powder
—	—	—	2000	Powder
106	—	—	1180	Liquid
85	127	190	1180	Liquid/prefilled
120	—	—	1000	Prefilled
67	—	—	1500	Powder
—	—	—	1500	Liquid/prefilled
16.67	—	—	2000	Powder

25

Parenteral Nutrition Products

George Melnik, Pharm. D.

Nutrition support is currently in a dynamic phase fostered by knowledge from molecular biology. New discoveries in molecular biology may "improve the efficiency and effectiveness of nutrition support."[1, 2] This premise consists of three parts: alteration of the stress response, provision of tissue-specific fuels (arginine, glutamine, etc.), and administration of growth factors. Future clinical nutrition trials will evaluate all aspects of this approach. However, the evaluation of clinical data in controlled studies awaits the approval and availability of tissue-specific fuels and growth factors and elucidation of the stress response.

Contemporary nutrition support of catabolic, critically ill patients requires knowledge of clinical evaluations of commercial parenteral nutrition products. These studies have concentrated on the approach to nutrition support, maintenance of body cell mass, and total nitrogen balance. The intent of this chapter is to present clinical data on the current, commercially available paren-

teral nutritional products used in catabolic, critically ill patients. We evaluate clinical studies of branched-chain amino acids (BCAAs), essential amino acids (EAAs), fat emulsions and volume aspects of parenteral nutrition solutions. Recommendations are made for appropriate use of parenteral nutrition products from the available information and cost criteria analysis.

Classically, the primary purpose of nutritional support is maintenance of the body cell mass.

> The cellular mass of the body is a pure culture of living cells. It is that component of body composition containing the oxygen-exchanging, potassium-rich, glucose-oxidizing, work-performing tissue. It is that entity with which one is primarily concerned in the consideration of the working, energy-metabolizing portion of the human body in relation to its supporting structures. In any anthropometric consideration of the energy conversion of foodstuffs, oxygen requirement, carbon dioxide production, or work performance of the

body cell mass is the basic reference entity. The controlling functional definition of the body cell mass is that these tissues obtain, convert, and use chemical energy (from food or tissue catabolism) to perform chemical, mechanical, and thermal work. The body cell mass is the body "engine."[3]

Catabolism mobilizes precursors for acute-phase reactant production and energy for metabolic function from the same pool, the body cell mass.

STANDARD AMINO ACIDS

The technique of subclavian vein catheterization and intravenous parenteral nutrition developed by Dudrick, Wilmore, Vars, and Rhoads opened new

frontiers of patient care and scientific investigation. Standard amino acid (STD AA) formulations (Table 25–1) based on egg protein were the workhorse for providing nutrients during the formative years of parenteral nutrition. This approach sought to provide nutrients for total-body nitrogen utilization. STD AA solutions provide essential and nonessential amino acids. Scientific inquiries used nitrogen balance as the benchmark for measuring efficacy.

BRANCHED-CHAIN AMINO ACIDS

Investigations into the composition of amino acids mobilized from lean body tissue during catabolism revealed increased concentrations of BCAAs in the

TABLE 25–1.

Standard Amino Acid Formulations

	Aminosyn II	Travasol	FreAmine III	Novamine	Novamine
AA concentration	10%	10%	10%	11.40%	15%
N (g/100 mL)	1.53	1.65	1.53	1.8	2.37
EAA (mg/100 mL)					
Isoleucine	660	600	690	570	749
Leucine	1000	730	910	790	1040
Lysine	1050	580	730	900	1180
Methionine	172	400	530	570	749
Phenylalanine	298	560	560	790	1040
Threonine	400	420	400	570	749
Tryptophan	200	180	150	190	250
Valine	500	580	660	730	960
NEAA (mg/100 mL)					
Alanine	993	2070	710	1650	2170
Arginine	1018	1150	950	1120	1470
Histidine	300	480	280	680	894
Proline	722	680	1120	680	894
Serine	530	500	590	450	592
Tyrosine	270	40		30	39
Glycine	500	1030	1400	790	1040
Glutamic acid	738			570	749
Aspartic acid	700			330	434
Cysteine			<24		
Electrolytes (mEq/L)					
Sodium	45.3		10		
Chloride		40	<3		
Acetate	71.8	60	89	114	151
Phosphate (mM/L)			10		
mOsm/L	873	970	950	1057	1388
Cost/500 mL cost per average wholesale price	$74.81	$70.72	$64.52	$90.61	$123.32

AA = amino acid; EAA = essential amino acid; NEAA = nonessential amino acid.

peripheral vascular system.[5] Initial data indicated that BCAA infusions may be beneficial to catabolic patients. Clinical observations in small numbers of catabolic patients showed favorable nitrogen balance results with BCAA solutions.[6, 7] The distinctive feature of BCAA solutions is greater concentrations of isoleucine, leucine, and valine in comparison to STD AA Formulations. These products (Table 25–2) include an exclusive BCAA formula (BranchAmin) and formulas enriched with 45% BCAAs (FreAmine HBC and Aminosyn HBC).

Rigorous prospective, randomized clinical trials comparing BCAA with STD AA formulas were performed after the appearance of commercial BCAA solutions (Table 25–3). The first two comparative trials produced diametrically opposite results. The initial trial was in ten polytrauma, septic, postoperative patients in a randomized, crossover, double-blind study.[8] Patients received either STD AA or BCAA total parenteral nutrition (TPN) for 4 days and crossed over to the other TPN solution for 4 days. The study revealed no statistical difference in nitrogen balance. Furthermore, seven out of the ten patients expired after completion of the investigation. Power analysis revealed that not enough patients were enrolled to detect a significant difference. Another criticism was the short infusion time of 4 days for each TPN solution. Some investigators think that 5 or more days is necessary to obtain a new plateau of urea nitrogen excretion when nitrogen intake is significantly altered.[9]

The next investigation was a multicenter, prospective, randomized, double-blind comparison for a minimum of 7 days.[10] It enrolled 87 poly-

TABLE 25–2.

Branched-Chain Amino Acids

	BranchAmin	FreAmine HBC	Aminosyn HBC
AA concentration	4%	6.90%	7%
N (g/100 mL)	0.443	0.97	1.12
EAA (mg/100 mL)			
Isoleucine	1380	760	789
Leucine	1380	1370	1576
Lysine		410	265
Methionine		250	206
Phenylalanine		320	228
Threonine		200	272
Tryptophan		90	88
Valine	1240	880	789
NEAA (mg/100 mL)			
Alanine		400	660
Arginine		580	507
Histidine		160	154
Proline		630	448
Serine		330	221
Tyrosine			33
Glycine		330	660
Cysteine		<20	
Electrolytes (mEq/mL)			
Sodium		10	7
Chloride		<3	
Acetate		57	72
Phosphate (mM/L)			
mOsm/L	316	620	665
Cost/500 mL cost per average wholesale price	$93.60	$87.48	$62.21

AA = amino acid; EAA = essential amino acid; NEAA = nonessential amino acid.

TABLE 25–3.

Comparison of Branched-Chain Amino Acid Studies

Study	Patients	N	Methods	TPN* Regimen	Deaths	Results
Vander Woude[8]	Septic, postoperative polytrauma	10	Randomized Double-blind Crossover Exclusion criteria 4 days STD AA 4 days BCAA	30 kcal/kg/day CHO:fat ratio: 70:30	7	BCAA increased plasma leucine and valine and decreased BCAA extraction by skeletal muscle STD AA increased BCAA extraction by skeletal muscle N balance NS between groups
Cerra[10]	Septic, postoperative polytrauma	87	Prospective Randomized Double-blind Exclusion criteria TPN × 7 days minimum STD AA vs. BCAA	114 CHO kcal/g N/day 1–2 g PRO/kg/day No fat	NA*	N balance: BCAA > STD at mid and end $P < .05$
Lenssen[11]	Allogeneic bone marrow transplantation	40	Prospective Randomized Double-blind Isocaloric Isonitrogenous STD AA vs. BCAA	155%–165% of BEE 0.24 g N/kg IBW/day 25%–30% kcal as fat	NA	N balance NS between groups Urinary 3-methylhistidine-to-creatinine ratio at wk 4 greater in BCAA, $P = .045$
Zaing[12]	Elective subtotal gastrectomy, hemicolectomy	16	Prospective Randomized STD AA vs. BCAA	16 CHO kcal/kg/day 14 fat kcal/kg/day 0.2 g N/kg/day	NA	N balance NS between groups 3-Methylhistidine NS between groups
Okada[13]	Subtotal gastrectomy	160	Prospective Randomized Isocaloric Isonitrogenous STD AA vs. BCAA	40 CHO kcal/kg/day 1.5 g PRO/kg/day No fat	NA	N balance NS between groups Total protein NS between groups Retinol binding NS between groups Prealbumin NS between groups Transferrin NS between groups

Study	N	Design	Nutrition regimen	Groups	Results
Chiarla[14]	16	Prospective Randomized Exclusion criteria STD AA vs. BCAA	1700 CHO kcal/day 650 fat kcal/day 17 g N as STD AA 16 g N as BCAA	1 STD AA 2 BCAA	BCAA > STD AA fibrinogen, $P < .0001$ BCAA > STD AA α_1-antitrypsin, $P < .001$ BCAA decreased proteolysis and ureagenesis, $P < .001$ C-reactive protein NS between groups Ceruloplasm NS between groups Transferrin NS between groups Fibrin NS between groups STD AA > BCAA α_2-macroglobulin, $P < .0001$
Scholten[16]	20	Prospective Randomized Double-blind Crossover Exclusion criteria STD AA vs. BCAA	30 kcal/kg/day With/without 30% fat 1.48 g PRO/kg/day	NA	N balance NS between groups BCAA had higher plasma levels of leucine, isoleucine, and valine
Brown[17]	20	Prospective Randomized Exclusion criteria STD AA vs. BCAA	1.5–1.7 × BEE CHO, 6 mg/kg/min 215 mg N/kg/day 25% fat IV adjusted for N equilibrium	4 BCAA 3 STD AA	N balance NS between groups Somatomedin C/insulin-like growth factor ↑ NS Fibronectin NS between groups Thyroxine-binding prealbumin NS Retinol-binding protein BCAA day 21, $P < .05$, but not at the end of the study Length of stay: BCAA, 56 ± 29 days; STD AA, 52 ± 42 days, NS between groups
Kuhl[18]	20	Prospective Randomized Exclusion criteria STD AA vs. BCAA	30 non-PRO kcal/kg/day 40% fat 250 mg N/kg/day IV adjusted for N equilibrium	1 BCAA 2 STD AA	N balance NS between groups Somatomedin C/insulin-like growth factor ↑ NS Fibronectin BCAA day 14, $P < 0.05$, but not at end Thyroxine-binding prealbumin NS

(Continued.)

TABLE 25–3 (CONT.).

Study	Patients	N	Methods	TPN* Regimen	Deaths	Results
von Meyenfeldt[20]	Septic, metabolically stressed	101	Prospective Randomized Double-blind Exclusion criteria Isonitrogenous Isocaloric STD AA vs. BCAA	1.1–1.6 × BEE 170 mg N/kg/day	31 BCAA 24 STD AA	N balance NS between groups 3-Methylhistidine NS between groups
Bruzzone[15]	Septic, polytrauma	16	Prospective Randomized Exclusion criteria STD AA vs. BCAA	See the Chiarla study	2 BCAA 1 STD AA	See the Chiarla study Daily urea production/g proteolysis decreased with BCAA, $P < .0001$
Jiminez-Jiminez[19]	Septic, postoperative	80	Prospective Randomized Exclusion criteria STD AA vs. BCAA	1.4 g PRO/kg/day 150:1 cal:N ratio 40% fat	12 BCAA 15 STD AA	BCAA N balance better at 7 days, $P < .005$ N balance NS at 15 days BCAA retinol-binding protein at 15 days better, $P < .005$ STD AA 3-methylhistidine excretion greater at 7 and 15 days, $P < .005$
Vente[21]	Trauma, septic	101	Prospective Randomized Double-blind Isocaloric Isonitrogenous STD AA vs. BCAA	34 kcal/kg/day 0.17 g N/kg/day Fat, 2×/wk	NA	N balance NS between groups STD AA total protein better, $P < .05$

TPN = total parenteral nutrition; STD AA = standard amino acid; BCAA = branched-chain amino acid; CHO = carbohydrate; NA = not available; PRO = protein; BEE = basal energy expenditure IBW = ideal body weight; MSOF = multiple systems organ failure; BSA = body surface area.

trauma, septic, postoperative patients. The results showed a statistically significant difference in nitrogen balance for BCAA formulas at the midpoint and conclusion of the study. The number of mortalities was not mentioned. It appeared that a BCAA formula was superior to an STD AA formula for maintaining the body cell mass in catabolic, critically ill patients.

This finding was not supported in additional studies. Lenssen and colleagues' randomized, prospective comparison in 40 allogeneic bone marrow transplant patients showed no difference in nitrogen balance.[11] The urinary 3-methylhistidine-to-urine creatinine ratio was greater in the BCAA-fed group at the end of the study. The study had adequate power to detect a difference of 2.5 g in nitrogen during week 1 and 4.0 g during week 2 of the study. No mortality data were reported.

Jaing and associates' prospective, randomized comparison of 16 elective subtotal gastrectomy or hemicolectomy patients showed no difference in nitrogen balance or in 3-methylhistidine production. Mortality data were not provided.[12] This study was small and subject to type II error. However, it did establish a trend of no difference in nitrogen balance and mortality between the two solutions in a prospective, randomized, clinical comparison.

Okada et al. studied 160 subtotal gastrectomy patients in a prospective, randomized, isocaloric, isonitrogenous comparison.[13] There were no significant differences in nitrogen balance, total serum protein, retinol-binding protein, prealbumin, or transferrin concentrations. No mortality data were reported.

Chiarla et al. investigated 16 septic, trauma patients in a prospective randomized comparison.[14] BCAA produced significantly greater serum concentrations of fibrinogen and α_1-antitrypsin and a significant decrease in proteolysis, ureagenesis, C-reactive protein, cerulopasm, transferrin, and fibrin concentrations. STD AA produced sig-

nificantly greater α_2-macroglobulin concentrations. Two BCAA- and 1 STD AA–fed patients died during the study. Bruzzone et al. reanalyzed the data for urea production per gram of proteolysis and found a significant decrease in BCAA-fed patients.[15] The clinical outcome was not improved with BCAA.

Scholten and coworkers investigated 20 septic, trauma, postoperative patients with multisystems organ failure in a prospective, randomized, double-blind, crossover study. The results indicated no difference in nitrogen balance. Mortality data were not reported.[16]

Brown et al. studied 20 burn patients with greater than 10% body surface area involvement in a prospective, randomized manner.[17] The length of hospitalization was not significantly different between formulas, 56 ± 29 days for the BCAA group and 52 ± 42 days for STD AA. Retinol-binding protein was significantly greater for BCAA on day 21 but not at the end of the study. Nitrogen balance, somatomedin C/insulin-like growth factor 1, fibronectin, and thyroxine-binding prealbumin were not significantly different. Deaths occurred in four BCAA-fed patients and three STD AA–fed patients. The same group studied 20 trauma patients in an identical manner.[18] Fibronectin was greater at day 14 for BCAA but not at the end of the study. There were no significant differences in nitrogen balance, somatomedin C/insulin-like growth factor 1, and thyroxine-binding prealbumin between groups. One BCAA- and 2 STD AA–fed patients died during the study.

Jimenez-Jimenez et al. investigated 80 septic, postoperative patients in a prospective, randomized manner.[19] The results indicated that nitrogen balance at day 7 was significantly greater for BCAA but not different at the end of the study. Retinol-binding protein was significantly greater in the BCAA group. 3-Methylhistidine excretion was significantly greater in the STD AA–fed group at days 7 and 15. There were 12 BCAA- and 15 STD AA–fed patients who died.

von Meyenfeldt et al. studied 101 septic, metabolically stressed patients in a prospective, randomized, double-blind, isocaloric, isonitrogenous comparison.[20] The results showed no differences in nitrogen balance and 3-methylhistidine excretion between groups. The mortality was 31 in BCAA-fed and 24 in STD AA–fed patients. The same results were also published in a follow-up article. Power calculation indicated that the study had adequate power to eliminate a type II error.[21, 22]

Recommendations

Ten studies compared BCAA and STD AA in metabolically stressed patients. Only one study indicated a positive effect on nitrogen balance with BCAA. Other studies indicated differences in fibrinogen, α_1-antitrypsin, proteolysis, ureagenesis, and retinol-binding protein, but none of these findings correlated with improved survival. It is difficult to justify the higher cost for BCAA from these results.

There were 570 patients enrolled in the ten studies. Assuming that the average weight was 60 kg and each patient received 220 mg of nitrogen/kg/day (1.375 g protein/kg/day) for 15 days, the total cost for amino acid solutions was $951,860 for STD AA and $2,035,669 for BCAA if all patients received one or the other amino acid solutions. This analysis used the published average wholesale price of $64.52 for STD AA and $87.48 for BCAA (many centers purchase parenteral products for less than this amount, but it indicates the price differential between the solutions). Stated another way, it would be difficult to justify an additional $127.00 per patient per day or a total of $1,083,809 more for BCAA for the entire study period with no improvement in mortality or improvement in nitrogen balance. Therefore, until further controlled comparative studies lead to different conclusions, the recommendation is to use STD AA solutions in catabolic, critically ill patients.

RENAL FAILURE FORMULA

Rose et al. described essential amino acid (EAA) requirements for man.[23] Giordano[24] and Giovanetti and Maffiore[25] administered oral EAA diets to ambulatory patients with chronic renal failure. These data demonstrated an improvement in serum urea concentrations and suggested a possible benefit for the treatment of acute renal failure in hospitalized patients.

A review of nutritional support in patients with acute renal failure reveals a mortality rate between 60% and 90%.[26–31] The first use of parenteral EAAs (Table 25–4) in hospitalized patients with acute renal failure was published in 1973.[26] Initial studies in this area compared EAA TPN with hypertonic dextrose alone in a prospective, randomized, blinded manner (Table 25–5). Two of three studies reported that EAA increased the survival rate in medical and surgical patients during hemodialysis.[26, 28] The other study reported no difference in survival rate during hemodialysis.[27]

A more important issue compares EAA with STD AA in acute renal failure. A retrospective study by Freund et al. in 22 surgical patients who received STD AA TPN reported a mortality rate of 91%. The investigators concluded that EAA TPN "may be better in acute renal failure."[29] However, this study did not directly compare STD AA with EAA.

Feinstein et al. in a prospective, randomized, double-blind investigation of 30 medical or surgical hemodialysis patients compared EAA TPN with STD AA TPN and hypertonic dextrose solution.[30] There were no significant differences in protein balance or mortality between groups. However, this study was of small size.

The final study by Mirtallo et al.[31] compared EAA TPN with STD AA TPN in nonhemodialysis patients with acute renal failure in a volume that provided an equal amount of EAA. There were no differences in nitrogen balance or mortality rates among the groups. This study

TABLE 25–4.

Amino Acid Nutritional Support in Renal Failure

	Aminosyn-RF	Aminess 5.2%	NephrAmine	RenAmin
AA concentration	5.20%	5.20%	5.40%	6.50%
N (g/100 mL)	0.79	0.66	0.65	1
EAA (mg/100 mL)				
Isoleucine	462	525	560	500
Leucine	726	825	880	600
Lysine	535	600	640	450
Methionine	726	825	880	500
Phenylalanine	726	825	880	490
Threonine	330	375	400	380
Tryptophan	165	188	200	160
Valine	528	600	640	820
Histidine	429	412	250	420
NEAA (mg/100 mL)				
Alanine				630
Arginine	600			560
Proline				350
Serine				300
Tyrosine				40
Glycine				300
Cysteine			<20	
Electrolytes (mEq/L)				
Sodium			5	
Chloride				31
Acetate	105	50	44	60
Phosphate (mM/L)				
Potassium	5.4			
mOsm/L	475	416	435	600
Cost/bottle cost per average wholesale price	$79.54	$102.96	$66.75	$75.00

AA = amino acid; EAA = essential amino acid; NEAA = nonessential amino acid.

lacked power to detect significant differences between groups because of the small sample size of the investigation. These studies suggest that patients with acute renal failure do better with protein supplementation.

Recommendations

On the basis of this information we recommend that patients in acute renal failure who are not receiving hemodialysis or peritoneal dialysis receive 0.5 g protein/kg/day as STD AA.[30–32] The amount of protein may be increased to 1.2 g protein/kg/day in hemodialysis and 1.5 g protein/kg/day in peritoneal dialysis patients.[32]

A cost analysis of EAA vs. STD AA (as above with BCAA) TPN studies of 299 patients with an average weight of 60 kg who received TPN for 15 days indicates costs of $173,659 for STD AA (0.5 g protein/kg/day) and $299,374 for EAA (250 mL/day). It would cost $125,715 more, or an additional $28.00 per patient per day to use EAA in acute renal failure.

INTRAVENOUS FAT EMULSIONS

Long-chain intravenous fat emulsions are approved by the U.S. Food and Drug Administration for the treatment of essential fatty acid deficiency (EFAD) and as a parenteral calorie source. EFAD is characterized by desquamative dermatitis, hair loss, thrombocytopenia, poor wound healing, abnormal plasma lipid patterns, and sparse hair growth.[33, 34] The accepted method for treatment is to provide 500 mL of a 10% intravenous fat emulsion two to three times weekly (Table 25–6).

TABLE 25–5.

Comparison of Renal Failure Studies

Study	Patients	N	Methods	TPN Regimen	Deaths	Results
Abel[26]	Medicine/surgery ARF* pts* Serum creatinine > 3.0 mg/dL BUN:Cr* ratio > 20:1 <200 mL urine/24 hr + no Rxn* to fluid/diuretics within 10 days of ARF 48 hr of TPN minimal	53	Randomized Prospective Double-blind	EAA + Dex vs. Dex alone	11 EAA 15 Dex	Hospital D/C NS Oliguric RF recovery: EAA > Dex, P = .05 Dialysis survival rate: EAA > Dex, P = .02 Nondialysis survival NS
Leonard[27]	Medicine/surgery ARF pts BUN > 80 mg/dL, dialysis required, GI ileus, TPN > 48 hr	20	Randomized Prospective Single-blind	EAA + Dex vs. Dex alone	7 EAA 5 Dex	Nitrogen balance NS Dialysis survival rate NS
Baek[28]	Postoperative ARF ICU* pts Oliguria, low urine specific gravity, increased BUN, increased creatinine, decreased water clearance, no Rxn to Lasix	129	Prospective Randomized	AA* + Dex Dex alone	30 AA 46 Dex	AA + Dex increased survival during hemodialysis (47% vs. 22% with Dex)
Freund[29]	Surgery ARF pts Increased Cr or urine < 200 mL/24 hr and no Rxn to IV fluids	22	Retrospective	STD AA* + Dex	20 STD AA	Longer interval between injury and TPN EAA may be better
Feinstein[30]	Medicine/surgery ARF pts Increased BUN and Cr, urine-to-plasma Cr ratio < 10, urine Na > 20 mEq/L, GI ileus	30	Randomized Prospective Double-blind	EAA + Dex Dex alone STD AA + Dex	5 EAA 5 Dex 9 STD AA	Mean protein balance NS
Mirtallo[31]	Medicine/surgery ARF pts: BUN > 30 mg/dL Cr > 1.8 mg/dL No Rxn to IV fluids	45	Prospective Randomized Double-blind	STD AA + Dex EAA + Dex	8 STD AA 6 EAA	Nitrogen balance NS

TPN = total parenteral nutrition; ARF = acute renal failure; pts = patients; BUN:Cr = blood urea nitrogen:creatinine; Rxn = reaction; EAA = essential amino acid; Dex = dextrose; ICU = intensive care unit; AA = amino acid; STD AA = standard AA; D/C = discharged.

TABLE 25–6.

Intravenous Fat Emulsions

	Intralipid	Liposyn	Liposyn II	Nutrilipid
Fat source	Soybean	Soy/safflower	Soy/safflower	Soybean
Linoleic (%)	50	66	55	49–60
Oleic (%)	26	18	22	21–26
Palmitic (%)	10	9	11	9–13
Linolenic (%)	9	4	8	6–9
Stearic (%)	3.50	3	4	3–5
Egg phospholipid (%)	1.2	1	1	1.2
Glycerin	2.25	3	3	2.21
kcal/mL 10%	1.1	1.1	1.1	1.1
kcal/mL 20%	2	2	2	2
mOsm/L 10%	260	276	284	280
mOsm/L 20%	260	258	292	315
pH	6–8.9	6–8.8	6–8.8	6–7.9
Manufacturer	Clintec	Abbott	Abbott	McGaw
$/500 mL 10%*	$49.11	$38.38	$57.27	$46.13
$/500 mL 20%*	$66.24	$61.03	$81.87	$70.89

*Cost per average wholesale price.

Intravenous fat emulsion provides a dense caloric source with minimal fluid volume to the patient. Recently, the practice of providing fat in three-in-one solutions (i.e., fat-carbohydrate-protein) or total nutrient admixtures (TNAs) has become standard. Clinical studies demonstrate no statistical difference in nitrogen balance in acutely ill patients given 50/50 lipid-based TPN vs. lipid-free TPN solution.[35] The mean nitrogen balance was -2 ± 38 mg N/kg/day for glucose-fat TPN and 11 ± 51 mg N/kg/day ($\pm$ SD) for fat-free TPN. However, this investigation had a small number of patients ($n = 23$) and is prone to type II error.

Recent clinical studies have characterized the kinetic properties of nutrient substrates in hypermetabolic patients. Isotope studies in a population of nine patients with acute pancreatitis indicate a decrease in the appearance rate of palmitate and free fatty acids (FFAs) when patients receive glucose. The appearance rate of palmitate (1.4 ± 1.2 μmol/kg/min) and FFA (4.2 ± 5.2 μmol/kg/min) decreased to 0.9 ± 0.9 μmol/kg/min and 3.0 ± 3.0 μmol/kg/min, respectively.[36]

Additional investigations in septic patients ($n = 12$, 6 of whom received TPN) and weight-losing cancer patients ($n = 14$, 8 of whom received TPN) studied FFA oxidation and recycling during basal and TPN conditions. TPN provided 3.7 ± 0.2 mg/kg/min of glucose, 7 ± 0.4 μL/kg/min of fat, and 1.6 ± 0.7 g/kg/day of protein. Basal FFA oxidation in weight-losing cancer patients was 1.2 ± 0.73 μmol/kg/min and increased to 2.5 ± 2.83 μmol/kg/min during TPN ($P < .05$). In septic patients the basal FFA oxidation rate was 4.0 ± 1.22 μmol/kg/min and increased to 5.2 ± 1.47 μmol/kg/min with TPN. The investigators reported increased FFA recycling during lipid-based TPN.[37]

A study of polytrauma patients provided data on fat fuel mobilization.[38] Patients were studied 48 to 96 hours after injury. TPN was administered as 300 mg N/kg/day (1.875 g protein/kg/day) and 25% dextrose equivalent to 1.5 times the basal energy expenditure. A 10% lipid emulsion was given on day 3 to prevent EFAD. The results of this study are reported in Table 25–7. The change in the respiratory quotient was due primarily to the use of endogenous fat at baseline. There was no significant correlation ($r = -0.11$) between FFA and fat oxidation. Fat oxidation decreased in six of nine patients.

Specific data concerning lipid kinetics and nutrition support in trauma patients was also presented (Table 25–8).[38] Fat oxidation was greater at baseline conditions when compared with TPN. FFA reesterification did not change. During baseline conditions two thirds of the energy expenditure was

TABLE 25–7.

Nutrition Influence on Energy Parameters in Trauma (Means + SD)

Parameter	Baseline	TPN	P
REE (kcal/kg/day)	37.7 ± 8.4	33.4 ± 8.1	
RQ	0.77 ± 0.06	0.83 ± 0.12	
VO_2	406 ± 81	359 ± 90	.025
N_2 balance (mg N/kg/day)	-215 ± 54	-105 ± 45	.001
Fat oxidation (kcal/kg/day)	25.2 ± 11.1	14.7 ± 8.7	.005
Percent REE	65.8 ± 20	40.7 ± 31	.025
Protein oxidation (kcal/kg/day)	5.5 ± 2.1	8.2 ± 3	.025
Percent REE	14.9 ± 5.4	25.2 ± 7.8	.01
CHO oxidation (kcal/kg/day)	7.1 ± 6.6	10.5 ± 9.9	
Percent REE	19.3 ± 6.8	34.1 ± 30.6	

TPN = total parenteral nutrition; REE = resting energy expenditure; RQ = respiratory quotient; CHO = carbohydrate.

TABLE 25–8.

Nutrition Effects on Lipid Kinetics (Means ± SD)

Parameter	Baseline	TPN	P
Glycerol clearance (L/min)	2.70 ± 1.2	3.46 ± 1.2	
Glycerol turnover (μmol/kg/min)	4.29 ± 1.9	3.46 ± 1.4	
Fat oxidation (kcal/kg/day)	25.2 ± 11	14.7 ± 8.7	.005
Percent REE	65.8 ± 20	40.7 ± 31	.025
Percent Tg hydrolyzed	53 ± 22	46 ± 24	
Tg hydrolysis (kcal/kg/day)	50 ± 22	40.6 ± 16.8	
Percent REE	130 ± 42	128 ± 57	
FFA reesterification (kcal/kg/day)	24.9 ± 16.5	25.9 ± 15.3	
Percent Tg hydrolyzed	46.7 ± 21.9	54 ± 26.7	
Tg/FFA cycle energy cost (kcal/kg/day)	0.47 ± 0.3	0.49 ± 0.3	
Percent REE	1.34 ± 0.8	1.64 ± 1.3	

TPN = total parenteral nutrition; REE = resting energy expenditure; Tg = triglyceride; FFA = free fatty acid.

provided by fat oxidation. However, some fat was diverted into triglyceride hydrolysis and FFA reesterification.

Nine papers in the nutritional literature address the immunologic effects of lipid emulsions (Table 25–9). Most studies are nonrandomized and unblinded. Jarstrand et al. provided 500 mL of 20% lipid emulsion by rapid intravenous administration to 14 postoperative meniscectomy patients.[39] The results indicated a significant decrease in granulocyte function and no affect on reticuloendothelial system (RES) clearance. Nördenstrom et al. studied healthy volunteers who received a 20% lipid emulsion in different dosing regimens over a period of 2 hours and showed a significant decrease in leukocyte chemotaxis and migration during and after the infusion of lipids when compared with baseline.[40] Palmbald and associates investigated the infusion of 500 mL of 10% lipid over a 6-hour period in ten hospitalized patients and found no significant change in neutrophil chemotaxis.[41] Wiernik et al. administered a 20% lipid emulsion at 100 mL/hr for 2 hours to eight healthy volunteers. The results showed an increase in monocyte motility and oxidation and a decrease in phagocyte motility and chemotaxis.[42] Ota et al., in a prospective, randomized clinical investigation

comparing lipid-free TPN with lipid-based TPN, reported no difference between groups for C3, C4, IgG, IgM, IgA, B cells, T cells, T-helper cells, T-suppressor cells, neutrophils, natural killer cells, chemotaxis, phagocytosis, and bactericidal index.[43] Lindh et al. gave an intravenous bolus of 0.1 g/kg (0.9 kcal/kg/day) of a 10% lipid emulsion to hospitalized patients. The study showed the following significant results: triglycerides increased, cholesterol decreased, and the fractional lipid removal rate decreased in stressed patients.[44] Robin and colleagues reported that neutrophil bactericidal activity significantly decreased in subjects who received 500 mL of a 10% lipid emulsion over a 4- to 6-hour period.[45] Seidner and associates' investigation showed that 3 consecutive days of 0.13 g/kg/day (1.2 kcal/kg/day) of lipid emulsion infused over a period of 10 hours each day significantly decreased RES fat clearance.[46] Gogos et al. compared medium-chain triglyceride TPN, long-chain triglyceride TPN, and lipid-free TPN. The study reported that long-chain triglyceride TPN decreased the T-helper:T-suppressor cell ratio.[47] In these studies, seven of nine papers showed that long-chain lipid emulsion infusions resulted in compromised immunologic effects.

The preceding discussion of the met-

TABLE 25-9.

Lipid Studies

Study	Patients	N	Methods	Administration	Results
Jarstrand[39]	Meniscectomy	14	Nonrandomized Unblinded Open protocol	20% lipid, 500 mL IV postoperative day 2	RES clearance not affected Granulocyte function decreased, $P < .05$
Nordenstrom[40]	Healthy volunteers	12	Nonrandomized Unblinded	20% lipids IV × 2 hr 100 mL/hr × 8 subjects 200 mL/hr × 2 subjects 50 mL/hr × 2 subjects	Decreased leukocyte chemotaxis and migration during and after lipids, $P < .05$
Palmblad[41]	Medical/surgical (2 orthopedic, 8 GI)	10	Nonrandomized Unblinded	10% lipids IV, 500 mL over 6 hr	NS neutrophil chemotaxis
Wiernik[42]	Healthy volunteers	8	Nonrandomized Unblinded	20% lipids, 100 mL/hr for 2 hr	Increased monocyte motility and oxidation Decreased phagocyte motility and chemotaxis
Ota[43]	Medical	40	Randomized Prospective Isonitrogenous Isovolemic Isocaloric Exclusion criteria CHO vs. CHO + FAT	120:1 cal:N ratio	NS intragroup or intergroup comparison of C3, C4, IgG, IgM, IgA, B cell, T cell, T-helper, suppressor, neutrophils, natural killer cells, chemotaxis, phagocytosis, bactericidal index
Lindh[44]	Medical/surgical	62	Nonrandomized Unblinded	0.1 g/kg IV bolus of 10% lipids	Tg significantly increased in stressed patients Cholesterol significantly lower in stressed patients Fractional lipid removal rate slower in stressed patients
Robin[45]	Medical/volunteers	35	Nonrandomized Unblinded Exclusion criteria	500-1000 mL of 10% lipids every week, then 500 mL of 10% lipids over 4-6 hr, then sample blood	Postlipid neutrophil bactericidal activity decreased, $P < .001$
Seidner[46]	Medical	10	Prospective Nonblinded Exclusion criteria	Fat on 3 consecutive days vs. one-time dose 0.13 g/kg/day	RES fat clearance decreased after 3-day regimen, $P < .05$
Gogos[47]	Medical	58	Randomized Prospective	Compare MCT-LCT vs. LCT vs. TPN alone	LCT decreased T-helper:T-suppressor ratio, $P < .01$

RES = reticuloendothelial system; CHO = carbohydrate; Tg = triglyceride; MCT-LCT = medium- and long-chain triglyceride.

abolic fate of lipid emulsions raises an issue of concern. Lipids are not completely oxidized. During stress there is increased reesterification of FFA into triglycerides and deposition into storage tissues. Large amounts of lipid emulsion at rapid infusion rates result in compromised function of granulocytes, leukocytes, neutrophils, and phagocytes and decreased T-helper:T-suppressor cell ratios. On the basis of this evidence, it is prudent to use lipid emulsions for prevention of EFAD in critically ill pa-

tients. This can be accomplished by infusing 500 mL of 10% lipids twice weekly. The optimal quantity and type of lipid fuel that maintains immune status requires further study.

For clinical situations requiring TNA, 4 to 7 kcal/kg/day should be provided as fat emulsion.[48, 49] A baseline serum triglyceride level should be obtained and triglycerides monitored biweekly. If triglyceride concentrations increase above normal levels, the TNA solution should be converted to a lipid-free TPN solution to enable triglycerides to clear the circulation. When serum triglyceride concentrations have normalized, lipid emulsions should be resumed twice weekly to prevent EFAD. The rationale is to minimize the accumulation of long-chain triglycerides and their potential aberrant white blood cell effects.

VOLUME ASPECTS OF PARENTERAL NUTRITION PRODUCTS

The critically ill patient presents a challenge in fluid management. Aside from the fluid received from TPN, other intravenous fluids are given for concurrent medical problems, i.e., antibiotic, cardiac, and pulmonary therapy. In order to minimize fluid overload, consideration should be given to using concentrated solutions to provide nonprotein kilocalories and protein.

Dextrose solutions are available in the following concentrations:

70% = 2.38 kcal/mL
50% = 1.70 kcal/mL
40% = 1.36 kcal/mL
30% = 1.02 kcal/mL

The following volumes are necessary to provide 2000 kcal/day:

841 mL of 70% dextrose
1177 mL of 50% dextrose
1471 mL of 40% dextrose
1961 mL of 30% dextrose

Providing kilocalories as 70% dextrose in TPN would save 336 mL of 50% dextrose, 630 mL of 40% dextrose, and 1120 mL of 30% dextrose.

Commercially available lipid emulsions provide 2 kcal/mL for 20% and 1.1 kcal/mL for 10% lipid emulsion. If patients receive 500 kcal of lipid in a TNA solution that provides 2000 kcal/day the following total volumes are possible:

250 mL of 20% lipid + 630 mL of 70% dextrose = 880 mL
250 mL of 20% lipid + 882 mL of 50% dextrose = 1132 mL
250 mL of 20% lipid + 1103 mL of 40% dextrose = 1353 mL
250 mL of 20% lipid + 1471 mL of 30% dextrose = 1721 mL

The use of 10% lipid would have the following total volumes:

455 mL of 10% lipid + 630 mL of 70% dextrose = 1085 mL
455 mL of 10% lipid + 882 mL of 50% dextrose = 1337 mL
455 mL of 10% lipid + 1103 mL of 40% dextrose = 1558 mL
455 mL of 10% lipid + 1471 mL of 30% dextrose = 1926 mL

It is evident that using the most concentrated solutions minimizes fluid intake.

Currently available STD AA formulations provide 10 g/100 mL (10%), 11.4 g/100 mL (11.4%), and 15 g/100 mL (15%). If a 70-kg individual were to receive 1.5 g protein/kg/day, 1050 mL, 921 mL, and 700 mL, respectively, are required to provide protein requirements. If fluid conservation is important, a 15% amino acid solution is preferred. However, the average wholesale cost of this solution is almost twice that of the least expensive 10% solution, $123.32 vs. $64.52 (see Table 25–1).

CONCLUSIONS

The classic approach to nutrition support centers around maintenance of body cell mass and nitrogen balance measurements to assess the effectiveness of nutrition support. The contemporary approach recognizes the multifactorial nature of illness. Alteration of the stress response, administration of tissue-specific nutrients, and stimulation or administration of growth factors are all goals of nutrition support. Maintenance of organ function and immune status and improvement in clinical outcome become more important than the maintenance of body cell mass or nitrogen balance. Future prospective, randomized, clinical trials will utilize elements of the contemporary, multifactorial approach to assess "the efficiency and effectiveness of nutrition support."

Current clinical data on commercially available parenteral nutrition solutions have not yet embraced this new approach. Comparison studies of BCAA to STD AA used nitrogen balance data to evaluate the ability of specific BCAAs to maintain body cell mass. Studies in acute renal failure also evaluated nitrogen balance. Lipid emulsions provide the essential fatty acid linoleic acid and calories to TPN patients. However, if given in large amounts or at rapid rates, they can compromise white blood cell activity. Finally, knowledge of the volume of parenteral nutrition solutions allows for minimizing potential fluid problems when providing nutrition support to the catabolic, critically ill patient.

REFERENCES

1. Wilmore DW: The practice of clinical nutrition: How to prepare for the future. *JPEN* 1989; 13:337–343.
2. Wilmore DW: Catabolic illness: Strategies for enhancing recovery. *N Engl J Med* 1991; 325:695–702.
3. Moore FD, Olesen KH, McMurrey JD, et al: *The body cell mass and its supporting environment,* in *Body Composition in Health and Disease.* Philadelphia, WB Saunders, 1963.
4. Author deleted reference in proof stage.
5. Sganga G, Siegel JH, Brown G, et al: Reprioritization of hepatic plasma protein release in trauma and sepsis. *Arch Surg* 1985; 120:187–199.
6. Freund H, Hoover HC, Atamian S, et al: Infusion of the branched chain amino acids in postoperative patients: Anticatabolic properties. *Ann Surg* 1979; 190:18–23.
7. Cerra FB, Upson D, Angelico R, et al: Branched chains support postoperative protein synthesis. *Surgery* 1982; 92:192–197.
8. Vander Woude P, Morgan RE, et al: Addition of branched-chain amino acids to parenteral nutrition of stressed critically ill patients. *Crit Care Med* 1986; 14:685–688.
9. Brennan MB, Cerra F, Daly JM, et al: Report of a research workshop: Branched-chain amino acids in stress and injury. *JPEN* 1986; 10:446–452.
10. Cerra F, Blackburn G, Hirsch J, et al: The effect of stress level, amino acid formula, and nitrogen dose on nitrogen retention in traumatic and septic stress. *Ann Surg* 1987; 205:282–287.
11. Lenssen P, Cheney CL, Aker S, et al: Intravenous branched chain amino acid in marrow transplant recipients. *JPEN* 1987; 11:112–118.
12. Jaing Z, Shang F, Zhu Y, et al: Evaluation of parenteral nutrition in the postoperative patient. *Surg Gynecol Obstet* 1988; 166:115–120.
13. Okada A, Mori S, Totsuka M, et al: Branched-chain amino acids metabolic support in surgical patients: A randomized, control trial in patients with subtotal or total gastrectomy in 16 Japanese institutions. *JPEN* 1988; 12:332–337.
14. Chiarla C, Siegel JH, Kidd S, et al: Inhibition of post-traumatic septic proteolysis and ureagenesis and stimulation of hepatic acute phase protein production by branched-chain amino-acid TPN. *J Trauma* 1988; 28:1145–1172.
15. Bruzzone P, Siegel JH, Chiarla C, et al: Leucine dose response in the reduction of urea production from septic proteolysis and in the stimulation of acute-phase proteins. *Surgery* 1991; 109:768–778.
16. Scholten DJ, Morgan RE, Davis AT, et al: Failure of BCAA supplementation to promote nitrogen retention in injured patients. *J Am Coll Nutr* 1990; 9:101–106.
17. Brown RO, Buonpane EA, Vehe KL, et al: Comparison of modified amino acids and standard amino acids in parenteral nutrition support of thermally injured patients. *Crit Care Med* 1990; 18:1096–1101.
18. Kuhl DA, Brown RO, Vehe KL, et al: Use of selected visceral protein measurements with the comparison of branched-chain amino acids with standard amino acids in parenteral nutrition support of injured patients. *Surgery* 1990; 107:503–510.
19. Jimenez-Jimenez FJ, Leyba CO, Mendez SM, et al: Prospective study on the efficacy of branched-chain amino acids in septic patients. *JPEN* 1991; 15:252–261.

20. von Meyenfeldt MF, Soeters PB, Vente JP, et al: Effect of branched-chain amino acid enrichment of total parenteral nutrition on nitrogen sparing and clinical outcome of sepsis and trauma: A prospective randomized double blinded trial. *Br J Surg* 1990; 77:924–929.

21. Vente JP, Soeters PB, von Meyenfeldt MF, et al: Prospective randomized double-blinded trial of branched chain amino acid enriched versus standard parenteral nutrition solutions in traumatized and septic patients. *World J Surg* 1991; 15:128–132.

22. Bessey PQ: Invited commentary. *World J Surg* 1991; 15:133.

23. Rose WC, Wixom RL, Lockhart HB, et al: The amino acid requirements of man. *J Biol Chem* 1955; 213:815–827, 913–922, 214:579–587, 215:101–110, 216:225–234, 287:987–995.

24. Giordano C: Use of exogenous and endogenous urea for protein synthesis in normal and uremic subjects. *J Lab Clin Med* 1963; 62:231.

25. Giovanetti S, Maffiore Q: A low-nitrogen diet with proteins of high biological value for severe chronic uremia. *Lancet* 1964; 1:1000.

26. Abel RM, Beck CH Jr, Abbott WM, et al: Improved survival from acute renal failure after treatment with intravenous essential L-amino acids and glucose. *N Engl J Med* 1973; 288:695–699.

27. Leonard CD, Luke RG, Seigel RR: Parenteral essential amino acids in acute renal failure. *Urology* 1975; 6:154–157.

28. Baek SM, Makabali GG, Byran-Brown CW, et al: The influence of parenteral nutrition on the course of acute renal failure. *Surg Gynecol Obstet* 1974; 141:405–408.

29. Freund H, Atamian S, Fischer J: Comparative study of parenteral nutrition in renal failure using essential and non-essential amino acid containing solutions. *Surg Gynecol Obstet* 1980; 151:652–656.

30. Feinstein EI, Blumenkrantz, MJ, Healey M, et al: Clinical and metabolic response to parenteral nutrition in acute renal failure. *Medicine (Baltimore)* 1981; 60:124–137.

31. Mirtallo JM, Schneider RJ, Mavko K, et al: A comparison of essential and general amino acid infusions in the nutritional support of patients with compromised renal function. *JPEN* 1982; 6:109–113.

32. Kopple JD: Nutritional therapy in kidney failure. *Nutr Rev* 1981; 39:193–206.

33. O'Neill JA Jr, Caldwell MD, Meng HC: Essential fatty acid deficiency in surgical patients. *Ann Surg* 1977; 185:535–542.

34. Bivins BA, Rapp RP, Record K, et al: Parenteral safflower oil emulsion (Liposyn 10%): Safety and effectiveness in treating or preventing essential fatty acid deficiency in surgical patients. *Ann Surg* 1980; 191:307–317.

35. Nördenstrom J, Askanazi J, Elwyn DH, et al: Nitrogen balance during total parenteral nutrition: Glucose vs. fat. *Ann Surg* 1983; 197:27–33.

36. Shaw JHF, Wolfe RR: Glucose, fatty acid, and urea kinetics in patients with severe pancreatitis. *Ann Surg* 1986; 204:665–672.

37. Shaw JHF, Wolfe RR: Fatty acid and glycerol kinetics in septic patients and in patients with gastrointestinal cancer: The response to glucose infusion and parenteral feeding. *Ann Surg* 1987; 205:368–376.

38. Jeevanandam M, Young DH, Schiller WR: Nutritional impact on the energy cost of fat fuel mobilization in polytrauma victims. *J Trauma* 1990; 30:147–154.

39. Jarstrand C, Berghem L, Lahnborg G: Human granulocyte and reticuloendothelial system function during Intralipid infusion. *JPEN* 1978; 5:663–670.

40. Nördenstrom J, Jarstrand C, Wiernik A: Decreased chemotactic and random migration of leukocytes during Intralipid infusion. *Am J Clin Nutr* 1979; 32:2416–2422.

41. Palmblad J, Brostrom O, Lahnborg et al: Neutrophil functions during total parenteral nutrition and Intralipid infusions. *Am J Clin Nutr* 1982; 35:1430–1436.

42. Wiernik A, Jarstrand C Julander I: The effect of Intralipid on mononuclear and polymorphonuclear phagocytes. *Am J Clin Nutr* 1983; 37:256–261.

43. Ota DM, Jessup JM, Babcock GF, et al:

Immune function during intravenous administration of a soybean oil emulsion. *JPEN* 1985; 9:23–27.

44. Lindh A, Lundholm M, Rossner S: Intralipid disappearence in critically ill patients. *Crit Care Med* 1986; 14:476–480.

45. Robin AP, Arian I, Phuangsab A, et al: Intravenous fat emulsion acutely suppresses neutrophil chemiluminescence. *JPEN* 1989; 13:608–613.

46. Seidner DL, Mascioli EA, Istfan NW, et al: Effects of long-chain triglyceride emulsion on reticuloendothelial system function in humans. *JPEN* 1989; 13:614–619.

47. Gogos CA, Kalfarentzos FE, Soumbos NC: Effect of different types of total parenteral nutrition on T-lymphocyte subpopulations and NK cells. *Am J Clin Nutr* 1990; 51:119–121.

48. Cerra FB, Shronts EP, Konstantinides NN, et al: Enteral feeding in sepsis: A prospective, randomized, double-blind trial. *Surgery* 1985; 98:632–639.

49. Cerra FB, Mazuski JE, Chute E, et al: Branched chain metabolic support: A prospective, randomized double-blind trial in surgical stress. *Ann Surg* 1984; 199:286–291.

26

Drug-Nutrient Interactions

Christine Mowatt-Larssen, Pharm.D.

Rex Brown, Pharm.D.

Drug effects on specialized nutrition support

    Electrolyte balance

    Vitamins

    Gastrointestinal

Nutritional effects on drug therapy

Alterations in pharmacokinetics and nutrient metabolism

The interactions between pharmacologic treatment and specialized nutrition support in the critically ill patient is becoming more important as more patients are being treated with extensive pharmacotherapy and nutrition support is being initiated sooner than in the past. There is now a substantial body of knowledge addressing these interactions, especially when one considers fluid and electrolyte therapy as part of specialized nutrition support. The population of elderly patients is growing, and these patients receive more medications than their younger counterparts. These patients are frequently treated in the intensive care unit and usually need specialized nutrition support during this stressed state. Therefore, drug-nutrient interactions are prevalent in this elderly population.[1]

Schneider and Mirtallo reported on drug therapy in over 600 patients receiving parenteral nutrition and found that 77% of the drugs taken by these patients had the potential for causing alterations in specialized nutritional support.[2] Recently, there has been a trend to feed critically ill patients via the gastrointestinal tract with enteral tube feeding. This is thought to prevent bacterial and endotoxin translocation, which may be important in preventing multiple organ failure syndrome. The increased use of enteral nutrition support in the critically ill patient who is often receiving several drugs has increased the probability of drug-nutrient interactions occurring in this patient population.[3] This chapter is divided into three parts: drug effects on specialized nutrition support, nutritional effects on drug therapy, and alterations in pharmacokinetics and nutrient metabolism. Interactions in the critical care setting will obviously be the focus of this chapter; however, it is very difficult to document cause-effect relationships between drugs and nutrients with all of the confounding variables in this patient population. Therefore, some clinical trials using normal subjects will be cited if they provide evidence of the drug or nutrient causing an interaction. There are also many potential drug-nutrient interactions that do not appear to be clinically important. These will not be addressed in this chapter.

DRUG EFFECTS ON SPECIALIZED NUTRITION SUPPORT

Pharmacotherapy may have significant effects on fluid and electrolyte balance, vitamin homeostasis, acid-base status, and gastrointestinal tract function. It is helpful if the critical care practitioner can predict potential problems and treat accordingly instead of correcting problems after they have occurred. This section will address drug effects on electrolyte balance, vitamin status, and gastrointestinal tolerance.

Electrolyte Balance

Some pharmacologic agents have a profound effect on electrolyte balance. This can be an intended effect like the expected natriuresis observed with loop diuretic therapy. Frequently, it is a side effect of the pharmacologic agent that may cause a metabolic disturbance.[4]

Sodium homeostasis is the most difficult of the electrolyte disorders to understand because the serum concentration of sodium must be interpreted along with a bedside assessment of the extracellular fluid compartment. Many drugs are marketed as sodium salts, or they are administered in normal saline piggybacks. Selected antibiotics and the sodium load they deliver with usual daily doses appear in Table 26–1. A patient receiving ticarcillin needs little if any sodium added to nutritional formulas unless the patient has substantial extrarenal losses. A patient in an edematous state who requires drugs like ticarcillin should have dietary sodium restricted. Alternatively, this drug may need to be changed to another antibiotic so that microbial coverage is similar without delivering the relatively high sodium load.

Renal wasting of sodium has been reported with both cisplatin[5] and

TABLE 26–1.

Sodium Content of Selected Antibiotics

Drug	Sodium Content (mEq/g)	Usual Daily Dose (g)	Sodium Delivery (mEq)
Carbenicillin	5.0	24	120.0
Ticarcillin	5.2	18	93.6
Azlocillin	2.2	18	39.6
Ceftizoxime	2.6	12	31.2
Metronidazole (ready-to-use vial)	14	2	28.0
Cephradine	6.0	4	24.0
Piperacillin	1.9	12	22.8
Cefamandole	3.3	6	19.8
Cefoxitin	2.3	8	18.4
Nafcillin	2.9	6	17.4
Mezlocillin	1.9	8	15.2
Moxalactam	3.8	4	15.2
Cefotetan	3.5	4	14.0
Ampicillin	3.0	4	12.0

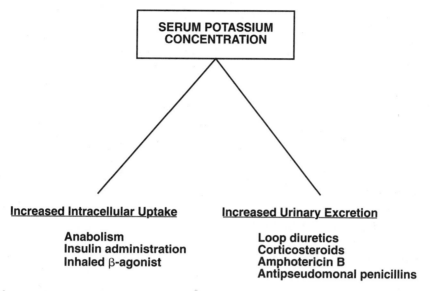

FIG 26–1.

The serum concentration of potassium can be decreased by pharmacologic agents that cause urinary wasting of potassium. Anabolism and other pharmacologic agents cause an intracellular shift of potassium that can also decrease the serum potassium concentration.

trimethoprim-sulfamethoxazole.[6] Patients receiving these drugs should be monitored closely for orthostatic hypotension because they may become salt depleted with these pharmacologic agents. Parenteral nutrition or enteral formulas should be supplemented with sodium chloride to maintain sodium balance in these situations. Sodium loading has been advocated to prevent renal toxicity from amphotericin B. This can be accomplished by administering normal saline as adjunctive therapy or by increasing the sodium load via the nutrition solution.

Overzealous use of lactulose in patients with liver failure and hepatic encephalopathy has been reported to result in hypernatremia, presumably from the loss of free water via loose stools.[7] The end point of dose titration with lactulose should be two to three soft stools per day, not frank diarrhea. Excessive lactulose administration should also be avoided in patients receiving enteral tube feeding because it will compromise the nutritional intake of this often undernourished population.

Maintenance of potassium homeostasis cannot be overemphasized in criti-

cally ill patients receiving specialized nutrition support. Many drugs can cause hypokalemia through urinary wasting of potassium or movement of this cation into the intracellular compartment (Fig 26–1). In fact, pharmacologic agents or failure to add potassium to intravenous solutions accounted for 50% of the patients in whom severe hypokalemia developed in one study.[8] Loop and thiazide diuretics, steroids, antipseudomonal penicillins, and amphotericin B have all been implicated in causing urinary potassium wasting. Kaliuresis results from diuretics that cause increased fluid and sodium delivery to the distal nephron and from the aldosterone effects of steroids. Antipseudomonal penicillins (e.g., ticarcillin) are sodium salts of nonreabsorbable anions. The drug is filtered at the glomerulus, and the sodium ions are primarily reabsorbed in the proximal convoluted tubule. The negatively charged anions create a gradient for positively charged ions (e.g., potassium) to be secreted in the distal convoluted tubule of the nephron and cause cation wasting.

Insulin and inhaled β-agonists cause

an intracellular shift of potassium that can also result in hypokalemia. Inhaled β-agonists stimulate β$_2$-adrenoceptor-linked receptor-bound sodium/potassium adenosine triphosphatase (ATPase). Hypokalemia from these agents has resulted in some morbidity and mortality.[9] Concomitant administration of pharmacologic agents that can cause hypokalemia and specialized nutrition support (which causes an intracellular shift of potassium as new tissue is being synthesized) results in supranormal requirements for potassium.

Other pharmacologic agents induce hyperkalemia and may require the critical care practitioner to modify the potassium content of nutrition solutions.[10] Angiotensin-converting enzyme inhibitors (e.g., captopril) and potassium-sparing diuretics (e.g., amiloride) cause natriuresis and potassium retention. Sodium heparin, which is structurally related to aldosterone, has been reported to antagonize the effects of aldosterone and cause hyperkalemia.[11] Nonsteroidal anti-inflammatory agents may also induce hyperkalemia by causing a hyporeninemic, hypoaldosterone state secondary to inhibition of prostaglandin synthetase.[12] Patients receiving any of the above drugs should have serum potassium concentrations monitored very closely. The potassium content of nutritional formulas may need to be decreased substantially if hyperkalemia develops. An enteral formula low in potassium may be indicated in patients who cannot tolerate the potassium in standard formulas.

Phosphorus homeostasis is extremely important in patients receiving specialized nutrition support. It also appears that pharmacotherapy is a major cause of severe hypophosphatemia in hospitalized patients.[13] Antacids (e.g., aluminum hydroxide) have long been known to be very effective phosphorus binders in the gastrointestinal tract. Sucralfate has also been shown to decrease serum phosphorus concentrations.[14, 15] Drugs such as theophylline have been impli-

cated in causing hypophosphatemia by either shifting phosphorus into the intracellular space or by reducing renal reabsorption of phosphorus.[16] Patients receiving these drugs and specialized nutrition support are particularly prone to the development of hypophosphatemia. Serum concentrations of phosphorus need to be monitored frequently. Phosphorus supplementation is frequently required in these patients and can be accomplished with intravenous bolus administration of phosphorus or by increasing its concentration in nutritional formulas. Patients receiving enteral nutrition can have phosphate salts (e.g., Fleets Phospho-soda) added to the enteral formula. Five to 10 mL of Fleets Phospho-soda added to each liter of enteral feeding is effective in treating mild to moderate hypophosphatemia. Parenteral phosphorus should be used to treat patients with serum phosphorus concentrations less than 1.5 mg/dL.

Hyperphosphatemia is relatively infrequent in patients without renal failure. Intravenous fat emulsions have been implicated as a cause of this disorder in one case.[17] The authors suggested that egg phospholipid in the intravenous fat emulsion provided elemental phosphorus to the patient and contributed to the hyperphosphatemia.[17] Hyperphosphatemia may also result from the use of phosphate-containing agents (e.g., KPO$_4$).

A number of drugs have been shown to cause renal wasting of magnesium resulting in profound hypomagnesemia. Magnesium is another predominately intracellular ion that is needed as new cells are synthesized during the administration of specialized nutrition support. Because of magnesium's effects on the sodium-potassium ATPase pump and parathyroid hormone, hypomagnesemia can result in hypokalemia and hypocalcemia. Therefore, it is particularly important for the critical care practitioner to understand magnesium homeostasis during the administration of specialized nutrition support. Amphotericin B, aminoglycosides, loop or thiazide diuretics, cyclosporine, and cisplatin have all been reported to cause urinary magnesium wasting following their administration.[18-21] Concurrent administration of these pharmacologic agents with specialized nutrition support will invariably result in moderate to severe hypomagnesemia if only standard doses of magnesium are given. These patients need to be monitored very carefully, and supplemental magnesium is usually required. This can be done by giving magnesium as an intravenous bolus, adding it to an intravenous solution, or increasing its concentration in the nutritional formula. Because the majority of total-body magnesium is not in the serum and the kidney has a low threshold for magnesium, some investigators have questioned the use of serum concentrations of this cation for assessment of magnesium homeostasis in clinical practice. Elin and Hosseini suggest that mononuclear cell magnesium is a better indicator of the total-body magnesium status than are traditional serum concentrations or the erythrocyte magnesium content.[22]

Vitamins

Although the potential for drugs to interfere with vitamin nutriture is great, there are only a few interactions that are clinically significant. The prevalence of tuberculosis is increasing, thus resulting in the increased use of isoniazid, especially since some drugs (e.g., streptomycin) previously used for tuberculosis are no longer commercially available. It is well known that peripheral neuropathy from isoniazid pharmacotherapy can be prevented by the administration of pyridoxine. Therefore, it is important that this vitamin be supplemented (10 to 50 mg/day) concurrently with isoniazid pharmacotherapy. Pyridoxine can be given in the parenteral nutrition solution if the patient does not have gastrointestinal access. Otherwise, it can be given orally or by feeding tube. Folic acid

deficiency secondary to sulfasalazine pharmacotherapy has been reported in patients with ulcerative colitis who are receiving this agent.[23] It appears that sulfasalazine interferes with the gastrointestinal absorption of folic acid.[24] Therefore, it is prudent to assess the folic acid status in patients who have been receiving long-term sulfasalazine pharmacotherapy. If the patient is receiving parenteral nutrition, folic acid (usually 1 mg/day) can be added to the parenteral nutrition solution. Patients receiving enteral nutrition can be given folic acid orally or by feeding tube. Seligmann et al. have reported a rather high prevalence of thiamine deficiency in patients with congestive heart failure who have received long-term furosemide.[25] The patients receiving furosemide had an inappropriately high urinary excretion of thiamine. Six patients were supplemented with intravenous thiamine (100 mg twice daily). Five of these patients were tested by echocardiography, and four demonstrated improved left ventricular ejection fraction after thiamine supplementation.[25]

Gastrointestinal

Diarrhea continues to be a problem in critically ill patients receiving enteral nutrition support. Multiple definitions of diarrhea during tube feeding exist, and they markedly influence the reported prevalence in various studies.[26] It is our observation that nursing tolerance of unformed stools has increased as the potential benefits of enteral feeding have been realized. The use of fiber-containing enteral formulas in critically ill patients may improve gastrointestinal tolerance. Drugs must be ruled out as a cause of diarrhea when gastrointestinal intolerance develops in a critically ill patient in association with enteral tube feeding (Table 26-2). In fact, Edes et al. suggest that pharmacotherapy is the most frequent cause of diarrhea in patients receiving enteral tube feeding.[27] Approximately 80% of diarrhea at

TABLE 26–2.

Selected Pharmacologic Agents Implicated in Causing Diarrhea Associated With Enteral Tube Feeding

Sorbitol
   Aminophylline solution
   Theophylline solution
   Acetaminophen elixir
Magnesium
   Magnesium-containing antacids
   Magnesium citrate
Electrolyte solutions
   Potassium chloride
   Sodium phosphate
   Potassium phosphate
Antibiotics

their institution was caused directly by medications or pseudomembraneous colitis (PMC) secondary to antibiotic pharmacotherapy. The authors reported a particularly high prevalence of diarrhea caused by sorbitol in aminophylline solution preparations.[27] Others have confirmed that pharmacotherapy is an important cause of enteral tube feeding–associated diarrhea.[28, 29] Sorbitol should always be considered because the concentration of this compound is not usually quantitated on the manufacturer's label. Our nutrition support service has observed gastrointestinal intolerance associated with the administration of acetaminophen elixir during enteral tube feeding. This is another preparation that contains a considerable amount of sorbitol. Changing the route of administration of acetaminophen to an oral tablet or rectal suppository resolves this problem in most cases. Sorbitol has also been implicated in causing diarrhea in diabetics who are restricting their carbohydrate intake.[30]

Magnesium administration (e.g., antacids) must also be assessed in patients in whom gastrointestinal intolerance develops in the critical care setting.[31] It is well known that excessive gastrointestinal magnesium can cause osmotic diarrhea. Changing to an aluminum-containing antacid or an H_2-receptor antagonist is an alternative to consider when the dose of magnesium must be

decreased or discontinued. Niemiec et al. suggest that hyperosmolar medications, in particular, electrolyte solutions, can induce diarrhea.[32] In 1988, 52 of 58 commercially available liquid pharmacologic agents had an osmolality of >1000 mOsm/kg H_2O.[33] Administration of these agents via feeding tube or jejunostomy could present the gastrointestinal tract with a large osmotic load. Changing formulations or diluting the liquid preparations can decrease the osmotic load in most cases.

Most antibiotics that are used for bacterial infections today have been implicated as a cause of PMC. Patients in whom loose, watery diarrhea develops during antibiotic therapy should have a stool sample tested for *Clostridium difficile* toxin. This will help differentiate the cause of the gastrointestinal intolerance. There is probably no absolute contraindication to administering enteral feeding to patients who have PMC. However, most practitioners withhold enteral feeding for 1 to 2 days while this disorder is being treated with oral vancomycin or metronidazole. Protein-losing enteropathy has been reported in patients who have PMC.[34]

Pharmacotherapy can be used to improve the tolerance to specialized nutrition support. For instance, several prokinetic agents have been used to treat gastroparesis.[35] Metoclopramide has been used to improve gastric emptying in critically ill patients receiving enteral nutrition support. Erythromycin, which has been shown to mimic the effects of motilin, can improve gastroparesis in diabetics.[36] Erythromycin has been used to enhance gastric emptying in critically ill patients receiving nasogastric feeding; however, it has not been studied in a randomized, controlled trial. Carlson et al. suggest that erythromycin enhances gastric emptying through a cholinergic pathway.[37]

Other pharmacologic agents have been implicated in causing diseases of the gastrointestinal tract, and these can interfere with the normal ingestion and

TABLE 26–3.

Drugs Implicated in Causing Pancreatitis or Esophagitis

Pancreatitis
    Conjugated estrogens
    Thiazide diuretics
    Azathioprine
    Furosemide
    Tetracycline
    Chlorthalidone
    Cisplatin
    L-Asparaginase
Esophagitis
    Doxycycline
    Potassium chloride
    Tetracycline
    Minocycline
    Aspirin

processing of nutrients. Drug-induced esophagitis or pancreatitis can cause substantial morbidity in patients in whom these disorders develop.[38–41] Drugs that have been reported to cause esophagitis or pancreatitis are listed in Table 26–3. Often, treatment with these pharmacologic agents can be stopped and another drug used to resolve the drug-induced process.

NUTRITIONAL EFFECTS OF DRUG THERAPY

The emphasis to enterally feed critically ill patients has facilitated the transition of medication administration from the intravenous to the enteral route. This route is both more cost-effective and advantageous in reducing the risk of infection and phlebitis. However, there are many factors that can impair enteral drug absorption and potentially result in subtherapeutic responses. Critically ill patients may have altered intestinal blood flow, enzyme secretion, intestinal transit time, and gut permeability. Additionally, some medications require an acidic milieu for absorption, which may not be present in patients who typically receive H_2-receptor antagonists or antacids for stress ulcer prophylaxis. Although the administration of drugs through feed-

ing tubes is common practice in the intensive care unit, minimal study has been done to evaluate the bioavailability of drugs delivered in this manner.

The delivery of medications through feeding tubes has many limitations. For example, some dosage formulations should not be crushed, which makes it virtually impossible to deliver these drugs through feeding tubes. These include buccal, sublingual, and enteric-coated tablets, as well as sustained-release tablets or capsules. Although liquid formulations are well suited for tube delivery, syrup preparations may be very acidic, and when added to enteral feedings, they increase the viscosity and particle size. This increases the chance of clogged feeding tubes.[42] Drug adherence to the feeding tubes decreases the amount of drug available for absorption. Suspensions have been reported to be physically compatible with enteral feedings. However, in vitro studies have reported significant losses of drug when delivered through nasogastric tubes.[42–44] This has been reported specifically with phenytoin and carbamazepine suspensions; therefore, it is recommended that these suspensions be diluted prior to delivery through nasogastric tubes.[43, 44] Conversely, an in vitro study with gastrostomy catheters reported no appreciable losses of phenytoin suspension when delivered undiluted followed by catheter irrigation.[45] Diluted phenytoin suspension followed by catheter irrigation demonstrated greater losses.[45] One additional in vitro study evaluated the administration of crushed ciprofloxacin tablets suspended in water through nasogastric feeding tubes and reported no significant decreases in recovery after delivery.[46] From these findings it can be concluded that these selected medications delivered through nasogastric feeding tubes should be diluted prior to administration to decrease the viscosity and drug contact with the tube. In addition, all feeding tubes should be irrigated before and after drug delivery to minimize contact between the medication and enteral formulation and to reduce the incidence of clogged feeding tubes.

A few studies have investigated the physical compatibility of medications with enteral feeding, but there has been minimal evaluation of the chemical stability of such mixtures.[47] Protein, fat, electrolytes, and vitamins in enteral feedings are thought to interact with some medications and result in bioavailability problems. Drugs that have been reported to be problematic include phenytoin, warfarin, theophylline, and ciprofloxacin.

In critically ill patients, phenytoin is often used acutely for seizure control and chronically for posttraumatic seizure prophylaxis. The oral route is preferred in patients requiring chronic prophylaxis because of the hypotensive risks associated with intravenous administration and because of the poor availability from intramuscular administration. Among the medications noted to interact with enteral feeding, phenytoin has been the most frequently reported. Bauer was the first to investigate this interaction in 20 neurosurgery patients requiring posttraumatic seizure prophylaxis.[48] During one phase of the study, 10 of the patients received phenytoin suspension for 1 week in a fasting state. Enteral feedings were introduced after this fasting period and given for 1 week. The mean phenytoin serum concentrations in these patients decreased approximately fourfold to a subtherapeutic concentration. In the other phase of the study, 10 patients received concurrent phenytoin suspension and enteral tube feeding for 1 week. During the second week, the enteral tube feedings were discontinued, and the mean phenytoin serum concentrations increased approximately fourfold from a subtherapeutic to a therapeutic concentration.[48] Since this study, there has been one additional study describing the interaction between oral phenytoin and enteral feedings.[49]

A significant amount of work has been done to investigate the mechanism of this interaction and the ways to minimize its occurrence. Bauer reported a fivefold increase in serum phenytoin concentration among ten patients when continuous enteral feeding was discontinued for 2 hours before and after phenytoin administration.[48] While this schedule is thought to allow for enhanced absorption of phenytoin suspension, one study conducted in patients and two in healthy volunteers have not been able to reproduce this result.[49–51] To compare the effects of an elemental diet and a complex diet on the absorption of phenytoin suspension, ten healthy volunteers completed a three-phase study including phenytoin suspension alone, phenytoin suspension with an elemental diet (Vivonex TEN, Norwich Eaton Pharmaceuticals, Inc.), and phenytoin suspension with a complex diet (Ensure, Ross Laboratories). Eight ounces of the enteral feeding was swallowed over a 15-minute period every 4 hours for six doses. The phenytoin suspension was administered 2 hours after the first enteral feeding bolus. No significant difference was found between any of the phases for area under the concentration-time curve, maximum concentration, or the time to reach the maximum concentration, thus suggesting that the type of substrate in enteral feeding had little effect on the rate or extent of phenytoin absorption.

The suspension formulation of phenytoin is inherent with bioavailability problems resulting from the small particle size, which leads to flocculation. Hence, investigators have evaluated the use of phenytoin capsules administered concomitantly with enteral feedings. Nishimura et al. conducted a randomized crossover study in six healthy volunteers.[52] During phase 1, subjects received phenytoin capsules with water. After a 1-week washout period the subjects began hourly bolus enteral feedings. Phenytoin capsules were administered with the second enteral feeding bolus. Similar to the previous studies in healthy volunteers, there was no significant difference between the two phases for area under the concentration-time curve, maximum concentration, or the time to reach the maximum concentration.[52] One additional pilot study with three head-injured patients reported a two-fold to threefold increase in phenytoin serum concentrations when phenytoin capsules were dissolved in hot water prior to delivery vs. phenytoin powder from capsules mixed with cold water.[53]

Although interactions between oral phenytoin and enteral feeding in patients continue to be reported in the literature, studies in healthy volunteers have not demonstrated significant decreases in phenytoin serum concentrations when administered concomitantly with enteral feeding. This may be due to a number of factors. In the studies with healthy normals, the enteral feedings were swallowed as a bolus at various intervals and not administered through feeding tubes as is done in patients. The phenytoin dose was given via feeding tube in the patients and swallowed by the normal volunteers. Also, in the studies with normal subjects, the duration of enteral feeding was shorter and the interaction evaluated only after single doses of phenytoin. Finally, the patients may have altered gastric emptying rates and absorptive capacities when compared with normal subjects.

There are several factors in critically ill patients that may lead to decreased total phenytoin concentrations regardless of whether the phenytoin is administered with enteral feeding. These include decreased protein binding and increased clearances of phenytoin. Phenytoin is approximately 90% protein bound, primarily to albumin. Therefore, during hypoalbuminemia and renal dysfunction there is an elevation of the free fraction of phenytoin that is thought to be responsible for the clinical effect. The total serum phenytoin concentration, which is most frequently reported, usu-

ally decreases in these situations because of increases in clearance of the drug.[54] Most reports addressing phenytoin pharmacokinetics do not provide information regarding the patients' serum albumin concentration or renal function. Additionally, it has been shown that critically ill trauma patients often have an increased phenytoin clearance over time. Therefore, without aggressive phenytoin dosing and monitoring, subtherapeutic concentrations are more likely to occur in this patient population.[55] None of the reports in patients have systematically examined phenytoin pharmacokinetics in detail.

A low phenytoin serum concentration requires careful investigation into all possible causes. Should the interaction between enteral feeding and phenytoin remain a possible cause of subtherapeutic concentrations, several options exist. The feedings may be withheld for 2 hours before and after phenytoin administration. If a liquid phenytoin preparation is desired other than the commercially available suspension, capsules may be dissolved in warm water, or the intravenous phenytoin product may be given via the feeding tube. Regardless of the phenytoin formulation utilized, nasogastric feeding tubes should be flushed with water following medication administration. The intravenous route for phenytoin administration may be necessary if therapeutic concentrations of the drug are not obtained with the above measures.

In mechanically ventilated patients with severe chronic obstructive pulmonary disease (COPD), theophylline is commonly used to enhance bronchodilation and improve diaphragmatic contractility. Many patients begin therapy with an intravenous theophylline infusion and are transitioned to oral therapy when an enteral feeding tube is available. Diets high in fat and low in protein have been reported to cause increases in theophylline absorption.[56] This is often refered to as "dose dumping" and may lead to toxic theophylline concentrations.[57] In contrast, patients receiving sustained-release theophylline products with therapeutic serum concentrations on admission may have a decrease in levels during enteral feeding.[58] The enteral feeding may cause theophylline malabsorption or increased drug clearance. These patients may attain therapeutic serum concentrations of theophylline when using a liquid preparation of this drug and having the feedings withheld 1 hour before and after the dose.[58] On the other hand, there have been two studies in healthy volunteers that demonstrate the lack of effects of enteral feedings on the absorption of sustained-release theophylline tablets.[59, 60] Likewise, in eight critically ill, mechanically ventilated patients who were receiving continuous enteral feedings via nasogastric or gastrostomy tubes, liquid theophylline was found to be completely bioavailable in all of the patients.[61]

Numerous cases have been reported in the literature that document warfarin resistance caused by the concomitant administration of enteral feedings. Initially, it was believed that the vitamin K content in enteral formulas was excessive and resulted in warfarin resistance. Subsequently, manufacturers decreased the amount of vitamin K content in their enteral formulas, yet the problem still exists.[62] It is now believed that the resistance develops as a result of warfarin sequestration by the enteral feeding formula rather than excessive vitamin K administration.[63] Patients receiving warfarin therapy with enteral feedings should have their prothrombin time monitored closely.

Ciprofloxacin, a quinolone antibiotic with broad-spectrum activity against organisms resistant to many other antibiotics, is available in both intravenous and oral formulations and is often considered for serious infections in critically ill patients. While crushed tablets may be the preferred route in patients with enteral feeding tubes, oral quinolones form chelate complexes with cations, which reduces quinolone absorp-

tion. Potential interactants include aluminum, calcium, magnesium, iron, and zinc.[64] Work investigating the bioavailability of quinolones when administered with enteral feedings has been limited and conflicting. An initial investigation in healthy volunteers concluded that ciprofloxacin is absorbed well after administration via a nasogastric tube, even with coadministration of enteral feedings.[65] In contrast, a second study of healthy volunteers reported significantly lower areas under the curve when ciprofloxacin was administered with enteral feeding formulas as compared with water.[66] A study conducted in critically ill patients receiving continuous enteral feedings reported that ciprofloxacin delivered through a nasoduodenal tube resulted in enhanced absorption when compared with delivery through a nasogastric or gastric tube.[67] Although these findings suggest that crushed ciprofloxacin tablets suspended in water and delivered to the gastric environment may result in increased degradation, additional work is necessary to evaluate its occurrence and clinical implications.

Critically ill patients usually receive parenteral opioids for pain management. However, oral formulations may be used when rapid titration is not required. Morphine sulfate solution (Roxanol, Roxane Laboratories, Inc., Columbus, Ohio) has been reported to be chemically and physically compatible with two enteral feedings, Isocal (Mead Johnson, Evansville, Ind) and Vivonex Standard (Norwich Eaton Pharmaceuticals, Norwich, NY).[68]

All medications should be diluted prior to administration to decrease viscosity and minimize drug contact with the tube. In addition, all feeding tubes should be flushed before and after drug delivery to minimize contact between drug and enteral feeding solutions and to decrease the incidence of clogged feeding tubes. Because modest research has been done in critically ill patients to assess the bioavailability of drugs administered enterally, clinicians should monitor the therapeutic response and, if indicated, obtain serum drug concentrations once the transition from intravenous to enteral delivery is made.

ALTERATIONS IN PHARMACOKINETICS AND NUTRIENT METABOLISM

Alterations in drug disposition or pharamacokinetics may be caused by changes in the nutritional status or nutritional supplementation. A majority of the work has been done in healthy volunteers and has focused on hepatic oxidative metabolism with antipyrine as a marker. This area of research requires further study to document the clinical significance as it pertains to specific drugs and patient populations.

Undernutrition has resulted in alterations in drug pharamacokinetics, including variations in hepatic metabolism and the volume of distribution. Studies conducted in children have found undernutrition to result in decreased hepatic metabolism.[69] A recent study evaluated the pharmacokinetics of metronidazole in children and found significantly decreased clearance in severely undernourished children as compared with nutritionally rehabilitated children.[70] In undernourished adults, hepatic oxidative metabolism is often normal or increased in mild to moderate undernutrition and decreased during severe protein-calorie undernutrition.[71] Tranvouez et al. conducted a study in 49 undernourished patients and 25 well-nourished control subjects.[72] The undernourished patients were further subdivided into those with energy undernutrition ($n = 26$) or protein-calorie undernutrition ($n = 23$). Hepatic oxidative metabolism was assessed by antipyrine clearance and found to be significantly lower in the protein-calorie–undernourished group when compared with the other two groups. In this study, 27 of the undernourished patients went on to receive nutritional rehabilitation with enteral or parenteral nutrition, and hepatic clearance returned toward normal in those patients who had protein-calorie undernutrition.[72]

The second pharmacokinetic parameter that has been shown to be altered in undernourished and critically ill patients is the volume of distribution. Zarowitz et al. combined hypoalbuminemia, reduced body weight, and an elevated ratio of exchangeable sodium to exchangeable potassium in a nutritional index and found that patients with high-risk undernutrition had significantly higher weight-adjusted volumes of distribution for gentamicin as compared with those who were not at high nutritional risk.[73] Critically ill surgical patients have also been shown to have increased volumes of distribution for aminoglycosides secondary to aggressive fluid therapy that expands the extracellular fluid compartment. Dasta and Armstrong reported a 40% increased volume of distribution for aminoglycosides in a group of 181 critically ill surgical patients.[74] The authors attributed this increase to fluid gain, which correlated with weight gain during the study.

Dietary constituents have been shown to have an influence on renal and hepatic drug metabolism. Dickson et al. conducted a study in healthy volunteers and found that protein supplementation (90 g/day) vs. a fasted state resulted in a significant increase in urinary excretion of gentamicin.[75] The amount of protein in the diet has also been shown to affect hepatically cleared drugs such as theophylline.[76] Juan et al. reported that a low-protein diet was associated with a 21% decrease in theophylline clearance when compared with a standard diet. A high-protein diet increased clearance 26% from baseline (with a standard diet). Theophylline clearance has been reported to be increased in both adults and children receiving high-protein diets.[77, 78] During administration of a high-carbohydrate, low-protein diet, theophylline clearance was decreased from normal.[78] The effects of diet composition have also been investigated for drugs with a high intrinsic clearance or low intrinsic clearance.[79] When the diet was changed from high carbohydrate/low protein to low carbohydrate/high protein, the clearance of propranolol increased approximately 74% while the clearance of theophylline increased approximately 32%, thus indicating that drugs with high intrinsic clearance may be more susceptible to dietary manipulations than drugs with low intrinsical clearance. Hamberg et al. evaluated the effects of energy and protein deficiency on drug metabolism and found that both a low-energy and a low-protein intake decreased the glucuronidation of oxazepam but did not affect the oxidative metabolism of antipyrine or metronidazole.[80]

The effects of parenteral nutrition on hepatic metabolism have also been investigated. In six healthy volunteers, the transition from a dextrose-only solution providing 440 kcal/day to an isocaloric regimen of standard amino acids resulted in a significant increase in antipyrine clearance.[81] A similar study in eight healthy volunteers compared a standard amino acid formula (23% branched-chain amino acids [BCAAs] with a high-BCAA formula (85% BCAAs) for their effects on hepatic metabolism. Antipyrine clearance was significantly increased with the standard amino acid formula but not with the high-BCAA formula, thus indicating that protein constituents may have an influence on hepatic oxidative metabolism. Additionally, the authors evaluated conjugative drug metabolism and reported that neither regimen affected it. To determine whether intravenous nutritional repletion can have an influence on oxidative drug metabolism, antipyrine pharmacokinetics were studied in six undernourished patients.[82] After a 2-day basal period that provided 440 kcal/day, all patients received two 8-day nutritional repletion periods. During the two reple-

tion periods all patients randomly received two regimens: one containing high dextrose (1.75 × baseline resting energy expenditure [REE]) and a second containing low dextrose (0.95 × baseline REE) in addition to nitrogen (20 mg/kcal of baseline REE). Although there was no significant difference in antipyrine clearance between the high- and low-dextrose periods, the initial 8-day period of nutritional repletion resulted in a significant increase in antipyrine clearance from baseline.

The effect of three parenteral nutrition regimens on antipyrine clearance has also been investigated in postoperative surgical patients.[83] All parenteral nutrition regimens provided 12 to 14 g of nitrogen with supplemental electrolytes, vitamins, and trace elements. The authors reported that the postoperative patients receiving 1600 or 2000 calories per day as dextrose (100% dextrose) for 7 days demonstrated a 34% decrease in antipyrine clearance when compared with the unfed control patients. The patients who received 2000 calories per day with 25% of the calories provided as lipid had antipyrine clearances similar to the unfed control group. The authors concluded that lipid should be included as a daily component of parenteral nutrition to preserve hepatic oxidative function.[83]

Although the pharmacokinetics of drugs are affected by nutritional status and supplementation, the clinical implications of these findings are difficult to interpret. Additional research, particularly in critically ill patients, needs to be conducted.

Pharmacotherapy may have substantial effects on nutrient metabolism. Some of these effects are beneficial (e.g., a decrease in nitrogen excretion) and can potentially be used to modulate nutrient metabolism. Other effects such as the increased catabolism observed during steroid administration may be detrimental. Some critically ill patients continue to lose body cell mass despite receiving what appears to be adequate doses of specialized nutrition support. It is not entirely clear whether long-term immobilization is the primary factor for the inability to attain nitrogen equilibrium. For this reason, there has been a significant amount of interest in using pharmacologic agents as adjunctive therapy to enhance the outcome of specialized nutrition support intervention. Advances in recombinant DNA technology have yielded many new biotechnological drugs that can be used to potentially enhance anabolism or decrease catabolism. Growth hormone and insulin-like growth factor 1 are two examples of these pharmacologic agents being investigated in clinical trials of critically ill patients. Because of the expense of these adjunctive drugs, it will be very important to identify which patient populations significantly benefit from them.

It is clear that patients with critical illness have an increased REE. It was once thought that this increase was two to three times the basal energy expenditure in most critically ill patients. However, indirect calorimetry has demonstrated that these increases in energy metabolism are modest (20% to 50% in most cases). Patients with severe thermal injury may have as much as a 100% increase in REE. There is some evidence that selected pharmacologic agents decrease the REE in humans.[84–86] Pentobarbital pharmacotherapy following acute head trauma has been shown to decrease the mean REE to 14% below that predicted by the basal energy expenditure equations. Control patients in this clinical study had a mean REE that was 26% above the predicted basal energy expenditure.[84] This drug results in a 30% to 40% decrease in REE in this patient population. Energy balance is much easier to attain in head-injured patients receiving pentobarbital. The effects of pharmacologic paralyzing agents (e.g., vecuronium bromide) on REE have not been studied in depth. Intravenous propranolol administration has been reported to decrease REE ap-

proximately 25% in patients with severe head injury.[85] This effect appears to be mediated through β-adrenergic receptor blockade.[86]

Trauma, thermal injury, and sepsis have all been shown to induce a hypercatabolic state. Some patients with these disorders remain in a markedly negative nitrogen balance despite receiving protein doses of 2 g/kg/day or greater as part of specialized nutrition support. Therefore, interest in adjunctive pharmacotherapy to decrease catabolism and potentially preserve the body cell mass has received much attention. Indomethacin, a prostaglandin synthetase inhibitor, has been used to decrease postoperative catabolism in patients undergoing elective gastrectomy.[87] Protein-sparing effects have also been reported in humans during parenteral nutrition and concomitant administration of phentolamine, somatostatin, ranitidine, and naloxone.[88, 89] More work in this area is definitely needed before any of these pharmacologic agents can be used routinely to reduce net protein catabolism.

Deleterious effects on nutrient metabolism may occur with the administration of cyclosporine or theophylline.[90, 91] In an animal model, cyclosporine has been shown to impair insulin synthesis and secretion and increase insulin clearance.[90] This could potentially contribute to the postoperative hyperglycemia that is commonly seen in patients receiving transplanted livers or kidneys. Patients with COPD have demonstrated increased urinary excretion of 3-methylhistidine in association with the administration of theophylline.[91] This interaction may be particularly important because patients with COPD are very prone to weight loss.

Drugs and nutrients can potentially interact in many different ways. It is prudent to be aware of medications that may interfere with fluid and electrolyte balance, vitamin homeostasis, or gastrointestinal tolerance when one is prescribing specialized nutrition support.

Knowledge of clinically significant interactions and close monitoring can help to identify trends so that early treatment can prevent these metabolic complications. Patients receiving drugs whose disposition is significantly altered by nutrients should be monitored closely so that the desired therapeutic outcome is achieved. This may include close monitoring of serum drug concentrations and dosage adjustments. Monitoring pharmacotherapy in patients receiving specialized nutrition support is part of optimal patient management.

REFERENCES

1. Roe DA: Drug-nutrient interactions in the elderly. *Geriatrics* 1986; 41:57−74.
2. Schneider PJ, Mirtallo JM: Medication profiles in TPN patients. *Nutr Supp Serv* 1983; 3:40−46.
3. Gora ML, Tschampel MM, Visconti JA: Considerations of drug therapy in patients receiving enteral nutrition. *Nutr Clin Pract* 1989; 4:105−110.
4. Driscoll DF: Drug-induced metabolic disorders and parenteral nutrition in the intensive care unit: A pharmaceutical and metabolic perspective. *Ann Pharmacother* 1989; 23:363−371.
5. Hutchison FN, Perez EA, Gandara DR, et al: Renal salt wasting in patients treated with cisplatin. *Ann Intern Med* 1988; 103:21−25.
6. Wofsy CB: Use of trimethoprim-sulfamethoxazole in the treatment of *Pneumocystis carinii* pneumonitis in patients with acquired immunodeficiency syndrome. *Rev Infect Dis* 1987; 9(suppl):184−191.
7. Nelson DC, McGrew WR, Hoyumpa AM: Hypernatremia and lactulose therapy. *JAMA* 1983; 249:1295−1298.
8. Lawson DH, Henry DA, Lowe JM, et al: Severe hypokalemia in hospitalized patients. *Arch Intern Med* 1979; 139:978−980.
9. Lipworth BJ, McDevitt DG, Struthers AD: Hypokalemic and ECG sequelae of combined beta-agonist/diuretic therapy. *Chest* 1990; 98:811−815.
10. Rimmer JM, Horn JF, Gennari J: Hyperkalemia as a complication of drug therapy. *Arch Intern Med* 1987; 147:867−869.
11. Gonzalez-Martin G, Diaz-Molinas MS, Martinez AM, et al: Heparin-induced hyperkalemia: A prospective study. *Int J Clin Pharmacol Ther Toxicol* 1991; 29:446−449.
12. Goldszer RC, Coodley EL, Rosner MJ, et al: Hyperkalemia associated with indomethacin. *Arch Intern Med* 1981; 141:802−824.
13. Halevy J, Bulvik S: Severe hypophosphatemia in hospitalized patients. *Arch Intern Med* 1988; 148:153−155.
14. Sherman RA, Hwang ER, Walker JA, et al: Reduction in serum phosphorus due to sucralfate. *Am J Gastroenterol* 1983; 78:210−211.
15. Johnston S, Simpson J: Medication-nutrient interactions: Hypophosphatemia associated with sucralfate in the intensive care unit. *Nutr Clin Pract* 1991; 6:199−201.
16. Brady HR, Ryan F, Cunningham J, et al: Hypophosphatemia complicating bronchodilator therapy for acute severe asthma. *Arch Intern Med* 1989; 149:2367−2368.
17. Vernon WB, Atkins JM, Stewart RD: Hyperphosphatemia from lipid emulsion in a patient on total parenteral nutrition. *JPEN* 1988; 12:84−87.
18. Zaloga GP, Chernow B, Pock A, et al: Hypomagnesemia is a common complication of aminoglycoside therapy. *Surg Gynecol Obstet* 1984; 158:561−565.
19. Sheehan J, White A: Diuretic-associated hypomagnesemia. *BMJ* 1982; 285:1157−1159.
20. Nozue T, Kobayashi A, Kodama T, et al: Pathogenesis of cyclosporine-induced hypomagnesemia. *J Pediatr* 1992; 120:638−640.
21. Schilsky RL, Anderson T: Hypomagnesemia and renal magnesium wasting in patients receiving cisplatin. *Ann Intern Med* 1979; 90:929−931.
22. Elin RJ, Hosseini JM: Magnesium content of mononuclear blood cells. *Clin Chem* 1985; 31:377−380.
23. Longstreth GF, Green R: Folate status in patients receiving maintenance doses of sulfasalazine. *Arch Intern Med* 1983; 143:902−904.
24. Halsted CH, Gandhi G, Tamura T: Sul-

fasalazine inhibits the absorption of folates in ulcerative colitis. *N Engl J Med* 1981; 305:1513–1517.

25. Seligmann H, Halkin H, Rauchfleisch S, et al: Thiamine deficiency in patients with congestive heart failure receiving long-term furosemide therapy: A pilot study. *Am J Med* 1991; 91:151–155.
26. Bliss DZ, Guenter PA, Settle RG: Defining and reporting diarrhea in tube-fed patients—what a mess! *Am J Clin Nutr* 1992; 55:753–759.
27. Edes TE, Walk BE, Austin JL: Diarrhea in tube-fed patients: Feeding formula not necessarily the cause. *Am J Med* 1990; 88:91–93.
28. Guenter PA, Settle RG, Perlmutter S, et al: Tube feeding-related diarrhea in acutely ill patients. *JPEN* 1991; 15:277–280.
29. Hill DB, Henderson LM, McClain CJ: Osmotic diarrhea induced by sugar-free theophylline solution in critically ill patients. *JPEN* 1991; 15:332–336.
30. Badiga MS, Jain NK, Casanova C, et al: Diarrhea in diabetics: The role of sorbitol. *J Am Coll Nutr* 1990; 9:578–582.
31. Fine KD, Santa Ana CA, Fordtran JS: Diagnosis of magnesium-induced diarrhea. *N Engl J Med* 1991; 324:1012–1017.
32. Niemiec PW, Vanderveen TW, Morrison JI, et al: Gastrointestinal disorders caused by medication and electrolyte solution osmolality during enteral nutrition. *JPEN* 1983; 7:387–389.
33. Dickerson RN, Melnik G: Osmolality of oral drug solutions and suspensions. *Am J Hosp Pharm* 1988; 45:832–834.
34. Rybolt H, Laughon BE, Greenough WB, et al: Protein-losing enteropathy associated with *Clostridium difficile* infection. *Lancet* 1989; 1:1353–1355.
35. Brown CK, Khankeria U: Use of metoclopramide, domperidone, and cisapride in the management of diabetic gastroparesis. *Clin Pharm* 1990; 9:357–365.
36. Janssens J, Peeters TL, Tack J, et al: Improvement of gastric emptying in diabetic gastroparesis by erythromycin. *N Engl J Med* 1990; 322:1028–1031.
37. Carlson RG, Hocking MP, Sninsky CA, et al: Erythromycin acts through a cholinergic pathway to improve canine-

38. Bannerjee AK, Patel KJ, Grainger SL: Drug-induced acute pancreatitis. A critical review. *Med Toxicol Adverse Drug Exp* 1989; 4:186–198.
39. Eckhauser ML, Dokler MA, Imbembo AL: Diuretic-associated pancreatitis: A collective review and illustrative cases. *Am J Gastroenterol* 1987; 82:865–870.
40. Bonavina L, Demeester TR, McChesney L, et al: Drug-induced esophageal strictures. *Ann Surg* 1987; 206:173–183.
41. Ovartlarnporn B, Kulwichit W, Hiranniramol S: Medication-induced esophageal injury: Report of 17 cases with endoscopic documentation. *Am J Gastroenterol* 1991; 86:748–750.
42. Cutie AJ, Altman E, Lenkel L: Compatibility of enteral products with commonly employed drug additives. *JPEN* 1983; 7:186–191.
43. Cacek AT, DeVito JM, Koonce JR: In vitro evaluation of nasogastric administration methods for phenytoin. *Am J Hosp Pharm* 1986; 43:689–692.
44. Clark-Schmidt AL, Garnett WR, Lowe DR, et al: Loss of carbamazepine suspension through nasogastric feeding tubes. *Am J Hosp Pharm* 1990; 47:2034–2037.
45. Splinter MY, Seifert CF, Bradberry JC, et al: Recovery of phenytoin suspension after in vitro administration through percutaneous endoscopic gastrostomy Pezzer catheters. *Am J Hosp Pharm* 1990; 47:373–377.
46. Druckenbrod RW, Healy DP: In vitro delivery of crushed ciprofloxacin through a feeding tube. *Ann Pharmacother* 1992; 26:494–495.
47. Cutie AJ, Holtz L, Milton J, et al: Compatibility of medications with enteral feedings. *JPEN* 1987; 11:183–186.
48. Bauer LA: Interference of oral phenytoin absorption by continuous nasogastric feedings. *Neurology* 1982; 32:570–572.
49. Ozuna J, Friel P: Effect of enteral tube feeding on serum phenytoin levels. *J Neurosurg Nurs* 1984; 12:289–291.
50. Krueger KA, Garnett WR, Comstock TJ, et al: Effect of two administration schedules of an enteral nutrient for-

mula on phenytoin bioavailability. *Epilepsia* 1987; 28:706–712.

51. Marvel ME, Bertino JS: Comparative effects of an elemental and a complex enteral feeding formulation on the absorption of phenytoin suspension. *JPEN* 1991; 15:316–318.

52. Nishimura LY, Armstrong EP, Plezia PM, et al: Influence of enteral feedings on phenytoin sodium absorption from capsules. *Ann Pharmacother* 1988; 22:130–133.

53. Schraeder PL, Cordas MR, Daxon M: Enteral tube feeding and phenytoin levels: The hot water solution (abstract). *Epilepsia* 1986; 27:593.

54. Levine M, Chang T: Therapeutic drug monitoring of phenytoin; rationale and current status. *Clin Pharmacokinet* 1990; 19:341–358.

55. Boucher BA, Rodman JH, Jaresko GS, et al: Phenytoin pharmacokinetics in critically ill trauma patients. *Clin Pharmacol Ther* 1988; 44:675–683.

56. Jonkman JHG: Food interactions with sustained-release theophylline preparations: A review. *Clin Pharmacokinet* 1989; 16:162–179.

57. Hendeles L, Weigberger M, Milavetz G, et al: Food-induced "dose dumping" from once-a-day theophylline product as a cause of theophylline toxicity. *Chest* 1985; 6:758–765.

58. Gal P, Layson R: Interference with oral theophylline absorption by continuous nasogastric feedings. *Ther Drug Monitor* 1986; 8:421–423.

59. Plezia PM, Thornley SM, Kramer TH, et al: The influence of enteral feedings on sustained-release theophylline absorption. *Pharmacotherapy* 1990; 10:356–361.

60. Schaaf LJ, Bhargava VO, Berlinger WG, et al: Effect of an enteral formula on sustained-release theophylline absorption (abstract). *Pharmacotherapy* 1989; 9:185.

61. Shalansky KF, Vaughan LM, Ustad C, et al: Absolute bioavailability of aminophylline liquid administered enterally in adults requiring mechanical ventilation. *Clin Pharm* 1992; 11:428–432.

62. Martin JE, Lutomski DM: Warfarin resistance and enteral feedings. *JPEN* 1989; 13:206–208.

63. Kuhn TA, Garnett WR, Wells BK, et al:

Recovery of warfarin from an enteral nutrient formula. *Am J Hosp Pharm* 1989; 46:1395–1399.

64. Lomaestro BM, Bailie GR: Quinolone-cation interactions: A review. *Ann Pharmacother* 1991; 25:1249–1258.

65. Yuk JH, Nightingale CH, Sweeney KR, et al: Relative bioavailability in healthy volunteers of ciprofloxacin administered through a nasogastric tube with and without enteral feeding. *Antimicrob Agents Chemother* 1989; 33:1118–1120.

66. Noer BL, Angaran DM: The effect of enteral feedings on ciprofloxacin pharmacokinetics (abstract). *Pharmacotherapy* 1990; 10:58.

67. Yuk, JH, Nightingale CH, Quintiliani R, et al: Absorption of ciprofloxacin administered through nasogastric or a nasoduodenal tube in volunteers and patients receiving enteral nutrition. *Diagn Microbiol Infect Dis* 1990; 13:99–102.

68. Michelini TJ, Bhargava VO, Dube JE: Stability of oral morphine sulfate solutions in two enteral tube feeding products. *Am J Hosp Pharm* 1988; 45:628–630.

69. Buchanan N: Effect of protein-energy malnutrition on drug metabolism in man. *World Rev Nutr Diet* 1984; 43:129–139.

70. Lares-Asseff I, Cravioto J, Santiago P, et al: Pharmacokinetics of metronidazole in severely malnourished and nutritionally rehabilitated children. *Clin Pharmacol Ther* 1992; 51:42–50.

71. Anderson KE: Influences of diet and nutrition on clinical pharmacokinetics. *Clin Pharmacokinet* 1988; 14:325–346.

72. Tranvouez JL, Lerebours E, Chretien P, et al: Hepatic antipyrine metabolism in malnourished patients: Influence of the type of malnutrition and course after nutritional rehabilitation. *Am J Clin Nutr* 1985; 41:1257–1264.

73. Zarowitz BJ, Pilla AM, Popovich J: Expanded gentamicin volume of distribution in patients with indicators of malnutrition. *Clin Pharm* 1990; 9:40–44.

74. Dasta JF, Armstrong DK: Variability in aminoglycoside pharmacokinetics in critically ill surgical patients. *Crit Care Med* 1988; 16:327–330.

75. Dickson, CJ, Schwartzman MS, Bertino JS: Factors affecting aminoglycoside disposition: Effects of circadian rhythm and dietary protein intake on gentamicin pharmacokinetics. *Clin Pharmacol Ther* 1986; 39:325–328.

76. Juan D, Worwag EM, Schoeller DA, et al: Effects of dietary protein on theophylline pharmacokinetics and caffeine and aminopyrine breath tests. *Clin Pharmacol Ther* 1986; 40:187–194.

77. Kappas A, Anderson KE, Conney AH, et al: Influence of dietary protein and carbohydrate on antipyrine and theophylline metabolism in man. *Clin Pharmacol Ther* 1976; 20:643–653.

78. Feldman Ch, Hutchinson VE, Sher TH, et al: Interaction between nutrition and theophylline metabolism in children. *Ther Drug Monito* 1982; 4:69–76.

79. Fagan TC, Walle T, Oexmann MJ, et al: Increased clearance of propranolol and theophylline by high-protein compared with high-carbohydrate diet. *Clin Pharmacol Ther* 1987; 41:402–406.

80. Hamberg O, Ovesen L, Dorfeldt A, et al: The effect of dietary energy and protein deficiency on drug metabolism. *Eur J Clin Pharmacol* 1990; 38:567–570.

81. Pantuck EJ, Pantuck CB, Weissman C, et al: Effects of parenteral nutritional regimens on oxidative drug metabolism. *Anesthesiology* 1984; 60:534–536.

82. Pantuck EJ, Weissman C, Pantuck C, et al: Effects of parenteral amino acid nutritional regimens on oxidative and conjugative drug metabolism. *Anesth Analg* 1989; 69:727–731.

83. Burgess P, Hall RI, Bateman DN, et al: The effect of total parenteral nutrition on hepatic drug oxidation. *JPEN* 1987; 11:540–543.

84. Dempsey DT, Guenter P, Mullen JL, et al: Energy expenditure in acute trauma to the head with and without barbiturate therapy. *Surg Gynecol Obstet* 1985; 160:128–134.

85. Chiolero RL, Breitenstein E, Thorin D, et al: Effects of propranolol on resting metabolic rate after severe head injury. *Crit Care Med* 1989; 17:328–334.

86. Welle S, Schwartz RG, Statt M: Reduced metabolic rate during β-adrenergic blockade in humans. *Metabolism* 1991; 40:619–622.

87. Asoh T, Shiraska C, Uchida I, et al: Effects of indomethacin on endocrine responses and nitrogen loss after surgery. *Ann Surg* 1987; 206:770–776.

88. Shaw JH, Holdaway CM, Humberstone DA: Metabolic intervention in surgical patient: The effect of α or β-blockade on glucose and protein metabolism in surgical patients receiving total parenteral nutrition. *Surgery* 1988; 103:520–525.

89. Shaw JH, Wolfe RR: Metabolic interventions in surgical patients. *Ann Surg* 1988; 207:274–282.

90. Dresner LS, Adnersen DK, Kahng KU, et al: Effects of cyclosporine on glucose metabolism. *Surgery* 1989; 106:163–170.

91. Wei IW, McFadden ER, Hoppel CL: Effect of theophylline on urinary excretion of 3-methylhistidine in patients with lung disease. *Metabolism* 1991; 40:702–706.

27

Effect of Nutrition on Inflammatory Mediators

William A. Thompson, III, M.D.

Stephen F. Lowry, M.D.

It is well documented that nutritional status influences the clinical outcome following injury, surgery, or infection. Malnourished patients subjected to such inflammatory insults have higher morbidity and mortality rates than their adequately nourished cohorts. Rhoades and Alexander in 1955 demonstrated the association between increased infectious complications and patients with hypoproteinemia.[1] Such a relationship between nutrition and inflammation has generally been assumed to be exerted through the availability of substrates to repair damaged tissue and support a functional immune system. However, recent evidence has suggested that nutritional support, in addition to preventing specific nutrient deficiencies, also exerts some influence over the endogenous production of inflammatory mediators. This chapter will focus on nutrition as a modulating influence upon several components of the inflammatory mediator cascade currently believed responsible for both initiating and perpetuating the host response to injury and infection.

CYTOKINES AS INFLAMMATORY MEDIATORS

The Role of Cytokines in Maintaining Physiologic Homeostasis

Present data support a role for endogenous cytokine peptides as important mediators of the local as well as systemic manifestations of severe injury or infection.[2, 3] These inflammatory mediators are produced by both myeloid[4] as well as nonmyeloid cells[5] in response to appropriate stimuli, including endotoxins, exotoxins, and viral particles.[6, 7]

Cytokines appear to be critical in modulating a number of beneficial responses to injury and infection by promoting wound healing,[8–11] prioritizing substrates for acute-phase protein synthesis,[12, 13] and eradicating invading microorganisms.[14, 15] As can be inferred from their cellular origin and stimuli for production, cytokines also exert significant control over immunocellular function and production. C3H/HeJ mice incapable of producing tumor necrosis factor α (TNF-α) to endotoxin challenge are more susceptible to infection with a virulent *Escherichia coli* strain than are their TNF-α–producing congenic cohorts. Pretreatment of such TNF-α–deficient mice with TNF-α and interleukin-α (IL-1α) confers protection against a subsequent bacterial challenge with an inoculum of greater than 20 times the median lethal dose (LD_{50}) of *E. coli*.[16] It is also evident that some degree of cytokine activity is necessary for long-term host recovery from severe injury because severely diminished host cytokine production correlates adversely with the ultimate outcome.[17] By inference, nutritional status may influence this capacity for cytokine production, not only in the acute situation but perhaps more importantly over longer periods of stressful illness.

The Role of Cytokines in Disease Processes

Despite the apparent necessity of cytokine-mediated immunocompetence, an exaggerated cytokine response has been implicated in the development of such divergent clinical entities as the chronic wasting syndrome of cancer cachexia[18] as well as the more acute cardiovascular collapse and multiorgan failure syndrome of gram-negative sepsis.[19] Most recent efforts have sought to alter the acutely exaggerated cytokine influence that presumptively underlies many adverse sequelae of trauma, shock, and infection.

Sepsis

It is increasingly evident that an exaggerated cytokine response is responsible for the initiation and some aspects of the perpetuation of organ system dysfunction following inflammatory stimuli.[2] The acute administration of TNF-α to experimental animals at doses presumably similar to those achieved endogenously mimics the cardiovascular collapse, organ failure, and death seen in gram-negative sepsis.[19, 20] Similarly, an IL-1α infusion in primates may replicate the hemodynamic and some but not all of the metabolic changes of sublethal endotoxemia.[21] Additionally, the administration of anti–TNF-α monoclonal antibodies to baboons 2 hours prior to the administration of an LD_{100} of intravenous *E. coli* afforded complete protection from the hemodynamic instability, organ system dysfunction, and death that uniformly appeared in the control animals.[22] However, unlike TNF-α blockade, neutralization of IL-1 activity by a continuous infusion of an IL-1 receptor antagonist only moderately attenuated the fall in arterial pressure and cardiac output but significantly improved survival in this model of gram-negative sepsis.[23]

Circulating cytokine levels following experimental bacterial or endotoxin infusion suggest that cytokine production and expression follow a reproducible temporal pattern. TNF-α has been shown to appear within 30 minutes of a bacterial infusion, peak at 90 minutes, and become undetectable at 4 hours. IL-1β and IL-6 appear somewhat later than TNF-α with IL-1β reaching a broad monophasic peak at 4 hours while IL-6 levels continue to rise for up to 8 hours following bacterial challenge.[3] We have observed similar patterns of cytokine appearance following experimental human endotoxemia, although IL-1 is not readily detectable in human endotoxemia or sepsis.[24] Moreover, TNF-α blockade prior to a bacteremic challenge not only neutralized the systemic manifestations of sepsis but also significantly abrogated the appearance of IL-1β and IL-6.[25]

An important feature of the proinflammatory cytokines TNF-α and IL-1 is their capacity to elicit significant tissue responses, even though they are not detectable through routine peripheral blood sampling. Through the demonstration of a high–molecular-weight cell-associated form of TNF-α[26] as well as through the demonstration of significant cytokine compartmentalization,[27] it is apparent that a majority of cytokine-cellular interactions occur locally. The balance of this chapter will focus on the contribution of varying nutritional parameters on the production of cytokine as well as noncytokine inflammatory mediators.

Cancer Cachexia

Chronic TNF-α administration to experimental animals reproduces many of the features of cachexia, including anorexia,[18] weight loss,[12] and a decline in nitrogen balance.[28] In a rat sarcoma model, tumor burden exhibited a direct correlation with TNF-α levels, the degree of anorexia, and weight loss.[29] Following tumor resection in these animals, TNF-α levels became undetectable upon a return of food intake and body weight.[30] Despite the detection of circulating levels of TNF-α in some humans with malignancies,[31] a strong correlation between circulating cytokine levels and the degree of cachexia is currently lacking. A similar lack of correlation between circulating cytokine levels and cachexia of benign inflammatory disease is also apparent.[32]

THE EFFECT OF THE ROUTE OF FEEDING ON INFLAMMATORY MEDIATORS

Dudrick and associates pioneering work[33] appeared to solve the dilemma of an ineffective means of nutritional support in populations desperately in need of protein and caloric repletion. Parenteral nutrition has unquestionably benefited patients with short-gut syndrome[34, 35] or high-output fistulas.[36, 37] On the other hand, parenteral nutrition has not proved to be of major benefit in patients with trauma[38] or cancer[39] or in patients receiving surgery.[40, 41]

Sepsis remains the most common problem in the care of the critically ill. Intuitively, the restoration of depleted energy and nitrogen stores in this population should render the host less susceptible to infection. However, a relationship between aggressive nutritional support and diminutions in septic complications has remained tenuous. Moore et al.[42] in a group of 75 patients with abdominal trauma randomized to either a parenteral or enteral regimen noted that despite equivalent protein and caloric intake, the parenterally fed patients experienced a higher incidence of major septic complications (20%) than did the enterally fed patients (3%). Kudsk et al.[38] also noted that enterally fed patients with severe trauma had significantly fewer infections than did their parenterally fed cohorts. These clinical observations linking the parenteral route of feeding with a maladaptive response to an inflammatory insult have been emphasized experimentally through work performed on the etiology and consequences of bacterial translocation.

The Pathophysiology of Bacterial Translocation and Cytokine Activation

Bacterial translocation has been defined as the passage of viable indigenous bacteria from the intact gastrointestinal tract into the mesenteric lymph nodes and beyond.[43] For bacterial translocation to activate inflammatory mediators and participate in disease processes two conditions must occur. Most importantly, there must be a loss of *functional* mucosal integrity leading to translocation of antigens in the form of bacteria or toxins to the splanchnic immune system. Second, this interaction of gut-derived antigens with splanchnic immune tissue must result in an enhanced state of cytokine production.

In addition to the administration of parenteral nutrients, or a state of negligible enteral intake, bacterial translocation has been shown to occur following immunosuppression, hemorrhagic shock, burns, malnutrition, intestinal obstruction, broad-spectrum antibiotic administration, and endotoxin exposure. In each of these experimental settings the development of bacterial translocation has been attributed to three pathologic mechanisms. These mechanisms include a physical or physiologic loss of the mucosal barrier function,[44, 45] bacterial overgrowth,[46, 47] and impaired host defense.[48]

The bacterial translocation hypothesis presumes that pathophysiolgoic processes can induce either systemic bacteremia/endotoxemia or the release of inflammatory mediators by antigen-exposed leukocytes of the splanchnic immune system. The clinical correlate to the first part of this hypothesis may explain why no septic focus is often identified at autopsy in more than 30% of patients succumbing to *bacteremic* multisystem organ failure.[49] The second part of this hypothesis may further explain the paradox of a septic-like syndrome (hyperdynamic circulation and systemic inflammation) when cultures are negative in greater than 50% of such cases.[50]

Both experimental animal and human studies have documented that antecedent nutritional manipulation has a profound influence on the metabolic and inflammatory response to subsequent traumatic and infectious insults. Many clinical trials comparing enteral and parenteral feedings have documented an increased susceptibility to infection in parenterally fed patients, perhaps implying some form of immunosuppression. Still unanswered is whether enteral feedings decrease the risk of infection or alternatively whether parenteral nutrition increases this risk.

Although not readily demonstrable in human studies, animal models have clearly shown that parenteral nutrition is associated with bacterial translocation.[51] However, human studies have shown that parenteral nutrition is able to invoke a differential inflammatory response to infectious stimuli ranging from tolerance in the neutrophil and complement cascade[52] to priming of the macrophage/monocyte system with enhanced cytokine production.[53] These findings are *"consistent with"* the general concept of endotoxin translocation and subsequent immunomodulation. Clinically, these divergent immune states may be represented by increased infectious complications (immunosuppression) or multisystem organ failure and septic shock secondary to an exaggerated or dysregulated tissue cytokine response. In healthy volunteers receiving 1 week of isocaloric and isonitrogenous regimens of either enteral or parenteral nutrition, we have shown how this paradoxical response within the immune system can coexist. Endotoxin administration in such normal subjects promotes a clinical condition similar to sepsis by producing an abbreviated systemic appearance of cytokines as well as self-limited systemic signs of sepsis.[54]

Parenteral Nutrition and Impaired Neutrophil Responsiveness

Using the above-described model, we have noted a blunting of both the neutrophilia and rise in C3a levels of the complement system, as well as diminished neutrophil chemotaxis to leukotriene B_4 (LTB$_4$) following endotoxin administration in parenterally fed normal subjects. No differences were noted between enterally and parenterally fed groups regarding neutrophil chemotaxis to N-formyl-methionyl-leucyl-phenylalanine—and zymosan-activated serum.[55] This apparent suppression of the neutrophil arm of the immune system in the parenterally fed volunteers was observed despite an intake of protein and calories similar to their orally fed cohort group. These data imply some potential tolerance to endotoxin activity, perhaps secondary to prior enterically derived endotoxin exposure.

Parenteral Nutrition and Enhanced Cytokine Responsiveness

In the same model, examination of the monocyte/macrophage system of parenterally fed volunteers also revealed some aspects of an exaggerated immunologic and metabolic response to endotoxin exposure. This is reminiscent of the physiologic derangements noted with multiorgan system failure and sepsis. Parenterally fed volunteers experience higher peak levels of systemic and hepatic vein TNF-α, arterial glucagon, and epinephrine, as well as increased symptomatology and febrile response following endotoxin administration (Fig 27–1). Additional findings in the subjects receiving total parenteral nutrition (TPN) included a significantly higher extremity efflux of lactate and amino acids.[56] Hence, the splanchnic cytokine and counterregulatory hormonal response to lipopolysaccharide (LPS) was enhanced following 1 week of TPN and bowel rest.

From these observations it is possible to construct a hypothesis explaining the effect of parenterally administered nutrients on inflammatory mediators.[57] As illustrated in Figure 27–2, under conditions of enteral nutrition the gut barrier remains intact, and there is minimal antigenic presentation to the reticuloendothelial cells of the splanchnic immune system and hence little cytokine expression. However, with TPN administration, conditions become more favorable (mucosal atrophy, bacterial overgrowth, and gastrointestinal immunosuppression) for the translocation of either gut-derived bacteria or bacterial products to the mononuclear cells of the submucosa, mesenteric lymphatics, or splanchnic tissue. This increased Kupffer/mononuclear cell antigenic exposure results in increased cytokine expression, particularly of the cell-associated forms.[26] Under these conditions there may be little if any cytokine activity evident within the systemic circulation. However, this increased cytokine expression not only influences neighboring hepatocytes through paracrine mechanisms to produce acute-phase proteins but may also prime local immune cells, such as the Kupffer cell, for future antigenic exposure. When a subsequent antigenic challenge occurs, whether experimentally with LPS administration or clinically with infectious complications, an exaggerated cytokine response is elicited from these primed mononuclear cells within the splanchnic system. With this level of cytokine production, soluble inflammatory mediators spill into the hepatic venous effluent and allow both detection in the systemic circulation as well as manifestations of the classic immunologic and counterregulatory endocrine hormonal features of sepsis. (Fig 27–3)

SPECIFIC NUTRIENT INFLUENCES

Although considerable clinical data support the route of feeding as a critical factor in determining the cytokine response and ultimate clinical outcome to an inflammatory stress, both cell culture and animal models suggest that specific amino acid and lipid moieties may have a similar influence on the inflammatory response. These specific nutrient influences may also modulate immune function regardless of the route of administration and may additively have

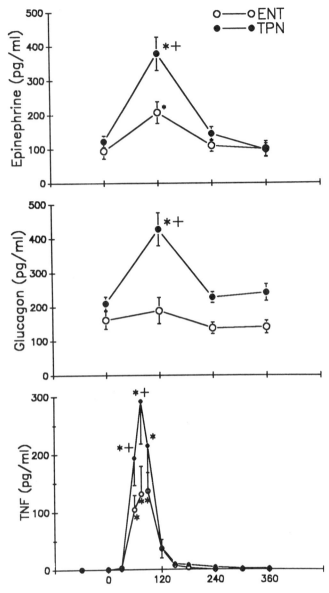

FIG 27–1.
Hormonal and tumor necrosis factor (TNF) levels in response to endotoxin. Epinephrine, glucagon, and TNF levels in arterial blood before (t = 0) and after intravenous endotoxin administration. Subjects were studied 12 hours after the cessation of 7 days of enteral (ENT) feedings (open circles) or total parenteral nutrition (TPN, closed circles). Points are means with their standard errors represented by vertical bars. * P < .05 vs. t = 0. + P < .05 vs. TPN.

an influence on noncytokine inflammatory mediators.

Glutamine

Glutamine, the most abundant free amino acid in both the circulation and intracellular pools,[58] is an important precursor for amino acids, proteins, and nucleotides. Not surprisingly, although

a nonessential amino acid,[59] when provided as a parenteral nutritional supplement, glutamine has been shown to attenuate the nitrogen loss following major surgery.[60, 61] Glutamine's effect, however, on the immune system in general and on inflammatory mediators specifically has not been entirely elucidated.

Glutamine may potentially exert an

NORMAL   **LOSS OF ENTERAL
                                                      NUTRIENT STIMULATION**

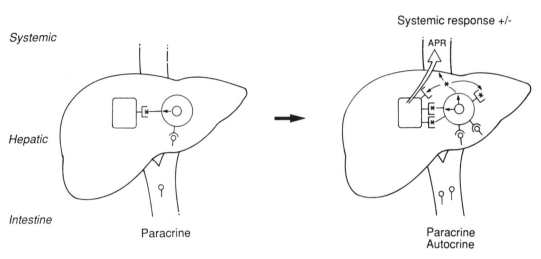

FIG 27–2.
A proposed mechanism for alterations in hepatic Kupffer cell *(large circle)* and hepatocyte *(rectangle)* function during loss of enteral nutrient stimulation. Under normal conditions *(left panel)* there is minimal inciting antigen (♀). There is evidence of constitutive Kupffer cell cytokine production. This low level of activation likely produces a cell-associated form of cytokine (∗—) that interacts with specific receptors on the hepatocyte (⊣). During conditions of loss of enteral nutrient stimulation *(right panel)*, mechanisms operative within the intestinal tract permit increased exposure to the inciting antigens of the liver. This increased antigen exposure enhances the production of cell-associated as well as soluble forms of cytokine (∗). These interact directly with the hepatocytes to alter cellular function, including the production of acute-phase proteins *(APR)*, some of which may be detectable in the peripheral circulation. Soluble cytokine also serves to alter Kupffer cell capacity for further cytokine production by autocrine mechanisms. During such conditions, there may be little if any cytokine evident in the systemic circulation.

immunomodulatory influence both as a direct rate-limiting substrate for metabolically active cells of the immune system as well as an intestinal trophic stimulus capable of attenuating gut atrophy and subsequent bacterial translocation. Ardawi and Newsholme[62] have shown that when glutamine is added to cultured lymphocytes from rat mesenteric lymph nodes, a marked incorporation of ^{3}H-thymidine into concanavalin A–stimulated lymphocytes occurs. Arginine, asparagine, aspartate, glutamate, glycine, histidine, proline, or serine stimulates lymphocyte proliferation only 10% to 20% of that produced by equimolar concentrations of glutamine. Similar findings have been noted in terminally differentiated, nondividing macrophages. Wallace and Keast[63] demonstrated that decreasing glutamine concentrations in culture medium lead to a decrease in phagocytosis of opso-

nized sheep erythrocytes by macrophages. These authors also noted that glutamine availability was essential in the synthesis of RNA and IL-1 production by LPS-stimulated macrophages.

Considerable interest has also focused on glutamine's potential to prevent gut atrophy and bacterial translocation. Glutamine has been shown to be a preferred fuel by the enterocyte.[64, 65] Animal models have shown that supplementation of parenteral formulas with glutamine results in increased intestinal mucosal height[66] and decreased bacterial translocation.[51] Alverdy has shown that glutamine's benefits to gut immune function may exceed that attributed to direct trophic effects on the intestinal mucosa.[51] A 50% decrease in biliary s-IgA and enhanced bacterial translocation to mesenteric lymph nodes developed in rats fed glutamine-free TPN. When glutamine

LOSS OF ENTERAL NUTRIENT STIMULATION
AND INJURY

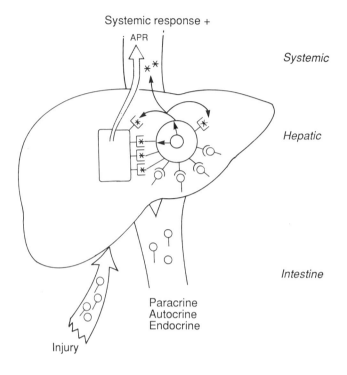

FIG 27–3.

A proposed mechanism for enhanced hepatic responses in patients experiencing loss of enteral nutrient stimulation and an associated or secondary injury. Under these conditions the predisposition to enhanced cytokine production by Kupffer cells is amplified by inciting antigen exposure from intestinal and injury sites. Demonstrable evidence of increased hepatic injury responses, such as acute-phase protein *(APR)* production, is evident in the circulation. With this level of cytokine production, soluble mediator is detectable in the circulation, and systemic responses consistent with cytokine appearance are observed. (See Fig 27–2 for definitions of symbols.)

was added to the TPN, both IgA levels and translocation of bacteria were similar to the control animals eating chow.[66] We have shown that glutamine was able to maintain small-bowel mass and preserve jejunal mucosal architecture in animals fed a defined formula diet[47, 67] and have also demonstrated such an influence during parenteral feedings.[68] However, glutamine had no effect on preventing cecal bacterial overgrowth or spontaneous bacterial translocation. Additionally, although glutamine-supplemented animals had a lower incidence of bacteremia than did rats fed a defined formula diet, there was no effect on cytokine response (TNF-α, IL-6), acute-phase response, or 24-hour mortality following endotoxin challenge. [47, 67]

Arginine

Arginine, a semiessential dibasic amino acid, plays a role in protein synthesis, biosynthesis of other amino acids, and the urea cycle when present in physiologic concentrations.[69] This amino acid exhibits potential benefits as a specific immunostimulant[70, 71] and inducer of growth hormone secretion.[72, 73] However, these benefits may be tempered by in vitro studies implicating arginine as an indispensable substrate in the formation of the inflammatory mediator nitric oxide (NO).

Oral arginine supplementation, when administered at 1% and 2% of the total energy intake in burned guinea pigs, decreased the mortality rate from 56% to 29% and 22%, respectively. In these studies, no nutritional indices were improved with arginine supplementation, whereas arginine did increase the ear thickness response to dinitrofluorobenzene, a T-lymphocyte–dependent delayed hypersensitivity test.[74] Other investigators[75–78] have been able to demonstrate a net reduction in protein loss in arginine-supplemented rats following experimental injury. Such a beneficial response may be mediated through the secretagogue activities (stimulation of growth hormone, prolactin, and insulin secretion) of arginine or its active metabolite ornithine.[79] Sitren and Fisher[78] have postulated that the anabolic properties of arginine during stress may be secondary to an injury-associated increase in the hepatic influx of amino acids. This increased metabolic demand increases amino acid deamination, urea cycle activity, and the demand for arginine.

Arginine has also been shown to possess strong thymotrophic actions, as demonstrated by increases in thymic weight in both injured and uninjured rats[70] and increased lymphocyte blastogenesis to concanavalin A and phytohemagglutinin in rats,[80] healthy volunteers,[81] and cancer patients.[82] In the latter study by Daly et al., there were also notable increases in the number of T-helper lymphocytes. Despite these apparent immunologic benefits to surgical cancer patients, there were no clinical differences between the arginine-supplemented patients and controls regarding postoperative respiratory, infectious, or gastrointestinal complications.

Controversy remains as to the role of arginine as potential substrate in the formation of the inflammatory mediator NO.[83, 84] NO formation, via the conversion of L-arginine to NO and L-citrulline by NO synthase, is now widely felt to be one of the common final pathways in the pathophysiology of septic shock.[83–85] NO, initially characterized as endothelial-derived relaxing factor,[86] causes vasodilatation by activating soluble guanylate cyclase of vascular smooth muscle cells, increasing cyclic guanosine monophosphate (cGMP), and thus decreasing intracellular calcium levels and inducing vascular relaxation.[87] Endotoxin and cytokines such as TNF-α have also been shown in vitro to stimulate NO production by endothelial cells,[88] macrophages,[89] Kupffer cells,[90] and hepatocytes.[91] Animals made hypotensive by endotoxin[92] and cytokine,[93] as well as two patients with vasopressor-resistant septic shock,[94] had a reversal of their hypotension by the administration of a competitive inhibitor of arginine, N^G-monomethyl-L-arginine (L-NMMA). Cobb et al.,[95] however, have shown that some potential adverse sequelae exist when NO synthase is inhibited. Although vascular resistance is elevated in endotoxemic canines by N^G-amino-L-arginine administration, these animals also exhibit a decrease in cardiac output and oxygen delivery and increased mortality. Conversely, Aisaka et al.[96] demonstrated that the in vivo administration of L-NMMA results in hypertension that is fully reversible with arginine administration. Moncada et al.[97] speculated that the supply of arginine is the rate-limiting step for the formation of NO by NO synthase. Although this relationship between L-arginine and NO may hold true in vitro, it is not known whether the same holds true in vivo. Although NO_2/NO_3 levels, the stable end products of NO, are higher in patients with sepsis, L-arginine concentrations are not significantly different from controls without sepsis.[98] Thus, although arginine may possess beneficial thymotrophic and secretagogue properties, its use in the critically ill may be limited by its potential to form NO.

DIETARY LIPIDS

ω-3 and ω-6 Polyunsaturated Fatty Acids

Eicosanoid generation is influenced by the enzymatic activity of phospholipase, lipooxygenase, and cyclooxygenase, as well as by the availability of the substrate arachidonic acid.[99] The balance of this section will focus on the diminution of eicosanoid and cytokine synthesis by altering the eicosanoid precursor pool through the dietary supplementation of ω-3 fatty acids. The primary substrates for eicosanoid inflammatory mediators are the ω-6 class of polyunsaturated fatty acids such as linoleic acid and its metabolite arachidonic acid.[100] The ω-6 class of fatty acids, found in soybean, corn, sunflower, and safflower oil, is the primary fat source for most nutritional formulations. Following appropriate activation of phospholipases, arachidonic acid is cleaved from the cell membrane where it is converted to prostaglandins by enzymes of the cyclooxygenase pathway or thromboxanes by the 5-lipooxygenase pathway.[100] Macrophages are the principal source of prostaglandins and leukotrienes and produce arachidonic acid by phospholipase A_2 enzymatic conversion of phosphotidylcholine and phosphotidylethanolamine.[101] Lymphocytes to a lesser degree also contain high concentrations of arachidonic acid cleaved from phosphotidylinositol by phospholipase C.[102] The biological activity of these mediators includes vasoconstriction and platelet aggregation by thromboxane A_2, vasodilation and decreased platelet aggregation by prostaglandin I_2, and increased neutrophil chemotaxis and aggregation by LTB_4.[99]

Diets rich in ω-3 fatty acids, found in high concentrations in fish oils, have correlated with a low incidence of cardiovascular and inflammatory diseases.[103, 104] Structurally, ω-3 fatty acids differ from their ω-6 counterpart by the location of the double bonds. The ω-6 fatty acids have their last double bond six carbons away from the methyl end of the chain, while it is located only three carbons away from the methyl end in ω-3 fatty acids. The ω-3 fatty acids, eicosapentaenoic acid (EPA) and docosahexaenoic acid (DHA), are incorporated into membrane phospholipids and exert anti-inflammatory effects not only by inhibiting cyclooxygenase activity but also by forming less potent prostaglandin and leukotriene products. With EPA as substrate, platelets synthesize TxA_3, which unlike its arachidonic acid counterpart TxA_2, has only mild vasoconstrictor properties and will not aggregate platelets. LTB_5, also derived from EPA, has only 12% of the neutrophil chemotactic properties and 5% of the aggregatory potency of LTB_4.[105-107]

Mascioli et al.[108] have shown that guinea pigs fed fish oil for 6 weeks had an 87% survival rate at 20 hours when challenged with an LD_{50} of LPS as compared with a 47% survival rate in animals maintained on safflower oil ad libitum. Pomposelli et al.,[109] in a similar model, noted improvements in microvascular perfusion, lactate levels, and lung morphology following LPS infusion in fish oil–supplemented animals. There were no improvements in cardiac output, Pao_2, or mean arterial pressure. The rapid and preferential incorporation of ω-3 fatty acids into membrane phospholipids was demonstrated by repeating the study with only a 3½-day period of prior ω-3 fatty acid supplementation. Again fish oil treatment improved the metabolic acidosis, lactic acidemia, and mixed venous oxygen content.[110] Pscheidl et al.[111] demonstrated improved splanchnic blood flow as well as decreased glucose, lactate, and pyruvate levels in an endotoxemic rat model following 40 hours of intravenous ω-3 fatty acid supplementation. Murray et al.,[112] by supplementing pigs with ω-3 fatty acids for 8 days, decreased the platelet membrane ratio of EPA to arachidonic acid from 1:20 to 1:1. A subsequent E. coli infusion, although yielding minimal cardiovascular improvements or changes in core temperature in the treatment group, improved oxygenation as well as significantly decreased pulmonary edema.

Although many of the benefits of ω-3 supplementation are secondary to alterations in the eicosanoid mediators, the dietary fat source can also have an influence on the cytokine class of mediators. Billiar et al.[113] demonstrated that Kupffer cells isolated from rats following 6 weeks of fish oil supplementation released less IL-1 and TNF when triggered by LPS than did corn oil–fed animals. A similar influence of dietary fat source on cytokine generation has also been demonstrated in normal volunteers.[114] Nine healthy volunteers added 18 g of fish oil concentrate to their diet daily for 6 weeks. Peripheral blood mononuclear cells (PBMCs) isolated from these volunteers and stimulated in vitro with LPS had decreased generation of TNF and IL-1 when compared with pre–ω-3 supplementation. These findings were in concert with a decrease in the arachidonic acid-to-EPA ratio in PBMC membranes, as well as a decrease in neutrophil chemotaxis to LTB_4. These findings may be partially explained by the finding that LTB_4 enhances PBMC IL-1 production following LPS exposure.[115]

By contrast, some studies have not demonstrated significant improvements with dietary lipid modulation during sepsis. Griswold et al.[116] in an endotoxemic rat model found no benefit upon mortality or neutrophil function following 2 weeks of fish oil supplementation. Similar findings were noted in a mouse *Pseudomonas* peritonitis model.[117] It is becoming apparent that the interaction of dietary lipids, eicosanoid, and cytokine mediators with the clinical outcome is a complex relationship influenced by the experimental model, as well as the amount and length of lipid administration. It is also apparent that some dietary ω-6 fatty acids are essential to maintain normal immune function. Animals rendered essential fatty acid deficient exhibit decreased antibody production and delayed-type hypersensitivity.[118]

Long-Chain Triglycerides

In addition to the double bond location, the absolute length of the fatty acid moiety may also have an influence on immune function. The long-chain triglycerides (LCTs) contain 16- and 18-carbon fatty acids and are found in high concentrations in soybean and safflower oil as well as the standard parenteral lipid emulsions. Data can be cited to both support as well as raise concern regarding the utilization of these lipid emulsions. Tovar et al.[119] noted that endotoxin clearance was enhanced in 6 to 8-week old white rabbits following a rapid infusion of 10% Intralipid whereas endotoxin clearance was unaffected in animals following a 1-week Intralipid infusion.

Most investigators, however, have noted immunosuppressive effects following LCT administration. Robin et al.[120] investigated the acute effects of a 4- to 6-hour Intralipid infusion in chronically ill patients and noted a decrease in neutrophil bactericidal indices as determined by neutrophil chemiluminescence. Nordenstrom et al.[121] demonstrated that an acute Intralipid infusion also impaired neutrophil chemotaxis and random migration. In these healthy subjects receiving a 2-hour Intralipid infusion, however, there was no effect on granulocyte counts. Furthermore, migration indices had returned to baseline values 22 hours postinfusion.

Chronic LCT administration has been shown to impair reticuloendothelial system (RES) function to an extent similar to the influence of acute lipid infusion on neutrophil function. Seidner et al.[122] noted that a 3-day infusion of soybean emulsion in malnourished patients depressed RES function as determined by ^{99m}Tc-sulfur colloid. These immunosuppressive effects were not apparent following a single 10-hour lipid infusion.

It has been proposed that some of the potential deleterious effects of LCTs can be circumvented by administering a mixed lipid system composed of both LCTs and medium-chain triglycerides (MCTs). MCTs, which contain 8- and 10-carbon fatty acids, are found in high concentrations in coconut and palm oils. Although MCTs are unable to prevent essential fatty acid deficiency, they are cleared more rapidly from the blood and more readily oxidized than LCTs.[123] Hamawy et al.[123] studied the effects of varying lipid emulsions on the RES in rats with *E. coli*–inoculated femur fractures. Animals were alimented parenterally for 3 days with nonprotein calories as either 100% dextrose, 50% dextrose/50% LCT, or 50% dextrose/50% mixed lipid system. The mixed lipid system was composed of 75% MCTs and 25% LCTs. Three days following septic femur fracture and hyperalimentation, the dextrose- and LCT-fed animals had blood cultures exhibiting greater than 10^2 colony-forming units (CFUs) of *E. coli* per milliliter, whereas the blood from MCT-fed animals was sterile. The MCT-fed animals were also noted to sequester fewer radiolabeled bacteria in the lungs as compared with the dextrose- and LCT-alimented animals.

Lipoproteins

Recent evidence also supports the concept that *endogenous* lipoproteins (chylomicrons, very low-density lipoprotein [VLDL], low-density lipoprotein [LDL], and high-density lipoprotein [HOL]) are capable of altering the physiologic response to LPS administration. The lipoprotein-induced attenuation of LPS responses has been postulated to result from a direct lipoprotein interaction with endotoxin. The specific lipoprotein component or the precise mechanism of this interaction awaits further characterization.

Ulevitch et al.[124] observed that HDL cause conformational changes in LPS that resulted in abrogation of some but not all of the biological responses to LPS. Those responses influenced by HDL included the pyrogenic response, rapid neutropenia, and anticomplement activity. However, in rabbits, this complex was still able to induce shock, disseminated intravascular coagulation, and death. The finding that this

HDL-LPS complex retained its original electrophoretic mobility on sodium dodecylsulfate–polyacrylamide gel electrophoresis (SDS-PAGE) suggested that major degradation did not occur. Abdelnoor et al.[102] also concluded that HDL was the lipoprotein responsible for LPS neutralization; they also noted that HDL in the absence of other components of Cohn fraction IV of the serum was ineffective in preventing LPS-induced hypotension in rabbits.

Weinstock et al.[125] also described a cholesterol-rich lipoprotein capable of neutralizing LPS. These investigators utilized sera from patients with familial hypercholesterolemia to inactivate five times more endotoxin, as determined by an endotoxin-induced in vitro monocyte assay, than after LDL was removed by apheresis. This LPS-inactivating component could be retrieved in the LDL-rich eluate. Navab et al.,[126] using cultured monolayers of rabbit aortic endothelial cells, noted that the integrity of these cells could be disrupted with as little as 2 ng/mL of LPS. When LPS was complexed to LDL, it required a 1000-fold increase in LPS concentration to disrupt the monolayer. This LPS-LDL complex, however, was able to be rapidly transported across the monolayer and maintain its biological activity. Flegel et al.[127] noted that HDL possessed some LPS-inactivating capacity but that this was small in comparison to that observed with LDL. These investigators observed that all lipoproteins, but specifically LDL, neutralized LPS by impairing monocyte recognition of LPS and subsequent TNF, IL-1, and IL-6 elaboration.

Harris et al.[128] observed that all lipoprotein fractions could protect mice against an endotoxin-induced death. By incubating LPS with varying concentrations of triglyceride-rich VLDL and chylomicrons, as well as cholesterol-rich LDL and HDL, survival rates following LPS exposure were increased from 7% to 100%, depending on the quality of lipoprotein administered as well as the duration of LPS/lipoprotein incubation.

These results, unlike those previously reported, suggested that cholesterol is not essential or necessary for lipoprotein neutralization of LPS.

Summary

Recent evidence suggests that nutritional modulation during critical illness may have an impact on survival through mechanisms far more complex than the maintenance of mere caloric and nitrogen balance. Provision of nutrients through parenteral routes to normal volunteers paradoxically promotes both an exaggerated cytokine response as well as diminished neutrophil chemotaxis and complement activation following an endotoxin challenge. These divergent immune responses following parenteral nutritional support may, by implication, be associated with the appearance of multiorgan system failure and increased infectious complications. This latter experimental observation has been replicated in several clinical trials comparing enteral and parenteral support. Similarly, alterations in the specific nutrient intake of amino acids such as arginine and glutamine as well as the ω-3 fatty acid and lipoprotein content in septic animal models can have a dramatic influence on the elaboration of inflammatory mediators to septic stimuli and thereby attenuate the deleterious physiologic manifestations of such an insult. Unfortunately, the theoretical advantages of such specific nutrient modulation have not fully withstood the rigors of human investigation or clinical trials, and their routine application cannot be fully endorsed at present. It is therefore essential that further studies be directed toward defining the role of specific nutrient modulation in the critical care arena.

REFERENCES

1. Rhoads JE, Alexander CE: Nutritional problems of surgical patients. *Ann N Y Acad Sci* 1955; 63:268–270.

2. Fong Y, Moldawer LL, Shires GT, et al: The biological characteristics of cytokines and their implication in surgical injury. *Surg Gynecol Obstet* 1990; 170:363–378.

3. Fong Y, Lowry SF: Cytokines and the cellular response to injury and infection, in Wilmore DW, Brennan MF, Harken AH, et al (eds): *Care of the Surgical Patient*, vol 1. New York, Scientific American, 1990, pp 1–17.

4. Hesse DG, Davatelis G, Felsen D, et al: Cachectin/tumor necrosis factor gene expression in Kupffer cells. *J Leukoc Biol* 1987; 42:422.

5. Warner SJC, Libby P: Human vascular smooth muscle cells: Target for and source of tumor necrosis factor. *J Immunol* 1989; 142:100.

6. Beutler B, Krochin N, Milsark IW, et al: Control of cachectin (tumor necrosis factor) synthesis: Mechanisms of endotoxin resistance. *Science* 1986; 232:977.

7. Wong GHW, Goeddal DV: Tumor necrosis factor α and β inhibit virus replication and synergize with interferons. *Nature* 1986; 323:819.

8. Nawroth PP, Stern DM: Modulation of endothelial cell hemostatic properties by tumor necrosis. *J Exp Med* 1986; 163:740.

9. Frater Schroder M, Risau W, Hallmann R, et al: Tumor necrosis factor type alpha, a potent inhibitor of endothelial cell growth in vitro, is angiogenic in vivo. *Proc Natl Acad Sci U S A* 1987; 84:5277–5281.

10. Sugarman BJ, Aggarwal BB, Hass PE, et al: Recombinant human tumor necrosis factor-alpha: Effects on proliferation of normal and transformed cells in vitro. *Science* 1985; 230:943–945.

11. Bertolini DR, Nedwin GE, Bringman TS, et al: Stimulation of bone resorption and inhibition of bone formation in vitro by human tumour necrosis factors. *Nature* 1986; 319:516–518.

12. Moldawer LL, Andersson C, Gelin J, et al: Regulation of food intake and hepatic protein synthesis by recombinant derived monokines. *Am J Physiol* 1988; 254:450.

13. Perlmutter DH, Dinarello CA, Punsal PI, et al: Cachectin/tumor necrosis factor regulates hepatic acute-phase gene expression. *J Clin Invest* 1986; 78:1349–1354.

518 Feeding

14. Shalaby MR, Aggarwal BB, Rinderknecht E, et al: Activation of human polymorphonuclear neutrophil functions by interferon-gamma and tumor necrosis factors. *J Immunol* 1985; 135:2069–2073.
15. Djeu JY, Blanchard DK, Halkias D, et al: Growth inhibition of *Candida albicans* by human polymorphonuclear neutrophils: Activation by interferon-gamma and tumor necrosis factor. *J Immunol* 1986; 137:2980–2984.
16. Cross AS, Sadoff JC, Kelly N, et al: Pretreatment with recombinant murine tumor necrosis factor alpha/cachectin and murine interleukin 1 alpha protects mice from lethal bacterial infection. *J Exp Med* 1989; 169:2021–2027.
17. Munoz C, Carlet J, Fitting C, et al: Dysregulation of in vitro cytokine production by monocytes during sepsis. *J Clin Invest* 1991; 88:1747–1754.
18. Tracey KJ, Wei H, Manogue KR, et al: Cachectin/tumor necrosis factor induces cachexia, anemia, and inflammation. *J Exp Med* 1988; 167:1211–1227.
19. Tracey KJ, Beutler B, Lowry SF, et al: Shock and tissue injury induced by recombinant human cachectin. *Science* 1986; 234:470–474.
20. Tracey KJ, Lowry SF, Fahey TJ III, et al: Cachectin/tumor necrosis factor induces lethal shock and stress hormone responses in the dog. *Surg Gynecol Obstet* 1987; 164:415–422.
21. Fischer E, Marano MA, Barber AE, et al: Comparison between effects of interleukin-1 alpha administration and sublethal endotoxemia in primates. *Am J Physiol* 1991; 261:442–452.
22. Tracey KJ, Fong Y, Hesse DG, et al: Anti-cachectin/TNF monoclonal antibodies prevent septic shock during lethal bacteremia. *Nature* 1987; 330:662–664.
23. Fischer E, Marano MA, Van Zee KJ, et al: Interleukin-1 receptor blockade improves survival and hemodynamic performance in *Escherichia coli* septic shock, but fails to alter host responses to sublethal endotoxemia. *J Clin Invest* 1992; 89:1551–1557.
24. Fong Y, Moldawer LL, Marano MA, et al: Endotoxemia elicits increased circulating β2-IFN/IL-6 in man. *J Immunol* 1989; 142:2321–2324.
25. Fong Y, Tracey KJ, Moldawer LL, et al: Antibodies to cachectin/tumor necrosis factor reduce interleukin-1β and interleukin-6 appearance during lethal bacteremia. *J Exp Med* 1989; 170:1627–1633.
26. Keogh CV, Fong Y, Marano MA, et al: Identification of a novel tumor necrosis factor-α/cachectin from the livers of burned and infected rats. *Arch Surg* 1990; 125:79–85.
27. Fong Y, Marano MA, Moldawer LL, et al: The acute splanchnic and peripheral tissue metabolic response to endotoxin in humans. *J Clin Invest* 1990; 85:1896–1904.
28. Michie HR, Spriggs DR, Rounds J, et al: Does cachectin cause cachexia? *Surg Forum* 1987; 38:38.
29. Stovroff MC, Fraker DL, Norton JA: Cachectin activity in the serum of cachectic, tumor bearing rats. *Arch Surg* 1989; 124:94.
30. Stovroff MC, Fraker DL, Travis WD, et al: Altered macrophage activity and tumor necrosis factor: Tumor necrosis and host cachexia. *J Surg Res* 1989; 46:462.
31. Saarinen UM, Koskelo EK, Teppo AM, et al: Tumor necrosis factor in children with malignancies. *Cancer Res* 1990; 50:592.
32. Coyle SM, Barber AE, Fong Y, et al: Hormone-cytokine responses to total parenteral nutrition in humans (abstract). *Clin Nutr* 1990; 9:20.
33. Dudrick SJ, Wilmore DW, Vars HM, et al: Can intravenous feeding as the sole means of nutrition support growth in the child and restore weight loss in an adult? An affirmative answer. *Ann Surg* 1969; 169:974–984.
34. Jeejeebhoy KN, Zohrab WJ, Langer B, et al: Total parenteral nutrition at home for 23 months, without complication, and with good rehabilitation. A study of technical and metabolic features. *Gastroenterology* 1973; 65:811–820.
35. Broviac JW, Scribner BH: Prolonged parenteral nutrition in the home. *Surg Gynecol Obstet* 1974; 139:24–28.
36. Dudrick SJ, Wilmore DW, Steiger E,

et al: Spontaneous closure of traumatic pancreatoduodenal fistulas with total intravenous nutrition. *J Trauma* 1970; 10:542–553.

37. Thomas RJ, Rosalion A: The use of parenteral nutrition in the management of external gastrointestinal tract fistulae. *Aust N Z J Surg* 1978; 48:535–539.

38. Kudsk KA, Croce MA, Fabian TC, et al: Enteral versus parenteral feeding. Effects on septic morbidity after blunt and penetrating abdominal trauma. *Ann Surg* 1992; 215:503–511.

39. Zaren H, Lerner H: Review of 100 consecutive parenteral nutritional support patients on an oncology unit. *Proc Am Soc Clin Oncol* 1982; 23:228.

40. Bower RH, Talamini MA, Sax HC, et al: Postoperative enteral vs parenteral nutrition. A randomized controlled trial. *Arch Surg* 1986; 121:1040–1045.

41. McArdle AH, Palmason C, Morency I, et al: A rationale for enteral feeding as the preferable route for hyperalimentation. *Surgery* 1981; 90:616–623.

42. Moore FA, Moore EE, Jones TN, et al: TEN versus TPN following major abdominal trauma–reduced septic morbidity. *J Trauma* 1989; 29:916–922.

43. Hildebrand GJ, Wolochow H: Translocation of bacteriophage across the intestinal wall of the rat. *Proc Soc Exp Biol Med* 1962; 109:183–185.

44. Vagianos C, Karatzas T, Scopa CD, et al: Neurotensin reduces microbial translocation and improves intestinal mucosa integrity after abdominal radiation. *Eur Surg Res* 1992; 24:77–83.

45. Deitch EA, Bridges W, Berg R, et al: Hemorrhagic shock–induced bacterial translocation: The role of neutrophils and hydroxyl radicals. *J Trauma* 1990; 30:942–951.

46. Barber AE, Jones WG II, Minei JP, et al: Bacterial overgrowth and intestinal atrophy in the etiology of gut barrier failure in the rat. *Am J Surg* 1991; 161:300–304.

47. Barber AE, Jones WG II, Minei JP, et al: Glutamine or fiber supplementation of a defined formula diet: Impact on bacterial translocation, tissue com-

position, and response to endotoxin. *JPEN* 1990; 14:335–343.

48. Alverdy J, Chi HS, Sheldon GF: The effect of parenteral nutrition on gastrointestinal immunity. The importance of enteral stimulation. *Ann Surg* 1985; 202:681–684.

49. Goris RJ, van Bebber IP, Mollen RM, et al: Does selective decontamination of the gastrointestinal tract prevent multiple organ failure? An experimental study. *Arch Surg* 1991; 126:561–565.

50. Sprung CL: Definitions of sepsis—have we reached a consensus? *Crit Care Med* 1991; 19:849–851.

51. Alverdy JC: Effects of glutamine-supplemented diets on immunology of the gut. *JPEN* 1990; 14(suppl):109–113.

52. Tracey KJ, Lowry SF, Beutler B, et al: Cachectin/tumor necrosis factor mediates changes of skeletal muscle plasma membrane potential. *J Exp Med* 1986; 164:1368–1373.

53. Tracey KJ, Lowry SF, Beutler B, et al: Cachetin/tumor necrosis factor participates in reduction of skeletal muscle membrane potential: Evidence for bioactivity in plasma during critical illness. *Surg Forum* 1986; 37:13–15.

54. Richardson RP, Rhyne CD, Fong Y, et al: Peripheral blood leukocyte kinetics following in vivo lipopolysaccharide (LPS) administration to normal human subjects: Influence of elicited hormones and cytokines. *Ann Surg* 1989; 210:239–245.

55. Meyer JD, Yurt RW, Duhaney R, et al: Differential neutrophil activation before and after endotoxin infusion in enterally versus parenterally fed volunteers. *Surg Gynecol Obstet* 1988; 167:501–509.

56. Fong Y, Marano MA, Barber AE, et al: Total parenteral nutrition and bowel rest modify the metabolic response to endotoxin in humans. *Ann Surg* 1989; 210:449–457.

57. Lowry SF: The route of feeding influences injury responses. *J Trauma* 1990; 30:510–515.

58. Bergstrom J, Furst P, Noree LO, et al: Intracellular free amino acid concentration in human muscle tissue. *J Appl Physiol* 1974; 36:693–697.

59. Rose WC: The nutritive significance of

the amino acids. *Physiol Rev* 1938; 18:109–136.

60. Stehle P, Zander J, Mertes N, et al: Effect of parenteral glutamine peptide supplements on muscle glutamine loss and nitrogen balance after major surgery. *Lancet* 1989; 1:231–233.

61. Hammarqvist F, Wernerman J, Ali R, et al: Addition of glutamine to total parenteral nutrition after elective abdominal surgery spares free glutamine in muscle, counteracts the fall in muscle protein synthesis, and improves nitrogen balance. *Ann Surg* 1989; 209:455–461.

62. Ardawi MM, Newsholme EA: Glutamine metabolism in lymphocytes. *Biochem J* 1983; 212:835–842.

63. Wallace C, Keast D: Glutamine and macrophage function. *Metabolism* 1992; 41:1016–1020.

64. Souba WW, Klimberg VS, Plumley DA, et al: The role of glutamine in maintaining a healthy gut and supporting the metabolic response to injury and infection. *J Surg Res* 1990; 48:383–391.

65. Klimberg VS, Souba WW: The importance of intestinal glutamine metabolism in maintaining a healthy gastrointestinal tract and supporting the body's response to injury and illness. *Surg Ann* 1990; 22:61–76.

66. Grant JP, Snyder PJ: Use of L-glutamine in total parenteral nutrition. *J Surg Res* 1988; 44:506–513.

67. Barber AE, Jones WG II, Minei JP, et al: Composition and functional consequences of fiber and glutamine supplementation of enteral diets. *Surg Forum* 1989; 40:15–17.

68. Rock CS, Barber AE, Ng E-H, et al: TPN vs. oral feeding: Bacterial translocation, cytokine response and mortality after *Escherichia coli* LPS administration. *Surg Forum* 1990; 41:14–16.

69. Kirk SJ, Barbul A: Role of arginine in trauma, sepsis, and immunity. *JPEN* 1990; 14(suppl):226–229.

70. Barbul A, Rettura G, Prior E, et al: Supplemental arginine, wound healing, and thymus: Arginine-pituitary interaction. *Surg Forum* 1978; 29:93–95.

71. Barbul A, Rettura G, Levenson SM, et al: Arginine: A thymotropic and wound-healing promoting agent. *Surg Forum* 1977; 28:101–103.

72. Merimee TJ, Burgess JA, Rabinowitz D: Arginine infusion in maturity-onset diabetes mellitus. Defective output of insulin and of growth hormone. *Lancet* 1966; 1:1300–1301.

73. Merimee TJ, Lillicrap DA, Rabinowitz D: Effect of arginine on serum-levels of human growth-hormone. *Lancet* 1965; 2:668–670.

74. Saito H, Trocki O, Wang SL, et al: Metabolic and immune effects of dietary arginine supplementation after burn. *Arch Surg* 1987; 122:784–789.

75. Seifter E, Rettura G, Barbul A, et al: Arginine: An essential amino acid for injured rats. *Surgery* 1978; 84:224–230.

76. Barbul A, Wasserkrug HL, Yoshimura N, et al: High arginine levels in intravenous hyperalimentation abrogate post-traumatic immune suppression. *J Surg Res* 1984; 36:620–624.

77. Sitren HS, Fisher H: Nitrogen retention in rats fed on diets enriched with arginine and glycine. 2. Effect of diethyl ether anaesthesia on N retention. *Br J Nutr* 1977; 37:209–214.

78. Sitren HS, Fisher H: Nitrogen retention in rats fed on diets enriched with arginine and glycine. 1. Improved N retention after trauma. *Br J Nutr* 1977; 37:195–208.

79. Evain Brion D, Donnadieu M, Roger M, et al: Simultaneous study of somatotrophic and corticotrophic pituitary secretions during ornithine infusion test. *Clin Endocrinol* 1982; 17:119–122.

80. Barbul A, Wasserkrug HL, Seifter E, et al: Immunostimulatory effects of arginine in normal and injured rats. *J Surg Res* 1980; 29:228–235.

81. Barbul A, Sisto DA, Wasserkrug HL, et al: Arginine stimulates lymphocyte immune response in healthy human beings. *Surgery* 1981; 90:244–251.

82. Daly JM, Reynolds J, Thom A, et al: Immune and metabolic effects of arginine in the surgical patient. *Ann Surg* 1988; 208:512–523.

83. Hibbs JB Jr, Taintor RR, Vavrin Z: Macrophage cytotoxicity: Role for L-arginine deminase and imino nitro-

gen oxidation to nitrate. *Science* 1987; 235:473–476.

84. Hibbs JB Jr, Vavrin Z, Taintor RR: L-arginine is required for expression of the activated macrophage effector mechanism causing selective metabolic inhibition in target cells. *J Immunol* 1987; 138:550–565.

85. Nava E, Palmer RM, Moncada S: Inhibition of nitric oxide synthesis in septic shock: How much is beneficial? *Lancet* 1991; 1:1555–1557.

86. Furchgott RF, Zawadzki JV: The obligatory role of endothelial cells in the relaxation of arterial smooth muscle by acetylcholine. *Nature* 1980; 228:373–376.

87. Gerzer R, Radany EW, Garbers DL: The separation of the heme and apoheme forms of soluble guanylate cyclase. *Biochem Biophys Res Commun* 1982; 108:678–686.

88. Kilbourn RG, Gross SS, Lodato RF, et al: Inhibition of interleukin-1-alpha–induced nitric oxide synthase in vascular smooth muscle and full reversal of interleukin-1-alpha–induced hypotension by N omega-amino-L-arginine. *J Natl Cancer Inst* 1992; 84:1008–1016.

89. Ding AH, Nathan CF, Stuehr DJ: Release of reactive nitrogen intermediates and reactive oxygen intermediates from mouse peritoneal macrophages. Comparison of activating cytokines and evidence for independent production. *J Immunol* 1988; 141:2407–2412.

90. Billiar TR, Curran TR, Ferrari FK, et al: Kupffer cell:hepatocyte cocultures release nitric oxide in response to bacterial endotoxin. *J Surg Res* 1990; 48:349–353.

91. Curran RD, Billiar TR, Stuehr DJ, et al: Multiple cytokines are required to induce hepatocyte nitric oxide production and inhibit total protein synthesis. *Ann Surg* 1990; 212:462–469.

92. Kilbourn RG, Jubran A, Gross SS, et al: Reversal of endotoxin-mediated shock by N^G-methyl-L-arginine, an inhibitor of nitric oxide synthesis. *Biochem Biophys Res Commun* 1990; 172:1132–1138.

93. Kilbourn RG, Gross SS, Jubran A, et al: N^G-methyl-L-arginine inhibits tumor necrosis factor–induced hypotension: Implications for the involvement of nitric oxide. *Proc Natl Acad Sci USA* 1990; 87:3629–3632.

94. Petros A, Bennett D, Vallance P: Effect of nitric oxide synthase inhibitors on hypotension in patients with septic shock. *Lancet* 1991; 1:1557–1558.

95. Cobb JP, Natanson C, Hoffman WD, et al: N(G)-amino-L-arginine, an inhibitor of nitric oxide synthase, raises vascular resistance but increases mortality rates in awake canines challenged with endotoxin. *J Exp Med* 1992; 176:1175–1182.

96. Asaika K, Gross SS, Griffith OW, et al: N(G)-methylarginine, an inhibitor of endothelium-derived nitric oxide synthesis, is a potent pressor agent in the guinea pig: Does nitric oxide regulate blood pressure in vivo? *Biochem Biophys Res Commun* 1989; 160:881–886.

97. Moncada S, Palmer RM, Higgs EA: Biosynthesis of nitric oxide from L-arginine. A pathway for the regulation of cell function and communication. *Biochem Pharmacol* 1989; 38:1709–1715.

98. Ochoa JB, Udekwu AO, Billiar TR, et al: Nitrogen oxide levels in patients after trauma and during sepsis. *Ann Surg* 1991; 214:621–626.

99. Kensella JE, Lokesh B: Dietary lipids, eicosanoids, and the immune system. *Crit Care Med* 1990; 18(suppl):94–113.

100. Ulevitch RJ, Tobias PS, Mathison JC: Regulation of the host response to bacterial lipopolysaccharides. *Fed Proc* 1984; 43:2755–2759.

101. Parker CW: Lipid mediators produced through the lipoxygenase pathway. *Annu Rev Immunol* 1987; 5:65–84.

102. Abdelnoor AM, Harvie NR, Johnson AG: Neutralization of bacteria- and endotoxin-induced hypotension by lipoprotein-free human serum. *Infect Immun* 1982; 38:157–161.

103. Robertson TL, Kato H, Gordon T, et al: Epidemiologic studies of coronary heart disease and stroke in Japanese men living in Japan, Hawaii, and California. *Am J Cardiol* 1977; 39:244–249.

104. Kromhout D, Bosscheiter EB, Cou-

lander C: The inverse relation be-tween fish consumption and 20 year mortality from coronary heart disease. *N Engl J Med* 1985; 312:1205–1209.

105. Seiss W, Scherer B, Bohlig B, et al: Platelet-membrane fatty acids, platelet-aggregation, and throm-boxane formation during a mackeral diet. *Lancet* 1980; 1:441–444.

106. Stasser T, Fischer S, Weber PC: Leu-kotriene B_5 is formed in neutrophils after dietary supplementation with icosapentaenoic acid. *Proc Natl Acad Sci U S A* 1985; 82:1540–1543.

107. Lee TH, Hoover RL, Williams JD, et al: Effect of dietary enrichment with eicosapentaenoic and docosahexa-enoic acids on in vitro neutrophil and monocyte leukotriene generation and neutrophil function. *N Engl J Med* 1985; 312:1217–1224.

108. Mascioli EA, Iwasa Y, Trimbo S, et al: Endotoxin challenge after menhaden oil diet: Effects on survival of guinea pigs. *Am J Clin Nutr* 1989; 49:277–282.

109. Pomposelli JJ, Flores EA, Blackburn GL, et al: Diets enriched with N-3 fatty acids ameliorate lactic acidosis by improving endotoxin-induced tis-sue hypoperfusion in guinea pigs. *Ann Surg* 1991; 213:166–176.

110. Pomposelli JJ, Flores E, Hirschberg Y, et al: Short-term TPN containing n-3 fatty acids ameliorate lactic acidosis induced by endotoxin in guinea pigs. *Am J Clin Nutr* 1990; 52:548–552.

111. Pscheidl EM, Wan JM, Blackburn GL, et al: Influence of omega-3 fatty acids on splanchnic blood flow and lactate metabolism in an endotoxemic rat model. *Metabolism* 1992; 41:698–705.

112. Murray MJ, Svingen BA, Holman RT, et al: Effects of a fish oil diet on pigs' cardiopulmonary response to bactere-mia. *JPEN* 1991; 15:152–158.

113. Billiar TR, Bankey PE, Svingen BA, et al: Fatty acid intake and Kupffer cell function: Fish oil alters eicosanoid and monokine production to endo-toxin stimulation. *Surgery* 1988; 104:343–349.

114. Endres S, Ghorbani R, Kelley VE, et al: The effect of dietary supplementa-tion with n-3 polyunsaturated fatty acids on the synthesis of interleukin-1 and tumor necrosis fac-tor by mononuclear cells. *N Engl J Med* 1989; 320:265–271.

115. Rola-Plezczynski M: Differential effects of leukotriene B_4 and T4+ and T8+ lymphocyte phenotype and immuno-regulatory functions. *J Immunol* 1985; 135:1357–1360.

116. Griswold J, Grogan J, Metcalf J, et al: The impact of dietary fish oil in endotoxin-induced stress. *Surg Fo-rum* 1991; 42:9–11.

117. Clouva Molyvdas P, Peck MD, Alex-ander JW: Short-term dietary lipid manipulation does not affect survival in two models of murine sepsis. *JPEN* 1992; 16:343–347.

118. DeWille JW, Fraker PJ, Romsos DR: Essential fatty acids and immunity: Influence of culture conditions and duration on lymphocyte activation (abstract). *Fed Proc* 1981; 40:344.

119. Tovar JA, Mahour GH, Miller SW, et al: Endotoxin clearance after in-tralipid infusion. *J Pediatr Surg* 1976; 11:23–30.

120. Robin AP, Arain I, Phuangsab A, et al: Intravenous fat emulsion acutely sup-presses neutrophil chemilumines-cence. *JPEN* 1989; 13:608–613.

121. Nordenstrom J, Jarstrand C, Wiernik A: Decreased chemotactic and random migration of leukocytes during In-tralipid infusion. *Am J Clin Nutr* 1979; 32:2416–2422.

122. Seidner DL, Mascioli EA, Istfan NW, et al: Effects of long-chain triglyceride emulsions on reticuloendothelial sys-tem function in humans. *JPEN* 1989; 13:614–619.

123. Hamawy KJ, Moldawer LL, Georgieff M, et al: The effect of lipid emulsions on reticuloendothelial system function in the injured animal. *JPEN* 1985; 9:559–565.

124. Ulevitch RJ, Johnston AR, Weinstein DB: New function for high density li-poproteins. Their participation in in-travascular reactions of bacterial lipo-polysaccharides. *J Clin Invest* 1979; 64:1516–1524.

125. Weinstock C, Ullrich H, Hohe R, et al: Low density lipoproteins inhibit endo-toxin activation of monocytes. *Arterio-scler Thromb* 1992; 12:341–347.

126. Navab M, Hough GP, Van Lenten BJ, et al: Low density lipoproteins trans-

fer bacterial lipopolysaccharides across endothelial monolayers in a biologically active form. *J Clin Invest* 1988; 81:601–605.

127. Flegel WA, Wolpl A, Mannel DN, et al: Inhibition of endotoxin-induced activation of human monocytes by human lipoproteins. *Infect Immun* 1989; 57:2237–2245.

128. Harris HW, Grunfeld C, Feingold KR, et al: Human very low density lipoproteins and chylomicrons can protect against endotoxin-induced death in mice. *J Clin Invest* 1990; 86:696–702.

28

Nutrition and Wound Healing

Pamela R. Roberts, M.D.

Physiology of wound healing

Metabolic effects of injury

Timing of nutritional support

General nutritional status

Protein

Peptides

Amino acids

Carbohydrates

Fats

Water-soluble vitamins

Vitamin C (absorbic acid)

Vitamin B complex

Fat-soluble vitamins

Vitamin A

Vitamin E

Trace elements

Zinc

Iron

Copper

Hormones/growth factors

Many hospitalized patients, especially trauma and surgical patients, sustain injuries that result in wounds. These wounds may originate from burns, fractures, trauma, surgery, intestinal anastomoses, or decubiti. The wound serves as a source of morbidity and mortality secondary to tissue inflammation and infection. Infection and inflammation, via release of cytokines and other mediators, are capable of causing the metabolic and physiologic changes that constitute the sepsis syndrome and may lead to multiple-system organ failure and death. Unhealed wounds are rapidly colonized by bacteria from the environment. In addition, wounds may serve as a primary source of bacteria (e.g., bowel perforation).[1] Long-term effects of the healing process such as contractures and scar formation may have both cosmetic and functional significance. The pulmonary fibrosis formed secondary to acute lung injury and the formation of intra-abdominal adhesions after abdominal surgery are examples of the increased morbidity and mortality that may be caused by the healing process. A major goal of medical therapy must therefore be directed at understanding and promoting healing, especially in intensive care units, since the presence of infection or inflammation can perpetuate critical illness.

Metabolic and nutritional factors have pronounced effects on wound healing. These effects vary with the systemic and local factors involved in healing. Frequently the illness or injury itself leads to metabolic or nutritional disorders that impair wound healing. Clinicians need to be aware of the parameters that affect the clinical course of patients and what preventive or corrective therapies can be administered to decrease the adverse effects of these metabolic or nutritional changes. In this chapter, we review current information regarding the influence of nutrition and specific nutrients on wound healing (Table 28–1).

PHYSIOLOGY OF WOUND HEALING

Wound healing involves a complex sequence of events that begin with bleeding, coagulation, and thrombosis. The "inflammatory phase" of healing begins as platelets are deposited in the wound; this activates the complement cascade and causes the release of a variety of vasoactive and chemotactic mediators. Initially, local vasoconstriction occurs as a result of the release of thromboxane A_2 and other metabolites. This is followed by vasodilatation secondary to the presence of mediators such as prosta-

glandins, histamine, and serotonin.[2] Increased vascular permeability develops and permits leakage of fluid and macromolecules. Endothelial cells become more adherent to leukocytes, and margination occurs, with white cells migrating to the site of injury in response to chemotactic agents. Neutrophils are the first to arrive at the wound and begin phagocytizing and killing bacteria; proteases that lyse devitalized tissue are released. Neutrophils require an adequate supply of oxygen in order to generate the oxygen radicals used to kill microorganisms. These neutrophils live only a few hours before releasing their intracellular contents into the wound area and forming part of the wound exudate. Impairment in blood flow or oxygen supply at this early stage of healing can weaken local defenses and allow bacteria to invade. Fibrin degradation products serve as chemoattractants for macrophages, which soon (within a few hours) become the predominant cell in the injured tissue. They are capable of killing bacteria and can direct healing activity via the release of monokines

TABLE 28–1.

Nutrients Involved in Wound Healing

Protein	Supplies building blocks for angiogenesis, fibroblast proliferation, collagen synthesis/remodeling; maintains tissue oncotic pressure/prevents excess edema
Peptides	Source of amino acids; some may have biological activity; enhanced healing vs. amino acid diets
Amino acids	Needed for protein synthesis; arginine may enhance healing and immune function
Carbohydrates	Provide energy for cellular metabolism and healing; hyperglycemia decreases leukocyte function
Fats	Essential components of cell membranes; required for synthesis of prostaglandins; intraluminal short-chain fatty acids may improve colonic anastomotic healing
Vitamin C	Required for angiogenesis, collagen synthesis, fibroblast maturation; important in immune function—bactericidal activity and complement production
Vitamin B complex	Essential cofactors in enzyme systems and normal metabolism; needed for leukocyte function/antibody production
Vitamin A	Prevents poor healing of multiple pathologic states; increases the rate of collagen synthesis; may improve the early inflammatory response; needed for intact immune function
Vitamin E	No known specific role in healing; its role as antioxidant has been questioned
Zinc	Required for normal healing; a component of metalloenzymes needed for DNA, RNA, and protein synthesis
Iron	Required for collagen synthesis and oxygen delivery
Copper	Required for collagen cross-linking (lysyl oxidase) and other metalloenzymes
Insulin	Mitigates diabetic-induced healing impairment; appears to be a necessary component of healing
Growth hormone	Causes anabolism and better nitrogen balance; enhances wound strength in malnutrition; improved healing in burned children and decreased hospital stay
Growth factors	Modulate events of wound response; may be useful adjunctive therapy in the future

or growth factors. Activated platelets also release growth factors, including platelet-derived growth factor (PDGF) and transforming growth factor β (TGF-β). Growth factors, chemoattractants, and hormones such as insulin, insulin growth factor-1 (IGF-1), and growth hormone (GH) modulate wound healing.[3]

In the first few days after an injury, angiogenesis or neovascularization is stimulated by local hypoxia and lactic acid. Endothelial cells proliferate and form capillary buds at the wound surface in response to cytokines. During the same period fibroblasts begin to appear in the wound. The presence of lactic acid, ascorbic acid, and growth factors from platelets and macrophages is thought to be the stimulus for fibroblast mitosis and proliferation as well as collagen synthesis. Fibroblasts are metabolically active cells and depend on an adequate oxygen supply and therefore adequate angiogenesis in order to continue to proliferate. Epithelial cells migrate toward and across the wound area to form a single cell layer, which forms the framework for other cell layers.

Lactate levels and growth factors stimulate fibroblasts to synthesize collagen. Fibroblasts cannot produce collagen without an adequate supply of molecular oxygen, ascorbic acid, ferrous iron, copper, and pyridoxal. The rate of collagen synthesis is maximal during the first to second week following wounding, and deposition of collagen is maximal by the third to fourth week of repair. The tensile strength of the wound is only 10% by the second week and about 25% by the fourth week; after several months the wound has about 70% to 80% of the tissue's ultimate strength.[4] The strength increases over time secondary to continued cross-linking of collagen fibers and remodeling. Collagenolysis, deposition of new collagen, and more effective cross-linking allow for refining of weaker areas. Fibroblasts and other mesenchymal cells produce an intracellular matrix composed of proteoglycans that provides architectural support. Wound contraction results from the activation of contractile elements in fibroblasts and myofibroblasts. This process lasts for weeks to months and can result in contractures that result in a loss of mobility. Scar maturation or wound remodeling usually begins about the third week after injury and lasts for months to years. Wound remodeling results from increased collagen cross-linking, breakdown of excess collagen by collagenase, regression of the increased vascular bed supplying the wound as metabolic demands decrease, and a decrease in the proteoglycan and water content of the wound. In general, the collagenase activity is in equilibrium with the deposition and remodeling of collagen, thereby preventing a net gain in collagen. Wound strength usually continues to increase beyond a year; however, skin and fascia never regain full strength.

METABOLIC EFFECTS OF INJURY

Following injury or during periods of severe illness, changes occur in energy, protein, carbohydrate, fat, vitamin, mineral, and water metabolism. These physiologic changes are dynamic and relate to the severity of injury. Patients with burns or septic shock have some of the most dramatic changes in metabolism seen in the clinical arena. These metabolic changes are modified by many factors (i.e., age, gender, previous nutritional status, the type and severity of injury, and nutrient intake) and have effects on nutrition, wound healing, the immune response, and other defense mechanisms. A major function of the altered metabolism is the provision of nutrients such as amino acids for the healing of wounds at a time when the organism is unable to find food. Metabolic studies performed in burned animals show that anabolism and catabolism are increased after injury.

TIMING OF NUTRITIONAL SUPPORT

The effects of varying the timing of initiation of nutritional support on wound healing responses have been evaluated in several studies. Delany et al.[5] reported improved 7-day colonic anastomotic healing and decreased weight loss in normally nourished rats given total parenteral nutrition (TPN) from the first day after celiotomy and colon reanastomosis as compared with rats with delayed TPN (i.e., begun on the third postoperative day) and rats given only intravenous fluids with vitamins. However, they found no significant differences in skin wound breaking strength among the three groups. Moss and associates[6, 7] evaluated the effect of early enteral feeding on colonic anastomotic healing in dogs. Dogs fed enterally immediately following wounding had improved colonic anastomotic bursting pressure and wound collagen synthesis when compared with nonfed controls. Zaloga et al.[8] reported a doubling of abdominal wound strength at 1 week in rats fed early after surgery vs. animals not fed until day 3 after surgery. Zaloga et al.[9] found no difference in wound healing strength in rats with early postoperative administration of TPN as compared with enteral nutrients (isocaloric/isonitrogenous diets). These two reports suggest that the timing of nutritional support is more important than the route of administration in effecting wound healing.

GENERAL NUTRITIONAL STATUS

Patients with protein-calorie malnutrition may have impaired wound healing, a decreased immune response, increased susceptibility to infection, longer hospitalization, and increased morbidity and mortality rates.[10] Malnutrition results from a variety of causes such as malabsorption, decreased intake of nutrients, and hypermetabo-

lism. Malnutrition can interfere with wound healing by either delaying or inhibiting healing. Haydock and Hill[11] studied the effect of preoperative nutritional status (determined by an assessment of recent weight loss, dietary history, and anthropometric measurements) on wound healing. Patients were assigned to one of three groups: normally nourished, mild protein-energy malnutrition (PEM), and moderate to severe PEM. Patients underwent elective gastrointestinal surgery and subcutaneous implantation of Gore-tex tubing. After 1 week the implants were removed and assayed for hydroxyproline content. Patients with both mild and moderate to severe PEM had decreased wound healing responses when compared with normally nourished patients. However, there were no significant differences in wound healing between patients with mild and severe PEM despite differences in the state of malnutrition between the groups. The group with mild PEM was not anthropometrically different from normally nourished patients, but they had significant recent weight loss. The authors concluded that changes in wound healing may occur even with states of mild malnutrition and that these changes may be related to the organism's overall recent metabolic state instead of the degree of tissue loss.

Windsor et al.[12] assessed the effect of preoperative food intake on the hydroxyproline content of Gore-tex implants. Patients with adequate food intake before surgery had improved wound healing when compared with patients with poor preoperative food intake. Haydock and Hill[13] also assessed the wound healing response with Gore-tex implants in surgical patients and reported increased 7-day wound healing in normally nourished controls vs. malnourished patients receiving TPN. However, after 2 weeks of TPN the malnourished group had wound healing responses significantly improved over the control group. Healing improved in patients treated preoperatively with intravenous nutrition when compared with patients given intravenous nutrition only postoperatively. The improved deposition of hydroxyproline was evident after 1 week of TPN and before other signs of improved nutritional status were measurable. The data suggest that there is a greater improvement in wound healing if TPN is given before rather than after the surgical procedure.

Alterations in protein metabolism vary between organs. For example, the metabolically active liver has an increased protein content after severe injury despite increased protein turnover rates. At the same time, injured animals have a net loss of lean body mass/protein, which suggests that some organ function is preserved at the expense of other tissue such as skeletal muscle. Disturbances in the metabolism of one metabolite may result in changes in function or quantity of other metabolites and effect alterations in target tissues such as healing wounds. In the following sections, individual nutrients will be discussed separately, but their effects on wound healing are related. These interrelationships need to be considered when treating wounded patients.

PROTEIN

The idea that disturbed protein metabolism and nutrition impairs wound healing has been explored for over 50 years. Among early experiments were those of Thompson and associates,[14-16] who found that chronically protein-depleted dogs had impaired fibroplasia and a 72% incidence of wound dehiscence after laparotomy. Transfusions of a colloid during and after surgery in these hypoproteinemic dogs improved their edema and wound healing. Irvin[17] studied rats starved of protein and found significant reductions in the breaking strength of skin and abdominal wounds after 7 weeks of protein depletion. He reported a decrease in co-

lonic anastomotic strength with severe protein depletion but that the changes were less remarkable than those in skin and abdominal wounds. Irvin also supplemented a group of severely protein-depleted rats with an enteral amino acid preparation beginning 1 week before surgery. Supplemented rats had greater abdominal wound strength and increased deposition of collagen in abdominal wounds as compared with protein-depleted animals. The study did not find significant differences in the breaking strength or collagen deposition in skin or colonic wounds in the amino acid–supplemented group vs. the protein-depleted animals. The studies of both Irvin[17] and Delany et al.[5] suggest that wound healing in various tissues responds to malnutrition differently and that changes in wound healing reflect the underlying nutritional status.

Normal protein synthesis and cell multiplication cannot occur without an adequate supply of proteins and amino acids. Animal studies show that chronic protein deficiency leads to impaired angiogenesis, decreased fibroblastic proliferation, and diminished reparative collagen synthesis, accumulation, and remodeling in healing wounds.[18] Modolin et al.[19] reported decreased wound contraction in protein-depleted rats as compared with normal controls and protein–depleted-repleted rats (fed a standard diet including protein after skin wounds were inflicted). They found no significant difference in wound contraction between control rats and the protein–depleted-repleted rats. The mechanism for the disturbance in wound contraction is currently unknown but may be secondary to a decreased ability of fibroblasts to manufacture proteoglycans or changes in contractile functions of myofibroblasts that are stimulated by protein mediators.

Previous studies of wound healing used models with hypoproteinemia induced by severe protein depletion or plasmapheresis so that animals had low oncotic pressures and tissue edema. Recently, Felcher and associates[20] used a strain of genetically analbuminemic rats to study the isolated effect of hypoproteinemia on wound healing. They found no significant differences in wound breaking strength or collagen content in polyvinyl alcohol sponges in normal control rats vs. analbuminemic rats and concluded that isolated hypoalbuminemia had no detrimental effect on wound healing. These results suggest that the plasma oncotic pressure and resultant tissue edema rather than hypoalbuminemia may play an important role in wound healing.

Healing of bone fractures may be improved with nutrient supplementation. In a prospective, randomized controlled study,[21] administration of an oral protein-containing supplement resulted in fewer complications and deaths and decreased length of hospitalization in elderly patients with femoral neck fractures. Bastow et al.[22] also reported improved outcome after hip fractures in patients given protein-containing supplements (enterally or parenterally). The major nutrient improving healing was protein.[23] In addition, protein supplementation was associated with improved osteocalcin levels (a marker of osteoblastic activity).

PEPTIDES

Partially hydrolyzed proteins or more refined peptides have recently been used as the nitrogen source in enteral nutrition products. The advantages of these products have been reported to include beneficial effects on wound healing. We[24] reported significant improvement in abdominal wound bursting pressure in rats fed isocaloric, isonitrogenous enteral diets containing peptides as compared with amino acids. Previously, our laboratory[25] reported higher levels of IGF-1 (a growth factor) in animals receiving peptide vs. amino acid diets. From these data, it appears that peptides have unique anabolic activities

and that there may be a role for luminal peptides in wound healing. Further studies are needed to determine the mechanism by which peptides stimulate wound healing.

AMINO ACIDS

Protein synthesis must be increased at the wound site in order for normal healing to occur. Deficiencies of amino acids may impair protein synthesis and wound healing. All amino acids are required for normal protein synthesis whether or not there is a dietary requirement for them. Generally, the body can synthesize most amino acids. However, in stressed states it may not be able to synthesize some of them fast enough to meet body needs. Amino acids that can be synthesized but that may become deficient are termed "semiessential." Only lysine and threonine cannot be synthesized by the body. These amino acids must be provided in the diet and are termed "essential."

Many years ago, Williamson and Fromm[26] and Localio et al.[27] reported that administration of the sulfur-containing amino acids (methionine, cystine, and cysteine) to protein-depleted rats improved wound healing. However, Caldwell et al.[28] could not confirm these findings. It seems unlikely that supplementation of a single amino acid will correct the healing impairment during protein deficiency.

On the other hand, during injury states some amino acids may become relatively deficient, and a dietary supply of these may be beneficial. A series of studies by Barbul and colleagues[29, 30] demonstrated that rats ingesting an arginine-free diet sustained weight loss and delayed healing of skin wounds following injury. They also reported an accelerated rate of healing (over normal control rates) when rats were fed commercial rat chow (containing 1.8% arginine) supplemented with 1% arginine.[30] They measured wound healing by wound strength and accumulation of collagen in polyvinyl alcohol sponges. The beneficial effects of supplemental arginine were not seen in animals after hypophysectomy. The authors concluded that the arginine effect required an intact hypothalamic-pituitary-adrenal axis. Supplemental arginine also prevented thymic involution and enhanced lymphocyte stimulation.[31, 32] Recently, Barbul et al.[33] demonstrated improved collagen deposition in polytetrafluoroethylene tubes and increased lymphocyte mitogenesis in healthy humans ingesting substantial amounts of supplemental arginine. At this time, the mechanisms for enhanced wound healing and immune responses with supplemental arginine remain unknown. Further studies are needed to determine the mechanism and clinical utility of supplemental arginine therapy in injured humans.

The effect of local application of specific amino acids on healing of open burn wounds has produced mixed results.[34] Others report that a mixture of 19 amino acids applied to guinea pig burns enhanced granulation and scar formation.[35] Nagai et al.[36] showed that the local injection of a dipeptide, carnosine, in steroid-treated wounded animals improved wound healing (overcoming the steroid-induced healing impairment). The authors suggested that the dipeptide increased local histamine levels via the metabolism of histidine (a component of the dipeptide). In animal studies, wound strength after abdominal surgery was inferior with amino acid vs. peptide diets.[24] The mechanisms and clinical significance of these findings require further study.

CARBOHYDRATES

Alterations in carbohydrate metabolism have direct and indirect effects on wound healing. Unless adequate glucose is available (produced via glycolysis and gluconeogenesis) and its metabolism normal, the energy requirements of cells involved in wound healing cannot be met. Indirect effects of abnormal carbohydrate metabolism include the excessive oxidation of amino acids to provide caloric needs when the supply of carbohydrates and fats is inadequate. The impairment in wound healing and susceptibility to infection that occur in patients with diabetes mellitus have been recognized for many years. The clinical significance is obvious since the incidence of diabetes is high and most diabetics undergo surgery at some point. The disturbance in wound healing in these patients is multifactorial and not fully understood.

Animal studies of acute experimental diabetes (usually induced by streptozotocin) have shown an impaired early inflammatory response to injury, decreased endothelial cell proliferation, decreased accumulation of collagen, and diminished gain in wound strength.[18] Studies have also shown decreased leukocyte chemotaxis associated with hyperglycemia. Another factor in long-standing diabetes is the frequent complication of vascular insufficiency, which may compromise the wound supply of oxygen and other necessary cells and nutrients. Some studies[37] of streptozotocin-induced diabetes showed that early postoperative (days 1 to 11) treatment with insulin corrected the hyperglycemia and alleviated the impaired wound healing measured on day 21. In contrast, if the diabetic rats were treated with insulin later (days 11 to 21), wound healing remained impaired. Weringer et al.[38] studied dermal wound healing in normal controls, diabetic treated, and diabetic untreated mice. They reported significantly improved healing with insulin treatment of diabetic mice vs. untreated animals. Insulin treatment of the diabetic mice appeared to mitigate the diabetes-induced wound healing impairment (as compared with normal controls). Weringer et al.[39] further evaluated the effects of hyperglycemia on the wound healing response by treating normal mice with insulin antisera or 2-deoxyglucose (both cause an acute hyperglycemia: insulin antisera by extracellular effects on insulin levels and 2-deoxyglucose via an intracellular-mediated decrease in glucose uptake by cells). The mice treated with antisera to insulin manifested impaired wound healing, whereas the 2-deoxyglucose–treated mice had a wound healing response similar to controls. The investigators concluded that hyperglycemia alone did not induce poor healing in diabetic mice and that insulin appeared to be a necessary component for the wound healing response. This conclusion is supported by data from Hanam et al.,[40] who reported improved wound healing after the topical application of insulin to infected skin wounds of diabetic mice. Similarly, Saragas et al.[41] reported a reversal of impaired wound healing induced by corticosteroid therapy in corneal wounds of rabbits with supplemental subconjunctival insulin.

Other studies failed to find disturbances in wound epithelialization in diabetics vs. nondiabetics. Snip et al.[42] reported similar corneal wound epithelialization rates in patients with and without diabetes. Similar observations were reported by Hatchell et al.[43] in corneal wounds of diabetic and nondiabetic rabbits. In addition, Seifter et al.[44] reported nearly normal healing rates in diabetic rats with hyperglycemia, without insulin therapy, when supplemented with vitamin A. They concluded that the action of supplemental vitamin A on the defects in wound healing seen in streptozotocin-induced diabetes is independent of effects on carbohydrate metabolism.

Impairment of wound healing in diabetics is complicated. Some of the indirect effects of hyperglycemia and insulin deficiency on wound healing are dehydration, acidosis, and decreased tissue perfusion. Associated diabetic immunodeficiency may lead to severe wound infection and an inability to heal. The interrelationships between all of these disturbances in carbohydrate metabolism are not well understood. Studies are currently under way to evaluate the potential benefits of treating wounds in diabetic patients with growth factors. Although the preliminary results warrant optimism, more data must be evaluated before recommendations regarding their use are made.

FATS

The effects of fats on wound healing have not been studied as extensively as carbohydrate and protein sources. Both linoleic and linolenic acid are essential in the diet. They are components of the phospholipids and triglycerides that compose cellular membranes. Unsaturated fatty acids are needed for the synthesis of prostaglandins, which regulate aspects of inflammation and cellular metabolism. Hulsey et al.[45] performed an extensive study demonstrating a significant impairment in wound healing with essential fatty acid deficiency in rats. The most significant effects were on healing of skin wounds, with less remarkable effects on colon anastomotic healing. Rolandelli et al.[46] reported enhanced rat colon anastomotic strength after intraluminal infusion of short-chain fatty acids. The same investigators[47] supplemented an elemental enteral diet with pectin and found improved healing of colon anastomoses upon the addition of pectin. The pectin-supplemented animals had decreased intracolonic pH, and they postulated that the beneficial effects were secondary to local increases in short-chain fatty acids derived from pectin fermentation.

WATER-SOLUBLE VITAMINS

Vitamin C (Ascorbic Acid)

As early as the 1500s, sailors with scurvy were observed to have abnormal wound healing. In the 1700s, citrus fruits were recognized to cure scurvy, and in the 1930s the active ingredient ascorbic acid was discovered. Over the years, many studies have demonstrated impairment of wound healing in vitamin C–deficient animals[48] and humans.[49, 50] The abnormalities include increased wound hemorrhage, decreased angiogenesis and reparative collagen formation, and delayed gain in wound strength. In patients with depleted levels of vitamin C, the incidence of wound dehiscence is eight times higher than in vitamin C–replete individuals.[10] In 1940, Crandon et al.[51] published a landmark report of controlled vitamin C deficiency in an otherwise healthy young man. Crandon himself ate a diet nutritionally complete except for vitamin C for 6 months. By day 42, his plasma vitamin C level was undetectable, but the white blood cell ascorbic acid level did not drop to the zero range until day 122. By that time he experienced a moderate loss of weight and had a decreased basal metabolic rate but was clinically well. Three months after the start of the experiment, a 2-in. skin incision was made, and it healed normally. Petechiae were noted on his limbs at 161 days. At the end of 6 months, a second skin incision was made, and healing failed to occur (gross failure of the wound edges to unite under the skin surface). A biopsy specimen of the wound was obtained, and histologic examination showed a lack of intercellular substance and vascular elements. After the biopsy, Crandon ingested 1 g of ascorbic acid per day, and 10 days later a second biopsy sample revealed good healing and evidence of capillary formation. In 1947, Wolfer et al.[52] studied wound healing in nine volunteers (medical students) who ate a diet that was extremely low in vitamin C and in 5 normal medical students who ate the same diet but were supplemented with 75 to 150 mg of vitamin C per day. After 7 months on the diet, the tensile strength of wounds in the vitamin C–deficient students was markedly decreased when compared with the controls.

Ascorbic acid plays a key role in the synthesis of collagen. It is required for the hydroxylation of proline and lysine. Fibroblast proliferation is not believed to be altered, but fibroblast maturation is impaired in vitamin C deficiency. Vitamin C also has important roles in maintaining immune function, which is necessary for normal wound healing to occur. Collagen is used to wall off the infected area and aids in limiting infection. Vitamin C is required for production of the complement and neutrophil superoxide used for antibacterial functions. Extensive reviews of the biological actions of ascorbic acid[53] and collagen biosynthesis have been published previously.[54–56]

Wounds are metabolically more active than normal connective tissue. Therefore, more ascorbic acid is required to maintain wound integrity than to maintain developmental collagen. Previously healed scars have been reported to break down in states of vitamin C deficiency.[57] Guinea pig abdominal wounds that healed normally for 6 weeks failed to synthesize adequate collagen when dietary ascorbic acid was withheld. The dynamic relationship between collagen production and collagenolysis was disrupted, and the wounds reverted to an immature state with weakness and hernia formation.

Primates (including humans) and guinea pigs are unable to synthesize ascorbic acid. Healthy young men have a total body pool of about 2.3 g of vitamin C and can maintain this pool by ingesting 10 to 20 mg/day. Elderly humans (men more than women) appear to need more ascorbic acid, around 60 to 70 mg/day, to maintain their total-body pool.[18] Today, vitamin C deficiency is rare. When evaluating patients for vitamin C deficiency, interpretation of plasma vitamin C levels alone is difficult because a low plasma level does not necessarily indicate tissue vitamin C deficiency. White blood cell ascorbic acid levels and tissue saturation tests are better indices of vitamin C deficiency.

Vitamin C metabolism is altered following acute trauma or severe burns. Plasma ascorbic acid levels and urinary ascorbic acid excretion may fall dramatically, and tissue saturation tests may indicate marked depletion. Indeed, a syndrome of "biochemical scurvy" has been described in which patients with severe injuries act biochemically like uninjured patients with chronic vitamin C deficiency from prolonged inadequate intake. Patients with "biochemical scurvy" require huge doses (2 g/day) of vitamin C before their biochemical indices return to normal.[57, 58] Abnormalities in wound healing in burned guinea pigs are overcome by giving them supplemental vitamin C.[59] The underlying mechanism for altered vitamin C metabolism after injury is not known, but the abnormalities may persist for long periods. Despite evidence that vitamin C is required for normal wound healing, there is no evidence that wound healing can be enhanced by the administration of more vitamin C than is needed to maintain normal tissue levels. Vitamin C is not stored to a great extent in the body, and physiologically significant deficiency in injured patients may develop rapidly. Therefore, patients with severe injuries and burns should be treated with 1 to 2 g of ascorbic acid daily after injury and treatment continued at least until the wounds have healed.[18]

Vitamin B Complex

There are few data on specific effects of the B-complex vitamins on wound repair. These vitamins are cofactors in multiple enzyme systems. They participate in antibody production and are needed for proper white blood cell function. Deficiencies of the B-complex vitamins could cause problems in protein, carbohydrate, and fat metabolism. Interference with wound healing is possible by a variety of mechanisms. Patients with severe injuries are reported to have disturbances in the metabolism of thia-

min, riboflavin, and nicotinic acid.[57, 59] These vitamins are not stored in significant quantities in the body, and some supplementation is warranted in states of severe illness. Clinical studies have not evaluated actual metabolic requirements of the B-complex vitamins in seriously ill patients. However, enteral nutritional products are expected to contain adequate amounts of these vitamins. Multiple vitamin preparations are routinely added to parenteral nutrition formulations, and this is believed to meet the needs of seriously ill or injured patients.

FAT-SOLUBLE VITAMINS

Vitamin A

The role vitamin A plays in cell differentiation and epithelialization was described by Wolbach and Howe in 1925.[18] These findings supported the use of liver oil as a folk remedy. In 1941, Brandaleone and Papper[60] reported that local and oral administration of cod liver oil overcame the impaired wound healing seen in vitamin A–deficient rats. Later, Ehrlich et al.[61–63] reported that supplemental vitamin A reversed or prevented the cortisone-induced healing impairment.

The role of vitamin A in wound healing has been extensively studied in recent years. Rats maintained on a diet low in vitamin A but sufficient to support nearly normal growth lost weight after minor wounding had impaired healing, and developed hypoglycemia. Histologic examination revealed decreased reparative collagen synthesis and diminished cross-linking. Rats with marginal vitamin A intake had a mortality rate of about 50% (vs. no deaths in the control group). Postoperative administration of vitamin A to these rats prevented these effects.[18]

Healthy wounded rats eating standard rat chow supplemented with vitamin A demonstrated increased inflammation, angiogenesis, and collagen accumulation. Demetriou et al.[64] found that mice undergoing peritoneal ligation that were supplemented with vitamin A had an increased incidence and severity of postoperative intra-abdominal adhesions. These investigators also treated some mice with citral, a vitamin A antagonist, and reported that citral decreased the formation of adhesions as compared with controls. Others reported increased hydroxyproline content and bursting pressures of normal colon and colon anastomotic sites after supplementation with vitamin A. Niu et al.[65] found increased breaking strength and reparative collagen accumulation in rat aorta anastomoses upon supplementation with vitamin A.

Supplemental vitamin A mitigates the poor healing associated with numerous pathologic states. Acute radiation- and tumor-induced defects in wound healing are prevented by supplemental vitamin A.[66, 67] The impaired wound healing of rats with femoral fracture(s) is also improved with vitamin A therapy.[68] Supplemental vitamin A prevents impairment of wound healing in rats with streptozotocin-induced diabetes.[44] In these diabetic rats, supplemental vitamin A also prevents thymic involution, peripheral lymphocytopenia, and adrenal hyperplasia (typically found in the streptozotocin-treated diabetic rats). These effects are independent of an effect on disturbed carbohydrate metabolism. The investigators postulate that the beneficial effects of vitamin A on wound healing in diabetic animals are due to an improved early inflammatory response.

Effects of vitamin A on gastrointestinal ulcerations have been evaluated by several laboratories. Chernov et al.[69] reported that vitamin A prevented or decreased stress ulcers. Dietary supplementation of vitamin A decreased the incidence of aspirin-induced gastric ulcers.[70] Mahmood et al.[71] induced duodenal ulcerations in rats with intragastric cysteamine HCI (which enhances gastric acid secretion) and showed that dietary supplementation of vitamin A prevented ulcerations in this model without altering gastric acid secretion.

Specific mechanisms for the wound healing effects of vitamin A remain to be elucidated. In general, it is believed that an improved early inflammatory response is the primary reason for these effects. This theory proposes an increased influx of macrophages, an increased release of growth factors by the macrophages, and an increase in the rate of fibroblast differentiation and collagen synthesis. Alternatively, vitamin A may have a direct influence on the effects of growth factors. This mechanism is supported by data obtained from cell cultures in which vitamin A increased fibroblast receptors for epidermal growth factor and increased fibroblast multiplication.[72] Others suggest that effects on cell membranes may play a role. Vitamin A antagonizes glucocorticoid-induced impairment of wound healing. Investigators postulate that vitamin A reverses the glucocorticoid effects on cell membranes. Further studies are needed to establish the mechanisms of action of vitamin A in the process of wound healing.

Vitamin A deficiency is associated with an increased incidence of infections. Supplemental vitamin A increases the cell-mediated immune response in normal, injured, and tumor-inflicted animals. Most of the immunologic effects are thymic dependent, and changes in T-lymphocyte subsets are present. However, humoral defense mechanisms are also affected by vitamin A. Several investigators have reported decreased numbers of antibody-producing cells and decreased antibody production in vitamin A–deficient rats. In contrast, these responses are increased in normally nourished rats supplemented with vitamin A. Barbul et al.[73] reported that supplemental vitamin A increased the number of white blood cells (monocytes/macrophages) migrating into the wound area in rats with femoral fractures. Vitamin A caused a temporary leukocytosis characterized by lymphocytosis, monocytosis, and a relative neutropenia.

Overt vitamin A deficiency is rare in developed countries but fairly common in third-world countries. Subclinical deficiencies are common in the United States. Large amounts of vitamin A are stored in the liver. Well-nourished patients undergoing elective uncomplicated surgery should have adequate amounts of vitamin A in storage. However, after serious injury, vitamin A requirements increase. Decreases in serum vitamin A, retinol binding protein, prealbumin, and β-carotene have been documented after burns, fractures, and elective surgery. In such patients the urinary excretion of vitamin A and retinol binding protein is increased.[74, 75] Deficiencies may develop in cases of prolonged interference with oral intake or gastrointestinal malabsorption. The American Medical Association (AMA) Nutrition Advisory Group Guidelines for Multivitamin Preparations for Parenteral Use recommends 3300 IU of vitamin A per day. However, no specific reference is made to patients with serious injury. Levenson and Demetriou advocate supplementing vitamin A in malnourished patients with gastrointestinal dysfunction before and after surgery (25,000 IU/day).[18] Patients with good nutritional status who undergo surgery and cannot eat for long periods should also be supplemented postoperatively. The daily dose of 25,000 IU recommended by Levenson and Demetriou is about seven to eight times the recommended dietary allowance (RDA) for healthy uninjured adults. Very large doses of vitamin A (100,000 IU/day) have been given to cancer patients for periods of 1 year with only isolated instances of mild toxicity. More data are needed to determine how vitamin A affects the metabolic response to injury, the immune response, and wound healing.

Vitamin E

There is a lack of evidence for alterations in vitamin E metabolism after injury. It is believed that vitamin E deficiency may develop in seriously ill patients if they are maintained on long-term TPN without parenteral vitamin E supplementation. In humans, vitamin E deficiency has been described in premature infants receiving a diet high in polyunsaturated fats but no vitamin E. Parenteral vitamin E is available in multivitamin preparations, which typically contain 25 mg of vitamin E. Alterations of vitamin E metabolism or requirements after injury have not been reported.

Little is known regarding a specific role for vitamin E in normal wound healing, and few studies have addressed the issue. Since deficiency of vitamin E is rare in humans, studies in vitamin E–deficient animals seem of little value. In some reports, excessive vitamin E supplementation has caused delayed wound healing. Vitamin E has also been reported to interfere with the beneficial effects of vitamin A on wound healing.[76] Others have reported decreased formation of experimental postoperative adhesions with excess dietary vitamin E.[77]

Vitamin E has antioxidant properties, and several groups have questioned whether it or other agents with free radical scavenging ability might be of benefit in wound healing. In one of the reports, intraperitoneal vitamin E resulted in increased breaking strength of wounds exposed to preoperative irradiation.[78] In another, Hayden et al.[79] found improved skin flap survival with supplemental vitamin A, C, or E (which all have free radical scavenging ability). Further studies are needed to determine the clinical utility and potential risks and benefits of supplemental vitamin E therapy in view of conflicting reports of delayed vs. enhanced healing.

TRACE ELEMENTS

The body does not require large stores of most trace minerals. In healthy individuals the body is efficient at retaining these elements during metabolism. Trace mineral deficiency (with the exception of iron) was not recognized as a clinical problem until the widespread use of long-term TPN. Some pathologic states such as serious injury, diabetes, alcoholism, and gastrointestinal disorders may induce deficiencies of trace minerals. However, it is rare to find a patient with an isolated deficiency of a trace mineral, and therefore it is hard to correlate alterations in the wound healing process with a specific deficit. In spite of these difficulties, three minerals (zinc, iron, and copper) appear to be important in wound healing.

Zinc

Chronic dietary zinc deficiency causes low plasma zinc levels, growth retardation, hypogonadism, mild anemia, and poor wound healing.[80] Zinc deficiency in humans was first reported in the 1950s. It appeared to be more prevalent in countries where the population consumed a diet that consisted primarily of cereal proteins. During the 1970s in the United States, nutritional zinc deficiency was observed in infants and children. This led to routine zinc supplementation of infant milk formulas. Zinc deficiency is known to be associated with alcoholism, gastrointestinal disorders such as inflammatory bowel disease, burns, and chronic renal disease.

Zinc is required for normal wound healing. Rats with zinc deficiency have impaired healing of skin wounds. Collagen and noncollagen protein levels are decreased in the connective tissue of these rats. In normal rats, zinc supplementation does not enhance healing. Pories et al.[81] reported that the oral administration of zinc sulfate to military personnel caused a twofold increase in the rate of reepithelialization of wounds formed from pilonidal sinus excision. They postulated that patients with healing problems may have zinc stores inadequate to meet the demands of healing tissues.

Zinc is an essential component of many metalloenzymes such as DNA and RNA polymerase and is required for protein synthesis, DNA synthesis, mitosis, and cell proliferation (all of which are required for healing). These processes are interfered with by zinc deficiency. Zinc also stabilizes cell membranes and in this capacity has effects counter to vitamin A. A number of host defense mechanisms are impaired in zinc deficiency, thus causing greater susceptibility to wound infection, which may interfere with healing.

Zinc is primarily absorbed in the small intestine and is excreted mainly in the feces. Gastrointestinal tract dysfunction can result in decreased absorption of zinc and increased losses of zinc, especially with diarrhea. Normal urinary excretion of zinc is low, but it is increased after severe injury. Patients with severe burns have a marked zinc deficit beginning shortly after injury and lasting as long as several months.[80] During the acute-phase response there is a dramatic decrease in plasma zinc levels, thought to be due to accumulation in the liver. Postoperative patients have shown a marked zincuria with a fall in zinc stores after surgery.[81] Intestinal absorption of zinc appears to be variable between individuals and dependent on the nutritional status of the individual. Zinc absorption is related to the associated protein and phosphate intake. The mean dietary zinc requirement of healthy American men, determined by metabolic balance studies, is around 12 mg/day on a moderate protein diet (80 to 100 g/day). The National Regulatory Commission (NRC) RDA of zinc for healthy adults is 15 mg. No studies have evaluated zinc requirements for seriously ill patients. The AMA Food and Nutrition Board has recommended that stable adult patients receiving TPN, without enteral feeding, be given 2.5 to 4.0 mg of zinc daily; adults in an acute catabolic state should receive 4.5 to 6.0 mg daily; stable adults with extensive intestinal losses should get an additional 12.2 mg/L of upper small-bowel loss and 17.1 mg/kg of stool or ileostomy output. Excess zinc can interfere with copper metabolism and the activity of lysyl oxidase. Therefore, excess zinc can interfere with wound healing. Zinc administration to patients without zinc deficiency does not enhance wound healing.

Iron

Ferrous iron (Fe^{2+}) is required for the hydroxylation of proline and lysine in collagen synthesis and is a component of a variety of cellular enzymes. Iron deficiency has not been noted to cause changes in connective tissue synthesis in man. Only when iron deficiency anemia is severe and acute may it impair wound healing by adversely affecting oxygen transport. Oxygen is required at the wound site for the healing process to occur. If blood loss renders the patient unable to deliver an adequate supply of oxygen to the tissues, transfusion of red blood cells should be considered. Iron deficiency can interfere with the bactericidal activity of leukocytes and increase the likelihood of infection, which could also interfere with healing.

Copper

Copper is a constituent of a number of metalloenzymes important in wound healing. It is a component of the enzyme lysyl oxidase, which catalyzes collagen cross-linking. It is also part of Zn-Cu superoxide dismutase, which helps to contain toxic oxygen free radicals. Copper deficiency became clinically apparent during long-term TPN therapy. Severe copper deficiency is characterized by anemia, neutropenia, hypercholesterolemia, and scorbutic bone changes.[82]

Copper is excreted into the bile and feces; urinary copper excretion is normally small. Copper absorption may be decreased and excretion increased in patients with gastrointestinal disorders. The absorption or excretion of copper has not been reported to change secondary to serious illness. The acute-phase response to injury includes a sharp rise in the level of ceruloplasmin, the major transport protein for copper. The administration of penicillamine to patients with Wilson's disease and to animals causes a decrease in healing secondary to depletion of copper stores.[83]

Copper should be supplied to patients who are seriously ill. Serum copper levels are not helpful in assessing copper needs of patients. If the gastrointestinal tract is functional, copper supplementation is accomplished by providing a standard diet or enteral nutrition. If prolonged parenteral nutrition is necessary, copper supplementation should be administered. The adult human body contains 70 to 100 mg of copper. The daily copper requirements of healthy adults are unknown, so there is no published RDA for copper. Instead the NRC has recommended a safe and adequate daily dietary intake for copper of 2 to 3 mg. For patients receiving TPN as their sole nutrition, the AMA Food and Nutrition Board recommends 0.5 to 1.5 mg daily for stable adults. No specific recommendations are made regarding patients in catabolic states or in those with increased intestinal losses.

HORMONES/GROWTH FACTORS

Wound healing is a complex process that involves many interrelated steps. For successful healing to occur proper balance and control of competing phases of the wound healing response must be maintained. Recent research suggests that hormones (the role of insulin was previously discussed) and growth factors have important roles in modulating the wound healing response.

In 1958, Prudden et al.[84] reported that bovine GH increased wound breaking strength and postoperative anabolism in rats. The clinical utility of the observed effect in rats was limited because bovine GH was inert in humans unless used at very high doses. Availability was a major issue. Today, biotechnology has made synthetic recombinant human GH available. Studies have shown improved wound strength[85, 86] and increased collagen formation[87] in normal or tumor-bearing rats treated perioperatively with human GH. Studies by Jiang et al.[88] showed that in patients receiving hypocaloric nutrition, the postoperative catabolic response was modified by treatment with GH. Patients treated with GH had better nitrogen balances as compared with controls. Zaizen et al.[89] administered rat GH perioperatively to malnourished rats and reported increased wound breaking strength with GH. Wound strength improved to levels that exceeded normally nourished controls. They suggested that GH could provide an adjunctive therapy for use in malnourished patients to enhance wound healing. On the other hand, feeding protein-depleted rats with chow for 3 days preoperatively resulted in better wound healing than administering GH alone.[90] The wound-healing effects of GH combined with aggressive nutritional support have not been adequately studied. Preliminary studies in our laboratory have failed to detect an added advantage of GH. In a prospective, randomized, double-blind controlled study, daily administration of recombinant human GH to severely burned children accelerated healing of donor sites and shortened hospital stay as compared with controls.[91] Further studies are required to define the clinical efficacy of recombinant human GH in addition to aggressive nutritional support in the seriously ill.

Some of the growth factors most likely to have important roles in wound healing are PDGF, fibroblast growth factors (FGFs), epidermal growth factor (EGF), TGF-α and TGF-β, and IGF-1 and IGF-2. The ability of cells to respond to growth factors is dependent on the presence of receptors on a given cell. In addition, some growth factors have been found to have chemoattractant properties and may have a dual mechanism for wound repair modulation. There is a long history of attempting to stimulate healing by applying extracts from various tissues to wounds. For example, pulverized earthworm is advocated for topical use on boils and cellulitis in some Indian cultures. Yegnanarayan et al.[92] report a decrease in carrageenan-induced edema in rats after the administration of earthworm extract. Perhaps some of these extracts have efficacy in improving wound healing by virtue of growth factors.

Many of these growth factors are now manufactured by techniques of biotechnology. Previously, they were available only by harvest from animal tissues. Recently, studies have been initiated to evaluate their therapeutic utility. Grotendorst et al.[93] report stimulation of granulation tissue by PDGF in normal and diabetic rats. Knighton et al.[94] report improved healing of nonhealing chronic ulcers in diabetic patients with the application of platelet extracts. Laato et al.[95] report a stimulatory, dose-dependent effect of locally applied EGF on granulation tissue formation in rats. In a prospective, randomized, double-blind clinical trial in humans, topical EGF accelerates the rate of healing of partial-thickness skin grafts.[96] In diabetic rats, EGF and insulin have synergistic effects on collagen synthesis above the effects seen with either EGF or insulin alone.[97] Others report enhanced wound healing in animals with TGF-α, vaccinia growth factor, and FGF.[98–100] Better understanding of the regulation and specific roles of growth factors may provide new therapeutic tools for enhancing wound repair and decreasing morbidity and mortality secondary to injuries.

REFERENCES

1. Robson MC: Disturbances of wound healing. *Ann Emerg Med* 1988; 17:1274–1278.
2. Hunt TK: The physiology of wound healing. *Ann Emerg Med* 1988; 17:1265–1273.
3. Ehrlichman RJ, Seckel BR, Bryan DJ, et al: Common complications of wound healing: Prevention and management. *Surg Clin North Am* 1991; 71:1323–1351.
4. Orgill D, Demling RH: Current concepts and approaches to wound healing. *Crit Care Med* 1988; 16:899–908.
5. Delany HM, Demetriou AA, Teh E, et al: Effect of early postoperative nutritional support on skin wound and colon anastomosis healing. *JPEN* 1990; 14:357–361.
6. Greenstein A, Rogers P, Moss G: Doubled fourth day colorectal anastomotic strength with complete retention of intestinal mature wound collagen and accelerated deposition following immediate full enteral nutrition. *Surg Forum* 1978; 29:78–81.
7. Moss G, Greenstein A, Levy S, et al: Maintenance of GI function after bowel surgery and immediate enteral full nutrition. I. Doubling of canine colorectal anastomotic bursting pressure and intestinal wound mature collagen content. *JPEN* 1980; 4:535–538.
8. Zaloga GP, Bortenschlager L, Black KW, et al: Immediate postoperative enteral feeding decreases weight loss and improves wound healing after abdominal surgery in rats. *Crit Care Med* 1992; 20:115–118.
9. Zaloga GP, Bortenschlager L, Black K: Early administration of enteral or parenteral nutrients improves wound healing. *JPEN* 1992; 16(suppl):28.
10. Young ME: Malnutrition and wound healing. *Heart Lung* 1988; 17:60–67.
11. Haydock DA, Hill GL: Impaired wound healing in surgical patients with varying degrees of malnutrition. *JPEN* 1986; 10:550–554.
12. Windsor JA, Knight GS, Hill GL: Wound healing response in surgical patients: Recent food intake is more important than nutritional status. *Br J Surg* 1988; 75:135–137.
13. Haydock DA, Hill GL: Improved wound healing response in surgical patients receiving intravenous nutrition. *Br J Surg* 1987; 74:320–323.
14. Thompson WD, Radvin IS, Frank IL: Effect of hypoproteinemia on wound disruption. *Arch Surg* 1938; 26:500–508.
15. Thompson WD, Radvin IS, Rhoads JE, et al: The use of lyophile plasma in correction of hypoproteinemia and prevention of wound disruption. *Arch Surg* 1938; 26:509–518.
16. Rhoads JE, Fliegelman MT, Panzer LM: The mechanism of delayed wound healing in the presence of hypoproteinemia. *JAMA* 1942; 118:21–25.
17. Irvin TT: Effects of malnutrition and hyperalimentation on wound healing. *Surg Gynecol Obstet* 1978; 146:33–37.
18. Levenson SM, Demetriou AA: Metabolic factors, in Cohen K, Diegelman RF, Lindblad WJ (eds): *Wound Healing: Biochemical and Clinical Aspects.* Philadelphia, WB Saunders, 1992, pp 248–273.
19. Modolin M, Bevilacqua RG, Margarido NF, et al: Effects of protein depletion and repletion on experimental open wound contraction. *Ann Plastic Surg* 1985; 15:123–126.
20. Felcher A, Schwartz J, Shechter C, et al: Wound healing in normal and analbuminemic (NAR) rats. *J Surg Res* 1987; 43:546–549.
21. Delmi M, Rapin CH, Bengoa JM, et al: Dietary supplementation in elderly patients with fractured neck of the femur. *Lancet* 1990; 1:1013–1016.
22. Bastow MD, Rawlings J, Allison SP: Benefits of supplementary tube feeding after fractured neck of femur: A randomized controlled trial. *BMJ* 1983; 287:1589–1592.
23. Tkatch L, Rapin CH, Rizzoli R, et al: Benefits of oral protein supplementation in elderly patients with fracture of the proximal femur. *J Am Coll Nutr* 1992; 11:519–525.
24. Roberts P, Black K, Zaloga G: Peptide-based enteral diets improve wound healing after abdominal surgery in rats. *JPEN* 1993; 17(suppl):32.

25. Zaloga GP, Ward KA, Prielipp RC: Effect of enteral diets on whole body and gut growth in unstressed rats. *JPEN* 1991; 15:42–47.

26. Williamson MB, Fromm HJ: The incorporation of sulfur amino acids into the proteins of regenerating wound tissue. *J Biol Chem* 1955; 212:705–712.

27. Localio SA, Morgan ME, Hinton JW: The biological chemistry of wound healing: I. The effect of *dl*-methionine on the healing of wounds in protein-depleted animals. *Surg Gynecol Obstet* 1948; 86:582–590.

28. Caldwell FT, Rosenberg IK, Rosenberg BF, et al: Effect of single amino acid supplementation upon the gain of tensile strength of wounds in protein-depleted rats. *Surg Gynecol Obstet* 1964; 119:823–830.

29. Barbul A, Rettura G, Levenson SM, et al: Arginine: A thymotropic and wound-healing promoting agent. *Surg Forum* 1977; 28:101–103.

30. Seifter E, Rettura G, Barbul A, et al: Arginine: An essential amino acid for injured rats. *Surgery* 1978; 84:224–230.

31. Barbul A, Rettura G, Levenson SM, et al: Wound healing and thymotropic effects of arginine: A pituitary mechanism of action. *Am J Coll Nutr* 1983; 37:786–794.

32. Barbul A, Fishel RS, Shimazu S, et al: Intravenous hyperalimentation with high arginine levels improves wound healing and immune function. *J Surg Res* 1985; 38:328–334.

33. Barbul A, Lazarou SA, Efron DT, et al: Arginine enhances wound healing and lymphocyte immune responses in humans. *Surgery* 1990; 108:331–337.

34. Harvey SG, Gibson JR: The effects on wound healing of three amino acids—a comparison of three models. *Br J Dermatol* 1984; 111(suppl):171–173.

35. Kaufman T, Levin M, Hurwitz DJ: The effect of topical hyperalimentation on wound healing rate and granulation tissue formation of experimental deep second degree burns in guinea pigs. *Burns* 1984; 10:252–256.

36. Nagai K, Suda T, Kawasaki K, et al: Action of carnosine and beta-alanine on wound healing. *Surgery* 1986; 100:815–821.

37. Goodson WH, Hunt TK: Studies of wound healing in experimental diabetes mellitus. *J Surg Res* 1977; 22:221–227.

38. Weringer EJ, Kelso JM, Tamai IY, et al: Effects of insulin on wound healing in diabetic mice. *Acta Endocrinol* 1982; 99:101–108.

39. Weringer EJ, Kelso JM, Tamai IY, et al: The effect of antisera to insulin, 2-deoxyglucose–induced hyperglycemia, and starvation on wound healing in normal mice. *Diabetes* 1981; 30:407–410.

40. Hanam SR, Singleton CE, Rudek W: The effect of topical insulin on infected cutaneous ulcerations in diabetic and nondiabetic mice. *J Foot Surg* 1983; 22:298–301.

41. Saragas S, Arffa R, Rabin B, et al: Reversal of wound strength by addition of insulin to corticosteroid therapy. *Ann Ophthalmol* 1985; 17:428–430.

42. Snip RC, Thoft RA, Tolentino FI: Similar epithelial healing rates of the corneas of diabetic and nondiabetic patients. *Am J Ophthalmol* 1980; 90:463–468.

43. Hatchell DL, Ubels JL, Stekiel T, et al: Corneal epithelial wound healing in normal and diabetic rabbits treated with tretinoin. *Arch Ophthalmol* 1985; 103:98–100.

44. Seifter E, Rettura G, Padawer J, et al: Impaired wound healing in streptozotocin diabetes. *Ann Surg* 1981; 194:42–50.

45. Hulsey TK, O'Neill JA, Neblett WR, et al: Experimental wound healing in essential fatty acid deficiency. *J Pediatric Surg* 1980; 15:505–508.

46. Rolandelli RH, Koruda MJ, Settle RG, et al: Effects of intraluminal infusion of short-chain fatty acids on the healing of colonic anastomosis in the rat. *Surgery* 1986; 100:198–203.

47. Rolandelli RH, Koruda MJ, Settle RG, et al: The effect of enteral feedings supplemented with pectin on the healing of colonic anastomoses in the rat. *Surgery* 1986; 99:703–707.

48. Bartlett MK, Jones CM, Ryan AE: Vitamin C and wound healing: I. Experimental wounds in guinea pigs. *N Engl J Med* 1942; 226:469–473.

49. Lanman TH, Ingalls TH: Vitamin C deficiency and wound healing. *Ann Surg* 1937; 105:616–625.

50. Bartlett MK, Jones CM, Ryan AE: Vitamin C and wound healing: II. Ascorbic acid content and tensile strength of healing wounds in human beings. *N Engl J Med* 1942; 226:474–481.

51. Crandon JH, Lund CC, Dill DB: Experimental human scurvy. *N Engl J Med* 1940; 223:353–369.

52. Wolfer JA, Farmer CJ, Carroll WW, et al: An experimental study in wound healing in vitamin C depleted human subjects. *Surg Gynecol Obstet* 1947; 84:1–15.

53. Englard S, Seifter E: The biochemical functions of ascorbic acid. *Annu Rev Nutr* 1986; 6:365–406.

54. Prockop DJ, Kivirikko KI, Tuderman L, et al: The biosynthesis of collagen and its disorders. *N Engl J Med* 1979; 301:13–23.

55. Miller EJ, Gay S: Collagen structure and function, in Cohen IK, Diegelmann RF, Lindblad WJ (eds): *Wound Healing: Biochemical and Clinical Aspects.* Philadelphia, WB Saunders, 1992, pp 130–151.

56. Phillips C, Wenstrup RJ: Biosynthetic and genetic disorders of collagen, in Cohen IK, Diegelmann RF, Lindblad WJ (eds): *Wound Healing: Biochemical and Clinical Aspects.* Philadelphia, WB Saunders, 1992, pp 152–176.

57. Levenson SM, Green RW, Taylor FLH, et al: Ascorbic acid, riboflavin, thiamin, and nicotinic acid in relation to severe injury, hemorrhage, and infection in the human. *Ann Surg* 1946; 124:840–856.

58. Lund CC, Levenson SM, Green RW, et al: Ascorbic acid, thiamin, riboflavin, and nicotinic acid in relation to acute burns in man. *Arch Surg* 1947; 55:557–583.

59. Levenson SM, Upjohn HL, Preston JA, et al: Effect of thermal burns on wound healing. *Ann Surg* 1957; 146:357–368.

60. Brandaleone H, Papper E: The effect of local and oral administration of cod liver oil on the rate of wound healing in vitamin A deficient and normal animals. *Ann Surg* 1941; 114:791–798.

61. Ehrlich HP, Hunt TK: Effects of cortisone and vitamin A on wound healing. *Ann Surg* 1968; 167:324–328.

62. Hunt TK, Ehrlich HP, Garcia JA, et al: Effect of vitamin A on reversing the inhibitory effect of cortisone on healing of open wounds in animals and man. *Ann Surg* 1969; 170:633–641.

63. Ehrlich HP, Tarver H, Hunt TK: Effects of vitamin A and glucocorticoids upon inflammation and collagen synthesis. *Ann Surg* 1973; 177:222–227.

64. Demetriou AA, Seifter E, Levenson SM: Effect of vitamin A and citral on peritoneal adhesion formation. *J Surg Res* 1974; 17:325–329.

65. Niu XT, Cushin B, Reisner A, et al: Effect of dietary supplementation with vitamin A on arterial healing in rats. *J Surg Res* 1987; 42:61–65.

66. Levenson SM, Gruber CA, Rettura G, et al: Supplemental vitamin A prevents the acute radiation-induced defect in wound healing. *Ann Surg* 1984; 200:494–512.

67. Weinzweig J, Levenson SM, Rettura G, et al: Supplemental vitamin A prevents the tumor-induced defect in wound healing. *Ann Surg* 1990; 211:269–276.

68. Seifter E, Crowley LV, Rettura G, et al: Influence of vitamin A on wound healing in rats with femoral fracture. *Ann Surg* 1975; 181:836–841.

69. Chernov MS, Hale HW, Wood M: Prevention of stress ulcers. *Am J Surg* 1971; 122:674–677.

70. Seifter E, Seifter J, Levenson SM, et al: Aspirin (A) toxicity: Antidotal action of vitamin A (VA) and β-carotene (BC) but not of transretinoic acid (RA) (abstract). *J Am Coll Nutr* 1982; 3:412.

71. Mahmood T, Tenenbaum S, Niu XT, et al: Prevention of duodenal ulcer formation in the rat by dietary vitamin A supplementation. *JPEN* 1986; 10:74–77.

72. Jetten AM: Modulation of cell growth by retinoids and their possible mecha-

nisms of action. *Fed Proc* 1984; 43:134–139.

73. Barbul A, Thysen B, Rettura G, et al: White cell involvement in the inflammatory, wound healing, and immune actions of vitamin A. *JPEN* 1978; 2:129–138.

74. Ramsden DB, Prince HP, Burr WA, et al: The inter-relationship of thyroid hormones, vitamin A and their binding proteins following acute stress. *Clin Endocrinol* 1978; 8:109–122.

75. Kuroiwa K, Trocki O, Alexander JW, et al: Effect of vitamin A in enteral formulae for burned guinea-pigs. *Burns* 1990; 16:265–272.

76. Ehrlich HP, Tarver H, Hunt TK: Inhibitory effects of vitamin E on collagen synthesis and wound repair. *Ann Surg* 1972; 175:235–240.

77. Kagoma P, Burger SN, Seifter E, et al: The effect of vitamin E on experimentally induced peritoneal adhesions in mice. *Arch Surg* 1985; 120:949–951.

78. Taren DL, Chvapil M, Weber CW: Increasing the breaking strength of wounds exposed to preoperative irradiation using vitamin E supplementation. *Int J Vitam Nutr Res* 1987; 57:133–137.

79. Hayden RE, Yeung CST, Paniello RC, et al: The effect of glutathione and vitamins A, C, and E on acute skin flap survival. *Laryngoscope* 1987; 97:1176–1179.

80. Prasad AS: Clinical, endocrinological and biochemical effects of zinc deficiency. *Clin Endocrinol Metab* 1985; 14:567–589.

81. Pories WJ, Henzel JH, Rob CG, et al: Acceleration of healing with zinc sulfate. *Ann Surg* 1967; 165:432–436.

82. Delves HT: Assessment of trace element status. *Clin Endocrinol Metab* 1985; 14:725–760.

83. Geever EF, Youssef SA, Seifter E, et al: Penicillamine and wound healing in young guinea pigs. *J Surg Res* 1967; 7:160–166.

84. Prudden JF, Nishihara G, Ocampo L: Studies on growth hormone III. The effect on wound tensile strength of marked postoperative anabolism induced with growth hormone. *Surg Gynecol Obstet* 1958; 107:481–482.

85. Hollander DM, Devereux DF, Marafino BJ, et al: Increased wound breaking strength in rats following treatment with synthetic human growth hormone. *Plast Surg Wound Heal* 1984; 35:612–614.

86. Pessa ME, Bland KI, Sitren HS, et al: Improved wound healing in tumor-bearing rats treated with perioperative synthetic human growth hormone. *Surg Forum* 1985; 36:6–8.

87. Jorgensen PH, Andreassen TT: A dose-response study of the effects of biosynthetic human growth hormone on formation and strength of granulation tissue. *Endocrinology* 1987; 121:1637–1641.

88. Jiang ZM, He GZ, Zhang SY, et al: Low-dose growth hormone and hypocaloric nutrition attenuate the protein-catabolic response after major operation. *Ann Surg* 1989; 210:513–525.

89. Zaizen Y, Ford EG, Costin G, et al: The effect of perioperative exogenous growth hormone on wound bursting strength in normal and malnourished rats. *J Pediatr Surg* 1990; 25:70–74.

90. Zaizen Y, Ford EG, Costin G, et al: Stimulation of wound bursting strength during protein malnutrition. *J Surg Res* 1990; 49:333–336.

91. Herndon DN, Barrow RE, Kunkel KR, et al: Effects of recombinant human growth hormone on donor-site healing in severely burned children. *Ann Surg* 1990; 212:424–431.

92. Yegnanarayan R: Anti-inflammatory effect of two earthworm potions in carrageenan pedal oedema test in rats. *Indian J Physiol Pharmacol* 1988; 32:72–74.

93. Grotendorst GR, Martin GR, Pencev D, et al: Stimulation of granulation tissue formation by platelet-derived growth factor in normal and diabetic rats. *J Clin Invest* 1985; 76:2323–2329.

94. Knighton DR, Fiegel VD, Austin LL, et al: Classification and treatment of chronic nonhealing wounds: Successful treatment with autologous platelet-derived wound healing factors (PD-WHF). *Ann Surg* 1986; 204:322–330.

95. Laato M, Niinikoski J, Gerdin B, et al: Stimulation of wound healing by epi-

dermal growth factor. *Ann Surg* 1986; 203:379–381.

96. Brown GL, Nanney LB, Griffen J, et al: Enhancement of wound healing by topical treatment with epidermal growth factor. *N Engl J Med* 1989; 321:76–79.

97. Hennessey PJ, Black CT, Andrassy RJ: Epidermal growth factor and insulin act synergistically during diabetic healing. *Arch Surg* 1990; 125:926–929.

98. Schultz GS, White M, Mitchell R, et al: Epithelial wound healing enhanced by transforming growth factor-α and vaccinia growth factor. *Science* 1987; 235:350–352.

99. Tsuboi R, Rifkin DB: Recombinant basic fibroblast growth factor stimulates wound healing in healing-impaired db/db mice. *J Exp Med* 1990; 172:245–251.

100. Hebda PA, Klingbeil CK, Abraham JA, et al: Basic fibroblast growth factor stimulation of epidermal wound healing in pigs. *J Invest Dermatol* 1990; 95:626–631.

29

Nutrition and Immunity

John C. Alverdy, M.D.

Elisabet M. Faber, Pharm. D.

Mucosal defense system

Stress and the IgA response: The link to sepsis of gut origin

Effects of nutrients on mucosal immune function

Gut-specific nutrition

  Enteral stimulation by foodstuffs

  Neuroendocrine immune control of the gut

  Gut-specific nutrients

Clinical application

  Enteral nutrition: Which diet?

The mucosal immune system is among the largest immune organs in man and higher mammals.[1] This system has ostensibly developed to such a high degree because of evolutionary pressure from a changing and potentially threatening microecologic unit that colonizes most of the mucosal surfaces in man. The mucosal immune system, also known as the mucosa-associated lymphatic tissue (MALT), must deal with continuous antigenic exposure at epithelial surfaces, including the lung (bronchus-associated lymphatic tissue [BALT]), the gastrointestinal tract (gut-associated lymphatic tissue [GALT]), the conjunctival-lacrimal system (LALT), and the genitourinary tract. These surfaces are continually exposed to the hostile microbial environment of unsanitary living conditions, environmental pollutants, and more recently the protean microbiology of modern intensive care units. Indeed, the most commonly acquired infections in intensive care units today occur on mucosal surfaces such as the sinobronchial tree, urinary tract, and gastrointestinal mucosa. Significant mechanical and immunologic breakdown in barrier function occurs in these areas as a result of direct injury (endotracheal tubes, nasogastric suction, ischemic injury, etc.) and pharmacologic immunosuppression (vasoactive pressors, steroids, broad-spectrum antibiotics, and parenteral nutrition). While research over the last 10 years has advanced our understanding of the effect of critical illness on the systemic immune compartment, virtually no work has been accomplished that deals with the effect of injury and infection on the separate and independently functioning mucosal immune compartment. Therefore, the following discussion reviews (1) the immunophysiology of the mucosal defense system, (2) the influence of injury and infection on this system, and (3) the mechanisms by which nutrients regulate mucosal immune function. Recognition of specific nutritional strategies that preserve and enhance mucosal immune function during infection and injury are likely to result in a decrease in infection-related morbidity in the critical care setting.

MUCOSAL DEFENSE SYSTEM

The principal function of the mucosal defense system is to confine potentially toxic substances (bacteria, viruses, fungi, and toxins) to the local colonized surface. If these toxic substances breach the mucosal barrier, a second backup system exists to further prevent access to the interior milieu and includes submucosal inflammatory cells, lymph nodes, the liver, spleen, etc. Mucosal defense is therefore the first line of resistance against local environmental pathogens. Mucosal immunity encompasses two basic functions: neutralization of luminal toxins and prevention of microbial attachment to the epithelial cell surface. The crucial initiating event for microbial pathogenicity is the attachment of the bacteria or fungus to the mucosal epithelial cell. The importance of bacterial adherence to mucosal cells as a crucial initiating step for alterations in intestinal barrier function is underscored by several important observations. First, bacterial attachment protects the bacteria from being swept away by the cleansing action of peristalsis. Second, penetration of the mucosal barrier must be preceded by adherence of the invading microbe onto the cell surface. Finally, there is direct evidence that secreted toxic products may reach their cell target more efficiently when secreted by adherent bacteria than when secreted by nonadherent bacteria. Therefore, microbial pathogens that lack the capacity to attach are simply swept away and elimi-

nated by the local mechanical forces for particulate clearance, such as the hydrokinetic urinary stream, the mucociliary escalator of the tracheobronchial tree, or the forces of peristalsis in the gastrointestinal tract.

In order to prevent bacterial adherence, a repertoire of both nonimmune and immune mechanisms is available at the mucosal surface. Nonimmune mucosal defense factors include mucus production, which physically prevents bacterial adherence; cell desquamation, which occurs when cells become heavily colonized with bacteria; the mechanical cleansing forces of peristalsis; the mucociliary escalator; and water secretion. While these physical barriers are important, the only immune-specific mucosal defense factor is the production of secretory IgA (s-IgA), the most abundant immunoglobulin in external secretions.

S-IgA, a 360,000−molecular-weight glycoprotein, is the most abundant immunoglobulin in the body and constitutes more than 60% of all immunoglobulins produced each day.[2] Up to 10 g of newly synthesized s-IgA is produced daily, thus underscoring the enormous requirement of the mucosal surface for immune-specific defense. S-IgA can neutralize toxins as well as coat bacteria and prevent their adherence to the mucosal cell—a pivotal event for pathogenicity. In this manner, s-IgA effectuates the process of "immune exclusion" at the mucosal surface, thereby shielding the host from further activation of the systemic immune compartment. The generation of s-IgA in external secretions functions largely independently of the systemic production of immunoglobulins such as IgG, IgE, IgM, or monomeric serum IgA, a distinct immunoglobulin from s-IgA.[3] Clinical and experimental states of low mucosal IgA concentration are associated with significant mucosal barrier dysfunction. This is especially evident at the gastrointestinal level, where s-IgA deficiency is associated with significant perturbation in gut barrier function and poor outcome following severe catabolic stresses such as bone marrow transplantation or liver transplantation.

The ontogeny of s-IgA begins in Peyer's patches, where ingested luminal antigens are taken up into these lymphoid aggregates (GALT) via specialized epithelial cells called M cells. Once antigen is incorporated within Peyer's patches, B cells committed to antigen-specific IgA production leave this area and enter the general circulation via the mesenteric lymph. These IgA-committed cells then home to various secretory immune sites such as the breast, salivary glands, lacrimal glands, tracheobronchial tree, and the lamina propria of the intestine, where under the influence of local T-cell factors they mature to IgA-producing plasma cells. These local IgA-producing plasma cells release their dimeric IgA, and binding to the basolateral secretory component receptor takes place (Fig 29–1). By a process of reverse pinocytosis (Fig 29–2), this newly formed molecule, s-IgA, is released into the appropriate secretion.[3] One can see by the schema in Figure 29–2 that GALT is an organ of central trafficking for s-IgA pro-

duction not only within the gut itself but also at remote organs of s-IgA production such as the liver, spleen, breast, lung, and genitourinary tract. Therefore, nutritional strategies in critically ill patients that impair GALT integrity may significantly impair mucosal immune function in the lung, liver, and gut.

STRESS AND THE IGA RESPONSE: THE LINK TO SEPSIS OF GUT ORIGIN

Significant immunosuppression can be demonstrated following both experimental and clinical catabolic stress.[5-7] While these studies have generally focused on the systemic immune system, only recently have laboratories examined the effect of injury and infection on the mucosal immune system. As mentioned previously, systemic immunity and mucosal immunity function rather independently of one another. Normal systemic indices of immunity can be present during states of mucosal immunosuppression. This is of special con-

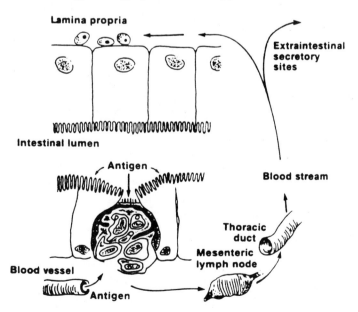

FIG 29–1.
Stimulation of secretory IgA (s-IgA) synthesis begins in a Peyer's patch in which antigen is sampled and processed and antigen-specific s-IgA–producing B cells are released into the circulation. These cells home to their secretory sites, where s-IgA is released into secretions.

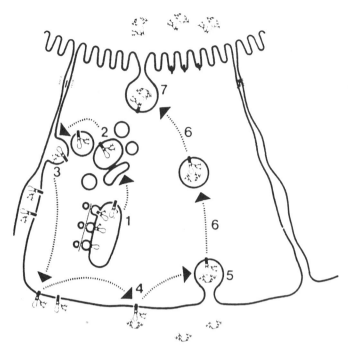

FIG 29–2.
Basolateral-membrane-to-brush-border transport of IgA occurs through secretory component receptors by reverse pinocytosis. This occurs in all secretory organs, including the liver, intestine, lung, and mammary gland.

cern to critically ill patients, whose most common infectious morbidity has been demonstrated to occur at mucosal sites, particularly the lung and gastrointestinal tract.[8]

Significant and dramatic decreases in s-IgA concentration in various external secretions have been demonstrated following experimental burns, femur fracture, cecal ligation and puncture, and after endotoxin administration.[5-7] Furthermore, significant disruption in mucosal barrier function to bacteria has been demonstrated in these models. For example, in experimental burn injury s-IgA concentrations in bile are decreased by 80% below normal as early as 18 hours following injury.[5] Burn injury results in significant disruption in intestinal barrier function to bacteria and alterations in intestinal permeability.[9] Inadequate production of s-IgA is associated with significant adherence of intestinal bacteria to the mucosal epithelial cell—an event that perturbs epithelial permeability.[10] This intestinal immunodeficient state may promote the absorption of luminal toxins or bacteria that activate and perpetuate disordered inflammation. Persistent intestinal permeability to endotoxin or other luminal proinflammatory mediators has been hypothesized to be the cause of the multiple organ failure syndrome.[11] In a recent report by LeVoyer et al., alterations in intestinal permeability following burn injury were associated with postburn septic morbidity.[12] Work from Tinsley and others has demonstrated a strong association between low s-IgA levels in burn patients and poor outcome.[13] Work from our laboratory on experimental models of stress suggests that under conditions of low IgA synthesis, bacterial adherence significantly perturbs epithelial permeability.[14] Therefore, nutritional strategies that maintain the IgA response and promote preservation of intestinal integrity may significantly limit the development of multiple organ failure.

Experimental stress has also been demonstrated to result in the depletion of s-IgA in pulmonary secretions. Robinson and Abraham in a murine model of hemorrhagic shock and resuscitation demonstrated persistent depletion of IgA-producing plasma cells in bronchoalveolar lavage samples.[15] Niederman and others have demonstrated significant alterations in IgA coating of bacteria in the pulmonary secretions of critically ill patients with pneumonia. Pneumonia did not develop in patients with normal pulmonary IgA levels and bronchial mucosa, which is less predisposed to bacterial adherence; this contrasts with the high incidence of pneumonia in patients with impairment in bronchial bacterial barrier function.[16] Again, an association between perturbed IgA secretion and mucosal infection is demonstrated. We can infer from these data that strategies that preserve IgA homeostasis may result in fewer infectious complications in the pulmonary circuit.

EFFECTS OF NUTRIENTS ON MUCOSAL IMMUNE FUNCTION

The traditional end points used to measure the efficacy of nutritional support in hospitalized patients include an improvement in body composition and visceral protein mass. More recently, several immune parameters have been studied that appear to correlate with improvements in overall nitrogen economy during the feeding of commercially available nutritional formulas.[17] These immune parameters have included delayed cutaneous hypersensitivity reactions, T-lymphocyte subpopulations (helper and suppressor), and mitogenic responses to harvested cells (B lymphocytes) from patients. Studies that have focused on the effects of nutrition on immune function have clearly demonstrated that immunosuppressed patients who are also malnourished tend to have worse outcomes than their well-nourished immunocompetent cohorts.[17] One common problem with the interpretation of these studies is that

while a strong association of malnutrition with immunosuppression can be demonstrated in these studies, association does not mean causation. Many of these patients have underlying problems such as cancer and infection, and while malnutrition alone can cause immunoincompetence, more often infection, injury, or cancer is the principal cause of the immunosuppression, while malnutrition exacerbates the problem. The important point is that correction of malnutrition without treating the natural history of the underlying disorder is unlikely to result in significant patient benefit. Furthermore, correction of malnutrition with diets that only replete body composition and visceral protein stores may not necessarily reestablish immune competence. Therefore, the efficacy of current formulations for nutritional support of hospitalized patients must be evaluated for their immune-enhancing properties and must be correlated to outcome variables. In addition, studies must be carefully interpreted so that direct comparisons are only made in those subjects who are age matched, disease matched, and treatment matched.

Study of the nutritional requirements of the immune system following the stress response has led to the concept of conditionally essential nutrients. Conditionally essential nutrients can be defined as those dietary elements that are required during certain conditions of stress for immune and physiologic homeostasis that are otherwise either not required or required in lesser amounts. For example, recent advances in our understanding of the metabolism of stress suggest that glutamine and arginine are conditionally essential amino acid sources for maintaining immune function during infection and injury.[18] Glutamine is a nonessential amino acid, the biosynthesis of which occurs normally without exogenous sources during states of health. However, during critical illness, glutamine stores are rapidly depleted, and biosynthesis is impaired. This situation can result in significant end-organ dysfunction. The following discussion will focus on the nutrient requirements of the critically ill patient, with particular attention to gut-specific nutrients as they relate to the stress response.

GUT-SPECIFIC NUTRITION

Enteral Stimulation by Foodstuffs

The gut has been traditionally viewed as an organ of quiescence during the postoperative period and following stress resulting from the presence of an adynamic ileus. Furthermore, the concept of bowel rest has been perpetuated by clinicians as an appropriate response for a passive metabolic organ during critical illness. However, it has been recently recognized that the gut is an active metabolic and immune organ participating in substantial interorgan nitrogen transfer and immune output following injury and infection.[19] The gut's epithelial cell mass undergoes cell turnover every 2 to 3 days and has specific requirements during the catabolic response to stress. Furthermore, the stress response results in significant splanchnic vasoconstriction both from endogenously released vasoactive mediators as well as from the use of pressor agents in the intensive care unit setting. If metabolic and immune breakdown occurs in the gastrointestinal tract during critical illness because of a failure to provide appropriate nutrition to the gastrointestinal tract, then loss of mucosal integrity and function may occur. Since there are enough toxins within the gastrointestinal tract to kill man many millions of times, loss of gastrointestinal barrier function following injury and infection can lead to a state of gut-derived sepsis characterized by culture-negative generalized inflammation. The development of sequential organ dysfunction, the most common cause of death in modern intensive care units, may result from inadequate attention to the gastro-

intestinal tract as an active metabolic organ and a functioning microecologic unit.

Data from our laboratory and others have clearly demonstrated that the enteral presentation of foodstuffs is an absolute requirement for maintenance of gut metabolic and immune function.[20] This point is underscored by clinical data from several randomized prospective trials that have demonstrated better outcome with enteral than parenteral feedings.[21, 22] In a prospective randomized study comprising trauma patients who were age matched and similar with respect to the severity of injury, Moore and associates tested this hypothesis by comparing infection rates between those receiving total parenteral nutrition (TPN) and those receiving total enteral nutrition (TEN).[21] Infections developed in 11 patients (37%) fed parenterally as compared with 5 (17%) fed enterally, and there was a statistically significant difference in the incidence of major septic complications. Abdominal abscess and/or pneumonia developed in 6 TPN patients (20%) while an abdominal abscess developed in only 1 patient (3%) fed by TPN. The authors concluded that early enteral feedings helped to decrease the possibility of septic complications in patients suffering from posttraumatic stress.

In a similar study comprising 98 patients who had sustained abdominal trauma, Kudsk and associates compared enteral feeding with parenteral feeding within 24 hours of injury and their effect on septic morbidity.[22] Patients were randomized to receive essentially identical formulations of fat, carbohydrate, and protein by one of the two routes of nutrient administration. Results showed that patients receiving enteral feeding within 24 hours of injury had significantly fewer pneumonias, intra-abdominal abscesses, and catheter-related sepsis as compared with the TPN group. The enteral group also had significantly fewer infections per patient and fewer complications per infected patient. The authors concluded that when compared with TPN, enteral feeding was significantly more beneficial for seriously ill patients. To date, however, the most convincing evidence that TPN results in significant alteration in intestinal permeability can be found in a study of human volunteers by Fong and associates.[23] Twelve healthy adults were randomized to receive either a chemically defined diet (Sustacal) orally or TPN without enteral feeding for 7 days. At the end of this course, each subject was given a sublethal (20 μg/kg) intravenous injection of *Escherichia coli* lipopolysaccharide, followed by a 6-hour metabolic study period. Results revealed that the TPN group had a statistically significant increase in both counterregulatory hormones and splanchnic-derived tumor necrosis factor as compared with the enterally fed cohorts. Lactate and C-reactive protein levels were also found to be greater in the TPN group. The data in this study suggest that an exaggerated counterregulatory hormone response as well as increased systemic and splanchnic cytokine release occurs during TPN and may lead to excessive systemic inflammation. This situation may predispose patients to multiple organ failure states and adversely affect outcome.

Neuroendocrine Immune Control of the Gut

The specific mechanisms by which intraluminal nutrition enhances immune function may relate to the link between nerves and neuropeptides and their regulation of mucosal immune response. Nerves are widely distributed throughout the mucosal lymphoid tissues of the gastrointestinal tract, and many of them contain multiple neuroendocrine immune mediators such as substance P, somatostatin, vasoactive intestinal polypeptide, and calcitonin-related peptide.[24]

It has been widely recognized that TPN feeding results in significant atrophy of the gastrointestinal tract and loss of barrier function to bacteria. Gastrointestinal hormones (e.g., cholecystokinin [CCK], neurotensin [NTN], epidermal growth factor [EGF], gastrin, secretin) administered exogenously are trophic to the intestinal mucosa and attenuate TPN-induced mucosal atrophy.[25-27] However, there is a significant disparity with respect to the morphologic effect of these hormones and their ability to regulate gut immune function and mucosal integrity. EGF, for example, results in significant attenuation of TPN-induced mucosal atrophy but does not maintain IgA function.[28, 29] CCK, another mucoproliferative hormone, plays an important role in lymphocyte proliferation and function. In vivo and in vitro studies demonstrate that CCK modulates the flux of calcium into lymphocytes by enhancing their activation and proliferation.[30] Exogenous administration of CCK also directly increases the concentration of IgA in secretions by unknown mechanisms.[31] The administration of NTN during parenteral nutrition in rats has been shown to maintain IgA concentrations in bile and attenuate the intestinal permeability defect associated with TPN.[30] CCK and NTN therefore appear to be key hormones in the neuroendocrine immune axis of the gut. Parenteral nutrition, with its attendant absence of enteral stimulation, does not activate the neuroendocrine immune axis, and serum concentrations of gastrointestinal hormones such as CCK and NTN remain suppressed with this therapy.[32] Despite the addition of newly recognized stress nutrients to the basic formula of TPN, its "bowel rest" effect on the gut may preclude it from maintaining normal gut integrity and function. Minimal enteral nutrition in conjunction with TPN has been shown to result in the release of many of the important gut neuropeptides that participate in the maintenance of gut integrity and function.[33] Therefore, some stimulation of the gut by intraluminal nutrition, albeit minimal, may be helpful. Trials are under way to establish whether a beneficial effect in terms of patient outcome can be achieved with minimal enteral nutrition.

Gut-Specific Nutrients

Specific fuel sources for the gastrointestinal tract are L-glutamine and short-chain fatty acids (SCFAs). L-glutamine is the most abundant amino acid in blood and is the preferred respiratory fuel for the small bowel. Severe catabolic stress such as sepsis results in impaired intestinal uptake of glutamine as well as intracellular glutamine depletion. Prolonged glutamine deprivation during catabolic stress may lead to critical deficiencies in small-bowel glutamine stores and significant compromise of gut integrity and function.[19] Commercial TPN solutions do not contain any glutamine because of problems with storage and degradation. Experimentally available parenteral solutions containing either free glutamine or the dipeptide alanyl glutamine significantly reduce nitrogen excretion, maintain water balance, and result in decreased hospital length of stay in bone marrow transplant patients.[34] Glutamine feeding during severe catabolic stress appears to have several beneficial effects, including a decrease in nitrogen excretion and protein conservation, enhancement of lymphocyte function, improvement in gut barrier function, maintenance of IgA synthesis, and maintenance of tissue glutathione concentration (an important intracellular antioxidant that prevents tissue damage from oxidant-induced injury in both the liver and lung).[35] Intravenous glutamine administration results in increased gut glutamine uptake. Since gut glutamine uptake may be impaired following stress, provision of glutamine may prevent functional changes in metabolic and immune function following injury and infection.

Other gut-specific nutrients include the SCFAs: butyrate, propionate, and acetate. Ingested dietary fiber is fermented to the SCFAs under the influence of the anaerobic colonic flora. SCFAs are the preferred respiratory fuel for colonocytes and directly suppress coliform overgrowth.[36] Removal of fiber from the diet and feeding by standard TPN result in small intestinal mucosal atrophy.[37] Findings by Koruda and associates demonstrate that SCFA-supplemented TPN reduces the atrophy associated with administration of TPN after massive small-bowel resection and that this therapeutic approach may facilitate adaptation to small-bowel resection.[38]

In a similar study, Kripke and associates[37] investigated whether continuous colonic infusion of butyrate or a combination of SCFAs would stimulate intestinal mucosal growth in animals deprived of their normal source of SCFAs (i.e., fiber fermentation in the cecum). After adult male Sprague-Dawley rats were fed a fat- and fiber-free elemental liquid diet, they underwent a cecectomy, ileocolic anastomosis, and insertion of a proximal colonic infusion catheter. Rats were then assigned to one of four treatment groups or three control groups. Treatment groups received either a continuous infusion of 20mM, 40mM, or 150mM butyrate or a mixture of 70mM acetate, 35mM propionate, and 20mM butyrate designed to approximate intracecal concentrations of SCFAs in a rat fed a regular chow diet. The control groups received saline or no infusion or underwent proximal colonic transection and reanastomosis. The colonic mucosal growth parameters analyzed included mucosal weight, protein, RNA, and DNA.

The 20mM butyrate infusion stimulated colonic mucosal DNA as effectively as the SCFA combination. However, raising the concentration of butyrate to 150mM (7.5 times the normal intracecal level) did not significantly increase growth when compared with the 20mM infusion. Mucosal growth was substantially enhanced following the 40mM butyrate infusion as compared with the control groups. In addition, mucosal DNA content in the jejunum and ileum was significantly greater in the SCFA-fed group than in the butyrate or control groups. The study's findings indicate that SCFA trophic effects are found throughout the intestinal tract while butyrate trophic effects are primarily localized to the colon.

Clausen and associates[39] have demonstrated that the administration of certain antibiotics reduces the fecal concentration of SCFAs in humans and that antibiotic-induced diarrhea is always associated with reduced levels of colonic SCFAs. Results from their study suggest that antibiotic-induced diarrhea may be secondary to impaired colonic fermentation by anaerobic bacteria and result in an accumulation of osmotically active saccharides in the lumen. Because SCFAs provide a powerful stimulus for electrolyte and fluid reabsorption in the colon, diminished levels of SCFAs will lead to a subsequent decrease in SCFA-stimulated absorption of sodium and water and resultant diarrhea.

Many current solutions available to critically ill patients for intravenous or enteral nutritional support do not contain these important colon fuels. If one imagines the gut as a "wound" in the intensive care unit resulting from insults such as pressor agents, antibiotics, surgery, ileus, drug-induced motility disorders, and pharmacologic immunosuppression, then nutritional regimens that promote gut wound healing may be reasonable end points upon which to choose a diet.

CLINICAL APPLICATION

The merging of theory, animal data, clinical data, and personal anecdotes can often create confusion as to what is an appropriate diet to choose for the critically ill patient. As mentioned previously, newly accepted criteria for dietary efficacy include length of intensive care unit stay, infectious morbidity, and survival. Laboratory parameters that predict nutrient efficacy remain elusive. In intensive care units during the first 5 days of severe catabolic stress, a positive nitrogen balance may be an unrealistic expectation. Furthermore, the use of urinary urea to calculate nitrogen balance may be inaccurate, total nitrogen excretion being a more precise measurement of total nitrogen economy.[40] Immunologic markers may be directly affected by the underlying inflammatory response and are impractical in the clinical arena. Therefore, the informed clinician may have substantial difficulty in translocating current nutritional discoveries to the patient bedside.

Enteral Nutrition: Which Diet?

When choosing an appropriate diet for a stressed patient, the following questions commonly arise:

1. Are there any advantages of polymeric vs. elemental diets in the critically ill patient?
2. Are there clinically measurable differences between diets that contain stress nutrients such as glutamine and arginine in whole protein form rather than as free amino acids?
3. If inadequate nitrogen and calories are delivered enterally because of limitations in gastrointestinal function, should parenteral nutrition be added?
4. If parenteral nutrition is being used, is there any advantage to minimal enteral nutrition? If certain stress nutrients are unavailable for parenteral use, can they be delivered enterally?
5. Should fiber or SCFAs be used in the critically ill?

Prevention of erosion of lean body mass during critical illness is an important therapeutic end point regardless of whether attenuation of inflammation occurs. No specific disease process appears to benefit from starvation, and therefore adequate delivery of calories and nitrogen to critically ill patients is important. When the enteral route is chosen, it must be recognized that statistically only 60% to 70% of ordered calories will be delivered to the patient in most critical care units.[41] The ostensible reason for this is the interruption of tube feeding inherent in the critical care setting. Interruption of tube feedings are due to tube displacements, tube occlusions, oral medication deliveries, cessation of tube feeding because of sudden changes in residual volume, and delays in feeding because of radiologic confirmation of tube placements. While many of these problems are not insurmountable, personnel changes often prevent assurance of nutrient delivery despite continuous efforts. For this reason the use of enteral and parenteral nutrition may be the most reasonable assurance against inadequate calorie and nitrogen delivery.

When choosing an enteral diet, a balanced polymeric diet is probably the most cost-effective. Elemental diets may offer an advantage to patients who have altered gastrointestinal tract physiology such as patients with biliopancreatic diversions or liver dysfunction. Peptide-based or whole protein–based diets result in the greatest stimulation of neuroendocrine release. Therefore, theoretically these diets may be more physiologic. Work by Shou and Daly have demonstrated that by enhancing gut barrier function polymeric diets protect against experimental infections better than elemental diets do.[42] However, some patients, such as those with radiation enteritis or inflammatory bowel disease, may tolerate elemental diets better. Each case must be individualized. However, all things being equal, there is no documented advantage to elemental feeding vs. polymeric feeding in the critically ill setting. If the diet is balanced, then the amount of available glutamine and arginine ought to be suffi-cient. While theoretically there may be an advantage to the provision of free, conditionally essential amino acids to patients, there are no clinical data to substantiate this. If an essential amino acid deficiency exists, such as following prolonged starvation with severe catabolic injury, repletion of the amino acid pool may require amino acid delivery in its free form. The only randomized prospective trial showing a clear outcome advantage in critically ill patients with a specialized enteral formula used a high arginine, RNA, and fish oil–containing diet.[43] Further trials are under way to confirm these findings.

The benefit of minimal enteral nutrition in the critically ill has not been studied. Our protocol is that all patients who must receive TPN have some enteral stimulation with elemental feedings. Our practice is to use 30 mL/hr of full-strength elemental feeding delivered postpylorically. The fact that these patients are receiving TPN implies that their gastrointestinal tract is unusable. We have found that this amount of elemental feeding is easily absorbed in most TPN-dependent patients, ileus or obstruction notwithstanding. Because cost and complications are minimal, the theoretical benefit makes the effort worthwhile.

Diets that maintain immune function following acute catabolic stress are likely to result in significant reductions in septic morbidity and significant patient benefits. Enteral provision of a balanced, well-tolerated diet that provides adequate stress nutrients is a reasonable approach to a complex and often confusing metabolic problem. Newly formulated parenteral diets with high concentrations of conditionally essential nutrients may offer significant benefits over existing parenteral formulations. A rethinking of the effect of nutrition on mucosal immune function may lead to further insights into the mechanisms by which nutrients improve outcome following injury and infection.

REFERENCES

1. McGhee JR, Mestecky J, Elson CO, et al: Regulation of IgA synthesis and immune response by T-cells and interleukins. *J Clin Immunol* 1989; 9:3.
2. Pockley AG, Montgomery PC: In vitro adjuvant effects of interleukin 5 and 6 on rat tear IgA antibody response. *Immunology* 1991; 73:19.
3. Langkamp-Henken B, Gletzer JA, Kudsk KA: Immunologic structures and function of the gastrointestinal tract. *Nutr Clin Pract* 1992; 7:99.
4. Van Thiel DH, Finkel R, Friedlander L: The Association of IgA deficiency but not IgG or IgM deficiency with a reduced patient and graft survival following liver transplantation. *Transplantation* 1992; 54:269–273.
5. Harmantz PR, Carter EA, Sullivan D, et al: Effect of thermal injury in the rat on transfer of IgA proteins into bile. *Ann Surg* 1989; 210:203.
6. Wira CR, Sandoe CP, Steele MG: Glucocorticoid regulation of the humoral immune system. *J Immunol* 1990; 144:142.
7. Alverdy JC, Aoys E: IgA deficiency: A common finding in models of bacterial translocation. *J Surg Res* 1992; 53:450.
8. Fiddian-Green RG, Baker S: Nosocomial pneumonia in the critically ill: Product of aspiration or translocation. *Crit Care Med* 1991; 19:763.
9. Dietch EA: Intestinal permeability is increased in burn patients shortly after injury *Surgery* 1990; 107:411–416.
10. Krogfelt KA: Bacterial adhesion: Genetics, biogenesis, and role in pathogenesis of fimbrial adhesins of *Escherichia coli*, *Rev Infect Dis* 1991; 13:721–735.
11. Carrico CJ, Meakins JL, Marshall JC, et al: Multiple organ failure syndrome. *Arch Surg* 1986; 121:196–209.
12. LeVoyer T, Cioffi WG, Pratt L, et al: Intestinal permeability following thermal injury (abstract). Presented at the annual meeting of the Surgical Infection Society, 1991.
13. Tinsley EX, Jackson AL, Alverdy JC: Salivary secretory IgA in burned patients (abstract). Presented at the Annual Symposium on Burn Therapy, Honolulu, 1992.
14. Spitz J, Taveras M, Hecht G, et al: The effect of dexamethasone administration on intestinal permeability. The role of bacterial adherence. *Gastroenterology*, in press.
15. Robinson A, Abraham E: Effects of hemmorrhage and resuscitation on bacterial antigen specific pulmonary plasma cell function. *Crit Care Med* 1991; 19:1285–1293.
16. Niederman MS, Merrill WW, Polomsky LM, et al: Influence of sputum IgA and elastase on trachial cell bacterial adherence. *Am Rev Respir Dis* 1986; 144:253–260.
17. Burby GP, Mullen JH, Matthews DC, et al: Prognostic nutritional index in gastrointestinal surgery. *Am J Surg* 1980; 139:160–170.
18. Barbul A: Arginine and immune function. *Nutrition* 1990; 6:53–58.
19. Souba WW, Klimberg SV, Plumley DA, et al: The role of glutamine in maintaining a healthy gut and supporting the metabolic response to injury and infection. *J Surg Res* 1990; 48:383.
20. Alverdy, JC, Chi HS, Sheldon GF: The effect of parenteral nutrition on gut immunity: The importance of enteral stimulation. *Ann Surg* 1985; 292:681.
21. Moore FA, Moore EE, Jones TN, et al: TEN vs. TPN following major abdominal trauma: Reduced septic morbidity. *J Trauma* 1989; 29:916.
22. Kudsk KA, Crole MA, Fabian TC, et al: Enteral versus parenteral feeding: Effects on septic morbidity following blunt and penetrating abdominal trauma. *Ann Surg* 1992; 215:503–513.
23. Fong Y, Marano MA, Barber A, et al: Total parenteral nutrition and bowel rest modify the metabolic response to endotoxins in humans. *Ann Surg* 1989; 210:449.
24. Furness JB, Costa M: *The Enteric Nerve System*. New York, Churchill Livingstone, 1987.
25. Hughes CA, Bates T, Dowling RH: Cholecystokinin and secretin prevent the intestinal mucosal hypoplasia of total parenteral nutrition in the dog. *Gastroenterology* 1978; 75:34.
26. Wood JG, Hoang HD, Bussjaeger LJ, et al: Neurotensin stimulates growth of small intestine in rats. *Am J Physiol* 1988; 255:813.
27. Jacobs DO, Evans DA, Mealy K, et al:

Combined effects of glutamine and epidermal growth factor on the rat intestine. *Surgery* 1988; 104:358.

28. Burke DA, Alverdy JC, Aoys E, et al: The effect of neurotensin and epidermal growth factors on TPN-induced IgA deficiency. *Surg Forum* 1990; 41:70.

29. Helton WS, Scheltinga MR, Hong RW, et al: Neurotensin attentuates increased intestinal permeability during intravenous feedings in rats (abstract). *Gastroenterology* 1991; 100:525.

30. Ferrara A, McMillen MA, Schaefer HC, et al: Effect of cholecystokinin receptor blockade on human lymphocyte proliferation. *J Surg Res* 1990; 48:354.

31. Freier S, Eran M, Faber J: Effect of cholecystokinin and its antagonist, of atropine, and food on release of IgA and IgG specific antibodies in the rat intestine. *Gastroenterology* 1987; 93:1242.

32. Aynsley-Green A, Lucas A, Lawson GR, et al: Gut hormones and regulatory peptides in relation to enteral feeding, gastroenteritis, and necrotizing entercolitis in infancy. *J Pediatr* 1990; 17(suppl):24.

33. Lucas A, Bloom SR, Aynsley-Green A: Gut hormones and "minimal enteral feeding." *Act Paediatr Scand* 1986; 75:719.

34. Ziegler TR, Young LS, Benfell K, et al: Clinical and metabolic efficacy of glutamine supplement parenteral nutrition after bone marrow transplantation: A randomized double blind controlled study. *Ann Intern Med* 1992; 116:821–828.

35. Lawrence HL, Hagen TH, Jones DP, et al: Exogenous glutamine protects intestinal epithelial cells from oxidative injury. *Proc Natl Acad Sci U S A* 1986; 83:4641–4646.

36. Lee A, Gemmell E: Changes in the mouse intestinal microflora during weaning: Role of volatile fatty acids. *Infect Immun* 1972; 5:1.

37. Kripke SA, Fox AD, Berman JM, et al: Stimulation of intestinal mucosal growth with intracolonic infusion of short-chain fatty acids. *JPEN* 1989; 13:109.

38. Koruda MJ, Rolando H, Rolandelli R, et al: Effect of parenteral nutrition supplemented with short-chain fatty acids on adaptation to massive bowel resection. *Gastroenterology* 1988; 95:715.

39. Clausen MR, Bonnen H, Tvede M, et al: Colonic fermentation to short-chain fatty acids is decreased in antibiotic associated diarrhea. *Gastroenterology* 1991; 101:1497.

40. Konstantinides FN: Nitrogen balance studies in clinical nutrition. *Nutr Clin Pract* 1992; 7:231.

41. Montecalvo MA, Steger KA, Farber HW: Nutritional outcome and pneumonia in critical care patients randomized to gastric versus jejunal tube feedings. *Crit Care Med* 1992; 20:1377–1387.

42. Shou J, et al: Effects of enteral nutrition on pulmonary macrophage function (abstract). Presented at the 26th Annual Meeting of the Association for Academic Surgery.

43. Bower R: A unique enteral formula as adjunctive therapy for septic and critically ill patients. Multicenter study—design and rationale. *Nutrition* 1990; 6:92–95.

30

The Gut Barrier

Mark R. Mainous, M.D.

Edwin A. Deitch, M.D.

The gut barrier

Relationship of nutrition to gut barrier function

The gut is a complex organ, the primary function of which is the digestion and absorption of nutrients. Another equally important function, one that is often not fully appreciated, is that of a barrier in preventing the spread of intraluminal bacteria and endotoxin to systemic organs and tissues, a process termed bacterial translocation.[1] When one considers the enormous concentrations of bacteria present in the distal portion of the small bowel and colon (10^{10} anaerobes and 10^5 to 10^8 each of gram-positive and gram-negative aerobic and facultative organisms), it is quite remarkable that in normal, healthy individuals gut-origin sepsis does not occur. Nevertheless, under certain basic pathophysiologic conditions, gut barrier function may be impaired to such an extent that bacterial translocation does occur. These basic conditions include (1) disruption of the ecologic balance of the indigenous gut flora and consequent overgrowth of gram-negative enteric bacilli, (2) impairment of host immune defenses, and (3) physical disruption of the gut mucosal barrier. The severity of the resultant bacterial translocation is proportional to the number of condi-

tions contributing to loss of gut barrier function, as well as to the magnitude of each insult. The phenomenon of bacterial translocation has been well described in numerous animal models and has recently assumed increasing clinical importance. The loss of intestinal barrier function and the subsequent translocation of intestinal bacteria and/or endotoxin have been implicated in the potential development of sepsis or multiple organ failure in selected patients[2, 3]

The importance of maintaining normal gut barrier function is obvious. Nevertheless, in the critically ill or injured patient at risk of the development of sepsis or multiple organ failure, maintenance of gut barrier function may be exceedingly difficult. These patients have frequently experienced major blood loss or hypotension and may be receiving vasoactive drugs, each of which may result in splanchnic vasoconstriction and gut mucosal injury. In addition, they usually have impaired immune function, and the antibiotic, antiulcer, and dietary regimens they receive may disrupt the normal ecology of the gut flora and result in the overgrowth of certain indigenous or exogenous organisms. The need to optimize gut barrier function in these critically ill patients presents a severe challenge to all who are involved in their care. In order to develop strategies to maintain normal gut barrier function, one must first understand each of the components that, functioning together, make up what is referred to as the gut barrier.

THE GUT BARRIER

The initial step in the translocation of bacteria from the intestinal tract is the adherence of the translocating bacteria to the epithelial cell surface or to ulcerated areas of the intestinal mucosal surface. Bacteria contain adhesive structures on their surfaces, called adhesins, that bind to specific receptor sites on epithelial cells.[4] The epithelial receptors are, in general, single or complex carbohydrates for gram-negative rods and glycoproteins for gram-positive organisms. In addition to native receptors on host cells, there is evidence that new receptors may be formed by virally infected cells, particularly by those infected with the influenza virus. Bacterial adherence is a prerequisite for infectivity. Once adherence occurs, the bacteria must then cross the mucosal barrier and reach the lamina propria in a viable state, at which point bacterial translocation has technically occurred. However, unless these bacteria can successfully spread from the lamina propria to systemic organs, the process is of no clinical significance. The host has developed a complex series of defense mechanisms to prevent bacteria from adhering to the intestinal mucosa and translocating to systemic organs. These defense mechanisms of the gut barrier provide four generalized levels of protection: the stabilizing influence of the normal intestinal microflora, mechanical and immunologic defenses, and the gut-liver axis (Table 30–1).

One major component of the gut bar-

TABLE 30–1.

Components of the Gut Barrier

Microbial
Contact inhibition
Colonization resistance
Mechanical
Peristalsis
Mucus layer
Epithelial barrier
Junctional complexes
Desquamation
Immunologic
GALT*
Secretory immunoglobulins
Gut-liver axis
Bile salts
Reticuloendothelial function

*GALT = gut-associated lymphoid tissue.

rier is the indigenous intestinal microflora. The protective role of the normal intestinal microflora in preventing intestinal infections and bacterial translocation has been well described by van der Waaij and associates[5–7] who showed that the resistance of the gut to infection by potential pathogens may be altered by the administration of various nonabsorbable oral antibiotic preparations and that overgrowth of pathogens is related to disruption of the normal gut microflora. They coined the term *colonization resistance* to describe the protective role of the normal intestinal microflora in preventing overgrowth by potential pathogens. It is now clear that the obligate anaerobic bacteria are largely responsible for the phenomenon of colonization resistance. They outnumber the enteric gram-negative and aerobic gram-positive bacteria by a factor of 1000 to 10,000 and associate closely with the intestinal epithelium to form, in effect, a physical barrier limiting the direct attachment or intimate association of potential translocating bacteria to the intestinal mucosa. This anaerobic barrier is lost when broad-spectrum antibiotics are administered because the obligate anaerobic bacteria are much more sensitive to antibiotic suppression than is the remainder of the gut flora.[8] Loss of the anaerobic barrier thus facilitates the direct attachment of potential pathogens to the intestinal epithelium.

In addition to colonization resistance, the normal intestinal microflora also maintains communal stability within itself by a series of complicated interactions termed *bacterial antagonism*, which includes such diverse processes as contact inhibition, the production of various antimicrobial factors such as colicins or volatile fatty acids, and competition for nutrients and attachment sites. Although the means by which the normal intestinal microflora maintains stability are not well understood, it is clear that disruption of the normal ecology of the gut microflora may promote the overgrowth of potential pathogens and lead to bacterial translocation.

A second component of the gut barrier involves the mechanical defenses of the gut. The intestinal epithelium is coated by a mucus gel layer 30 to 50 μm thick. This gel layer functions to prevent the adherence of bacteria to epithelial cell surface receptors and also provides a favorable environment for the anaerobic bacteria, by which it is densely colonized. The presence of a normal, continuous, heavily colonized mucus layer prevents tissue colonization by potential pathogens.[9] Elimination of this mucus layer has been shown to result in bacterial overgrowth and in increased numbers of bacteria adhering directly to the intestinal epithelium.[10]

In the small intestine, normal peristalsis prevents prolonged stasis of bacteria in close proximity to the intestinal mucosa and thereby reduces the possibility that bacteria may have adequate time to penetrate the mucus gel layer and attach to epithelial cell surface receptors. If the peristaltic clearing of bacteria is impaired, either by mechanical small-bowel obstruction or by the development of an ileus, bacterial stasis will occur. Under these circumstances, bacterial overgrowth occurs rapidly, and penetration of the mucus gel layer and

bacterial adherence to the mucosal epithelial cells can occur.

The intestinal epithelium consists of a variety of cells, including the columnar epithelial cells, or enterocytes, which function to absorb nutrients; goblet cells, which secrete mucus; intraepithelial leukocytes, which play an active role in the immune function of the gut; and amine precursor uptake decarboxylation (APUD) cells, which secrete gastrointestinal hormones and other regulatory peptides. These cells are tightly bound by junctional complexes consisting of a tight junction, an intermediate junction, and a belt desmosome. The tight junction surrounds each cell and joins the plasma membranes of the entire epithelium together. The junctional complexes allow the diffusion of small molecules and ions but, under normal circumstances, prevent the paracellular migration of macromolecules and bacteria.[11]

The epithelial cells at the villus tips are constantly being desquamated and replaced by newer cells migrating up from the crypts. The few bacteria that have adhered to the epithelial cells are expelled into the intestinal lumen along with the desquamated epithelial cells to which they are attached. Epithelial cell migration and desquamation are an extremely rapid process that results in complete renewal of the epithelial surface every 2 to 3 days in rodents and every 4 to 5 days in man. Although desquamation of epithelial cells creates an area of denudation and a potential portal for the translocation of bacteria or endotoxin, the defect shrinks rapidly in size, aided in part by an adenosine triphosphate (ATP)-dependent, neurally mediated subepithelial shortening of the villi to reduce the surface area in need of resurfacing.[12] In addition, the tight junctional elements undergo rapid rearrangement and expansion at the basolateral surfaces of the cell extrusion zone. As the extruding cell extends into the lumen, existing junctional elements expand along the periphery while maintaining contact with neighboring cells. The neighboring cells also extend their basal processes to close the space vacated by the extruded cell and establish new junctional complexes.[13] In this way, access by bacteria to the basement membrane is severely limited during the process of normal epithelial cell turnover.

The intestinal immune system, also known as the gut-associated lymphoid tissue (GALT), regulates the local immune response to soluble and particulate antigens within the gastrointestinal tract. The GALT consists of five populations of cells: lamina propria lymphocytes, intraepithelial lymphocytes, lymphoid follicles, Peyer's patches, and cells of the mesenteric lymph node complex. The Peyer's patches are the major site of antigen sensitization in the gastrointestinal tract. Peyer's patches are aggregates of lymphoid tissue scattered throughout the lamina propria of the small intestine, predominantly in the ileum. B lymphocytes present in the germinal center of the Peyer's patch, once exposed to gut antigens, migrate to the mesenteric lymph node complex and then to lymphoid sites within the lamina propria where they differentiate into plasma cells that produce IgA. Transport of IgA into the gut lumen is facilitated by its binding with secretory component, which is a prerequisite for pinocytic transport and also prevents proteolytic degradation of IgA within the gut lumen. Secretory IgA binds to bacteria to prevent adherence and also neutralizes toxins and prevents the absorption of various other antigens. Secretory IgA is unique in that it does not activate the effector arms of the immune system and therefore does not create a local inflammatory response that might impair the normal absorptive processes of the gut.[14]

M cells are a recently described subpopulation of specialized cells located in the epithelial layer of the gut mucosa overlying the lymphoid follicles. M cells originate from epithelial cell precursors and occur as single cells scattered among the enterocytes and attached to them by tight junctions. They contain numerous pinocytic vesicles and have a poorly developed glycocalyx and sparse, broad microvilli. On their antiluminal surface they are indented by adjacent lymphocytes and macrophages. Particulate antigens and bacteria bind to the M-cell membrane and are taken up in pinocytic vesicles. The vesicles transport their contents to the antiluminal border of the cell, where they are transferred to the macrophage unaltered. The macrophage processes the antigens and presents them to the neighboring lymphocytes. M cells do not appear to engage significantly in the uptake of normal gut flora, possibly due to the lack of surface adhesins on the commensal bacteria for binding to specific receptors on the M-cell membrane.[15]

Once the bacteria enter the lamina propria, they may be transported to the mesenteric lymph node complex by macrophages or freely in the lymph. The mesenteric lymph node complex is able to contain and eliminate intestinal bacteria under normal circumstances, but if overwhelmed, bacteria could conceivably escape the mesenteric lymph node complex and enter the systemic circulation via the thoracic duct. Alternatively, bacteria and endotoxin may enter the portal blood and be processed by the reticuloendothelial cells of the liver.

Although much less is known about the antiendotoxin defenses of the gut, most investigators believe that bile salts play a major role in preventing the escape of endotoxin from the gut. Bile salts are thought to prevent endotoxemia by binding to intraluminal endotoxin and forming poorly absorbed detergent-like complexes.[16] Although small amounts of endotoxin may enter the portal circulation even under normal circumstances, the reticuloendothelial cells of the liver are normally very efficient in clearing endotoxin from the portal blood, and systemic endotoxemia does not occur unless the reticuloendothelial function of the liver has been severely impaired.[17]

A clinically important relationship appears to exist between the state of intestinal barrier function and hepatic reticuloendothelial cell activity. Furthermore, this relationship may be beneficial or deleterious, depending on the circumstances.[18] The presence of gut-derived endotoxin appears to play an important physiologic role in maintaining reticuloendothelial system phagocytic activity, thereby increasing the host's resistance to various insults such as hemorrhagic shock.[19] Endotoxin at low levels is a normal constituent of human portal blood,[20] and may serve to maintain a primed reticuloendothelial system in order to protect the host. However, higher levels of portal endotoxin may actually increase the susceptibility of the liver to certain types of injury.[21] In addition, in the presence of hepatic dysfunction, endotoxin clearance is impaired, and the systemic resistance to endotoxin is decreased.[22]

Since the clearance of translocating bacteria and endotoxin from the portal blood is dependent on normal Kupffer cell phagocytic activity, impaired hepatic reticuloendothelial system function could conceivably potentiate the systemic effects of gut barrier failure by allowing gut-derived bacteria or endotoxin to reach the systemic circulation. In addition, the presence of bacteria and endotoxin in the portal blood may induce hepatic macrophages to secrete numerous factors that may directly injure or alter hepatocyte function, and in concert with other soluble or cellular factors, may lead to distant organ injury. Therefore, normal hepatic reticuloendothelial system function is an essential component of the gut barrier.

RELATIONSHIP OF NUTRITION TO GUT BARRIER FUNCTION

As stated earlier, gut barrier failure may result from one or more of the following three basic pathophysiologic conditions: disruption of the normal ecologic balance of the indigenous gut microflora, with resultant overgrowth of gram-negative enteric bacilli; impaired host immune defenses; and physical disruption of the gut mucosal barrier. Each of these variables may be affected by various dietary factors or the host's nutritional status. For example, starvation and protein malnutrition have been documented to impair host immune and antibacterial defenses, disrupt the normal ecology of the gut microflora, and lead to mucosal atrophy. Thus, there is good indirect evidence to suggest that nutritional variables may have a profound impact on gut barrier function. Additionally, Alexander et al.[23] showed that total parenteral nutrition (TPN)-fed human volunteers have a greater splanchnic and systemic cytokine response to parenteral endotoxin than do enterally fed volunteers. This study and the results of other human and animal studies[23, 25–29] indicate that the route by which patients are fed may influence the immuno-inflammatory and metabolic response to injury[24–26] as well as affect the incidence of infectious complications[27, 28] and modulate clinical outcome.[23, 29, 30] One hypothesis to explain the observation that enteral feeding appears clinically superior to parenteral feeding is that parenteral feeding predisposes to an exaggerated cytokine response because of the loss of intestinal barrier function.[24, 31, 32] As will be discussed shortly, the composition of the diet as well as the route of administration may have profound effects on intestinal morphology and function as well as on the incidence and susceptibility to systemic infection and the development of hypermetabolism. Thus, since nutritional problems are relatively common in severely traumatized or critically ill patients, the resultant alterations in intestinal barrier function are likely to be of extreme clinical importance.

The main focus of our laboratory over

the past decade has been directed toward defining the mechanisms of gut barrier failure and its potential relationships to systemic sepsis and multiple organ failure. Some of our early studies on nutrition were performed to determine the influence of prolonged protein malnutrition on gut barrier function. In these studies[33, 34] mice received either a normal chow diet or an equicaloric protein-deficient diet. Animals fed the protein-deficient diet for 21 days lost 30% of their original body weight and 75% of their gut mucosal height. Nevertheless, bacterial translocation did not occur. However, when challenged with a nonlethal dose of endotoxin, the protein-malnourished mice had a significantly increased incidence of bacterial translocation to systemic organs when compared with the chow-fed controls, as well as a 66% mortality rate.[33] These experiments were repeated with the inflammatory stimulant zymosan, with similar results.[34] The major conclusion from these studies was that protein malnutrition leads to profound gut mucosal atrophy and renders the animals more susceptible to the lethal effects of endotoxemia or systemic inflammation. However, these studies also indicate that mucosal atrophy alone was not sufficient to promote the loss of gut barrier function, measured as bacterial translocation.

The pioneering work from Rhoads' laboratory in the 1960s introduced parenteral feeding as a viable means of nutritional support for those patients unable to be fed enterally.[35] Although TPN has benefited innumerable critically ill patients, recent evidence suggests that parenteral nutrition may in fact be deleterious to gut barrier and host immune function when compared with enteral nutritional support. Kudsk and colleagues have demonstrated that parenterally fed rodents tolerate a septic insult far worse than do rodents fed an identical diet enterally.[29] Alverdy and associates have shown that enterally fed rats maintain levels of secretory IgA far

better than do rats fed the same diet parenterally.[36] Several other animal studies have demonstrated that immediate enteral feeding following thermal injury reduces the hypermetabolic response by maintaining gut mucosal mass and preventing the excessive release of catabolic hormones.[25, 37] Moreover, Fong and associates, using human volunteers, have shown an exaggerated response of glucagon, epinephrine, and cytokine production to endotoxin challenge following 7 days of bowel rest and TPN as compared with enteral feedings. This was associated with an enhanced acute-phase protein response, peripheral amino acid mobilization, and increased peripheral lactate production. Their conclusion was that TPN may exacerbate the metabolic derangements seen in sepsis through an enhancement of cytokine production as well as an exaggerated response by counterregulatory hormones.[24]

The ability of high-protein enteral feedings to improve the clinical outcome was demonstrated conclusively by Alexander and associates in a prospective study of burned children randomized to receive nutritional support either enterally or parenterally. The enterally fed children had less impairment of their systemic immune defenses, fewer infectious complications, and an increase in survival as compared with those children maintained on a total parenteral diet.[23] Similar results have been reported in trauma victims, where the incidence of major infectious complications was less in enterally than parenterally fed patients.[27, 28] However, simply providing nutrients via the enteral route does not necessarily guarantee normal gut barrier function. Alverdy and colleagues have shown that either enteral or parenteral administration of a TPN solution will promote bacterial translocation in rats.[31] Using Alverdy's model, our laboratory has demonstrated that enteral administration of a TPN solution not only promotes bacterial translocation but is also associated with in vivo and in vitro depression of T-cell—mediated immune function, all of which may be reversed by refeeding the rats a normal chow diet.[38] Therefore, the composition of the diet seems to be just as important as the route by which it is administered.

Wilmore et al. have suggested that current methods of parenteral nutrition are not capable of adequately supporting the structural and functional integrity of the gut largely because of the lack of glutamine in these solutions.[26] The rationale for this conclusion is based on several facts. First, glutamine appears to be the primary respiratory fuel of the gut since the uptake of glutamine by the gut far exceeds that of any other nutrient. In fact, glutaminase, the enzyme required for glutamine metabolism, is found in its highest concentration in the enterocytes of the jejunum. Not only does the metabolism of glutamine provide energy for the enterocytes, but it also results in the release of alanine to be utilized in gluconeogenesis by the liver. Second, in certain stress states, glutamine uptake and utilization by the gut as well as other tissues is markedly increased, thus indicating that glutamine may be a conditionally essential nutrient of the gut during stress.[26] Although there appears to be nearly uniform agreement that glutamine promotes small intestinal growth and limits mucosal atrophy, its beneficial effects on gut barrier function are less clear. Souba and colleagues have shown that in animals receiving abdominal radiation, a diet supplemented with glutamine was associated with an increase in villus height and weight, a decrease in the incidence of bacterial translocation, and an improvement in survival.[39] Burke and associates have demonstrated that a parenteral diet supplemented with glutamine was associated with a decrease in the incidence of bacterial translocation and the prevention of secretory IgA deficiency seen in association with the administration of a glutamine-free parenteral diet.[40]

In contradistinction to these studies, Barber et al. demonstrated that an enteral defined diet (Criticare HN) promoted bacterial translocation that could not be prevented by the supplementation of this diet with glutamine, although the glutamine-supplemented diet did prevent the loss of gut mucosal mass to a large extent.[41] In addition, studies from our laboratory have shown that an enteral, elemental glutamine—free diet fed to rats promotes bacterial translocation and impaired lymphocyte blastogenesis, both of which could not be reduced by the addition of glutamine to the diet.[42] Moreover, Wells and colleagues have shown that the addition of glutamine to an enteral diet failed to prevent endotoxin-induced or antibiotic-induced bacterial translocation.[43] Therefore, although glutamine clearly supports intestinal mucosal growth, its effects on bolstering gut barrier function remain in question.

Recent work by Zaloga and associates suggests that the source of protein in the enteral formula is important in maintaining gut mucosal mass. They fed unstressed rats enteral diets that contained a protein source consisting of either amino acids, peptides, or complex proteins. The enteral diet containing complex proteins was much more effective in stimulating gut mucosal growth than were the diets containing peptides or amino acids as their protein source. They propose that complex proteins may be more effective in stimulating the generation of various trophic factors in the gut than are the simpler protein formulations.[44]

Other substrates besides protein may also be important in maintaining gut structure and function. Short-chain fatty acids, particularly butyrate, are produced by the fermentation of fiber by the enteric bacteria and are the preferred respiratory fuel of the colonocytes. Delivery of short-chain fatty acids to the gut has been shown to result in increased colonic mucosal height and DNA content,[45] and may exert trophic effects on the small bowel as well.[46] Koruda and associates have demonstrated that the addition of short-chain fatty acids to parenteral nutrition solutions results in a reduction in the degree of mucosal atrophy associated with TPN following massive small-bowel resection.[47] Nevertheless, the effect of short-chain fatty acids on gut barrier function remains unclear since its effects on barrier function have not been directly tested.

Since dietary fiber is important in maintaining the normal ecologic balance of the gut microflora and the end products of bacterial fermentation are trophic for intestinal epithelial cells, our laboratory has become interested in studying the effects of dietary fiber on gut barrier function. Initially, we tested the hypothesis that the bacterial translocation induced by the administration of a TPN solution either enterally or parenterally could be reduced by the addition of fiber to the diet. The results of our initial study verified the data of Alverdy et al.[31] that either intravenous or enteral administration of a TPN solution will induce bacterial translocation in rats. Furthermore, the ingestion of cellulose, a dietary fiber with both fermentable and bulk-forming properties, prevented bacterial translocation in the enterally or parenterally fed rats.[32] Interestingly, although the addition of cellulose prevented bacterial translocation, it did not prevent atrophy of the jejunal and ileal mucosa.

Our next study was carried out to determine which properties of dietary fiber are important in helping to maintain the gut mucosal barrier: fermentability, bulk, or both.[48] Enteral administration of a TPN solution again resulted in bacterial translocation. The administration of cellulose or kaolin (a pure bulk-forming agent) prevented bacterial translocation, while citrus pectin (a fully fermentable, nonresidue fiber) failed to prevent bacterial translocation. This study suggests that the bulk-forming properties of dietary fiber are more im-

portant than fermentability in supporting gut barrier function.

The mechanism by which dietary fiber supports gut barrier function could not be determined by these studies. However, dietary fiber is known to exert a trophic effect on the intestinal mucosa and is necessary for the maintenance of normal mucosal cell turnover. The fact that diets lacking in fiber may lead to a loss of gut barrier function is not surprising since the addition of dietary fiber to a low-residue enteral diet has been shown to exert a beneficial effect on the preservation of intestinal structure and function.[49] Whether fiber exerts this protective effect by direct stimulation of the gut mucosa or by stimulating the release of various gut hormones or growth factors is not clear. If fiber protected against parenteral or oral elemental diet–induced bacterial translocation by stimulating trophic hormones, then inhibition of hormone secretion should negate its protective effects. Conversely, stimulation of appropriate intestinal hormones, in the absence of fiber, should protect against diet-induced bacterial translocation. We tested this hypothesis by using octreotide acetate (Sandostatin) to inhibit and bombesin to stimulate intestinal hormone secretion. The results of this study documented that bombesin significantly reduced diet-induced bacterial translocation while Sandostatin abrogated the protective effects of fiber in elemental diet–fed and parenterally fed rats (unpublished data).

A new and exciting area of research involves the use of specific growth factors and gut hormones as nutritional supplements to support intestinal structure and function. Epidermal growth factor is a potent mitogen for a large number of cells, including liver parenchymal cells and enterocytes. The major source of epidermal growth factor is the salivary glands, although Brunner's glands in the small intestine are also known to synthesize and secrete large amounts of epidermal growth factor. Jacobs and associates have demonstrated in rats that the addition of epidermal growth factor to the diet results in an increase in the DNA content and protein content of the small intestinal mucosa and that its effects are dose dependent.[50]

Evers and colleagues studied the effects of various gut hormones administered concurrently with an enteral elemental diet on the structure of the rat small intestinal mucosa.[51] Whereas the enteral elemental diet alone resulted in mucosal atrophy throughout the small intestine, the addition of bombesin prevented jejunal mucosal atrophy and actually increased ileal mucosal growth. The addition of neurotensin prevented jejunal but not ileal mucosal atrophy. Pentagastrin had no effect on either the jejunal or the ileal mucosa. Their conclusion from this study was that gut hormones trophic for the small-bowel mucosa may some day prove useful as nutritional adjuncts in helping maintain normal gut structure and function during periods of physiologic stress.

One of the major problems with many of the published studies examining the relationships between nutritional modulation and gut barrier function is that many of these studies have not measured gut barrier function per se but instead have measured changes in certain parameters related to mucosal atrophy, such as intestinal weight, gut mucosal protein content, or villus height, assuming that a decrease in one or more of these parameters would correlate with impaired gut barrier function. However, to equate mucosal atrophy with impaired gut barrier function is much too simplistic since studies from our laboratory indicate that there is no direct correlation between intestinal mucosal atrophy and the loss of gut barrier function.[32, 33] In fact, although intestinal mucosal atrophy and loss of gut barrier function often coexist, the presence of mucosal atrophy in and of itself does not necessarily imply a loss of gut barrier function, and conversely, the prevention of intestinal mucosal atrophy does not guarantee the prevention of gut barrier failure.

The gut barrier, when intact, functions to prevent the spread of intraluminal bacteria and endotoxin to systemic organs and tissues. Loss of gut barrier function has been theoretically implicated in the potential development of systemic sepsis and multiple organ failure. Maintenance of normal gut barrier function requires the complex interaction of numerous defense mechanisms, including the normal ecologic balance of the indigenous gut microflora, peristalsis, an intact mucus layer, an intact epithelial cell barrier, normal epithelial cell turnover, normal immune function, and the gut-liver axis. Numerous factors that complicate the care of the critically ill or injured patient may result in impairment of gut barrier function. Therapeutic measures that may aid in the support of gut barrier function include maintenance of an effective circulating blood volume, early definitive surgery, prompt recognition and control of infectious processes, the judicious use of antibiotics, and optimal nutritional support.

It is now clear that enteral nutrition is superior to parenteral nutrition in supporting gut barrier function. This conclusion is based on clinical studies indicating that enteral feedings improve systemic immunity, reduce the incidence of major infectious complications, and improve survival, as well as on laboratory studies showing that enteral nutrition improves the host immune response, attenuates the hypermetabolic response to injury, helps to maintain gut mucosal mass, and helps to maintain the normal ecologic balance of the indigenous gut microflora. In the future, it is likely that enteral feedings will be formulated to provide specific nutrients, as well as mucosal trophic factors, in order to maintain mucosal structure, optimize intestinal function, and prevent gut barrier failure in the critically ill patient.

REFERENCES

1. Berg RD, Garlington AW: Translocation of certain indigenous bacteria from the gastrointestinal tract to the mesenteric lymph nodes and other organs in a gnotobiotic mouse model. *Infect Immun* 1979; 23:405–411.

2. Deitch EA: Gut failure: Its role in the multiple organ failure syndrome, in Deitch EA (ed): *Multiple Organ Failure: Pathophysiology and Basic Concepts of Therapy.* New York, Thieme Medical, 1990.

3. Mainous MR, Deitch EA: Bacterial translocation and its potential role in the pathogenesis of multiple organ failure. *J Intensive Care Med* 1992; 7:101–108.

4. Beachey EH: Bacterial adherence: Adhesin-receptor interactions mediating the attachment of bacteria to mucosal surfaces. *J Infect Dis* 1981; 143:325–345.

5. van der Waaij D, Berghuis-deVries JM, Lekkerkerk–van der Wees JEC: Colonization resistance of the digestive tract in conventional and antibiotic treated mice. *J Hyg (Camb)* 1971; 69:405–411.

6. van der Waaij D, Berghuis-deVries JM, Lekkerkerk–van der Wees JEC: Colonization resistance of the digestive tract and the spread of bacteria to the lymphatic organs in mice, *J Hyg (Camb)* 1972; 70:335–342.

7. van der Waaij D, Berghuis-deVries JM, Lekkerkerk–van der Wees JEC: Colonization resistance of the digestive tract of mice during systemic antibiotic treatment. *J Hyg (Camb)* 1972; 70:605–609.

8. Berg RD: Promotion of the translocation of enteric bacteria from the gastrointestinal tracts of mice by oral treatment with penicillin, clindamycin, or metronidazole. *Infect Immun* 1981; 33:854–861.

9. Rozee KR, Cooper D, Lam K, et al: Microbial flora of the mouse ileum mucus layer and epithelial surface. *Appl Environ Microbiol* 1982; 43:1451–1463.

10. Banwell JG, Howard R, Cooper D, et al: Intestinal microbial flora after feeding phytohemagglutinin lectins *(Phaseolus vulgaris)* to rats. *Appl Environ Microbiol* 1985; 50:68–80.

11. Madara JL: Pathobiology of the intestinal epithelial barrier. *Am J Pathol* 1990; 137:1273–1281.

12. Moore R, Collins S, Madara JL: Villus contraction aids repair of intestinal epithelium after injury. *Am J Physiol* 1989; 257:274–283.

13. Madara JL: Maintenance of the macromolecular barrier at cell extrusion sites in intestinal epithelium: Physiologic rearrangement of tight junctions. *J Membr Biol* 1991; 116:177–184.

14. Tomasi TB Jr: Mechanisms of immune regulation at mucosal surfaces. *Rev Infect Dis* 1983; 5(suppl 4):785–792.

15. Sneller MC, Strober W: M cells and host defense. *J Infect Dis* 1986; 154:737–741.

16. Bertok L: Physico-chemical defense of vertebrate organisms: The role of bile acids in defense against bacterial endotoxins. *Perspect Biol Med* 1977; 21:70–76.

17. McCuskey RS, McCuskey PA, Urbaschek R, et al: Kupffer cell function in host defense. *Rev Infect Dis* 1987; 9(suppl 15):616–619.

18. Nolan JP: Intestinal endotoxins as mediators of hepatic injury: An idea whose time has come again. *Hepatology* 1989; 10:887–891.

19. Altura BM: Hemorrhagic shock and reticuloendothelial system phagocytic function in pathogen-free animals. *Circ Shock* 1974; 1:295–300.

20. Jacob AI, Goldberg PK, Bloom N, et al: Endotoxin and bacteria in portal blood. *Gastroenterology* 1977; 72:1268–1270.

21. Nolan JP, Camara DS: Intestinal endotoxins as cofactors in liver injury. *Immun Invest* 1989; 18:325–337.

22. Formal SB, Noyes HE, Schneider H: Experimental *Shigella* infections III: Sensitivity of normal, starved, and carbon tetrachloride treated guinea pigs to endotoxin, *Proc Soc Exp Biol Med* 1960; 103:415–418.

23. Alexander JW, MacMillan BG, Stinnett JD, et al: Beneficial effects of aggressive protein feeding in severely burned children. *Ann Surg* 1980; 192:505–517.

24. Fong Y, Marano MA, Barber A, et al: Total parenteral nutrition and bowel rest modify the metabolic response to endotoxin in humans. *Ann Surg* 1989; 210:449–457.

25. Mochizuki H, Trocki O, Dominioni L: Mechanism of prevention of post-burn hypermetabolism and catabolism by early enteral feeding. *Ann Surg* 1984; 200:297–310.
26. Wilmore DW, Smith RJ, O'Dwyer ST, et al: The gut: A central organ after surgical stress. *Surgery* 1988; 104:917–923.
27. Moore FA, Moore EE, Jones TN, et al: TEN versus TPN following major torso trauma: Reduced septic morbidity. *J Trauma* 1989; 29:916–923.
28. Kudsk KA, Croce MA, Fabian TC, et al: Enteral versus parenteral feeding: Effects on septic morbidity after blunt and penetrating abdominal trauma. *Ann Surg* 1992; 215:503–513.
29. Kudsk KA, Stone JM, Carpenter G, et al: Enteral and parenteral feeding influences mortality after hemoglobin–*E. coli* peritonitis in normal rats. *J Trauma* 1983; 23:605–609.
30. Border JR, Hasset JM, LaDuca J, et al: Gut origin septic states in blunt multiple trauma (ISS = 40) in the ICU. *Ann Surg* 1987; 206:427–448.
31. Alverdy JC, Aoys E, Moss GS: Total parenteral nutrition promotes bacterial translocation from the gut. *Surgery* 1988; 104:186–190.
32. Spaeth G, Berg RD, Specian RD, et al: Food without fiber promotes bacterial translocation from the gut. *Surgery* 1990; 108:240–247.
33. Deitch EA, Winterton J, Li M, et al: The gut as a portal of entry for bacteremia: Role of protein malnutrition. *Ann Surg* 1987; 205:681–692.
34. Deitch EA, Ma WJ, Ma L, et al: Protein malnutrition predisposes to inflammatory-induced gut-origin septic states. 1990; *Ann Surg* 211:560–568.
35. Dudrick SJ, Wilmore DW, Vars HM, et al: Can intravenous feeding as the sole means of nutrition support growth in the child and restore weight loss in an adult? An affirmative answer. *Ann Surg* 1968; 169:974–984.
36. Alverdy J, Chi HS, Sheldon GF: The effect of parenteral nutrition on gastrointestinal immunity: The importance of enteral stimulation. *Ann Surg* 1985; 202:681–684.
37. Saito H, Trocki O, Alexander JW, et al: The effect of route of nutrient administration on the nutritional state, catabolic hormone secretion, and gut mucosal integrity after burn injury. *JPEN* 1987; 11:1–7.
38. Mainous MR, Xu D, Lu Q, et al: Oral TPN-induced bacterial translocation and impaired immune defenses are reversed by refeeding. *Surgery* 1991; 110:277–284.
39. Souba WW, Klimberg VS, Hautamaki RD, et al: Oral glutamine reduces bacterial translocation following abdominal radiation. *J Surg Res* 1990; 48:1–5.
40. Burke D, Alverdy JC, Aoys E, et al: Glutamine-supplemented total parenteral nutrition improves gut immune function. *Arch Surg* 1989; 124:1396–1400.
41. Barber AE, Jones WG, Minei JP, et al: Glutamine or fiber supplementation of a defined formula diet: Impact on bacterial translocation, tissue composition, and response to endotoxin. *JPEN* 1990; 14:335–343.
42. Xu D, Lu Q, Thirstrup C, et al: Elemental diet–induced bacterial translocation and immunosuppression is not reversed by glutamine. *J Trauma*, in press.
43. Wells CL, Jechorek RP, Erlandsen SL, et al: The effect of dietary glutamine and dietary RNA on ileal flora, ileal histology, and bacterial translocation in mice. *Nutrition* 1990; 6:70–75.
44. Zaloga GP, Ward KA, Prielipp RC: Effect of enteral diets on whole body and gut growth in unstressed rats. *JPEN* 1991; 15:42–47.
45. Friedel D, Levine GM: Effect of short chain fatty acids on colonic function and structure. *JPEN* 1992; 16:1–4.
46. Kripke SA, Fox AD, Berman JM, et al: Stimulation of intestinal mucosal growth with intracolonic infusion of short chain fatty acids. *JPEN* 1989; 13:109–116.
47. Koruda MJ, Rolandelli RH, Settle RG, et al: Effect of parenteral nutrition supplemented with short chain fatty acids on adaptation to massive small bowel resection. *Gastroenterology* 1988; 95:715–720.
48. Spaeth G, Specian RD, Berg RD, et al: Bulk prevents bacterial translocation induced by the oral administration of total parenteral nutrition solution. *JPEN* 1990; 14:442–447.

49. Hosoda N, Nishi M, Nakagawa M, et al: Structural and functional alterations in the gut of parenterally or enterally fed rats. *J Surg Res* 1989; 47:129–133.

50. Jacobs DO, Evans DA, Mealy K, et al: Combined effects of glutamine and epidermal growth factor on the rat intestine. *Surgery* 1988; 104:358–364.

51. Evers BM, Izukura M, Townsend CW, et al: Differential effects of gut hormones on pancreatic and intestinal growth during administration of an elemental diet. *Ann Surg* 1990; 211:630–638.

PART IV

Specific Disease States

31

Trauma

Frederick A. Moore, M.D.

Ernest E. Moore, M.D.

Rationale for early nutritional support

  Background information

  Clinical investigation

Early enteral nutritional support

  Background information

  Clinical investigation

Current recommendations

There is an emerging consensus that early nutritional support benefits moderately and severely injured patients, but the optimal route of substrate delivery (enteral vs. parenteral) continues to be debated.[1-16] Enteral nutrition is cheaper and safer, but an inappropriate fear of gastrointestinal intolerance has discouraged its use in the immediate postinjury period.[17] Recent basic and clinical research, however, offers compelling physiologic reasons for considering early enteral feeding. Substrates delivered via the enteral route appear to be better utilized than those administered parenterally.[18-21] Additionally, enteral nutrition prevents gastrointestinal mucosal atrophy, attenuates the injury stress response, maintains immunocompetence, and preserves normal gut flora.[9-12, 22-28] Despite these considerations, there is a paucity of controlled clinical trials that assess the impact of early total enteral nutrition (TEN) vs. total parenteral nutrition (TPN) on the clinical outcome of critically ill patients.[2, 11, 14, 16, 29, 30] The purpose of this chapter is to review the available ba-

sic and clinical research data to specifically address whether early TEN, when compared with TPN, provides an outcome advantage following major injury.

RATIONALE FOR EARLY NUTRITIONAL SUPPORT

Background Information

Before discussing the optimal route of substrate administration, a brief review of the rationale of early nutritional support is necessary. Until recently, conventional therapy has been to wait 5 days and then to start TPN if the patient is intolerant of oral intake. However, it is now believed that unless exogenous nutrients are provided early, the inexorable hypermetabolism induced by the injury stress response can seriously deplete endogenous substrate stores. The injury stress response is well characterized metabolically. Energy expenditure peaks in 3 to 4 days and then subsides by 7 to 10 days unless driven by a delayed septic insult. The degree to which energy expenditure rises depends on the mechanism of injury as well as the magnitude of trauma. Energy expenditure typically increases 80% to 100% after major burns, 50% to 60% after severe closed-head injury, and 30% to 50% after multisystem trauma. Net somatic muscle proteolysis occurs as protein catabolism exceeds synthesis.[31] The branched-chain amino acids leucine, isoleucine, and valine become important oxidative fuel,[32, 33] while the glucogenic amino acids, principally alanine, are taken up by the liver to produce greater quantities of glucose. Glutamine becomes the preferred oxidative fuel for the gastrointestinal tract and an important energy source for the immune system and is critical for glutathione synthesis in the liver.[34] Circulating amino acids also provide the necessary substrate for hepatic acute-phase proteins, wound healing, and maintenance of other vital organ functions.[35, 36] Abnormal glucose tolerance exists, but insulin levels are normal or even elevated. Insulin no longer has the predominate role in glucose kinetics; instead hyperglycemia is the net result of persistent hepatic gluconeogenesis.[37] Overall, glucose utilization is elevated because of increased demands by the central nervous system and hematopoietic system as well as injured tissue, while clearance by skeletal muscle and adipose tissue is blunted. The kinetics of fat metabolism after injury is not well defined, but in general, lipolysis is enhanced, fatty acid oxidation accelerated, and ketosis relatively suppressed.[38–41]

The traditional teaching has been that the injury stress response is primarily a neuroendocrine reflex that activates the hypothalamic-pituitary-adrenal axis to produce elevated plasma levels of catecholamines, glucocorticoids, and glucagon. Bessey et al.,[42, 43] however, showed that while simultaneous infusion of epinephrine, cortisol, and glucagon into normal healthy volunteers produced the hypermetabolism observed following major injury, these counterregulatory hormones did not induce the obligatory catabolism. Subsequently, this group showed that sterile inflammation caused by intramuscular injection of etiocholanolone produced systemic signs of inflammation (e.g., fever, leukocytosis, increased C-reactive protein) but again did not induce protein breakdown.[44] However, when this sterile inflammatory insult was combined with the above triple-hormone infusion, this produced the hypermetabolic catabolic state that characterizes the early postinjury period.[45] More recently, other investigators have implicated interleukin-1 and tumor necrosis factor as being the primary signals for postinjury protein breakdown, but there appear to be other critical elements.[46–48] In sum, the injury stress response is the net result of neuro-mediated counterregulatory hormone secretion and a complex cascade of cell-generated inflammatory mediators. These driving mechanisms are continuously being redefined. Consequently, modulating the injury stress response is not a current clinical option. The only recourse is to support it and to avoid late septic complications.[3, 49, 50]

Hypercatabolism is the prominent feature of the early postinjury stress response. The obligatory rate of protein turnover parallels the rise in metabolic rate. The ultimate fate of catabolized amino acid carbon skeletons is energy production via the Krebs' cycle, while the resultant ammonia is detoxified in the liver and excreted primarily as urea. Thus, the magnitude of protein degradation is reflected in the urinary excretion of urea nitrogen (N_2). In our experience, patients sustaining multisystem trauma lose 13 to 18 g/day of N_2; if compounded by closed-head injury with increased intracranial pressure or long-bone pelvic fractures, N_2 excretion is frequently greater than 25 g/day.[2, 14, 15, 51–53] If exogenous amino acids are not supplied, then amino acids must be diverted from endogenous sources.[3, 32, 35, 46, 50, 54] At first, oxidative amino acid demands are met by skeletal muscle proteolysis. However, in a short period of time, this autocannibalism progress erodes crucial visceral structure elements and circulating proteins and results in acute protein malnutrition. Additionally, animal studies and clinical observations indicate that acute protein malnutrition is associated with cardiac, pulmonary, hepatic, gastrointestinal, and immunologic dysfunction.[55-63] In essence, subclinical multiple organ dysfunction evolves, and the patient becomes progressively more immunocompromised. Delayed infection can then cause persistent hypermetabolism and eventually multiple organ failure.[3, 49, 50] Thus, it is conceivable that failure to provide adequate nutritional support in the first 5 days after major trauma has an adverse impact on patient outcome.

Clinical Investigation

The first clinical suggestion that this is true came from Alexander and associates in 1980.[1] They noted that severely burned children (average burn size, 60%) randomized to receive an early high-protein diet vs. a normal low-protein diet had better immunologic parameters, fewer bacteremic days, and significantly improved survival. Stimulated by this report as well as the success of Page et al.[64] with needle catheter jejunostomy (NCJ) after elective gastrointestinal surgery, we first completed a prospective trial that confirmed the feasibility of early NCJ feeding in patients who had sustained major abdominal trauma.[53] Convinced of the efficacy and safety of early jejunal feeding, our next step was to identify a high-risk group of patients who might benefit by receiving early nutritional support. Because standard nutritional indices developed for elective surgical patients are unreliable in the early postinjury period, we devised the Abdominal Trauma Index (ATI).[51, 52, 65] This is an anatomic score that quantitates the severity of organ injury found at laparotomy. Each

organ system is assigned a complication risk factor (range, 1 to 5) based on the reported morbidity of that specific organ injury. This is multiplied by an organ severity of injury estimate to obtain an individual organ score. The individual organ severity of injury estimate is graded (range, 1 to 5) on a scale modified from the Abbreviated Injury Scale: 1 = minimal, 2 = minor, 3 = moderate, 4 = major, and 5 = maximal. The final ATI score is the sum of the individual organ scores. Despite its simplicity, the ATI has proved to be sensitive and reasonably specific in predicting morbidity after major abdominal trauma. ATI scores less than 16 reflect low risk of septic morbidity; 16 to 25, moderate risk; and greater than 25, high risk.[66]

Prepared with the ATI to identify a relatively homogeneous group of high-risk patients, we then conducted a prospective randomized trial to investigate immediate postinjury nutritional support.[2] Over a 30-month period ending November 1983, 75 (20%) of 371 injured patients requiring emergent laparotomy at the Denver General Hospital (DGH) had an ATI score greater than 15 and were enrolled in a prospective study that randomized patients to either a control or enteral-fed group. Control patients received conventional 5% dextrose in water (D_5W) (approximately 10 g/day) intravenously during the first 5 postoperative days, and TPN with a nonprotein calorie-to-nitrogen ratio ($NPC:N_2$) of 133:1 was started if they were not tolerating a regular diet at that time. The enterally fed group had an NCJ placed just before abdominal closure. Infusion of an elemental diet (Vivonex HN, Norwich Eaton Pharmaceuticals, Norwich, NY; $NPC:N_2$ = 150:1) was begun via the NCJ within 12 hours postoperatively and advanced to meet the metabolic demands at 72 hours.

Twelve patients were excluded from analysis within the first 72 hours because of reoperation (6), death (4), or transfer to another hospital (2). The remaining study groups (32 TEN patients vs. 31 control patients) were comparable with respect to age (31 ± 2 vs. 31 ± 2 years), injury mechanism (31% vs. 23% blunt), shock (34% vs. 29%), and ATI (30.6 ± 2.2 vs. 29.0 ± 2.1). The groups were also equivalent according to initial nutritional assessment. Results are outlined in Table 31−1. The only significant changes in nutritional parameters occurred in the enterally fed group. The total lymphocyte count increased at day 7, and nitrogen balance improved at days 4 and 7. Septic morbidity was significantly greater in the control group. Major septic complications (i.e., abdominal abscess or pneumonia) developed in 9 (29%) patients in the control group vs. 3 (9%) in the enterally fed group. Moreover, the mean ATI score of patients in whom complications developed in the control group was 31, while in the enterally fed group it was 48. Finally, the cost savings based on a review of actual hospital bills exceeded $3000 per patient in the enterally fed group. Thus, this prospective randomized study demonstrated a statistically significant reduction in septic morbidity after major abdominal trauma as a result of immediate postinjury nutritional support.

EARLY ENTERAL NUTRITIONAL SUPPORT

Background Information

After acknowledging the benefit of early postinjury nutrition, the next is-

sue was the optimal route of substrate delivery, i.e., enteral vs. parenteral. There has been a reluctance to administer enteral feeding after major injury because of an inappropriate fear of gastrointestinal intolerance. However, our work, as well as that of others, has shown that roughly 85% of high-risk patients will tolerate early full-dose enteral feeding.[2, 8, 11, 14−17, 53] On the other hand, with two decades of experience and the establishment of monitoring protocols, TPN has become a convenient option in the critical care setting. Now, however, basic and clinical research offers compelling physiologic benefits for considering early enteral feeding. Substrates absorbed from the gut appear to be better utilized, presumably because they first pass through the liver. Although TPN can be advanced more quickly than TEN, this is accompanied by increased nitrogen excretion.[15] Piccone et al.[19] demonstrated a similar nitrogen-sparing effect when delivering TPN via the portal vein. Glucose intolerance is a frequent problem with TPN. Comparative trials have documented significant hyperglycemia in the face of high insulin levels in TPN patients, while TEN patients have only mild elevations in the levels of glucose and insulin.[14, 20] Moreover, in comparative trials TPN patients gain more weight while TEN patients, despite receiving fewer nutrients, have higher end-of-study nutritional protein markers (total protein, albumin, and transferrin) as

TABLE 31−1.

Clinical Benefits of Early Postinjury Nutritional Support

Study Group	Total Lymphocyte Count (Cells/mm³)	N₂ Balance (g/Day)	Sepsis	Hospital Cost/Patient
Control (n = 31)				
Day 1	1408 ± 158*	−13.2 ± 0.5	9	$19,636
Day 4	1175 ± 176	−11.4 ± 0.7	(29%)	
Day 7	1482 ± 138	−11.1 ± 0.7		
Enteral (n = 32)				
Day 1	1831 ± 206	−13.7 ± 0.7	3	
Day 4	1344 ± 166	−3.9 ± 1.6†	(9%)	$16,280
Day 7	2054 ± 164†	−5.2 ± 1.3†		

*Data are means ± SEM.
†P < .05.

well as similar total lymphocyte counts.[14, 15]

Recent work has established the gut to be metabolically active in stressed patients. The intestinal mucosa undergoes rapid turnover and is vulnerable to starvation.[67] It derives nutrients from both the luminal contents and the circulating blood. Gut atrophy is well documented in animals fed long-term by vein.[68-70] Standard TPN avoids the trophic stimulating effects of enteral feeding and lacks gut-specific nutrients.[71-73] For example, glutamine, normally considered a nonessential amino acid, becomes an essential substrate for the enterocyte during critical illness.[34, 54, 74] Systemic levels of gut-derived hormones such as gastrin, glucagon, insulin, and gastric inhibitory peptide are altered during parenteral nutrition.[75] Saito et al.[12] reported an attenuated stress response in burned animals that were fed through the gut vs. the central vein.

The gastrointestinal tract appears to have important immune regulatory functions. Kudsk et al.[9, 10] showed that enteral feeding as compared with TPN in both malnourished and well-nourished rats improved survival following *Escherichia coli* hemoglobin peritonitis. In a rat model, Alverdy et al.[22] documented that enteral feeding maintains normal biliary levels of secretary IgA while TPN is associated with a precipitous fall. Similarly, Birkhahn and Renk have shown that TPN fails to maintain lymphocyte function when compared with enteral feeding in rats.[76] In more recent human comparisons of TEN and TPN, Meyer et al.[27] showed that TPN adversely affects neutrophil responses, whereas Lowry[28] observed that parenterally fed patients exhibit an exaggerated cytokine response to an endotoxin challenge.

While the gut is metabolically active and appears to be an important effector organ for immunologic function during critical illness, recent research interests have focused upon its barrier function. Transmural migration of viable gastrointestinal tract organisms (bacterial translocation) was demonstrated experimentally 40 years ago.[77] Most recently, the animal models of Deitch et al.[23] and others[78, 79] have comprehensively addressed the factors that govern this phenomenon. While these animal studies are logical, consistent, and compelling, clinical evidence that bacterial translocation is a pathologic event in critically injured patients is sparse. We recently reported the results of a prospective trial where 20 severely injured patients with known risk factors for multiple organ failure (MOF) had portal vein catheters placed for sequential blood sampling up to 5 days postoperatively.[80] Only 8 (2%) of 212 portal cultures were positive; 7 were presumed contaminants. The only positive systemic culture (total, 212) was *Staphylococcus aureus* on day 5 in a patient with a concurrent staphylococcal pneumonia. While this does not exclude the lymphatics as an early route of translocation, the lack of positive systemic cultures suggests that it is well contained. In another study, we obtained ileocolic mesenteric lymph node (MLN) cultures at emergent laparotomy in 54 trauma patients; 8 (15%) were positive.[81] Four of these patients had an associated hollow-viscus injury. Seven patients with positive MLN cultures were not in shock and had negative concurrent blood cultures, postoperative sepsis or MOF did not develop, and all survived. The remaining patient arrived in profound shock, had the same organism cultured in the blood, and died on the operating room table. Consequently, bacterial translocation to the MLNs occurs in patients sustaining abdominal trauma, but with the exception of 1 patient, it was not associated with an adverse outcome. Of course, bacterial translocation to the MLNs may be a normal event in healthy humans. In fact, Wells et al.[82] propose that translocation is a part of the antigen-sampling process of gut-associated lymphoid tissue. They have shown that suppression of cell-mediated immunity does not itself promote translocation but does permit greater numbers of translocated bacteria to survive in the MLN. Thus, delayed translocation via a disrupted mucosal barrier in an immunocompromised host may allow for systemic spread of gut bacteria. Although there is no direct clinical evidence to support bacterial translocation as a delayed pathologic event, the epidemiologic studies of Marshal et al.[83] and Border et al.[5] strongly implicate the gut as the occult source of bacteremias found in late sepsis. Indeed, Driks and associates'[84] analysis of various stress ulcer prophylaxis regimens, Cerra and colleagues'[85] recent trial of selective decontamination of the gut, and our previous study addressing the optimal route of nutritional support document significant reductions in nosocomial pneumonia rates attributed to various gut-specific therapies.[14] Presumably, in the first study, normal gastric acidity and, in the second study, topical antibiotics prevented digestive tract colonization by hospital-acquired bacteria that were subsequently aspirated into the compromised lung. In our study, it is tempting to assume that enteral nutrition prevented systemic bacterial translocation by maintaining gut barrier function or enhancing immunity; however, it is plausible that the observed decreased incidence of pneumonia with enteral feeding is simply due to maintenance of normal gut flora. In sum, the available clinical data strongly implicate the gut as the source of bacteria found in late nosocomial infections, but whether or not bacterial translocation is the prime pathway for bacterial dissemination is speculative.

Clinical Investigation

Our initial clinical investigation demonstrating a significant reduction in septic complications as a result of immediate postinjury TEN prompted further study asking whether early TPN would produce equivalent benefits.[2, 14] Over a 28-month period ending August 1988, 75 (18%) of 407 patients requiring emergent laparotomy at DGH who had an ATI over 15 but less than 40 were randomized at initial laparotomy to receive either TEN (Vivonex TEN) or TPN (Freamine HBC, 6.9%, and Trophamine, 6%; Kendall-McGaw Laboratories, Irvine, Calif); both regimens contained 2.5% fat and 33% BCAAs and had an NPC:N_2 ratio of 150:1. Nutritional support was initiated within 12 hours postoperatively in both groups and infused at a rate sufficient to render the patients in positive N_2 balance within 48 hours. TEN was delivered via NCJ. Sixteen patients were subsequently excluded from the study, which left 59 evaluable subjects. Reasons for exclusion were early death (4 patients), reoperation within 72 hours (3 patients), significant chronic medical disease (3 patients), an ATI score greater than 40 (2 patients), head injury requiring fluid restriction (2 patients), mechanical failure of TEN delivery (1 patient), and early transfer (1 patient). The study groups (29 TEN patients vs. 30 TPN patients) were comparable at presentation with respect to age (28 ± 2 vs. 32 ± 2 years), injury mechanism (28% vs. 36% blunt injury), Injury Severity Score [ISS] (28.7 ± 2.3 vs. 25.1 ± 1.0), ATI (24.7 ± 1.1 vs. 24.0 ± 1.0), and Revised Trauma Score (6.9 ± 0.2 vs. 6.9 ± 0.31). Of the evaluable TEN patients, 4 (14%) subjects failed to tolerate the protocol increments in the enteral diet, 3 patients responded to manipulation in the feeding schedule, and the remaining patient underwent transition to TPN on day 7 due to severe intolerance in the face of persistent hypermetabolism. All were retained in the TEN group for analysis. On day 5, calorie and N_2 intake were higher in TPN patients vs. patients receiving TEN. Despite this slight advantage in protein-calorie intake via the parenteral route, no significant differences for N_2 balance were noted between the two groups at day 5 (−0.3 ± 1.0 vs. 0.1 ± 0.8 g/day). Of note, albumin, transferrin, and retinol-binding protein levels increased throughout the study in patients receiving TEN (Table 31−2): on day 5, the dif-

TABLE 31–2.

Laboratory Results of Total Enteral Nutrition vs. Total Parenteral Nutrition Study Groups Following Major Abdominal Trauma*

Test	TEN ($n = 29$)	TPN ($n = 30$)	P Value
Total protein (g/dL)			
Day 1	5.0 ± 0.1†	5.2 ± 0.1	NS
Day 5	5.9 ± 0.1	5.2 ± 0.1	.03
Day 10‡	6.3 ± 0.2	5.5 ± 0.3	NS
Albumin (g/dL)			
Day 5	3.3 ± 0.1	3.1 ± 0.2	.01
Day 10	3.4 ± 0.1	2.7 ± 0.2	.01
Transferrin (mg/dL)			
Day 1	190 ± 10	192 ± 7	NS
Day 5	190 ± 10	170 ± 5	NS
Day 10	216 ± 25	150 ± 18	.05
Retinol-binding protein (mg/dL)			
Day 1	2.8 ± 0.1	2.7 ± 0.1	NS
Day 5	2.5 ± 0.1	2.2 ± 0.3	NS
Day 10	3.1 ± 0.3	2.0 ± 0.3	.06
Bilirubin (mg/dL)			
Day 1	1.6 ± 0.2	1.2 ± 0.1	NS
Day 5	0.9 ± 0.1	1.4 ± 0.2	.03
Day 10	0.8 ± 0.3	2.9 ± 1.2	NS
Alkaline phosphatase (units)			
Day 1	61 ± 4	59 ± 4	NS
Day 5	83 ± 5	92 ± 6	NS
Day 10	135 ± 29	220 ± 96	NS
Glucose (mg/dL)			
Day 1	152 ± 8	162 ± 10	NS
Day 5	144 ± 10	190 ± 17	NS
Insulin (μU/mL)§			
Day 1	23.5 ± 3.2	29.3 ± 5.3	NS
Day 5	66.0 ± 9.3	93.3 ± 8.3	.02
Glutamine (nmol/mL)‖			
Day 1	275 ± 31	266 ± 18	NS
Day 5	241 ± 31	178 ± 20	NS
Alanine (nmol/mL)¶			
Day 1	370 ± 40	372 ± 35	NS
Day 5	472 ± 52	490 ± 39	NS

*Data from Moore FA, Moore EE, Jones TN, et al: J Trauma 1989, 22:916.
†Means ± SEM.
‡Day 10 data based on 10 patients in each group.
§Normal fasting insulin level, 20 μU/mL
‖Normal fasting glutamine level, 400 to 500 nmol/mL.
¶Normal fasting alanine level, 350 to 370 nmol/mL.

ference between treatment groups reached statistical significance for albumin, and day 10 albumin and transferrin levels were significantly higher in TEN patients. Abnormalities in liver function were observed and, of note, bilirubin and alkaline phosphatase levels were higher in patients receiving TPN. Glucose levels also tended to be higher in TPN patients, but this failed to reach statistical significance. However, glucose levels were maintained at acceptable levels by exogenous insulin in 5 (17%) of the TPN group as compared with 1 (3%) of the TEN group, and insulin levels by day 5 were significantly elevated in patients receiving TPN.

Complications occurred in 10 TEN patients (34%) as compared with 17 TPN patients (57%). Seven patients in the TPN group and 6 patients in the TEN group experienced nonseptic complications including pancreatitis (5 patients), atelectasis (3 patients), recurrent pneumothorax (1 patient), biliary fistula (1 patient), breakdown of exteriorized colon repair (1 patient), and cerebrospinal fluid leak (1 patient). Septic complications are summarized in Table 31–3. The overall incidence of septic morbidity was 17% (5 patients) in the TEN group vs. 37% (11 patients) in the TPN group. There was a significant difference with respect to major infections (pneumonia and intra-abdominal abscess), i.e., 1 (3%) patient in the TEN group vs. 6 (20%) in the TPN group. All 6 pneumonia cases were in the TPN group.

More recently, Kudsk et al.[16] have confirmed these observations in a prospective study that randomized 98 patients with an ATI of 15 or greater to receive TEN (Vital HN, Ross laboratories, Columbus, Ohio; NPC:N_2, 150:1), or TPN (Travasol, Clintec Nutrition, Deerfield, Ill; NPC:N_2, 150:1), which was initiated within 24 hours of injury. Two patients died early, which left 96 evaluable subjects, and the groups (51 TEN patients vs. 45 TPN patients) were comparable at presentation with respect to age (30 ± 2 vs. 31 ± 1 years), injury mechanisms (31% vs. 22% blunt injury), and ISS (25.1 ± 1.8 vs. 29.1 ± 1.4). Two (4%) patients failed to tolerate TEN. There were no significant differences in N_2 between the groups on any day, but

the TEN patients received significantly less N_2 per kilogram per day than did the TPN patients. As in our trial, patients randomized to receive TEN experienced significantly fewer septic complications than did patients receiving TPN (Table 31–4). TEN patients sustained significantly fewer infections per patient (TEN = 0.25 ± 0.06 vs. TPN = 0.71 ± 0.14, $P < .03$) as well as fewer infections per infected patients (TEN = 1.08 ± 0.08 vs. TPN = 1.6 ± 08, $P = .04$).

On reviewing the literature, there is only one other prospective randomized trial (PRT) comparing early postinjury TEN vs. TPN in which septic complications are recorded as an outcome variable. In this study by Adams et al.,[11] over a 30-month period ending June 1984, 46 patients with "two or more body system injuries" were randomized to receive TEN (Isocal HCN in the first 5 patients, NPC:N_2 = 145; Traumacal in the remaining 18 patients, NPC:N_2 = 90) vs. TPN (Travasol, NPC:N_2 = 150). The groups (23 TEN patients vs. 23 TPN patients) were comparable with respect to age (30 ± 2 vs. 29 ± 2 years) and ISS (39 ± 3 vs. 36 ± 3), but the TEN group had more bluntly injured patients (87% vs. 56%). The TEN patients received significantly fewer calories because of discontinuation of feedings before and after secondary operative procedures. Additionally, 3 (13%) patients failed to tolerate TEN. Consequently, the TPN

TABLE 31–3.

Septic Complications of Total Enteral Nutrition vs. Total Parenteral Nutrition Study Groups*

Complications	Group		P Value
	TEN (n = 29)	TPN (n = 30)	
Major infections			
Abdominal abscess	1 ⎫	2 ⎫	
Pneumonia	0 ⎬ 1 (3%)	6 ⎬ 6 (20%)	.03
Minor infections			
Wound	3 ⎫	1 ⎫	
Catheter	0 ⎪	2 ⎪	
Urinary	0 ⎬ 4 (14%)	0 ⎬ 5 (17%)	NS
Miscellaneous	1 ⎭	0 ⎭	
Total patients	5 (17%)	11 (37%)	

*Data from Moore FA, Moore EE, Jones TN, et al: *J Trauma* 1989, 29:916.

TABLE 31–4.

Septic Complications of Total Enteral Nutrition vs. Total Parenteral Nutrition Study Groups*

Complication	TEN	TPN	P Value
Pneumonia	6/51 (11.8%)	14/45 (31%)	<.2
Intra-abdominal abscess	1/51 (1.9%)	6/45 (13.3%)	<.4
Empyema	1/51 (1.9%)	4/45 (8.9%)	NS
Line sepsis	1/51 (1.9%)	6/45 (13.3%)	<.5
Fasciitis/dehiscence	3/51 (5.9%)	4.5 (8.9%)	NS

*Data from Kudsk KA, Croce MA, Fabian TC, et al: *Ann Surg,* 1992, 215:503.

group had better nitrogen balance than did the TEN patients. While septic morbidity was not a focus of this study, the recorded incidence of major septic complications (i.e., pneumonia, abscess, and wound infection) was 61% (14 patients) in the TEN group vs. 43% (10 patients) in the TPN group.

In summary, there are three published PRTs that (1) compare early TEN vs. TPN in high-risk trauma patients and (2) have septic morbidity recorded as an outcome variable. Two demonstrated a significant reduction in septic morbidity in patients receiving early enteral feeding, but the third study did not. While PRTs are the gold standard for assessing this type of clinical question, nutrition research is not well suited for this methodology. By necessity nutritional PRTs are frequently open label, and therefore, with the exception of measuring a definitive end point (e.g., mortality), study outcome indices are vulnerable to biased interpretation. But if mortality were to be used as the primary end point, an exceptionally large number of patients would need to be studied. Additionally, randomization cannot adequately control the confounding variables present in complex patient scenarios. Therefore, strict inclusion/exclusion criteria are necessary (e.g., ATI greater than 15 but less than 40), but this can severely limit subject enrollment. Typically a single institution does not have the patient volume necessary for timely completion of a large study, and even when well designed, the resulting small PRTs are

prone to generate misleading conclusions by type I (false positive) or type II (false negative) statistical error.[86, 87] Multicenter trials are viable alternatives but are pragmatically difficult to organize and require substantial funding.

Recently, meta-analysis has become a popular option.[88–90] Meta-analysis is a statistical method for combining data from multiple protocols to provide evidence of overall statistical significance where individual study results are inconclusive.[91, 92] We have recently completed a meta-analysis that combined data from eight PRTs that were conducted to assess the nutritional equivalence of the same enteral formula (Vivonex TEN) vs. nutritionally similar TPN solutions. In each study, complications were prospectively recorded as an outcome variable. Two of these trials are published, and both attest to patient tolerance of early postoperative enteral feeding.[14, 29] One trial demonstrated a significant reduction in major septic complications in those patients receiving early postinjury TEN.[14] Review of the six unpublished PRTs showed a similar trend toward decreased sepsis. The original intent was to combine these trials as a multicenter experience, but variability in individual protocol implementation (e.g., nontrauma vs. trauma entry criteria, timing of measurements, TPN composition, etc.) precluded this type of data pooling. By using meta-analysis, these data were rigorously evaluated for combinability, and sufficient patient numbers (statistical power) were obtained to adequately assess whether TEN was associated with decreased septic complications. A literature review revealed that no other published trials met the inclusion criteria for this meta-analysis. The eight studies contributing data enrolled 230 patients; 118 were randomized to receive TEN, and 112 were randomized to receive TPN. Thirty-six patients were classified as dropouts for non–diet-related reasons, including protocol violations (10 TEN, 3 TPN), patient/primary physician preference (8 TEN, 1 TPN), reoperation within 72 hours (4 TEN, 2 TPN), death within 72 hours (2 TEN, 3 TPN), and other miscellaneous reasons (2 TEN, 1 TPN). Of the 92 completed TEN patients, 15 (16%) were classified as treatment failures because of gastrointestinal intolerance (distension/cramping in 8, high gastric residuals in 6, and diarrhea in 1). Of the 102 TPN patients, 3 (3%) failed treatment because of metabolic problems (hyperglycemia in 2, ascites in 1).

This was a two-part meta-analysis. Phase I meta-analysis assessed 194 patients (including treatment failures and excluding study dropouts) and demonstrated that (1) the data were homogeneous across the study sites; (2) the combined treatment groups (92 TEN patients vs. 102 TPN patients) were comparable with regard to age, sex, race, injury/surgery type, and initial level of stress (ATI, ISS, basal energy expenditure, urinary nitrogen); and (3) significantly fewer TEN patients experienced one or more septic complications (TEN = 17% vs. TPN = 44%). After-the-fact power calculations indicated that this observed difference in septic complications was detectable at the $P < .05$ significance level with power in excess of 80%.

Based on highly significant differences in septic complications between the TEN and TPN treatment groups in the first analysis, a second analysis was conducted to more rigorously evaluate septic complication differences. Phase II was an intent-to-treat analysis (i.e., dropouts were included) and made comparisons of five patient subgroups: all patients, all trauma patients, penetrating trauma patients, blunt trauma patients, and all nontrauma patients. Table 31–5 depicts the phase II septic complication data. One or more infections developed in twice as many TPN as TEN patients (TEN = 16%, TPN = 35%; $P = .01$), and there was no difference in the number of infectious complications per patient. The most significant differences in the number of patients with septic complications between sub-

TABLE 31–5.

Patients With Postoperative Septic Complications by Surgery/Injury Type and Phase II Meta-analysis (Including Dropouts)

Complications	Blunt Trauma TEN (n = 48)	Blunt Trauma TPN (n = 44)	Penetrating Trauma TEN (n = 38)	Penetrating Trauma TPN (n = 40)	Nontrauma Surgery TEN (n = 32)	Nontrauma Surgery TPN (n = 28)	Total Patients TEN (n = 118)	Total Patients TPN (n = 112)
Abdominal abscess	2	1	2	6	1	0	5	7
Pneumonia	4	10	1	2	1	3	6	15
Wound infection	0	2	3	1	1	0	4	3
Bacteremia	1	4	0	1	1	0	2	5
Urinary tract infection	1	1	0	1	0	1	1	3
Catheter sepsis	0	4	0	1	0	2	0	7
Other*	5	4	1	1	0	1	6	6
Total events	13	26	7	13	4	7	24	46
No. of patients	10	22	6	11	3	6	19	39
% of patients	21	50†	16	27.5	9	21	16	35†

*Other infections included clinical sepsis in 8 and meningitis, empyema, sinusitis, and not specified in 1.
†$P < .05$ for patients; $P < .05$ excluding patients with line sepsis (incidence of infections for total patients, $P = .03$; all trauma patients, $P = .04$; and blunt trauma patients, $P < .05$).

groups were observed among all trauma (i.e., blunt and penetrating) patients (P = .02) and among blunt trauma patients (P = .02). Because differences observed between the TEN and TPN groups in septic complications could have been due to catheter sepsis, the differences in septic morbidity were also assessed for significance, excluding patients with catheter sepsis. A significant difference between groups in the number of patients with septic complications remained when catheter sepsis patients were excluded in (1) all patients combined (TEN = 16% vs. TPN = 29%; P = .03), (2) all trauma patients (TEN = 19% vs. TPN = 33%; P = 0.04), and (3) blunt trauma patients (TEN = 21% vs. TPN = 41%; P = < 0.05).

CURRENT RECOMMENDATIONS

This review of current basic and clinical research data indicates that early postinjury enteral feeding, when compared with TPN, reduces septic morbidity following major injury. The gut is now recognized to be a metabolically active, immunologically significant, and bacteriologically decisive organ during critical illness, and we assume that patients receiving early TPN have higher septic morbidity because this therapy does not maintain one or more of these vital gut functions. It is conceivable that early TPN could by itself be immunosuppressive or by some other means promote bacterial infection. However, this is not a cogent issue if one acknowledges the need for early nutrition in high-risk patients. Our nutritional support protocol for patients sustaining major torso trauma is as follows (see Fig 31–1). An ATI score greater than 17 should prompt placement of an NCJ at the initial laparotomy unless reexploration is planned within 24 hours. In the latter situation, this catheter is placed more safely at the second operation. An NCJ is also warranted in patients with less severe abdominal injuries if they have significant extraabdominal trauma (i.e., ISS greater

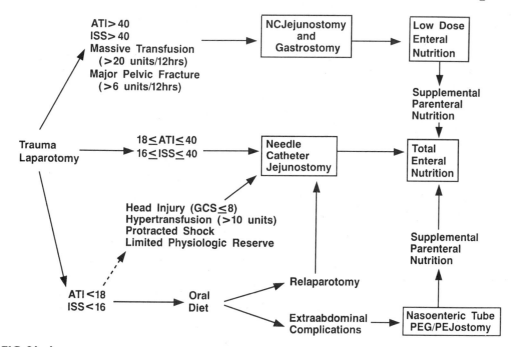

FIG 31–1.
Nutritional support protocol for patients sustaining major abdominal trauma at the Denver General Hospital. *ATI* = Abdominal Trauma index; *ISS* = Injury Severity Score; *GCS* = Glasgow Coma Scale; *NC* = needle catheter; *PEG* = percutaneous endoscopic gastrostomy; *PEJostomy* = percutaneous endoscopic jejunostomy.

than 15) or postoperative septic complications and organ dysfunction are anticipated (e.g., transfusion of more than 10 units, protracted shock, or patients with limited physiologic reserve). Of note, an NCJ and a gastrostomy are placed in massively injured patients (e.g., ATI greater than 40, ISS greater than 40, transfusion of more than 20 units, or a bleeding pelvic fracture), but because of anticipated intolerance to aggressive, early TEN, these patients receive low-dose enteral feeding with supplemental TPN for the first 3 postinjury days. The enteral feeding is then advanced as tolerated to full dose levels as the TPN is weaned. The gastrostomy is initially used to decompress the stomach but later will be used to deliver cheaper polymeric diets. For multisystem injured patients who do not require an early laparotomy, nasoduodenal or nasogastric feeding is initiated early, but these patients are likewise maintained on low-dose enteral feeding with supplemental TPN for 3 days to minimize the risk of pulmonary aspiration.[93, 94] If the need for long-term enteral access is anticipated, a percutaneous endoscopic gastrostomy (PEG) is placed at the bedside in the intensive care unit.[95] While passing a long tube through the PEG into the small bowel (i.e., PEG jejunostomy) may reduce the risk of aspiration, the currently available commercial kits are not ideal.[96, 97]

Acknowledgment

The writers gratefully acknowledge Jacqueline D. Ward and Susan E. Padilla for their excellent preparation of the manuscript.

REFERENCES

1. Alexander JW, MacMillian BG, Stinnett JD, et al: Beneficial effects of aggressive protein feeding in severely burned children. *Ann Surg* 1980; 192:505.
2. Moore EE, Jones TN: Benefits of immediate jejunal feeding after major abdominal trauma—a prospective randomized study. *J Trauma* 1986; 26:874.
3. Cerra FB: Hypermetabolism, organ failure, and metabolic support. *Surgery* 1987; 101:1.
4. Law NW, Ellis H: The effect of parenteral nutrition on the healing of abdominal wall wounds and colonic anastomoses in protein-malnourished rats. *Surgery* 1990; 107:449.
5. Border JR, Hassett J, LaDuca J, et al: The gut origin septic states in blunt multiple trauma (ISS = 40) in the ICU. *Ann Surg* 1987; 206:427.
6. Mochizuki H, Trocki O, Dominioni L, et al: Mechanism of prevention of postburn hypermetabolism and catabolism by early enteral feeding. *Ann Surg* 1984; 200:297.
7. Wilmore DW, Smith RJ, O'Dwyer ST, et al: The gut: A central organ after surgical stress. *Surgery* 1988; 104:917.
8. Page CP: The surgeon and gut maintenance. *Am J Surg* 1989; 158:485.
9. Kudsk KA, Carpenter G, Peterson SR, et al: Effect of enteral and parenteral feeding in malnourished rats with hemoglobin–E. coli adjuvant peritonitis. *J Surg Res* 1981; 31:105.
10. Kudsk KA, Stone JM, Carpenter G, et al: Effect of enteral and parenteral feeding influences mortality after hemoglobin–E. coli peritonitis in normal rats. *J Trauma* 1983; 23:605.
11. Adams S, Dellinger EP, Wertz MJ, et al: Enteral versus parenteral nutritional support following laparotomy for a trauma: A randomized prospective trial. *J Trauma* 1986; 26:882.
12. Saito H, Trocki O, Alexander JW, et al: The effect of route of nutrient administration on the nutritional state, catabolic hormone secretion, and gut mucosal integrity after burn injury. *JPEN* 1987; 11:1.
13. Peterson VM, Moore EE, Jones TN, et al: Total enteral nutrition versus total parenteral nutrition after major torso injury: Attenuation of hepatic protein reprioritization. *Surgery* 1988; 104:199.
14. Moore FA, Moore EE, Jones TN, et al: TEN versus TPN following major abdominal trauma—reduced septic morbidity. *J Trauma* 1989; 29:916.
15. Moore FA, Feliciano DV, Andrassy RJ,

et al: Early enteral feeding, compared with parenteral, reduces postoperative septic complications—The results of a meta-analysis. *Ann Surg* 1992; 216:62.

16. Kudsk KA, Croce MA, Fabian TC, et al: Enteral versus parenteral feeding: Effects on septic morbidity following blunt and penetrating abdominal trauma. *Ann Surg* 1992; 215:503.

17. Jones TN, Moore FA, Moore EE, et al: Gastrointestinal symptoms attributed to jejunostomy feeding after major abdominal trauma—a critical analysis. *Crit Care Med* 1989; 17:1146.

18. Lickley HLA, Track NS, Vranic M, et al: Metabolic responses to enteral and parenteral nutrition. *Am J Surg* 1978; 135:172.

19. Piccone VA, LeVeen HH, Glass P: Prehepatic hyperalimentation. *Surgery* 1980; 87:263.

20. McArdle AH, Palmason C, Morency I, et al: A rationale for enteral feeding as the preferred route for hyperalimentation. *Surgery* 1981; 90:616.

21. Enrione EB, Gelfand MJ, Morgan D, et al: The effects of rate and route of nutrient intake on protein metabolism. *J Surg Res* 1986; 40:320.

22. Alverdy J, Chi HS, Sheldon GF: The effect of parenteral nutrition on gastrointestinal immunity. *Ann Surg* 1985; 202:681.

23. Deitch EA, Winterton J, Li M, et al: The gut as a portal of entry for bacteremia. *Ann Surg* 1987; 205:681.

24. Souba WW, Smith RJ, Wilmore DW: Glutamine metabolism by the intestinal tract. *JPEN* 1985; 9:608.

25. Alverdy JC, Aoys E, Moss GS: Total parenteral nutrition promotes bacterial translocation from the gut. *Surgery* 1988; 104:185.

26. Burke DJ, Alverdy JC, Aoys E, et al: Glutamine-supplemental total parenteral nutrition improves gut immune function. *Arch Surg* 1989; 124:1396.

27. Meyer J, Yurt RW, Duhaney R: Differential neutrophil activation before and after endotoxin infusion in enterally versus parenterally fed volunteers. *Surg Gynecol Obstet* 1988; 167:50.

28. Lowry SF: The route of feeding influences injury responses. *J Trauma* 1990; 30(suppl):10.

29. Bower, RH, Talamini MA, Sax HC, et al: Postoperative enteral vs parenteral nutrition. A randomized controlled trial. *Arch Surg* 1986; 121:1040.

30. Cerra FB, McPherson JP, Konstantinides FN, et al: Enteral nutrition does not prevent multiple organ failure syndrome (MOFS) after sepsis. *Surgery* 1988; 104:727.

31. Birkhahn RH, Long CL, Fitkin D: Effect of major skeletal trauma on whole body protein turnover in man measured by L-1, ^{14}C-leucine. *Surgery* 1980; 88:294.

32. Cerra R, Blackburn G, Hirsch J, et al: The effect of stress level, amino acid formula and nitrogen dose on nitrogen retention in traumatic and septic stress. *Ann Surg* 1987; 205:282.

33. Sax HC, Talamini MA, Fischer JE: Clinical use of branched-chain amino acids in liver disease, sepsis, trauma, and burns. *Arch Surg* 1986; 121:358.

34. Souba WW, Smith RJ, Wilmore DW: Glutamine metabolism by the intestinal tract. *JPEN* 1981; 9:608.

35. Askanazi J, Carpenter YA, Michelsen CB, et al: Muscle and plasma amino acids following injury. *Ann Surg* 1980; 192:78.

36. Barbul A: Arginine: Biochemistry, physiology, and therapeutic implications. *JPEN* 1986; 10:227.

37. Black PR, Brooks DC, Bessey PQ, et al: Mechanisms of insulin resistance. *Ann Surg* 1982; 196:420.

38. Birkhahn RF, Long CL, Fitkin DL, et al: A comparison of the effects of skeletal trauma and surgery on the ketosis of starvation in man. *J Trauma* 1981; 21:513.

39. Harris RL, Frenkel RA, Cotton GL, et al: Lipid mobilization and metabolism after thermal trauma. *J Trauma* 1982; 204:194.

40. Robin AP, Askanazi J, Greenwood TC, et al: Lipoprotein lipase activity in surgical patients: Influence of trauma and infection. *Surgery* 1981; 90:401.

41. Shaw JHF, Wolfe RR: An integrated analysis of glucose, fat, and protein metabolism in severely traumatized patients. *Ann Surg* 1989; 209:63.

42. Bessey PQ, Watters JM, Aoki TT, et al: Combined hormonal infusion simulates the metabolic response to injury. *Ann Surg* 1984; 200:264.

43. Bessey PQ, Jiang Z, Johnson DJ, et al: Posttraumatic skeletal muscle proteoly-

sis: The role of hormonal environment. *World J Surg* 1989; 13:465.

44. Watters JM, Bessey PQ, Dinarella CA, et al: The induction of interleukin 1 in humans and its metabolic effects. *Surgery* 1985; 98:298.

45. Watters, JM, Bessey PQ, Dinarella CA, et al: Both inflammatory and endocrine mediators stimulate host responses to sepsis. *Arch Surg* 1986; 121:179.

46. Clowes GHS, Hirsch E, George BC, et al: Survival from sepsis. The significance of altered protein metabolism regulated by proteolysis inducing factor, the circulating cleavage product of interleukin-1. *Ann Surg* 1985; 202:446.

47. Fong Y, Moldawer LL, Shires GT, et al: The biologic characteristics of cytokines and their implications in surgical injury. *Surg Gynecol Obstet* 1990; 170:363.

48. Moldawer LL, Svaninger G, Gelin J: Interleukin-1 and tumor necrosis factor do not regulate protein balance in skeletal muscle. *Am J Physiol* 1987; 253:766.

49. Cerra FB, Siegel JH, Coleman, et al: Septic autocannibalism. A failure of exogenous nutritional support. *Ann Surg* 1980; 192:570.

50. Border JR, Chenier R, McMenamy RH, et al: Multiple systems organ failure: Muscle fuel deficit with visceral protein malnutrition. *Surg Clin North Am* 1976; 56:1147.

51. Moore EE, Jones TN: Nutritional assessment and preliminary report on early support of the trauma patient. *J Am Coll Nutr* 1983; 2:45.

52. Jones TN, Moore EE, Van Way CW: Factors influencing nutritional assessment in abdominal trauma patients. *JPEN* 1983; 7:115.

53. Moore EE, Dunn EL, Jones TN: Immediate jejunostomy feeding: Its use after major abdominal trauma. *Arch Surg* 1981; 116:681.

54. Souba WW, Klinberg VS, Plumley DA, et al: The role of glutamine in maintaining a healthy gut and supporting the metabolic response to injury and infection. *J Surg Res* 1990; 48:383.

55. Abei RM, Grimes JB, Alonso D: Adverse hemodynamic and ultrastructural changes in dog hearts subjected to protein-calorie malnutrition. *Am Heart J* 1979; 97:734.

56. Arora NS, Rochester DF: Respiratory muscle strength and maximal voluntary ventilation in undernourished patients. *Am Rev Respir Dis* 1982; 126:5.

57. Clark RM: The time-course of changes in mucosal architecture and epithelial cell production and cell shedding in the small intestine of the rat fed after fasting. *J Anat* 1975; 120:321.

58. Drakik MD, Schnure FC, Mok KT: Effect of protein depletion and short-term parenteral refeeding on the host response to interleukin-1 administration. *J Clin Lab Med* 1987; 109:509.

59. Eastwood GL: Small bowel morphology and epithelial proliferation in intravenously alimented rabbits. *Surgery* 1977; 82:613.

60. Goodlad RA, Wright NA: The effects of starvation and refeeding on intestinal cell proliferation in the mouse. *Cell Pathol* 1984; 45:63.

61. Krishnaswamy K, Naidu AN: Microsomal enzymes in malnutrition as determined by plasma half-life of antipyrine. *BMJ* 1977; 1:538.

62. Vazquez JA, Morse El, Adibi SA: Effect of starvation on amino acid and peptide hydrolysis in humans. *Am J Physiol* 1985; 249:563.

63. Law DK, Dudrick SJ, Abdow NI. Immunocompetence of patients with protein-calorie malnutrition—the effects of nutritional repletion. *Ann Intern Med* 1973; 79:545.

64. Page CP, Carlton PK, Andrassey RJ, et al: Safe, cost-effective postoperative nutrition: Refined formula diet via needle catheter jejunostomy (NCJ). *Am J Surg* 1979; 133:939.

65. Moore EE, Dunn EL, Jones TN, et al: Penetrating abdominal trauma index. *J Trauma* 1982; 21:439.

66. Borlase BC, Moore EE, Moore FA: The abdominal trauma index—a critical reassessment and validation. *J Trauma* 1990; 30:1340.

67. Clark RM: The time-course of changes in mucosal architecture and epithelial cell production and cell shedding in the small intestine of the rat fed after fasting. *J Anat* 1975; 120:321.

68. Johnson LR, Capeland EM, Durdick SJ, et al: Structural and hormonal al-

terations in the gastrointestinal tract of parenterally fed rats. *Gastroenterology* 1975; 68:1177.

69. Thompson JS, Vaughan WP, Forst CF, et al: The effect of the route of nutrient delivery on gut structure and diamine oxidase levels. *JPEN* 1987; 11:28.

70. Hosada N, Nishi M, Nakaguwa M, et al: Strutural and functional alterations in the gut of parenterally or enterally fed rats. *J Surg Res* 1989; 47:129.

71. Gleesan MH, Dawleng, RH, Peters TJ: Biochemical changes in intestinal mucosa after experimental small bowel bypass in the rat. *Clin Sci* 1972; 43:743.

72. Clark RM: Evidence for both luminal and systemic factors in the control of rat intestinal epithelial replacement. *Clin Sci Mol Med* 1976; 50:139.

73. Sagor GR, Ghatei MA, Al-Mukhtar MY, et al: Evidence for a humoral mechanism after small bowel resection. Exclusion of gastrin but not enteroglucagon. *Gastroenterology* 1983; 84:902.

74. Sanba WW, Wilmore DW: Postoperative alteration of arteriovenous exchange of amino acids across the gastrointestinal tract. *Surgery* 1983; 94:342.

75. Gimman Z, Murphy RF, Chen MH, et al: The effect of parenteral and enteral nutrition on portal and systemic glucogon and vasoactive intestinal polypeptide (VIP). *Ann Surg* 1982; 196:571.

76. Birkhahn RH, Renk CM: Immune response and leucine oxidation in oral and intravenous fed rats. *Am J Clin Nutr* 1984; 39:45.

77. Schweinberg FR, Seligman AM, Fine J: Transmural migration of intestinal bacteria. *N Engl J Med* 1950; 242:747.

78. Alverdy JC, Aoys E, Moss GS: Total parenteral nutrition promotes bacterial translocation from the gut. *Surgery* 1988; 104:185.

79. Rush BF, Sori AJ, Murphy TF, et al: Endotoxemia and bacteremia during hemorrhagic shock. *Ann Surg* 1988; 207:549.

80. Moore FA, Moore EE, Poggetti R, et al: Gut bacterial translocation via the portal vein: A clinical prospective with major torso trauma. *J Trauma* 1991; 31:629.

81. Moore FA, Moore EE, Poggetti RS, et al: Postinjury shock and early

bacteremia—a lethal combination. *Arch Surg* 1992; 127:893.

82. Wells CL, Maddaus MA, Simmons RL: Proposed mechanisms for the translocation of intestinal bacteria. *Rev Infect Dis* 1988; 10:958.

83. Marshall JC, Christou NV, Horn R, et al: The microbiology of multiple organ failure. *Arch Surg* 1988; 123:309.

84. Driks MR, Craven DE, Celli BR, et al: Nosocomial pneumonia in intubated patients given sucralfate as compared with antacids or histamine type 2 blockers. *N Engl J Med* 1987; 317:1376.

85. Cerra FB, Maddaus MA, Dunn DL, et al: Selective gut decontamination reduces nosocomial infections and length of stay but not mortality or organ failure in surgical intensive care unit patients. *Arch Surg* 1992; 127:163.

86. Horwitz RI: Complexity and contradiction in clinical trial research. *Am J Med* 1987; 82:498.

87. Freeman JA, Chalmers TC, Smith H, et al: The importance of beta, the type II error and sample size in the design and interpretation of randomized control trials. *N Engl J Med* 1978; 299:690.

88. Detsky AS, Baker JP, O'Rourke K, et al: Perioperative parenteral nutrition: A meta-analysis. *Ann Intern Med* 1987; 107:195.

89. Naylor CD, Detsky AS, O'Rourke K, et al: Does treatment with essential amino acids and hypertonic glucose improve survival in acute renal failure? A meta-analysis. *Renal Failure* 1987; 10:141.

90. Naylor CD, O'Rourke K, Detsky AS, et al: Parenteral nutrition with branched-chain amino acids in hepatic encephalopathy—A meta-analysis. *Gastroenterology* 1989; 97:1033.

91. Sacks HS, Berrier J, Reitman D, et al: Meta-analysis of randomized controlled trials. *N Engl J Med* 1987; 316:450.

92. L'Abbe KA, Detsky AS, O'Rourke K: Meta-analysis in clinical research. *Ann Intern Med* 1987; 107:224.

93. Weltz CR, Morris JB, Mullen JL: Surgical jejunostomy in aspiration risk patients. *Ann Surg* 1992; 215:140.

94. Strong RM, Condan SC, Solinger MR, et al: Equal aspiration rates from post-

pylorus and intragastric feeding tubes: A randomized, prospective study. *JPEN* 1992; 16:59.

95. Moore FA, Haenel JB, Moore EE, et al: Percutaneous tracheostomy/ gastrostomy in the brain injured patient—a minimally invasive alternative. *J Trauma* 1992; 33:435.

96. Disario JA, Fouth PG, Sanowski RA: Poor results with percutaneous endoscopic jejunostomy. *Gastrointest Endosc* 1990; 36:257.

97. Woolfsen HC, Kozarek RA, Ball TJ, et al: Tube dysfunction following percutaneous endoscopic gastrostomy and jejunostomy. *Gastrointest Endosc* 1990; 36:261.

32

Burns

Angelo Chiarelli, M.D.

Luca Siliprandi, M.D.

Pathophysiology of burn injury

Assessment of nutritional status and caloric need in the burned patient

Nutrient composition

Carbohydrates

Proteins

Lipids

Methods of nutrient delivery

Oral diet

Tube feeding

Parenteral nutritional support

Evaluation of the effectiveness of nutritional support

Complications of nutritional care

PATHOPHYSIOLOGY OF BURN INJURY

Major burn injury is the most severe form of stress documented in humans. The postburn period is characterized by a hypermetabolic and hypercatabolic state that results in visceral protein loss, weight loss, impaired antibacterial host defenses, and delayed wound healing.[1-4] In severely burned patients, *energy expenditure* increases to support wound healing, hyperdynamic circulation, accelerated respiratory drive, and protein flux.[5] Exposed wounds, relative environmental hypothermia and dryness, pain, anxiety, muscle activity, surgical procedures, vomiting, diarrhea, excessive sweating, sepsis, and bone fractures contribute to the increased metabolic rate in burn patients.[5] In addition, the daily fluid loss

from large burns can reach 6 to 8 L.[6] Despite these large demands for increased energy, burn patients appear to be internally warm,[7] thus suggesting that there is an increase in energy production relative to energy demands. Burns covering 10% to 15% of the body surface rarely show significant increases in the metabolic rate. However, in more extended lesions a close relationship exists between burn size and increased metabolic rate. The metabolic rate may increase 2 to 2.25 times the normal values.[8, 9] These values are close to the maximum increase possible. In fact, patients with greater than 50% body burns are not capable of further increases in metabolic rate.[4]

Fluid and protein losses must be controlled to limit energy dissipation and consequently the hypermetabolic response and weight loss. These goals can be partially reached through control of the above-mentioned stressful events, but nutrition must receive priority among the many aspects of burn care. To provide burn patients with optimal nutritional support the following steps must be considered[8]:

- Assessment of the nutritional and metabolic status and caloric need
- Formulation of an adequate nutritional plan, with consideration of both the amount of calories and the nutrient's composition
- Determination of the best method for nutrient delivery
- Monitoring and evaluation of the effectiveness of the nutritional support

ASSESSMENT OF NUTRITIONAL STATUS AND CALORIC NEED IN THE BURNED PATIENT

Nutrient administration in burn patients must be optimized. Energy loss must be restored while avoiding insufficient caloric intake as well as caloric or fluid excess (to limit the risk of hepatic steatosis and impaired ventilatory function). Accurate assessment of the patient's nutritional status on admission and during hospitalization is essential to ensure a good nutritional regimen both quantitatively and qualitatively. Pre-existing malnutrition and its etiologies must be assessed on admission, particularly in infant and elderly patients.[10] The clinical, dietary, and weight history as well as physical examination are valuable tools. A premorbid weight of less than 90% of the desirable weight for height reflects a significant decrement in energy stores.[5] A number of clinical, biochemical, anthropometric, and immunologic reference parameters may be used to assess nutritional status. However, these traditional parameters are relatively inaccurate in burn patients (Table 32-1), and their results can be distorted by medical/sur-

TABLE 32-1.

Parameters for Assessing the Nutritional Status of the Burned Patient: Pitfalls

Anthropometric indices
  Presence of third-degree burn
  Edema
  Donor sites
Body weight
  Edema
  Dressing and casts
  Escharectomies, amputations
  Technical difficulties of weighing
  Scarce precision of the balance
Visceral protein concentration
  Increased space of distribution
  Increased rates of synthesis and catabolism
  Intravenous fluid and transfusion
  Exudative wound loss
  Infection
  Renal or hepatic failure
Hematologic and immunologic indices
  Pre-existing anemia
  Hepatic impairment
  Infection
  Stress response
Nitrogen balance
  Burn exudation
  Immobility
  Variability in the total urinary nonurea nitrogen

gical treatments.[11] Therefore, assessment of energy expenditure remains the fundamental means of evaluating the caloric requirement in these patients.[1] The total energy expenditure can be *estimated* by using formulas or directly *measured* by indirect calorimetry. Among the several formulas proposed (Table 32-2), Curreri's formula[1] is the most widely used and also the one preferred by the authors. The advantages of using a formula include virtually no cost, simplicity, and reasonable accuracy.[1] Since this approach may overestimate the patient's nutritional needs,[12] effective monitoring of the patient is important during follow-up.[8] While direct calorimetry is of little use in routine clinical care,[1] the efficacy of *indirect calorimetry* in the nutritional care of burn patients has been demonstrated.[12] However, no study has demonstrated a clinical superiority of indirect calorimetry over formulas. Since metabolic changes occur more rapidly than clinical

TABLE 32–2.

Formulas Proposed for Energy Requirement Estimation in the Burned Patient

Reference	Age (yr)	BSAB* (%)	Calories per Day	Protein per Day
Curreri[1]	0–1	Any	BMR* + 15/%BSAB	
	1–3	Any	BMR + 25/%BSAB	
	4–15	Any	BMR + 40/%BSAB	
	16–59	Any	25/kg* + 40/%BSAB	
	>60	Any	20/kg + 65/%BSAB	
Modified Harris-Benedict[1]	Any		Calculated or measured RMR* × M (M range = 1.3–2.0)	
Wilmore[4]	Adult	>40	2,000/m²	94 g/m²
Davies and Liljedahl[5]	Adult	Any	20/kg + 70/%BSAB	1 g/kg + 3 g/% BSAB
	Child	Any	60/kg + 35/%BSAB	3 g/kg + 1 g/% BSAB
Burke and Wolfe[1]	Adult	Any	2 × BMR	2.5 g/kg
	Child	Any	2 × BMR	3–5 g/kg
Galveston I[1]	Any	Any	1,800/m² + 2,200/m² burn	
Galveston II[1]	Any	Any	1,800/m² + 1,300/m² burn	
RDA[5]	0.0–0.5	Any	115/kg	
	0.5–1.0	Any	105/kg	
	1–3	Any	100/kg	
	4–10	Any	85/kg	
	M: 11–14	Any	60/kg	
	F: 11–14	Any	48/kg	
Grotte[8]	0–1	<20	125/kg	0.45 g (N)/kg
		> 20	150/kg	0.5 g (N)/kg
	1–8	<20	100/kg	0.3 g (N)/kg
		>20	125/kg	0.45 g (N)/kg
	8–15	< 20	75/kg	0.23 g (N)/kg
		> 20	100/kg	0.3 g (N)/kg
O'Neil[7]	1–3	<20	110/kg	
		> 20	100/kg + 25/%BSAB	
	4–6	<20	85/kg	
		>20	70/kg + 35/%BSAB	
	7-10	< 20	80/kg	
		> 20	60/kg + 35/%BSAB	
	11–14	<20	55/kg	
		>20	50/kg + 35/%BSAB	
		<20	35/kg	
		>20	25/kg + 40/%BSAB	

*BSAB = body surface area burned; BMR = basal metabolic rate; Kg = kilograms of body weight; RMR = resting metabolic rate.

changes, we believe that formulas are more convenient in the less severe patients and in the later phases of illness. Indirect calorimetry may be more useful during the acute phase of illness and in the more critical patients.

NUTRIENT COMPOSITION

After calculating the total caloric requirement, the quality of the diet should be considered next.

Carbohydrates

Requirements of carbohydrates increase after burn injury. Anaerobic glycolysis is the major metabolic pathway for the synthesis of adenosine triphosphate (ATP). Adequate supply of carbohydrate provides energy and has major protein-sparing effects. Carbohydrate supply may be limited by glucose intolerance, excess CO_2 production and respiratory reserve, and the necessity for fluid restriction. These conditions are frequently observed in burn patients.[5]

It has been estimated that only 5 to 7 mg/kg/min of intravenously administered glucose can be completely oxidized to CO_2 and water[5] and 1500 to 1600 kcal/day is regarded as being the maximum calories that can be provided as carbohydrate in the burn patient.[10]

Proteins

The central nutritional problem in burn patients is the obligatory mobilization and oxidation of proteins, which diminish as wound healing occurs. Over 200 g of protein per day is lost by a fasting severely burned patient as a consequence of both wound exudation and skeletal muscle protein breakdown. Protein-calorie undernutrition results in rapid loss of skeletal muscle proteins, visceral and plasma protein wasting, impaired wound healing, and diminished host defense mechanisms. Even with aggressive protein feeding, it appears impossible to inhibit protein catabolism during the first week of burn injury. The goal of nutritional support is to achieve nitrogen balance by the third week and weight gain by the time the burn wound is nearly closed. It is important to minimize net protein losses during the early stages of illness and to maximize lean tissue synthesis during the convalescent period.[5] Even if treatment that includes aggressive protein feeding improves the survival of burn patients,[2] "the optimum amount of protein required for wound healing and maintenance of lean tissue mass is still a matter of speculation."[5] In general, 20 to 25 g of nitrogen per day is required during the first 2 weeks after a burn.[6] Several formulas have been suggested for calculating protein needs in burn patients (see Table 33–2). A nonprotein calorie-to-nitrogen ratio varying from a minimum of 100 to a maximum of 200 kcal/g N has been recommended.[6, 8–10] Intact proteins are preferred to free amino acids since the form of the nitrogen source may influence the hypermetabolic response.[13]

Lipids

Lipid administration is also important for the nutritional support of burn patients. Lipids can be infused as iso-osmolar emulsions. Their high caloric content allows for a reduction in glucose intake. In addition, large quantities of potential energy can be administered in relatively small volumes.[6] Furthermore, fat acts as a carrier for fat-soluble vitamins, protects hepatic microsomal enzyme function,[10] and prevents essential fatty acid (particularly linoleic acid) deficiency. These effects may have an influence on the response to stress, wound healing, and hypertrophic scar formation.[14] The amount of lipid administered and its composition have a profound influence on the metabolic, immunologic, and inflammatory responses.[12] However, the optimal amount of fat to be given in seriously burned patients is not yet established. In general, it is recommended that fat not provide more than 50% of energy needs. The primary caloric source should be carbohydrates.[6, 13, 14] During the last few years, some investigators have suggested that energy requirements be met by providing equal quantities of carbohydrate and lipid, particularly when parenteral nutrition is contemplated.[15] On the other hand, others recommend the use of enteral formulas with 30% to 45% consisting of lipid calories.[16–19] These suggestions differ from the traditional approach of administering 5% to 15% fat calories.[1, 14]

METHODS OF NUTRIENT DELIVERY

Five different methods of nutrient delivery are available for the nutritional support of critically ill patients. From the simple and more physiologic to the more invasive, these methods are oral diet with or without oral supplements, tube feeding, tube feeding plus peripheral or central vein nutrient supplementation, and total parenteral nutrition, (TPN). Patients may receive nutritional support via different routes during their stay in the burn unit. It is also common to simultaneously nourish a burn patient via two or even three routes. Aggressive nutritional support is always indicated. However, no rigid guidelines exist for determining the best method of nutrient delivery. The route of nutrient delivery must be individualized to maintain adequate intake and avoid malnutrition. Factors influencing nutrient delivery and the route of support include clinical management (surgery, medications), daily caloric and fluid requirements (preburn malnutrition, burn size and depth, the ideal-actual body weight ratio), fever and infection, physical activity (mental status, skeletal injuries), underlying disease (e.g., diabetes mellitus), gastrointestinal complications (diarrhea, vomiting, gastric residuals, ileus), rejected skin grafts, and renal, hepatic, or pulmonary failure.[12, 20]

Oral Diet

This is the most physiologic route for nutrient delivery and must be encouraged. A high-protein, high-calorie oral diet can be maintained in many severely burned patients (i.e., up to 60% of the body surface area) if they are able to masticate and swallow.[8, 9] Liquid or semiliquid supplements should be given to patients who do not meet 75% of their calorie requirements[8] and in those with pre-existing malnutrition.[10] However, 3000 kcal/day often represents the maximum amount that can be administered orally.[6] Lack of interest in food, anorexia, and the inability to transfer food from the plate to the mouth and then chew it (as in the case of hand burns, burns of the upper limbs and face) are all features that interfere with optimal oral nutrition and require some form of supplementation. Enteral nutrients can be delivered with fine-bore nasogastric or nasoduodenal tubes. These tubes allow the patient to eat around the tube.

Tube feeding supplements may be administered at night to permit normal activity, appetite, and feeding behavior during the day.[10] Supplemental nutrients may be administered through a peripheral vein (i.e., 5% glucose, amino acids, and lipids). Intravenous nutrients should be given when the daily caloric need cannot be satisfied by the sole use of enteral feeding. Such is the case when very high calorie requirements are needed or when nausea, vomiting, or an excessive, continuous gastric residual is present. We often use "mixed nutrition" in the most severely burned patients. We prefer to administer supplemental nutrients, enterally or intravenously, during the night to make up for the nutrients that the patient was unable to introduce orally during the day. The patient is fasted in the early morning to favor spontaneous food intake during the morning hours.

Tube Feeding (Enteral Nutrition)

Tube feeding is indicated for patients unable or unwilling to consume 75% of their calorie and protein requirements orally, provided that normal upper gastrointestinal function is present.[8] We never exceed the limit of 2000 mL/24 hr and 7.5 kJ/mL, which respectively represent the maximum volume and concentration tolerated by most adult patients.[9] An infusion rate of 125 mL/hr represents the maximum tolerated rate in the adult burn patient on the fourth postburn day.[8] Intravenous supplements should be given whenever gastrointestinal complications ensue or when enteral feeding is insufficient to meet daily caloric needs.

Traditionally, enteral feeding is not begun until gastrointestinal function has returned to normal after the acute fluid resuscitation period (i.e., by the fourth postburn day) because of the fear that immediate feeding will cause more complications than delayed feeding.[6, 9] However, increasing experimental evidence indicates that *immediate*[20] and

A

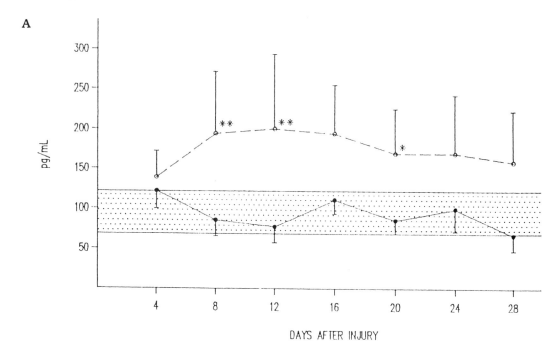

B

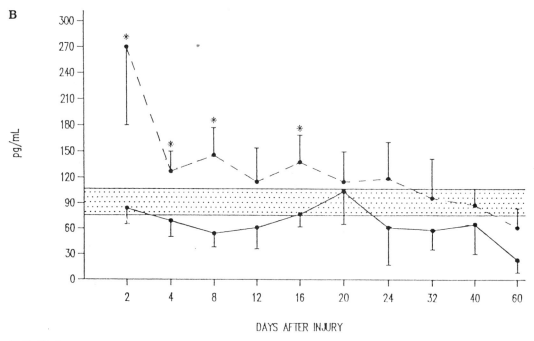

FIG 32–1.
Effect of very early enteral nutrition on the plasma glucagon concentration (mean ± SEM) with proprietary **(A)** and commercially available **(B)** preparations. * $P < .05$; ** $P < .01$; *filled circles*, burn patients fed 5 hours postburn; *open circles*, control subjects (burned patients fed 48 hours postburn). The normal range is in the *shaded area*. (From Chiarelli A, Enzi G, Casadei A, et al: *Am J Clin Nutr* 1990; 51:1035.)

A

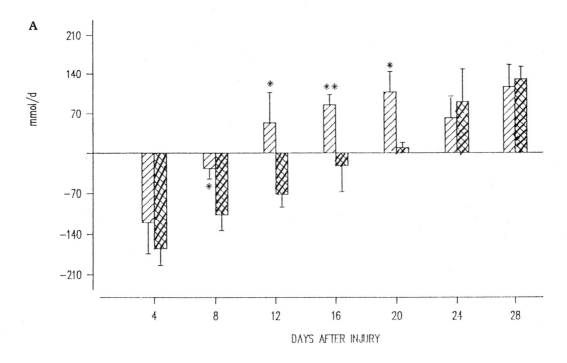

B

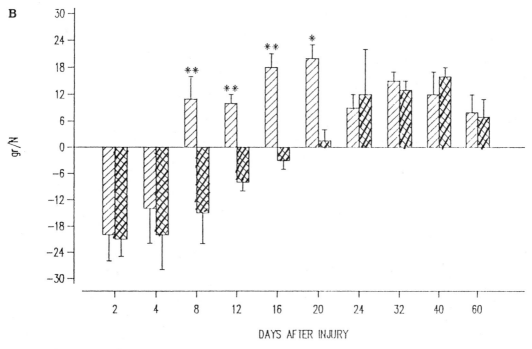

FIG 32–2.
Effect of very early enteral nutrition (5 hours postburn) on nitrogen balance (mean ± SEM) with proprietary **(A)** and commercially available **(B)** preparations. * $P < .05$; ** $P < .01$; *shaded bars,* burned patients fed 5 hours postburn; *cross-hatched bars,* control subjects (burned patients fed 48 hours postburn). (Redrawn from Chiarelli A, Enzi G, Casadei A, et al: *Am J Clin Nutr* 1990; 51:1035.

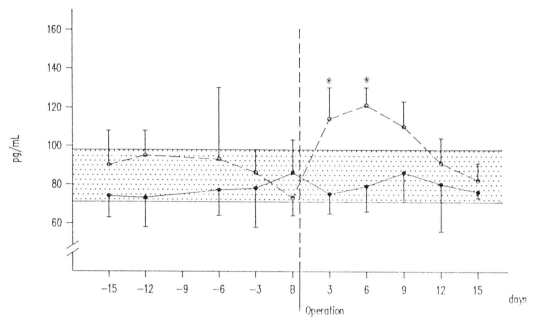

FIG 32–3.

Basal plasma glucagon levels (mean ± SEM) in burned patients before and after surgery for wound excision and autograft coverage. *Filled circles,* patients enterally fed 2 hours after surgery; *open circles,* control subjects (patients enterally fed on the second day after surgery; *P* < .05. (Adapted from Enzi G, Casadei A, Sergi G, et al: *Crit Care Med* 1990; 18:719.)

early[16, 21] nutrition is helpful in the control of the hypercatabolic and hypermetabolic responses to thermal trauma. It is hypothesized that decreased gut perfusion coupled with the lack of enteral feeding early after burn injury results in acute atrophy of the intestinal villi and in the translocation of bacteria, endotoxins, and other active substances into the lymphatic and portal circulation. The consequent activation of the complement cascade and the arachidonic pathway stimulates secondary rises in cortisol, glucagon, and catecholamine levels that contribute to the hypermetabolic response and to multiple organ failure.[13] Several clinical studies in severely burned patients fed orally or by nasogastric[16, 19] or nasoduodenal[21] tubes demonstrate beneficial effects of immediate or early enteral nutrition on nitrogen balance, serum protein levels, and immunocompetence. There is a reduction in the metabolic rate and catabolic processes. Adverse effects such as diarrhea or paralytic ileus are rare. The absorptive ability of the small intestine

early after thermal injury is not completely inhibited, even in the most critically ill patients.[19] In a study performed recently at the Padua Burn Unit,[20] patients fed within 5 hours of burn injury showed normal levels of urinary catecholamines. On the other hand, patients fed after 48 hours showed abnormally elevated levels of catecholamines that persisted until the 16th day after the burn. Furthermore, the early fed patients had lower glucagon (Fig 32–1) and higher insulin blood levels. Nitrogen balance became positive earlier (Fig 32–2), and there was reduced weight loss. The number of positive blood cultures was lower and the hospitalization time shorter with early feeding. Similar findings were obtained for early nutritional supplementation in burn patients after surgery[22] (Fig 32–3). We hypothesize that early supplementation of carbohydrates and other nutrients prevents a decrease in insulin secretion that enhances glucose utilization in burned tissues. Decreased gluconeogenesis from visceral and muscle protein results in a protein-sparing effect. These observations indicate that the 12- to 24-hour period after a burn injury is critical for the control of energy balance. Very early enteral nutrition represents a safe and well-tolerated therapeutic approach to prevent burn-induced increases in catecholamine and glucagon secretion and leads to improved control of the hypercatabolic state and an improved clinical course for burn patients. Additional advantages of immediate enteral feeding[16] include avoidance of anorexia and improved patient well-being. Our policy is to feed burn patients immediately after admission. A semiliquid ready-to-use food source containing 1 kcal/mL is given orally or through a nasogastric tube connected to refrigerated infusion pumps at a 50-mL/hr rate. Forty-eight hours after the injury the infusion rate is augmented to 80 mL/hr and progressively to higher rates according to patient requirements until a limit of 125 to 150 mL/hr is reached.

Parenteral Nutritional Support

Parenteral nutrition can be given either as supplementation to enteral nutrition or as TPN. Supplementation through a peripheral vein is required in patients unable to satisfy their daily energy requirements by enteral nutrition alone. Surgery imposes a further metabolic load on the burn patient, and may cause the loss of as much as a day's nutrition.[10] Pasulka and Wachtel[5] calculated that a maximum of 1400 to 1700 calories per day can be delivered by using a mixture of amino acids, 10% dextrose, and lipids as peripheral parenteral nutrition. The scarce availability of peripheral veins and their intolerance to hyperosmolar solutions limit the use of peripheral parenteral nutrition as the sole source of nutrition in patients unable to tolerate enteral feeding. Because of its disadvantages, TPN should be used as the sole nutritional support only as a last resort when the more physiologic method of enteral feeding is insuf-

ficient or contraindicated (as in the case of paralysis of the ileus) and when the utilization of peripheral veins is restricted. When TPN is used in burn patients, one must consider the unusually large need for nitrogen and calories, the restricted availability of unburned skin sites for line placement, and the high risk of sepsis resulting from central line contamination or infection. Daily protein requirements approach 140 g.[6] Carbohydrates and lipids are administered to meet the total daily caloric requirements. Glucose is limited to 5 to 7 mg/kg/min, and the remainder of the energy requirements are provided as lipids.[5] The antecubital vein is preferred. However, subclavian puncture often remains the only reliable venous access site, and sometimes it may even be necessary to perform the puncture through the burned area.[6] To diminish the risk of sepsis and suppurative thrombophlebitis, the line should be inserted with aseptic technique in the cleanest possible environment. The skin should be punctured as far as possible from vein entry.[10] Central lines should be changed every second or third day. Manipulations of the central venous catheter for blood sampling or transfusion should be avoided.[6] Catheters should be cultured upon removal to allow for identification of contaminated insertion sites.

EVALUATION OF THE EFFECTIVENESS OF NUTRITIONAL SUPPORT

In addition to assessment of the nutritional status on admission, it is important to monitor the quantity and quality of nutritional support. Many clinical, anthropometric, biohumoral, and immunologic parameters are available for this purpose. However, none of these are reliable alone, and they should be used in conjunction with others. Burn wound appearance must be frequently and meticulously monitored. Body weight should be measured twice weekly in severely burned patients to assess *weight change over time.* Several factors contribute to weight loss in severely burned patients. These include increased catabolism, hypermetabolism, protein loss from wound surfaces, immobilization, frequent surgery, sepsis, anorexia, nausea, diarrhea, and delayed wound closure.[9] Losses exceeding 10% to 15% of body weight result primarily from inadequate nutritional care. Body weight in the burned patient can be distorted by several factors (see Table 32–1). Weight elevations may result from resuscitative fluid administration. The premorbid weight[9] or the "dry" body weight measured immediately after admission[11] should be used for the calculation of nutritional needs. Correction of weight loss for escharectomy requires measurement of the total weight of excised tissue.[11] Overestimation of weight because of dressings can be avoided by weighing the patient at dressing changes.[10] Henley[10] suggests using the *body mass index* instead of body weight. *Anthropometric measurements* may be unreliable because of the presence of burns, donor sites, and interstitial edema.[10, 11] Blood transfusions, fluid shifts, direct protein losses from wounds, increased synthetic and catabolic rates, infection, and renal or hepatic failure may limit the significance of *serum proteins* and *creatinine-height index* determinations, especially during the early stage of illness.[5, 10, 11] Hemolysis, immunodepression, hepatic impairment, pre-existing anemia, and overhydration can distort the value of *hematologic and immunologic indices.* Evaluation of *nitrogen balance* may be troublesome because of a lack of precise measurements of nitrogen utilization for anabolism rather than for energy, the difficulty in evaluating nitrogen losses resulting from burn exudation or immobility, and the considerable variability in total urinary nonurea nitrogen.[10, 11] Furthermore, excessive protein intake can improve nitrogen balance without increasing net synthesis of lean tissue or benefiting the patient.[5] *Isotopes and neutron activation analysis, bioelectrical impedance analysis, total-body electrical conductivity,* and *near-infrared interaction* are new methods claimed to be useful in the assessment of nutritional status. However, each of them has limitations when applied to burned patients.[10]

COMPLICATIONS OF NUTRITIONAL CARE

Insufficient calorie and protein intake induces skeletal and visceral protein wasting and consequently immunodepression and impaired wound healing. However, overfeeding of patients may be as dangerous as underfeeding. The risk of feed-related complications can be diminished by the use of peristaltic pumps that allow for constant control of the infusion rate.

The side effects of early enteral nutrition on the gastrointestinal tract are generally mild and infrequent. They can be limited by modification of the amount and rate of nutrient administration.[20] The risk of septicemia resulting from long-term use of central venous catheters is higher in burn patients than in other critically ill patients because of heavy bacterial colonization of wounds, the frequency of bacteremias, and immunodepression. Catheter infections are usually caused by repeated bacteremias rather than by direct entry of bacteria during the puncture.[6]

REFERENCES

1. Curreri PW: Assessing nutritional needs for the burned patient. *J Trauma* 1990; 30:20.
2. McDonald WS, Sharp CW, Deitch EA: Immediate enteral feeding in burn patients is safe and effective. *Ann Surg* 1991; 213:177.
3. Wilmore DW: Pathophysiology of the hypermetabolic response to burn injury. *J Trauma* 1990; 30:4.

4. Davies JWL: *Physiological Responses to Burning Injury*. London, Academic Press, 1982, p 424.

5. Pasulka PS, Wachtel TL: Nutritional considerations for the burned patient. *Surg Clin North Am* 1987; 67:109.

6. Kauste A: Parenteral and enteral nutrition of the thermally injured patients. *Ann Chir Gynaecol* 1980; 69:197.

7. Wilmore DW, Aulick LH, Mason AD, et al: Influence of the burn wound on local and systemic response to injury. *Ann Surg* 1977; 186:444.

8. O'Neil C, Roeber J: Burn care protocols—nutritional support. *J Burn Care Rehabil* 1986; 7:351.

9. Jacobs LS, de Kock M, van der Merwe AE: Oral hyperalimentation and the prevention of severe weight loss in burned patients. *Burns* 1987; 13:154.

10. Henley M: Feed that burn. *Burns* 1989; 15:351.

11. Murphy M, Bell SJ: Assessment of nutritional status in burn patients. *J Burn Care Rehabil* 1988; 9:432.

12. Ireton-Jones CS: Use of indirect calorimetry in burn care. *J Burn Care Rehabil* 1988; 9:526.

13. Alexander JW: Nutrition and infection. New perspectives for an old problem. *Arch Surg* 1986; 121:966.

14. Gottschlich MS, Alexander JW: Fat kinetics and recommended dietary intake in burns. *JPEN* 1987; 11:80.

15. Macfie J: Towards cheaper intravenous nutrition. *BMJ* 1986; 292:107.

16. Kaufman T, Hirshowitz B, Moscona R, et al: Early enteral nutrition for mass burn injury: The revised egg-rich diet. *Burns* 1986; 12:260.

17. Klasen HJ, ten Duis HJ: Early oral feeding of patients with extensive burns. *Burns* 1987; 13:49.

18. Ioannovich J, Llakakos Th, Panayotou P, et al: Tolerance and complications of early enteral nutrition in burns. *Ann Mediterranean Burns Club* 1989; 3:95.

19. Sologub VK, Zaets TL, Tarasov AV, et al: Enteral hyperalimentation of burned patients: The possibility of correcting metabolic disorders by the early administration of prolonged high calorie evenly distributed tube feeds. *Burns* 1992; 18:245.

20. Chiarelli A, Enzi G, Casadei A, et al: Very early nutrition supplementation in burned patients. *Am J Clin Nutr* 1990; 51:1035.

21. McArdle AH, Palmason C, Brown RA, et al: Early enteral feeding in patients with major burns: Prevention of catabolism. *Ann Plast Surg* 1984; 13:396.

22. Enzi G, Casadei A, Sergi G, et al: Metabolic and hormonal effects of early nutritional supplementation after surgery in burn patients. *Crit Care Med* 1990; 18:719.

33

Sepsis

Michael D. Peck, M.D., Sc.D.

Deleterious effects of overfeeding

Route of feeding

Choice of nutrients for septic patient

  Lipids

  Glutamine

  Arginine

Review of current products

  Specialized enteral support of stressed patients

Recommendations

Guidelines for the use of enteral and total parenteral nutrition (TPN) in hospitalized patients have been established by the board of directors of the American Society of Parenteral and Enteral Nutrition.[1, 2] As noted in their introduction, "There is no disease process that benefits from starvation." The following are examples of clinical settings in which enteral or parenteral nutrition should be a part of routine care:

1. Normal nutritional status with less than 50% of the required nutrient intake for the previous 7 to 10 days
2. Protein-calorie malnutrition with inadequate intake of nutrients for the previous 5 days
3. Severely catabolic patients with or without malnutrition when adequate oral intake is not anticipated within 5 to 7 days

It can easily be appreciated that the septic patient qualifies for nutritional support for a variety of reasons. Some patients may have an acute infectious event complicating an underlying chronic condition, such as cancer, that has left them malnourished. In others, the progression of infection has been accompanied by anorexia, and oral intake for several days prior to admission may have been inadequate. Finally, patients with the sepsis syndrome, particularly those in septic shock, will be hypercatabolic and may be suffering from paralytic ileus or may have diarrhea, thus precluding use of the gastrointestinal tract.[3]

Although the hypercatabolism of sepsis and the consumption of lean body mass are concepts that are unchallenged, there have been few prospective studies that have investigated the therapeutic value of nutritional support during sepsis. The studies that have been done suggest that adequate nutritional support in a patient compromised by injury, malnutrition, cancer, or other stress will prevent the occurrence of septic episodes and lessen their severity. Since it has not been demonstrated that

WHAT IS SEPSIS?

It is important to establish a few definitions of common terms that overlap in meaning. In this chapter, *infection* is defined as proliferation and invasion of the host by microorganisms beyond what is commonly accepted as commensal colonization. *Sepsis* is the systemic evidence of infection, that is, tachypnea, tachycardia, and hypothermia or hyperthermia.[4] *Sepsis syndrome* is sepsis with evidence of altered organ perfusion, including hypoxemia, lactic acidosis, and oliguria.[4] *Septic shock* is the sepsis syndrome with hypotension.[4] *Multiple organ failure syndrome* (MOFS) is a group of signs and symptoms related to the failure of various organ systems, which may occur as sequelae to sepsis.[5, 6]

aggressive nutritional support during the septic state affects outcome, we should be directed by the adage *primum non nocere* and make sure that we are doing no harm to our septic patients with the formulas that we use.

What are the consequences of the hypercatabolic state that accompanies sepsis? Depletion of glycogen stores occurs early, as it does in other stressed patients, and the body is left to mobilize stored triglycerides for fuel. In addition, there is marked catabolism of skeletal muscle protein, and in an unfed patient up to 250 g of body protein will be broken down each day.[7, 8] Some of the freed amino acids provide fuel via gluconeogenesis, but even in the face of apparently adequate provision of glucose there is continued mobilization of amino acids.[9, 10] It has been suggested that the purpose of this response is to provide glutamine for enterocytes and leukocytes, thus explaining the persistence of what otherwise appears to be a nonadaptive response.[11, 12] Whatever the cause, prolonged catabolism of skeletal muscle protein leaves the patient debilitated, compromises respiratory function, impairs wound healing, exac-

erbates immunosuppression, accelerates the loss of strength and endurance necessary for recovery, and increases the risk of death.

As mentioned above, even apparently adequate nutritional support may not abrogate the hypermetabolic response. Eight surgical intensive care patients with both respiratory failure and septic shock had total-body water, protein, and fat measured before and after 10 days of TPN (Fig 33–1).[9] Intravenous nutrition support provided 34.1 kcal/kg nonprotein calories and 1.82 g/kg protein per day. Half of the nonprotein calories were given as carbohydrate and half as fat. Enteral feedings were not given during this period. Most changes in weight during the 10-day study period were due to changes in body water. However, there was a mean loss of 12.5% of total-body protein. In addition, there was a mean gain of 2.2 kg of fat. These results suggest that nutritional support in septic patients does not prevent the loss of total-body protein, although there is an increase in energy stores.

The beneficial effect of nutritional support may be due to increased synthetic rates rather than to diminished breakdown. Shaw and associates used isotopic techniques to estimate rates of whole-body protein synthesis and breakdown in septic patients and in normal human volunteers.[13] Twenty-two septic patients were studied, 14 with abscesses and 15 with associated organ dysfunction. Nonprotein calories were provided as 50% glucose and 50% lipid in the form of TPN. From the flux of radioisotopically labeled lysine, they observed that septic patients have increases in both protein catabolism and synthesis (41% and 15%, respectively, vs. controls). Neither glucose infusion (at a mean rate of 3.8 mg/kg/min) nor TPN altered the rate of protein catabolism. However, both glucose and TPN infusions significantly increased the rate of protein synthesis, thus reducing net protein catabolism. Interestingly, the

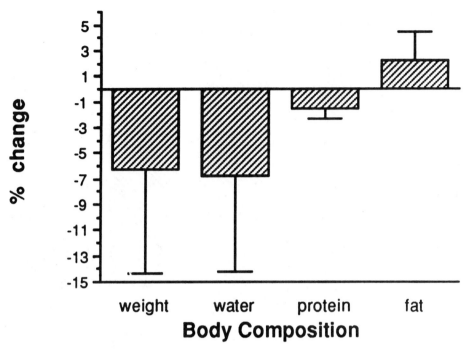

FIG 33–1.
Components of body composition were measured before and after 10 days of intravenous nutrition in eight septic patients. Despite aggressive nutritional support, there were significant losses of body weight and protein. (Data from Streat SJ, Beddoe AH, Hill GL: *J Trauma* 1987;27: 262–266.)

authors noted that increasing the protein infusion rate beyond 1.5 g/kg/day had no further effect on net protein catabolism.

Sepsis is associated with hypercatabolism, which in itself may prolong or intensify the response to infection. Previous attempts to prevent this hypercatabolism by using traditional methods of nutritional support have not been successful, although the degree of lean body wasting can be lessened. Perhaps more benefit can be derived from new approaches to nutritional support in the septic patient in such areas as estimation of caloric needs, route of feeding, and composition of formulas.

DELETERIOUS EFFECTS OF OVERFEEDING

Prior to the pioneering work of Dudrick,[14] there were no effective means by which sufficient quantities of carbohydrates and amino acids could be delivered to patients intolerant of oral intake. With the advent of TPN delivered via central venous catheters and managed by multidisciplinary teams, hyperalimentation could be safely administered to septic and other critically ill patients. The ease with which hypercaloric solutions could be administered to patients led some clinicians to enthusiastically prescribe several thousand calories per day along with 2 to 3 g of protein per kilogram. In our enthusiasm, we must remember that more is not always better.

There are risks to hypercaloric glucose infusions. It is well recognized that the administration of TPN may be complicated by hyperglycemia and hyperosmolality, which can lead to osmotic diuresis, dehydration, and ketotic acidosis. However, most nutritional support teams are vigilant about the management of hyperglycemia, and this problem is not nearly as common as it was in the early days of TPN.

There are other risks to hypercaloric

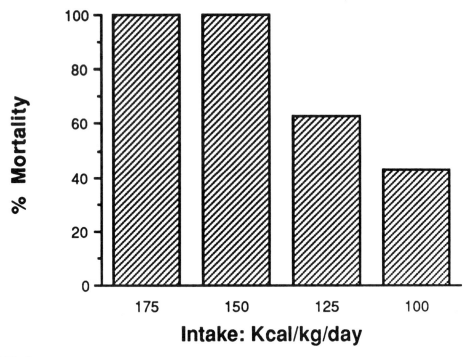

FIG 33-2.
Guinea pigs were fed enteral diets at various rates during episodes of bacterial peritonitis. Paradoxically, the animals fed the least amount (100 kcal/kg/day) had the best survival rates, although they were gaunt and emaciated by the end of the study.

feeding that are more subtle. Burke and associates studied the effect of TPN with hypercaloric glucose and amino acids administered to patients with severe burn injuries.[15] Beyond the infusion of 5 mg glucose/kg/min, there were no further increases in glucose oxidation or protein synthesis. Moreover, in nine patients who died after having received at least 3 weeks of TPN, there was evidence of severe hepatic steatosis, thus suggesting that the unoxidized glucose was stored as fat depots, possibly impairing liver function.

The hazards of overfeeding have been suggested in clinical studies. One reason for the increase in infectious complications seen in borderline or mildly malnourished adult patients receiving TPN prior to elective surgery in the Veterans Affairs (VA) TPN Cooperative Study may have been that they were fed 1000 kcal above the resting metabolic expenditure.[16]

However, animal studies have clearly established that there is a risk associated with overnutrition during infectious stress. Alexander and associates fed enteral diets to guinea pigs suffering from bacterial peritonitis (Fig 34-2).[17] In this study, guinea pigs fed pump-controlled feedings at 175 kcal/kg/day, which was a rate previously found to be optimal for restoration of immune function in burned animals,[18] had a 100% mortality rate after 2 weeks. In contrast, animals fed 100 kcal/kg/day, during which time the animals became emaciated and gaunt, had a dramatic decrease in the mortality rate to 43%. Thus, although high caloric feedings led to better maintenance of lean body mass, they had a deleterious effect on the response to infection.

Similarly, Yamazaki and associates studied the effect of overfeeding on survival and protein metabolism in rats.[19] Overfeeding was accomplished by supplying 175% of the rats' usual voluntary intake by a gastrostomy tube for 6 days prior to cecal ligation and puncture (CLP). Although the overfed rats had increased body weight gain and greater nitrogen balance before infection, they had a higher mortality rate from CLP than did controls, a lower leucine incorporation into whole-body protein, and a lower fractional synthetic rate of serum albumin. The authors suggested that

> Overnutrition, the reciprocal of undernutrition, may also be a risk factor in hospitalized patients in terms of susceptibility to infection as well as to altered protein metabolism. Because severely stressed patients have a reduced capacity to utilize exogenous energy sources, nutritional therapies that aim to maximize nitrogen balance may adversely affect host responses when given in excess of energy needs.[19]

Since in both of these animal studies overfeeding of all nutrients was performed, it is not clear which individual nutrients were responsible for the observed results. In follow-up to the experiments in septic guinea pigs performed in Alexander's laboratory,[17] my associates and I were able to demonstrate that underfeeding of protein improved survival in this model and that this effect may have been related to diminished levels of plasma ammonia.[20, 21] However, the degree to which protein was restricted was severe (roughly equivalent to 0.5 g/kg/day in adult humans), and these results, although intriguing, should not be used to guide clinical practice until further confirmatory work has been done.

It is clinically difficult to estimate the caloric needs of septic patients. In clinical research studies, a variety of experimental methods have been used, but the results are often contradictory. For example, Shizgal and Martin used body composition measurements determined by multiple isotopy dilution with radio-labeled sodium and water.[22] With this technique, they have estimated that the septic patient may require approximately 50 kcal/kg/day in order to maintain body cell mass. In a hypothetical 40-year-old male weighing 75 kg, this is equivalent to over 220% of the basal energy expenditure (BEE) estimated by the Harris-Benedict equation. In contrast, indirect calorimetry measurements made on 27 septic patients revealed a range of metabolic rates of 1027 to 2646 kcal/m^2/day (median, 1576 kcal/m^2/day), equivalent to 115% to 295% of the BEE (median, 176% of BEE) of our hypothetical male (body surface area [BSA], 1.92 m^2).[23] Indeed, measurements of energy expenditure by indirect calorimetry are often lower than estimates derived from standardized formulas such as the Curreri formula for burn patients.[24]

It is important to focus on the nutritional needs of the hypercatabolic patient who becomes further stressed by sepsis. Injury and major surgery are causes of hypermetabolism in critically ill patients; sepsis also induces a hypermetabolic response. The clinician is frequently faced with a patient recovering from severe injury who is already receiving hypercaloric solutions and then becomes septic. Should caloric and protein intake be increased even further in this setting?

Although certain aspects such as glucose uptake[25] do differ among patient populations, it is apparent that there is a universal stress response that characterizes both injury and infection.[10] Furthermore, once this stress response is established, further stress (such as an episode of sepsis in a patient with severe burn injuries) does not additionally increase caloric expenditure or protein catabolism (personal communication: Michele Gottschlich, Ph.D., and Robert Wolfe, Ph.D.). Thus, increased delivery of hypercaloric glucose and amino acid solutions to an injured patient who becomes septic will not provide any further benefit to the patient and may present some risk.

ROUTE OF FEEDING

Once its safety and efficacy were established, the utilization of intravenous

TPN grew rapidly. However, it is now well known that equal amounts of calories and protein can be delivered via the enteral route. Nonetheless, many physicians and surgeons believe that the parenteral route is preferred in critically ill patients, largely because the daily estimate of nutritional needs is more often met (see audience discussions of Kudsk et al.[26]). Although it is true that patients fed enterally do not always receive the prescribed number of calories because of interruptions in tube feedings or a lack of tolerance, there are several advantages to enteral feeding.

The route of administration may affect the immune response to infection. Clinical studies of enteral vs. parenteral nutrition in trauma patients have shown that septic complications and the elevation of levels of acute-phase proteins were lower in the group fed enterally.[26-28] The results of these well-designed studies show that enteral feeding in the injured patient will decrease the incidence of sepsis.

Animal studies confirm these findings. Rats that were fed protein-deficient diets for 2 weeks and then refed with either oral or intragastric diets had improved survival after intraperitoneal challenge of *Escherichia coli* and hemoglobin when compared with animals repleted with intravenous nutrition.[29, 30] Subsequent experiments showed that simply feeding previously well-nourished animals intravenously for 12 days increased mortality when compared with intragastrically fed animals.[31]

There are several reasons why enteral feedings may be optimal for resistance to infection.[32] Recent reports have documented that biliary levels of IgA are higher with enteral diets, although the significance of this finding is not clear.[33] More importantly, enteral feedings maintain gut mucosa integrity[33-35] and thus may limit bacterial translocation.

Bacterial translocation is the movement of bacteria and endotoxin from the lumen of the gut to the lymphatic and venous drainage systems and may contribute to multiple organ failure in injured or septic patients. Alverdy and associates have shown that rats fed intravenously have a significantly higher rate of bacterial translocation from the intestine to the mesenteric lymph nodes than did animals fed orally.[36]

Unfortunately, bacterial translocation can be studied only with great difficulty in humans. Nonetheless, carefully performed studies in human subjects emphasize the importance of the route of feeding. Fong and associates studied healthy human volunteers who were randomized to receive either enteral feedings or 7 days of TPN without oral intake (Fig 34–3).[37] They were then challenged with intravenous lipopolysaccharide. Subsequent peak levels of glucagon, epinephrine, and arterial and hepatic venous tumor necrosis factor (TNF) and the efflux of lactate and amino acids from peripheral muscle were all higher in the TPN group. In a similar study, neutrophil function was also impaired by TPN.[38] The authors concluded that antecedent TPN may influence the metabolic alterations seen in infection and sepsis via both an exaggerated counterregulatory hormone response as well as an enhanced systemic and splanchnic production of cytokines.

However, there is no evidence that the route of feeding has an effect on outcome once sepsis is established. Cerra and associates studied the efficacy of enteral nutrition in preventing the progression of the sepsis syndrome to multiple organ failure syndrome (MOFS).[39] Sixty-six patients with persistent hypermetabolism 4 to 6 days after the onset of the sepsis syndrome were prospectively randomized to receive isonitrogenous and isocaloric nutrition by either the enteral or parenteral route. There were no differences in the rate of progression to MOFS or in the mortality rate. Thus, if the initiation of enteral feeding is delayed until the patient is hypermetabolic, the benefits of enteral feeding, such as protection of the gut

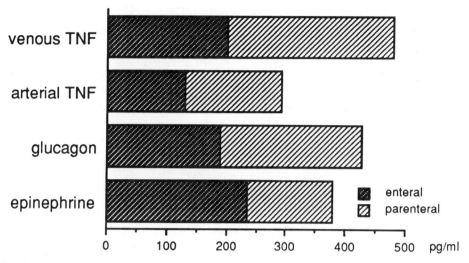

FIG 33–3.
Twelve healthy volunteers were randomized to receive 7 days of either enteral or parenteral feeding prior to challenge with endotoxin. Circulating levels of hormones and cytokines were significantly higher in the subjects treated with "bowel rest." TNF = tumor necrosis factor. (Data from Fong U, Marano MA, Barber A, et al: *Ann Surg* 1989; 210:449–457.)

against further bacterial translocation, will have no effect on outcome.

There is still merit to the adage that "if the gut works, use it," and there is sufficient evidence to support the use of enteral feeding to reduce septic morbidity in patients immunocompromised by injury or disease. Unfortunately, enteral feeding can be difficult once sepsis is established because of delayed gastric emptying and diarrhea, and there may be insufficient delivery of nutrients for these reasons. In addition, there are only sparse clinical data on the use of enteral feeding during sepsis, and what few data are available are not supportive of its use. Nonetheless, enteral feeding should be continued as long as possible in a patient who becomes septic, even if nutrient delivery has to be combined with peripheral parenteral hyperalimentation, for it is important to diminish the rate of bacterial translocation from the gut.

CHOICE OF NUTRIENTS FOR THE SEPTIC PATIENT

Once the decision has been made that nutritional support is indicated, once the calorie and nitrogen goals have been

established, and once the route of delivery has been decided upon, the clinician is faced with a variety of options of nutrient combinations with which to achieve these objectives. In the discussion that follows, emphasis will be placed on macronutrients such as lipids and amino acids, although there is abundant evidence that micronutrients such as vitamins A, E, and C, iron, and selenium also affect the immune response.[40]

Lipids

One of the first decisions to be made is whether the nonprotein calories are to be given primarily as carbohydrate or in combination with lipids. As with the increased catabolism of protein, there is general agreement that endogenous glucose production is elevated in sepsis, as evidenced by the hyperglycemia and increased requirements for exogenous insulin seen in many septic patients fed hypercaloric solutions. However, there have been concerns that glucose oxidation may be impaired.

Is there a preferred fuel source for septic patients? Although a number of well-designed studies have been performed, there is disagreement among the results. It appears that glucose oxidation is increased in sepsis and up to a certain point can provide the appropriate route of disposal for exogenously administered glucose.[41] However, above glucose administration rates of 5 to 7 mg/kg/min, there is evidence of lipogenesis, and the maximum contribution of glucose oxidation toward supplying energy needs is 50% to 60%.[41]

On the other hand, it it also known that exogenous lipids can be effectively utilized as a fuel source during sepsis.[42] Although originally intended to provide essential fatty acids to patients receiving total intravenous alimentation, lipid emulsions are now routinely used as secondary fuel sources in septic, injured, and other stressed patients. There have been concerns about their possible deleterious effects on host defense systems, but those concerns do not appear to have deterred utilization of lipid emulsions.[43] In our medical center, more than 7,500 L of 20% intravenous fat emulsion are used each year.

Despite the lack of clinical investigations on the effect of lipid emulsions on outcome in septic patients, their immunoregulatory effects should not be forgotten. For example, since lipid emulsions were designed to prevent essential fatty acid deficiency, they all are based on soybean or safflower oil, which are high in essential fatty acids such as linoleic acid. Since essential fatty acids are the sole precursors to eicosanoids, these products may alter the rate of eicosanoid production, which in turn modulates the immune response.

There have been major developments in the understanding of the role of eicosanoids (prostaglandins, thromboxanes, and leukotrienes) in the pathophysiology of illness and injury. There is also evidence that dietary fatty acid composition clearly affects eicosanoid metabolism.[44–50] Specifically, diets rich in linoleic acid result in increased amounts of dienoic prostaglandin and thromboxane production (such as prostaglandin E_2 [PGE_2] and thromboxane A_2 [TBA_2] and increased

amounts of tetraenoic leukotriene production (such as leukotriene B_4 [LTB_4]). On the other hand, diets enriched with fish oils are high in ω-3 fatty acids, the precursors to trienoic prostaglandins (e.g., PGE_3) and pentaenoic leukotrienes (e.g., LTB_5). This diversion of the metabolites of arachidonic acid has tremendous implications for modification of the immune response after injury, because PGE_2 has more potent immunosuppressive effects than its trienoic counterpart[51] and TBA_3 has much less biological potency than TBA_2.

In this regard, it is of interest to review the few studies that have been done on the relationship of dietary lipid to outcome from stress states. Parenteral feeding of fish oil emulsions to guinea pigs improved survival from a subsequent challenge with endotoxin when compared with animals fed safflower oil.[52] This beneficial effect was not as powerful when the animals were fed enterally.[53]

Manipulation of dietary fat can improve outcome parameters in burned guinea pigs. Previously gastrostomized guinea pigs were fed enteral diets with 10% of the total calories as fat, either safflower oil, linoleic acid, or fish oil, after a 30% total body surface area (TBSA) flame burn. Animals fed the fish oil diet had an improved delayed-type hypersensitivity response, smaller *Staphylococcus aureus* intradermal abscesses, larger spleens, lower resting metabolic rates, and lower serum cortisol levels.[54]

Contradictory results have come from experiments using burned mice that were subsequently infected. For 2 to 3 weeks mice were fed diets with different amounts and types of fats, including fish oil and safflower oil. They were then subjected to a 20% TBSA flame burn and challenged with *Pseudomonas aeruginosa* subeschar. Survival in the group fed a diet high in safflower oil (40% of the total calories) was significantly better than that in the group fed a diet high in fish oil.[55]

There have also been conflicting reports of the effect of lipids on survival in animal models of peritonitis. Barton and associates fed rats via gastrostomy for 5 days prior to challenge with an intra-abdominal abscess of defined bacterial content; the rats were continued on the diets for another week. The mortality rate was decreased in fish oil–fed rats when compared with safflower oil–fed animals (16% vs. 35%).[56] However, my associates and I found that guinea pigs fed by gastrostomy for 2 weeks after intraperitoneal implantation with bacteria-filled osmotic pumps showed no significant difference in survival when fish oil diets were compared with safflower oil diets. Interestingly, the optimal lipid source was an equal mixture of the two lipids (with an ω-6 to ω-3 ratio of approximately 2:1) and resulted in a statistically significant increase in survival from sepsis when compared with either lipid alone (Fig 34–4).[57]

There are few reports of the use of fish oil in clinical studies in stressed patients. Alexander and Gottschlich have reported clinical results with a modular diet containing 12% of the total calories as lipids, half fish oil and half safflower oil. The use of this diet in burn patients reduced wound infection and shortened hospital stay when compared with other standard enteral formulations.[58] However, other changes in nutrient composition (such as supplemental arginine) make it difficult to attribute these benefits to the lipid composition alone.

Similarly, Daly and associates have reported, in patients recovering from resection of upper gastrointestinal tract cancer, that an enteral preparation containing approximately 10% of the total calories as menhaden oil (Impact, Sandoz Nutrition, Minneapolis) reduced infections by 70% and the length of hospital stay by 22%.[59, 60] Again, as will be discussed below, there were other significant differences between the test diet and the control, such as amount of protein and arginine.

These studies suggest that manipulation of dietary lipids has the potential to alter the host response to infection. The choice of lipids in intravenous emul-

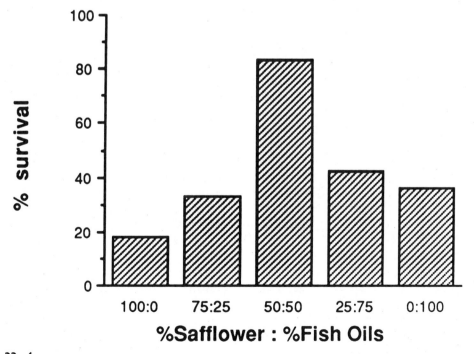

FIG 33–4.
Despite previous studies attesting to the immune-enhancing properties of fish oil, septic guinea pigs were more likely to survive bacterial peritonitis if fed an equal mixture of safflower and fish oils with an ω-6 to ω-3 ratio of 2:1.

sions or in enteral products has been limited up to now, but there will be a rapidly increasing diversity of choices available in the near future.

Glutamine

Preservation of the integrity of intestinal mucosa has become a topic of increasing importance since the implications of bacterial translocation have become evident, as mentioned above. Intestinal epithelial cells preferentially utilize glutamine and short-chain fatty acids for energy metabolism.[61] Whether the glutamine is absorbed from the gut lumen or from the bloodstream appears to have no effect on its metabolism by mucosal cells,[62] and indeed, glutamine-enriched parenteral solutions have led to increased mucosal mass.[63, 64] This may have important clinical significance because Fox and associates have shown that a glutamine-supplemented enteral diet significantly improved nutritional status, decreased intestinal injury, decreased bacterial translocation, and resulted in improved survival in a lethal model of enterocolitis in rats.[65] Others have confirmed the efficacy of glutamine supplementation in decreasing bacterial translocation in healthy[66] and irradiated[67] rats.

Sepsis reduces plasma and muscle glutamine concentrations.[68] Austgen and associates have examined the effects of endotoxin infusion on skeletal muscle glutamine metabolism in vivo.[69] Using hindquarter flux studies in anesthetized rats, the authors showed that endotoxin increased net hindquarter glutamine efflux and decreased the skeletal muscle intracellular glutamine concentration. The specific activity of glutamine synthetase increased significantly, while the activity of phosphate-dependent glutaminase, the major enzyme of glutamine degradation, was unchanged. The authors suggest that the accelerated release of muscle glutamine during sepsis is an adaptive response designed to supply glutamine to the liver, intestine, and lymphocytes during critical illness.

This intriguing hypothesis has been developed by Newsholme and associates.[11] They postulate that the purpose of increased protein catabolism during trauma, sepsis, surgery, and burns is to supply alanine to the liver and glutamine to the gut and leukocytes for energy and synthesis of nucleotide precursors. This theory attempts to develop a teleologic explanation for skeletal muscle consumption of branched-chain amino acids, the ketoacids of which provide the precursors for alanine and glutamine. In addition, it emphasizes the potential importance of glutamine to the cells of the immune system.

There are few clinical studies of glutamine supplementation to date, but those completed have shown impressive results. Ziegler and associates performed a double-blind, randomized, controlled clinical trial in adults receiving allogeneic bone marrow transplants for hematologic malignancies in order to determine whether glutamine-supplemented parenteral nutrition would improve the outcome.[70] Patients receiving the glutamine-supplemented formula benefited from improved nitrogen balance, attenuation of fluid retention, diminished expansion of the extracellular fluid compartment, reduction in the incidence of bacterial infections, and shortened hospital stay.[70, 71]

Arginine

Arginine has been described as a conditionally essential amino acid. Biological functions requiring arginine in adult humans can occur in the absence of dietary arginine, for arginine can be synthesized from ornithine, a urea cycle intermediate. However, under certain conditions the endogenous synthesis of arginine is apparently inadequate. The seminal work of Borman and colleagues showed that dietary arginine was necessary for normal growth in immature rats.[72] Barbul and associates subsequently demonstrated in a series of reports that dietary arginine supplementation improved weight gain in rats recovering from trauma, that it led to increased weight and cellularity of the thymus, and that lymphocytes from animals fed the arginine-supplemented diets had an enhanced proliferative response when stimulated by lectins in vitro.[73, 74]

Several studies, both in man and in rodents, confirmed the thymotropic effects of arginine.[75-78] In addition, two animal studies have produced results suggesting that dietary arginine supplementation may affect the outcome from infection. In one study, survival from CLP was improved by oral supplementation before or by intravenous supplementation after the onset of infection in rats.[79] In another, arginine supplementation after injury resulted in improved cell-mediated immunity and survival in burned guinea pigs.[80]

However, arginine is not beneficial in all models of sepsis, and in high concentrations it may be harmful. Supplementation of dietary arginine to septic guinea pigs at lower levels (i.e., 2% and 4% of the total calories) was not associated with higher survival rates than in controls.[81] Of concern, supplementation with a higher level (i.e., 6% of the total calories) was associated with decreased nitrogen retention and increased mortality.

The effect of supplemental arginine has also been tested in a murine model of infection in which malnourished mice were repleted with diets containing varying amounts of supplemental arginine prior to challenge with *Salmonella typhimurium*.[82] In this study there was evidence that high levels of dietary arginine supplementation (5% of the total calories) impaired weight gain and worsened mortality.

The mechanisms responsible for the increased mortality rates observed with high levels of dietary arginine are not understood. Arginine may affect the outcome by its effect on the hormonal milieu. Rats that were administered parenteral arginine (5 mg/kg) subsequent to the intravenous injection of endotoxin had significantly higher mortality rates than did controls.[83] This phenomenon was observed in association with hyperinsulinemia and hypoglycemia, thus suggesting a mechanism for the increased susceptibility to endotoxin. Burned guinea pigs also showed a marked elevation of plasma glucose levels during feeding with diets containing 4% of the total calories as arginine.[80]

Arginine also plays roles in the urea cycle, in polyamine synthesis, and in the production of reactive nitrogen intermediates, specifically nitric oxide. Reactive nitrogen intermediates are involved in macrophage cytotoxicity against target tumor cells and are also capable of mediating the effect of Kupffer cells on hepatocyte protein synthesis.[84, 85] In addition, nitric oxide, or endothelial-derived relaxing factor, is a potent vasodilator.[86, 87] The by-products of reactive nitrogen intermediates, nitrates and nitrites, are found in higher levels in the plasma of septic humans and may be responsible for the decrease in peripheral vascular resistance seen in septic shock.[88, 89] However, there was no evidence that serum NO_2^-/NO_3^- levels were affected by dietary arginine in septic, previously malnourished mice in the study cited above.[82] Although arginine may contribute to the complex cellular interactions evoked in septic animals via increased production of reactive nitrogen intermediates, this hypothesis, despite its attractiveness, remains unproved.

Arginine, like glutamine, is a specific example of the immunomodulatory potential of nutrients. Arginine has been shown to be efficacious at stimulating lymphocyte activity in animals and man and may prove to be useful clinically. However, animal studies attest to the importance of determining the appropriate dose of arginine, for excessive doses may be harmful.

REVIEW OF CURRENT PRODUCTS

Knowledge of the potential beneficial effects of immunomodulatory nutrients, which is a growing field of nutritional pharmacology, has resulted in the formulation of products to provide nutritional support to critically ill patients.

Nutritional Pharmacology

The concept of using nutrients to alter physiologic processes is not new and has its roots in the pioneering experiments done by early nutrition biochemists who investigated the functions of the newly isolated micronutrients. However, the emphasis of this early work was on establishing the minimum re-

quirements for nutrients to sustain normal metabolic processes.

Richard J. Wurtman, Professor of Brain and Cognitive Sciences at Massachusetts Institute of Technology, performed original studies on the effect of specific nutrients on neurotransmitters and the function of the nervous system in the early 1970s. These studies demonstrated that normal physiologic processes such as cognitive function and appetite could be affected by altering dietary components.[90] These studies were done on subjects of normal nutritional status, and the effects were not due simply to repletion of essential nutrients. This work, which showed that nutrients could affect function beyond simply supplying essential metabolic fuel and co-

TABLE 33–1.

Formulation of Impact, Immun-Aid, and Alitraq*

Component	Impact	Immun-Aid	Alitraq
Nitrogen source			
Caseinates	65.0	—	—
Lactalbumin hydrolysates	—	55.5	33.1
Whey protein	—	—	8.7
Arginine	15.0	21.0	6.7
Glutamine	—	13.5	21.3
Branched-chain amino acids	—	30.0	14.6
Total protein and amino acids	80.0	120.0	78.8
Carbohydrate source			
Maltodextrin	197.6	180.0	74.3
Lipid source			
Structured lipids (Captex 710-A)	25.0	—	—
Menhaden oil	16.75	—	—
MCT	—	16.5	12.3
Canola oil	—	16.5	—
Safflower oil	—	—	11
Total lipids	41.75	33.0	23.3
Typical fatty acid profile			
MCT	8–13	16.5	12.3
Monounsaturated fat	—	9.6	1.8
Linoleic acid (18:2 ω6)	2.5–4.5	4.3	10
Linolenic acid (18:3 ω3)	—	1.7	0.03
EPA (20:5 ω3)	1.0–2.0	—	—
DHA (2:6 ω3)	0.25–1.0	—	—
RNA source			
Yeast RNA	1.88	—	—
Caloric composition			
Carbohydrate	53%	48%	66%
Protein	22%	32%	21%
Lipid	25%	20%	13%

*Values are grams per 1,500 mL.
MCT = medium-chain triglycerides; EPA = eicosapentaenoic acid; DHA = docosahexaenoic acid.

factors, was the first demonstration of *nutritional pharmacology.*

More recently, J. Wesley Alexander, Professor of Surgery at the University of Cincinnati, has popularized this term to describe the therapeutic effects of nutrients on the immune system of injured and septic animals.[91] The concept of nutritional pharmacology has in fact become the rationale for the design of specific enteral formulas to support or stimulate the immune system while providing nutritional support in immunocompromised patients. The formulations of Impact (Sandoz Nutrition, Minneapolis), Immun-Aid (McGaw, Inc., Irvine, Calif), and Alitraq (Ross Laboratories, Columbus, Ohio) are presented in Table 33–1.

Specialized Enteral Support of Stressed Patients

Impact has been constructed to stimulate the immune response through the use of supplemental arginine, dietary nucleotides, medium-chain triglycerides, and ω-3 fatty acids. Immun-Aid has been similarly formulated, with supplemental arginine, glutamine, branched-chain amino acids, medium-chain triglycerides, and ω-3 fatty acids. In addition, Immun-Aid has increased amounts of vitamins E, C, and B_6 and copper and zinc. Alitraq has been formulated with supplemental glutamine and arginine and uses safflower oil and medium-chain triglycerides for lipids.

One subtle difference between Impact and Immun-Aid is the source of ω-3 fatty acids. Immun-Aid is constructed with canola oil, which has α-linolenic acid (ALA, 18:3 ω-3). Impact is constructed with menhaden oil, with eicosapentaenoic and docosahexaenoic acids (EPA, 20:5 ω-3, and DHA, 22:6 ω-3, respectively). There are concerns that ALA is not as efficient a precursor for eicosanoids as the longer-chain ω-3 fatty acids and thus the biologic effects of EPA/DHA-enriched diets may be more pronounced.[92, 93]

Another difference among the products is the presence of glutamine in Immun-Aid and Alitraq. Although clinical trials of glutamine supplementation in septic patients have not been published, glutamine supplementation has been shown to reduce the incidence of infections and to shorten hospital stay in allogeneic bone marrow transplant recipients.[70, 71]

Impact has been studied in clinical trials.[94] Daly and associates presented their preliminary experience with Impact in patients with upper gastrointestinal malignancies.[59, 60] In this trial, 85 surgical patients with upper gastrointestinal cancer were randomized to postoperatively receive either Impact or Osmolite HN. The mean hospital length of stay was reduced by 22% and infectious complications by 70% in the Impact-supplemented group.

Bower and associates have reported the results of a multicenter trial comparing Impact with Osmolite HN.[95] This study included critically ill adult intensive care unit patients with APACHE II (Acute Physiology, Age, and Chronic Health Evaluation II) scores of 10 or more or Trauma Injury Severity Score scores of 20 or more who were entered within 48 hours of injury or a septic event and who required 7 days of enteral nutrition. Both groups had similar tolerance to the formulas. As in the study cited above by Daly and associates,[59, 60] there was a reduction in the length of stay in the Impact-treated group (25.3 vs. 35.6 days). However, there was not a significant decrease in the incidence of all infectious complications. Those patients with pneumonia who received Impact had a decreased length of hospital stay from the onset of infectious complications to discharge (23 vs. 34 days). Thus the authors observed that "although Impact did not prevent the occurrence of complications, it reduced length of stay from onset of complication to discharge."[95]

The design of this study has been criticized because of the significant difference in nitrogen content between the two study formulas. Impact contains 53.6 g/1,000 mL of caseinates and free amino acids, whereas Osmolite HN contains only 42.2 g/1,000 mL of caseinates and soy protein isolates. The beneficial effect of increased protein supplementation after surgery or injury has long been recognized,[96] and there is concern that the observed differences in outcome may be related largely to differences in protein intake.

There is ample evidence that the composition of the diet can affect the immune response. However, there is not enough evidence at this point in time to describe the specific formulations that are appropriate for hospitalized patients. All three of the novel formulas described above have theoretical merit. As the results from prospective randomized trials are published and as both safety and efficacy can be demonstrated, these formulas can be evaluated and compared with other currently available products. However, it may be necessary to construct "disease-specific" diets; for example, dietary modifications that are important for the trauma patient may not be suitable for the septic patient.

Much work remains to be done in the field of nutritional pharmacology. Yet the hope remains that we now have another tool to use in the struggle against infection in the immunocompromised host.

RECOMMENDATIONS

1. Septic patients require nutritional support to abrogate the loss of lean muscle mass and to maintain other physiologic functions that depend on protein synthesis.

2. More is not better. Indirect calorimetry should be used to estimate energy expenditure in septic patients. If indirect calorimetry is not available, patients should be given 150% of BEE as estimated by the Harris-Benedict equations.

3. Enteral feeding is generally preferred to parenteral feeding. However, the septic patient may be intolerant of enteral feeding, and there is no evidence that the route of feeding has any effect on outcome once the septic state is established. The greatest value of enteral feeding is in a nonseptic critically ill patient immunocompromised by injury, cancer, or surgery; nourishment of the gut may prevent bacterial translocation and decrease the incidence of subsequent septic episodes.

4. It is unclear whether there is an optimal fuel source for septic patients, but since the rate of glucose administration should not exceed 5 mg/kg/min, intravenous fat emulsions will be needed in most patients to provide adequate delivery of calories.

5. Novel formulas based on nutrients with immunomodulatory properties are exciting alternatives for the future but as yet are of unproven safety and efficacy.

REFERENCES

1. ASPEN Board of Directors: Guidelines for use of total parenteral nutrition in the hospitalized adult patient. *JPEN* 1986; 10:441–445.
2. ASPEN Board of Directors: Guidelines for use of enteral nutrition in the adult patient. *JPEN* 1987; 11:435–439.
3. Chang RWS, Jacobs S, Lee B: Gastrointestinal dysfunction among intensive care unit patients. *Crit Care Med* 1987; 15:909–914.
4. Bone RC: Sepsis, the sepsis syndrome, multi-organ failure: A plea for comparable definitions. *Ann Intern Med* 1991; 114:332–333.
5. Baue A: Multiple, progressive, or sequential systems failure. *Arch Surg* 1975; 110:779–781.
6. Eiseman B, Beart R, Norton L: Multiple organ failure. *Surg Gynecol Obstet* 1977; 144:323–326.
7. Long CL, Jeevanandam M, Kim BM, et al: Whole body protein synthesis and catabolism in septic man. *Am J Clin Nutr* 1977; 30:1340–1344.

8. McDougal WS, Wilmore DW, Pruitt BA: Effect of intravenous near isosmotic nutrient infusions on nitrogen balance in critically ill injured patients. *Surg Gynecol Obstet* 1977; 145:408–414.

9. Streat SJ, Beddoe AH, Hill GL: Aggressive nutritional support does not prevent protein loss despite fat gain in septic intensive care patients. *J Trauma* 1987; 27:262–266.

10. Jahoor F, Shangraw RE, Miyoshi H, et al: Role of insulin and glucose oxidation in mediating the protein catabolism of burns and sepsis. *Am J Physiol* 1989; 257:323–331.

11. Newsholme EA, Newsholme P, Curi R, et al: A role for muscle in the immune system and its importance in surgery, trauma, sepsis and burns. *Nutrition* 1988; 4:261–268.

12. Herskowitz K, Souba WW: Intestinal glutamine metabolism during critical illness: A surgical perspective. *Nutrition* 1990; 6:199–206.

13. Shaw JHF, Wildbore M, Wolfe RR: Whole body protein kinetics in severely septic patients. The response to glucose infusion and total parenteral nutrition. *Ann Surg* 1987; 205:288–294.

14. Dudrick SJ: The genesis of intravenous hyperalimentation. *JPEN* 1977; 1:23.

15. Burke JF, Wolfe RR, Mullany CJ, et al: Glucose requirements following burn injury. *Ann Surg* 1979; 190:274–285.

16. The Veterans Affairs Total Parenteral Nutrition Cooperative Study Group: Perioperative total parenteral nutrition in surgical patients. *N Engl J Med* 1991; 325:525–532.

17. Alexander JW, Gonce SJ, Miskell PW, et al: A new model for studying nutrition in peritonitis. *Ann Surg* 1989; 209:334–340.

18. Dominioni L, Trocki O, Fang CH, et al: Enteral feeding in burn hypermetabolism: Nutritional and metabolic effects of different levels of calorie and protein intake. *JPEN* 1985; 9:269–279.

19. Yamazaki K, Maiz A, Moldawer LL, et al: Complications associated with overfeeding of infected animals. *J Surg Res* 1986; 40:152–158.

20. Peck MD, Alexander JW, Gonce SJ, et al: Low protein diets improve survival from peritonitis in guinea pigs. *Ann Surg* 1989; 209:448–454.

21. Peck MD, Ogle CK, Alexander JW, et al: High protein diets are associated with hyperammonemia in septic guinea pigs. *Surg Res Commun* 1991; 10:173–182.

22. Shizgal HM, Martin MF: Caloric requirement of the critically ill septic patient. *Crit Care Med* 1988; 16:312–317.

23. Stoner HB, Little RA, Frayn KN, et al: The effect of sepsis on the oxidation of carbohydrate and fat. *Br J Surg* 1983; 70:32–35.

24. Cunningham JJ: Factors contributing to increased energy expenditure in thermal injury: A review of studies employing indirect calorimetry. *JPEN* 1990; 14:649–656.

25. Shangraw RE, Jahoor F, Miyoshi H, et al: Differentiation between septic and postburn insulin resistance. *Metabolism* 1989; 38:983–989.

26. Kudsk KA, Croce MA, Fabian TC, et al: Enteral versus parenteral feeding: Effects on septic morbidity after blunt and penetrating abdominal trauma. *Ann Surg* 1992; 215:503–513.

27. Peterson VM, Moore EE, Jones TN, et al: Total enteral nutrition versus total parenteral nutrition after major torso injury: Attenuation of hepatic protein reprioritization. *Surgery* 1988; 104:199–207.

28. Moore FA, Moore EE, Jones TN, et al: TEN versus TPN following major abdominal trauma—reduced septic morbidity. *J Trauma* 1989; 29:916–923.

29. Kudsk KA, Carpenter G, Petersen S, et al: Effect of enteral and parenteral feeding in malnourished rats with E. coli–hemoglobin adjuvant peritonitis. *J Surg Res* 1981; 31:105–110.

30. Petersen SR, Kudsk KA, Carpenter G, et al: Malnutrition and immunocompetence: Increased mortality following an infectious challenge during hyperalimentation. *J Trauma* 1981; 21:528–533.

31. Kudsk KA, Stone JM, Carpenter G, et al: Enteral and parenteral feeding influences mortality after hemoglobin–E. coli peritonitis in normal rats. *J Trauma* 1983; 23:605–609.

32. Bragg LE, Thompson JS, Rikkers LF: Influence of nutrient delivery on gut structure and function. *Nutrition* 1991; 7:237–243.

33. Alverdy JC, Chi HS, Sheldon GF: The

effect of parenteral nutrition on gastro-intestinal immunity: The importance of enteral stimulation. *Ann Surg* 1985; 202:681−684.

34. Saito H, Trocki O, Alexander JW, et al: The effect of route of nutrient adminis-tration on the nutritional state, cata-bolic hormone secretion, and gut mu-cosal integrity after burn injury. *JPEN* 1987; 11:1−7.
35. Thompson JS, Vaughan WP, Forst CF, et al: The effect of the route of nutrient delivery on gut structure and diamine oxidase levels. *JPEN* 1987; 11:28−32.
36. Alverdy JC, Aoys E, Moss GS: Total parenteral nutrition promotes bacterial translocation from the gut. *Surgery* 1988; 104:185−190.
37. Fong U, Marano MA, Barber A, et al: Total parenteral nutrition and bowel rest modify the metabolic response to endotoxin in humans. *Ann Surg* 1989; 210:449−457.
38. Meyer J, Yurt RW, Duhaney R, et al: Differential neutrophil activation before and after endotoxin infusion in enter-ally versus parenterally fed volunteers. *Surg Gynecol Obstet* 1988; 167:501−509.
39. Cerra FB, McPherson JP, Konstan-tinides FN, et al: Enteral nutrition does not prevent multiple organ failure syn-drome (MOFS) after sepsis. *Surgery* 1988; 104:727−733.
40. Chandra RK: *Nutrition and Immunol-ogy.* New York, Alan R Liss, 1988.
41. Long CL: Fuel preferences in the septic patient: Glucose or lipid? *JPEN* 1987; 11:333−335.
42. Nordenstrom J, Carpentier YA, Askan-azi J, et al: Metabolic utilization of in-travenous fat emulsion during total parenteral nutrition. *Ann Surg* 1982; 196:221−231.
43. Palmblad J: Intravenous lipid emul-sions and host defense—a critical re-view. *Clin Nutr* 1991; 10:303−308.
44. Hwang DH, Carroll AE: Decreased for-mation of prostaglandin derived from arachidonic acid by dietary linolenate in rats. *Am J Clin Nutr* 1980; 33:590−597.
45. Ferretti A, Schoene NW, Flanagan VP: Identification and quantification of prostaglandin E_3 in renal medullary tissue of three strains of rats fed fish oil. *Lipids* 1981; 16:800−804.
46. Marshall LA, Szczesniewski A, Johns-ton PV: Dietary alpha-linoleic acid and prostaglandin synthesis: A time course study. *Am J Clin Nutr* 1983; 38:895−900.
47. Fischer S, Weber PC: Prostaglandin I_3 is formed in vivo in man after dietary eicosapentaenoic acid. *Nature* 1984; 307:165−168.
48. Holmer G, Beare-Rogers JL: Linseed oil and marine oil as sources of (ω-3) fatty acids in rat heart. *Nutr Res* 1985; 5:1011−1014.
49. Kelley VE, Ferretti A, Izui S, et al: A fish oil diet rich in eicosapentaenoic acid reduces cyclooxygenase metabo-lites, and suppresses lupus in MRL-1 pr mice. *J Immunol* 1985; 134:1914−1919.
50. Terano T, Salmon JA, Higgs GA, et al: Eicosapentaenoic acid as a modulator of inflammation: Effect on prostaglan-din and leukotriene synthesis. *Bio-chem Pharmacol* 1986; 35:779−785.
51. Needleman P, Raz A, Minkes MS, et al: Triene prostaglandins: Prostacyclin and thromboxane biosynthesis and unique biological properties. *Proc Natl Acad Sci U S A* 1979; 76:944−948.
52. Mascioli E, Leader L, Flores E, et al: Enhanced survival to endotoxin in guinea pigs fed IV fish oil emulsion. *Lipids* 1988; 23:623−625.
53. Mascioli EA, Iwasa Y, Trimbo S, et al: Endotoxin challenge after menhaden oil diet: Effects on survival of guinea pigs. *Am J Clin Nutr* 1989; 49:277.
54. Alexander JW, Saito H, Ogle CK, et al: The importance of lipid type in the diet after burn injury. *Ann Surg* 1986; 204:1−8.
55. Peck MD, Alexander JW, Ogle CK, et al: The effect of dietary fatty acids on re-sponse to *Pseudomonas* infection in burned mice. *J Trauma* 1990; 30:445−452.
56. Barton RG, Wells CL, Carlson A, et al: Dietary omega-3 fatty acids decrease mortality and Kupffer cell prostaglan-din E_2 production in a rat model of chronic sepsis. *J Trauma* 1991; 31:768−774.
57. Peck MD, Ogle CK, Alexander JW: Com-position of fat in enteral diets can in-fluence outcome in experimental peri-tonitis. *Ann Surg* 1991; 214:74−82.
58. Alexander JW, Gottschlich MM: Nutri-

tional immunomodulation in burn patients. *Crit Care Med* 1990; 18(suppl):149–153.

59. Daly JM, Lieberman M, Goldfine J, et al: Enteral nutrition with supplemental arginine, RNA and omega-3 fatty acids: A prospective clinical trial. *JPEN* 1991; 15(suppl):19.

60. Daly JM, Lieberman MD, Goldfine J, et al: Enteral nutrition with supplemental arginine, RNA, and omega-3 fatty acids in patients after operation: Immunologic, metabolic, and clinical outcome. *Surgery* 1992; 112:56–67.

61. Windmueller HG, Spaeth AE: Identification of ketone bodies and glutamine as the major respiratory fuels in vivo for the postabsorptive rat small intestine. *J Biol Chem* 1978; 253:69–76.

62. Windmeuller HG, Spaeth AE: Intestinal metabolism of glutamine and glutamate from the lumen as compared to glutamine from blood. *Arch Biochem Biophys* 1975; 171:662–672.

63. Hwang TL, O'Dwyer ST, Smith RJ, et al: Preservation of small bowel mucosa using glutamine-enriched parenteral nutrition. *Surg Forum* 1986; 37:56–57.

64. Jacobs D, Evans DA, O'Dwyer ST, et al: Trophic effects of glutamine-enriched parenteral nutrition on colonic mucosa. *JPEN* 1988; 12(suppl):6.

65. Fox AD, Kripke SA, Paula JD, et al: Effect of a glutamine-supplemented enteral diet on methotrexate-induced enterocolitis. *JPEN* 1988; 12:325–331.

66. Burke DJ, Alverdy JC, Aoys E, et al: Glutamine-supplemented total parenteral nutrition improves gut immune function. *Arch Surg* 1989; 124:1396–1399.

67. Souba WW, Klimberg S, Hautamaki RD, et al: Oral glutamine reduces bacterial translocation following abdominal radiation. *J Surg Res* 1990; 48:1–5.

68. Roth E, Funovics J, Muhlbacher F, et al: Metabolic disorders in severe abdominal sepsis: Glutamine deficiency in skeletal muscle. *Clin Nutr* 1982; 1:25.

69. Austgen TR, Chakrabarti R, Chen MK, et al: Adaptive regulation in skeletal muscle glutamine metabolism in endotoxin-treated rats. *J Trauma* 1992; 32:600–607.

70. Ziegler TR, Young LS, Benfell K, et al: Clinical and metabolic efficacy of glutamine-supplemented parenteral nutrition after bone marrow transplantation. A randomized, double-blind, controlled study. *Ann Intern Med* 1992; 116:821–828.

71. Scheltinga MR, Young LS, Benfell K, et al: Glutamine-enriched intravenous feedings attenuate extracellular fluid expansion after a standard stress. *Ann Surg* 1991; 214:385–393.

72. Borman A, Wood TR, Black HC, et al: The role of arginine in growth with some observations on the effects of arginine acid. *J Biol Chem* 1946; 166:585.

73. Barbul A, Wasserkrug HL, Seifter E, et al: Immunostimulatory effects of arginine in normal and injured rats. *J Surg Res* 1980; 29:228–235.

74. Barbul A, Wasserkrug HL, Yoshimura NN, et al: High arginine levels in intravenous hyperalimentation abrogate post-traumatic immune suppression. *J Surg Res* 1984; 36:620–624.

75. Barbul A, Wasserkrug HL, Sisto DA, et al: Thymic stimulatory actions of arginine. *JPEN* 1980; 4:446–449.

76. Barbul A, Sisto DA, Wasserkrug HL, et al: Arginine stimulates lymphocyte immune response in healthy human beings. *Surgery* 1981; 90:244–251.

77. Barbul A, Fishel RS, Shimazu S, et al: Intravenous hyperalimentation with high arginine levels improves wound healing and immune function. *J Surg Res* 1985; 38:328–334.

78. Daly JM, Reynolds J, Thom A, et al: Immune and metabolic effects of arginine in the surgical patient. *Ann Surg* 1988; 208:512–516.

79. Madden HP, Breslin RJ, Wasserkrug HL, et al: Stimulation of T cell immunity by arginine enhances survival in peritonitis. *J Surg Res* 1988; 44:658–663.

80. Saito H, Trocki O, Wang S, et al: Metabolic and immune effects of dietary arginine supplementation after burn. *Arch Surg* 1987; 122:784–789.

81. Gonce SJ, Peck MD, Alexander JW, et al: The effect of supplemental arginine on recovery from peritonitis in guinea pigs. *JPEN* 1990; 14:237–244.

82. Peck MD, Babcock GF, Alexander JW, et al: Effects of dietary arginine in mu-

rine models of infection. Submitted for publication.

83. Yelich MR, Filkins JP: Insulin hypersecretion and potentiation of endotoxin shock in the rat. *Circ Shock* 1982; 9:589–603.

84. Billiar TR, Curran RD, Stuehr DJ, et al: An L-arginine–dependent mechanism mediates Kupffer cell inhibition of hepatocyte protein synthesis in vitro. *J Exp Med* 1989; 169:1467–1472.

85. Hibbs JB, Taintor RR, Vavrin Z, et al: Nitric oxide: A cytotoxic activated macrophage effector molecule. *Biochem Biophys Res Commun* 1988; 157:87–94.

86. Rees DD, Palmer RMJ, Moncada S: Role of endothelium-derived nitric oxide in the regulation of blood pressure. *Proc Natl Acad Sci U S A* 1989; 86:3375–3378.

87. Vallance P, Collier J, Moncada S: Effects of endothelium-derived nitric oxide on peripheral arteriolar tone in man. *Lancet* 1989; 2:997–1000.

88. Ochoa JB, Udekwu AO, Billiar TR, et al: Nitrogen oxide levels in patients following trauma and during sepsis. *Ann Surg* 1991; 214:621–626.

89. Kilbourn RG, Gross SS, Jubran A, et al: L-N^G-methylarginine inhibits tumor necrosis factor–induced hypotension: Implications for the involvement of nitric oxide. *Proc Natl Acad Sci U S A* 1990; 87:3629–3632.

90. Wurtman RJ: Effects of foods and nutrients on brain neurotransmitters. *Curr Concepts Nutr* 1984; 13:103–112.

91. Alexander JW, Peck MD: Future considerations for nutrition, in Fischer JE (ed): *Total Parenteral Nutrition.* Boston, Little, Brown, 1991.

92. Nettleton JA: ω-3 fatty acids: Comparison of plant and seafood sources in human nutrition. *J Am Diet Assoc* 1991; 91:331–337.

93. Whelan J, Broughton KS, Kinsella JE: The comparative effects of dietary α-linolenic acid and fish oil on 4- and 5-series leukotriene formation in vivo. *Lipids* 1991; 26:119–126.

94. Bower RH: A uniquely enteral formula as adjunctive therapy for septic and critically ill patients. *Nutrition* 1990; 6:92–95.

95. Bower RH, Lavin PT, LiCari JJ, et al: A modified enteral formula reduces hospital length of stay in patients in intensive care units. *Clin Nutr* 1992; 11:(suppl).

96. Alexander JW, MacMillan BG, Stinnett JD, et al: Beneficial effects of aggressive protein feeding in severely burned children. *Ann Surg* 1980; 192:505–517.

34

Gut Disease

Donald F. Kirby, M.D.

Mark H. DeLegge, M.D.

In reviewing the present "state-of-the-art" data for nutrition in the critical care of gastrointestinal diseases, it must be immediately recognized that there are very few hard data for the clinician to call upon. Care must be exercised when extrapolating animal data to humans. Also, the human data in this particular area are composed of few double-blind, placebo controlled, randomized clinical trials, which are considered by many to be the gold standard. In addition, many other factors confound the true nutritional impact of a study, most notably the lack of specific markers that indicate that improved nutritional status yields reductions in morbidity and mortality.

The purpose of this chapter is to review the current role of nutrition support in patients who have gastrointestinal diseases. There may not be a clear-cut answer in the literature for many areas, but we will try to temper experience with facts to provide the intensivist with guidelines on how to deal with patients with the following problems: pancreatitis, ulcer disease, gastrointestinal fistulas, inflammatory bowel disease (IBD), hepatic failure, liver transplantation, and short-bowel syndrome (SBS).

PANCREATITIS

The majority of patients with acute or chronic relapsing pancreatitis are eating normally within a week. However, varying percentages (5% to 30%) of patients are referred for consideration of nutrition support. These patients may be critically ill, and others may have complications of pancreatitis where oral intake may be undesirable.[1] Controversy continues over whether parenteral or enteral nutrition is preferable, but individual circumstances must be considered carefully.

Acute Pancreatitis

In patients in whom severe pancreatitis develops as assessed by Ranson's criteria, APACHE II (Acute Physiology, Age and Chronic Evaluation II) scores, or computed tomography (CT) scan scores, fewer than a third of patients will require intensive care admission or urgent surgery. While the provision of parenteral nutrition has no immediate effect on the course of pancreatic inflammation, recent studies are divided on the risk and benefits of its use. Table 34–1 highlights some of the more classic and recent studies of pancreatitis and lists some of the major findings.

For parenteral nutrition, the issues that most concern its use in severe pancreatitis are whether it reduces the frequency of complications or mortality, whether there is a higher catheter infection rate, and whether hyperglycemia is a more serious problem or even prognostic in its severe forms in patients with pancreatitis who are receiving parenteral nutrition? Most studies have been retrospective, and many studies have included all evaluable patients who have received parenteral nutrition, including patient groups with moderate to severe pancreatitis.

Kalfarentzos et al.[8] reported on 67 patients with severe acute pancreatitis who were treated in a surgical unit. They found that with early institution of total parenteral nutrition (TPN) i.e., within 72 hours, there was a reduction

TABLE 34–|.

Use of Nutrition Support in Acute Pancreatitis

Study	Year	No. of Patients	ICU* Setting	R or P*	Major Findings
Feller[2]	1974	200	No	No	Mortality reduction from 21.6% to 14%
Goodgame[3]	1977	46	No	No	Increased catheter-related sepsis episodes to 17% of study patients
Van Gossum[4]	1988	18	Yes	No	Patients with persistent hypertriglyceridemia, hyperglycemia, hypoalbuminemia, and higher insulin requirements tended to have poorer outcome
Sax[5]	1987	54	No	P & R	No advantage in early TPN*; catheter-related sepsis, 10.4%
Sitzmann[6]	1989	73	No	P	Failure to achieve positive nitrogen balance associated with increased mortality
Robin[7]	1990	156	No	No	Early aggressive use of parenteral nutrition if patient malnourished; no increase in catheter-related infections
Kalfarentzos[8]	1991	67	Yes	P	TPN safe and effective: overall mortality rate, 24%; catheter-related sepsis, 8.9% in patients with pancreatitis vs. 2.9% in other ICU patients; reduction in complications and mortality rate if TPN begun within 72 hr of admission

*ICU = intensive care unit; R = randomized; P = prospective; TPN = total parenteral nutrition.

in complications and the mortality rate from 95.6% and 38% to 23.6% and 13%, respectively, when compared with patients who received TPN later in their treatment. They also noted a higher catheter-related sepsis rate of 8.9% vs. 2.9% for other patients treated in their unit. In this very sick population the incidence of hyperglycemia was 88% during the therapy.

Hyperglycemia may be an important issue in these particular patients since it has recently been reported that transient hyperglycemia may alter immune function. Hennessey et al.[9] have shown that hyperglycemia may impair the complement fixation function of Ig G. As further factors are unraveled about the immune system, more risk factors in patients with pancreatitis may emerge.

Another major issue in nutrition support for pancreatitis is whether the enteral route can be utilized. Certainly this route may have less potential complications as compared with TPN. Many investigators have demonstrated that duodenal feedings stimulate pancreatic secretion. However, conflicting data have emerged as to whether jejunal feeding in patients with pancreatitis stimulates the pancreas. Data from Ragins and coworkers[10] suggest that intrajejunal feeding may not stimulate the pancreas. From a practical standpoint, Kudsk et al.[11] placed feeding jejunostomies in 11 patients who underwent exploratory laparotomy for pancreatitis. It was possible to feed the majority of these patients. Catheter-related problems as well as hyperglycemia and glucosuria were important factors in this report. Also, it is not clear that the dogma stating that elemental diets must be utilized in jejunostomy tubes is justified (Kudsk KA, personal communication; see also Chapter 19).

Further research into the exact role of enteral feeding in acute, severe pancreatitis seems warranted. If an exploratory laparotomy is performed, it seems reasonable to place a feeding jejunostomy. Otherwise, newer nasoenteric tubes and techniques that allow for their placement past the ligament of Treitz seem to be an acceptable alternative to TPN in selected patients.

In acute severe pancreatitis, TPN and its components, including fat, appear to be safe.[1] For the intensive care patient, nutrition support should start as early as possible. If parenteral nutrition is used, hyperglycemia and catheter-related sepsis must be vigorously managed. If jejunal access is available, then enteral nutrition may be possible without further stimulating the pancreas.[11]

Chronic Pancreatitis

Patients with chronic pancreatitis may have pancreatic insufficiency resulting in maldigestion from a paucity of pancreatic enzymes, which in turn fosters malabsorption, particularly of fat due to the complexity of its digestion. Thus, steatorrhea and to a lesser extent azotorrhea may be the clinical result. The severity of these will depend on the level of pancreatic reserve and the type of diet ingested. A high-fat diet may exacerbate the patient's symptoms, while a low-fat diet may minimize them. In the most severe forms of chronic pancreatitis, peripheral edema, hypoalbuminemia, hypovitaminosis, and essential fatty acid deficiency may be evident. The treatment consists of providing commercially available pancreatic enzyme preparations that supply approximately 30,000 units of lipase activity per meal. Attention to fat-soluble vitamins must also be considered.

Another major problem for the patient with chronic pancreatitis is glucose intolerance. The incidence of glucose intolerance is variable from 40% to 90%, with insulin-requiring diabetes eventually developing in 20% to 30%. The onset of diabetes is usually 7 or more years after the diagnosis of chronic pancreatitis.[12]

Finally, the most potentially debilitating problem in patients with chronic pancreatitis is pain. While it is beyond the scope of this section to go into detail on this, it is important because many patients with alcohol-induced pancreatic disease will return to drinking to help alleviate the pain. Unfortunately, they may be faced with an acute exacerbation of pancreatitis and have other complications.

Complications of Pancreatitis

While the role of parenteral nutrition is unclear for acute pancreatitis, it has been found to be a useful adjunct for patients with complications of pancreatitis.[1] Table 34–2 shows a list of complications that have been treated by parenteral nutrition. Most of these studies have been small studies or case reports.

Pancreatic Ascites

Pancreatic ascites results from either a rupture in the pancreatic duct or leakage of a pancreatic pseudocyst into the peritoneal cavity. In 1983 Variyam[13] reported that pancreatic ascites was noted to regress in three patients while being managed by TPN. Of interest, at surgery on two of the patients, there was no ascites in one and 1.5 L in the second. The third patient refused surgery. Current options might include placing a pancreatic stent via endoscopic retrograde cholangiopancreatography (ERCP) or treatment with somatostatin, either individually or in combination with parenteral nutrition. Jejunal feeding might also be an option; however, more proximal feeding that could stimulate pancreatic secretions might be counterproductive.[14]

No controlled trials for optimal doses

TABLE 34–2.

Complications of Pancreatitis Where Total Parenteral Nutrition May Be a Useful Adjunct

Pancreatic ascites
Pancreatic fistulas
Hemosuccus pancreaticus
Pancreatic pseudocysts
Pleural effusions

of somatostatin, the optimal timing of endoscopic stenting, and/or their use in combination are presently available. However, several reports have suggested a benefit from the following: low-dose radiation,[15] peritoneovenous shunting,[16, 17] and the use of somatostatin.[18, 19] Oktedalen et al.[18] reported one patient who failed to resolve his ascites after repeated paracenteses, plasma infusions, diuretics, and TPN but improved dramatically after a 9-day continuous infusion of octreotide (Sandostatin; Sandoz, Basel, Switzerland). An infusion of 250 µg/hr was begun and given concurrently with plasma infusions and TPN. The patient had no further recurrence of the ascites in 9 months of follow-up.

Gislason and coworkers[19] reported two patients where TPN and H_2 blockers did not have an effect on the ascites after 2 weeks in one and 4 weeks in the other. There was rapid improvement when somatostatin infusion at 250 µg/hr was begun. They concluded that somatostatin infusion should be tried prior to any diagnostic or therapeutic intervention.

In the United States, Barritt[20] tried to treat a case of pancreatic ascites with 100 µg of somatostatin subcutaneously twice daily but did not have success in his patient. It is unclear whether a higher subcutaneous dose would have been effective or whether the continuous intravenous dose is superior. There was no comment on the use of TPN.

Pancreatic Fistulas

As with pancreatic ascites, pancreatic fistulas may also be managed by TPN. Several small case reports have studied the effect of TPN and its components on pancreatic output.[21–24] These studies suggested that there was a beneficial effect of TPN, but these are not data from large prospective randomized trials.

TPN's independent influence on pancreatic fistula closure may not have been rigorously studied because the introduction of somatostatin led to investigations with TPN and somatostatin, singularly or in combination. In an uncontrolled study from Finland, Saari et al.[25] reported on TPN and somatostatin treatment of 19 patients with pancreatic fistulas. Somatostatin was given as a bolus of 250 μg and followed by a continuous infusion of 250μg/hr. In this study 68% of the fistulas closed after an average of 10 days. They also identified that it was important to have unobstructed drainage of pancreatic secretions through the pancreatic duct into the bowel.

In a French study by di Costanzo and colleagues,[26] 37 patients with external fistulas were treated with TPN and somatostatin. Again, somatostatin was used as a continuous intravenous infusion at 250 μg/hr. Five of these fistulas were pancreatic, 2 healed on treatment, 1 required surgical closure, and 2 were failures. The main conclusion from this study was that if fistula output falls more than 50% on the first day of treatment, then it should be continued for at least 14 days.

In a recent study from Spain on the use of somatostatin in the treatment of gastrointestinal fistulas, Torres et al.[27] reported a multicenter, controlled, prospective randomized trial of 40 patients who were randomized to treatment with TPN or TPN and a continuous intravenous infusion of somatostatin (250 μg/hr with no bolus). Seven patients had pancreatic fistulas; however, data on site-specific closure were not given. They observed that there were no significant differences between the two groups in closure rate, 81.25% vs. 85%, but those patients treated with TPN and somatostatin had the fistulas close within a significantly shorter time with less morbidity.

Unfortunately, the last three studies represent European data using somatostatin as a continuous infusion. How this data would compare in the United States with intermittent therapy with somatostatin given subcutaneously is less clear and needs to be addressed.

Thus it seems that the conservative approach to closing fistulas with TPN and somatostatin warrants further investigation. It is key to know the amount of output as well as the anatomy of pancreatic duct drainage in these patients.

Hemosuccus Pancreaticus

Hemorrhage via the pancreatic duct, hemosuccus pancreaticus, is a rare cause of gastrointestinal bleeding. Morse et al.[28] treated one patient with TPN, with resolution of the bleeding. While major surgery is usually the treatment for such a condition, these authors concluded that TPN is worth a trial if bleeding is not life-threatening and not from a pseudoaneurysm. It is not known what effect somatostatin would have had if it had been added to this regimen.

Pancreatic Pseudocysts

With the advent of diagnostic radiographic techniques such as ultrasonography and CT scanning, the incidence of pancreatic pseudocysts is much higher than previously thought. While the incidence of pseudocysts has been estimated to be 10% with acute alcoholic pancreatitis, pseudocysts do occur with other etiologies of acute or chronic pancreatitis and with pancreatic trauma, either operative or external.[29, 30] In 1979 Bradley and coworkers[31] nicely documented the natural history of pseudocysts by ultrasonography. It was noted that pseudocysts present for less than 6 weeks had a 40% chance of spontaneous resolution with a 20% complication rate and pseudocysts present more than 12 weeks never resolved spontaneously and had a 67% complication rate. These data led to the practice of operative intervention for most pseudocysts that were present over 6 weeks and generally greater than 6 cm, which appears to be an important size over which the incidence of complications rises dramatically.

Yeo et al.[30] have recently reviewed the natural history of 75 patients with pseudocysts documented by CT scanning. Nonoperative management was possible in 48%, but 52% required operative management for persistent abdominal pain (62%), enlargement (18%), or complications attributable to the pseudocyst (20%). They suggested that (1) if a pseudocyst was found and the patient could eat, then follow-up with a repeat CT scan should occur monthly; (2) if there was continued pain with eating, then the patient should be given TPN, and it should be decided over several weeks whether operative management is necessary; (3) in an asymptomatic patient incidentally discovered to have a pseudocyst, the patient should be followed to see whether operative management is needed. It was again noted that pseudocysts greater than 6 cm required operative intervention more frequently. It must be noted that this study is heavily biased toward surgical approaches, and while it mentions percutaneous approaches to drainage, these authors did not utilize this approach often.

Other approaches that have been reported but not adequately controlled include percutaneous catheter drainage,[32-35] pancreatic stenting or nasopancreatic drainage via ERCP, internal drainage by cyst gastrostomy and cyst duodenostomy via ERCP,[36] and treatment with somatostatin.[37-39] The use of TPN is often discussed but has never been rigorously controlled.

Clinical management of pseudocysts is most likely to be highly influenced by local expertise in therapeutic radiology or endoscopy or surgery. A controlled trial of nonsurgical management including nutrition support, somatostatin, and catheter drainage either percutaneously or endoscopically vs. surgical management is badly needed.

Pleural Effusions

Pleural effusions caused by pancreatic disease do occur. Some will regress spontaneously with conservative treatment such as pancreatic rest, TPN, and repeated thoracentesis. Some patients will ultimately come to surgery if there is an obstructed duct, while some pleural effusions caused by pseudocysts may escape surgical repair.[40]

PEPTIC ULCER DISEASE AND STRESS GASTRITIS

In the United States peptic ulcer disease is a multibillion-dollar-a-year problem. The direct costs related to medical expense, indirect costs resulting from time lost from work, and the loss of potential lifetime earnings when an ulcer-related death occurs are of national concern.[41] By definition, an ulcer is a break in the mucosa that extends through the muscularis mucosa. In this section, peptic ulcer will refer to gastric and duodenal ulcers unless otherwise specified. This section will discuss nutrition and nutrition support as it relates to peptic ulcer disease, its complications, and stress ulceration in the critically ill patient.

Many tales are told about how certain foods cause ulcers. However, while certain spices, foods, and beverages may cause dyspeptic symptoms, they do not cause, perpetuate, or reactivate peptic ulcer disease.[41] It is not within the scope of this chapter to discuss the pathophysiology of this disorder, but Marotta and Floch[42] have nicely reviewed the subject of diet and nutrition in ulcer disease.

In this age of technological advances such as endoscopy, it has been discovered that symptoms alone, even seemingly classic ones,[43] may not be diagnostic of either the presence or location of disease.[41] Since the introduction of the H_2 antagonists, surgery for peptic ulcer disease has been markedly reduced. However, a change in symptoms may herald the development of complications.[41] Most patients who have an operation either have a complication of ulcer disease or have intractable pain. Common complications that must concern clinicians who manage them include the following: gastric outlet obstruction, hemorrhage, intractable pain, penetration, and perforation.

Nutrition support for the ulcer patient who has had surgery is the same as that for any postoperative patient. If the patient is not expected to regain gastrointestinal function quickly or if the patient was grossly malnourished preoperatively, then intravenous support may be appropriate. Table 34–3 lists complications that can occur after peptic ulcer surgery and complicate the return of function or use of the gastrointestinal tract. Nutrition in patients after gastric surgery, especially in treating the dumping syndrome and bezoars, has recently been reviewed and will not be covered here.[44] Appropriate evaluation and treatment will be important in returning the patient to a more normal eating pattern.

Stress Gastritis

In the critically ill patient stress-induced gastritis and ulceration are well recognized. Generally, the more severe the underlying disease, the greater the chance of gastric mucosal damage and subsequent bleeding. The actual incidence of mucosal damage is dependent on the method of evaluation. With endoscopic evaluation, 60% to 100% of patients may be found to have mucosal injury.[45] Also, with improvement in the care of the critically ill, more patients are surviving longer to have gastric mucosal damage develop. While this type of injury is common, patient mortality appears to be related to the severity and natural history of the underlying disease.[45]

Macroscopic damage can occur within hours of the stress, with submucosal petechiae and bleeding being the first abnormalities. These lesions begin in the gastric fundus and body but can then spread to the antrum, duodenum, or esophagus. These initial lesions can progress to erosions and ulcers and cause serious complications such as massive bleeding and perforation. The mortality rate can approach 80% if these latter complications require surgical intervention.[45]

Many treatments have been suggested for the treatment or prophylaxis of gastrointestinal bleeding. The pathophysiology of peptic ulcer disease and stress-induced mucosal injury is different, and they therefore require different treatment. Stress injury results from either the excess caustic effects of hydrochloric acid and pepsin or inadequate mucosal defenses. Table 34–4 lists the agents or modalities that have been studied.[46, 47] Of these agents, the ones most commonly used are antacids, H_2-receptor antagonists, and sucralfate. Omeprazole has been least studied for this indication because of the lack of an intravenous formulation in the United States. Daneshmend et al.[48] performed a large double-blind, randomized, placebo-controlled assessment of the effect of high-dose omeprazole vs. placebo

TABLE 34–3.

Postoperative Complications of Peptic Ulcer Surgery

Afferent loop syndrome
Bezoar formation
Bile reflux or gastritis
Delayed gastric emptying
Dumping syndrome
Efferent loop syndrome
Marginal ulcer
Small-pouch syndrome
Postvagotomy dysphagia
Postvagotomy diarrhea

TABLE 34–4.

Agents or Modalities Used in Treating Stress Gastritis

Allopurinol
Antacids
Epidermal growth factor
Glucagon
H_2-receptor antagonists
Nasoenteric feeding
Omeprazole
Prostaglandins
Somatostatin
Sucralfate
Tranexamic acid

on upper gastrointestinal hemorrhage. They found no difference in transfusion requirements, the need for emergency surgery, or mortality.

Cimetidine and ranitidine are the best studied of the H_2-receptor antagonists for the indication of stress gastritis. Most authorities suggest giving these drugs as continuous infusions to decrease the peak and trough levels that occur with bolus dosing.[49] There are fewer data on famotidine when used for this indication, but it has been studied for duodenal ulcer.[50] Cimetidine and ranitidine may be infused with TPN. This method of administration is cost-effective.[51] Famotidine is also compatible with TPN, but few data are available to support its use.[51, 52]

A continuing debate concerns the role of enteral feeding in the prevention or treatment of stress-induced gastritis. One of the greatest concerns is whether enteral feeding predisposes to the development of nosocomial pneumonia. Valentine et al.[53] showed in 20 critically ill patients that intragastric feeding controlled gastric pH much better than intraduodenal feeding. This study has been criticized for not having a control group and not performing serial endoscopies but still showed that maintaining the gastric pH over 5.0 was associated with a marked decrease in bleeding. While feeding by needle jejunostomy may be very effective in providing nutrition support for those patients who require surgery, gastric pH is not affected, and stress ulceration prophylaxis is still required.[54]

In a retrospective study, Kuric et al.[55] reviewed the clinical course of 166 patients. The first 66 patients were given enteral nutrition when "clinically ready," while the next 100 patients were fed with TPN within 4 days of admission if enteral nutrition could not be tolerated. The ulcer prophylaxis protocol was the same in both groups and consisted of cimetidine, nasogastric suction, hourly pH monitoring, and additional antacid therapy for pH less than 5.0.

There was a reduction in severe bleeding and perforation in the patients treated with early nutrition support. While some patients were fed enterally, the potential impact of this route of feeding on gastritis was not adequately discussed, and enteral complications were not mentioned.

A reduction in gastric bleeding with enteral nutrition does not appear to be solely based on using the tube feeding as a pH buffer.[56] It is known that gastric mucosa has low glycogen levels and is dependent on a continuous supply of nutrients for metabolism. However, Ephgrave and coworkers[57] showed that enteral feeding does not prevent stress ulceration by glucose's repletion of local glycogen stores; both glucose and lipid were equally protective of the gastric mucosa in a rat restraint model. Thus, feeding may improve the intrinsic mucosal defense system of the stomach but the mechanism by which it occurs is unclear.

While gastrointestinal bleeding and perforation are major complications at which treatment and prophylaxis are aimed, increasing the risk of pneumonia may be a serious consequence. Tryba[58] has recently reviewed the literature concerning this issue and has concluded that there is an increased risk of pneumonia associated with medication-induced increases in gastric pH. Table 34–5 lists those patients at highest risk.

Torres et al.[59] found that the supine position and length of time in that posi-

TABLE 34–5.

Patients at Increased Risk of Pulmonary Infections Due to the Gastropulmonary Route of Colonization*

Patients: Surgical, trauma
Ventilation: Mean duration, >4 days
Study period: >7 days
Pneumonia rate: ≥20% with antacids/H_2 antagonists
Antacids/H_2 antagonists: High dose, pH titration
Gastric colonization: Increase with antacids/H_2 antagonists
Nutrition: Enteral feeding (continuous)

*From Tryba M: Am J Med 1991; 91(suppl 2A):135–146. Used by permission.

tion were important factors contributing to pulmonary aspiration of gastric contents. They concluded that elevating the head of the bed was a simple, no-cost prophylactic measure for reducing aspiration (measured by radioactive means in a ventilated population).

An additional study implicated translocation as a significant factor in the pathogenesis of nosocomial pneumonia.[60]

GASTROINTESTINAL FISTULAS

Gastrointestinal fistulas are associated with increased morbidity and mortality as well as prolonged hospitalizations and increased resource utilization. Fluid and electrolyte disturbances, sepsis, and malnutrition are the three factors that have been associated with increased mortality.[61] We have previously discussed pancreatic fistulas and will not consider these further.

A high-output fistula has an output greater than 500 mL/day. The output will be partially dependent on the location of the fistula and oral intake. Table 34–6 details the contributions from gastrointestinal secretions that must be considered and rough estimates of total intestinal secretion at several anatomic areas.

Failure to adequately replace fistulous losses can result in dehydration, hypoperfusion, and ultimately multiple organ failure. Depending on the location of the fistula, there are significant vari-

ations in electrolyte composition. Thus, sending an aliquot of drainage fluid for sodium and potassium determinations can aid in determining replacement therapy.

Most fistulas occur after abdominal surgery when there is unrecognized trauma to the bowel or breakdown of an anastomosis. About 25% are caused by either extension of the bowel disease to surrounding structures or extension of disease from surrounding organs to the bowel. Examples of these latter etiologies include IBD, radiation therapy, benign or malignant tumors, and vascular processes (including ischemia of operated tissues).[61, 62]

The importance of nutrition support in the management of fistulas is credited to a 1964 report by Chapman et al.[63] These authors reported an increased fistula closure rate with decreased mortality when more than 1600 kcal/day were given. This study utilized early intravenous followed by enteral feedings. It was not until 1973 that MacPhayden et al.[64] reported achieving a 70.5% spontaneous closure rate with a 6.45% overall mortality rate when intravenous hyperalimentation was used to treat fistulas. Other studies have questioned the role of TPN in the treatment of fistulas. Table 34–7 lists our suggestions for management.

It seems prudent to support the patient with aggressive nutrition support. Initial nutrients are given intravenously, followed by the enteral route if fistulous drainage is not markedly in-

TABLE 34–6.

Input/Output in Normal Man

Approximate GI Tract Daily Contributions		Potential Output in Normal Man	
Source	Input (mL/Day)	Site	Approximate Fluid That Passes by the Site
Salivary juice	1500	Ligament of Treitz	7–9 L
Gastric juice	3000	Jejunum/ileum	3–4 L
Bile	500	Ileocecal valve	1–2 L
Pancreatic juice	2000	Rectum	100–200 cc
Oral intake	2000		

TABLE 34-7.

Fistula Therapy Checklist

1. Recognition and patient stabilization
   Correct fluid deficits
   Measure fistula output
   Decrease fistula output, NPO, complete bowel rest,
     ?somatostatin
   Begin TPN after fluid and electrolyte abnormalities
     corrected
   Drain abscesses
   Antibiotics when sepsis not controlled by drainage
   Local skin care
2. Nutrition support decisions
   TPN started—look for vitamin and mineral deficiencies
     that may affect healing
   Consider enteral nutrition if fistula output is low and
     enteral nutrition does not increase output; a
     nasoenteric tube may be placed beyond some fistulas
3. Define fistula anatomy after the patient is stabilized
4. Monitor fistula output
   Decide whether surgery is indicated sooner or
     conservative therapy indicated for 4–8 wk

creased. Enteral nutrition may decrease infectious complications by maintaining intestinal integrity and decreasing bacterial translocation. In proximal fistulas it may be possible to place a nasoenteric tube past the fistula or place a feeding jejunostomy.

While many uses of somatostatin have been proposed, its use in the treatment of fistulas has attracted much attention.[65] Several case reports and trials have utilized nutrition support and somatostatin to show a positive benefit.[26, 27, 66] As previously discussed, differences in the protocols are problematic since most have used continuous infusions of somatostatin. Nubiola et al.[67] published a study where they used SMS 201-995 (Sandostatin; Sandoz, Basel, Switzerland) subcutaneously, 100 µg every 8 hours. In their population of 27 patients with postoperative enterocutaneous fistulas, 11 had high-output fistulas (>1000 mL/48 h), 11 had low-output fistulas, and 5 patients had fistulas sitting in large abdominal wall defects. They observed a mean reduction of 55% in fistula output within 24 hours of treatment. The rate of spontaneous closure was 77%.

Sandostatin is the only available somatostatin formulation in the United States. Most clinicians underdose this medication. A typical dose is 50 to 100 µg every 12 hours. However, higher doses may be required to achieve the degree of success that has been noted by European investigators. Harris[65] has even suggested that Sandostatin be used postoperatively to prevent fistula formation; however, there are no prospective data that examine this issue or look at its cost-effectiveness. In addition, most insurance carriers are reluctant to reimburse for this medication as an outpatient, even if it means that the patient can go home.

Most of the adverse effects of Sandostatin are infrequent and transient. Discomfort at the site of injection may be bothersome to some patients. Also, there appears to be reports of gallstones. TPN may also cause gallstones. Messing et al.[68] reported that parenteral nutrition, continued for 6 weeks, was associated with 100% gallbladder sludge formation. Fifty percent (3/6) of patients in whom gallstones developed became symptomatic and required surgery. In addition, the antibiotic ceftriaxone (Rocephin; Roche Laboratories, Nutley, NJ) has been reported to cause a lithogenic state.[69]

In a study in dogs, Medeiros and Soares[70] showed that a high suction device placed into a fistulous tract could facilitate rapid healing and allow for a normal diet. This was in an uninfected and unobstructed model, and while a clinical trial in patients has not been published, the authors state that the preliminary results are favorable.

The treatment of fistulas continues to evolve, and the provision of nutrition support, either enterally or parenterally, is essential. Further studies are needed to better define the role and effectiveness of various therapies. The ultimate goal is more rapid, cost-efficient, and conservative therapy for this devastating problem.

INFLAMMATORY BOWEL DISEASE

Crohn's disease and ulcerative colitis are the major forms of idiopathic IBD. Crohn's disease is a transmural, nonconfluent inflammatory process that can involve any portion of the gastrointestinal tract from the mouth to the anus. A patient can have disease of the small intestine, the large intestine, or a combination of both; the rectum is usually spared. Ulcerative colitis is limited to the large intestine. It is predominantly a mucosal disease and usually involves the rectum. Lack of transmural inflammation makes fistula formation or perirectal abscess formation a rare complication of this disease.

Patients with severe Crohn's disease may require one or more intestinal resections during the course of the disease. Usually these resections involve the small bowel. These resections are not curative and often leave the patient with a reduced absorptive small-bowel surface in combination with ongoing inflammation in the remaining small intestinal segments. In contrast, the bowel disease associated with ulcerative colitis is cured by a total proctocolectomy, although extraintestinal manifestations of the disease may remain a problem. In both disease processes, multiple medications including corticosteroids, immunosuppressive agents, and sulfasalazine are used long-term for suppression of inflammation. These drug regimens promote catabolism and often inappropriate utilization of nutrients.

Malnutrition is prevalent among patients with IBD, although it is more prevalent in Crohn's disease. Two thirds of patients hospitalized with Crohn's disease are malnourished.[71] Protein-calorie malnutrition is the most common deficiency associated with IBD.[72] Table 34–8 lists a number of factors responsible for the development of malnutrition in this patient population. The most important mechanism is de-

TABLE 34–8.

Etiologies of Malnutrition in Inflammatory Bowel Disease

Decreased nutrient intake
  Anorexia
  Nausea
  Abdominal pain
Malabsorption
  Loss of absorptive surface
  Bacterial overgrowth
Protein-losing enteropathy
Maldigestion of fat
  Bile salt loss/ileal disease and resection
Drug-nutrient interaction
  Corticosteroids with calcium and protein
  Sulfasalazine with folate
  Cholestyramine with fats and fat-soluble vitamins
Increased caloric requirements
  Sepsis/fever
  Cell repair
  Steroid therapy

creased food intake.[73] Associated abdominal pain, diarrhea, multiple medication usage, and nausea amplify the generalized anorexia associated with a chronic inflammatory process. Restricted diets and associated lactose intolerance also add to the inadequate ingestion of adequate calories and nutrients.

Protein losses may be substantial and can approach 80 to 90 g/24 hr.[74] There is a loss of brush border and associated digestive enzymes that potentiates malabsorption. This malabsorption is worsened by the rapid transit of food through the small bowel secondary to the chronic mucosal irritation. Prior surgical resections may create SBS. Approximately 120 cm of small bowel is required for adequate protein digestion and absorption. An adequate reserve of small bowel is required to allow adequate mixing of food with bile and pancreatic secretions, especially important for fat absorption. Loss of ileal length results in bile salt depletion and eventual loss of the bile salt pool. Malabsorbed bile salts worsen diarrhea via an irritative mechanism. Interestingly, there is great reserve in the small bowel for the absorption of carbohydrates, except for lactose. Thus, we recommend diets that are high in both carbohydrate and protein calories and limited in fat calories. Prior surgery creates an environment for bacterial overgrowth by promoting stasis, especially in blind loops. Reduced gastric acid secretion or the use of proton pump inhibitors or H_2-receptor blockers also reduces gastric pH and propagates bacterial overgrowth. Resection of the ileocecal valve is responsible for colonization of the small bowel with large-bowel bacteria.

It is important to remember that all protein loss is not in the feces. An intra-abdominal abscess or other secretory process may account for a large share of protein loss.[75] Powell-Tuck[76] demonstrated an increase in the fractional loss of albumin in patients with both ulcerative colitis and Crohn's disease. Such losses correlated with the severity of the disease. Thus, the hypoalbuminemia associated with IBD may represent a combination of decreased production, increased catabolism, and intestinal leakage.

Protein malnutrition associated with IBD leads to immunologic impairment, a higher incidence of infection, poor wound healing, weight loss, and growth failure.[72] Several studies have shown that growth failure associated with IBD can be corrected by increasing the nutrient intake.[77] Motil et al.[78] demonstrated with ^{15}N tracer studies that nitrogen retention increases with increased protein delivery.

Deficiencies of vitamins and trace elements are common in IBD (Table 34–9). Minerals and trace elements are often lost in diarrheal fluids and fistula output. Loses include magnesium, potassium, selenium, and zinc. The small bowel is the major site of zinc uptake.[79] Steatorrhea produces a loss of calcium, magnesium, zinc, and copper in the form of soaps. Patients with zinc deficiency are prone to fistula formation and poor wound healing. Zinc, potassium, and calcium deficiency impairs protein

TABLE 34–9.

Common Nutrient Deficiency in Inflammatory Bowel Disease

Nutrient	Crohn's Disease	Ulcerative Colitis
Iron	Yes	Yes
Folate	Yes	Yes
Magnesium	Yes	No
Potassium	Yes	No
Vitamin A	Yes	No
Vitamin D	Yes	No
Vitamin B_{12}	Yes	Yes
Selenium	Yes	Yes
Zinc	Yes	No

synthesis.[80] Chronic occult blood loss leads to iron deficiency. If the duodenum is resected or bypassed, calcium and iron may be malabsorbed. Resection of the ileum leads to vitamin B_{12} deficiency.

Energy consumption is an important nutritional parameter to utilize in prescribing adequate nutritional therapy. Patients with diarrhea, bowel inflammation, abscesses, or other infectious complications have an increased caloric need. Patients with clinically mild IBD have calculated caloric needs by the Harris-Benedict equation similar to normal controls.[81] However, in severe disease processes, the use of the Harris-Benedict equation may be inadequate. Indirect calorimetry will better assess caloric needs in this group of patients.

SPECIFIC SUPPORT IN INFLAMMATORY BOWEL DISEASE

Considerable attention has been focused on the nutritional support of patients with IBD. These studies have examined both the utilization of enteral nutrition, especially elemental feedings, and the use of bowel rest and TPN. The end points of these studies have been varied, including morbidity, mortality, length of hospital stay, time to rehospitalization, medication usage, and disease activity scores, and this has resulted in a confusing mix of information. Although the cure for IBD remains elusive, what is clear is that adequate, aggressive nutritional support is a key adjuvant in the total treatment plan for patients with IBD.

Dietary manipulation in IBD has long been considered important in the treatment process. In general, no one specific diet is recommended. Dietary modification may assume many facets (Table 34–10). In certain patients either lactose or fat is restricted to limit malabsorption. Medium-chain triglycerides (MCTs) can be substituted for long-chain fatty acids if there is fat malabsorption to provide calories but not a source of essential fatty acids. Intolerance to certain foods has been well documented, and in one series, a strict elimination diet resulted in a cumulative remission rate of 45% over a period of 5 years.[82] Generally speaking, a diet consisting of 40 to 45 kcal/kg and 1.5 to 2 g/kg of protein is required in patients with active disease. Supplementation with a multivitamin containing one to five times the recommended dietary allowance is advised.[83] Certain patients will require iron, folate, and vitamin B_{12} additives. Special attention should be paid to fluid requirements, especially during an active flare. Recently, attention has been paid to the immunologic manipulations possible with dietary therapy. Neutrophils are attracted to sites of inflammation by chemoattractants such as leukotriene B_4 (LTB_4) and prostaglandin E_2 (PGE_2). Eicosapentae-noic acid (EPA), a polyunsaturated fat in fish oil, diminishes the effects of LTB_4 and PGE_2. O'Morain[84] treated a group of patients with ulcerative colitis with EPA and noted both clinical and histologic improvement and a decrease in neutrophil activity. However, further investigations are required in this area.

Dudrick et al.[85] describe inflammation of the bowel as similar to burns of the skin. During the early phases of disease or with modest inflammation of the mucosa, which they compare with a first-degree burn, there is minimal histologic disease and an intact absorptive function. This phase can be successfully treated with nutritional therapy. However, patients with transmural intestinal disease are similar to patients with third-degree burns. Normal intestinal mucosa is replaced with granulation tissue, often resulting in irreversible disease and elimination of absorptive capacity. This disease would not be expected to respond to even the most intensive nutritional therapy. Between these two extremes is a group of patients with moderate mucosal and submucosal damage, similar to a second-degree burn. The mucosal cells have been severely damaged but could regenerate in the proper environment if the basal cells in the villus crypts are protected from further damage. This is the group in which aggressive nutritional intervention could demonstrate the greatest efficacy.

Total Parenteral Nutrition in Inflammatory Bowel Disease

While the uses of TPN have expanded during the last two decades, it is known that long-term TPN is associated with decreased villus height, decreased gut thickness, and bacterial translocation through a thinned intestinal mucosa. The use of TPN could hypothetically potentiate the process of translocation by an associated reduction of mucosal growth factors or a reduction in IgA se-

TABLE 34–10.

Dietary Modifications in Complications Associated With Inflammatory Bowel Disease

Complication	Modification
None	Discourage generalized dietary restrictions
Steatorrhea/fat malabsorption	Low fat, medium-chain triglycerides
Calcium oxalate stones	Low oxalate/low fat
Strictures	Low fiber
Severe diarrhea	High fiber, bile-binding resins
Lactose intolerance	Lactose-free diet

cretion.[86, 87] The use of TPN in IBD is based on the concept that bowel rest is helpful, especially in the patient who is refractory to standard medical treatment. This would allow for nutrition support during total bowel rest, which could reduce mechanical trauma, thus decreasing both chemical and hormonal stimulation. It may also eliminate the antigenic stimulation of foods.[88]

Various studies are available that report an initial improvement of 40% to 90% in patients with Crohn's disease treated with TPN. Muller et al.[89] noted a return to work and a resumption of oral feedings in 83% of patients with Crohn's disease treated with TPN during a flare. However, the relapse rate at 2 years was 60%. Kushner et al.[90] also demonstrated a high relapse rate among patients with Crohn's disease treated with TPN. However, Ostro et al.[91] was able to maintain a 60% remission rate at 1 year in 100 patients with Crohn's disease treated with TPN that was refractory to other conventional medical treatment. All of these patients, however, continued to receive some drug therapy. TPN in the preoperative setting has only been shown to be effective in patients with significant malnutrition and results in decreased morbidity such as wound infection, anastomotic leaks, and prolonged ileus.[92] In conclusion, TPN as the sole therapy is effective in inducing remissions in patients with Crohn's disease; however, relapse rates are high. Concurrent drug therapy may be important for preventing relapses. The use of TPN in IBD should be reserved for those patients with Crohn's disease who have not responded to conventional medical therapy, including enteral nutrition. The cost and risk of this therapy should always be taken into consideration. Emergent surgery should not be delayed to correct nutritional deficiencies. Patients with ulcerative colitis generally respond poorly to TPN, but TPN may play a supportive role in maintaining nutritional needs that are not met with enteral therapy.

Enteral Diets in Inflammatory Bowel Disease

A number of studies have demonstrated long-term success with the administration of enteral diets.[93] Enteral feeding improves mucosal thickness, stimulates gut trophic hormones, stimulates IgA production, and potentiates generalized immune responses. It must be remembered that the gut is the largest lymphoid organ in the body. Preferred gut fuel sources such as glutamine reverse negative nitrogen balance and stimulate mucosal growth.[94]

Several prospective and retrospective trials have failed to demonstrate a clinical difference in the ability of total enteral nutrition (TEN) as compared with TPN to induce remission. Jones[95] noted an 84% in-hospital remission rate in patients with Crohn's disease who were fed an elemental diet vs. an 87.5% remission rate in those treated with TPN and bowel rest. Greenberg et al.[71] in a multicenter trial, reported that there was no difference in remission rates among patients with Crohn's disease unresponsive to medical therapy who were randomized to receive either TPN or a defined-formula diet (administered by nasoenteric tube). These data must be considered along with the reduced risk and cost of TEN. Recent changes in the formulation and palatability of elemental formulations have made it easier to administer enteral nutrition by the oral route, which may eliminate the need for nasoenteric tube placement. New enteral formulations are available that contain essential amino acids, specific gut fuels such as glutamine, and short-chain fatty acids.

Nutritional therapy for IBD continues to evolve. Recent years have shown a shift away from parenteral nutrition and bowel rest toward enteral elemental nutrition. Bacterial translocation, gut-stimulated immune response, and gut-specific fuels are emerging concepts driving research in enteral nutrition.

HEPATIC FAILURE

Nutritional deficiencies are common in liver disease. Decreased dietary intake is the principal cause. Additional factors include decreased absorption, decreased hepatic storage, altered nutrient metabolism, and increased requirements of nutrients. Alcoholism, a common cause of liver disease, can also be associated with severe nutritional deficiency.

Decreased dietary intake is often secondary to anorexia and nausea and has been recorded prospectively in 73% of 124 hospitalized alcoholic patients with cirrhosis and hepatic failure and in 21% of nonalcoholic hospitalized patients with hepatic failure.[96, 97] Ethanol may provide between 52% and 63% of the total calories in alcoholic patients with cirrhosis.[98] Both protein and vitamin intake are limited in these patients, and there is a propensity for carbohydrate calories.

Steatorrhea is the most common form of malabsorption in patients with cirrhosis. It occurs in 50% of these patients and is generally mild (<10 g/day), although in 10% of patients it may exceed 30 g/day.[98] The cause of the steatorrhea is a decrease in bile salt synthesis coupled with a decrease in biliary excretion, which can also result in malabsorption of the fat-soluble vitamins.[99] In addition, thickened mucosal folds secondary to hypoalbuminemia and bowel wall edema may contribute to carbohydrate and protein malabsorption. Hypoalbuminemia is secondary to decreases in hepatic synthesis, a decrease in small intestinal lymphatic drainage due to high portal pressures, and a generalized debilitated state of the patient.

Abnormalities in the metabolism of protein, carbohydrates, lipids, and vita-mins occur in liver disease. There may be marked depletion of muscle mass secondary to the lack of adequate glucose stores and an increased drain on protein for both gluconeogenesis and repair of liver injury.[100] An increase in plasma glucagon levels and a decrease in plasma insulin levels further drive gluconeogenesis. There is an alteration in the plasma amino acid pattern with a rise in the aromatic amino acids tyrosine, phenylalanine, and methionine and a fall in the branched-chain amino acids (BCAAs) valine, leucine, and isoleucine.[101] The aromatic amino acids (AAA) are normally removed by the liver, while the BCAAs are principally taken up by extrahepatic tissue. Some have speculated that BCAAs provide a better protein source in liver failure, although this remains a topic of controversy.

Glucose intolerance is found in 50% to 80% of patients with cirrhosis.[102] The primary cause is insulin resistance. In addition, there is a reduction of insulin binding to target tissues.[103] Patients with liver failure also have increased levels of free fatty acids and triglycerides. There is decreased lipolytic activity, decreased degradation of fatty acids, and decreased removal of fatty acids.[104]

Vitamin deficiencies are common in liver disease. A defect in the phosphorylation of thiamine leads to thiamine deficiency. Ethanol ingestion interferes with both the formation and excretion of 5-methyltetrahydrofolic acid and inhibits folate secretion into the bile.[105] There is increased degradation of pyridoxal-5-phosphate, the biologically active form of vitamin B_6.[106] Decreased liver synthesis of retinol-binding protein decreases plasma vitamin A levels. The conversion of vitamin D to 25-hydroxy vitamin D is slowed, with resultant progression of bone disease in patients with chronic liver failure. In addition, vitamins A, D, E, and K may be malabsorbed because of fat intolerance. Some of the increased risk for bleeding in patients with liver failure may be secondary to a decreased hepatic synthesis of the vitamin K–dependent coagulation factors, as well as malabsorption of vitamin K.

Nutritional Assessment in Liver Disease

The presence of liver disease, either acute, chronic, or acute-on-chronic, affects our ability to determine nutritional status by traditional methods. Anthropometric measurements provide a clue to current nutritional status by estimating both somatic protein stores (midarm circumference) and fat stores (triceps skin fold). However, these measurements may often be skewed because of the presence of subclinical edema.[107] The creatinine/height index may be useful in monitoring muscle mass breakdown. However, this measurement is not useful in the presence of concurrent renal disease. All four major circulating plasma proteins utilized to monitor visceral protein stores (albumin, transferrin, prealbumin, and retinol-binding protein) are synthesized largely by liver cells, and these markers do not correlate with the degree of malnutrition, but rather with the extent of liver injury.[108]

The presence of liver disease depresses immune function and invalidates the commonly used nutritional indices of delayed-hypersensitivity skin tests and total lymphocyte counts.[109] Appropriate interpretation of nutritional assessment techniques will be of primary importance in attempting to delineate adequate nutritional therapy.

Alterations in nitrogen metabolism are prominent in liver failure and result from active deamination and gluconeogenesis in the intestine and muscle, intraluminal bacterial degradation of protein in the gut, impaired urea generation, and inadequate delivery of nitrogen to the liver secondary to portalsystemic shunting; hyperammonemia is a common finding. These factors can result in an underestimation of negative nitrogen balance if urinary nitrogen excretion is relied on for protein repletion.[110]

Hypercatabolism often accompanies liver failure. Increased glucagon, cortisol, and epinephrine levels stimulate the basal metabolic rate.[111] Elevated counterregulatory hormones result from a decrease in hepatic metabolism of these hormones. Resting energy expenditure is usually increased in liver failure, and the traditional Harris-Benedict equation has little role in such metabolically altered patients. Indirect calorimetry measurements may be used to assess caloric needs. Examination of the respiratory quotient (RQ) also provides insight into substrate utilization. Patients with liver failure utilize fat as a primary fuel source after an overnight fast. The lack of sufficient glucose stores and the inability to utilize peripheral glucose effectively potentiate the need for alternative fuel sources. Additionally, the RQ can aid in determining whether a patient is being adequately fed. An RQ greater than 1.0 indicates overfeeding and lipogenesis, while an RQ less than 0.75 suggests underfeeding and lipolysis.

Nutrition Support in Severe Liver Disease

The objective of nutritional support in liver failure is to provide adequate calories and protein to support the energy requirements of the patient and to prevent protein-calorie malnutrition. However, care must be taken to prevent the precipitation of hepatic encephalopathy. The needs of the patient will change depending on the rate and amount of functional hepatic tissue loss and the presence of concurrent major diseases. In a well-compensated nonencephalopathic cirrhotic, protein administration of 0.8 to 1.0 g/day is adequate to maintain a neutral protein balance.

BCAAs are preferentially used for energy by the patient in liver failure because they do not require the liver to play a role in their metabolism. Specialized formulations low in aromatic amino acids and enriched with BCAAs are designed to normalize plasma amino acid profiles. Marchesini et al.[112] studied the anticatabolic effects of BCAAs in cirrhotic patients who had decreased levels of BCAAs but no muscle wasting or encephalopathy. They demonstrated a decrease in muscle catabolism measured by 3-methylhistidine urinary excretion. Two studies comparing BCAA parenteral solutions with a standard amino acid parenteral solution in stressed cirrhotic patients noted no improvement in nitrogen balance, morbidity, mortality, or hepatic encephalopathy in the BCAA-treated group.[113, 114] They did note an improvement in the amino acid profile in the BCAA-treated group.

α-Ketoanalogues of BCAA (BCKAs) are the nitrogen-free deaminated products of leucine, isoleucine, and valine. BCKAs are converted back to BCAAs by transamination, which theoretically results in the reduction of toxic amines and increases precursors for protein synthesis without the addition of a nitrogen source. Keto acids converted to amino acids are incorporated into the protein skeleton. BCKAs have also been shown to stimulate insulin secretion and decrease glucagon production, reduce glucocorticoid levels, and lead to protein sparing in liver failure.[115, 116] Although some studies substantiate the ability of BCKAs to improve nitrogen balance in cirrhotic patients, other studies have been disappointing.[117] Further large clinical trials will be necessary to evaluate the practicality and validity of BCKA supplementation in liver failure.

Vegetable protein is an alternative protein source that is better tolerated in encephalopathic patients.[118] This is due to increased incorporation of nitrogen in the stool secondary to high dietary fiber content. Casein-based diets are also antiencephalopathic. They have been found to improve encephalopathy to a greater extent than BCAAs.[119]

Cirrhotic patients have approximately the same daily energy needs as normal subjects, approximately 25 to 35 kcal/kg.[120] Underfeeding leads to protein-calorie malnutrition, increased morbidity and mortality, and immune dysfunction. Overfeeding potentiates hepatic steatosis, CO_2 retention, and immune dysfunction. Altered carbohydrate metabolism may present problems for supplying energy needs. Glucose intolerance is common in liver failure. Ultimately, dextrose solutions or oral glucose should provide 40% to 50% of the total calories. The addition of insulin may be necessary to control glucose intolerance. MCTs are a useful method of caloric supplementation in malnourished cirrhotics, especially those with steatorrhea. MCTs are directly absorbed into the portal vein and do not require biochemical transformation or chylomicron formation prior to intestinal absorption. The administration of large amounts of MCTs has not precipitated encephalopathy but can lead to diarrhea.[121] MCTs do not contain essential fatty acids, and prolonged use in the absence of other fats may contribute to fatty acid deficiency. Intravenous lipid emulsions are attractive nutritional formulations because they are calorie dense, contain little water, and depend little on the liver for metabolism.

The primary goal in liver failure is to prevent further injury and promote hepatic regeneration. One nutritional approach to a patient with liver failure is to start with a low protein intake of 0.6 g/kg body weight per day and to increase to 1.2 to 1.5 g/kg/day. If there is evidence of encephalopathy, standard medical therapy can be initiated. Due to their cost and controversial efficacy, BCAAs should be reserved for the treatment of encephalopathy not responsive to standard medical care. Adequate dextrose calories can prevent hypoglycemia secondary to impaired gluconeogenesis. Fat calories may be added to meet calorie needs. Both fat-soluble vitamin deficiency secondary to malabsorption and water-soluble vitamin deficiency secondary to diuretic-induced urinary losses need to be monitored and corrected.

Parenteral nutrition should be used cautiously in patients with liver failure. A dysfunctional gastrointestinal tract or the inability to gain enteral access favors the use of TPN. In addition to the metabolic complications previously described, TPN is associated with cholestasis, fatty liver metamorphosis, hepatocellular fibrosis, hepatocellular necrosis, and occasionally cirrhosis. Early conversion to enteral feedings is necessary to prevent the associated atrophy of small intestinal mucosa, bacterial translocation, and multiple organ failure.

The specific goals of nutrition support in patients with liver failure are to meet the increased requirements of hypercatabolism and hypermetabolism with substrates that produce minimal metabolic complications. Only with a clear understanding of the metabolic changes associated with liver failure can these nutritional goals be met.

Liver Transplantation

The majority of liver transplant patients are at high nutritional risk because of anorexia and altered metabolism associated with liver failure. The stress of a long surgical procedure combined with the many possible postsurgical complications amplifies the effect of nutritional deficiencies. Adequate pretransplantation nutritional assessment combined with appropriate preoperative and postoperative nutritional intervention may make a significant impact on the morbidity, mortality, and success of liver transplantation.

Nutritional status is an important determinant of operative morbidity and mortality. Mourkarzel et al.[122] noted a significant increase in surgical complications after liver transplantation and the need for increased numbers of retransplantations in a group of pediatric patients who were malnourished. Shaw

and coworkers[123] retrospectively analyzed the preoperative records of 160 adult liver transplant patients. Several clinical variables were assessed, and malnutrition was found to be highly correlated with patient survival.

An adequate nutritional assessment is imperative in identifying those liver failure patients with malnutrition. The reported incidence of malnutrition in liver failure is varied in the literature. Guarnieri et al.[124] studied a large number of nutritional parameters and found that 100% of 23 cirrhotic patients were malnourished. Franco and colleagues,[125] using anthropometric measurements and visceral protein levels, noted at least two abnormalities in 66% of patients with alcoholic liver disease.

Recently, DiCecco et al.[126] assessed the nutritional status of 100 patients prior to liver transplantation. Patients with cholestatic liver disease had significantly decreased midarm muscle circumferences, while the group with noncholestatic liver disease had significantly decreased triceps skin folds. Visceral protein markers were found to be reduced in a majority of the patients. Anergy and reduced total lymphocyte counts were also found in nearly all patients. Although most patients demonstrated fat malabsorption, there were no significant abnormalities in fat-soluble vitamin levels. Serum zinc levels were decreased because of decreased circulating protein levels, general malnutrition, and increased fecal and skin losses.

Orthotopic liver transplantation is associated with a state of hypermetabolism and hypercatabolism. Extra demand for substrate, if not supplied exogenously, must be met endogenously by muscle protein breakdown. Indirect calorimetric measurements of energy needs after liver transplantation are 33% higher than predicted based on controls. Liver transplantation is also associated with daily nitrogen losses of approximately 22 g/day in the early postoperative period.[127] High nitrogen losses in the early postoperative period were also confirmed by O'Keefe and William.[128] These investigators demonstrated that body protein losses could be reduced by providing adequate glucose and amino acid calories. However, they failed to provide the necessary mixed fuel source to completely prevent protein-calorie malnutrition in this patient population. Shanbhogue et al.[129] noted that a semistarved group of liver transplant patients had a 7-g negative nitrogen balance in the preoperative period that increased to 13-g negative nitrogen balance in the postoperative period, thus demonstrating the catabolic status of these individuals and underscoring the need for adequate nutritional therapy. This protein catabolic state is potentiated by the use of certain medications such as high-dose steroids in patients after liver transplantation. Cyclosporine inhibits T-lymphocyte function at the expense of increased release of interleukin-1, which is a principal metabolic mediator in states of stress.[130, 131] Even in previously well nourished patients, rapid protein turnover can erode critical visceral protein mass and set the stage for multiple organ failure.

The interrelationships between nutritional status and immunocompetence are complex and multifactorial. In some series, malnutrition is associated with an increased incidence of skin anergy.[132] Abnormalities of serum IgG, complement, lymphocyte counts, lymphocyte response, and neutrophil chemotaxis have been described in malnourished dogs.[133] Skin anergy is closely associated with body cell mass and therefore protein mass and underscores the close relationship between immune status and nutrition.[134] A failure to replenish body cell mass has been correlated with decreased skin anergy and poor prognosis in the general surgical literature. O'Keefe et al.[135] noted a close relationship between reduced triceps skin fold measurements and skin anergy in liver failure patients with malnutrition. Clearly, our ability to define

immunocompetence accurately in the liver failure population is poor; however, it is closely tied to the patient's nutritional status and carries a significant impact on postoperative morbidity and mortality. Because rejection of liver allografts is primarily mediated by recipient T lymphocytes, one could expect fewer rejection episodes after orthotopic liver transplantation in malnourished patients. However, this has not been shown and demonstrates that rejection is a much more complex process.

Pre–Liver Transplant Nutrition

Pre–liver transplantation nutritional therapy involves the provision of adequate protein and calories (Table 34–11). Liver failure is marked by endogenous protein breakdown. The primary nitrogenous load is derived from muscle breakdown.[136] Dietary protein restriction only worsens the protein deficit. Protein malnutrition also potentiates bacterial translocation from the gut

TABLE 34–11.

Nutritional Requirements Before Liver Transplantation

Energy/calories	35–45 kcal/kg or 150%–175% of basal energy expenditure Based on indirect calorimetry measurements 25%–40% provided as fat calories
Fluid/electrolytes	Sodium restriction: approximately 2 g/day Fluid restriction: 1000–1500 cc/day in appropriate patients
Protein	1.5 g/kg/day Use BCAA* if there is encephalopathy not responsive to medical therapy Adjust administered protein based on 24-hr urinary nitrogen excretion measurements
Vitamins/minerals/trace elements	Monitor and supplement Fat-soluble vitamins Magnesium Zinc

*BCAA = branched-chain amino acid.

to the periphery, which increases the risk for systemic infection.[135] Patients should consume 40 to 60 g of protein per day, increased at times of metabolic stress. Most patients require 35 to 40 kcal/kg/day and 150% to 175% of basal energy expenditure to achieve anabolism. Twenty-five percent to 40% of the total calories should be provided as fat calories, with the use of MCTs as a fat source if fat intolerance is present.[137] Sodium restriction for patients with liver failure should approximate 2 g/day. This will aid in preventing a rapid accumulation of ascities and edema. Fluid should be limited to 1000 to 1500 cc/day in patients at risk for fluid accumulation. Although clear evidence for fat-soluble vitamin deficiency has not been well documented in the literature, signs and symptoms of deficiency should be monitored, as well as zinc and magnesium deficiency. Zinc deficiency resulting from both increased urinary excretion and decreased intestinal absorption is well documented in liver disease.[138] Manifestations of zinc deficiency are numerous, and zinc levels should be monitored.

Post–Liver Transplant Nutrition

In the post–liver transplant patient, BCAAs are no more effective than standard amino acid solutions in improving nitrogen balance when compared with semistarved controls.[139] Nutritional supplementation seems to play no role in altering the preoperative AAA/BCAA ratio. However, successful liver transplantation results in an immediate improvement in this ratio. The AAA/BCAA ratio is predictive of liver graft survival if closely followed in the post-transplant period.[140] BCAAs also compete with AAAs for transport proteins in the central nervous system. A marked decrease of BCAA potentiates the influx of AAA into the central nervous system. AAAs may act as false neurotransmitters and potentiate hepatic encephalopathy. A review of multiple investigations notes that BCAAs may be beneficial in the protein-intolerant patient whose encephalopathy fails to respond to traditional medical therapy.[141]

After liver transplantation, the nutritional needs of the patient are determined both by the acceptance of the allograft with a return to normal metabolic status and by postoperative complications. Similar to other postoperative states, there is substantial nitrogen wasting and resultant high protein needs. There is an early daily nitrogen loss of approximately 22 g/day, with a continued nitrogen loss of approximately 12.5 g/day through the seventh postoperative day.[127, 128] Reilley et al.[140] demonstrated the importance of post–liver transplant nutritional therapy. Patients received either 35 kcal/kg of nonprotein calories and 1.5 g/kg/day of amino acids or an isotonic glucose solution of 400 kcal/day for 7 postoperative days. The patients fed isotonic glucose had poorer nitrogen balance and longer lengths of stay in the intensive care unit. Refeeding can be complicated by concurrent medical problems and medication usage. Corticosteroid, azothioprine, and cyclosporine use can alter nutrient metabolism.[136, 142]

Specific Support After Liver Transplantation

Table 34–12 shows our general suggestions for the first several days after liver transplantation; however, the feeding regimen for each patient after liver transplantation must be individualized. Generally, TPN should begin on day 1 after an adequate nutritional assessment has been obtained to aid in determining both protein and caloric needs. A liter of parenteral nutrition of standard amino acid/dextrose concentration should be initiated (e.g., 4.25% amino acid/25% dextrose). Serum glucose levels require frequent monitoring. Serum potassium, magnesium, and phosphorous levels need to be closely monitored to reduce the risk of refeeding syndrome.[143] The parenteral solution should be increased

TABLE 34–12.

Post–Liver Transplant Nutritional Regimen*

Preoperative:
  Indirect calorimetry and 24-hr total urinary urea
    excretion
  Baseline zinc measurement
  Baseline anthropometric measurements
  Baseline infrared spectroscopy measurement of fat
    store†
  Calorie count
Day 1:
  Total parenteral nutrition
    1 L 4.25% amino acids/25% dextrose
    Monitor serum glucose frequently
    Monitor for refeeding syndrome (potassium,
      phosphorous, magnesium)
Days 2–3:
  Total parenteral nutrition
    Increase amino acids and/or dextrose to meet
      caloric/protein needs
    Increase volume to meet fluid requirements, but do
      not increase TPN volume or amount of dextrose if
      the patient is hyperglycemic
    Addition of fats for
      Caloric source
      Prevention of fatty acid deficiency
      Reduction in CO_2 production
    Monitor serum potassium, phosphorous, magnesium,
      and renal function
    Daily calorie count
    Monitor for return of bowel function unless a
      jejunostomy was placed at surgery
Day 4 and on:
  Enteral nutrition—Begin as soon as possible
    Increase volume/osmolality as tolerated
    Monitor serum potassium, phosphorous, magnesium,
      and renal function
    Biweekly indirect calorimetry/24-hr urinary urea
      nitrogen excretion†
    Baseline handgrip dynanometry followed weekly†
    Baseline infrared spectroscopy followed every other
      week†
    Anthropometric measurements followed every other
      week
    Daily calorie count
  Total parenteral nutrition
    Reduce as enteral nutrition is increased; maintain
      protein/calorie needs

*This regimen should be altered to meet the special needs of each
particular patient.
†When available.

both in volume and, if needed, in dextrose and amino acid concentrations over the next 24 to 48 hours to meet both protein and caloric needs. Intravenous lipids are administered at least twice per week to prevent essential fatty acid deficiency and to act as a major ca-

loric source. The quantity of lipids may be increased to provide increased calories in a patient who cannot tolerate the volume needed to receive adequate dextrose. Lipids may also help decrease CO_2 production in ventilated patients who are retaining carbon dioxide secondary to dextrose metabolism. Lipid infusions should be administered at rates less than 3.0 mg/kg/min to minimize increases in thromboxane production, vasoconstriction, and resultant pulmonary shunting.[144] Controversy still exists over the potential for lipids to induce immune dysfunction. However, to date, studies have failed to demonstrate clinically significant immune dysfunction with intravenous lipids.[145] If available, the patient should have biweekly indirect calorimetry and 24-hour urea nitrogen excretion measurements for the first 2 weeks post–liver transplant to help direct nutritional therapy. Calorie counts should be monitored daily.

Post–liver transplant patients should be converted to enteral feedings as soon as possible. This will depend on the return of gastrointestinal tract function. There is no indication for the use of total parenteral nutrition in the patient with a functioning gastrointestinal tract who can tolerate enteral feedings. The continued use of parenteral feedings is associated with increased complications as compared with enteral feedings.[146, 147] Early enteral feeding will also maintain small-bowel mucosal depth and prevent bacterial translocation with its associated increased risk for systemic infection.[148, 149] Feedings should begin at low volumes and advanced to meet the desired needs based on the patient's tolerance and protein/caloric requirements. In the transitional phase, the calorie/protein load from TPN should be decreased as enteral feedings are increased.

The goal of nutritional support is to optimize the patient's nutrient and metabolic status so that it will have a favorable impact on liver transplant outcome. The nutrition support team should be involved early in the management of patients with liver failure who may proceed on to liver transplantation. Knowledge of the metabolic changes associated with liver failure and the ability to adequately assess the patient with reproducible tools will allow intensive nutritional therapy for the patient at risk. Aggressive post–liver transplant nutritional assessment and therapy should aid in reducing complications, shortening intensive care unit stay, and it is hoped, improving outcome. Nutrition is the foundation upon which other technical therapy must be built to ensure a positive transplant result.

SHORT-BOWEL SYNDROME

SBS represents a challenge to the management skills of the physician in both the early stages of the disease as well as the later, more chronic stages. SBS occurs in patients when there is less than 150 cm of small intestine. There is usually marked dysfunction of the remaining small and large (if present) bowel.[150] Table 34–13 lists etiologies of SBS.

The severity of SBS is dependent upon a number of factors that are listed

TABLE 34–13.

Etiologies of Short-Bowel Syndrome*

Massive surgical resection
  Congenital abnormalities
  Crohn's disease
  Malignancy
  Radiation injury
  Trauma
  Vascular catastrophes
    Embolism or thrombosis leading to infarction
  Volvulus and strangulated hernias
Intrinsic disease†
  Crohn's disease
  Radiation enteritis
Surgical bypass
Surgical error or obesity treatment

*From Purdum PP III, Kirby DF: *JPEN* 1991; 15:93–101. Used by permission.
†Varying degrees of diseased bowel, fistulization, and/or surgical resection.

in Table 34–14. Not only is the absolute extent of resection important, but also the health of the remaining bowel. Patients with Crohn's disease and radiation enteritis are particularly problematic since some of these patients have had multiple intestinal resections and the remaining intestine may still be diseased or develop disease.

The physician involved in the care of these patients may need to provide care in the early stages of the disease or later when complications develop. The early stages represent the first few weeks to months after the initial insult. Nutritional care hinges on providing appropriate fluid and electrolyte management and instituting nutritional repletion. Parenteral nutrition is frequently required due to inadequate gastrointestinal function. The initiation of some form of enteral feeding is important if the patient can tolerate it. Enteral nutrients provide essential fuels to the intestine, stimulate hypertrophy of the remaining gut, and decrease the incidence of bacterial translocation. While somatostatin has been shown to be useful in a number of gastrointestinal related conditions,[65] Rosen[151] has reviewed its role in SBS and found it to be of little value. A nutrition support team should be involved early in the management of these patients to optimize the patient's rehabilitation.

The provision of nutrition support, both enteral and parenteral, stimulates the process of intestinal adaptation. This process can take up to a year or more and determines whether a patient will be dependent on some form of intravenous support. A patient's intestinal mucosa, supported by TPN alone, will undergo atrophy. These changes occur in as few as 3 days of TPN support in the rat.[152] In humans, 3 weeks of TPN may cause only minor morphologic changes; however, enterocyte enzyme activities show marked decreases that are reversible with enteral feeding.[153] Biasco et al.[154] demonstrated intestinal hyperplasia during the refeeding phase in a pa-

TABLE 34–14.

Factors Affecting the Severity of Short-Bowel Syndrome*

Factor	Favorable	Unfavorable
Extent of resection	<80%	>80%
Site of resection	Jejunum	Ileum
Concomitant GI disease	Absent	Present
Time from onset	>1 yr	<1 yr
GI tract anatomy	Ileocecal valve present, nondiseased colon present	Stomach and/or colon resected

*From Purdum PP III, Kirby DF: *JPEN* 1991; 15:93–101. Used by permission.

tient who had been maintained on TPN following small-bowel resection.

While the actual mechanisms of adaptation have recently been challenged, the fact that it occurs in man is well documented.[155–157] A combination of bowel dilatation, lengthening, and cellular compensation with increases in the activity of brush border disaccharidases and other enzymes occurs.[157–159] While rapid adaptation may occur in the rat, it may take well over a year or more in man.[160–162]

Early management of SBS focuses on fluid and electrolyte management and diarrhea. Management concerns also include central venous catheter maintenance and its complications. Infection and sepsis are the most frequent problems in these patients. An interesting paper suggests that many of these infections may be related to bacterial translocation.[163] However, there have been rare case reports where patients have been maintained on a single intravenous catheter for 10 years or more.[164] Another serious management problem relates to venous thrombosis, which may be induced by the presence of a catheter or an underlying hypercoagulable state.[165] Patients who have multiple venous thromboses pose a significant problem in catheter placement and maintenance since they utilize all the standard locations for catheter placement. Femoral vein and right atrial placement have been performed in these patients.

A wide variety of other complications can occur and are listed in Table 34–15.

Emergent situations requiring urgent care include cholelithiasis, dehydration, mental status changes resulting from D-lactic acidosis or liver failure, and mineral deficiencies such as hypocalcemia or hypomagnesemia. Table 34–16 lists our suggestions for management both in the early stages as well as later during the adaptation phase.

Small-bowel transplantation is being performed at several centers in the United States. However, until more is understood about the mechanisms of immune suppression related to the small bowel, the technique may be best performed in conjunction with transplantation of other organs such as the

TABLE 34–15.

Complications of Short-Bowel Syndrome*

Metabolic
  Anemia
  Bile salt depletion
  Bone disease
  Cholelithiasis
  Dehydration
  Diarrhea (cholerrheic/steatorrheic)
  D-Lactic acidosis
  Hypocalcemia
  Hypomagnesemia
  Liver fibrosis
  Oxalate renal stones
  Protein-calorie malnutrition
  Trace mineral deficiencies
  Vitamin deficiencies (B_{12}, A, D, E, K)
Catheter (most common)
  Infection
  Thrombosis
  Breakage of catheter
  Air embolus

*From Purdum PP III, Kirby DF: *JPEN* 1991; 15:93–101. Used by permission.

TABLE 34-16.

Management Considerations*

Early
Fluid and electrolyte stabilization (attention to weight, input and output, and serum electrolytes)
Early initiation of TPN
Prophylaxis of hypersecretion of gastric acid (use of H_2 antagonists)
Early initiation of enteral feedings
Periodic nutritional assessment

Late
Dietary assessment of intake (all sources with an emphasis on oral)
Periodic nutritional assessment
Continued electrolyte surveillance (emphasis on potassium, phosphorus, and magnesium)
Monitoring and appropriate supplementation of trace elements (iron, copper, zinc, selenium, chromium,† and manganese†)
Supplementation of fat-soluble vitamins and vitamin B_{12}
Consideration of discontinuing H_2 antagonists
Monitoring drug levels, as appropriate
Consider medium-chain triglyceride (MCT) oil for calorie supplementation‡
If diarrhea persists: trial of cholestyramine (intact colon) or trial of somatostatin
Attempt to wean from TPN: first, by volume to I L/day; then, by frequency—every other day to every third day, etc.

*From Purdum PP III, Kirby DF: *JPEN* 1991; 15:93-101. Used by permission.
†Not routinely monitored in practice.
‡Too much MCT oil can cause or exacerbate diarrhea.

liver. Clearly, additional treatment options besides lifelong TPN are needed for patients with SBS.

REFERENCES

1. Kirby DF, Craig RM: The value of intensive nutritional support in pancreatitis. *JPEN* 1985; 9:353-357.
2. Feller JH, Brown RA, MacLaren-Toussant GP, et al: Changing methods in the treatment of severe pancreatitis. *Am J Surg* 1974; 127:196-201.
3. Goodgame JT, Fischer JE: Parenteral nutrition in the treatment of acute pancreatitis: Effect on complications and mortality. *Ann Surg* 1977; 186:651-658.
4. Van Gossum A, Lemoyne M, Greig PD, et al: Lipid-associated total parenteral nutrition in patients with severe acute pancreatitis. *JPEN* 1988; 12:250-255.
5. Sax HC, Warner BW, Talamini MA, et al: Early total parenteral nutrition in acute pancreatitis: Lack of beneficial effects. *Am J Surg* 1987; 153:117-124.
6. Sitzmann JV, Steinborn PA, Zinner MJ, et al: Total parenteral nutrition and alternate energy substrates in treatment of severe acute pancreatitis. *Surg Gynecol Obstet* 1989; 168:311-317.
7. Robin AP, Campbell R, Palani CK, et al: Total parenteral nutrition during acute pancreatitis: Clinical experience with 156 patients. *World J Surg* 1990; 14:572-579.
8. Kalfarentzos FE, Karavias DD, Karatzas TM, et al: Total parenteral nutrition in severe acute pancreatitis. *J Am Coll Nutr* 1991; 10:156-162.
9. Hennessey PJ, Black CT, Andrassy RJ: Nonenzymatic glycosylation of immunoglobulin G impairs complement fixation. *JPEN* 1991; 15:60-64.
10. Ragins H, Levenson SM, Singer R, et al: Intrajejunal administration of an elemental diet at neutral pH avoids pancreatic stimulation. *Am J Surg* 1973; 126:606-614.
11. Kudsk KA, Campbell SM, O'Brien T, et al: Postoperative jejunal feedings following complicated pancreatitis. *Nutr Clin Pract* 1990; 5:14-17.
12. Bank S: Chronic pancreatitis: Clinical features and medical management. *Am J Gastroenterol* 1986; 81:153-166.
13. Variyam EP: Central vein hyperalimentation in pancreatic ascites. *Am J Gastroenterol* 1983; 78:178-181.
14. Stabile BE, Borzatta M, Stubbs RS: Pancreatic secretory responses to intravenous hyperalimentation and intraduodenal elemental and full liquid diets. *JPEN* 1984; 8:377-380.
15. Kishore AT, Chan CH: Resolution of pancreatic ascites after low-dose radiation. *South Med J* 1991; 84:1364-1367.
16. De Waele B, Van der Spek P, Devis G: Peritoneovenous shunt for pancreatic ascites. *Dig Dis Sci* 1987; 32:550-553.
17. Giaffar MH, Isaacs PE: Treatment of

alcoholic pancreatic ascites by intravenous infusion of ascitic fluid. *J Clin Gastroenterol* 1989; 11:568–570.

18. Oktedalen O, Nygaad K, Osnes M: Somatostatin in the treatment of pancreatic ascites. *Gastroenterology* 1990; 99:1520–1521.

19. Gislason H, Gronbech JE, Soreide O: Pancreatic ascites: Treatment by continuous somatostatin infusion. *Am J Gastroenterol* 1991; 86:519–521.

20. Barritt SA III: Treating a patient with pancreatic ascites by an intravenous infusion of a somatostatin analog (letter). *Gastroenterology* 1991; 100:1784–1785.

21. Klein E, Shnebaum S, Ben-Ari G, et al: Effects of total parenteral nutrition on exocrine pancreatic secretion. *Am J Gastroenterol* 1983; 78:31–33.

22. Bivins BA, Bell RM, Rapp RP, et al: Pancreatic exocrine response to parenteral nutrition. *JPEN* 1984; 8:34–36.

23. Grundfest S, Steiger E, Selinkoff P, et al: The effect of intravenous fat emulsions in patients with pancreatic fistula. *JPEN* 1980; 4:27–31.

24. Dudrick SJ, Wilmore DW, Steiger E, et al: Spontaneous closure of traumatic pancreatoduodenal fistulas with total intravenous nutrition. *J Trauma* 1970; 10:542–553.

25. Saari A, Schroder T, Kivlaakso E, et al: Treatment of pancreatic fistulas with somatostatin and total parenteral nutrition. *Scand J Gastroenterol* 1989; 24:859–862.

26. di Costanzo J, Cano N, Martin J, et al: Treatment of external gastrointestinal fistulas by a combination of total parenteral nutrition and somatostatin. *JPEN* 1987; 11:465–470.

27. Torres AJ, Landa JI, Moreno-Azcoita M, et al: Somatostatin in the management of gastrointestinal fistulas: A multicenter trial. *Arch Surg* 1992; 127:97–100.

28. Morse JMD, Reddy KR, Thomas E: Hemosuccus pancreaticus: A cause for obscure gastrointestinal bleeding—diagnosis by endoscopy and successful management by total parenteral nutrition. *Am J Gastroenterol* 1983; 78:572–574.

29. O'Malley VP, Cannon JP, Postier RG: Pancreatic pseudocysts: Cause, therapy, and results. *Am J Surg* 1985; 150:680–682.

30. Yeo CJ, Bastidas JA, Lynch-Nyhan A, et al: The natural history of pancreatic pseudocysts documented by computed tomography. *Surg Gynecol Obstet* 1990; 170:411–417.

31. Bradley E III, Clements J Jr, Gonzalez A: The natural history of pancreatic pseudocysts: A unified concept of management. *Am J Surg* 1979; 137:135–141.

32. Banks PA, Gerzof SG: Pancreatic pseudocyst and abscess—is percutaneous drainage a reasonable option? in Barkin JS, Rogers AL (eds): *Difficult Decisions in Digestive Diseases.* St Louis, Mosby–Year Book, 1989, pp 181–191.

33. Korman SH, Lebensart P, Martin O, et al: Pancreatic pseudocyst: Successful treatment by percutaneous external catheter drainage. *J Pediatr Gastroenterol Nutr* 1991; 12:372–375.

34. Barkin JS, Smith FR, Pereiras RV, et al: Therapeutic percutaneous aspiration of pancreatic pseudocyst. *Dig Dis Sci* 1981; 26:585–586.

35. van Sonnenberg E, Wittich GR, Casola G, et al: Percutaneous drainage of infected pancreatic pseudocysts: Experience in 101 cases. *Radiology* 1989; 170:757–761.

36. Cremer M, Deviere J, Engelholm L: Endoscopic management of cysts and pseudocysts in chronic pancreatitis: Long-term follow up after 7 years of experience. *Gastrointest Endosc* 1989; 35:1–9.

37. Barkin JS, Reiner DK, Deutch E: Sandostatin for control of catheter drainage of pancreatic pseudocyst. *Pancreas* 1991; 6:245–248.

38. Gullo L, Barbara L: Treatment of pancreatic pseudocysts with octreotide. *Lancet* 1991; 338:540–541.

39. Morali GA, Braverman DZ, Shemesh D, et al: Successful treatment of pancreatic pseudocyst with somatostatin analogue and catheter drainage. *Am J Gastroenterol* 1991; 86:515–518.

40. Bedingfield JA, Anderson MC: Pancreatopleural fistula. *Pancreas* 1986; 1:283–290.

41. Soll AH: Duodenal ulcer and drug

therapy, in Sleisenger MH, Fordtran JS (eds): *Gastrointestinal Disease; Pathophysiology, Diagnosis, and Management*, ed 4. Philadelphia, WB Saunders, 1989, pp 814–879.

42. Marotta RB, Floch MH: Diet and nutrition in ulcer disease. *Med Clin North Am* 1991; 75:967–979.

43. Moynihan BGA: On duodenal ulcer: With notes of 52 operations. *Lancet* 1905; 1:340–346.

44. Jordan AJ, Hocking MP: Nutrition therapy for the postgastrectomy patient, in Hocking MP, Vogel SB (eds): *Postgastrectomy Syndromes*, ed 2. Philadelphia, WB Saunders, 1991, pp 183–187.

45. Peura DA: Stress-related mucosal damage: An overview. *Am J Med* 1987; 83(suppl 6A):3–7.

46. Zuckerman GR, Shuman R: Therapeutic goals and treatment option for prevention of stress ulcer syndrome. *Am J Med* 1987; 83(suppl 6A):29–35.

47. Knodell RG, Garjian PL, Schreiber JB: Newer agents available for treatment of stress-related upper gastrointestinal tract mucosal damage. *Am J Med* 1987; 83(suppl 6A):36–40.

48. Daneshmend TK, Hawkey CJ, Langman MJS, et al: Omeprazole versus placebo for acute upper gastrointestinal bleeding; Randomised double blind controlled trial. *BMJ* 1992; 304:143–147.

49. Critchlow JF: Comparative efficacy of parenteral histamine (H_2)-antagonists in acid suppression for the prevention of stress ulceration. *Am J Med* 1987; 83(suppl 6A):23–28.

50. Merki HS, Witzel L, Kaufman D, et al: Continuous intravenous infusions of famotidine maintain high intragastric pH in duodenal ulcer. *Gut* 1988; 29:453–457.

51. Baptista RJ: Role of histamine (H_2)-receptor antagonists in total parenteral nutrition patients. *Am J Med* 1987; 83(suppl 6A):53–57.

52. Bullock L, Fitzgerald JF, Glick MR, et al: Stability of famotidine 20 and 40 mg/L and amino acids in total parenteral nutrient solutions. *Am J Hosp Pract* 1986; 46:2321–2325.

53. Valentine RJ, Turner WM, Borman KR, et al: Does nasoenteral feeding afford adequate gastroduodenal stress prophylaxis? *Crit Care Med* 1986; 14:599–601.

54. Civil ID, Schwab CW: The effect of enteral feeding on gastric pH. *Am Surg* 1987; 53:688–690.

55. Kuric J, Lucas CE, Ledgerwood AM, et al: Nutritional support: A prophylaxis against stress bleeding after spinal cord injury. *Paraplegia* 1989; 27:140–145.

56. Pingleton SK: Gastric bleeding and/or (?) enteral feeding. *Chest* 1986; 90:2–3.

57. Ephgrave KS, Kleiman-Wexler RL, Adair CG: Enteral nutrients prevent stress ulceration and increase intragastric volume. *Crit Care Med* 1990; 18:621–624.

58. Tryba M: The gastropulmonary route of infection—fact or fiction? *Am J Med* 1991; 91(suppl 2A):135–146.

59. Torres A, Serra-Batlles J, Ros E, et al: Pulmonary aspiration of gastric contents in patients receiving mechanical ventilation: The effect of body position. *Ann Intern Med* 1992; 116:540–543.

60. Fiddian-Green RG, Baker S: Nosocomial pneumonia in the critically ill: Product of aspiration or translocation. *Crit Care Med* 1991; 19:763–769.

61. Benson DW, Fischer JE: Fistulas, in Fischer JE (ed): *Total Parenteral Nutrition*, ed 2. Boston, Little, Brown, 1991, pp 253–262.

62. Reber HA, Austin JL: Abdominal abscesses and gastrointestinal fistulas, in Sleisenger MH, Fordtran JS (eds): *Gastrointestinal Disease; Pathophysiology, Diagnosis, and Management*, ed 4. Philadelphia, WB Saunders, 1989, pp 392–397.

63. Chapman R, Foran R, Dunphy JE: Management of intestinal fistulas. *Am J Surg* 1964; 108:157–164.

64. MacPhayden BV Jr, Dudrick SJ, Rudberg RL: Management of gastrointestinal fistulas with parenteral hyperalimentation. *Surgery* 1973; 74:100–105.

65. Harris AG: Future medical prospects for sandostatin. *Metabolism* 1990; 39(suppl 2):180–185.

66. Garden OJ, Dykes EH, Carter DC: Surgical and nutritional management of postoperative duodenal fistulas. *Dig Dis Sci* 1988; 33:30–35.

67. Nubiola P, Badia JM, Martinez-Rodenas F, et al: Treatment of 27 postoperative enterocutaneous fistulas with the long half-life somatostatin analogue SMS 201-995. *Ann Surg* 1989; 210:56–58.

68. Messing B, Bories C, Kunstlinger F, et al: Does total parenteral nutrition induce gallbladder sludge formation and lithiasis? *Gastroenterology* 1983; 84:1012–1019.

69. Lopez AJ, O'Keefe P, Morrissey M, et al: Ceftriaxone-induced cholelithiasis. *Ann Intern Med* 1991; 115:712–714.

70. Medeiros Ada C, Soares CER: Treatment of enterocutaneous fistulas by high-pressure suction with a normal diet. *Am J Surg* 1990; 159:411–413.

71. Greenberg GR, Fleming CR, Jeejeebhoy KN, et al: Controlled trial of bowel rest and nutritional support in the management of Crohn's disease. *Gut* 1988; 29:1309–1315.

72. Perkal MF, Seashore JH: Nutrition and inflammatory bowel disease. *Gastroenterol Clin North Am* 1989; 18:129–155.

73. Sitrin MS: Nutrition support in inflammatory bowel disease. *Nutr Clin Pract* 1992; 2:53–60.

74. Fischer JE: Inflammatory bowel disease, in Fischer JE (ed): *Total Parenteral Nutrition*, ed 2. Boston, Little, Brown, 1991, pp 239–251.

75. Clark RG, Lauder NM: Undernutrition and surgery in regional enteritis. *Br J Surg* 1969; 56:736–738.

76. Powell-Tuck J: Protein metabolism in inflammatory bowel disease. *Gut* 1986; 27(suppl 1):67–71.

77. Kelts DG, Grand RJ, Sten G, et al: Nutritional basis of growth failure in children and adolescents with Crohn's disease. *Gastroenterology* 1979; 79:720–727.

78. Motil K, Grand RJ, Maletkos CJ, et al: The effects of drug and diet on whole body protein metabolism in adolescents with Crohn's disease and growth failure. *J Pediatr* 1982; 101:345–351.

79. Goldschmid S, Graham M: Trace element deficiencies in inflammatory bowel disease. *Gastroenterol Clin North Am* 1980; 78:272–279.

80. McClain C, Soutor C, Zieve L: Zinc deficiency: A complication of Crohn's disease. *Gastroenterology* 1980; 78:272–279.

81. Chan ATH, Fleming CR, O'Fallen WM, et al: Measured basal energy requirements in patients with Crohn's disease. *Gastroenterology* 1986; 91:75–78.

82. Alfonso JJ, Rombeau JL: Nutritional care for patients with Crohn's disease. *Hepatogastroenterology* 1990; 37:32–41.

83. Rosenberg IH: Nutrition and diet in the management of the gastrointestinal tract, in Shils ME, Young VR (eds): *Modern Nutrition in Healing and Disease*, ed 7. Philadelphia, Lea & Febiger, 1988, pp 1138–1143.

84. O'Morain C: Nutritional therapy in ambulatory patients. *Dig Dis Sci* 1987; 32(suppl):95–99.

85. Dudrick SJ, Latifi R, Schrager R: Nutritional management of inflammatory bowel disease. *Surg Clin North Am* 1991; 71:609–623.

86. Dean RF, Campos MM, Barrett B: Hyperalimentation in the management of chronic inflammatory intestinal disease. *Dis Colon Rectum* 1976; 19:601–609.

87. Alverdy J, Chi HS, Shelton GF: The effect of parenteral nutrition on gastrointestinal immunity: The importance of enteral stimulation. *Ann Surg* 1986; 202:681–687.

88. McIntyre PB, Powell-Tuck JM, Wood SR: Controlled trial of bowel rest in the treatment of severe acute colitis. *Gut* 1986; 27:481–485.

89. Muller JM, Keller HW, Erasmi H, et al: Total parenteral nutrition as the sole therapy in Crohn's disease: A prospective study. *Br J Surg* 1983; 70:40–43.

90. Kushner RF, Shapir J, Sitrin MD: Endoscopic, radiographic and clinical response to prolonged bed rest and home parenteral nutrition in Crohn's disease. *Gut* 1988; 29:1309–1315.

91. Ostro MJ, Greenberg GR, Jeejeebhoy KN: Total parenteral nutrition and complete bowel rest in the management of Crohn's disease. *JPEN* 1986; 10:274–278.

92. The Veteran's Affairs Total Parenteral Nutrition Cooperative Study Group.: Perioperative total parenteral nutrition in surgical patients. *N Engl J Med* 1991; 325:525–532.

93. Driscoll RH, Rosenberg IH: Total parenteral nutrition in inflammatory bowel disease. *Med Clin North Am* 1978; 62:185–201.

94. Stehle P, Zander J, Mertes N, et al: Effect of parenteral glutamine peptide supplements on muscle glutamine loss and nitrogen balance after major surgery. *Lancet* 1985; 1:231–239.

95. Jones VA: Comparison of total parenteral nutrition and elemental diet in induction of remission in Crohn's disease: Long term maintenance of remission by personalized food exclusion. *Dig Dis Sci* 1987; 32(suppl):1005–1075.

96. Russell RM, Morrison JA, Smith FR, et al: Vitamin A reversal of abnormal dark adaptation in cirrhosis. Study of the effects on the plasma retinol transport system. *Ann Intern Med* 1978; 88:622–628.

97. Morgan AG, Kelleher J, Walker BE, et al: Nutrition in cryptogenic cirrhosis and chronic active hepatitis. *Gut* 1976; 17:113–117.

98. Linschar WG: Malabsorption in cirrhosis. *Am J Clin Nutr* 1970; 23:488–493.

99. Baraona E, Orrego H, Fernadez O, et al: Absorptive function of the small bowel in liver cirrhosis. *Am J Dig Dis* 1962; 7:318–325.

100. Owen OE, Trapp VE, Reichard GA Jr, et al: Nature and quantity of fuels consumed in patients with alcoholic cirrhosis. *J Clin Invest* 1983; 72:1821–1824.

101. Soeters PD, Fisher JE: Insulin, glucagon, amino acid imbalance and encephalopathy. *Lancet* 1976; 2:880–886.

102. Megyes C, Samols E, Marks V: Glucose intolerance and diabetes in chronic liver disease. *Lancet* 1967; 2:1051–1057.

103. Latifi R, Killam RW, Dudrick SJ: Nutrition support in liver failure. *Surg Clin North Am* 1991; 71:567–578.

104. Lieber CS, Spritz N: Effects of prolonged ethanol intake in man: Role of dietary adipose and endogenously synthesized fatty acids in the pathogenesis of alcoholic fatty liver. *J Clin Invest* 1966; 45:1400–1410.

105. Paine CJ, Eichner ER, Dickson V: Concordance of radioassay and microbiologic assay in the study of the ethanol induced fall in serum folate level. *Am J Med Sci* 1973; 266:135–144.

106. Mitchell D, Wagner C, Stone WJ, et al: Abnormal regulation of plasma pyridoxal-5-phosphate in patients with liver disease. *Gastroenterology* 1976; 71:1043–1050.

107. Shronts EP: Nutritional assessments of adults with end stage hepatic failure. *Nutr Clin Pract* 1988; 3:113–119.

108. Merli M, Romiti A, Riggio O, et al: Optimal nutritional indexes in chronic liver disease. *JPEN* 1987; 11(suppl):130–134.

109. Dominioni L, Dionigi R: Immunologic function and nutritional assessment. *JPEN* 1987; 11(suppl):70–72.

110. Hiyama DT, Fisher JF: Nutritional support in hepatic failure. *Nutr Clin Pract* 1983; 3:96–105.

111. Eigler N, Sacca L, Sherwin RS: Synergistic interactions of physiologic infusions of glucose, epinephrine and cortisol in the dog: A model for stress induced hyperglycemia. *J Clin Invest* 1979; 63:114–123.

112. Marchesini G, Zoli M, Dondi C, et al: Anticatabolic effects of branched-chain amino acid–enriched solutions in patients with cirrhosis. *Hepatology* 1982; 2:420–425.

113. Okuno M, Nagayama M, Takai T, et al: Postoperative total parenteral nutrition in patients with liver disorders. *J Surg Res* 1985; 39:93–102.

114. Kanematsu T, Koyangi N, Matsumata T, et al: Lack of preventative effect of branched-chain amino acid solution on postoperative hepatic encephalopathy in patients with cirrhosis. A randomized, prospective trial. *Surgery* 1988; 104:482–488.

115. Lecleroq-Meyer V, Marchano J, Lecleroq R, et al: Ketoisocaproate, glucose and arginine in the secretion of glucagon and insulin from the perfused rat pancreas. *Diabetologia* 1979; 17:121–126.

116. Sapir DG, Stewart PM, Walser M, et al: Effects of alphaketoisocaproate and of leucine on nitrogen metabolism in postoperative patients. *Lancet* 1983; 1:1010–1014.

117. Herlong HF, Maddrey WC, Walser M: The use of ornithine salts of

branched-chain ketoacids in portal-systemic encephalopathy. *Ann Intern Med* 1980; 93:545–550.

118. McCullough AJ, Mullen KD, Smanik EJ, et al: Nutritional therapy and liver disease. *Gastroenterol Clin North Am* 1989; 18:619–643.

119. Egberts AH, Schomerus H, Manster W, et al: Branched-chain amino acids in the treatment of latent portosystemic encephalopathy. *Gastroenterology* 1985; 88:887–895.

120. Jhangiani SS, Agarwal N, Holmes R: Energy expenditure in chronic alcoholics with and without liver disease. *Am J Clin Nutr* 1986; 44:323–329.

121. Morgan MH, Bolton CM, Morris JJ: Medium chain triglycerides and hepatic encephalopathy. *Gut* 1974; 15:180–184.

122. Moukarzel AA, Najm I, Vargas J, et al: Effect of nutritional status on the outcome of orthotopic liver transplantation in pediatric patients. *Transplant Proc* 1990; 22:1560–1563.

123. Shaw BW Jr, Wood RP, Gordon RD, et al: Influence of selected patient variables and operative blood loss on 6 month survival following liver transplantation. *Semin Liver Dis* 1985; 5:385–393.

124. Guarnieri GF, Tolgo G, Situlin R, et al: Muscle biopsy studies on malnutrition in patients with liver cirrhosis, in Capocaccia L, Fisher JE (eds): *Hepatic Encephalopathy in Chronic Liver Failure*. New York, Plenum Publishing Corp, 1984, pp 193–208.

125. Franco D, Belghiti J, Cortesse A, et al: Nutrition et immunite du du cirrhotique alcoolique. *Gastroenterol Clin Biol* 1981; 5:839–846.

126. DiCecco SR, Wieners EJ, Wiesner RH, et al: Assessment of nutritional status with end-stage liver disease undergoing liver transplantation. *Mayo Clin Proc* 1989; 64:95–102.

127. Delafosse JL, Faure Y, Boufferd JP, et al: Liver transplantation—energy expenditure, nitrogen loss and substrate oxidation rate in the first two postoperative days. *Transplant Proc* 1989; 21:2453–2454.

128. O'Keefe SJD, William R: "Catabolic" loss of body protein after human liver transplantation. *BMJ* 1980; 280:1107–1108.

129. Shanbhogue RLK, Bistrian BR, Jenkins RL, et al: Increased protein catabolism without hypermetabolism after human orthotopic liver transplantation. *Surgery* 1987; 101:146–149.

130. Clowes GHA, Hirsch E, George B, et al: The significance of altered protein metabolism regulated by proteolysis inducing factor, the circulating cleavage product of interleukin-1. *Ann Surg* 1985; 202:446–458.

131. Kahan BD, Vanburen CT, Flechner SM, et al: Clinical and experimental studies with cyclosporine and renal transplantation. *Surgery* 1986; 97:125–140.

132. Meakins JL, Pietsch JB, Bubenick O: Delayed hypersensitivity: Indicator of acquired failure of host defense in sepsis and trauma. *Ann Surg* 1977; 186:241–250.

133. Dionigi R, Zonta A, Dominioni L: The effect of total parenteral nutrition on immunodepression due to malnutrition. *Ann Surg* 1977; 185:467–474.

134. Mullen JL, Buzby GP, Matthews DC, et al: Reduction of operative mortality by combined preoperative and postoperative nutritional support. *Ann Surg* 1979; 192:604–613.

135. O'Keefe SJD, Carraher TE, El-Zayadi AR, et al: Malnutrition and immunocompetence in patients with liver disease. *Lancet* 1980; 2:615–617.

136. Porayko MK, DiCecco S, O'Keefe SJD: Impact of malnutrition and its therapy on liver transplantation. *Semin Liver Dis* 1991; 11:305–314.

137. Shronts EP, Teasley KM, Thoele SL, et al: Nutrition support of the adult liver transplant candidate. *J Am Diet Assoc* 1987; 87:441–451.

138. Vallee BL, Wacker WEC, Bartholomay AF, et al: Zinc metabolism in hepatic dysfunction. Serum zinc concentration in Laënnec's cirrhosis and their validation by sequential analysis. *N Engl J Med* 1956; 255:403–408.

139. Reilley J, Mehta R, Teperman L, et al: Nutritional support after liver transplantation: A randomized, prospective study. *JPEN* 1990; 14:386–391.

140. Reilley J, Halow GM, Gerhardt AL, et al: Plasma amino acids in liver transplantation: Correlation with clinical outcome. *Surgery* 1985; 97:263–269.

141. Fischer JE: Branched-chain-enriched amino acid solution in patients with liver failure: An early example of nutritional pharmacology. *JPEN* 1990; 5(suppl):249–255.

142. Oates JA, Wood AJJ: Cyclosporine. *N Engl J Med* 1989; 321:1725–1738.

143. Solomon SM, Kirby DF: The refeeding syndrome: A review. *JPEN* 1990; 14:90–97.

144. Huang T-L, Huang S-I, Chen M-F: Effects of intravenous fat emulsion on respiratory failure. *Chest* 1990; 97:934–938.

145. Wan JM, Teo TC, Babayan VK, et al: Lipids and the development of immune dysfunction and infection. *JPEN* 1988; 12(suppl 6):43–52.

146. Moore EE: Benefits of immediate jejunostomy feeding after major abdominal trauma: A prospective randomized study. *J Trauma* 1986; 26:874–881.

147. Fischer JE: Hepatobiliary dysfunction associated with total parenteral nutrition. *Gastroenterol Clin North Am* 1989; 18:645–666.

148. Walker LCW: Changes in the gastrointestinal tract during enteral or parenteral feeding. *Nutr Rev* 1989; 47:193–198.

149. Page CP: The surgeon and gut maintenance. *Am J Surg* 1989; 158:485–490.

150. Purdum PP III, Kirby DF: Short-bowel syndrome: A review of the role of nutrition support. *JPEN* 1991; 15:93–101.

151. Rosen GH: Somatostatin and its analogs in the short bowel syndrome. *Nutr Clin Pract* 1992; 7:81–85.

152. Hughes CA, Dowling RH: Speed of onset of adaptive mucosal hypoplasia and hypofunction in the intestine of parenterally fed rats. *Clin Sci* 1980; 59:317–327.

153. Guedon C, Schmitz J, Lerebours E, et al: Decreased brush border hydrolase activities without gross morphologic changes in human intestinal mucosa after prolonged total parenteral nutrition of adults. *Gastroenterology* 1986; 90:373–378.

154. Biasco G, Callegari C, Lami F, et al: Intestinal morphologic changes during oral refeeding in a patient previously treated with total parenteral nutrition for short bowel resection. *Am J Gastroenterol* 1984; 79:585–588.

155. O'Keefe SJD, Shorter RG, Bennet WM, et al: Villous hyperplasia is uncommon in patients with massive intestinal resection (abstract). *Gastroenterology* 1992; 102:231.

156. Senn N: An experimental contribution to intestinal surgery with special reference to the treatment of intestinal obstruction: II. Enterectomy. *Ann Surg* 1888; 7:99–115.

157. Flint JM: The effect of extensive resections of the small intestine. *Bull Johns Hopkins Hosp* 1912; 23:127–144.

158. Chaves M, Smith M, Williamson RCN: Increased activity of digestive enzymes in ileal enterocytes adapting to proximal small bowel resection. *Gut* 1984; 28:981–985.

159. McCarthy DM, Nicholson JA, Kim VS: Intestinal enzyme adaptation to normal diets of different composition. *Am J Physiol* 1980; 239:445–451.

160. Dowling RH, Booth CC: Functional compensation after small bowel resection in man: Demonstration by direct measurement. *Lancet* 1966; 2:146–147.

161. Williamson RC, Chir M: Intestinal adaptation: Structural, functional, and cytokinetic changes. *N Engl J Med* 1978; 298:1393–1402.

162. Gouttebel MC, Saint Aubert B, Colette C, et al: Intestinal adaptation in patients with short bowel syndrome: Measurements by calcium absorption. *Dig Dis Sci* 1984; 34:709–715.

163. Kurkchubasche AG, Smith SD, Rowe MI: Catheter sepsis in short-bowel. *Arch Surg* 1992; 127:21–25.

164. Heimburger DC: Ten-year survival of a Broviac catheter. *Nutr Clin Pract* 1992; 7:74–76.

165. Mailloux R, DeLegge MH, Kirby DF: Pulmonary embolism as a complication of long term total parenteral nutrition. JPEN in press.

35

Respiratory Failure

Diana S. Dark, M.D.

Susan K. Pingleton, M.D.

Respiratory failure has many causes, including both pulmonary and extrathoracic diseases. Pulmonary diseases such as chronic obstructive lung disease (COPD) and interstitial lung disease (ILD) can lead to respiratory failure. Chest wall abnormalities and extrathoracic conditions including many neurologic disorders are also associated with the development of respiratory failure. Malnutrition can cause or worsen respiratory failure by several mechanisms, including impairment of respiratory muscle function and decreased ventilatory drive.[1] Other adverse effects on thoracorespiratory function include alteration of pulmonary defense mechanisms.[1] This chapter will focus on the effects of protein-calorie malnutrition and nutritional support on the respiratory system. Nutritional complications that affect the respiratory system will be discussed, as well as the effects of nutritional repletion on the respiratory system.

MALNUTRITION AND THE RESPIRATORY SYSTEM

Malnutrition is a common problem of hospitalized patients overall. In patients with chronic illness, underlying malnutrition may be compounded by an acute severe illness. Failure to adequately feed a hospitalized patient can also worsen underlying malnutrition. Patients with chronic respiratory problems are prone to the development of malnutrition. Investigators in the late 1960s first noted the association between weight loss and increased mortality in COPD.[2, 3] A more recent study demonstrated that weight loss was found in 70% of patients hospitalized with COPD; abnormal anthropomorphic measurements were documented in half of these patients.[4] Hospitalized patients may also experience deterioration in nutritional status during their stay. In a retrospective study of 26 patients, Driver and LeBrun found inadequate nutritional support in 23 patients (89%).[5] Body weight, anthropomorphic measurements, and visceral measurements of nutritional status were less in patients with respiratory failure when compared with a control group of 18 patients without respiratory failure. They concluded that malnutrition should be suspected in any patient with COPD and respiratory failure. Similar results were found when nutritional therapy was retrospectively assessed in respiratory intensive care unit (ICU) patients over a 1-year period of time.[6] Calorie, carbohydrate, and protein requirements were met in only 70%, 51%, and 26% of ICU days, respectively. These data suggest that inadequate nutrition on an iatrogenic basis occurs in mechanically ventilated patients.

Malnutrition may have an impact on the morbidity of the patient. In a preliminary study, the nutritional status of 80 consecutive respiratory ICU patients was evaluated.[7] Weight loss (less than 80% of ideal body weight) was noted in 24%. Anthropomorphic measurements of triceps skin fold thickness and midarm muscle circumference were abnormal in almost half of the patients. Although poor nutritional status did not appear to predispose to the need for mechanical ventilation, malnourished patients who required mechanical ventilation had significantly higher mortality than did well-nourished patients requiring mechanical ventilation.

EFFECT OF MALNUTRITION ON RESPIRATORY FUNCTION

Malnutrition affects the respiratory system by several different mechanisms. Poor nutritional status can adversely affect thoracopulmonary function by impairment of respiratory muscle function, ventilatory drive, and pulmonary defense mechanisms.[1] The adverse effects of malnutrition occur independently of the presence or absence of primary lung disease. However, the adverse effects of malnutrition may be additive in some patients with acute respiratory failure, such as those with respiratory failure associated with COPD. In COPD, primary abnormalities of decreased inspiratory pressure and increased work of breathing are found. Inspiratory muscle weakness, as assessed by maximal inspiratory pressure, results from both a mechanical disadvantage to inspiratory muscles consequent to hyperinflation as well as generalized muscle weakness.[8, 9] Inspiratory muscle weakness must be severe for hypercapnia to occur. For example, in patients with myopathy, hypercapnia does not occur until inspiratory pressures are less than one third of normal.[10] However, hypercapnia was found in 13 of 18 patients with COPD when inspiratory pressures were just less than half normal.[11] Thus, hypercapnia occurs with much less respiratory muscle weakness when other mechanical abnormalities are present that increase the work of breathing, i.e., in patients with COPD. While none of these studies have addressed the COPD patient with respiratory failure, they do suggest that inspiratory muscle weakness from malnutrition may further compromise already compromised lung function. Hypercapnic respiratory failure and/or difficulty in weaning from mechanical ventilation may be more easily precipitated in the malnourished patient with COPD than in the normally nourished patient with COPD.

In simple starvation or undernutrition, fat and protein are lost, but the loss of protein is minimized by the lesser need to use it as a source of energy.[12] Nitrogen loss is modified by mobilization of fat; enhanced fat oxidation is the principal source of energy in a starving but otherwise normal individual. Some protein wasting does occur despite the availability of fat as a source of energy; it becomes markedly accelerated when fat stores are depleted. In critical illness, protein catabolism may occur to provide energy. With inadequate caloric intake in critically ill patients, energy sources are derived from protein breakdown and gluconeogenesis. One of the protein "pools" available is the muscle protein pool, which is susceptible to catabolism to provide fuel.[13] Inspiratory and expiratory respiratory muscles, primarily the diaphragm and intercostal muscles, are skeletal muscles and therefore susceptible to this catabolic effect. Because the diaphragm is a critical respiratory muscle, the following discussion will focus on it, although these considerations may be valid for all respiratory muscles. It is important to note that few if any data exist that directly examine respiratory muscle function and malnutrition in the critically ill patient with respiratory failure.

Malnutrition reduces diaphragmatic muscle mass in health and disease. Thurlbeck correlated low diaphragmatic mass with low body weight in patients with emphysema.[14] The diaphragmatic weight was lower than predicted from body weight, which suggests that additional factors are involved. In an autopsy study, Arora and Rochester evaluated diaphragmatic muscle mass, thickness, and area in normal-weight patients dying suddenly and underweight patients dying of a variety of diseases.[15] Body weight and diaphragmatic muscle mass were reduced to 70% and 60% of normal in poorly nourished patients. Animal studies confirm the loss of diaphragmatic strength in prolonged nutritional deprivation.[16-19]

Isolated mineral and electrolyte deficiencies can also impair respiratory muscle function. Hypophosphatemia reduces diaphragmatic contractile strength as measured by transdiaphragmatic pressure (Pdi) in mechanically ventilated patients with acute respiratory failure (ARF).[20] The development of hypophosphatemia in nonventilated patients has been shown to precipitate ARF, probably via a similar mechanism.[21] Hypocalcemia is also associated with decreased diaphragmatic function.[22] When hypocalcemia was induced in dogs by infusion of ethyleneglycol-*bis*-(β-aminoethylether)-N, N'-tetraacetic acid (EGTA), a chelating agent that forms soluble complexes with calcium and results in hypocalcemia, Pdi decreased to 74% ± 5% and 79% ± 6% for low- and high-frequency electrical stimulation as compared with controls. Maintenance of blood pressure and cardiac output with dextran infusions did not ameliorate the decrease in diaphragmatic function. Thus, extracellular calcium plays a role in diaphragmatic strength generation, and the decreased diaphragmatic strength is not related to changes in cardiac output. Hypomagnesemia can also cause a decrease in respiratory muscle strength.[23] Improvement in respiratory muscle function was found in 17 hypomagnesemic patients after institution of magnesium replacement.

Ventilatory drive is altered by malnutrition. In general, conditions that reduce the metabolic rate reduce the ventilatory drive. A decrease in metabolic rate has been shown to occur with starvation.[24] Zwillich et al. suggested that the interaction of nutrition and ventilatory drive was a direct function of the influence of nutrition on the metabolic rate.[25] Doekel et al. demonstrated, in seven healthy volunteers, a parallel fall in the metabolic rate and hypoxic ventilatory response that returned toward normal with refeeding.[26] A study of hospitalized patients suffering from long-term semistarvation (greater than 15% weight loss) who received total parenteral nutrition (TPN) demonstrated a marked effect of protein intake on the ventilatory response to CO_2.[27] This effect could be detrimental, however, in patients who have limited pulmonary reserve and lead to an unnecessary increase in respiratory effort.

Malnutrition has been shown to alter immune function and is the most frequent cause of acquired immunodeficiency in humans.[28] Polymorphonuclear leukocytes are normal in number in malnutrition; chemotaxis, opsonic function, and phagocytic function usually remain normal or are mildly depressed while intracellular killing decreases.[29] The thymus, spleen, and lymph nodes become markedly atrophic, and lymphocyte numbers may decrease. While immunoglobulin concentrations remain normal or slightly increased, the antibody response may be depressed.[29]

Although death from starvation is frequently accompanied by pneumonia, it is unclear whether the cause is from an immune deficit or from an alteration in pulmonary function predisposing the patient to infection. Rosenbaum et al. demonstrated a marked decrease in "sighing" in hospitalized patients with malnutrition.[30] Studies of patients with chest wall weakness due to muscle disease or from submaximal paralyzing doses of curare have demonstrated a decrease in functional residual capacity.[31, 32] These changes may predispose the patient to atelectasis and infection and provide one possible explanation for the increased respiratory morbidity associated with malnutrition.

EFFECTS OF REFEEDING ON THE RESPIRATORY SYSTEM

The goals of nutritional support include reversing or improving many of the possible alterations discussed above. Ventilatory drive has been shown to return to normal with refeeding of a malnourished patient. Immune deficits can be corrected, at least in part, by correction of the malnutrition. Nutritional repletion can also improve diminished respiratory muscle strength in some patients. Kelly et al. showed a 37% increase in maximal inspiratory pressure; a 12% increase in body cell mass was noted in 21 of 29 hospitalized patients given parenteral nutrition for 2 to 4 weeks.[33] The other 8 patients had a 10% decrease in body cell mass and a similar

but not significant decrease in maximum inspiratory pressure. Improvement in respiratory muscle function with orally administered nutritional supplementation in patients with COPD appears to depend on the presence of weight gain. Wilson et al. studied six malnourished patients with emphysema during a 3-week admission to a clinical research unit. Body weight increased by 6%, while maximum inspiratory pressures and maximum transdiaphragmatic pressures increased by 41%.[34] In contrast, another study showed that when 8 weeks of nutritional supplementation in 21 malnourished patients with COPD produced no change in weight, no change in respiratory muscle function was found.[35] Short-term refeeding of malnourished patients with COPD can also improve respiratory muscle function. With the administration of nocturnal, nasoenterally administered calories in a controlled study, Whittaker et al. found significant weight gain and improved maximum expiratory pressures after just 16 days of refeeding.[36] Maximum inspiratory pressures increased by 19% after feeding, but this was not statistically significant. Refeeding has also been found to improve diaphragmatic contractility in patients with anorexia nervosa.[37] After 1 month of enteral nutrition and weight gain of 15%, stimulated Pdi increased from 16 ± 5 cm H_2O to 23 ± 7 cm H_2O. This suggested that compromised diaphragmatic function is reversible with nutritional support.

The mechanism of improved respiratory muscle performance with renutrition is not completely understood. It has been shown in both animal and human studies that long-term hypocaloric dieting produces changes in skeletal muscle that may be important in the genesis of muscle dysfunction. In addition to protein catabolism, these changes include depletion of glycolytic and oxidative enzymes, a reduction in high-energy phosphate stores, and an increase in intracellular calcium. Severe malnutrition depresses muscle glycolytic energy activity, thus reducing the availability of energy from glycolysis during contraction.[38] One study showed that succinate dehydrogenase, phosphofructokinase, and hydroxyacyl-CoA-dehydrogenase levels were reduced in skeletal muscle homogenates of malnourished rats.[39] Energy stores are also decreased in severe undernutrition. Pichard et al. demonstrated that creatine phosphate levels fell in a 2-day fasting rat model and were associated with a loss of muscle total creatinine.[40] Thus, the reserves of energy phosphorus were decreased, and the calculated free adenosine diphosphate (ADP) increased, thus suggesting deficient oxidative phosphorylation. These findings suggest that reduced glycolytic and oxidative enzymes such as phosphofructokinase and succinate dehydrogenase may limit the flux of glycolytic and oxidative pathways.

Succinate dehydrogenase activity, when quantified in individual muscle fibers, does not appear to be altered in diaphragmatic muscle in chronic undernutrition.[41] Oxidative muscle activity may depend in part on the fiber type and exercise activity of a particular muscle. The electrophysiologic properties of the muscle can also be altered by modification of the cell membrane properties. This decreases the sodium-potassium pump activity, alters ionic permeability, and thus unbalances the intracellular electrolyte composition.[42] These data suggest that alterations in muscle contractile and endurance properties are not simply or solely due to changes in lean tissue. Indeed, refeeding studies in hypocaloric dieting and fasting, as well as severe starvation of anorexia nervosa patients, document improvement in muscle performance at a time when significant changes in body composition could not be detected.[43] In patients with anorexia nervosa, maximal peripheral muscle force (adductor pollicis) increased significantly by 18% and muscle fatigability decreased to normal after 4

weeks of refeeding. In contrast, body weight, although significantly increased by 11% at 4 weeks and 19% after 8 weeks, was still only 76% of the mean ideal body weight at 8 weeks. Three of four aspects of muscle function were restored at a time when body weight was only 71% of the ideal body weight; total-body nitrogen was less than 85% of normal, and anergy was still observed in half of the six patients with anorexia nervosa. Refeeding restored muscle function at a time when other aspects of body composition were still markedly abnormal. The authors suggest that changes in intracellular electrolytes may be responsible for early improvement in muscle contractile and endurance properties.

Appropriate nutritional support requires information regarding energy needs in malnourished patients with weight loss. On the basis of starvation studies in normal individuals, weight loss has been proposed to be an adaptive mechanism to decrease oxygen consumption ($\dot{V}o_2$) and lessen metabolic demands.[24] Recent data suggested that in malnourished patients with COPD, weight loss results from a hypermetabolic state due, in part, to an increased work of breathing. Wilson et al. measured resting energy expenditure (REE) in normal individuals, in adequately nourished patients with COPD, and in undernourished patients with COPD by indirect calorimetry.[44] Measured REE was higher (1.15 ± 0.02) in malnourished patients with COPD as compared with the adequately nourished patients with COPD (0.99 ± 0.03) and normal groups (0.93 ± 0.02). They concluded that malnourished patients with COPD are hypermetabolic in comparison to normally nourished controls. Further work from the same group evaluated the oxygen cost of augmenting ventilation (O_2 cost) in controls, normally nourished, and malnourished COPD patients.[45] Oxygen cost was significantly elevated in the malnourished group with COPD (4.28 ± 0.98 ml O_2/L) relative to the normally nourished COPD group (2.61 ± 1.07) and the normal controls (1.23 ± 0.51). The malnourished population was characterized by a greater degree of hyperinflation and inspiratory muscle weakness than in the other two groups. Thus, malnourished patients with COPD are hypermetabolic and require increased energy expenditure because of an increased mechanical work load associated with severe COPD and a reduced ventilatory muscle efficiency.

NUTRITIONAL NEEDS OF PATIENTS WITH RESPIRATORY FAILURE

Energy Needs in Respiratory Failure

ICUs are well established and their services available even in many smaller community hospitals. Charts and formulas applying to most procedures and practices are readily available and accessible for nursing and paramedical personnel. What is not as easily defined and readily accessible are dictates for nutritional supplementation. Guidelines are available, however, as is the expertise of the hospital dietician to help direct the physician's nutrition orders. Many hospitals now have nutrition support teams available for consultation. Standardized nutritional regimens are also available in most institutions, and because of cost and time savings, physicians are encouraged to utilize these products. Caution must be used, however, because these standardized regimens will fail to meet some patients' needs and may exceed the needs of others. Thus, it is imperative that the physician be knowledgeable about the fundamentals of nutritional support.

The optimal caloric needs of the patient must first be determined. This may be done by one of several different ways. Levels of energy expenditure can be estimated, calculated with formulas or nomograms, or determined by using measurements of energy expenditure.

TABLE 35–1.

Accepted Estimates for Daily Energy Requirements

Population	Requirement (kcal/kg of Body Weight)
Minimally ill patients	20–30
Moderately stressed patients	30–40
Critically ill patients	40–50

Accepted guidelines for estimating daily energy requirements are listed in Table 35–1. Alternatively, REE is probably better estimated by using a formula based on age, sex, and body size and then adjusting this value for the patient's physical activity and severity of illness. There are more than 190 equations utilizing such variables as weight, height, and age to predict energy needs. The most frequently used formula for determining REE is the Harris-Benedict equation (Table 35–2). This equation was developed from oxygen consumption measurements and established standard basal metabolic rates for both men and women.[46] A "stress factor," or percent increase in energy requirement, is then added to this determination based on the severity of the patient's illness. The stress factor guidelines have been determined, to a large degree, by indirect calorimetry studies done primarily in the surgical patient population.[47] Stress factors are based on *estimated* metabolic needs over and above basal needs and will vary with respect to body temperature, degree of physical activity and agitation, extent of injury, etc.[48]

While estimates for burned and traumatized patients may be fairly reliable, few good studies exist to determine the

TABLE 35–2.

Harris-Benedict Equation

Males:	BMR (kcal/24 hr) = 66.5 + 13.8W + 5.OH − 6.8A
Females:	BMR (kcal/24 hr) = 655 + 9.6W + 1.9H − 4.7A

BMR = basal metabolic rate; W = weight (kg); H = height (cm); A = age (yr).

degree of stress factor needed in medical ICU patients with respiratory failure. Because caloric requirements can be affected by many factors, estimates and predictive equations may not be accurate for severely ill patients; indirect calorimetry can be performed to actually measure the energy expenditure of these patients. Indirect calorimetry measures the rate of oxygen consumption, each liter representing approximately 4 to 5 kcal.[49–51] Stand-alone metabolic measurement charts can be used to measure oxygen consumption in both mechanically ventilated and spontaneously breathing patients but are expensive ($40,000 and above) and require technical expertise. Although there are limitations, when used on a regular basis, accurate information can usually be reliably obtained.[51] Energy expenditure has also been measured by using a pulmonary artery catheter to determine the oxygen consumption from the measured thermodilution cardiac output and the O_2 content differences between arterial and mixed venous blood.[52] With this method, there is good correlation with the estimated caloric needs as determined by the Harris-Benedict equation unless sepsis is present.[53]

Protein, Carbohydrate, and Fat Requirements in Respiratory Failure

Once energy needs are established, the proportions of protein, carbohydrate, and fat are then determined. It is estimated that a 70- to 80-kg person has 10 to 13 kg of protein, approximately half of which is intracellularly located.[54] The average person stores approximately 20,000 kcal as protein, 1000 as carbohydrates, and over 140,000 as fats.[12, 55] A malnourished patient with COPD may have decreased stores. In otherwise normal starvation, it takes only a few days of inadequate nutrition to begin depletion of these stores. In the presence of prolonged or severe trauma or sepsis, the continued demand for amino acids will exceed the supply from endogenous protein sources. The response of body protein to injury is characterized by mobilization of amino acids from skeletal muscle and connective tissue to more active tissues involved in host defense and recovery.[56] One of the goals of nutritional supplementation is to provide adequate calories and protein to meet endogenous requirements, thus avoiding loss of body protein and preventing alterations in respiratory muscle function, as detailed above. In general, large protein intakes (> 2 g/kg/day) can maintain a positive nitrogen balance with only minimal caloric intake.[57] However, a positive *energy* balance is also important since nonprotein energy spares utilization of protein for energy.

There is some controversy surrounding the proportions of nutritional supplementation given to carbohydrates vs. fat, particularly concerning the effects on the respiratory system. Carbohydrates have traditionally been considered a more efficient source of energy in acute illness. However, seriously ill patients may have a decreased ability to utilize carbohydrates.[58] Because of this, it has been suggested that fat may be a preferable source of energy in critically ill patients.[59] The respiratory quotient (RQ) is the ratio of carbon dioxide production to oxygen consumption during substrate utilization. Proteins yield 4 kcal/g using about 1 L of oxygen and have an RQ of 0.8. Metabolism of carbohydrates yields approximately 4 kcal/g with an RQ of 1.0. Fats yield 9 kcal/g with an RQ of 0.7. When excess energy is delivered to the patient, it is stored as fat; storage of fat, or lipogenesis, is accompanied by a high RQ (~8.0) and, therefore, a proportionally higher production of CO_2. This can lead to hypercapnia, particularly in patients with fixed minute ventilation such as those with chronic obstructive lung disease. Some advocate the use of a low-carbohydrate/high-fat solution in patients with respiratory disease in order to avoid carbohydrate-associated lipogenesis. The importance of this remains controversial; there is some question as to whether the total carbohydrate load or the total caloric load is more important in producing excessive CO_2. One recent study compared carbon dioxide production ($\dot{V}co_2$) from isocaloric nutritional regimens with varying concentrations of carbohydrates with $\dot{V}co_2$ from low and high caloric nutritional regimens with constant concentrations of carbohydrates in 20 stable mechanically ventilated patients.[60] The study showed that high caloric feeding, as opposed to high-percentage carbohydrate formulation feeding, increases $\dot{V}co_2$. Moderate caloric intake appears to be more important in avoiding nutritionally related increases in $\dot{V}co_2$ in stable mechanically ventilated patients. Clinical sequelae of nutritionally associated hypercapnia in critically ill patients include precipitation of hypercapnic respiratory failure or difficulty in weaning from mechanical ventilation.[61, 62] As demonstrated above, avoiding nutritionally associated increases in carbon dioxide production in critically ill patients is best accomplished by avoiding high or excess total calories.

Quantitation of carbon dioxide production can be easily accomplished by analyzing a timed collection of expired air as well as by indirect calorimetry measurements. If identified, nutritionally associated excessive CO_2 production can be remedied by altering the feeding solution. Unfortunately, definite guidelines are not yet established for proportional administration of carbohydrates and fats; once the necessary amino acids are provided, the remaining nonprotein calories are usually delivered in equal proportions plus or minus 20%.

Route of Administration of Nutritional Supplementation

The route of administration by which nutritional support is administered is of major biological importance. Enteral nutrition has significant advantages over TPN. The rationale for enterally feeding a patient as opposed to parenteral feeding is based on the physiologic effects of digestion, absorption, and hormone substrate. In addition to the well-accepted primary roles of digestion and absorption of nutrients, the gastrointestinal tract also has important defense mechanisms. The intestinal mucosa functions as a major local defense barrier to prevent bacteria colonizing the gut from invading systemic organs and tissues. Thus, the normal intestine protects the host from intraluminal bacteria and their toxins. The structural maintenance of normal intestinal epithelial cells prevents the transepithelial migration of bacteria. A variety of immunologic mechanisms complement this barrier function. The intestinal wall contains immunologically active cells such as lymphocytes and macrophages, and the mesentery is filled with regional lymph nodes. Secretory IgA intraluminally prevents adherence of bacteria to mucosal cells and is the principal component of the gut mucosal defense system. Kupffer cells of the liver and spleen provide a backup barrier to trap and detoxify bacteria and their toxic products if penetration of the epithelium and regional lymph nodes does occur. It has been shown that when the same nutrient mix is administered enterally or parenterally, enterally fed animals are more resistant to an infectious challenge.[63, 64] Thus, the gut can be described as a metabolically active, immunologically important, and bacteriologically decisive organ in any critical illness including respiratory failure.

After an insult to the intestinal epithelium, indigenous bacteria colonizing the gastrointestinal tract pass through the epithelial mucosa to infect the mesenteric lymph nodes and systemic organs. This microbial migration has been termed *bacterial translocation*.[65] Three major mechanisms promote bacterial translocation, any of which may be present in patients with respiratory failure: altered permeability of the intestinal mucosa as caused by hemorrhagic shock, sepsis, or endotoxemia; decreased host defense mechanisms such as immunosuppression; and increased bacterial numbers within the intestine from bacterial overgrowth or intestinal stasis. Enterally administered nutrients do appear to preserve the structure[66] and function[67] of the intestine to a greater degree than do the same nutrients administered parenterally. Parenteral nutrition has been shown, in animals, to promote bacterial translocation from the gut by increasing the cecal bacterial count and impairing intestinal defense.[68] Some data suggest that diets lacking bulk or fiber may not maximally support intestinal antibacterial barrier function.[69, 70] Much of the data evaluating bacterial translocation has been gathered in animals, but because the factors that facilitate bacterial translocation occur frequently in critically ill patients, these patients may be vulnerable to the invasion of enteral bacteria. The clinical significance of these observations remains uncertain in humans. However, infection remains a major cause of morbidity and mortality in critically ill patients with respiratory failure. Further justification for enteral feeding includes its safety, convenience, and economy of nutrient delivery.

Modification of amino acid formulations may improve the clinical and metabolic efficacy of parenteral nutrition. Glutamine is a nonessential amino acid that is undergoing intensive study and evaluation to determine its role in nutritional supplementation of critically ill patients, including patients with respiratory failure. Endothelial cells in the lungs have been shown to avidly consume glutamine as a key precursor for nucleotide biosynthesis.[71] Additionally, the lungs have been shown to play an important role in glutamine metabolism in the body.[72, 73] Souba et al. showed that cytokines accelerate glutamine uptake by pulmonary artery endothelial cells (PAECs), a response that may be required to support endothelial metabolism, structure, and function

during infection and inflammation.[74] Hinshaw et al. showed that glutamine supplementation in cultured PAECs significantly enhanced adenosine triphosphate synthesis and improved survival after hydrogen peroxide injury.[75] These data suggest that glutamine supplementation prior to or at the time of injury might be beneficial.

In other animal studies, glutamine-enriched TPN has been associated with decreased bacterial translocation when compared with standard formulas. This decrease in translocation was associated with a normalization of secretory-IgA levels and a decrease in bacterial adherence to enterocytes, thus suggesting that glutamine-supplemented TPN may enhance gut immune function. Additional studies have shown that both glutamine-enriched enteral and parenteral formulas accelerate intestinal glutamine uptake.[76, 77] Thus, in various stress states (shock, sepsis, trauma) associated with bacterial translocation, the provision of diets that are glutamine supplemented may reduce the incidence of bacterial translocation, promote "bowel rescue," and possibly improve overall survival.[74] Ziegler et al. showed, in a recent prospective, randomized, double-blind study of 45 adults receiving allogeneic bone marrow transplants, significant effects of glutamine supplementation. Those patients receiving glutamine-supplemented parenteral nutrition had improved nitrogen balance, a diminished incidence of clinical infection, lower rates of microbial colonization, and shortened hospital stays when compared with patients receiving standard parenteral nutrition.[78] These effects occurred despite no differences between groups in the incidence of fever, antibiotic requirements, or time to neutrophil engraftment. Although these data suggest that glutamine-supplemented diets may have a significant impact in some clinical settings, it should be emphasized that additional carefully designed studies are necessary before the use of glutamine-enriched enteral or parenteral solutions in critically ill patients can be advocated.

Disorders of nutrition, especially prolonged protein-calorie malnutrition, can precipitate or worsen ventilatory failure. Respiratory muscle strength and ventilatory drive are decreased with malnutrition. Immune function may be altered and the patient more susceptible to infection. Electrolyte abnormalities, notably hypophosphatemia, hypocalcemia, and hypomagnesemia, also diminish respiratory muscle strength independent of malnutrition. Nutritional repletion improves respiratory muscle strength, although the mechanism of recovery is not known with certainty. Much work remains, especially in critically ill patients, to directly examine and study the effect of malnutrition and refeeding on ventilatory failure.

REFERENCES

1. Rochester DF, Esau SA: Malnutrition and respiratory system. *Chest* 1984; 85:411–415.
2. Vandenburgh E, Van de Woestigne K, Gyselen A: Weight changes in the terminal stages of chronic obstructive lung disease. *Am Rev Respir Dis* 1967; 96:556–565.
3. Renzetti AD, McClement JH, Litt BD: The Veterans Administration Cooperative Study of Pulmonary Function. Mortality in relation to respiratory function in chronic obstructive pulmonary disease. *Am J Med* 1966; 41:115–129.
4. Hunter AMB, Carey MA, Larsh HU: The nutritional status of patients with chronic obstructive pulmonary disease. *Am Rev Respir Dis* 1981; 124:376–381.
5. Driver AG, LeBrun M: Iatrogenic malnutrition in patients receiving ventilatory support. *JAMA* 1980; 244:2195–2196.
6. Harmon G, Pingleton SK, Hanson FN, et al: Computer-assisted nutritional therapy (CANT) in the intensive care unit (abstract). *Am Rev Respir Dis* 1985; 131:152.
7. Pingleton SK, Eulberg M: Nutritional analysis of acute respiratory failure (abstract): *Chest* 1983; 84:343.
8. Weiner P, Suo J, Fernandes E, et al: The effect of hyperinflation on respiratory muscle strength and efficiency in healthy subjects and patients with asthma. *Am Rev Respir Dis* 1990; 141:1501–1505.
9. Lands L, Desmond KJ, Demizio D, et al: The effects of nutritional status and hyperinflation on respiratory muscle strength in children and young adults. *Am Rev Respir Dis* 1990; 141:1506–1509.
10. Braun NMT, Arora NS, Rochester DF: Respiratory muscle and pulmonary function in proximal myopathies. *Thorax* 1983; 38:616–623.
11. Rochester DF, Braun NMT: Determinants of maximal inspiratory pressure in chronic obstructive pulmonary disease. *Am Rev Respir Dis* 1985; 132:42–47.
12. Cahill G: Starvation in man. *N Engl J Med* 1970; 282:668–675.
13. Long CL, Birkham RH, Geiger JW: Contribution of skeletal muscle protein in elevated rates of whole body protein catabolism in trauma patients. *Am J Clin Nutr* 1981; 34:1087–1093.
14. Thurlbeck WM: Diaphragm and body weight in emphysema. *Thorax* 1978; 33:483–487.
15. Arora NS, Rochester DF: Effect of body weight and muscularity on human diaphragm muscle mass, thickness and area. *J Appl Physiol* 1982; 52:64–70.
16. Kelsen SG, Ference M, Kapoor S: Effects of prolonged undernutrition on structure and function of the diaphragm. *J Appl Physiol* 1985; 58:1354–1359.
17. Lewis MI, Sieck GC, Fournier M, et al: Effect of nutritional deprivation on diaphragm contractility and muscle fiber size. *J Appl Physiol* 1986; 60:596–603.
18. Lewis MI, Sieck GC: Effect of acute nutritional deprivation on diaphragm structure and function. *J Appl Physiol* 1990; 68:1938–1944.
19. Drew JS, Farkas GA, Pearson RD, et al: Effects of a chronic wasting infection on skeletal muscle size and contractile properties. *J Appl Physiol* 1988; 64:460–468.

20. Aubier M, Murciano D, Lecoguic Y, et al: Effects of hypophosphatemia on diaphragmatic contractility in patients with acute respiratory failure. *N Engl J Med* 1985; 313:420–424.

21. Newman JH, Neff TA, Ziporin P: Acute respiratory failure associated with hypophosphatemia. *N Engl J Med* 1977; 296:1101–1103.

22. Aubier M, Viires N, Piquet J, et al: Effects of hypocalcemia on diaphragmatic strength generation. *J Appl Physiol* 1985; 58:2054–2061.

23. Molloy DW, Shingra S, Solven F, et al: Hypomagnesium and respiratory muscle power. *Am Rev Resp Dis* 1984; 129:497–498.

24. Keys A, Brozek J, Henschel A, et al: *Biology of Human Starvation*. Minneapolis, University of Minnesota, 1950.

25. Zwillich CW, Sahn SA, Weil JV: Effects of hypermetabolism on ventilation and chemosensitivity. *J Clin Invest* 1977; 60:900–906.

26. Doekel RC Jr, Zwillich CW, Scoggin CH: Clinical semi-starvation: Depression of hypoxic ventilatory response. *N Engl J Med* 1976; 295:358–361.

27. Askanazi J, Rosenbaum SH, Hyman AI, et al: Effects of parenteral nutrition on ventilatory drive. *Anesthesiology* 1980; 53(suppl 1):185.

28. Chandra RK: Malnutrition, in Chandra RK (ed): *Primary and Secondary Immunodeficiency Disorders*. New York, Churchill Livingston, 1983, p 187.

29. Shizgal HM: Nutrition and immune function. *Surg Ann* 1981; 12:15–29.

30. Rosenbaum SH, Askanazi J, Hyman AI, et al: Respiratory patterns in profound nutrition depletion. *Anesthesiology* 1979; 51(suppl):366.

31. De Troyer A, Bastenier-Geens J: Effects of neuromuscular blockade on respiratory mechanics in conscious man. *J Appl Physiol* 1979; 47:1162–1168.

32. Gibson GJ, Pride NB, Newsom Davis J: Pulmonary mechanics in patients with respiratory muscle weakness. *Am Rev Respir Dis* 1978; 118:373.

33. Kelly SM, Rosa A, Field S, et al: Inspiratory muscle strength and body composition in patients receiving total parenteral nutrition therapy. *Am Rev Respir Dis* 1984; 130:33–37.

34. Wilson DO, Rogers RM, Sanders MH, et al: Nutritional intervention in malnourished patients with emphysema. *Am Rev Respir Dis* 1986; 134:672–677.

35. Lewis MI, Belman MJ, Dorr-Uyemura L: Nutritional supplementation in ambulatory patients with chronic obstructive pulmonary disease. *Am Rev Respir Dis* 1987; 135:1062–1068.

36. Whittaker JS, Ryan CF, Buckley PA, et al: The effects of refeeding on peripheral and respiratory muscle function in malnourished chronic obstructive pulmonary disease patients. *Am Rev Respir Dis* 1990; 142:283–288.

37. Murciano D, Armengauk MH, Rigaud D, et al: Effect of renutrition on respiratory and diaphragmatic function in patients with severe mental anorexia (abstract). *Am Rev Respir Dis* 1990; 141:547.

38. Layman DKM, Merdian-Bender M, Hegarty PVJ, et al: Changes in aerobic and anaerobic metabolism in rat cardiac and skeletal muscles after total or partial dietary restrictions. *J Nutr* 1981; 111:994–1000.

39. McRussell DR, Atwood HL, Whittaker JS, et al: The effect of fasting and hypocaloric diets on the functional and metabolic characteristics of rat gastrocnemius muscle. *Clin Sci Lond* 1984; 67:185–194.

40. Pichard C, Vaughan C, Struk R, et al: Effect of dietary manipulations (fasting, hypocaloric feeding and subsequent refeeding) on rat muscle energetics as assessed by nuclear magnetic resonance spectroscope. *J Clin Invest* 1988; 82:895–901.

41. Dieck GC, Lewis MI, Blanco CE: Effects of under-nutrition on diaphragm fiber size, SDH activity, and fatigue resistance. *J Appl Physiol* 1989; 66:2196–2205.

42. Pichard C, Jeejeebhoy KN: Muscle dysfunction in malnourished patients. *Q J Med* 1988; 260:1021–1045.

43. McRussell DR, Pendergast PJ, Darby PL, et al: A comparison between muscle function and body composition in anorexia nervosa; the effect of refeeding. *Am J Clin Nutr* 1983; 38:229–237.

44. Wilson DO, Donahoe M, Rogers RM, et al: Metabolic rate and weight loss in chronic obstructive lung disease. *JPEN* 1990; 14:7–11.

45. Donahoe M, Rogers RM, Wilson DO, et al: Oxygen consumption of the respiratory muscles in normal and malnourished patients with chronic obstructive lung disease. *Am Rev Respir Dis* 1989; 140:385–391.

46. Harris JS, Benedict FG: *A Biometric Study of Basal Metabolism in Man.* Washington, DC, Carnegie Institute of Washington, 1919, Publication 297.

47. Kinney JM, Duke JH Jr, Long CL, et al: Tissue fuel and weight loss after injury. *J Clin Pathol* 1970; 23(suppl):65–69.

48. Long CL, Schaffel N, Geiger JW, et al: Metabolic response to injury and illness: Estimation of energy and protein needs from indirect calorimetry and nitrogen balance. *JPEN* 1979; 3:452–456.

49. Bartlett RH: Assessment and management of nutrition in critical illness, in Bone RC (ed): *Critical Care: A Comprehensive Approach,* ed 1. Park Ridge, Ill, American College of Chest Physicians, 1984, pp 60–81.

50. Feurer ID, Crosby LO, Mullen JL: Measured and predicted resting energy expenditure in clinically stable patients. *Clin Nutr* 1987; 3:27–34.

51. Damask MC, Schwarz Y, Weissman C: Energy measurements and requirements of critically ill patients. *Crit Care Clin* 1987; 3:71–96.

52. Liggett SB, St John RE, Lefrak SS: Determination of resting energy expenditure utilizing the thermodilution pulmonary artery catheter. *Chest* 1987; 91:562–566.

53. Liggett SB, Renfro AD: Energy expenditures of mechanically ventilated nonsurgical patients. *Chest* 1990; 98:682–686.

54. Moore FD: Surgical care and metabolic management of the postoperative patient, in Winters RW, Greene HL (eds): *Nutritional Support of the Seriously Ill Patient.* Bristol-Myers Nutrition Symposia series, vol 1. New York, Academic Press, 1983, pp 5–12.

55. Blackburn GL, Flatt JP, Hensle TW: Peripheral amino acid infusions, in Fischer JE (ed): *Total Parenteral Nutrition.* Boston, Little, Brown, 1976, pp 363–394.

56. Blackburn GL: Protein metabolism and nutritional support. *J Trauma* 1981; 21(suppl):707–711.

57. Elwyn DH: Protein metabolism and requirements in the critically ill patient. *Crit Care Clin* 1987; 3:57–69.

58. Wolfe RR: Carbohydrate metabolism in the critically ill patient: Implications for nutritional support. *Crit Care Clin* 1987; 3:11–23.

59. Wiener M, Rothkopf MM, Rothkopf G, et al: Fat metabolism in injury and stress. *Crit Care Clin* 1987; 3:25–56.

60. Talpers SS, Romberger DJ, Bunce SB, et al: Nutritionally-associated increased carbon dioxide production: Excess total calories versus high proportion of carbohydrate calories. *Chest* 1992;102:551–555.

61. Dark DS, Pingleton SK, Kerby GR: Hypercapnia during weaning: A complication of nutritional support. *Chest* 1985; 88:141–143.

62. Covelli HD, Black JW, Olsen MS, et al: Respiratory failure precipitated by high carbohydrate loads. *Ann Intern Med* 1981; 95:579–581.

63. Kudsk KA, Stone JM, Carpenter G, et al: Enteral and parenteral feeding influence mortality after hemoglobin–*E. coli* peritonitis in normal rats. *J Trauma* 1983; 23:605–609.

64. Kudsk KA, Stone JM, Carpenter G, et al: Effects of enteral versus parenteral feeding on body composition of malnourished animals. *J Trauma* 1982; 22:904–906.

65. Berg RD: Translocation of indigenous bacteria from the intestinal tract, in Hentges DJ (ed): *Human Intestinal Microflora in Health and Disease.* New York, Academic Press, 1983.

66. Johnson LR, Copeland EM, Dudrick SJ, et al: Structural and hormonal alterations in the gastrointestinal tract of parenterally fed rats. *Gastroenterology* 1975; 68:1177–1183.

67. Levine GM, Deren JJ, Steiger E, et al: Role of oral intake in maintenance of gut mass and disaccharidase activity. *Gastroenterology* 1974; 67:975–982.

68. Alverdy JC, Aoys E, Moss GS: Total parenteral nutrition promotes bacterial translocation from the gut. *Surgery* 1988; 104:185–190.

69. Spaeth G, Specian RD, Berg RD, et al: Bulk prevents bacterial translocation

induced by the oral administration of total parenteral nutrition solution. *JPEN* 1990; 14:442–447.

70. Alverdy JC, Aoys E, Moss GS: Effect of commercially available chemically defined liquid diets on the intestinal microflora and bacterial translocation from the gut. *JPEN* 1990; 14:1–6.

71. Frissell WR: Synthesis and catabolism of nucleotides, in Frissell WR (ed): *Human Biochemistry.* New York, Macmillan, 1982, pp 292–304.

72. Austgen TR, Souba WW: The effects of endotoxin on lung glutamine metabolism in vivo. *J Trauma,* 1991; 31:742–751.

73. Plumley DA, Austgen TR, Salloum RM, et al: The role of the lungs in maintaining amino acid homeostasis. *JPEN* 1990; 14:569–573.

74. Souba WW, Herskowitz K, Austgen TR, et al: Glutamine nutrition: Theoretical considerations and therapeutic impact. *JPEN* 1990; 14(suppl 1):237–243.

75. Hinshaw DB, Burger JM, Delius RE, et al: Mechanism of protection of oxidant-injured endothelial cells by glutamine. *Surgery* 1990; 108:298–305.

76. Klimberg VS, Souba WW, Sitren H, et al: Glutamine-enriched total parenteral nutrition supports gut metabolism. *Surg Forum* 1989; 40:175–177.

77. Salloum RM, Souba WW, Klimberg VS, et al: Glutamine is superior to glutamate in supporting gut metabolism, stimulating intestinal glutaminase activity, and preventing bacterial translocation. *Surg Forum* 1989; 40:6.

78. Ziegler TR, Young LS, Benfell K, et al: Clinical and metabolic efficacy of glutamine-supplemented parenteral nutrition after bone marrow transplantation. *Ann Intern Med* 1992; 116:821–828.

36

Renal Failure

Michael Y. Suleiman, M.D.

Gary P. Zaloga, M.D.

Metabolic abnormalities

Nutritional consequences of renal failure

Protein metabolism

Fluid and electrolyte disorders

Carbohydrate and lipid metabolism

Vitamins

Clinical approach to patient with acute renal failure

General principles of nutritional support

Energy requirements

Low-protein diets

Protein intake

Fluid, electrolyte, vitamin, and trace element requirements

Routes of feeding

Nutritional formulations

Form of renal replacement therapy

Monitoring of nutritional support

Future studies

The metabolic/nutritional care of acute renal failure patients is of paramount importance in the total body concept whilst that of dialysis is of secondary importance. Thus, if a patient's nutritional/metabolic requirements are of a certain magnitude then these should not be curtailed to reduce the frequency of dialysis but, on the contrary, dialysis be undertaken as frequently as is necessary to accomodate a patient's requirements. Lee, 1980

Acute renal failure is characterized by a sudden reduction in the glomerular filtration rate (GFR) and loss of renal tubular function. Common etiologies include shock, sepsis/infection, trauma, drugs, urinary tract obstruction, and glomerulonephritis. In spite of improvements in intensive care, nursing, nutritional support, respiratory support, and dialysis, mortality rates for critically ill patients with acute renal failure remain high. Overall, mortality rates have changed little over the past 20 years. However, we are treating a more elderly and sicker patient population today. Some argue that we have improved the outcome over the past years since we have obtained similar mortality rates in a more severely ill population. Some deterioration in renal function develops in approximately 5% of hospitalized patients.[1] Roughly 20% of these patients progress to fulminant acute renal failure.[1] The overall hospital mortality rate of acute renal failure ranges from 40% to 70% and has remained essentially the same for the last two decades despite major advances in dialysis and intensive care.[1-7] Death usually results from the underlying disease rather than uremia. Some studies suggest that survival in acute renal failure could be improved by specific nutritional regimens.[8, 9] However, the severity of the underlying illness is obviously the most important prognostic determinant of survival from acute renal failure in patients supported by modern intensive care. Single-organ acute renal failure has an overall mortality rate of about 30%. On the other hand, when it occurs as part of multiple organ failure, the mortality rate is 70% to 80%. Today, most acute renal failure seen in the intensive care unit (ICU) occurs as part of multiple organ failure syndromes. The kidney may be considered a victim of the disease rather than the cause of the disease.

Patients with acute renal failure are frequently catabolic and can succumb to rapid nutritional deterioration. This catabolic state is characterized by protein breakdown, lipolysis, water retention, and disorders of electrolyte and acid-base balance. A number of factors are responsible for the hypercatabolic state and malnutrition in acute renal failure. First, many toxic metabolic products are retained by the body. These products stimulate catabolism, impair anabolism, impair nutritional intake, and alter the digestion/absorption of nutrients. Second, elevated concentrations of catabolic hormones (e.g., cortisol, epinephrine, glucagon, and parathyroid hormone) contribute to net catabolism.[10, 11] Third, proteolytic activity may be released from cells, tissues, and biological fluids.[12, 13] Forth, catabolic agents may be released by microorganisms (e.g., endotoxin) or as part of the inflammatory response (e.g., cytokines). Fifth, inadequate food intake may be caused by nausea and vomiting or impaired gastrointestinal function.[14] Sixth, losses of fluids rich in protein may result from fistulas, diarrhea, wound drainage, ascites, hemofiltration, or hemodialysis.[15] Seventh, blood loss may occur from bleeding, multiple blood drawings, or sequestration of blood in the hemodialyzer. In addition, dietary protein restriction in these patients introduces further insult to their already compromised nutritional status. Malnutrition in acute renal failure can result in serious complications. These include compromised immune status, increased susceptibility to infections, impaired healing, and increased morbidity and mortality. These complications may result in further worsening of the nutritional status.[15, 16]

It remains unclear whether current techniques of nutritional support (as well as other ICU therapies) have improved the outcome in critically ill patients with acute renal failure. Despite this, we believe that nutrition is an integral part of the comprehensive supportive therapy of patients with acute renal failure. Attention to metabolic and nutritional details can help avoid complications while awaiting the return of renal function. Over the past few years, there has been a move away from parenteral toward enteral nutrition and a move away from protein restriction and the use of essential amino acid (EAA) formulas in the treatment of this disease. This chapter discusses the nutritional management of acute renal failure. It is important to note that the nutritional management of chronic renal failure differs from that of acute renal failure.

METABOLIC ABNORMALITIES

The kidney possesses a variety of metabolic functions. It synthesizes a number of hormones, including renin, 1,25-dihydroxyvitamin D, prostaglandins, and erythropoietin. The kidney also degrades insulin, glucagon, parathyroid hormone, thyrotropin, and gastrin. The kidney synthesizes and catabolizes amino acids, peptides, and proteins. For example, it produces serine from glycine and converts glutamine to glutamate and ammonia. Excretory functions include the regulation of water, electrolyte balance, and acid-base status and the removal of metabolic wastes. These functions are altered when renal function is impaired.

Malnutrition alters renal function. There is a decrease in the GFR secondary to decreases in extracellular fluid volume, blood volume, renal plasma flow, and circulating protein concentrations. There is reduced capacity to concentrate urine because of decreased protein and urea synthesis, which results in decreased hypertonicity of the renal medulla. Urine acidification is also impaired as a result of lowered phosphorus levels and ammonia generation. Malnutrition also diminishes the secretion of catecholamines and other hormones that can affect renal function.

Acute renal failure develops in the majority of cases as a consequence of severe illness or injury.[1-9] Accordingly, the metabolic changes caused by failing renal function are superimposed on the metabolic effects of the primary illness and are often indistinguishable. Increased catabolism, whether resulting from the primary illness or acute renal failure, worsens the underlying disease and renal function. Renal failure leads to changes in the metabolism of proteins, amino acids, carbohydrates, lipids, electrolytes, minerals, trace elements, and vitamins.[17-27]

NUTRITIONAL CONSEQUENCES OF RENAL FAILURE

Not only does nutrition affect renal function, but renal function also affects nutritional status. Changes in renal function alter protein, carbohydrate, and lipid metabolism. There are changes in fluid and electrolyte balance,

acid-base status, vitamin levels, food intake, hormone secretion, and organ function (Table 36-1).

Protein Metabolism

Protein is a vital component for the structural and biochemical/physiologic

TABLE 36-1.

Nutritional Consequences of Renal Failure

Protein metabolism
  Decreased protein synthesis
  Decreased amino acid synthesis (i.e., serine, glycine)
  Increased protein catabolism
  Altered amino acid metabolism (i.e., glutamine)
  Altered peptide metabolism
  Azotemia
  Elevated creatine, creatinine
  Protein-calorie malnutrition
Lipid metabolism
  Increased lipolysis
  Hyperlipidemia
    Hypertriglyceridemia
    Hypercholesterolemia
  Reduced clearance of intravenous fat
    Decreased lipase activity
  Altered prostaglandin synthesis and metabolism
Carbohydrate metabolism
  Hyperglycemia
  Insulin resistance
  Decreased glucose utilization
  Decreased insulin metabolism
Fluid and electrolytes
  Fluid retention
  Hyponatremia
  Hypocalcemia
  Hyperphosphatemia
  Hyperkalemia
  Hypermagnesemia
  Aluminum toxicity
Gastrointestinal
  Altered digestion and absorption
  Impaired nutritional intake
  Loss of fluid and nutrients via fistulas, diarrhea, etc.
Others
  Vitamin deficiencies (i.e., B_6, C, folate)
  Elevated vitamin A levels
  Acidosis
  Altered hormone levels (i.e., renin, erythropoietin, calcitriol, thyroid hormone)
  Anemia
  Osteodystrophy
  Muscle weakness and wasting
  Decreased mentation
  Effects of dialysis
    Loss of protein, vitamins, minerals
    Increased catabolism and energy expenditure

integrity of cells. Excessive loss of body protein can compromise the organism and, if severe, result in death. In acute renal failure, protein synthesis is decreased and protein degradation increased.[28-32] Investigators have described reduced protein synthesis and enhanced protein degradation in peripheral tissues of acutely uremic rats.[28, 30, 32] Grossman et al.[31] found decreased hepatic protein synthesis in uremic rats. Decreased protein synthesis may partially relate to impaired amino acid transport[33] or diminished insulin-stimulated protein synthesis.[34] Most patients have net protein breakdown (synthesis minus degradation), with losses of 150 to 200 g/day reported.[14, 35] This amount of loss can quickly compromise organ function. Catabolism is further increased with underlying shock, sepsis, trauma, or rhabdomyolysis. Abnormal enzyme activities may contribute to this catabolic state. Animals studies of acute renal failure reveal increased activity of liver glutamate oxaloacetic aminotransferase (GOT) and ornithine aminotransferase.[36] These enzymes catalyze the transformation of glutamine to ornithine in the urea cycle. Arginase activity is increased and catalyzes the formation of urea and ornithine from arginine. In addition, serine dehydratase and tyrosine aminotransferase activities are elevated. Tyrosine aminotransferase is the key enzyme in hepatic tyrosine metabolism.

No "toxin" has been identified to account for the clinical disturbances of uremia. However, uremic symptoms usually occur when blood urea nitrogen (BUN) levels exceed 100 to 150 mg/dL. Urea is the major nitrogenous product of protein and amino acid metabolism. Nitrogen from dietary and body protein is converted to urea and appears in body fluids and urine. This fraction of the total urea production is defined as urea appearance.[37]

Urea synthesis increases following the onset of acute renal failure because of increased hepatic uptake of amino acids.[38, 39] The main determinants of urea appearance are nitrogen intake, dietary nitrogen utilization, and the rate of body protein breakdown. The nitrogen in urea is derived from ammonia and aspartate. Ammonia is generated from transamination of amino acids (to glutamate), urea degradation in the gastrointestinal tract, and purine metabolism. Aspartate is synthesized from oxaloacetate in the liver by transamination from glutamate. Urea appearance is usually increased in acute renal failure because of both increased protein breakdown and decreased urea excretion. Urea degradation does not contribute significantly to protein nutrition since urea is poorly reutilized. Many individuals tolerate elevated urea levels without difficulties. The accumulation of urea is not directly responsible for uremic symptoms but rather indicates the degree of uremia. Urea production can be reduced by limiting catabolism with exogenous calories (i.e., glucose) and protein.

Protein intake affects renal function. Protein increases renal plasma flow, the GFR, and creatinine clearance.[40-43] Protein may alter renal hemodynamics through stimulation of hormonal (i.e., glucagon) and vasoactive factors (i.e., prostaglandins).[42, 43] The quality of protein (as well as quantity) also affects glomerular filtration. Vegetarian diets (lacking meat proteins) are associated with lower renal plasma flow, GFR, and creatinine clearance as compared with meat-containing diets.[40, 44] Glomerular hyperfiltration has been proposed to accelerate glomerular injury and progression of renal failure.[45] This theory forms the basis for the use of low-protein diets in long-term therapy for chronic renal failure.

Creatine arises from endogenous synthesis (from arginine and glycine) and from the diet (meat contains 4.2 mg of creatine per gram). Creatine is synthesized and concentrated in muscle (stored as creatine and creatine phosphate). Creatinine is formed from the metabolism of creatine. The rate of formation is related to muscle mass and is 1.7% per day of the creatine pool in normal individuals. Thus, the serum level of creatinine depends upon the muscle mass of the patient. Since creatinine is primarily cleared by the kidney, serum levels correlate inversely with renal function (i.e., glomerular filtration). Wasted individuals may have a normal or slightly elevated creatinine level in the face of significant renal insufficiency.

Fluid and Electrolyte Disorders

Acute renal failure is characterized by a sudden reduction in GFR. The acute reduction can cause substantial fluid, electrolyte, and acid-base derangements. Substances cleared by the kidney are retained. These include metabolic acids, potassium, phosphorus, and magnesium (see Table 36–1). The presence of oliguria and catabolism significantly increases the risk for these disorders. Acidosis develops as a result of decreased renal excretion of acid and is accentuated when tissue ischemia and catabolism are present.[46] Hyperkalemia and hyperphosphatemia develop as a consequence of acidosis, tissue catabolism, and decreased renal excretion of potassium and phosphate. The tendency to hyperkalemia is less marked in patients without oliguria since an increase in tubular secretion of potassium can partially compensate for the decrease in GFR.[46] The increase in plasma phosphate levels is often associated with decreased plasma calcium concentrations.[27, 46] Plasma calcium levels may also be decreased because of a failure of the kidney to synthesize 1,25-dihydroxyvitamin D, the active form of vitamin D. Hypermagnesemia may also occur[46] and, when severe, may suppress the parathyroid glands and accentuate hypocalcemia. The reduced excretion of water predisposes the patient to fluid overload and dilutional hyponatremia. Strict monitoring of fluid and electrolyte balance and treatment of abnormalities is the key for maintenance of body ho-

meostasis. There have been few studies of trace element metabolism in patients with acute renal failure. Some studies report a decrease in zinc.

Carbohydrate and Lipid Metabolism

Changes in carbohydrate and lipid metabolism have been studied extensively in chronic renal failure but very little in acute renal failure.[18, 19, 21, 22, 25, 27] Hyperlipidemia (both hypertriglyceridemia and hypercholesterolemia) and glucose intolerance are characteristic findings in chronic renal failure.[18, 19, 22, 25] Hypertriglyceridemia and low cholesterol levels have been observed in acute renal failure, although the mechanisms are not clear.[21] Clearance of intravenous fat emulsions is reduced. There are also decreases in the activity of lipoprotein lipase and hepatic triglyceride lipase.[21]

Glucose intolerance may result in hyperglycemia. Associated hyperinsulinemia suggests the presence of insulin resistance. Glucose utilization is reduced in several tissues (i.e., muscle, fat) in the critically ill patient with acute renal failure.[34] Although detailed studies are not available, this phenomenon is most likely related to insulin resistance (postreceptor type), particularly in the presence of associated sepsis or trauma.[47, 48] In addition, increased gluconeogenesis associated with injury or sepsis can increase the tendency to hyperglycemia. Hepatic glucose output is normal or increased.

Insulin requirements may be increased because of insulin resistance in patients with severe stress. On the other hand, daily insulin requirements may be decreased because of decreased insulin removal (from renal injury). Weinrauch et al.[49] reported that the daily insulin requirements of diabetic patients with acute renal failure were diminished by as much as 40% and led to hypoglycemia. The requirements for insulin depend upon the degree of insulin resistance, stress hormone secretion, and residual renal function. Blood glucose should be monitored, especially in patients receiving insulin or unable to communicate (i.e., sedation, intubation, decreased mentation).

Vitamins

Many patients with acute renal failure have a low vitamin intake. The water-soluble vitamins are most affected. Decreased absorption and increased losses (especially during dialysis) contribute to vitamin deficiency states. Vitamin B_6 and folate requirements are usually elevated. Synthesis of 1,25-dihydroxyvitamin D is impaired, while clearance of vitamin A is diminished. Vitamin E levels are reported to be normal.

The value of vitamin supplementation in patients with acute renal failure is unclear. We do not usually supplement these patients. Instead, we initiate early nutritional support with standard amounts of vitamins (i.e., quantities that meet the recommended dietary allowances [RDAs]). We believe that there is little harm to vitamin supplementation in normal amounts.

CLINICAL APPROACH TO THE PATIENT WITH ACUTE RENAL FAILURE

General Principles of Nutritional Support

The goals of nutritional therapy for acute renal failure are to maintain good nutritional status, promote recovery of renal function (i.e., healing), prevent further renal damage, and prevent or minimize toxicity and metabolic derangements. A definitive protocol that meets these goals does not exist. The available data regarding the optimal nutritional management of acute renal failure are limited and conflicting. The administration of nutritional support often creates problems with intravascular volume overload and worsening uremia. Nevertheless, a failure to provide adequate nutrients for prolonged periods will ultimately allow malnutrition to become an independent risk factor affecting survival. Because the clinical status of patients with acute renal failure is so diverse, the prescribed nutrient intake may vary greatly from patient to patient and should depend on the underlying nutritional status, catabolic rate, associated disease processes, residual GFR, and intensity of dialysis or hemofiltration therapy. As a rule, nutrients should be administered as needed to meet the demands of severely catabolic patients. The development of fluid and electrolytes abnormalities or the accumulation of metabolic waste products can be prevented by adjusting the intensity of renal replacement therapy. For patients with lower degrees of stress and catabolism, reduced water, mineral, and protein intake might be feasible to reduce the need for renal replacement therapy as long as it does not impair nutritional status or organ function. Since it is often difficult to predict the length of time that a patient will be unable to tolerate spontaneous feeding, nutritional supplementation should be initiated early after injury, even if hemodialysis or ultrafiltration becomes necessary. Hemofiltration is an ideal method for fluid removal since it enables the clinician to provide full nutritional supplementation.

Energy Requirements

Energy requirements for patients with acute renal failure are determined by the same factors that affect non-uremic individuals, including weight, sex, age, associated diseases (i.e., sepsis, trauma), and physical activity. There is no appreciable increase in the energy requirement that is due to renal insufficiency alone.

In a nonrandomized comparison, patients with positive energy balance had improved survival as compared with those with negative energy balance (38% vs 9%).[50, 51] Feinstein et al.[52] also reported similar results where they found that patients with acute renal failure who survived had higher energy intake than those who died. Forsberg et al.[53] observed that patients with acute renal failure and lower energy intake were at greater risk for fatality. Although these findings reflect the importance of high energy intake in patients with acute renal failure, one should note that patients with greater negative energy and nitrogen balance were significantly sicker. They had more serious underlying conditions, which in turn may have contributed to the increased mortality in this group of patients.

The standard method for assessing energy needs is based on the Harris-Benedict equation,[54] which estimates basal energy expenditure (BEE) as a function of age, sex, body weight, and height.

Men: BEE = 66.5 + (13.8 × weight [kg])
  + (0.5 × height [cm]) − (6.8 × age [yr])

Women: BEE = 65.5 + (9.6 × weight [kg])
  + (1.8 × height [cm]) − (4.7 × age [yr])

BEE can be adjusted for the level of stress by using a variety of factors (Table 36−2). The energy requirement is

TABLE 36−2.

Stress-Induced Increases in Energy Expenditure (Factors)

Type of Stress	Fraction of Basal Energy Expenditure
Malnutrition	0.70
Chronic renal failure, nondialyzed	1.00
Maintenance hemodialysis	1.00−1.05
Elective surgery, uncomplicated	1.00
Peritonitis	1.15
Soft-tissue trauma	1.15
Fractures	1.20
Infections	
Mild	1.00
Moderate	1.20−1.30
Severe	1.40−1.50
Burns	
0%−20%	1.00−1.50
20%−40%	1.50−1.80
40%−100%	1.80−2.00

frequently increased by 25% to cover individual variability in energy needs and the specific dynamic action of nutrients. Many investigators have reported that energy expenditure calculated by using the Harris-Benedict equation with an activity factor overestimates energy expenditure in the critically ill patient. The increased energy requirements of critical illness are frequently compensated for by decreased energy needs resulting from bed rest, sedation, paralyzation, and mechanical ventilation. Thus, the Harris-Benedict equation without the activity factor may be a better estimate of energy needs in critically ill patients with renal failure.

One may also determine energy needs by indirect calorimetry. These studies report normal energy expenditures in patients with isolated chronic renal failure. We have found that patients with acute renal failure have similar energy expenditures to other critically ill patients without renal failure (matched for underlying illness). Energy expenditure is usually 30 to 35 kcal/kg/day in most critically ill patients with acute renal failure[50, 55−57] (Table 36−3). In another study, patients with acute renal failure requiring mechanical ventilation showed a median energy expenditure of 124% of the BEE (range, 90% to 148%) predicted by the Harris-Benedict equation.[58] In addition, Bouffard et al. reported that energy expenditure in mechanically ventilated patients with acute renal failure was 1.19 times the predicted BEE (range, 0.7 to 1.7).[59] The major factor increasing energy expenditure above resting levels was the presence of underlying disease (i.e., sepsis).

Renal deterioration may be influenced by carbohydrate intake as well as protein intake (see the section on low-protein diets). Renal injury in rats was reduced by decreasing carbohydrate intake and calories (at a constant protein intake).[60] Lowering the carbohydrate and energy intake reduced weight gain and renal deterioration and prolonged survival in uremic rats.[61] Clinical stud-

TABLE 36–3.

Recommended Protein and Energy Intake

Critically Ill Acute Renal Failure, No Dialysis	Noncatabolic Chronic Renal Failure	Noncatabolic Chronic Renal Failure, Dialysis
Protein: 1.0–1.3 g/kg/day	GFR > 70 mL/min/m² No restriction GFR < 70 mL/min/m² 0.6–0.8 g/kg/day	Hemodialysis 1.0–1.2 g/kg/day Peritoneal dialysis 1.2–1.4 g/kg/day
Energy: 30–35 kcal/kg/day (30% fat)	Same	Same

ies are needed to further address these issues.

We advocate administering a mixture of lipid and carbohydrate as the energy source (i.e., approximately 70% carbohydrate, 30% lipid). Insulin may be required to control blood glucose levels. Carnitine levels may be low in patients with acute renal failure as a result of losses with dialysis.[62, 63] Lipid metabolism may be improved in these patients by carnitine supplementation.[62]

Overfeeding may have a variety of detrimental effects in critically ill patients with underlying systemic inflammatory conditions (i.e., sepsis, multiple trauma, rhabdomyolysis). Overfeeding increases the metabolic demand (oxygen consumption), CO_2 production, and fatty infiltration (especially of the liver) and may precipitate ventilatory failure. Recent experimental studies also indicate that overfeeding causes increased mortality in animal models of sepsis and organ failure. Thus it is important to avoid overfeeding while simultaneously administering adequate nutrients.

Low-Protein Diets

Low-protein diets have been used traditionally in the support of patients with chronic renal failure. These diets were designed to ameliorate the symptoms of uremia and slow progression of renal disease. In the 1970s and 1980s, studies in both humans and animals indicated that low-protein diets (also low in phosphorus) could slow the progression of renal failure.[61, 64–71] These studies restricted protein intake to 0.4 to 0.6

g/kg/day.[64–67] However, many of these studies suffered from a lack of proper controls, retrospective review, poor documentation of actual nutrient intake, and lack of data related to malnutrition. Other investigators failed to find a benefit of dietary protein restriction on the course of renal disease in many patient groups.[72, 73]

The exact role of protein in altering the loss of glomerular filtration is unclear. Most diets restricted protein and phosphorus. Females did not benefit from the protein restriction.[66, 72] The results were frequently disease specific.[66, 72] Patients with glomerulonephritis and interstitial nephritis did better than those with renal failure from other causes (i.e., diabetes, hypertension). In addition, many patients suffered adverse nutritional consequences from these diets. Brodsky et al.[74] reported protein undernutrition when diabetic patients with early nephropathy were fed diets containing 0.6 g/kg/day protein. It is also unclear whether the quantity or quality of protein was more important. Vegetarian diets produce less effect on glomerular filtration than do meat-containing diets.[40, 44]

Some investigators suggest that renal function deterioration can be slowed by using very low protein diets supplemented with EAAs (15 to 20 g mixed protein plus EAA supplements) or keto acids.[71, 75–78] Others doubt the efficacy of these diets on the progression of renal disease.[79, 80] Overall, these diets have little advantage over conventional low-protein diets.

Overall, it would appear that reducing

protein intake in patients with chronic renal failure to the minimum required for adequate nutrition can slow the progression of renal disease in "selected" patient groups. A similar effect can be seen with very low protein diets supplemented with EAAs or keto acids. However, careful attention is required to maintain protein nutrition with these diets.

There are no data to indicate that low-protein diets decrease the loss of renal function or improve the recovery of renal function in patients with acute renal failure. Some studies suggest that protein depletion can decrease renal recovery and outcome. Several investigators have shown an inverse relationship between dietary protein consumption and morbidity/mortality in maintenance hemodialysis patients. The lower the protein intake, the higher the morbidity/mortality. However, there are no prospective randomized trials addressing these issues.

Dietary protein restriction reduces nitrogenous waste products and the intake of sodium, potassium, and phosphorus (found in foods rich in protein). In the past, protein intake has been reduced in patients with acute renal failure in an attempt to reduce uremic toxicity and the need for dialysis. However, this treatment can result in the loss of lean body mass, immune compromise, organ dysfunction, increased infections, and reduced recovery of renal function. It is important to remember that the kidney is frequently only one component of multiple organ failure in these patients. Protein intake is important for the recovery of renal and other organ function. Abel et al.[8] reported improved renal recovery in patients receiving protein and glucose vs. glucose alone. Twenty-one of 28 patients treated with amino acids recovered renal function as compared with 11 of 25 treated with glucose alone. In rats with acute renal failure, amino acid supplementation also enhanced renal recovery.[81, 82] Waste products continue to accumulate

because of the degradation of endogenous protein stores. In summary, there is no place for restriction of protein intake in acutely stressed patients with acute renal failure. The goal is to limit waste product accumulation while simultaneously preserving body nuriture.

Protein Intake

Nutritional support (i.e., protein and calories) has improved outcome in patients with acute renal failure in some[8, 9, 83] but not all studies.[35, 84] Abel et al.[8] compared outcome in patients receiving amino acids plus glucose vs. glucose alone in a prospective double-blind randomized trial. Survival was better in the amino acid groups (75% vs. 44%). In an uncontrolled study, Baek et al.[9] compared hypertonic glucose alone ($n = 66$) with fibrin hydrolysate plus hypertonic glucose ($n = 63$). The mortality rate was 70% with glucose alone vs. 46% in the peptide group.

Critically ill patients with acute renal failure catabolize endogenous and exogenous protein as rapidly as patients with similar disease processes who have intact renal function.[35, 52] Nitrogen balance studies in noncatabolic adult patients with chronic renal failure indicate a neutral or positive nitrogen balance with 40 g/day of high-quality protein.[85] The minimum daily protein requirement of noncatabolic patients with chronic renal failure is approximately 0.6 g/kg/day of high-quality protein (see Table 36−3). The daily protein requirement of hemodialysis patients is higher at 1 to 1.2 g/kg/day. Protein needs are even larger during peritoneal dialysis.[86, 87] Protein requirements of dialysis patients are higher because of the stimulation of catabolism by dialysis and the loss of nutrients in the dialysate. These deficits can result in protein depletion unless dietary protein intake is increased. Available data suggest that highly catabolic patients with acute renal failure require 1.25 to 1.5 g/kg/day of high–biological value protein for maintenance of nitrogen equilibrium. These requirements are even higher in critically ill patients receiving dialysis.

Previously, many advocated protein restriction in patients with acute renal failure to reduce the frequency of dialysis and to prevent the appearance of uremic symptoms (see the section on low-protein diets). Current dictum indicates that protein should not be restricted but should be administered in amounts to satisfy needs. On the other hand, excessive quantities should be avoided. Dialysis and hemofiltration therapy can be used to treat azotemia and electrolyte disorders if they should develop. Moreover, achieving adequate nutritional status has more impact on the overall outcome in patients with acute renal failure than does preventing the evolution of metabolic complications (which can easily be treated with dialysis). Improved protein synthesis is important for survival and renal recovery.

Some have advocated the use of EAA diets in the treatment of renal failure. Initially, it was suggested that by providing EAAs only, nitrogen from endogenous and exogenous sources would be utilized to synthesize the nonessential amino acids required for protein formation. This would result in sufficient amino acids for the synthesis of body proteins and would minimize urea generation from endogenous amino acid catabolism.[29, 88] Subsequently, Varcoe et al.[89] showed that urea generation from nonessential amino acid metabolism was small in patients receiving general amino acid (GAA) diets. In addition, there is little evidence that urea nitrogen is reutilized for amino acid or protein synthesis.[29, 89] The rate of protein synthesis depends on the availability of essential and nonessential amino acids. If these are limited, protein synthesis will be impaired. By increasing the quantity of nonessential amino acids there is less need for de novo synthesis and transamination, which might deplete the free amino acid pool. The net result is an improvement in nitrogen balance despite a slight increase in urea production.[90]

Intravenous amino acid formulas containing only EAAs were developed and tested clinically in patients with renal failure over the past 20 years (Table 36–4). These formulas improved nutritional status when compared with hypertonic glucose alone.[8, 83, 84, 91–93] However, overall they did not improve renal function. Only two studies demonstrated improved survival with amino acid–supplemented formulas.[8, 83] These results were not unexpected since the control groups did not receive adequate nutritional support and were placed on protein-depleted diets. Subsequent studies[35, 52, 94–97] compared EAA solutions with GAA solutions (Table 36–5). The three studies that evaluated outcome reported no differences between diet groups.[35, 96, 97] Both solutions maintained "nutritional

TABLE 36–4.

Essential Amino Acids vs. Glucose

Study	Description	N	Renal Recovery or Nitrogen Balance	Nutritional Status	Outcome
Wilmore[91]	EAA* (case report)	1	No controls	Improved	No controls
Dudrick[92]	EAA in glucose	10	No controls	Improved	No controls
Abel[93]	EAA in glucose	17	No controls	Improved	No controls
Abel[8]	EAA + glucose vs. glucose	53	Improved renal function with EAA	Improved	Improved survival with EAA
Leonard[84]	EAA + glucose vs. glucose	20	Decreased urea with EAA	N/A*	No effect
Milligan[83]	EAA + glucose vs. glucose	76	N/A	Improved	Improved survival with EAA

*EAA = essential amino acid solutions; N/A = not available.

TABLE 36–5.

Essential Amino Acids vs. General Amino Acids

Study	Description	N	Renal Recovery or Nitrogen Balance	Nutritional Status	Outcome
Wassner[94]	EAA* vs. GAA* in malnourished patients with normal renal function	6	Urea nitrogen lower with EAA	N/A*	N/A
Blackburn[95]	EAA vs. GAA	19	No difference	N/A	N/A
Feinstein[35]	Glucose vs. EAA + glucose vs. GAA + glucose	30	No difference	No difference	No difference
Mirtallo[96]	EAA + glucose vs. GAA + glucose	45	No difference	N/A	No difference
Feinstein[52]	EAA + glucose vs. GAA + glucose	11	Urea nitrogen lower with EAA	No difference	N/A
Tempel[97]	EAA + glucose vs. GAA + glucose (trauma and surgery, normal renal function)	61	No difference	N/A	N/A

*EAA = essential amino acid solutions; GAA = essential plus nonessential amino acid solutions; N/A = not available.

status" to the same degree. There were no differences between groups for recovery of renal function.

Several studies where EAA solutions were used as the sole amino acid source for patients with acute renal failure demonstrated a slowing of the rate of rise in BUN[84, 91, 92] or a decrease in urea nitrogen appearance.[52] However, dialysis was not initiated in these studies, and renal function remained unchanged. On the other hand, a number of controlled studies have not uniformly confirmed these observations. A meta-analysis[98] questioned the efficacy of these solutions. In addition, EAA therapy does not alter the course of renal insufficiency in experimental acute renal failure.[99]

In the past, many patients with acute renal failure were treated with EAA formulas. These formulas do not meet the needs of these patients and are no longer recommended. These formulas were designed to reduce urea formation; however, they fail to support the protein metabolism required for healing, immune function, organ function, and other important determinants of recovery/survival. Experiments in normal and uremic animals indicate that mixtures of essential and nonessential amino ac-

ids promote better growth than do EAAs alone.[100, 101]

The EAAs represent those amino acids that are not synthesized by the body (hence the term "essential") and are required for protein synthesis in normal individuals. Normal individuals are capable of synthesizing the remaining amino acids from the "essential" amino acids. A number of "nonessential" amino acids are now recognized as being essential during severe stress, growth, and critical illness. Synthetic pathways for the synthesis of these "conditionally essential" amino acids are depressed (i.e., hepatic or renal dysfunction) or limited during critical illness such that insufficient quantities are produced for optimal protein synthesis. These amino acids include arginine, glutamine, histidine, serine, taurine, cysteine, and tyrosine[102] and should be supplied during nutritional support (especially to patients with renal insufficiency). Interestingly, when only EAAs are administered for nutritional support, hyperammonemia may develop. Hyperammonemia probably results from a deficiency of arginine, an important amino acid in the production of urea from ammonia.[103, 104] Arginine administration can correct EAA-induced hyperammonemia.[104] High-quality protein contains a high ratio of EAAs to total amino acids and better supports nitrogen balance. Examples of such protein include eggs, milk, and lean meat. In conclusion, it is now recognized that patients with renal failure require both "essential" and "nonessential" amino acids.

Some have also advocated the use of branched-chain amino acid (BCAA) formulas in patients with organ failure (including renal failure). Initial clinical studies compared BCAA-supplemented hypertonic glucose with hypertonic glucose alone in patients with hepatic failure. Some studies found that patients had reduced encephalopathy and improved outcome. However, when all studies were analyzed, there was no significant improvement in encephalopathy or outcome with the high-BCAA formulas. It is important to note that these studies compared glucose alone with glucose supplemented with BCAAs. They did not compare two nutritionally complete formulas. When normal vs. high-BCAA formulas were compared, no significant differences in encephalopathy or outcome were found. When high-BCAA formulas were administered to metabolically stressed patients (i.e., trauma, sepsis), there was a reduction in BUN concentration, and nitrogen balance was achieved with lower protein quantities. There was no difference in outcome or organ failure. The overall cost of administering the formulas was higher than with standard formulas. Thus, high-BCAA formulas can support the nutritional needs of stressed patients and patients with organ failure; however, they do not appear to be superior to standard and cheaper formulas.

Keto acid–supplemented diets have been used to support patients with chronic renal failure. Keto acids are converted to EAAs in the body and reduce the production of urea. These compounds have not been well studied in acute renal failure. The same problems that exist with EAAs also exist with keto acids.

Fluid, Electrolyte, Vitamin, and Trace Element Requirements

Fluid status must be closely monitored in patients with acute renal failure. Fluid requirements depend on residual excretory capacity (i.e., oliguric vs. nonoliguric), gastrointestinal fluid losses, and insensible water losses (i.e., fever, sweating). Patients with acute renal failure demonstrate impaired water excretory capacity. Thus they are susceptible to water overload, which may manifest itself as peripheral edema, pulmonary edema, congestive heart failure, or hyponatremia. Many patients with acute renal failure require 1500 to 2000 mL of water per day to replace residual urinary, gastrointestinal, and insensible losses. This fluid is best replaced

TABLE 36–6.

Enteral Renal Formulas

Component	Nepro (Ross)	Suplena (Ross)	Travasor Renal (Clintec)	Nutren-2 (Clintec)	TwoCal HN (Ross)	Magnacal (Sherwood)
kcal/mL	2	2	1.35	2	2	2
Protein (g/L)	69.9, intact	30, intact	22.9, amino acids	80, intact	83.7, intact	70, intact
Fat (g/L)	95.6	95.6	17.7	106	90.0	80
Carbohydrate (g/L)	215	255	270	196	217	250
mOsm/kg H_2O	635	600	590	710	690	590
Na (mg/L)	830	784	None	1000	1057	1000
K (mg/L)	1056	1116	None	2500	2325	1252
PO_4 (mg/L)	686	728	None	1400	1057	1000
Mg (mg/L)	210	210	None	680	423	400
Ca (mg/L)	1372	1386	None	1400	1057	1000

with an enteral nutritional formula that supplies both water and needed nutrients. Enteral nutritional formulas are available as standard (1 kcal/mL) and double-strength (2 kcal/ml) solutions. One thousand milliliters per day of a double-strength formula can supply 2000 kcal and 70 to 80 g of protein (Table 36–6). Parenteral nutritional formulas can also supply nutrients in concentrated form (i.e., using 70% hypertonic glucose, 20% lipid) to avoid excess water ad-ministration. Nutrient administration should not be limited in an attempt to avoid fluid administration. If fluid retention develops, it can be managed with dialysis or continuous hemofiltration techniques.

Dietary administration of potassium, phosphorus, and magnesium should be restricted in acute renal failure since these minerals are normally excreted by the kidney. Patient requirements for these elements change according to the metabolic status. In highly catabolic patients, intracellular electrolytes escape from cells and cause significant elevations in their serum levels. However,

during anabolism the opposite occurs and may render the patient hypokalemic, hypophosphatemic, and/or hypomagnesemic. Protein synthesis requires adequate quantities of potassium, phosphorus, and magnesium. Therefore, while it may be appropriate to withhold certain electrolytes at the time that nutritional support is initiated, monitoring and adjustment of electrolyte intake are essential during therapy to avoid life-threatening electrolyte imbalances.

The vitamin and mineral needs of patients with acute renal failure are not well defined. Needs vary with the patient's clinical status (i.e., metabolic state), underlying disease, gastrointestinal losses, residual renal/excretory function, and use of dialysis. Vitamin and mineral requirements in patients with acute renal failure usually exceed those of patients with chronic renal failure because of increased metabolic needs and greater losses (Table 36–7). We usually begin with these levels and adjust after clinical/laboratory assessment (i.e., serum levels). With the exception of iron and zinc, trace elements are infre-

TABLE 36–7.

Daily Mineral and Vitamin Requirements

Component	Acute Renal Failure	Chronic Renal Failure	Chronic Renal Failure—Dialysis
Na (mg/day)	ND*	1000–3000	1500–2000
K (mg/day)	ND	1600–2800	1600–2800
PO$_4$ (mg/kg/day)	ND	4–10	8–17
Ca (mg/day)	ND	1400–1600	1400–1600
Mg (mg/day)	ND	200–300	200–300
Fe (mg/day)	ND	10–18	10–18
Zn (mg/day)	ND	15	15
Trace	ND	Unknown	Unknown
Thiamine (mg/day)	ND	1.5	1.5
Riboflavin (mg/day)	ND	1.8	1.8
Pantothenic acid (mg/day)	ND	5	5
Niacin (mg/day)	ND	20	20
Pyridoxine (mg/day)	ND	5	10
Vitamin B$_{12}$ (μg/day)	ND	3	3
Vitamin C (mg/day)	ND	60–100	100
Folate (mg/day)	ND	1	1
Vitamin A	None	None	None
Vitamin D	Monitor Ca	Monitor Ca	Monitor Ca
Vitamin E (IU/day)	ND	15	15
Vitamin K	Monitor the patient	Monitor the patient	Monitor the patient

*ND = not defined.

quently required during the first 2 to 3 weeks of therapy. Patients receiving chronic hemodialysis may also have low plasma selenium levels.[105]

Several studies of chronic renal failure suggest a relationship between phosphorus intake and the rate of decrease in renal function.[61] Excess phosphorus intake induces nephropathy with calcification of the renal parenchyma. However, most studies of reduced phosphorus intake also restricted protein intake. Improved outcome likely resulted from protein restriction.

Calcium should not be restricted since calcium mobilization from bone may be impaired because of the loss of 1,25-dihydroxyvitamin D synthesis. Many prefer to administer extra calcium in the presence of diminished gut calcium absorption (vitamin D–dependent process). Enteral calcium also binds with luminal phosphorus, decreases its absorption, and prevents hyperphosphatemia. Persistent ionized hypocalcemia should be avoided since it can result in tertiary hyperparathyroidism and osteodystrophy.

Patients with acute renal failure require less sodium than do patients with normal renal function. However, they still require sodium replacement as a result of obligatory losses from the gastrointestinal tract and skin. Sodium intake should be matched to output. Obviously, fluid and electrolyte requirements vary with the type of renal replacement (i.e., dialysis, continuous hemofiltration).

Vitamin requirements have not been well defined for patients with acute renal failure, and much of the recommended intake is based on data from patients with chronic renal failure and normal individuals. Vitamin A is probably best avoided because in chronic renal failure serum vitamin A levels are elevated. Even small doses of vitamin A have been reported to cause toxicity within a few days. It is unlikely that deficiency of this fat-soluble vitamin will

occur. If patients require nutritional support for more than 2 weeks, then the RDA for vitamin A should be provided. Although vitamin D is fat soluble and vitamin D stores should not become depleted during a few days to weeks of the onset of acute renal failure, the synthesis of its most active form, 1,25-dihydroxyvitamin D, is significantly impaired. The requirement for this vitamin D analogue in acute renal failure has not been defined. We do not usually administer vitamin D analogues to patients with acute renal failure. We prefer to monitor blood ionized calcium levels and maintain normal levels with calcium supplementation. If blood ionized calcium levels are difficult to maintain within normal levels, we do administer vitamin D once the renal failure has stabilized. Vitamin K is another fat-soluble vitamin. Deficiencies have been reported in nonuremic patients receiving inadequate intake and/or antibiotics.[106] Vitamin K is normally synthesized by gut bacteria. We monitor the prothrombin time/partial thromboplastin time (PT/PTT) and give vitamin K if these times become prolonged or evidence of bleeding develops. We also recommend a daily dose of pyridoxine hydrochloride (10 mg) because studies in patients undergoing maintenance hemodialysis indicate that this amount may be necessary to prevent or correct vitamin B_6 deficiency. Enteral nutritional formulas contain vitamins at amounts that meet RDAs for normal individuals. We believe these amounts to be safe in patients with acute renal failure.

In summary, nutritional requirements must be evaluated on a daily basis in patients with acute renal failure. Recommended amounts of electrolytes in all nutritional solutions should be considered tentative because these patients may undergo rapid changes in their metabolic and clinical status that mandate modifications of the nutritional formulations.

ROUTES OF FEEDING

Whenever feasible, patients should ingest nutrients. Because of anorexia, nausea, vomiting, altered mentation, or impaired swallowing, oral feeding may not always be an option. These patients should receive nutritional support via enteral feeding tubes. If gastric emptying is adequate (i.e., gastric residuals are less than 100 to 150 mL in adults) and the patient is not known to reflux, feedings are best initiated in the stomach. When gastric emptying is impaired, enteral nutrients are best administered postpylorically in the small bowel. Patients should be inclined with the head elevated to minimize reflux and aspiration.

Accumulating data indicate that enteral nutrition is superior to parenteral nutrition (see the chapter on timing and the route of nutritional support). It is associated with improved gut mass and function, reduced bacterial translocation, improved liver function, enhanced immune function, reduced infection rates, and better survival in many critically ill patients.

There are no prospective randomized trials comparing enteral with parenteral nutrition in patients with renal failure. Bihari et al.[107] recently reported their experience with enteral and parenteral nutrition in patients with combined acute respiratory and renal failure. The investigators performed an audit study of prospectively collected data over a 2-year period. During the first year, patients received primarily total parenteral nutrition (TPN) followed by enteral nutrition when "traditional" criteria of gut function returned (i.e., bowel sounds, absence of diarrhea, small gastric residual). During the second year, the primary mode of nutritional support was enteral feeding. There were 42 patients studied in the first year and 79 in the second year. Patient groups had similar age, diagnoses, and APACHE II (Acute Physiology, Age, and Chronic Health

Evaluation II) scores. In the first year, 17% of patients received enteral nutrition alone, while 71% received parenteral nutrition (12% received no feedings). In the second year, 73% received enteral nutrition alone, and 11% received parenteral feeding (16% received no feedings). Mortality rates decreased from 76% in the first year to 43% in the second year ($P < .01$). The cost per survivor fell from 61,180 pounds in the first year to 20,545 pounds in the second year. The feeding cost per patient also fell from 676 pounds to 145 pounds. These data suggest that enteral feeding may also be associated with improved outcome in acute renal failure (similar to other critically ill patients). However, definitive results await a prospective randomized trial.

NUTRITIONAL FORMULATIONS

Many standard, commercially available enteral formulas containing high-quality protein, vitamins, and minerals can be employed in patients with acute and chronic renal failure (see the chapter on enteral nutritional products). However, these formulas may deliver larger quantities of minerals (such as potassium, phosphorus, and magnesium) than required in patients with acute renal failure. Several enteral formulas meet the caloric and metabolic needs of patients with acute renal failure (see Table 36–6). These formulas provide variable quantities of protein, carbohydrate, fat, fluid, and minerals. Some of these formulas are lower in potassium, phosphorus, and magnesium as compared with standard formulas.

As previously discussed, EAA formulas do not supply the needed nitrogen sources for patients with renal failure and should be avoided. Patients who are stressed and in catabolic renal failure require a high-nitrogen formula. One may use a 2-kcal/mL formula if fluid retention is a problem. If fluid and electrolyte balance is not a problem, a standard enteral formula is adequate (and cheap). If gastrointestinal digestion/absorption is impaired, we prefer to use a peptide-based formula.

FORM OF RENAL REPLACEMENT THERAPY

The form of renal support alters the nutritional requirements. Peritoneal dialysis leads to peritoneal inflammation and loss of proteins into the dialysate.[108, 109] Amino acid losses are frequently in the range of 30 to 40 g/day.[86, 87] Some add amino acids and albumin to the dialysate in an attempt to minimize protein losses. Minerals and vitamins are also lost into the peritoneal fluid. Absorption of glucose from peritoneal dialysate can be substantial (i.e., 1000 to 1500 kcal/day) and may result in overfeeding.[110]

Intermittent hemodialysis continues to be the major form of renal replacement therapy used in critical care units.[111] The metabolic effects of hemodialysis vary with the type of membrane (i.e., cuprophane vs. polyacrylonitrile) and buffer (i.e., acetate vs. bicarbonate) used. Bicarbonate buffers are preferred over acetate buffers since acetate dialysis has been associated with hypotension. Cuprophane membranes result in the activation of complement, kinins, coagulation factors, platelets, and white blood cells. Polyacrylonitrile membranes are more biocompatible and do not activate cells (releasing cytokines) or complement. Cuprophane membranes are associated with enhanced release of amino acids from skeletal muscle, an effect not seen with polyacrylonitrile membranes.[112] There is a loss of nutrients (i.e., amino acids, vitamins, minerals, glucose) during hemodialysis.[113–115] Ten to 15 g of amino acids and 10 to 25 g of glucose are normally lost during a 4- to 6-hour hemodialysis treatment (using glucose-free dialysate). Hemodialysis is also re-

ported to increase catabolism[116–118] and energy expenditure.[119]

Continuous renal support (i.e., continuous arteriovenous or venovenous hemofiltration with or without dialysis) is being increasingly used in critical care units. These techniques also remove nutrients (i.e., amino acids) but have been less well studied. Continuous arteriovenous hemofiltration has been reported to facilitate the nutritional management of critically ill patients with acute renal failure by allowing for the delivery of adequate quantities of nutrients.[51]

MONITORING OF NUTRITIONAL SUPPORT

It is important that patients receive monitoring during nutritional support to avoid nutritional depletion syndromes and overfeeding. Fluid status can be assessed by using a combination of vital signs (i.e., blood pressure, heart rate), serum sodium concentration, hemoglobin level, central venous pressure, and body weight. Serum electrolytes can be measured and treated accordingly.

The optimal method for monitoring calorie/protein repletion in patients with acute renal failure remains unclear. Ideally, the clinician wants a monitor that predicts outcome. Anthropometric measurements (i.e., skin folds, weight), total lymphocyte counts, and skin test hypersensitivity responses have not been useful.

Current monitoring is best accomplished by using serial visceral protein levels, nitrogen balance, or indirect calorimetry. We have found serial changes in serum prealbumin and transferrin concentrations to best correlate with outcome in critically ill patients. The direction of change over time is more important than an isolated value. Serum albumin is slow to change (because of its long half-life and preferential catabolism). Retinol binding protein and insulin growth factor 1 (IGF-1) levels are more variable and difficult to measure. Decreases in prealbumin reflect a reprioritization of hepatic protein synthesis during systemic inflammatory states such as sepsis and trauma. The liver switches its synthetic pathways to acute-phase proteins and away from prealbumin. Thus, serial increases in prealbumin suggest resolution of the systemic inflammatory state coupled with adequate nutrient intake. Levels may also be altered as a result of the hydration status and hepatic function.

Nitrogen balance is less useful in patients with renal failure because of the loss of urinary nitrogen excretion. The goal of therapy is to produce a decrease in negative nitrogen balance over the first 3 to 5 days of illness and eventually to obtain a positive nitrogen balance. The attainment of these goals indicates resolution of the underlying inflammatory/catabolic state and provision of adequate nutrients. Nitrogen balance can be calculated as follows:

$$\text{Urea nitrogen appearance (UNA) (g/day)} = \\ \text{Urinary urea nitrogen (UUN) (g/day)} \\ + \text{dialysate urea nitrogen (DUN) (g/day)} \\ + \text{Change in body urea nitrogen (CBUN) (g/day),}$$

$$\text{where CBUN (g/day)} = SUN_f - SUN_i \text{ (g/L)} \times BW_i \\ \text{(kg/day)} \times (0.6 \text{ L/kg}) + (BW_f - BW_i, \text{ kg/day}) \\ \times SUN_f \text{ (g/L)} \times (1.0 \text{ L/kg}),$$

where f and i are the final and initial values, SUN = serum urea nitrogen, and BW = body weight

$$\text{Total nitrogen output (g/day)} = UNA + 2$$

$$\text{Nitrogen balance} = \text{Total nitrogen output} \\ - \text{Nitrogen input}$$

FUTURE STUDIES

Animal studies evaluating the use of growth factors in the treatment of acute renal failure are under way. Growth factors such as erythropoietin are commonly used in patients with established renal failure to support erythrocyte synthesis. Growth hormone has shown promise in improving nitrogen balance

and protein synthesis. IGF-1, atrial natriuretic hormone, and epidermal growth factor may be useful in speeding recovery from renal failure. Speeding recovery of renal function may have a significant impact upon both morbidity and mortality. Faster return of renal function may spare patients the ordeal and complications of dialysis. Small improvements may be clinically very important. Improving the GFR from 8 to 15 mL/min may make the difference between dialysis and no dialysis.

Nutritional studies evaluating the effects of various nutrients (i.e., peptides, amino acids, lipids) on renal function are also under way. These studies include evaluation of renal blood flow, GFR, renal tubular function, renal metabolic activity, cytokine response, and immune function.

Several reports suggest a role for lipids in the progression of renal disease. High-cholesterol diets have been reported to accelerate glomerular sclerosis.[61, 120] In addition, high–linoleic acid diets prevent the development of renal lesions in remnant kidneys of animals,[120, 121] which suggests a beneficial role for prostaglandins (i.e., PGE_2). Renal prostaglandin synthesis is necessary for the maintenance of GFR in the face of renal disease.[120]

Animals with subtotal nephrectomy fed diets rich in the ω-3 long-chain fatty acid eicosapentaenoic acid (EPA) have lower PGE_2 excretion, lower creatinine clearances, and higher mortalities than do rats fed standard diets.[122, 123] Suppression of PGE_2 may result in deleterious renal effects in these animals. On the other hand, EPA-enriched diets prevent proteinuria and prolong survival in experimental glomerulonephritis.[124] This effect may relate to the reduced production of inflammatory mediators (i.e., arachidonic acid metabolites). The role of lipid modulation on the development and progression of renal disease requires further study.

The quantity as well as the quality (i.e., protein, carbohydrate, lipids) of nutrient intake may affect renal function. Many studies have shown that nutrient restriction lengthens the life span of normal animals.[61, 125-127] Nutrient restriction increases the life span and ameliorates the development of renal lesions during aging.[127] Protein restriction improves survival in animals with experimental immunologic nephropathy (injection of nephrotoxic serum).[128] Restriction of food intake decreases progression of lupus and renal lesions in mice.[129, 130] On the other hand, protein supplementation increases the severity of experimental glomerulonephritis in rats, even when introduced after the induction of disease.[131] It is known that immunologic reactions are modified by dietary intake. Excessive restriction (starvation) increases complications and worsens outcome. However, moderate restriction of a well-balanced diet reduces morbidity and mortality in experimental animals. Some day, specific nutritional manipulations may be useful for protecting the kidney from damage during critical illness and shock states.

The administration of nutritional support to patients with acute renal failure creates perplexing management problems. Clinicians have often pondered the benefits of nutritional supplementation and have weighed this against the risks of uremia, electrolyte imbalance, and volume overload. The goal of nutritional support in acute renal failure has shifted away from its use for preventing uremic symptoms to maintaining good nutritional status. Several decades ago it was believed that dietary protein restriction in patients with acute renal failure helped to minimize uremic symptoms and reduced the accumulation of nitrogenous waste products. On the other hand, maintenance of good nutrition was a secondary aim.[48] Subsequent studies indicated that low-protein diets contribute to net catabolism in acute renal failure. The availability of dialysis and hemofiltration therapies to treat severe azotemia

and electrolyte abnormalities has reduced the need for low-nitrogen diets in patients with acute renal failure. Since dialysis is not free of complications, requires large-bore central venous catheters and anticoagulation, and can cause intermittent hypotension as well as fluid and electrolyte shifts, a major issue is whether malnutrition or dialysis is of greater risk to survival. No data are currently available that determine which risk, malnutrition or hemodialysis, puts the patient at a greater risk. However, continuous hemofiltration is safer for the patient and has allowed for optimal nutritional repletion. New trials are needed to evaluate the effects of nutrition on outcome. The clinical course of patients with acute renal failure is so variable and so complex that it may be necessary to study large numbers of patients in a randomized prospective fashion to show statistically significant advantages to nutritional therapy. The optimal composition of diets, TPN solutions, or tube feeding formulas in patients with acute renal failure has not been defined.

The following conclusions are based upon the available data:

1. Acute renal failure usually occurs as part of multiple organ failure in critically ill patients and substantially increases the mortality in these patients.

2. Acute renal failure is associated with hypermetabolism and hypercatabolism.

3. Protein intake should not be limited in patients with acute renal failure. Protein intake should meet metabolic needs.

4. Avoid the use of EAA formulas. GAA formulas better meet the protein needs of the patient. There is no evidence that high-BCAA formulas provide any advantage over GAA formulas.

5. Patients with acute renal failure are at risk for fluid overload, hyperkalemia, hyperphosphatemia, and hypermagnesemia. Frequent monitoring of fluid and electrolyte status is essential.

6. Enteral nutrition is the preferred route for delivery of nutrients to patients with acute renal failure. The majority of patients can be fed by enteral nutrition.

7. Dialysis is associated with increased catabolism and energy expenditure. It also results in the loss of protein, minerals, and vitamins.

REFERENCES

1. Hou SH, Bushinsky Da, Wish JB et al: Hospital-acquired renal insufficiency: A prospective study. *Am J Med* 1983; 74:243.

2. Balsloy JT, Jorgensen HE: A survey of 499 patients with acute anuric renal insufficiency. *Am J Med* 1963; 34:753.

3. Bluemle LW, Webster GD, Elkinton JR: Acute tubular necrosis. *Arch Intern Med* 1959; 104:190.

4. Karatson A, Juhasz J, Hubler J, et al: Factors influencing the prognosis of acute renal failure. *Int Urol Nephrol* 1978; 10:321.

5. Kleinknecht D, Jungers P, Chanard J, et al: Factors influencing immediate prognosis in acute renal failure, with special reference to prophylactic hemodialysis. *Adv Nephrol* 1971; 1:207.

6. McMurry SD, Luft FE, Kirschbaum BB, et al: Amino acid therapy in the treatment of experimental acute renal failure in the rat. *Kidney Int* 1980; 17:14.

7. Merill JP: Acute renal failure (editorial). *N Engl J Med* 1975; 295:220.

8. Abel RM, Beck CH Jr, Abbott WM, et al: Improved survival from acute renal failure after treatment with intravenous essential L-amino acids and glucose. Results of a prospective, double-blind study. *N Engl J Med* 1973; 288:695.

9. Baek SM, Makabali GG, Bryan-Brown CW et al: The influence of parenteral nutrition on the course of acute renal failure. *Surg Gynecol Obstet* 1975; 141:405.

10. Bessey P, Watters JM, Aoki T, et al: Combined hormonal infusion stimulates the metabolic response to injury. *Ann Surg* 1984; 200:264–281.

11. Eigler N, Sacca L, Sherwin R: Synergistic interactions of physiologic increments of glucagon, epinephrine and cortisol in the dog. A model for stress induced hyperglycemia. *J Clin Invest* 1979; 63:114.

12. Horl W, Heidland A: Enhanced proteolytic activity—cause of protein catabolism in acute renal failure. *Am J Clin Nutr* 1980; 33:1423.

13. Horl W, Stepinski J, Schaefer R, et al: Role of proteases in hypercatabolic patients with acute renal failure. *Kidney Int* 1983; 24(suppl 16):37.

14. Leonard C, Luke R, Siegell R: Parenteral essential amino acids in acute renal failure. *Urology* 1975; 6:154.

15. Lindholm B, Bergstrom J: Nutritional management of patients undergoing peritoneal dialysis, in Nolph K (ed): *Peritoneal Dialysis*, ed 3. Boston, Kluwer, 1989, pp 230–260.

16. Kratka R, Shuler C, Wolfson M: Nutrition in hemodialysis and peritoneal dialysis patients, in Nissenson AR, Fine RN, Gentile DE (eds): *Clinical Dialysis*, ed 2. Norwalk, Conn, Appleton & Lange, 1990, pp 350–365.

17. Alfrey AC, Rudolph H, Smythe WR: Mineral metabolism in uremia. *Kidney Int* 1975; 7(suppl):85.

18. Cohen BD: Interaction of protein, carbohydrate, and fat in uremia, in *Proceedings of 6th International Congress of Nephrology, Florence, 1975*, Basel, Switzerland, S Karger, 1976, pp 204–211.

19. De Fronzo RA, Alvestrand A, Smith D, et al: Insulin resistance in uremia. *J Clin Invest* 1981; 67:563.

20. Delaporte C, Gros F, Anagnostopoulos C: Inhibitory effects of plasma dialysate on protein synthesis in vitro: Influence of dialysis and transplantation. *Am J Clin Nutr* 1980; 33:1407.

21. Druml W, Laggner A, Widhalm K, et al: Lipid metabolism in acute renal failure. *Kidney Int* 1983; 24(suppl):139.

22. Frolich J, Schollmeyer P, Gerok W: Carbohydrate metabolism in renal failure. *Am J Clin Nutr* 1978; 131:1541.

23. Kopple JD, Jones M, Fukuda S, et al: Amino acid and protein metabolism in renal failure. *Am J Clin Nutr* 1978; 31:1532.

24. Kopple JD, Swendseid ME: Vitamin nutrition in patients undergoing maintenance hemodialysis. *Kidney Int* 1975; 7(suppl):79.

25. Reaven GM, Swenson RS, Sanfelippo ML: An inquiry into the mechanism of hypertriglyceridemia in patients with chronic renal failure. *Am J Clin Nutr* 1980; 33:1476.

26. Sandstead HH: Trace elements in uremia and hemodialysis. *Am J Clin Nutr* 1980; 33:1501.

27. Walser M: Nutrition in renal failure. *Annu Rev Nutr* 1983; 3:125.

28. Clark A, Mitch W: Muscle protein turnover and glucose uptake in acutely uremic rats. Effect of insulin and the duration of renal insufficiency. *J Clin Invest* 1983; 72:836.

29. Mitch WE, Wilmore DW: Nutritional considerations in the treatment of acute renal failure, in Brenner BM, Lazarus JM (eds): *Acute Renal Failure*, ed 2. New York, Churchill Livingstone, 1988, pp 743–765.

30. Mitch WE: Amino acid release from the hindquarter and urea appearance in acute uremia. *Am J Physiol* 1982; 241:226.

31. Grossman SB, Yap SH, Shafritz DA: Influence of chronic renal failure on protein synthesis and albumin metabolism in rat liver. *J Clin Invest* 1977; 59:869.

32. Flugel-Link RM, Salusky IB, Jones MR, et al: Protein and amino acid metabolism in posterior hemicorpus of acutely uremic rats. *Am J Physiol* 1983; 244:615.

33. Arnold WC, Holliday MA: Tissue resistance to insulin stimulation of amino acid uptake in acutely uremic rats. *Kidney Int* 1979; 16:124.

34. May RC, Clark AS, Goheer A, et al: Identification of specific defects in insulin mediated muscle metabolism in acute uremia. *Kidney Int* 1985; 28:490.

35. Feinstein E, Blumenkrantz M, Healy M, et al: Clinical and metabolic responses to parenteral nutrition in acute renal failure. A controlled double-blind study. *Medicine (Baltimore)* 1981; 60:124.

36. Sapico V: Enzyme alterations and subcellular translocation of inducible tyrosine aminotransferase in acute uremia (abstract). *Fed Proc* 1973; 32:505.

37. Walser M: Determinants of ureagenesis, with particular reference to renal failure. *Kidney Int* 1980; 17:709.

38. Lacy WW: Effect of acute uremia on amino acid uptake and urea production by perfused rat liver. *Am J Physiol* 1969; 216:1300.

39. Lacy WW: Uptake of individual amino acids by perfused rat liver: Effect of acute uremia. *Am J Physiol* 1970; 219:649.

40. Bosch JP, Saccaggi A, Lauer A, et al: Renal functional reserve in humans—Effect of protein intake on glomerular filtration rate. *Am J Med* 1983; 75:943.

41. Graf H, Stummvoli HF, Luger A, et al: Effect of amino acid infusion on glomerular filtration rate correspondence. *N Engl J Med* 1983; 308:159.

42. Ando A, Kawata T, Hara Y, et al: Effects of dietary protein intake on renal function in humans. *Kidney Int* 1989; 36(suppl):64.

43. Winchester JF, Chapman AB: Effect of dietary constituents on renal function. *Kidney Int* 1989; 36(suppl):68.

44. Kontessis P, Jones S, Dodds R, et al: Renal, metabolic, and hormonal responses to ingestion of animal and vegetable proteins. *Kidney Int* 1990; 38:136.

45. Brenner MB, Meyer TW, Hostetter TH: Dietary protein intake and the progressive nature of kidney disease: The role of hemodynamically mediated glomerular injury in the pathogenesis of progressive glomerular sclerosis in aging, renal ablation, and intrinsic renal disease. *N Engl J Med* 1982; 307:652.

46. Kopple JD: Nutritional therapy in kidney failure. *Nutr Rev* 1981; 39:193.

47. Black PR, Brooks DC, Bessey PQ, et al: Mechanisms of insulin resistance following injury. *Ann Surg* 1982; 196:420.

48. Mitch WE, May RC, Clark AS, et al: The influence of insulin resistance and amino acid supply on muscle protein turnover in uremia. *Kidney Int* 1987; 22:5104.

49. Weinrauch LA, Healy RW, Leland OS,

et al: Decreased insulin requirement in acute renal failure in diabetic nephropathy. *Arch Intern Med* 1978; 138:399.

50. Mault J, Bartlett R, Dechert R, et al: Starvation—a major contribution to mortality in acute renal failure? *Trans Am Soc Artif Intern Organs* 1983; 29:390.

51. Bartlett RH, Mault JR, Dechert RE, et al: Continuous arteriovenous hemofiltration—improved survival in surgical acute renal failure? *Surgery* 1986; 100:400.

52. Feinstein E, Kopple J, Siberrman H, et al: Total parenteral nutrition with high or low nitrogen intake in patients with acute renal failure. *Kidney Int* 1983; 16(suppl):319.

53. Forsberg E, Carlsson M, Thorne A, et al: Energy expenditure in long-term critically ill patients with acute renal failure (abstract). Presented at the Fourth International Congress of Nutrition and Metabolism in Renal Disease, Williamsburg, Va, 1985.

54. Harris J, Benedict F: *A Biometric Study of Basal Metabolism in a Man.* Washington, DC, Carnegie Institute, Publication No 279, 1919.

55. Kopple JD, Monteon FJ, Shaib JK: Effect of energy intake on nitrogen metabolism in nondialyzed patients with chronic renal failure. *Kidney Int* 1986; 29:734.

56. Monteon FJ, Laidlaw SA, Shaib JK, et al: Energy expenditure in patients with chronic renal failure. *Kidney Int* 1986; 30:741.

57. Slomowitz LA, Monteon FJ, Grosvenor M, et al: Effect of energy intake on nutritional status in maintenance hemodialysis patients. *Kidney Int* 1989; 35:704.

58. Little RA, Campbell IT, Green CJ, et al: Nutritional support in acute renal failure in critically ill, in Bihari D, Neild G (eds): *Acute Renal Failure in the Intensive Therapy Unit.* Heidelburg, Springer-Verlag, 1990, pp 347–357.

59. Bouffard Y, Viale JP, Annat G, et al: Energy expenditure in the acute renal failure patient mechanically ventilated. *Intensive Care Med* 1987; 13:401.

60. Bras G, Ross MH: Kidney disease and nutrition in the rat. *Toxicol Appl Pharmacol* 1964; 6:247.

61. Laouari D, Kleinknecht C: The role of nutritional factors in the course of experimental renal failure. *Am J Kidney Dis* 1985; 5:147.

62. Lacour B, Guilio SD, Chanard J, et al: Carnitine improves lipid anomalies in hemodialysis patients. *Lancet* 1980; 2:763.

63. Bohmer T, Bergrem H, Eiklind K: Carnitine deficiency induced during intermittent hemodialysis for renal failure. *Lancet* 1978; 1:126.

64. Maschio G, Oldrizzi L, Tessitore N, et al: Early dietary protein and phosphorus restriction is effective in delaying progression of chronic renal failure. *Kidney Int* 1983; 24:272.

65. Maschio G, Oldrizzi L, Tessitore N, et al: Effects of dietary protein and phosphorus restriction on the progression of early renal failure. *Kidney Int* 1982; 22:371.

66. Rosman JB, Meijer S, Sluiter WJ, et al: Prospective randomized trial of early dietary protein restriction in chronic renal failure. *Lancet* 1984; 2:1291.

67. Ihle BU, Becker GJ, Whitworth JA, et al: The effect of protein restriction on the progression of renal insufficiency. *N Engl J Med* 1989; 321:1773.

68. Klahr S, Buerkert J, Purkerson ML: Role of dietary factors in the progression of chronic renal disease. *Kidney Int* 1983; 24:579.

69. Mitch WE: The influence of the diet on the progression of renal failure. *Annu Rev Med* 1984; 35:249.

70. Lumlertgul G, Burke TJ, Gillum DM, et al: Phosphate depletion arrests progression of chronic renal failure independent of protein intake. *Kidney Int* 1986; 29:658.

71. Mitch WE, Walser M, Steinman TI, et al: The effect of a keto acid amino acid supplement to a restricted diet on the progression of chronic renal failure. *N Engl J Med* 1984; 311:623.

72. Rosman JB, Langer K, Brandl M, et al: Protein-restricted diets in chronic renal failure: A four year follow-up shows limited indications. *Kidney Int* 1989; 36(suppl):96.

73. Bergstrom J, Alvestrand A, Bucht H, et al: Stockholm clinical study on progression of chronic renal failure—an interim report. *Kidney Int* 1989; 36(suppl):110.

74. Brodsky IG, Robbins DC, Hiser E, et al: Effects of low protein diets on protein metabolism in insulin-dependent diabetes mellitus patients with early nephropathy. *J Clin Endocrinol Metab* 1992; 75:351.

75. Alvestrand A, Ahlberg M, Bergstrom J: Retardation of progression of renal insufficiency in patients treated with low protein diets. *Kidney Int* 1983; 24(suppl):268.

76. Alvestrand A, Ahlberg M, Furst P, et al: Clinical experience with amino acid and keto acid diets. *Am J Clin Nutr* 1980; 33:1654.

77. Alvestrand A, Ahlberg M, Furst P, et al: Clinical results of long term treatment with a low protein diet and a new amino acid preparation in patients with chronic uremia. *Clin Nephrol* 1983; 19:67.

78. Gretz N, Korb E, Strauch M: Low protein diet supplemented by keto acids in chronic renal failure: A prospective controlled study. *Kidney Int* 1983; 24(suppl):263.

79. Bergstrom J, Alvestrand A, Bucht H, et al: Stockholm clinical study on progression of chronic renal failure—an interim report. *Kidney Int* 1989; 36(suppl):110.

80. Kampf D, Fischer HC, Kessel M: Efficacy of an unselected protein diet (25 g) with minor oral supply of essential amino acids and keto analogs compared with a selected protein diet (40 g) in chronic renal failure. *Am J Clin Nutr* 1980; 33:1673.

81. Toback FG: Amino acid enhancement of renal regeneration after acute tubular necrosis. *Kidney Int* 1977; 12:193.

82. Toback FG, Teegarden DE, Havener LJ: Amino acid mediated stimulation of renal phospholipid biosynthesis after acute tubular necrosis. *Kidney Int* 1979; 15:542.

83. Milligan S, Luft FC, McMurray S, et al: Intra-abdominal infection and acute renal failure. *Arch Surg* 1978; 113:467.

84. Leonard CD, Luke RG, Siegel RR: Par-

enteral essential amino acids in acute renal failure. *Urology* 1975; 6:154.

85. Kopple JD, Coburn JW: Metabolic studies of low protein diets in uremia: I. Nitrogen and potassium. *Medicine (Baltimore)* 1973; 52:583.

86. Young GA, Parsons FM: The effect of peritoneal dialysis upon the amino acids and other nitrogenous compounds in the blood and dialysates from patients with renal failure. *Clin Sci* 1969; 37:1.

87. Blumenkrantz MJ, Gahl GM, Kopple JD, et al: Protein losses during peritoneal dialysis. *Kidney Int* 1981; 19:593.

88. Giordano C: Use of exogenous and endogenous urea for protein synthesis in normal and uremic subjects. *J Lab Clin Med* 1963; 62:231.

89. Varcoe R, Halliday D, Carson R, et al: Efficiency of utilization of urea nitrogen for albumin synthesis by chronically uremic and normal man. *Clin Sci Mol Med* 1975; 48:379.

90. Wassner SJ, Sanders R, Orloff SH, et al: A comparison of essential and general amino acid infusions in protein-depleted patients receiving parenteral alimentation. *Am J Clin Nutr* 1979; 32:1497.

91. Wilmore DW, Dudrick SJ: Treatment of acute renal failure with intravenous essential L-amino acids. *Arch Surg* 1969; 99:669.

92. Dudrick SJ, Steiger E, Long JM: Renal failure in surgical patients: Treatment with intravenous essential amino acids and hypertonic glucose. *Surgery* 1970; 68:180.

93. Abel R, Abbott W, Fischer J: Intravenous essential L-amino acids and hypertonic dextrose in patients with acute renal failure. *Am J Surg* 1972; 123:632.

94. Wassner SJ, Sanders R, Orloff S, et al: Comparison of essential amino acids and general amino acids for hyperalimentation. *Fed Proc* 1977; 36:1164.

95. Blackburn GL, Etter G, Mackenzie T: Criteria for choosing amino acid therapy in acute renal failure. *Am J Clin Nutr* 1978; 31:1841.

96. Mirtallo JM, Schneider PJ, Mavko K, et al: A comparison of essential and

general amino acid infusions in the nutritional support of patients with compromised renal function. *JPEN* 1982; 6:109.

97. Tempel G, Jelen S, Jekat F: Investigation of protein metabolism with respect to amino acid administration. *JPEN* 1985; 9:725.

98. Naylor CD, Detsky AS, O'Rourke K, et al: Does treatment with essential amino acids and hypertonic glucose improve survival in acute renal failure? A meta-analysis. *Renal Failure* 1987; 10:141.

99. Oken DE, Sprinkel FM, Kirschbaum BB, et al: Amino acid therapy in the treatment of experimental acute renal failure in the rat. *Kidney Int* 1980; 17:14.

100. Pennisi AJ, Wang M, Kopple JD: Effects of protein and amino acid diets in chronically uremic and control rats. *Kidney Int* 1978; 13:472.

101. Ranhotra GS, Johnson BC: Effect of feeding different amino acid diets on growth rate and nitrogen retention of weanling rats. *Proc Soc Exp Biol Med* 1965; 118:1197.

102. Furst P, Stehle P: Are we giving unbalanced amino acid solutions? in Wilmore D, Carpentier Y (eds): *Metabolic Support of the Critically Ill Patient.* Berlin, Springer-Verlag, 1993, in press.

103. Motil KJ, Harmon WE, Grupe WE: Complications of essential amino acid hyperalimentation in children with acute renal failure. *JPEN* 1980; 4:32.

104. Fahey JL: Toxicity and blood ammonia rise resulting from intravenous amino acid administration in man: The protective effect of L-arginine. *J Clin Invest* 1957; 36:1647.

105. Saint-Georges M, Bonnefont DJ, Bourely BA, et al: Correction of selenium deficiency in hemodialyzed patients. *Kidney Int* 1989; 36(suppl):274.

106. Kopple JD: Renal failure and nutrition. Presented at the American Society of Enteral and Parenteral Nutrition, San Diego, 1993.

107. Bihari DJ, Mitchell I, Chang R, et al: Acute renal failure in the intensive care unit—approaches to nutritional support, in Wilmore D, Carpentier Y (eds): *Metabolic Support of the Critically Ill Patient.* Berlin, Springer-Verlag, 1993, in press.

108. Blumenkrantz MJ, Kopple JD, Moran JK, et al: Nitrogen and urea metabolism during continuous ambulatory peritoneal dialysis. *Kidney Int* 1981; 20:78.

109. Blumenkrantz MJ, Gahl GM, Kopple JD, et al: Protein losses during peritoneal dialysis. *Kidney Int* 1981; 19:593.

110. Manji S, Shikora S, McMahon M, et al: Peritoneal dialysis for acute renal failure—overfeeding resulting from dextrose absorbed during dialysis. *Crit Care Med* 1990; 18:29.

111. Bihari DJ, Beale RJ: Renal support in the intensive care unit. *Curr Opin Anesthesiol* 1991; 4:272.

112. Gutierrez A, Alvestrand A, Wahren J, et al: Effect of in vivo contact between blood and dialysis membranes on protein catabolism in humans. *Kidney Int* 1990; 38:487.

113. Feinstein EI: Nutritional hemodialysis. *Kidney Int* 1987; 32(suppl):167.

114. Young GA, Parsons FM: Amino nitrogen loss during hemodialysis: Its dietary significance and replacement. *Clin Sci* 1966; 31:299.

115. Ganda OMP, Aoki TT, Soeldner JS, et al: Hormone-fuel concentrations in anephric subjects. Effect of hemodialysis (with special reference to amino acids). *J Clin Invest* 1976; 57:1403.

116. Borah MF, Schoenfeld PY, Gotch FA, et al: Nitrogen balance during intermittent dialysis therapy of uremia. *Kidney Int* 1978; 14:491.

117. Gutierrez A, Alvestrand A, Weiland I, et al: Blood-membrane interaction without dialysis induces increased protein catabolism in normal man. *Proc E D T A* 1985; 22:223.

118. Mitch WE, Sapir DG: Evaluation of reduced dialysis frequency using nutritional therapy. *Kidney Int* 1981; 20:122.

119. Mault JR, Dechert RE, Bartlett RH, et al: Oxygen consumption during hemodialysis for acute renal failure. *Trans Am Soc Artif Intern Organs* 1982; 28:510.

120. Klahr S, Harris K: Role of dietary lip-

ids and renal eicosanoids on the progression of renal disease. *Kidney Int* 1989; 36(suppl):27.

121. Barcelli UO, Weiss M, Pollak VE: Effects of dietary prostaglandin precursor on the progression of experimentally induced renal failure. *J Lab Clin Med* 1982; 100:786.

122. Hirshberg R, Herrath D, Klaus H, et al: Effect of diets containing varying concentrations of essential fatty acids and triglycerides on renal function in uremic rats and NZB/NZW F1 mice. *Nephron* 1984; 38:233.

123. Scharschmidt LA, Gibbons NB, McGarry L, et al: Effects of dietary fish oil on renal insufficiency in rats with subtotal nephrectomy. *Kidney Int* 1987; 32:700.

124. Prickett JD, Robinson DR, Steinberg AD: Dietary enrichment with polyunsaturated fatty acid eicosapentaenoic acid prevents proteinuria and prolongs survival in NXB × NZW F1 mice. *J Clin Invest* 1981; 68:556.

125. Laouari D, Kleinknecht C, Cournot-Witmer G, et al: Beneficial effect of low phosphorus diet in uremic rats. A reappraisal. *Clin Sci* 1982; 63:539.

126. Berg BN, Simms HS: Nutrition and longevity in the rat. III. Food restriction beyond 800 days. *J Nutr* 1961; 74:23.

127. Nolen GA: Effect of various restricted dietary regimens on the growth, health and longevity of albino rats. *J Nutr* 1972; 102:1477.

128. Farr LE, Smadel JE: The effect of dietary protein in the course of nephrotoxic nephritis in rats. *J Exp Med* 1939; 70:615.

129. Fernandes G, Yunis EJ, Good RA: Influence of diet on survival of mice. *Proc Natl Acad Sci USA* 1976; 73:1279.

130. Friend PS, Fernandes G, Good RA, et al: Dietary restrictions early and late. Effects on the nephropathy of the NZB × NZW mouse. *Lab Invest* 1978; 38:629.

131. Neugarten J, Feiner HD, Schacht RG, et al: Amelioration of experimental glomerulonephritis by protein restriction. *Kidney Int* 1983; 24:595.

37

Cardiac Surgery

Loren F. Hiratzka, M.D.

Karl S. Ulicny, Jr., M.D.

Nutrition and cardiac physiology

Malnutrition and cardiac surgery

Nutritional repletion

Patients currently undergoing cardiac surgery are generally older and have more associated operative risk factors than in the past. Often these patients have lengthy hospitalizations preoperatively for diagnostic and therapeutic interventions and come to the operation acutely or chronically malnourished.[1, 2] The myocardium is not spared in malnourished states.[3] Furthermore, severe cardiac dysfunction results in worsening nutrition. Thus, as these patients undergo more complex and higher-risk cardiac surgical procedures, clinicians must better understand the importance of nutrition in this setting.

NUTRITION AND CARDIAC PHYSIOLOGY

Prolonged heart failure can lead to a specific form of protein and calorie malnutrition, cardiac cachexia. It can be seen in older patients with long-standing valvular heart disease or in patients with end-stage cardiomyopathy

who are awaiting heart transplantation. The pathogenesis of cardiac cachexia was described by Pittman and Cohen[4] as being secondary to congestive heart failure in conjunction with tissue hypoxia, anorexia, and hypermetabolism with resultant wasting of muscle protein and adipose tissue. Excessive protein requirements have been demonstrated in such patients.[5]

Anorexia may be aggravated by dietary restrictions of salt and fat as well as the administration of medications, many of which adversely affect the appetite. Cachexia may lead to gastrointestinal hypomotility, decreased gastric capacity, and further anorexia.[5] Splanchnic congestion may lead to malabsorption and protein-losing enteropathy.[1] Dyspnea related to heart failure can increase oxygen consumption, particularly of the respiratory musculature.[6] Thus, energy supply may be reduced and demand increased.

Voit[7] in 1866 found that the heart of starved felines was only slightly smaller than the heart of normal animals. He concluded that the heart was "spared" the effects of malnutrition. More recently, autopsy data suggest that myocardial mass reduction is proportionate to total-body mass reduction.[3] Myocardial atrophy has been described in patients with cardiac cachexia,[3] anorexia nervosa,[8] low-energy diets,[9] and kwashiorkor.[3, 10] Keys et al.[3] showed that after 6 months of a low-energy, low-protein diet with a loss of 25% of body weight, roentgenographic dimensions of the heart were markedly decreased and the calculated decrease in cardiac volume was 70% of the loss of body weight. Structurally, myocardial atrophy is associated with vacuolization as well as a decrease in size and sometimes fragmentation of myofibrils.[11] Kuykendall et al.[12] showed that protein depletion produced a reduction in total cardiac mass with decreased nitrogen and glycogen contents and increased fat content. Protein repletion restored normal cardiac mass but not liver mass.

Decreased myocardial mass in malnourished states is associated with decreased mechanical properties of the heart. Information is conflicting with regard to changes in cardiac output and stroke volume. The stroke volume index and cardiac index usually remain the same or slightly increase due to a decrease in overall body mass.[11, 13, 14] However, a decrease in cardiac index has also been described.[15] In an animal model, protein malnutrition appeared to decrease both left ventricular stroke work and stroke volume when left atrial pressures exceeded 10 cm H_2O.[16] Further increases in left atrial pressure in excess of 25 cm H_2O resulted in a reduction in cardiac output and aortic blood flow. The protein-depleted group was unable to match the increases in heart rate seen in the control group at high left atrial pressures.[16] Protein and calorie malnutrition can lead to both structural and functional myocardial impairment.[15-17] Contractility is also reduced by electrolyte deficiencies.[18] Fa-

tal myocardial dysfunction has been ascribed to selenium deficiency after long-term parenteral nutrition.[19] Thus, severe malnutrition leads not only to decreased baseline performance but also to the inability of the heart to respond to increased metabolic demands.

In response to these changes, a variety of compensatory mechanisms occur.[1] Blood pressure, heart rate, blood volume, and oxygen demand decrease in malnourished states.[3, 10, 13] Plasma catecholamine levels are affected by fat and carbohydrate consumption,[20] and a hypoadrenergic state in the fasting individual results in bradycardia.[3, 21] Low catecholamine levels and decreased activity of the renin-angiotensin-aldosterone axis can result in decreased blood pressure due to loss of sodium and vasodilatation.[3, 21] An impairment of deiodination of thyroxine to triiodothyronine leads to further decreases in the metabolic rate and cardiac work.[14]

The association of malnutrition and cardiac dysrhythmias has also been noted. Investigation of sudden deaths reported among patients following a strict low-calorie "liquid protein" diet concluded that electrolyte or mineral deficiencies might have been the cause of the dysrhythmias.[22] Another study in such patients noted electrocardiographic abnormalities, including ventricular tachycardia and prolongation of the QT interval prior to death.[9] Autopsy examination showed myocardial atrophy with myofibril attenuation and excessive lipofucsin production.[9]

MALNUTRITION AND CARDIAC SURGERY

Malnutrition has been demonstrated to be a significant risk factor for patients undergoing major surgical procedures. Morbidity and mortality are greater in cachectic patients than in normally nourished patients undergoing similar operative procedures.[5, 15, 23-25] Abel et al.[26] reported a 16% mortality rate for 44 malnourished patients undergoing cardiac surgery as compared with no mortality for matched well-nourished patients. Morbidity, including respiratory failure, pneumonia, renal failure, and sternal wound complications, was more frequent in malnourished patients. Herreros et al.[15] in a retrospective review found malnutrition in 28% of 60 patients undergoing cardiac valve surgery. In the malnourished patients, postoperative complications including sternal infection, ventricular arrhythmias, or pulmonary infection that prolonged the hospital stay developed in 58%, while such complications occurred in only 6% of the well-nourished patients.

A variety of immune defects are seen with protein and protein-calorie deficiencies in both experimental animals and patients. These include low levels of individual complement components, impaired opsonic and neutrophil function, impaired delayed hypersensitivity, decreased lymphoid mass and function, and an associated increased susceptibility to infection.[21] Delayed-hypersensitivity testing has been used as a marker for cell-mediated immunity. Anergic responses to a standard battery of recall antigens have been associated with greater morbidity,[27, 28] sepsis,[29] and mortality[30] in postoperative and posttrauma patients and have been proposed as a method to identify which patients are at risk for increased morbidity and mortality.[31] Prospective studies by Abel et al.[27] and Ulicny et al.[32] have not, however, demonstrated the usefulness of delayed hypersensitivity testing to predict the occurrence of sternal wound infection or other postoperative infective complications in cardiac surgical patients.

NUTRITIONAL REPLETION

Nutritional repletion has been successful in reversing some chemical and cellular abnormalities associated with malnutrition. Spanier et al.[33] showed that reconstitution of total-body cellular mass by total parenteral nutrition is followed by a return of the normal delayed-hypersensitivity response. Forse et al.[34] demonstrated a 43% conversion from anergy to a normal delayed-hypersensitivity response after 2 weeks of total parenteral nutrition.

Improved nutrition can reverse starvation-induced myocardial atrophy.[3, 13] Heymsfield et al.[13] noted, in five chronically malnourished patients following nutritional repletion, a 12% total-body weight gain associated with a 59% increase in diastolic volume (by echocardiography), a 31% increase in left ventricular mass, and a 90% increase in cardiac output. Reactivation of the renin-angiotensin-aldosterone system and release of catecholamines led to increases in plasma volume and blood pressure.[20] Nutritional repletion also reversed starvation-associated natriuresis.[35]

Although nutritional repletion reverses many abnormalities related to starvation and in some patients reduces heart failure, hypermetabolism and increased plasma volume with subsequent heart failure have also been described.[1, 36, 37] Enteral nutritional supplementation appears to have a lower risk for subsequent heart failure.[38]

Whether nutritional repletion can have a beneficial impact on malnourished cardiac surgical patients is not clear. Abel et al.[24] did not demonstrate any improvement after a 5-day postoperative course of parenteral nutrition. In an early clinical study, Gibbons et al.[25] suggested that a minimum of 3 weeks of preoperative nutritional repletion would be required to reverse severe malnutrition.

Malnutrition has detrimental effects on myocardial mass and function. The immune defects seen with protein-calorie malnutrition are associated with increased morbidity and mortality following surgery and trauma. Nutritional repletion can reverse myocardial abnormalities as well as immune defects, but the role of nutritional repletion in preoperative and postoperative cardiac surgical patients is not clear.

REFERENCES

1. Webb JG, Kiess MC, Chan Yan CC: Malnutrition and the heart. *Can Med Assoc J* 1986; 135:753–758.
2. Weinsier RL, Hunker EM, Krumdieck CL, et al: Hospital malnutrition: A prospective evaluation of general medical patients during the course of hospitalization. *Am J Clin Nutr* 1979; 32:418–426.
3. Circulation and cardiac function, in Keys A, Brosek J, Henschel A, et al (eds): *The Biology of Human Starvation*. Minneapolis, University of Minnesota, 1950, pp 607–634.
4. Pittman JG, Cohen P: The pathogenesis of cardiac cachexia. *N Engl J Med* 1964; 271:403–409.
5. Blackburn GL, Gibbons GW, Bothe A, et al: Nutritional support in cardiac cachexia. *J Thorac Cardiovasc Surg* 1977; 73:489–496.
6. Field S, Kelly SM, Macklem PT: The oxygen cost of breathing in patients with cardiorespiratory disease. *Am Rev Respir Dis* 1982; 126:9–13.
7. Voit C: Ueber die Verschiedenbeiten der Eiwesszersetzung beim Hungern. *Z Biol* 1866; 2:309–365.
8. Isner JM, Roberts WC, Heymsfield SB, et al: Anorexia nervosa and sudden death. *Ann Intern Med* 1985; 102:49–52.
9. Isner JM, Sours HE, Paris AL, et al: Sudden, unexpected death in avid dieters using the liquid-protein-modified-fast diet: Observations in 17 patients and the role of the prolonged QT interval. *Circulation* 1979; 60:1401–1412.
10. Bloom WL, Azar G, Smith EG Jr: Changes in heart size and plasma volume during fasting. *Metabolism* 1966; 15:409–413.
11. Abel RM, Paul J: Failure of short-term nutritional convalescence to reverse the adverse hemodynamic effects of

12. Kuykendall RC, Rowlands BJ, Taegtmeyer H, et al: Biochemical consequences of protein depletion in the rabbit heart. *J Surg Res* 1987; 43:62–67.
13. Heymsfield SB, Bethel BA, Ansley JD, et al: Cardiac abnormalities in cachectic patients before and during nutritional repletion. *Am Heart J* 1978; 95:584–594.
14. Heymsfield SB, Head CA, McManus CB III, et al: Respiratory, cardiovascular, and metabolic effects of enteral hyperalimentation: Influence of formula dose and composition. *Am J Clin Nutr* 1984; 40:116–130.
15. Herreros J, De Oca J, Sanchez R, et al: Etat nutritionnel et immunologique des patients operes de chirurgie cardiaque valvularie. *J Chir (Paris)* 1985; 122:707–710.
16. Kyger ER, Block WJ, Roach G, et al: Adverse effects of protein malnutrition on myocardial function. *Surgery* 1978; 84:147–156.
17. Abel RM, Grimes JB, Alonso D, et al: Adverse hemodynamic and ultrastructural changes in dog hearts subjected to protein-caloric malnutrition. *Am Heart J* 1979; 97:733–744.
18. Frustaci A, Penniestri F, Scoppetta C: Myocardial damage due to hypokalemia and hypophosphatemia. *Postgrad Med J* 1984; 60:679–681.
19. Quercia RA, Korn S, O'Neill D, et al: Selenium deficiency and fatal cardiomyopathy in a patient receiving long-term home parenteral nutrition. *Clin Pharm* 1984; 3:531–535.
20. Landsberg L, Young JB: The role of the sympathetic nervous system and catecholamines in the regulation of energy metabolism. *Am J Clin Nutr* 1983; 38:1018–1024.
21. Sowers JR, Nyby M, Stern N, et al: Blood pressure and hormone changes associated with weight reduction in the obese. *Hypertension* 1982; 4:686–691.
22. Frank A, Graham C, Frank S: Fatalities on the liquid-protein diet: An analysis of possible causes. *Int J Obes* 1981; 5:243–248.
23. Mullen JL, Buzby GP, Matthews DC, et al: Reduction of operative morbidity and mortality by combined preopera-

tive and postoperative nutritional support. *Ann Surg* 1980; 192:604–613.

24. Abel RM, Fischer JE, Buckley MJ, et al: Malnutrition in cardiac surgical patients: Results of a prospective randomized evaluation of early postoperative parenteral nutrition. *Arch Surg* 1975; 111:45–50.

25. Gibbons GW, Blackburn GL, Harken DE, et al: Pre and postoperative hyperalimentation in the treatment of cardiac cachexia. *J Surg Res* 1975; 19:439–444.

26. Abel RM, Fischer JE, Buckley MJ, et al: Hyperalimentation in cardiac surgery: A review of 64 patients. *J Thorac Cardiovasc Surg* 1974; 67:294–300.

27. Abel RM, Fisch D, Horowitz J, et al: Should nutritional status be assessed routinely prior to cardiac operation? *J Thorac Cardiovasc Surg* 1983; 85:752–757.

28. Meakins JL, Pietsch JB, Bubenick O, et al: Delayed hypersensitivity: Indicator of acquired failure of host defenses in sepsis and trauma. *Ann Surg* 1977; 186:241–250.

29. Cainzos M, Potel J, Puente JL: Anergy in patients with biliary lithiasis. *Br J Surg* 1989; 76:169–172.

30. MacLean LD, Meakins JL, Taguchi K, et al: Host resistance in sepsis and trauma. *Ann Surg* 1975; 182:207–217.

31. Meakins JL, Christou NV, Shezgal HM, et al: Therapeutic approaches to anergy in surgical patients. *Ann Surg* 1979; 190:286–296.

32. Ulicny KS, Hiratzka LF, Williams RB, et al: Sternotomy infection: Poor prediction by acute phase response and delayed hypersensitivity. *Ann Thorac Surg* 1990; 50:949–958.

33. Spanier AH, Pitesch JB, Meakins JL, et al: The relationship between immune competence and nutrition. *Surg Forum* 1976; 27:332–336.

34. Forse RA, Christou N, Meakins JL, et al: Reliability of skin testing as a measure of nutritional state. *Arch Surg* 1981; 116:1284–1288.

35. Wright HK, Gann DS, Albertsen K: Effect of glucose on sodium excretion and renal concentrating ability after starvation in man. *Metabolism* 1963; 12:804–811.

36. Wharton BA, Howells GR, McCance RA: Cardiac failure in kwashiorkor. *Lancet* 1967; 2:384–387.

37. Edozien JC, Rahim Khan MA: Anaemia in protein malnutrition. *Clin Sci* 1986; 34:315–326.

38. Bougle D, Iselin M, Kahyat A, et al: Nutritional treatment of congenital heart disease. *Arch Dis Child* 1986; 61:799–801.

38

Neurosurgery

Linda Ott, M.S.

Byron Young, M.D.

Global viewpoint

Head injury

  Hypermetabolism

  Hypercatabolism

  The acute-phase response

  Hyperglycemia/hypoglycemia

  Immunology

  Altered gastric function

Spinal cord injury

  Decreased energy expenditure

  Increased urinary nitrogen loss

  Hypoalbuminemia

  Altered mineral levels

Cellular approach

Nutrient modification

  Humans

  Animals

Pharmacologic intervention

  Humans

  Animals

Physiologic intervention

  Animals

Growth factors

  Animals

  Humans

Provision of nutrition

Following neurologic insult, a cascade of events occurs in both the brain and the systemic circulation; these events can have deleterious effects that lessen the individual's chances for survival.[1, 2] Advances in medical management such as control of intracranial pressure, swift patient transport, traction, and intensive care unit (ICU) treatment have improved the outcome of these patients.[3, 4] Biochemical and physiologic events still ensue and can adversely affect outcome by causing secondary injury to the neurologic system and/or initiating systemic events (e.g., compromised immune status, increased vascular permeability) that can increase morbidity and mortality (Fig 38–1).

Over 100,000 individuals sustain central nervous system (CNS) trauma in the United States each year.[5] Approximately half of those individuals eventually die, and half of the survivors are left permanently disabled.[2, 6] The emotional and monetary costs of these injuries are difficult to estimate; many of the victims are healthy young males. It is estimated that the monetary loss is approximately

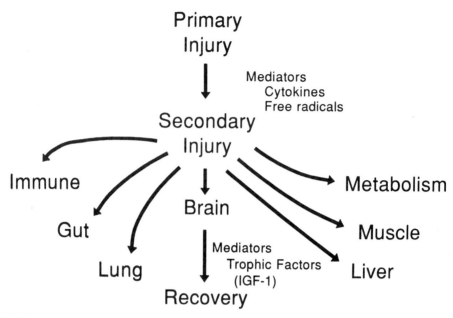

FIG 38–1.
Biochemical and physiologic events ensue that can adversely affect the outcome by causing secondary injury to the neurologic system and/or initiating systemic events. *IGF-1* = insulin-like growth factor 1.

15 to 30 billion dollars each year.[7] Thus, determining ways to improve the outcome of these patients and reintegrate them into society is very important. Study and manipulation of the metabolic events that follow these injuries may be an important way to improve the outcome of these patients.

Basic studies have determined that neurons can regain function.[8] Thus, if the patient can be maintained in a physiologic state that provides an optimal environment for survival and repair of the damaged neuron, the outcome from neurologic injury could be further improved.

Work is currently being directed toward decreasing the secondary effects of injury. Articles describing the use of nutrient modification, pharmacologic agents, growth factors, and physiologic modification have been published in the neurologic field in the past few years. In the past, lack of an adequate animal model has hindered progress in these fields. Such models are being improved, and work toward finding the optimal mode of improving the outcome from this injury is forthcoming.

This chapter will delineate the current global viewpoint of metabolic management of these patients and will describe the work that has been done in manipulating the secondary metabolic events that occur after CNS injury.

GLOBAL VIEWPOINT

Head Injury

In addition to brain injury, the patient with head injury suffers a prominent systemic metabolic response to stress. After brain injury, catabolic hormones and cytokine levels increase.[9–12] Clifton et al. found that patients with head injury alone have norepinephrine levels as high as seven times normal.[13] Chiolero et al. found that isolated head injury induces a full response in the secretion of the counterregulatory hormones, including serum glucagon, insulin, cortisol, and urinary adrenaline and noradrenaline.[14] Goodman et al. found significantly elevated tumor necrosis factor (TNF) levels in the serum of head-injured patients during the first week postinjury.[15] We observed increases in plasma and ventricular interleukin-1, interleukin-6, and interleukin-8 levels in head-injured patients.[10, 11] Hypothalamic-pituitary axis regulation is altered following brain injury. There are alterations in feedback mechanisms, excesses in catabolic hormones, and deficiencies in follicle-stimulating hormone, luteinizing hormone, and growth hormone.[16, 17] The metabolic response to head injury is speculated to be induced in part by this systemic and central surge of metabolites. This response is characterized by hypermetabolism, hypercatabolism, the acute-phase response, hyperglycemia, depressed immunocompetence, altered vascular permeability, and altered gastrointestinal function.[18–25] The effects or specific purposes of these responses for the patient with head injury are unclear, but investigators have attempted to determine the causative agents and block the response.

Hypermetabolism

Energy expenditure following head injury has been extensively studied.[26–38] It is generally agreed that patients with severe head injury have increased oxygen consumption postinjury. There is an average increase in the metabolic rate of 40% above that calculated for an uninjured person of equal sex, age, and size.[19] Investigators disagree as to how long this metabolic rate stays elevated. Haider et al. suggest that the metabolic rate stays elevated in some patients for approximately 1 year postinjury.[31] Deutchman et al. suggest that the increase in metabolic rate lasts for only 5 to 7 days postinjury and that prolonged elevations are due to the administration of steroids, infection, the thermic effect of nutrient administration, or patient activity.[27, 28] This debate has not been settled; however, investigators agree that this increase in metabolic rate is a negative effect and that slowing or decreasing the rate would be beneficial to patient outcome.

Toward this end, Dempsey et al.

showed that head-injured patients in barbiturate coma have energy expenditure levels that are much lower than that of head-injured patients not in coma.[36] Chiolero et al. showed that propranolol administration (100 µg/kg) produces a decrease in the metabolic rate (and heart rate) accounting for 25% of the hypermetabolism.[39] This latter study was performed 3 to 12 days following injury in head-injured patients no longer requiring mechanical ventilation. Robertson et al. correlated the severity of head injury (Glasgow Coma Scale [GCS]), temperature, catecholamine levels, resting muscle tone, spontaneous muscle activity, and drugs such as barbiturates and musculoskeletal blocking agents with the metabolic rate.[19] Bucci et al. found that an increased metabolic rate was related to increased intracranial pressure.[40] Clifton et al. reported that the severity of head injury and days postinjury were the most potent predictive factors for estimating the degree of elevation in the metabolic rate after head injury.[41] They also found that patients with head injury continued to have increased energy expenditure despite paralysis, which suggests that muscle tone alone could not fully explain hypermetabolism. Although certain investigators have suggested that steroid administration, infection, and nutrient intake contribute to an increased metabolic rate, studies that have specifically studied these variables have found that they have no significant impact on the metabolic rate.[19, 29, 42–44] The current medical therapy for an increased metabolic rate is to increase the nutrient intake to achieve caloric balance. Despite increased calorie and protein administration and achievement of caloric balance, however, a negative nitrogen balance and weight loss persist in this population.

Hypercatabolism

Increased urinary nitrogen loss occurs in patients with severe head injury.* The cause of this increased nitrogen loss is greatly debated. Urinary nitrogen excretion in critically ill patients has been used as an indicator of increased protein turnover. Investigators suggest that nitrogen loss in head-injured patients is secondary to immobilization, steroid administration, and nutrient intake.[27, 28] Four separate investigators have found that fasting urinary nitrogen excretion is higher in head-injured patients treated with steroids as compared with those who are not.[4, 30, 31, 42] When patients were fed, the difference disappeared. On the other hand, Zagara et al. found (in a prospective, randomized trial) no difference in weight, blood glucose, albumin, creatinine, and urinary urea nitrogen loss in 12 head-injured patients who received steroids vs. 12 who did not.[50]

Complete immobilization with casts increases urinary nitrogen excretion in healthy young men after a period of 5 to 6 days.[51] Thus, the immediate increase in urinary nitrogen in head-injured patients cannot be explained by immobilization. A paralyzed or flaccid patient could fit into the immobilization theory; however, other patients might not. In addition, Fried et al. found that barbiturates (which cause immobility) improved nitrogen balance in head-injured patients.[52] Clifton et al. found that the level of calorie and protein intake influences nitrogen excretion. At 140% above predicted energy expenditure, 50% of the administered nitrogen is excreted.[41]

Positive nitrogen balance is difficult to achieve in head-injured patients for the first 2 weeks postinjury. As early as 1959, McLaurin et al. suggested that these patients have decreased nitrogen efficiency.[53] Increased nitrogen output occurs despite adequate nitrogen intake. Urinary nitrogen loss following head injury can be increased by steroid administration, immobility, and nutrient intake. Increased nitrogen excretion

*References 1–4, 6–9, 14, 15, 17–19, 22, 24, 41, 42, and 45–49.

occurs, however, even without these confounding variables. This increase is secondary to muscle loss and increased protein turnover. The current method of decreasing nitrogen loss in these patients is to increase nitrogen intake. Negative nitrogen balance can be improved, but a positive nitrogen balance is not achieved during the first 2 weeks following head injury despite increasing input of nitrogen.

The Acute-Phase Response

The acute-phase response is a common phenomenon following head injury and is identified by fever without evidence of infection, increased levels of positive acute-phase proteins, decreased levels of negative acute-phase proteins, hypozincemia, hyperzincuria, and hypoferremia. This response has been attributed to increased levels of interleukin-1 and interleukin-6.[10, 11, 54] Interleukin-6 causes a dose- and time-dependent increase in the synthesis of serum α_2-macroglobulin, fibrinogen, cysteine proteinase inhibitor, C-reactive protein, and α_1-acid glycoprotein and a decrease in albumin.[54] Some of these responses are probably favorable for host survival, while others may be detrimental. Hypozincemia and hyperzincuria may indicate an increased requirement for zinc. In a prospective, randomized trial, we found that zinc supplementation increased visceral protein levels and improved the GCS score.[22, 55]

Albumin depression is detrimental since albumin is important in a number of processes, including maintenance of oncotic pressure, drug transport, and tolerance of enteral feedings.[23] Hypoalbuminemia is probably mediated by cytokine elevation. Intravenous injection of recombinant TNF into normal rabbits causes a dose-dependent depression of serum albumin levels.[23, 56] In vitro exposure to murine interleukin-1 and TNF increases endothelial permeability to albumin and causes a time- and dose-dependent albumin leakage.[23] Interleukin-1 and interleukin-6 decrease the synthesis of mRNA for albumin. Thus, albumin depression probably occurs because of increased vascular permeability and decreased synthesis. The current therapy for hypoalbuminemia is to increase nutrient administration and give exogenous albumin. Albumin supplementation has not been investigated in patients with severe head injury. In other critically ill patients, despite an increase in the serum albumin level secondary to albumin supplementation, Foley et al. found no difference in the complication rate, duration of hospital and ICU stay, mechanical ventilation, or tolerance of enteral feeding.[57] Brown et al. found that albumin supplementation in critically ill patients caused a twofold reduction in complication rates, and Ford et al. found that albumin supplementation improved enteral feeding tolerance in pediatric patients.[58, 59]

Other acute-phase response reactants may play important roles in host function.[25] α_1-Antitrypsin and α_2-macroglobulin may be required because they are proteinase inhibitors of leukocytes and lysosomes released from destroyed cells. Fibrinogen may be necessary for the formation of blood coagulation products at the wound site. C-reactive protein may play a role in immune status. Some proteins such as α_1-acid glycoprotein decrease interleukin-1 activity in vivo, thus suggesting that they play a regulatory role in the stress response.[60] Current medical therapy is aimed at replacing substrate deficiencies (e.g., albumin depression, zinc depression) in an effort to maintain host function.

Hyperglycemia/Hypoglycemia

Hyperglycemia is common following head injury in both animal and human studies.[61–63] In head injury with ischemia, hyperglycemia may worsen the outcome by causing secondary damage to ischemic cells.[64] The mechanisms for this damage are unclear, but investigators suggest that lactate accumulation

and acidosis may play a role.[65, 66] In animal studies, hyperglycemia before and during ischemic head injury is correlated with cell damage and death.[64] Clinical studies of head-injured and stroke patients have established a relationship between outcome and the level of hyperglycemia. However, a prospective, randomized, controlled trial in which hyperglycemia is treated or untreated has not been done.[61, 62] Robertson et al. randomly assigned 21 patients with severe head injury to alimentation with or without glucose.[67] There were no differences in blood or cerebrospinal fluid glucose concentrations in the two groups, but ketone bodies (i.e., β-hydroxybutyrate and acetoacetate) were used more extensively by the brain in the saline group. The cerebrospinal fluid lactate concentration was lower in the patients treated with saline. Since hyperglycemia occurs as part of the stress response, it is not surprising that withholding a small amount of glucose (5%) does not affect the serum glucose level. Of interest is the speculation that glucose administration may affect cerebral metabolism of glucose, ketones, and lactate. Current therapy for hyperglycemia in head-injured patients consists of insulin administration when the glucose level is elevated above 200 mg/dL. In most cases, insulin effectively decreases blood glucose levels. The effect of insulin on cerebral metabolism is unknown. Its effects should become known in the next few years as more investigators measure the cerebral metabolic rate of oxygen and lactate in patients with head injury.

Severe hypoglycemia also has negative effects on the CNS. In animal and human studies, hypoglycemia may evoke a stress response and may alter cerebral blood flow and metabolism.[68] Thus, both hypoglycemia and hyperglycemia may produce neurologic changes.

Immunology

Approximately 60% of severely head-injured patients become infected, with

35% of late deaths attributed to infection.[69, 70] Rapp et al., Imhoff et al., Quattrocchi et al., and Miller et al. found a high incidence (almost 100%) of anergy in these patients.[71–74] Imhoff et al. found that the anergy rate was related to the severity of injury.[72] Miller et al. found that lymphocyte activation and interleukin-2 receptor production were suppressed after head injury.[73] Quattrocchi et al. found that interferon-γ production (another necessary component of cell-mediated immunity) was also depressed in these patients.[75] This same group found that lymphocyte-blastogenesis, T-cell expression, helper T-cell expression, interleukin-2 production, and interferon-γ production were significantly depressed in head-injured patients. They found no significant decrease in immunoglobulin and complement levels. Hoyt et al. found a reduction in the proliferative response of T cells to mitogen stimulation in 27 patients with severe head injury.[76] The B-cell response was unaffected. They also found a diminished expression of early activation antigens (interleukin-2 receptor and transferrin receptor) and late antigen (HLA-DR). In 20 patients with severe head injury, Maerker et al. found no decrease in IgG, IgA, IgM, and the complement factors.[77] The cause of the depression in immune function is speculated to result from a nutrient, mineral, or cytokine deficit. Miller et al. found that lymphokine-activated killer T-cell cytotoxicity following incubation with interleukin-2 was diminished.[73] Cellular dysfunction of suppressor cells may also be involved in immune depression. The current medical therapy for depressed immune function after head injury involves provision of optimal nutrients. The above studies do not delineate the quantity or types of nutrients that are deficient. Whether nutrient therapy improves immune status remains unproved.

Altered Gastric Function

Gastric function has long been thought to be depressed following head injury.[78] In 12 patients with severe head injury, gastric emptying was found to be prolonged. There was an altered biphasic response, similar to that often found in patients who undergo pyloroplasty or vagotomy.[79] This alteration in gastric function is correlated with the inability to tolerate gastric enteral feedings. The cause of the altered gastric function is unknown. Increased intracranial pressure, head injury, opioids, corticotropin-releasing factor, and cytokines have all been speculated to play a role. The current medical therapy for altered gastric function is to bypass the stomach and feed into the small intestine.[80] The function of the small intestine following head injury is unknown.

Spinal Cord Injury

The metabolic response to spinal cord injury has not been studied in as much detail as head injury. The hormonal and cytokine response to spinal cord injury has not been well elucidated. Some of the metabolic changes observed in this patient population include negative nitrogen balance, hypoalbuminemia, mineral alterations, and decreased energy expenditure.

Decreased Energy Expenditure

The metabolic rate in spinal cord–injured patients is widely variable; however, several studies have found the metabolic rates to be lower than those predicted for a person of equal size, sex, and age without injury.[81–84] Kolpek et al. found that metabolic rates average 94% of those predicted by the Harris-Benedict equation.[82] The higher the lesion, the lower the energy expenditure measurement. Since these patients do have lower-than-predicted energy expenditure, it is easy to overfeed them. Indirect calorimetry and measurement of energy expenditure are ideal; however, Cox and coworkers found that quadriplegics require approximately 23 kcal/kg and paraplegics require 28 kcal/kg/day.[83] In spite of low energy expenditure rates, these patients progressively lose weight after injury. It is speculated that this weight loss is secondary to muscle loss and body composition changes.

Increased Urinary Nitrogen Loss

Increased urinary nitrogen loss is observed after spinal cord injury.[81, 82, 85, 86] Kaufman et al. found urinary nitrogen excretions of 15 to 27 g/day in spite of negligible nitrogen intake.[85] Rodriguez et al. found that a positive nitrogen balance is not possible in spinal cord–injured patients during the first 7 weeks after injury.[86] In these patients, increased urinary nitrogen loss is speculated to occur secondary to muscle atrophy. The current medical therapy for increased nitrogen loss in these patients is to provide nutrients and physical therapy. Weight loss and muscle atrophy continue to occur despite these efforts.

Hypoalbuminemia

Hypoalbuminemia is often found during the acute period of spinal cord injury.[87, 88] Ring et al. suggest that the half-life of albumin decreases in these patients secondary to increased elimination of albumin.[89] It is also possible that increased vascular permeability may be causing the depression in albumin levels. The current medical therapy is to treat hypoalbuminemia with nutrient intake, possibly with exogenous albumin supplementation. Whether this method increases albumin levels in these patients is unclear.

Altered Mineral Levels

Hypercalcemia, hypercalciuria, and hyponatremia may occur in the acute period of spinal cord injury.[81, 90–92] Hypercalcemia occurs in approximately 5% of patients.[90] Mobilization is most effective at controlling hypercalcemia. Other methods include the administration of steroids, furosemide, calcitonin, mithramycin, and bisphosphanate.[81, 93–97] Hypercalciuria increases over the first 4 weeks after injury. Calcium balance is negative in all bones during this period.

The long-term effects of these calcium changes include osteoporosis, fractures, and nephrolithiasis.[91–93] During the chronic period, osteoporosis is present below the level of injury in 88% of patients.[98] There are metabolic changes that make supplementation of calcium ineffective. These include a decrease in gastrointestinal calcium absorption, low levels of vitamin D, and high levels of parathyroid hormone and calcitonin. The best method of managing these problems is unclear. Hyponatremia occurs secondary to difficulties with free water excretion (elevated antidiuretic hormone [ADH] levels) during the acute period.[99] Fluid restriction is the current method of medical management.

CELLULAR APPROACH

After brain and spinal cord injury, a number of changes occur in both the systemic circulation and the nervous system. Many of the systemic changes have been discussed above. Some of the changes that occur in the nervous system include increased lipid peroxidation, intracellular calcium influx, lactate accumulation, increased potassium release, excitatory amino acid excess, neu-

TABLE 38–1.

Mediators of Neural Secondary Injury

Alterations
  Lipid peroxidation
  Cell calcium influx
  Cell potassium release
  Lactate accumulation/acidosis
  Cellular swelling
  Excitatory amino acid excess
  Neurotransmitter release
  Increase in catabolic hormones
  Increase in cytokine levels
  Ionic destabilization
  Prostaglandin synthesis
  Decreased immune status
  Increased systemic metabolic requirements
  Opioid release
Deficiencies
  Trophic factors
  Anabolic hormones
  Intracellular magnesium
  Intracellular zinc

TABLE 38–2.

Methods Used to Improve Neurologic Outcome After Brain and Spinal Cord Injury

Nutritional
  Provision of adequate nutrients
  Enrichment of amino acid solutions with branched-chain
    amino acids
  Zinc supplementation
  Withholding of glucose
  Vitamin E supplementation
  Ascorbic acid supplementation
  Magnesium supplementation
Growth factors
  Insulin-like growth factor I
  Nerve growth factor
  Fibroblast growth factor
  Growth hormone
Physiologic
  Administration of norepinephrine
  Hypothermia
  Thyrotropin-releasing hormone (opioid antagonist)
Pharmacologic agents
  Opioid antagonists (naloxone, naimefene, Win 44,
    441-3)
  Catecholamine blockers (p-chlorophenolalanine,
    amphetamine, serotonin blockade)
  Lipid peroxidation (glucocorticoids, methlyprednisolone,
    indomethacin, superoxide dismutase and catalase,
    lazeroids, dimethyl sulfoxide)
  Bradykinin antagonists (aprototin)
  Calcium channel blockers (cobalt, flunarizine)
  Excitatory amino acid blockers (kynurenic acid,
    phencyclidine, scopolamine, NMDA
    (N-methyl-D-aspartate) antagonists, baclofen)
  Receptor antagonists of neurotransmitter release
    (serotonin blockers, scopolamine, dicyclomine, A-4,
    A-5)
  Anion transport inhibitors (L-644.711, ethacrynic acid)
  Monosialic gangliosides
  Inhibitors of arachidonic metabolism (cyclooxygenase)
  Systemic metabolic blockers (propranolol, barbiturates,
    tromethamine)

rotransmitter excess, opioid release, ionic destabilization, and prostaglandin synthesis (Table 38–1). There is also a deficiency of trophic factors, anabolic hormones, and intracellular magnesium after neural injury. These metabolic instabilities have been linked to nerve cell damage and death, hypotension, poor brain perfusion, increased blood-brain barrier damage, depressed brain metabolism, membrane instability, depressed synthesis of DNA, RNA, and protein, increased inflammation and edema, and increased vascular permeability. During the past 10 years, a

host of studies have attempted to define ways to correct the metabolic derangements. These will be discussed in the following section and categorized by nutrient modification, physiologic intervention, pharmacologic intervention, and growth factor administration (Table 38–2).

Nutrient Modification

Humans

Six trials have studied the effect of nutrient administration on the outcome of patients with severe head injury. The study by Rapp et al. in 1983 prospectively randomized patients with severe head injury to receive parenteral or enteral nutrition.[71] Intolerance to gastric feedings rendered the enteral group a semistarved group. Mortality in the enteral group was significantly higher than in the parenteral group. The authors attributed this increased mortality rate to a lack of adequate feedings in the enteral group. In a later prospective, randomized, controlled trial, the same authors attempted to reproduce these study results.[100] Improved nutrient delivery was observed in the enteral group. The parenteral group had a more rapid improvement in neurologic outcome. Hadley et al. also randomized patients with head injury to receive parenteral and enteral nutrition.[101] An improved protein balance was observed in the parenteral group. No difference was observed in caloric intake, morbidity, or mortality between groups. Kaufman et al., in a retrospective analysis, found no relationship between nutrient intake and patient outcome.[102] Waters et al. and Balzola et al. found better neurologic outcome in head-injured patients provided with higher nutrient intake.[103, 104] It seems that nutrient intake may affect neurologic outcome after severe head injury. The mechanisms whereby this occurs are not known. Nutrient supplementation may provide substrates that are essential for immune system function, cellular membrane integrity, cellular repair, neural reorganization, and other restorative functions necessary for host survival.

High protein intake has been compared in a prospective, randomized fashion in two head injury trials. Clifton et al. and Twyman et al. found that high protein intake improved nitrogen balance in these patients.[105, 106] Whether high protein administration has an effect on morbidity and mortality is unresolved.

In prospective, randomized trials of humans with head injury, Rowlands et al. and Ott et al. found improved nitrogen retention following the administration of intravenous amino acid formulas enriched with branched-chain amino acids.[107, 108] Branched-chain amino acids are oxidized by the skeletal muscle. Infusion of amino acids that supply the skeletal muscle with nutrients may decrease catabolism. Most clinicians do not use this therapy since branched-chain amino acid therapy is expensive and has no proven effect on morbidity and mortality. Plasma amino acid levels may also affect cerebral influx of excitatory amino acids such as glutamate and aspartate or the necessary metabolites required for neural repair.[109] Work in this area should be forthcoming.

In a prospective, randomized trial, patients supplemented with zinc demonstrated improved retinol-binding protein and thyroxine-binding protein levels and a more rapid improvement in GCS score.[55] Cerebral metabolism of glucose and lactate is affected by glucose administration; the effect on patient morbidity and mortality remains unclear.[67]

Animals

In animals with severe head injury and those with spinal cord injury, administration of vitamin E improves neurologic outcome.[110, 111] Vitamin E may act as an antioxidant and ameliorate lipid peroxidation. Selenium and ascorbic acid have the same effects.[111, 112] Magnesium administration decreases mortality and improves motor function.[113] A trial of magnesium supplementation in humans with head injury is currently being conducted. The viability of using selenium, vitamin E, or ascorbic acid in patients with head injury has not been tested.

Pharmacologic Intervention

Humans

Propranolol and barbiturates have been administered to humans with head injury to decrease energy expenditure and urinary nitrogen excretion. These agents have had limited effects. In addition, the opioid antagonist naloxone has been given to humans with spinal cord injury without beneficial effects. On the other hand, methylprednisolone administration significantly improved recovery in a recent randomized, controlled trial of patients with spinal cord injury.[114] The drug was given within 8 hours of injury. Another promising therapy in patients with spinal cord injury is monosialic ganglioside.[115] This therapy, given for weeks after injury, significantly improved recovery. In a small series of patients, scopolamine and ethacrynic acid also demonstrated positive results.[116, 117]

Animals

In animal models, investigators have administered opioid antagonists, catecholamine blockers, lipid peroxidation inhibitors, bradykinin antagonists, calcium channel blockers, excitatory amino acid inhibitors, acetylcholine antagonists, anion transport inhibitors, and inhibitors of arachidonic metabolism.[113, 118–121] All of these drugs (see Table 39–2) have had success in blocking their respective metabolic pathways and improving neurologic outcome. The optimal dose for human intervention must now be determined. Future therapy will likely utilize a combination of these metabolic blockers at different time points following injury.

Physiologic Intervention

Animals

Hypothermia has been used to decrease neuronal death after both spinal cord and brain injury. Its effects include a reduction of excitotoxic processes and decreased permeability of the blood-brain barrier.[122] Thyrotropin-releasing hormone (TRH) has been used because of its known role in antagonizing endogenous opioid peptides.[123, 124] Indeed, TRH physiologically reduces many of the effects of opioids on blood flow after spinal cord injury. Motor recovery was improved in animals with fluid percussion injury after the administration of norepinephrine.[113, 125] Future work is needed to determine whether these agents are viable options for use in humans with head injury.

Growth Factors

Animals

In vivo work with exogenous nerve growth factor demonstrated a decrease in injury-induced neural cell death in rats with septohippocampal lesions.[126] Gluckman et al. infused insulin-like growth factor 1 into the brains of rats following ischemic injury and found a decrease in neuronal loss.[127] In vitro work found that fibrocytic growth factor promoted the survival of neurons.[128] Growth factors provide a promising avenue of research for human work. Not only do they decrease neuronal loss, but they also improve the systemic effects of brain injury such as negative nitrogen balance and depressed immune status.[129]

Humans

Growth hormone has been administered to patients with severe head and spinal cord injuries.[130] A decrease in the acute-phase response was observed in patients infused with growth hormone. Insulin-like growth factor 1 is currently being infused in patients with severe head injury in a phase II trial.

PROVISION OF NUTRITION

A topic currently being debated is whether patients with severe head injury require parenteral nutrition or whether early enteral nutrition can be achieved in these patients. As early as 1976, Lutz et al. suggested that parenteral nutrition was often not tolerated in these patients.[131] In 1983, Rapp et al. brought attention to the fact that the then-standard enteral feeding regimen was inadequate with an average caloric intake of approximately 685 kcal/day.[71] Norton et al.,[24] Hunt et al.,[132] Twyman et al.,[106] and Clifton et al.[105] found that 35% to 50% of patients could not tolerate enteral nutrition until 10 days to 2 weeks following injury. Turner suggested that these patients could tolerate enteral feeding if the feeding tube was placed in the small bowel.[133] We showed that these patients often experienced inappropriate gastric emptying similar to patients with vagotomy. Grahm et al. and Kirby et al. found that feeding into the small bowel significantly improved enteral feeding tolerance in these patients and decreased the requirement for parenteral feeding.[80, 134]

As technology improves and intensive care clinicians dedicate time to placing feeding tubes in the patient with head injury, improved nutrient delivery can occur. A person dedicated to placing these tubes is instrumental for successful early enteral support in these patients. Another factor is the risk of aspiration. The above studies suggest that aspiration is not a problem; however, several studies suggest that the aspiration rate is no different in patients fed prepylorically vs. postpylorically.[135] The risk of aspiration has not yet been adequately determined. In the event that enteral nutrition cannot be provided within 24 hours postinjury, the parenteral route should be used. Some neurosurgeons are reluctant to provide parenteral nutrition because of the risk of hyperglycemia or exacerbation of cerebral edema. Using an animal model,

Waters et al. suggested that parenteral nutrition with high dextrose concentrations worsened vasogenic edema.[136] In our laboratory, studies in both animals and humans indicate that parenteral nutrition can be safely administered. We prospectively randomized 96 patients with severe head injury to receive parenteral or enteral nutrition.[137] Parenteral nutrition could be safely administered without causing hyperglycemia, increased intracranial pressure, or increased serum osmolality. Combs et al. found, in rats with cold injury, that infusion of parenteral nutrition did not increase specific gravity values in brain areas.[138]

The patient with brain or spinal cord injury suffers from a series of metabolic events that cause systemic effects and secondary brain injury. Investigators have defined these metabolic events and have attempted to block them with nutrient modification, pharmacologic intervention, physiologic modification, and growth factor administration. Future research is aimed at determining the optimal mode of treatment to improve the outcome of patients with neural injury.

REFERENCES

1. Hovda DA, Becker DP, Katayama Y: Secondary injury and acidosis. *J Neurotrauma* 1992; 9(suppl):47–60.
2. Feldman Z, Narayan RK, Robertson CS: Secondary insults associated with severe closed head injury. *Contemp Neurosurg* 1992; 14:1–8.
3. Marshall LF, Gautille T, Klauber MR: The outcome of severe closed head injury. *J Neurosurg* 1991; 75(suppl):28–36.
4. Woosley RM: Modern concepts of therapy and management of spinal cord injuries. *Crit Rev Neurobiol* 1988; 4:137–156.
5. Committee on Trauma Research, Commission on Life Sciences, National Research Council and Institute of Medicine: *Injury in America.* Washington, DC, National Academy Press, 1985.
6. Roye WP Jr, Dunn EL, Moody JA: Cervical spinal cord injury—a public catastrophe. *J Trauma* 1988; 28:1260–1264.
7. Anderson DW, McLaurin RL: Report on the national head and spinal cord injury survey. *J Neurosurg* 1980; 53:35.
8. Davis JN: *Neuronal Rearrangements after Brain Injury: A Proposed Classification.* Central Nervous System Trauma Status Report. Bethesda, Md, National Institutes of Health, National Institute of Neurological and Communicative Disorders and Stroke, 1985.
9. Haider W, Benzer H, Krystof G, et al: Urinary catecholamine excretion and thyroid hormone bloc level in the course of severe acute brain damage. *Eur J Intensive Care Med* 1975; 1:115–123.
10. McClain CJ, Cohen D, Ott L, et al: Ventricular fluid interleukin-1 activity in patients with head injury. *J Lab Clin Med* 1987; 110:48–54.
11. McClain CJ, Cohen D, Phillips R, et al: Increased plasma and ventricular fluid interleukin-6 levels in patients with head injury. *J Lab Clin Med* 1991; 118:225–231.
12. Bouzarth NF, Shenkin HA, Feldman W: Adrenocortical response to craniocerebral trauma. *Surg Gynecol Obstet* 1986; 126:995–1001.
13. Clifton GL, Ziegler MG, Grossman RG: Circulating catecholamines and sympathetic activity after head injury. *Neurosurgery* 1991; 8:10–14.
14. Chiolero R, Schutz Y, Lemerch T, et al: Hormonal and metabolic changes following severe head injury or noncranial injury. *JPEN* 1989; 13:5–12.
15. Goodman JC, Robertson CS, Grossman RG, et al: Elevation of tumor necrosis factor in head injury. *J Neuroimmunol* 1990; 30:213–217.
16. Clark JDA, Raggatt PR, Edwards OM: Hypothalamic hypogonadism following major head injury. *Clin Endocrinol* 1988; 29:153–165.
17. Edwards OM, Clark JDA: Post-traumatic hypopituitarism. Six cases and a review of the literature. *Medicine (Baltimore)* 1986; 65:281–290.

18. Clifton GL, Robertson CS, Grossman RG, et al: The metabolic response to severe head injury. *J Neurosurg* 1984; 60:687–696.

19. Robertson CS, Clifton GL, Grossman RG, et al: Oxygen utilization and cardiovascular function in head-injured patients. *J Neurosurg* 1984; 15:307–314.

20. Young B, Ott L, Norton J, et al: Metabolic and nutritional sequelae in the non–steroid treated head injury patient. *Neurosurgery* 1985; 17:784–791.

21. Gadisseux P, Ward J, Young H, et al: Nutrition and the neurosurgical patient. *J Neurosurg* 1984; 60:219–232.

22. McClain CJ, Twyman DL, Ott LG, et al: Serum and urine zinc response in head-injured patients. *J Neurosurg* 1986; 64:244–230.

23. McClain CJ, Hennig B, Ott L, et al: Mechanisms and implications of hypoalbuminemia in head-injured patients. *J Neurosurg* 1988; 69:386–392.

24. Norton J, Ott L, McClain C, et al: Intolerance to enteral feeding in the brain injured patient. *J Neurosurg* 1988; 68:62–66.

25. Young B, Ott L, Beard D, et al: The acute phase response of the brain-injured patient. *J Neurosurg* 1988; 69:375–380.

26. Long CL, Schaffel N, Geiger JW, et al: Metabolic response to injury and illness: Estimation of energy and protein needs from indirect calorimetry and nitrogen balance. *JPEN* 1979; 3:452–456.

27. Deutschman CS, Konstantinides FN, Raup S, et al: Physiological and metabolic response to isolated closed-head injury. Part 1: Basal metabolic state: Correlations of metabolic and physiological parameters with fasting and stressed controls. *J Neurosurg* 1986; 64:89–98.

28. Deutschman CS, Konstantinides FN, Raup S, et al: Physiological and metabolic response to isolated closed-head injury. Part 2: Effects of steroids on metabolism. Potentiation of protein wasting and abnormalities of substrate utilization. *J Neurosurg* 1987; 66:388–395.

29. Fruin AH, Taylor C, Pettis S: Caloric requirements in patients with severe head injuries. *Surg Neurol* 1986; 25:25–28.

30. Bruder N, Dumon JC, Francois G: Evolution of energy expenditure and nitrogen excretion in severe head-injured patients. *Crit Care Med* 1991; 19:43–48.

31. Haider W, Lackner F, Schlick W, et al: Metabolic changes in the course of severe acute brain damage. *Eur J Intensive Care Med* 1975; 1:91–96.

32. Kahn RC, Koslow M, Butcher S: Metabolic studies in head injured patients (abstract). *JPEN* 1987; 11(suppl):9.

33. Long CL, Schaffel N, Geiger JW, et al: Metabolic response to injury and illness: Estimation of energy and protein needs from indirect calorimetry and nitrogen balance. *JPEN* 1979; 3:452–456.

34. Durr D, Hunt D, Rowlands B, et al: Energy supply and demand following head injury: Balancing the metabolic budget (abstract). *JPEN* 1987; 11(suppl):5.

35. Touho H, Karasawa J, Nakagawara J, et al: Measurement of energy expenditure in the acute stage of head injury (Part 1). *No To Shinkei* 1987; 39:739.

36. Dempsey DT, Guenter P, Mullen JL, et al: Energy expenditure in acute trauma to the head with and without barbiturate therapy. *Surg Gynecol Obstet* 1985; 160:128–134.

37. Gerold K, Frankenfield D, Turney S, et al: Energy expenditure in acute severe head injury (abstract). *JPEN* 1989; 13(suppl):20.

38. Moore R, Najarian P, Konvolinka C: Measured energy expenditure in severe head trauma. *J Trauma* 1989; 29:1633–1666.

39. Chiolero RL, Breitenstein E, Thorin D, et al: Effects of propranolol on resting metabolic rate after severe head injury. *Crit Care Med* 1989; 17:328–334.

40. Bucci MN, Dechert RE, Arnoldi DK, et al: Elevated intracranial pressure associated with hypermetabolism in isolated head trauma. *Acta Neurochir* 1988; 93:133–136.

41. Clifton GL, Robertson CS, Choi SC: Assessment of nutritional requirements of head-injured patients. *J Neurosurg* 1986; 64:895–901.

42. Robertson CS, Clifton GL, Goodman

JC: Steroid administration and nitrogen excretion in the head injured patient. *J Neurosurg* 1985; 63:714–718.

43. Greenblatt SH, Long CL, Blakemore RS, et al: Catabolic effect of dexamethasone in patients with major head injuries. *JPEN* 1989; 13:372–376.

44. Young B, Ott L, Phillips R, et al: Metabolic management of the patient with head injury. *Neurosurg Clin North Am* 1991; 2:301–320.

45. Boop FA, Andrassy RJ, Brown WE, et al: Excessive nitrogen losses in severe brain injury (abstract). *Neurosurgery* 1985; 16:725.

46. Miller SL: The metabolic response to head injury. *S Afr Med J* 1984; 65:90–91.

47. Piek J, Lumenta CH, Bock WJ: Amino acid metabolism in patients with severe head injury (abstract). *Acta Neurochir* 1983; 68:165.

48. Schiller WR, Long CL, Blackmore WS: Creatinine and nitrogen excretion in seriously ill and injured patients. *Surg Gynecol Obstet* 1979; 149:561–566.

49. Hausmann D, Mosebach O, Caspari R, et al: Effects of steroid on nitrogen loss and plasma amino acid profiles after head injury (abstract). *JPEN* 1987; 11(suppl):10.

50. Zagara G, Scaravilli R, Bellucci CM, et al: Effect of dexamethasone on nitrogen metabolism in brain-injured patients. *J Neurosurg Sci* 1987; 31:207–212.

51. Schonheyder F, Heilskov NSC, Olesen K: Isotopic studies on the mechanism of negative nitrogen balance produced by immobilization. *Scand J Clin Lab Invest* 1954; 6:178–188.

52. Fried R, Dempsey D, Guenter P, et al: Barbiturates improve nitrogen balance in patients with severe head trauma (abstract). *JPEN* 1984; 8:86.

53. McLaurin RL, King L, Tutor FT, et al: Metabolic response to intracranial surgery. *Surg Forum* 1959; 10:770–773.

54. Castell JV, Andus T, Kunz D, et al: Interleukin-6. The major regulator of acute-phase protein synthesis in man and rat. *Ann N Y Acad Sci* 1988; 557:87–101.

55. Ranseen JD, Schmitt FA, Holt K, et al: Zinc supplementation and early outcome following severe brain injury (abstract). *J Clin Exp Neuropsychol* 1990; 12:34.

56. Hennig B, Honchel R, Goldblum SE, et al: Tumor necrosis factor–mediated hypoalbuminemia in rabbits. *J Nutr* 1988; 118:1586–1590.

57. Foley EF, Borlase BC, Dzik WH: Albumin supplementation in the critically ill. *Arch Surg* 1990; 125:739–742.

58. Brown RO, Bradley JE, Bekemeyer WB, et al: Effect of albumin supplementation during parenteral nutrition on hospital morbidity. *Crit Care Med* 1988; 16:1177–1182.

59. Ford EF, Jennings LM, Andrassey R: Serum albumin (oncotic pressure) correlates with enteral feeding tolerance in pediatric surgical patients. *J Pediatr Surg* 1987; 22:597.

60. Bories PN, Guenounou M, Feger J, et al: Human alpha 1-acid glycoprotein–exposed macrophages release interleukin 1 inhibitory activity. *Biochem Biophys Res Commun* 1987; 147:710–715.

61. Rosner MJ, Newsome HH, Becker DP: Mechanical brain injury: The sympathoadrenal response. *J Neurosurg* 1984; 61:76–86.

62. Young B, Ott L, Dempsey R, et al: Relationship between admission hyperglycemia and neurologic outcome of severely brain-injured patients. *Ann Surg* 1989; 210:466–473.

63. Lam AM, Winn R, Cullen BF, et al: Hyperglycemia and neurological outcome in patients with head injury. *J Neurosurg* 1991; 75:545–551.

64. Marie C, Bralet J: Blood glucose level and morphological brain damage following cerebral ischemia. *Cerebrovasc Brain Metab Rev* 1991; 3:29–38.

65. Kraig RP, Petito CK, Plum F, et al: Hydrogen ions kill brain at concentrations reached in ischemia. *J Cereb Blood Flow Metab* 1987; 7:379–386.

66. Siesjo BK, Wieloch T: Cerebral metabolism in ischaemia: Neurochemical basis for therapy. *Br J Anaesth* 1985; 57:47–62.

67. Robertson CS, Goodman JC, Narayan RK, et al: The effect of glucose administration on carbohydrate metabolism after head injury. *J Neurosurg* 1991; 74:43–50.

68. Sieber FE, Traystman RJ: Special is-

sues: Glucose and the brain. *Crit Care Med* 1992; 20:104–114.

69. Clifton GL, McCormick WF, Grossman RG: Neuropathology of early and late deaths after head injury. *Neurosurgery* 1981; 8:309–314.

70. Helling RS, Evans LL, Fowler DL, et al: Infectious complications in patients with severe head injury. *J Trauma* 1988; 28:1575–1577.

71. Rapp RP, Young B, Twyman D, et al: The favorable effect of early parenteral feedings on survival in head-injured patients. *J Neurosurg* 1983; 58:906–912.

72. Imhoff M, Gahr RH, Hoffmann P: Delayed cutaneous hypersensitivity after multiple injury and severe burn. *Ann Ital Chir* 1990; 61:525–528.

73. Miller CH, Quattrocchi KB, Frank EH, et al: Humoral and cellular immunity following severe head injury: Review and current investigations. *Neurol Res* 1991; 13:117–124.

74. Quattrocchi KB, Frank EH, Miller CH, et al: Suppression of cellular immune activity following severe head injury. *J Neurotrauma* 1990; 7:77–87.

75. Quattrocchi KB, Frank EH, Miller CH, et al: Impairment of helper T-cell function and lymphokine-activated killer cytotoxicity following severe head injury. *J Neurosurg* 1991; 75:766–773.

76. Hoyt DB, Ozkan AN, Hansbrough JF, et al: Head injury: An immunologic deficit in T-cell activation. *J Trauma* 1990; 30:759–766.

77. Maerker AG, Beckmann H, Richard KE, et al: Humoral immunodeficiency syndrome in patients with severe head injury. *Neurosurg Rev* 1989; 12:420–428.

78. Stanghellini V, Malagelada JR, Zinsmeister AR, et al: Stress-induced gastroduodenal motor disturbances in humans: Possible humoral mechanisms. *Gastroenterology* 1983; 85:83–91.

79. Ott L, Young B, Phillips R, et al: Altered gastric emptying in the head-injured patient: Relationship to feeding intolerance. *J Neurosurg* 1991; 74:738–742.

80. Grahm TW, Zadrozny DB, Harrington T: The benefits of early jejunal hyperalimentation in the head-injured pa-

tient. *Neurosurgery* 1989; 25:729–735.

81. Chin DE, Kearns P: Nutrition in the spinal-injured patient. *Nutr Clin Pract* 1991; 6:213–222.

82. Kolpek J, Ott LG, Record KE, et al: Comparison of urinary urea nitrogen excretion and measured energy expenditure in spinal cord injured and nonsteroid-treated severe head trauma patients. *JPEN* 1989; 13:277–280.

83. Cox SAR, Weiss SM, Posuniak EA, et al: Energy expenditure after spinal cord injury: Evaluation of stable rehabilitating patients. *J Trauma* 1985; 25:419–423.

84. Kearns PJ, Pipp TL, Quirk M, et al: Nutritional requirements in quadriplegics (abstract). *JPEN* 1982; 6:577.

85. Kaufman HH, Rowlands BJ, Stein DK, et al: General metabolism in patients with acute paraplegia and quadriplegia. *Neurosurgery* 1985; 16:309–313.

86. Rodriguez DJ, Clevenger FW, Osler TM, et al: Obligatory negative nitrogen balance following spinal cord injury. *JPEN* 1991; 15:319–322.

87. Arieff AJ, Pyzik JW, Tigay EL, et al: Some metabolic studies in quadriplegia following SCI. *Ill Med J* 1960; 117:219–223.

88. Robinson R: Serum protein changes following spinal cord injuries. *Proc R Soc Med* 1954; 47:1109–1113.

89. Ring J, Seifert J, Lob G, et al: Elimination rate of human serum albumin in paraplegic patients. *Paraplegia* 1974; 12:139–144.

90. Maynard FM, Imai K: Immobilization hypercalcemia in spinal cord injury. *Arch Phys Med Rehabil* 1977; 58:16–24.

91. Bildsten C, Lamid S: Nutritional management of a patient with brain damage and spinal cord injury. *Arch Phys Med Rehabil* 1983; 64:382–383.

92. Whedon GD: Disuse osteoporosis: Physiological aspects. *Calcif Tissue Int* 1984; 37(suppl):146–150.

93. Claus-Walker J, Halstead LS, Rodriguez GP, et al: Spinal cord injury hypercalcemia: Therapeutic profile. *Arch Phys Med Rehabil* 1982; 63:108–115.

94. Stewart AF, Adler M, Byers C, et al:

Calcium homeostasis in immobilization: An example of resorptive hypercalciuria. *N Engl J Med* 1982; 306:1136–1140.

95. Schneider AB, Sherwood LM: Calcium homeostasis and pathogenesis and management of hypercalcemic disorders. *Metabolism* 1974; 23:975–1007.

96. Boris A, Hurley JF, Tramal T, et al: Inhibition of disphosphonate-blocked bone mineralization: Evidence that calcitonin promotes mineralization. *Acta Endocrinol (Copenh)* 1979; 91:351–361.

97. McCagg CM: Postoperative management and acute rehabilitation of patients with spinal cord injuries. *Orthop Clin North Am* 1986; 17:171–182.

98. Chantraine A: Actual concept of osteoporosis in paraplegia. *Paraplegia* 1978; 116:51–58.

99. Leehey DJ, Picache AA, Robertson GL: Hyponatraemia in quadriplegic patients. *Clin Sci* 1988; 75:441–444.

100. Young B, Ott L, Twyman D, et al: The effect of nutritional support on outcome from severe head injury. *J Neurosurg* 1987; 67:668–676.

101. Hadley MN, Grahm TW, Harrington T, et al: Nutritional support and neurotrauma: A critical review of early nutrition in forty-five acute head injury patients. *Neurosurgery* 1986; 19:367–373.

102. Kaufman HH, Bretaudiere JP, Rowlands BJ, et al: General metabolism in head injury. *Neurosurgery* 1987; 20:254–265.

103. Waters DC, Dechert R, Bartlett R: Metabolic studies in head injury patients: A preliminary report. *Surgery* 1986; 100:531–534.

104. Balzola F, Boggio BD, Solerio A, et al: Dietetic treatment with hypercaloric and hyperproteic intake in patients following severe brain injury. *J Neurosurg Sci* 1980; 24:131–140.

105. Clifton GL, Robertson CS, Contant CF: Enteral hyperalimentation in head injury. *J Neurosurg* 1985; 62:186–193.

106. Twyman D, Young B, Ott L, et al: High protein enteral feedings: A means of achieving positive nitrogen balance in head-injured patients. *JPEN* 1985; 9:679–684.

107. Rowlands B, Hunt D, Roughneen P, et al: Intravenous and enteral nutrition with branched chain amino acid enriched products following multiple trauma with closed head injury, (abstract). *JPEN* 1986; 10(suppl):4.

108. Ott L, Schmidt J, Young B, et al: Comparison of administration of two standard intravenous amino acid formulas to severely brain-injured patients. *Drug Intell Clin Pharm* 1988; 22:763–768.

109. Robertson CS, Clifton GL, Grossman RG, et al: Alterations in cerebral availability of metabolic substrates after severe head injury. *J Trauma* 1988; 28:1523–1532.

110. Travis MA, Hall ED: The effects of chronic twofold dietary vitamin E supplementation on subarachnoid hemorrhage–induced brain hypoperfusion. *Brain Res* 1987; 418:366–370.

111. Kirsch JR, Helfaer MA, Lange DG, et al: Evidence for free radical mechanisms of brain injury resulting from ischemia/reperfusion-induced events. *J Neurotrauma* 1992; 9(suppl):157–163.

112. Braughler JM, Hall ED: Involvement of lipid peroxidation in CNS injury. *J Neurotrauma* 1992; 9(suppl): 1–7.

113. McIntosh TK: Pharmacologic strategies in the treatment of experimental brain injury. *J Neurotrauma* 1992; 9(suppl):201–209.

114. Bracken MB, Shepard JJ, Collins WF, et al: A randomized controlled trial of methylprednisolone or naloxone in the treatment of acute spinal cord injury. *N Engl J Med* 1990; 322:1405–1411.

115. Geisler FH, Dorsey FC, Coleman WP: GM-1 ganglioside in human spinal cord injury. *J Neurotrauma* 1992; 9(suppl):407–416.

116. Hayes RL, Lyeth BG, Jenkin SLW: Neurochemical mechanisms of mild and moderate head injury: Implications for treatment, in Levin HS, Eisenberg HM, Benton AL (eds): *Mild Head Injury.* New York, Oxford University Press, 1989, pp 54–79.

117. Cragoe EJ: Drugs for the treatment of

traumatic brain injury. *Med Res Rev* 1987; 7:271–305.

118. Young W: Role of calcium in central nervous system injuries. *J Neurotrauma* 1992; 9(suppl):9–26.

119. Francel PC: Bradykinin and neuronal injury. *J Neurotrauma* 1992; 9(suppl):27–46.

120. Hayes RL, Jenkins LW, Lyeth BG: Neurotransmitter-mediated mechanisms of traumatic brain injury: Acetylcholine and excitatory amino acids. *J Neurotrauma* 1992; 9(suppl):173–188.

121. Nockels R, Young W: Pharmacologic strategies in the treatment of experimental spinal cord injury. *J Neurotrauma* 1992; 9(suppl):211–218.

122. Clifton GL, Jiang JY, Lyeth BG, et al: Marked protection by moderate hypothermia after experimental traumatic brain injury. *J Cereb Blood Flow Metab* 1991; 11:114–121.

123. McIntosh TK, Vink R, Faden AI: An analogue of thyrotropin-releasing hormone improves outcome after brain injury:^{31}P-NMR studies. *Am J Physiol* 1988; 257:785–792.

124. Faden AI: TRH analog YM-14673 improves outcome following traumatic brain and spinal cord injury in rats: Dose-response studies. *Brain Res* 1989; 486:228–235.

125. Romhanyi RS, Tandian D, Hovda DA, et al: Catecholaminergic stimulation enhances recovery of function following concussive brain injury. *J Neurotrauma* 1990; 9:164.

126. Rich KM: Neuronal death after trophic factor deprivation. *J Neurotrauma* 1992; 9(suppl):61–69.

127. Gluckman P, Klempt N, Guan J, et al: A role for IGF-1 in the rescue of CNS neurons following hypoxic-ischemic injury. *Biochem Biophys Res Commun* 1992; 182:593–599.

128. Walicke PA, Baird A: Neurotropic effects of basic and acidic fibroblast growth factors are not mediated through glial cells. *J Dev Brain Res* 1986; 40:171–179.

129. Froesch ER, Guler HP, Schmid C, et al: Therapeutic potential of insulin like growth factor 1. *Trends Endocrinol Metab* 1990; 1:254–260.

130. Behrman SW, Wojtysiak S, Brown RO, et al: The effect of growth hormone on nutritional markers in enterally fed, immobilized trauma patients. *Surg Forum* 1990; 41:20–22.

131. Lutz H, Peter K, Van Ackern K: Total parenteral alimentation in neurosurgical and neurological patients, in Manni C, Magalina SI, Scrascio E, editors: *Total Parenteral Alimentation.* Amsterdam, Excerpta Medica, 1976; pp 214–217.

132. Hunt D, Rowlands B, Allen S: The inadequacy of enteral nutritional support in head injury patients during the early post-injured period (abstract). *JPEN* 1985; 9:121.

133. Turner WW Jr: Nutritional considerations in the patient with disabling brain disease. *Neurosurgery* 1985; 16:707–713.

134. Kirby D, Turner J, Barrett J, et al: Early enteral feeding with PEG/J's in severe head injury. *JPEN* 1991; 15:298–302.

135. Strong RM, Namihas N, Matsuyama R, et al: Random, prospective assessment of aspiration risk for percutaneous endoscopic gastrojejunostomy and percutaneous endoscopic gastrostomy (abstract). *JPEN* 1990; 14(suppl):18.

136. Waters DC, Hoff JT, Black KL: Effect of parenteral nutrition on cold-induced vasogenic edema in cats. *J Neurosurg* 1986; 64:460–465.

137. Young B, Ott L, Haack D, et al: Effect of total parenteral nutrition upon intracranial pressure in severe head injury. *J Neurosurg* 1987; 67:76–80.

138. Combs DJ, Ott L, McAninch PS, et al: The effect of total parenteral nutrition on vasogenic edema development following cold injury in rats. *J Neurosurg* 1989; 70:623–627.

39

Cancer

Michael H. Torosian, M.D.

John M. Daly, M.D.

Tumorigenesis and tumor growth

Cancer cachexia

Clinical efficacy of nutrition support

Protein-calorie malnutrition is a common problem in the cancer patient. Both disease- and treatment-related factors contribute to the malnourished state of cancer patients. Widespread nutritional and metabolic abnormalities, including derangements in protein, carbohydrate, lipid, and energy metabolism, have been documented in patients with malignancy.[1-3] Malnutrition in the cancer patient is associated with increased morbidity and mortality from surgery, chemotherapy, and radiation therapy and a shortened duration of survival.[4, 5]

Malnutrition is an important prognostic factor, and the association between weight loss and increased mortality in cancer patients has been known for several decades. Although nutrition support can significantly alter nutritional status and immune function, objective clinical trials have shown limited efficacy of parenteral or enteral nutrition to reduce patient morbidity.[1, 2, 6] Furthermore, the potential to stimulate tumor growth and metastasis exists in cancer patients receiving nutrition support.[7, 8] Thus, controversy continues regarding the effectiveness of nutrition support to significantly influence clinical outcome parameters in the cancer patient undergoing antineoplastic therapy.

TUMORIGENESIS AND TUMOR GROWTH

Spontaneous and carcinogen-induced tumors are influenced by nutrient administration. Numerous laboratory studies have demonstrated that protein-calorie deprivation significantly inhibits spontaneous and carcinogen-induced tumorigenesis as well as establishment and growth of transplanted tumors.[9-11] As early as 1953, Tannenbaum and Silverstone reported that protein-calorie restriction significantly inhibited spontaneous tumorigenesis in a variety of tumor-bearing animal models.[12] In the majority of tumor systems, refeeding rapidly reverses this trend and stimulates spontaneous tumorigenesis and the development of transplanted tumors.[13]

Once established, tumor growth and metastases can be significantly altered by nutrient intake. Restriction of protein and calorie intake causes decreased tumor growth in numerous tumor systems. In 1978 Daly et al. reported significant reduction of tumor growth in malnourished tumor-bearing animals.[14] Within 48 hours of initiating oral nutritional repletion, significant growth stimulation of the Walker 256 carcinosarcoma was observed in Sprague-Dawley rats.[15] A similar rate of increase in tumor volume was found in the Morris hepatoma of orally repleted Buffalo rats. A disproportionate increase in tumor vs. host growth was not found in these studies as evidenced by a constant tumor-to-host weight ratio in nutritionally repleted and depleted animals.

Parenteral nutrients similarly accelerate tumor growth in the majority of animal models studied. In 1975 Steiger et al. demonstrated increased growth of the AC-33 mammary adenocarcinoma in Lewis/Wistar rats receiving total parenteral nutrition (TPN).[16] Parenteral amino acids with or without hypertonic dextrose stimulated tumor growth in this system. Stimulation of tumor protein and DNA synthesis occurred in animals given parenteral nutrients. In 1981, Cameron reported increased ^{3}H-thymidine uptake in tumor cells of animals receiving TPN.[17] In this study, the significant increase in tumor: host weight upon parenteral nutrition indicated preferential growth of the Morris hepatoma cells. In 1983, Popp et al. reported similar results in methylcholanthrene induced sarcomas in Fischer 344 rats.[18] A direct correlation was observed between tumor weight and the rate of parenteral nutrient infusion in this study. With higher levels of parenteral nutrient infusion, tumor growth was

stimulated out of proportion to host lean body mass. Torosian et al. documented an increase in S-phase, or DNA synthesizing, tumor cells after only 2 hours of parenteral nutrient infusion.[7] Improved tumor response to cycle-specific chemotherapy (methotrexate, doxorubicin [Adriamycin]) but not cycle-nonspecific chemotherapy (cyclophosphamide) was observed as predicted by this perturbation in tumor growth kinetics by TPN.[19] Selective potentiation of tumor cytotoxicity occurred as no increase in host toxicity was detected.

Recent studies have suggested that TPN may similarly affect tumor metastasis. In 1987 Bryant et al. and Mahaffey et al. reported an increase in spontaneous pulmonary metastases in animals with Lewis lung carcinoma implants that received parenteral infusions.[20, 21] However, increased pulmonary metastases were also observed in animals receiving parenteral electrolyte infusions in this model. Thus, parenteral fluid load and not nutrient intake significantly stimulated the development of metastases, and it was hypothesized that alterations in circulating prostaglandin levels might be responsible for this phenomenon. In two different animal models, Torosian et al. reported an increase in spontaneous pulmonary metastasis in tumor-bearing, Lewis/Wistar rats receiving TPN. In Lobund rats with PA-III prostate carcinoma implants and Lewis/Wistar rats bearing MAC-33 tumors, combined TPN with glucose, amino acids, and long-chain triglycerides stimulated the development of tumor metastases to the greatest extent.[22, 23] Substitution of medium- for long-chain triglycerides, however, reduced the incidence of pulmonary metastasis in the MAC-33 mammary carcinoma model.[23] Other studies have suggested that structured lipids and ω-3 fatty acids may similarly inhibit tumor growth and metastasis.[24] Thus, although the majority of nutrients tested have been found to stimulate tumor growth, specific nutrients may be identified that inhibit primary tumor growth or spontaneous metastasis.

Controversy exists regarding the phenomenon of nutrient-induced acceleration of tumor growth in human tumors. In 1980 Mullen et al. studied fractional rates of protein synthesis in upper gastrointestinal cancers of patients receiving TPN as compared with patients nourished orally.[25] Tumor protein synthesis rates were determined by ^{15}N-glycine infusion and were found to be identical in these two groups of patients. In 1981, Nixon et al. found no direct clinical or biochemical evidence of tumor stimulation with TPN in patients with metastatic colon cancer vs. patients fed orally.[26] In contrast, two recent reports have suggested that TPN may stimulate the growth of head and neck cancers. In 1986, Baron et al. reported an increase in the percentage of hyperdiploid cancer cells in patients after receiving 7 to 10 days of TPN.[27] In a similar patient population, Frank et al. in 1991 reported increased bromodeoxyuridine (BrdU) incorporation into tumor cells of patients after 10 days of TPN.[28] These nutrient-induced changes in the growth kinetics of head and neck cancers indicate increased DNA synthesis following parenteral nutrient administration.

Significant differences in animal and human tumors justify the concern of directly extrapolating results from animal research to clinical populations. The most significant differences between animal and human tumors include differences in tumor doubling time, tumor burden, and host immunity. Animal tumors characteristically exhibit a doubling time of several days as compared with weeks, months, or years in human tumors. At the time of study, tumor burden in animal models may reach levels greater than 50% to 60% of body weight, whereas human tumors typically amount to less than 1% of host weight. Finally, animal tumor

models exhibit variable degrees of immunogenicity depending on tumor- and host-specific factors. In contrast, the vast majority of human tumors exhibit weak tumor-specific transplantation antigens and, therefore, elicit weak antitumor immune responses.

CANCER CACHEXIA

Cancer cachexia is the clinical syndrome that develops as a consequence of the nutritional and metabolic abnormalities of the tumor-bearing host. This symptom complex consists of anorexia, body weight loss, severe tissue wasting, asthenia, and organ dysfunction. Despite uncertainty regarding the etiology of cancer cachexia, this syndrome develops almost uniformly in patients with advanced malignancies.

The relationship of cachexia to tumor burden, stage of disease, and tumor histology is inconsistent, and no single theory satisfactorily explains the catabolic state characteristic of cancer cachexia.[29] Undoubtedly the cause of cachexia in cancer patients is multifactorial. Both disease- and treatment-related factors contribute to the development of cancer cachexia. This syndrome is not simply a local effect of the tumor but results from distant metabolic effects induced by malignancy, i.e., a type of paraneoplastic syndrome.[29, 30]

Extensive changes in energy, carbohydrate, lipid, and protein metabolism have been demonstrated in the cancer patient. Abnormalities in energy expenditure and inefficient energy utilization are frequently cited causes of malnutrition in tumor-bearing hosts. In 1977, Young reported increased resting energy expenditure in leukemia and lymphoma patients with rapidly progressing disease.[31] However, energy expenditure was not consistently elevated in patients with other malignancies. Knox et al. in 1983 measured resting energy expenditure in 200 malnourished cancer patients.[32] Only 41% of cancer patients exhibited normal resting energy expenditure in this study. Decreased and increased energy expenditure was documented in 33% and 26% of patients, respectively. Subsequently, Shike et al. found increased energy expenditure in patients with small-cell lung carcinoma, whereas Heber et al. reported no clear evidence of hypermetabolism in noncachectic lung cancer patients.[33, 34] Thus, although abnormalities in energy expenditure have been documented, elevated energy expenditure does not occur uniformly in cancer patients to account for progressive catabolism and weight loss.

Inefficient energy utilization by the tumor-bearing host may occur due to several mechanisms. Holroyde and Reichard reported increased Cori cycle activity in patients with cancer.[35] This futile cycle in which glucose is converted to lactic acid and subsequently reconverted to glucose by hepatocytes is an energy-wasting process. The highest level of Cori cycle activity was observed in patients with the greatest energy expenditure and weight loss in this study.

Abnormalities in carbohydrate metabolism include glucose intolerance, impaired whole-body insulin sensitivity, abnormal glucose oxidation, and increased rates of gluconeogenesis and glucose cycling.[35] Glucose intolerance is documented by hyperglycemia and delayed clearance of blood glucose in patients after oral or intravenous glucose administration.[35, 36] Glucose intolerance is due, in part, to decreased peripheral tissue sensitivity to insulin but may also involve blunted insulin release from pancreatic islet cells. Furthermore, feedback control mechanisms for glucose production may be impaired in the cancer patient. For instance, gluconeogenesis and Cori cycle activity occur at increased rates in cancer patients and are not inhibited by normal mechanisms such as exogenous glucose administration.[35–37]

Aberrations in lipid metabolism occur in patients with malignancy. The most significant changes in lipid metabolism include an increased rate of lipolysis with accelerated catabolism of body fat stores.[29, 37] Increased plasma clearance of endogenous fat stores and exogenously administered fat emulsions has been documented in cancer patients in both the fasting and fed states.[37] During periods of glucose administration, normal individuals suppress lipid mobilization and preferentially oxidize glucose. In the cancer patient, glucose administration fails to suppress endogenous lipid mobilization, and persistent oxidation of free fatty acids occurs. Finally, lipid depletion in the tumor-bearing host occurs in a nonuniform manner with resultant abnormalities in total-body lipid profiles.[38] Relative changes in the proportions of specific lipids contribute to further body compositional and metabolic derangements.

Abnormalities of protein metabolism present in cancer patients include host nitrogen depletion, decreased synthesis and increased catabolism of muscle protein, increased gluconeogenesis, and abnormal plasma aminograms.[2, 39] Nitrogen depletion in the tumor-bearing host is evidenced by severe wasting of lean body mass. Negative nitrogen balance and skeletal muscle wasting are common in patients with progressive malignancy at a time when tumor growth is progressing. Increased rates of gluconeogenesis contribute to skeletal muscle breakdown and are not suppressed by normal feedback mechanisms.[39] Tumor growth at the expense of host tissues has led to the concept of the tumor as a "nitrogen trap."

Although the etiology of cancer cachexia remains unknown, two classes of cachexia mediators believed to be important in the development of this catabolic state are cytokines and regulatory hormones. Cytokines are soluble proteins secreted by host tissues in response to cancer, sepsis, inflammation, starvation, and other pathophysiologic insults. Cytokines function by autocrine, paracrine, or systemic mechanisms of action. Specific cytokines implicated in the development of cancer cachexia include tumor necrosis factor (TNF, cachectin), interleukin-1 (IL-1), IL-6, and the interferons.[40, 41] TNF is a 17,000-dalton protein secreted by macrophages in response to malignancy or endotoxin.[42] TNF administration to animals causes anorexia, weight loss, depletion of fat stores, loss of lean body mass, and increased total-body water. Although some of the effects characteristic of cancer cachexia can be reproduced by TNF, this cytokine is certainly not the sole mediator of cancer cachexia. In fact, it is difficult to detect circulating levels of TNF in cancer patients even with advanced disease.[43]

IL-1 is secreted by macrophages exposed to endotoxin and causes anorexia, pyrexia, hypotension, decreased systemic vascular resistance, and increased cardiac output.[44] Genetic amplification of the IL-1 locus has been documented in one cachectic, tumor-bearing model, and IL-1–induced alterations in hepatic protein synthesis are similar to those seen in the tumor-bearing state.[45] IL-6 is secreted by macrophages stimulated by TNF or IL-1.[46] Many of the activities of IL-6 are similar to those of TNF and IL-1. Elevated levels of circulating IL-6 have been documented in tumor-bearing animals and do correlate with the hepatic acute-phase response to cancer. However, the precise roles of TNF, IL-1, and IL-6 as biological mediators of cancer cachexia remain undetermined.

CLINICAL EFFICACY OF NUTRITION SUPPORT

Numerous retrospective and prospective studies have evaluated the role of perioperative nutrition support on post-operative morbidity and mortality.[2, 5, 6] In general, retrospective studies in surgical patients have indicated reduced morbidity and mortality in patients receiving perioperative nutrition support.[5, 47] However, prospective, randomized trials of perioperative nutrition support have shown limited success.[2, 6] It is now generally accepted that preoperative TPN results in a significant reduction in postoperative morbidity only in severely malnourished patients, i.e., those at high risk for the development of nutritionally related complications.[48] There is no benefit to administering perioperative TPN to well-nourished or moderately malnourished patients or to patients undergoing low-risk procedures. In fact, numerous studies have demonstrated an increased incidence of infectious complications in mild or moderately malnourished patients receiving perioperative TPN (Table 39–1).[2, 6]

The use of nutrition support in cancer patients receiving chemotherapy and radiation therapy remains controversial. This controversy continues to exist because of major flaws in the majority of published clinical trials evaluating the efficacy of nutrition support in patients receiving antineoplastic therapy. Inadequate patient sample size, inadequate duration or amount of nutrition support, heterogeneous tumor types, and inappropriate study populations render the results of many trials inconclusive. Similar to surgical studies, several retrospective studies suggested improved tolerance to chemotherapy in patients receiving nutrition support. However, prospective, randomized trials have failed to confirm this initial finding (Table 39–2).[1, 2, 6]

The clinical outcome regarding toxicity and tumor response to chemotherapy is similar between patients receiving parenteral nutrition and control groups with one exception. In 1987 Weisdorf et al. demonstrated improved overall survival, improved disease-free survival, and decreased rates of relapse in bone marrow transplant recipients receiving TPN as compared with control patients.[49] This single prospective study demonstrates the possibility of using

TABLE 39–1.

Prospective Randomized Trials of Preoperative Total Parenteral Nutrition in Surgical Patients*

Author	No. of Patients	Preoperative TPN Duration (Days)	Complication Rate (%): TPN vs. Control	Mortality Rate (%): TPN vs. Control
Holter	56	3	13 vs. 19	7 vs. 8
Heatley	74	7–10	28 vs. 25	15 vs. 22
Holter	26	2	16 vs. 18	ND
Moghissi	15	5–7	30 vs. 50	ND
Preshaw	47	1	33 vs. 17	ND
Simms	40	7–10	ND	0 vs. 10
Lim	19	21–28	30 vs. 50	10 vs. 20
Schildt	15	14	38 vs. 57	0 vs. 0
Thompson	41	5–14	17 vs. 11	0 vs. 0
Sako	69	8–32	50 vs. 56	50 vs. 25
Mueller	125	10	11 vs. 19†	3 vs. 11
Burt	18	14	ND	ND
Jenson	20	2	Significant in TPN group	ND
Starker	59	5–42	12.5 vs. 45†	0 vs. 10†
Foschi	64	20	18 vs. 47	3.5 vs. 12.5
Bellantone	100	7	5.3 vs. 22	5.3 vs. 6.6

*Adapted from Redmond HP, Daly JM: Preoperative nutritional therapy in cancer patients is beneficial, in Simmons R (ed): *Debates in Clinical Surgery*, vol 2. St Louis, Mosby, 1991.
†Number of control patients vs. patients who received TPN.
ND = not determined.

TPN to support patients through extremely aggressive chemotherapy regimens. As chemotherapy regimens become more aggressive, new indications for TPN may be evident.

Radiation therapy has significant side effects, including xerostomia, decreased taste sensation, esophagitis, stricture formation, and enteritis, which can aggravate pre-existing nutritional deficits. However, the only consistent finding in prospective, randomized trials in patients receiving radiation therapy is an increase in the body weight of TPN-treated groups.[50] This increase in weight gain has little clinical significance because the majority of studies demonstrate no improvement in

TABLE 39–2.

Effect of Parenteral Nutrition on Chemotherapy Toxicity*

Tumor Type	N	Gastrointestinal	Hematologic	Infections
Lymphoma	41	—	ND	—
Colorectal	45	ND	↓	—
Testicular	30	ND	↑	↓
Metastatic sarcoma	27	—	ND	ND
Childhood metastatic	19	—	—	↓
Acute leukemia	23	—	ND	—
Lung, small cell	39	ND	ND	—
Lung, small cell	39	↓	ND	ND
Lung, small cell	31	—	ND	—
Lung, adenocarcinoma	43	↓	ND	ND
Lung, non–small cell	27	—	ND	—
Lung, squamous cell	—	↑	↑	—

*Adapted from Koretz RL: *J Clin Oncol* 1984; 2:535.
— = information not provided; ND = no difference; ↑ = TPN group had reduced toxicity vs. control group; ↓ = TPN group had increased toxicity vs. control group.

TABLE 39-3.

Total Parenteral Nutrition and Radiation Therapy*

Cancer	N	Weight	Toxicity	X-ray Therapy Given (%)		Survival
				TPN	Control	
Pelvic	32	↑ TPN	ND	—	—	—
Abdominal pelvic	20	↑ TPN	ND	92	I00	ND
Abdominal pelvic	40	↑ TPN	—	—	—	↑
Ovarian	8I	—	—	—	—	ND
Abdominal pelvic	25	—	ND	I00	I00	ND
Abdominal pelvic	29	↑ TPN	ND	9I	82	ND

*Adapted from Daly JM, Torosian M: In DeVita VT, Hellman S, Rosenberg SA (eds): *Cancer—Principles and Practice of Oncology,* ed 4. Philadelphia, JB Lippincott, in press.
ND = not determined.

morbidity or tumor response to radiation therapy in patients receiving TPN. However, few clinical trials have been performed to adequately evaluate the efficacy of nutrition support in patients undergoing radiation therapy (Table 39-3).[51, 52]

In summary, malnutrition is common in the cancer patient. Although the etiology of cancer cachexia is unknown, multiple factors including cytokines and regulatory hormones may play an etiologic role. Conventional nutrition support has been found to significantly reduce morbidity only in severely malnourished patients undergoing major surgery or intense antineoplastic therapy. In the future, specific nutrients such as glutamine, arginine, and ω-3 fatty acids may play a more direct role in preventing the occurrence of organ- or site-specific morbidity. The successful treatment of cancer cachexia requires an innovative, metabolic approach to cancer cachexia to selectively reverse the progressive catabolic effects of the tumor-bearing state.

REFERENCES

1. Torosian MH, Daly JM: Nutritional support in the cancer-bearing host. *Cancer* 1986; 58:1915-1929.
2. Brennan MF: Total parenteral nutrition in the cancer patient. *N Engl J Med* 1981; 305:375-381.
3. Lundholm K, Edstron S, Ekman L, et al: Metabolism in peripheral tissues in cancer patients. *Cancer Treat Rep* 1981; 65(suppl):79-83.
4. Studley HO: Percentage of weight loss: A basic indicator of surgical risk in patients with chronic peptic ulcer. *JAMA* 1936; 106:458.
5. Mullen JL: Consequences of malnutrition in the surgical patient. *Surg Clin North Am* 1981; 61:465-473.
6. Loretz RL: Parenteral nutrition: Is it oncologically logical? *J Clin Oncol* 1984; 2:534-538.
7. Torosian MH, Tsou KC, Daly JM, et al: Alteration of tumor cell kinetics by total parenteral nutrition: Potential therapeutic implications. *Cancer* 1984; 53:1409-1415.
8. Popp MB, Wagner SC, Brito OJ: Host and tumor responses to increasing levels of intravenous nutritional support. *Surgery* 1983; 94:300-308.
9. Begg RW, Dickinson TE: Systemic effects of tumors in force-fed rats. *Cancer Res* 1951; 11:409-412.
10. Ross MH, Bras G: Lasting influence of early caloric restriction on prevalence of neoplasms in the rat. *J Natl Cancer Inst* 1971; 51:1095-1113.
11. Moore C, Tittle PW: Muscle activity, body fat, and induced rat mammary tumors. *Surgery* 1973; 73:329-332.
12. Tannenbaum A, Silverstone H: Nutrition in relation to cancer. *Adv Cancer Res* 1953; 1:451-501.
13. Daly JM, Copeland EM, Dudrick SJ, et al: Nutritional repletion of malnourished tumor-bearing and nontumor-bearing rats: Effects on body weight, liver, muscle and tumor. *J Surg Res* 1980; 28:507-518.
14. Daly JM, Reynolds HM, Rowlands BJ, et al: Nutritional manipulation of

tumor-bearing animals: Effects of body weight, serum protein levels, and tumor growth. *Surg Forum* 1978; 29:143−144.

15. Daly JM, Copeland EM, Dudrick SJ: Effect of intravenous nutrition on tumor growth and host immunocompetence in malnourished animals. *Surgery* 1978; 84:655−658.

16. Steiger E, Oram-Smith J, Miller E, et al: Effects of nutrition on tumor growth and tolerance to chemotherapy. *J Surg Res* 1975; 18:455−461.

17. Cameron JL: Effect of total parenteral nutrition on tumor-host responses in rats. *Cancer Treat Rep* 1981; 65(suppl):93−99.

18. Popp MB, Wagner SC, Brito OJ: Host and tumor responses to increasing levels of intravenous nutritional support. *Surgery* 1983; 94:300−308.

19. Torosian MH, Mullen JL, Miller EE, et al: Enhanced tumor response to cycle-specific chemotherapy by parenteral amino acid administration. *JPEN* 1983; 7:337−345.

20. Bryant MS, Copeland EM III, Sinclair KGA, et al: Causative factors for decreased pulmonary metastasis in parenterally fed mice. *J Surg Res* 1987; 42:467−474.

21. Mahaffey SM, Copeland EM III, Conomides E, et al: Decreased lung metastasis and tumor growth in parenterally fed mice. *J Surg Res* 1987; 42:159−165.

22. Torosian MH, Donoway RB: Total parenteral nutrition and tumor metastasis. *Surgery* 1991; 109:597−601.

23. Bartlett D, Charland S, Torosian M: Differential effect of medium- and long-chain triglycerides on tumor growth and metastasis. *JPEN* 1992; 16(suppl): 30.

24. Ling PR, Istfan NW, Lopes SM, et al: Structured lipid made from fish oil and medium-chain triglycerides alters tumor and host metabolism in Yoshida-sarcoma−bearing rats. *Am J Clin Nutr* 1991; 53:1177−1184.

25. Mullen JL, Buzby GP, Gertner MH, et al: Protein synthesis dynamics in human gastrointestinal malignancies. *Surgery* 1980; 87:331−338.

26. Nixon DW, Moffitt S, Lawson DH, et al: Total parenteral nutrition as an adjunct to chemotherapy of metastatic colorectal cancer. *Cancer Treat Rep* 1981; 65(suppl):121−128.

27. Baron PL, Lawrence W Jr, Chan WMY, et al: Effect of parenteral nutrition on cell cycle kinetics of head and neck cancer. *Arch Surg* 1986; 121:1831−1886.

28. Frank JL, Lawrence W Jr, Banks WL Jr, et al: Modulation of cell cycle kinetics in human cancer with total parenteral nutrition. *Proc Assoc Acad Surg* 1991; 25:128.

29. Theologides A: Cancer cachexia. *Cancer* 1979; 43:2004−2012.

30. van Eys J: Nutrition and cancer: Physiologic interrelationships. *Annu Rev Nutr* 1985; 5:435−461.

31. Young VR: Energy metabolism and requirements in the cancer patient. *Cancer Res* 1977; 37:2336−2347.

32. Knox LS, Crosby LO, Feurer ID, et al: Energy expenditure in malnourished cancer patients. *Ann Surg* 1983; 197:152−162.

33. Shike M, Russell D, Detsky A, et al: Changes in body composition in patients with small-cell lung cancer: The effect of TPN as an adjunct to chemotherapy. *Ann Intern Med* 1984; 101:303−309.

34. Heber D, Chlebowski RT, Ishibashi DE, et al: Abnormalities in glucose and protein metabolism in non-cachectic lung cancer patients. *Cancer Res* 1982; 42:4815−4819.

35. Holroyde CP, Reichard GA: Carbohydrate metabolism in cancer cachexia. *Cancer Treat Rep* 1981; 65(suppl):55−59.

36. Schein PS, Kesner D, Haller D, et al: Cachexia of malignancy: Potential role of insulin in nutritional management. *Cancer* 1979; 43:2070−2076.

37. Waterhouse C, Kemperman JH: Carbohydrate metabolism in subjects with cancer. *Cancer Res* 1971; 31:1273−1278.

38. Waterhouse C, Nye WH: Metabolic effects of infused triglyceride. *Metabolism* 1961; 10:403−414.

39. Brennan MF, Burt ME: Nitrogen metabolism in cancer patients. *Cancer Treat Rep* 1981; 65(suppl):67−78.

40. Nakahara W: A chemical basis for tumor host relations. *J Natl Cancer Inst* 1960; 24:77–86.

41. Langstein H, Fraker D, Norton JA: Reversal of cancer cachexia by antibodies to interferon-gamma but not cachectin/tumor necrosis factor. *Surg Forum* 1989; 40:408–410.

42. Beutler B, Cerami A: Cachectin and tumor necrosis factor as two sides of the same biological coin. *Nature* 1986; 320:584–588.

43. Beutler B, Cerami A: Cachectin: More than a tumor necrosis factor. *N Engl J Med* 1987; 316:379–385.

44. Woloski BMRNJ, Fuller GM: Identification and partial characterization of hepatocyte stimulating factor from leukemia cell lines: Comparison with interleukin 1. *Proc Natl Acad Sci USA* 1985; 82:1443–1447.

45. Dinarello CA: Interleukin 1 and the pathogenesis of the acute phase response. *N Engl J Med* 1984; 311:1413–1418.

46. Powanda MC, Beisel WR: Hypothesis: Leukocyte endogenous mediator/endogenous pyrogen/lymphocyte activating factor modulates the development of nonspecific and specific immunity and affects nutritional status. *Am J Clin Nutr* 1982; 35:762–768.

47. Daly JM, Massar E, Giacco G, et al: Parenteral nutrition in esophageal cancer patients. *Ann Surg* 1982; 196:96–99.

48. The Veterans Affairs Total Parenteral Nutrition Cooperative Study Group: Perioperative total parenteral nutrition in surgical patients. *N Engl J Med* 1991; 325:525–532.

49. Weisdorf SA, Lysne J, Wind D: Positive effect of prophylactic total parenteral nutrition on long-term outcome of bone marrow transplantation. *Transplantation* 1987; 43:833.

50. Donaldson SS: Nutritional support as an adjunct to radiation therapy. *JPEN* 1984; 8:302–309.

51. Bothe A Jr, Valerio D, Bistrian BR, et al: Nutritional support of cancer patients receiving abdominal and pelvic radiotherapy: A randomized prospective, clinical experiment of intravenous versus oral feeding. *Surg Forum* 1978; 29:145–148.

52. Solassol C, Joyeuz H, Dubois JB: Total parenteral nutrition (TPN) with complete nutritive mixtures: An artificial gut in cancer patients. *Nutr Cancer* 1979; 1:13–18.

40

Geriatrics

John E. Morley, M.B., B.Ch.

Energy balance and aging

Macronutrient metabolism

Protein energy malnutrition

Complications of nutritional support in older individuals

Growth hormone and malnutrition

Hypodipsia and aging

Vitamin D

Over 12% of the U.S. population is 65 years and older. Eighty-five percent of older persons living at home have at least one chronic condition and 45% have some limitation of activity due to chronic disease. The most common causes of death in older persons in order of frequency are heart disease, cancer, stroke, chronic obstructive pulmonary disease, lung infections, diabetes mellitus, and accidents. Thus, it is not surprising that older persons utilize a disproportionate amount of acute hospital care. Sixteen percent of community-dwelling persons older than 60 years of age ingest fewer than 1,000 calories per day, a situation incompatible with maintenance of adequate nutrition.[1] Malnutrition is present in 17% to 65% of elderly persons in acute hospitals and from 26% to 59% of older individuals living in long-term care institutions.[2] A number of studies have demonstrated that with advancing age, being underweight places the person at much greater risk for death than does being overweight.[3-5] Thus, it is not surprising that the nutritional status of older persons plays an important role in determining both the morbidity and mortality associated with critical care in older persons.

ENERGY BALANCE AND AGING

Between the ages of 20 and 50 years, the average human increases body weight, due mainly to increased accumulation of body fat. This situation then remains stable until about 65 years of age, after which there is a tendency to lose weight due to a loss of both lean and adipose body mass.[6] The changes in energy balance that result in these anthropometric changes involve both changes in energy expenditure and alterations in the control of food intake. There is little evidence that altered digestion and absorption with aging play a role in the changes in energy balance in the majority of older persons. The total energy expenditure is approximately 20% lower in older men (1.58 times the resting metabolic rate [RMR]) as compared with younger men (1.85 times

717

RMR).[7] However, older women do not differ significantly from younger women (1.43 vs. 1.50 times RMR). Vo_2 max is the best predictor of total energy expenditure in older persons. However, it is important to realize that in healthy older persons there is large interindividual variability in total energy expenditure.

The RMR is reduced by approximately 20% in males and 13% in females between the ages of 30 and 75 years.[8] The causes of the reduction in RMR have not been clearly determined. Twenty percent to 40% of the RMR is due to the energy cost of the "sodium pump," but erythrocyte Na^+ K^+ adenosine triphosphatase (ATPase) activity does not decline with age in men and is only slightly reduced in women.[9] There is a mild reduction in triiodothyronine levels and a reduced responsiveness to norepinephrine, both of which would reduce the RMR.[10] Muscle tone activity is certainly slightly reduced with aging (secondary to the loss of muscle tissue) in the majority of older persons. With aging there is a selective loss of type II fibers in muscle, which leads to a reduced strength of contraction.[11] The RMR has been demonstrated to be increased in older persons with Parkinson's disease as a result of continuous muscular activity.[12] Finally, the reduction in food intake seen in many older persons may, itself, reduce the RMR, although it is often stated that the aging-associated reduced RMR leads to reduced food intake.

There is a small reduction in the thermic response to meals with advancing age.[13] The ability to disperse excess calories following a meal (diet-induced thermogenesis) is reduced in rodents with aging, most probably due to decreased brown adipose tissue responsiveness to norepinephrine.[14] This appears to be of minor significance in humans. Older persons decrease their physical activity, and maximal exercise capacity is reduced by 10% per decade between the ages of 25 and 65 years .[11] As alluded to above, this decrease in

physical activity and Vo_2 max appear to be the major factors involved in the reduction of total energy expenditure with age. However, it needs to be recognized that because of altered mechanical efficiency of movement, especially in the lower limbs, older persons expend more energy during simple exercises such as walking.[11]

Food intake clearly decreases in the majority of older persons. The physiologic reasons for this are poorly delineated in humans. Some of the decrease appears to be a result of the decrease in physical activity. Age-associated decreases in the ability to taste have been reported in older persons, although some of these changes appear to be due to lifelong cigarette smoking and the lack of dental hygiene.[15] Olfactory ability is clearly decreased with age and appears to play a more important role in decreased food intake than does taste. Older subjects have been found to prefer higher concentrations of sugar and salt.[16]

Animal studies have shown that food intake is regulated by both a peripheral satiety system and a central food drive system.[17] With advancing age, there is a deficit in the ability of the endogenous opioid dynorphin to increase food intake.[18] Dynorphin is predominantly involved in driving the appetite for fat foods. Besides this deficit in the food drive system, the gastrointestinal peptide cholecystokinin appears to be a more efficient satiety agent in older animals.[19] Older, malnourished persons have elevated levels of circulating cholecystokinin as compared with older, well-nourished persons and younger persons.[20] These studies point to a possible role of these peptides in the pathogenesis of the anorexia of aging.

Both tumor necrosis factor and interleukin-1 have been demonstrated to produce an anorectic effect.[21] They appear to produce this effect by activating the release of corticotropin-releasing factor (CRF) within the hypothalamus. CRF, which is also activated by a variety of other stresses, is a potent anorectic agent.[22] These findings provide a possible biological explanation for the anorexia seen in older persons with repeated infections and those in critical care situations.

MACRONUTRIENT METABOLISM

There is a decrease in protein synthesis with aging. This is offset by a decreased protein breakdown such that protein balance is not altered in healthy older persons.[23] Gersovitz et al.[24] have reported that the ingestion of 0.8 g of egg protein per kilogram of body weight per day is insufficient to maintain nitrogen balance in older persons. While serum essential amino acid levels tend to be lower in older than younger persons, they appear to be more than sufficient. While serum albumin levels may be slightly lower in the old-old (80 + years), it would appear that the majority of older persons maintain albumin levels greater than 4.0 g/dL.

Serum cholesterol and triglyceride levels both increase by about 60 mg/dL between the ages of 20 to 50 years in males and 20 to 65 years in females.[25] They then tend to fall by approximately 15 mg/dL between the ages of 65 to 80 years. The increase in cholesterol is mainly in the low-density lipoprotein (LDL) fraction. With advancing age, the production rate of LDL apoprotein B is unchanged, while there is a clear fall in the fractional catabolic rate. Similarly, the major factor for the increased triglyceride levels with age appears to be a decrease in the fractional rate of very low density lipoprotein (VLDL) lysolysis. A number of studies have suggested that with advancing age low cholesterol levels are more predictive of subsequent mortality than are elevated cholesterol levels.[26] This appears to be due to the effect of malnutrition and cytokines on cholesterol metabolism.

When compared with younger persons, older persons have decreased lipol-ysis per unit of adipose tissue when exposed to a prolonged fast.[27] In addition, traumatized older persons, in comparison to traumatized younger persons, have reduced triglyceride/free fatty acid cycling and energy metabolism.[28] These studies suggest that the older person with limited fat stores may be particularly at risk for the development of malnutrition in the intensive care unit.

With advancing age, there is a decrease in the effectiveness of insulin to drive glucose into peripheral tissues.[29] This is due to both receptor and postreceptor deficits. In addition, the islets of Langerhans of the pancreas are less effective at releasing insulin for a given glucose concentration. This combination of factors results in the hyperglycemia of aging and puts older persons at increasing risk of the development of diabetes mellitus. This may be unmasked in critical care situations due to an increase in stress hormones (i.e., cortisol and growth hormone) antagonizing the effect of insulin. A newly isolated pancreatic islet cell hormone, amylin, may also play an important role in carbohydrate metabolism in older persons. It antagonizes the functions of insulin and appears to delay the return of glucose to basal levels following a meal.

PROTEIN ENERGY MALNUTRITION

A number of studies that included substantial numbers of older patients have examined the relationship of serum albumin levels to death (Table 40–1). These studies clearly indicate that low albumin levels are highly predictive of death in the intensive care unit[30, 31] following surgery,[32–34] or during a hospital admission.[35–37]

Foster et al.[38] studied 40 older persons with an average age of 78.2 years (range, 45 to 97 years) who had sustained a hip fracture. Within 11 months of follow-up, those who died had a mean albumin level of 2.8 g/dL as compared

TABLE 40–1.

Role of Albumin as a Predictor of Mortality in Older Hospitalized Patients

Author	Age (yr)	n	Mean Albumin (g/dL)		Comments
			Died	Survived	
Intensive Care Unit					
Boosalis et al.[30]	32–88	78	3.1	3.5	
Murray et al.[31]	20–91	111	3.0	3.2	
Surgical					
Lai et al.[32]	67 ± 14	96	3.1	3.6	Preoperative
Christou et al.[33]	64.9 ± 12.8	245	2.9	3.6	Preoperative
Rich et al.[34]	75–90	92	—	—	Cardiac surgery: With albumin < 3.5 g/dL, 31% died With albumin > 3.5 g/dL, 13% died
General hospital					
Agarwal et al.[35]	85–100	80	—	—	Albumin < 3.0 g/dL predicts mortality
Herrman et al.[36]	67 ± 14	15, 511	—	—	With albumin < 3.4 g/dL, 14% died; with albumin > 3.4 g/dL, 4% died
Constans et al.[37]	M 78.8 ± 5.4	128	3.2	3.6	
	F 81.3 ± 6.8	196	3.3	3.5	

with 3.5 g/dL for those who lived. Transferrin, prealbumin, delayed hypersensitivity, and the total lymphocyte count did not predict outcome. Patterson et al.[39] found that following hip fracture, patients who were protein depleted had a higher mortality within 1 year of the fracture, had longer hospital stays, and were less likely to return to their prefracture environment. In a larger British series of 744 women with femoral neck fracture, food intake and serum albumin were correlated with subsequent mortality.[40] Barstow et al.[41] have demonstrated that enteral tube feeding enhances outcome in malnourished older persons with hip fractures. Two small studies have suggested that oral supplementation of patients with hip fractures may be equally efficacious at reducing subsequent mortality and morbidity.[42, 43]

Delirium is an important cause of prolonged hospital admission in older persons. Dickson[44] and Levkoff et al.[45] have reported that hypoalbuminemia is a major predictive factor of delirium. Low albumin levels result in an increase in unbound drug concentrations, and this results in greater concentrations of drug crossing the blood-brain barrier. Drugs are commonly the cause of delirium in older persons.

Constans et al.[37] reported that in addition to albumin, midarm circumference is a useful predictor of mortality in older persons in the hospital. Because this measure is relatively independent of fluctuations in water balance, it may be particularly useful to identify the nutritional status of older persons in the intensive care unit.

Protein energy malnutrition occurs in older persons for a variety of reasons. Poverty, the inability to shop for oneself or to adequately prepare food, and social isolation can all play a role in making the older person extremely vulnerable to the development of malnutrition. This section will concentrate on the major causes of malnutrition in hospitalized older persons (Table 40–2).[46, 47]

Multiple drugs result in nausea or anorexia. Digoxin commonly produces anorexia and weight loss in older persons without serum levels being in the toxic range.[48] Mild theophylline toxicity can lead to anorexia and perhaps a mild increase in the metabolic rate. Antibiotics commonly produce mild nausea and anorexia. Hyperparathyroidism can be manifested as anorexia. When serum albumin levels are decreased, a high-normal calcium level may not be noticed. Abscesses in the mouth or lack of dentition leads to decreased food intake. Patients with stroke often aspirate and develop a conditioned aversion to eating. Persons with tremors often have difficulty getting the food to their mouth and spill more food than they ingest. Intestinal ischemia can be manifested as early satiety.

Depression is commonly missed in older persons. Older persons with depression are more prone to the development of anorexia and weight loss than are younger persons. Persons with dementia may forget to eat. In the hospital, insufficient time is often spent on feeding these individuals. Weight maintenance may take up to 90 minutes per day of feeding time. Persons with late-life paranoia may believe that their food is poisoned and refuse to eat. Recurrence of anorexia nervosa in older

women who had this disorder when young is being more commonly recognized. Older males often have abnormal attitudes to food ingestion that result in a decreased food intake even in the face of malnutrition.[49] This condition is called anorexia tardive. It needs to be recognized that some older persons become overwhelmed with the burden of their disease and refuse to eat as a rational response to their life situation.

Hyperthyroidism may be difficult to diagnose in an older person with multiple disease processes.[10] Often the clinical presentation is masked, with the major initial features being weight loss, muscle weakness, cardiac failure, and atrial fibrillation. Malnutrition can decrease triiodothyronine and thyroxine levels into the normal range, even when the values are corrected for throxine-binding globulin levels.[50] For this reason, severely ill persons with triidothyronine levels above the midnormal range should have the diagnosis of hyperthyroidism entertained. Recently, it has been demonstrated that pheochromocytoma occurs as commonly in old persons as it does in young persons, but that the diagnosis is rarely made before death.[51] Severely malnourished older persons whose hypertension persists in the presence of malnutrition should have a diagnostic workup for pheochromocytoma.

Patients with chronic obstructive pulmonary disease expend excess calories because of their use of accessory muscles when breathing. In addition, food intake can result in a marked drop in oxygen saturation and cause dyspnea and the inability to finish a meal.

In occasional patients with severe cardiac failure, a condition known as cardiac cachexia develops.[52] This condition appears to be secondary to multiple factors. These include decreased food intake due to gastric and liver congestion, drug therapy, and general malaise. Calories can be lost because of malabsorption secondary to small-bowel congestion and protein loss from the kidneys and gut. Energy consumption is in-

TABLE 40–2.

Causes of Malnutrition in Hospitalized Older Persons

Decreased food intake
  Medical causes
    Drugs, e.g., digoxin, theophylline, psychotropic agents
    Hyperparathyroidism
    Poor dentition
    Swallowing problems, i.e., stroke, candidal esophagitis
    Zinc deficiency
    Physical causes, e.g., severe tremor
    Intestinal ischemia
    Infection
  Psychological causes
    Depression
    Dementia
    Late-life paranoia
    Anorexia nervosa (tardive)
    Overwhelming burden of life
Increased metabolism
  Hyperthyroidism
  Pheochromocytoma
  Parkinson's disease
Mixed
  Chronic obstructive pulmonary disease
  Cancer
  Cardiac cachexia
Malabsorption
  Celiac disease
  Lactase deficiency

creased secondary to the increased work of breathing. Energy delivery is impaired as a result of poor cardiac function. Overall, approximately one in seven older persons with cardiac failure will have some degree of protein energy malnutrition. Treatment on the whole requires correction of the underlying heart failure. There are no data suggesting that enteral or parenteral feeding has a positive benefit in this unique group of older persons with extremely precarious fluid balance.

Malabsorption due to late-life onset of cardiac disease is not a rare cause of malnutrition in older persons. This condition occurs more commonly in older persons with diabetes mellitus.

In our experience, scheduling of multiple tests resulting in overnight food abstention often aggravates a borderline nutritional status. Similarly, an acutely ill older person with borderline nutritional status may be allowed to eat poorly for a number of days before the need for aggressive nutritional support is recognized. Finally, we have seen a number of older persons who, having been told to lower their cholesterol intake to protect their heart, present with infection secondary to hypoalbuminemia and malnutrition. Cholesterol mania can be an important cause of malnutrition. Dietary counseling often begins in the critical care situation, and these evangelical crusaders often fail to modify their advice to older persons in whom the benefit is questionable.[26] Finally, the use of restraints has been associated with anorexia and weight loss as well as dehydration in older persons.[53]

COMPLICATIONS OF NUTRITIONAL SUPPORT IN OLDER INDIVIDUALS

Complications of enteral feeding in older persons include gastrointestinal (diarrhea, poor gastric emptying, vomiting, and gastrointestinal bleeding), mechanical (aspiration pneumonia and tube misplacement), and metabolic abnormalities (hyperkalemia and hypokalemia, prerenal azotemia, hypophosphatemia, hyperglycemia, and liver failure). The available literature does not clearly allow a delineation of which of these occur more commonly in older vs. younger persons. In one study of the development of pneumothorax due to nasogastric feeding tubes, four of the five patients were over 60 years of age.[54] Mullan et al.[55] reported that the major risk of pulmonary aspiration among patients receiving enteral nutritional support is advancing age.

A relatively unique complication of feeding for older persons is postprandial hypotension. Carbohydrate meals can cause a drop in both systolic and diastolic blood pressure by at least 10 mm Hg for up to 3 hours following a meal. This effect is further aggravated by the administration of nitrates. Our studies have suggested that the fall in blood pressure in older persons following glucose ingestion is due to release of the vasodilatory peptide calcitonin gene-related peptide.

GROWTH HORMONE AND MALNUTRITION

With advancing age, there is a decrease in growth hormone secretion from the pituitary.[56] This appears to be predominantly due to an increase in hypothalamic somatostatin secretion. The decrease in growth hormone with aging is associated with a decrease in insulin growth factor 1 (IGF-1). IGF-1 levels are even further decreased in malnourished older persons.[57] Growth hormone has been administered to healthy older persons with a resultant increase in IGF-1 and a decrease in body fat.[58] Growth hormone has also resulted in a positive effect on parameters associated with aging.[59]

Kaiser et al.[60] demonstrated that severely malnourished older persons had a positive response to recombinant growth hormone with an increase in

IGF-1. When compared with control subjects, growth hormone–treated subjects had an increase in weight and enhanced nitrogen retention. A shorter-term study reported similar results in a group of older persons.[61] These and other studies in critically ill malnourished older persons suggest the potential use of recombinant growth hormone in the management of these individuals.

HYPODIPSIA AND AGING

Older persons often fail to recognize the need to drink adequately so as to rehydrate themselves.[62] Silver and Morley[63] demonstrated in humans that this is due to a deficit in the mulcopioid drinking drive. Stroke may further reduce the recognition of the need for fluid intake. This situation may be aggravated for older persons in the hospital, by physical restraints and/or bed rails that prevent the patient from reaching water on the bedside table. This problem may be aggravated by the excessive use of diuretics to treat pedal edema in an old person. Thus, it is not surprising that dehydration is a common problem in older persons.

Hyponatremia is commonly observed in older persons. Common causes are a low-salt diet and diminished free water excretion. Lack of adequate salt content of tube feedings has also been associated with hyponatremia. The syndrome of inappropriate antidiuretic hormone secretion (SIADH) is common in older persons and leads to hyponatremia in the face of continued sodium excretion. The role of elevated atrionatriuretic factor levels in the pathogenesis of dehydration and/or hyponatremia remains to be determined.[64]

VITAMIN D

Up to one in five older persons has been demonstrated to be vitamin D deficient.[65] Older persons are less capable of synthesizing cholecalciferol in their skin in response to ultraviolet light. They also have decreased conversion of 25-(OH)-vitamin D to $1,25(OH)_2$-vitamin D by α-hydroxylase in the kidneys and often have decreased oral intake of vitamin D. Vitamin D deficiency leads to an increased risk of hip fracture due to osteomalacia and decreased muscle strength. In addition, there is evidence that vitamin D deficiency may result in macrophage malfunction and an increased propensity to the development of tuberculosis. In addition to vitamin D deficiency, many older persons have secondary hyperparathyroidism associated with mild renal insufficiency. For these reasons, vitamin D replacement may be appropriate in the majority of older persons with total serum calcium levels of 9 mg/dL or less.

SUMMARY

There is increasing evidence that nutritional problems are extremely important in the pathogenesis of morbidity and mortality in older persons. However, only the studies in patients with hip fractures and one study of nutritional supplementation in a geriatric hospital[66] have clearly demonstrated positive effects of nutritional support in the elderly. There is a paucity of information specifically examining the nutritional needs and the complications associated with nutritional support of older persons in the critical care situation. Clearly, more attention needs to be paid to the unique nutritional needs of older persons receiving critical care.

REFERENCES

1. Abrahamson S, Carroll MD, Dresser CM, et al: *Dietary Intake of Persons 1–74 Years of Age in the United States.* Advance data from Vital and Health Statistics of the National Health Center for Health Statistics, No 6, Rockville, Md, US Department of Health, Education and Welfare, Health Resources Administration, Public

Health Services, DHEW Publication No (HRA) 77–1647, 1977.

2. Morley JE: Nutrition and aging, in Hazzard WR, Andres R, Bierman EL, et al (eds): *Principles of Geriatric Medicine and Gerontology.* New York, McGraw-Hill, 1990, pp 48–59.

3. Tayback M, Kumanyika S, Chei E: Body weight as a risk factor in the elderly. *Arch Intern Med* 1990; 150:1065–1072.

4. Harris T, Cook F, Garrison R, et al: Body mass index and mortality for non-smoking older persons. *JAMA* 1988; 259:1520–1524.

5. Waaler M: Height, weight and mortality: The Norwegian experience. *Acta Med Scand* 1983; 679(suppl):1–56.

6. Glick Z: Energy balance, in Morley JE, Glick Z, Rubenstein LZ (eds): *Geriatric Nutrition.* New York, Raven Press, 1990, pp 27–40.

7. Goran MI, Poehlman ET: Total energy expenditure and energy requirements in healthy elderly persons. *Metabolism* 1992; 41:744–753.

8. Durnin JVGA: Energy metabolism in the elderly, in Munro H, Schlierf G (eds): *Nutrition of the Elderly.* New York, Raven Press, 1992, pp 51–63.

9. Simat B, Morley JE, From AHL, et al: Variables affecting measurement of human red cell Na$^+$ K$^+$ ATPase. *Am J Clin Nutr* 1984; 40:339–345.

10. Mooradian AD, Morley JE, Korenman SG: Endocrinology in aging. *Dis Mon* 1988; 34:395–461.

11. Shephard RJ: *Physical Activity and Aging,* ed 2. London, Croom Helm, 1987.

12. Levi S, Cox M, Lugon M, et al: Increased energy expenditure in Parkinson's disease. *BMJ* 1990; 301:1256–1257.

13. Schwartz RS, Jaeger LF, Veith RC: The thermic effect of feeding in older men: The importance of the sympathetic nervous system. *Metabolism* 1990; 39:733–737.

14. Scarpace PJ, Mooradian AD, Morley JE: Age associated decrease in beta-adrenergic receptors and adenylate cyclase activity in rat brown adipose tissue. *J Gerontol* 1988; 45:65–70.

15. Murphy C: Age associated changes in taste and odor sensation, perception and preference, in Munro H, Schlierf G (eds): *Nutrition of the Elderly.* New York, Raven Press, 1992, pp 79–88.

16. Murphy C, Withee J: Age-related differences in the pleasantness of chemosensory stimuli. *Psychol Aging* 1986; 1:312–318.

17. Morley JE: Neuropeptide regulation of appetite and weight. *Endocr Rev* 1987; 8:256–287.

18. Gornell BA, Levine AS, Morley JE: The effects of aging on opioid modulation of feeding in rats. *Life Sci* 1983; 32:2793–2799.

19. Silver AJ, Flood JF, Morley JE: Effect of gastrointestinal peptides on ingestion in young and old mice. *Peptides* 1988; 9:221–226.

20. Berthelemy P, Bouisson M, Vellas B, et al: Postprandial cholecystokinin secretion in elderly with protein energy under nutrition. *J Am Geriatr Soc* 1992; 40:365–369.

21. Morley JE: Appetite regulation: The role of peptides and hormones. *J Endocrinol Invest* 1989; 12:135–147.

22. Morley JE, Levine AS: Corticotropin-releasing factor; grooming and ingestive behavior. *Life Sci* 1982; 31:1459–1464.

23. Kritchevsky D: Protein requirements of the elderly, in Munro H, Schlierf G (eds): *Nutrition of the Elderly.* New York, Raven Press, 1992, pp 109–118.

24. Gersovitz M, Motel K, Munro HM, et al: Human protein requirements: Nitrogen assessment of the adequacy of the current recommended dietary allowance for dietary protein in elderly men and women. *Am J Clin Nutr* 1982; 35:6–14.

25. Miller NE, Nanjee MN: Hyperlipidemia in the elderly: Metabolic changes underlying increases in plasma cholesterol and triglycerides during aging. *Cardiovasc Risk Factors* 1992; 2:158–169.

26. Kaiser FE, Morley JE: Cholesterol can be lowered in older persons: Should we care? *J Am Geriatr Assoc* 1990; 38:239–253.

27. Klein S, Young VR, Blackburn GL, et al: Palmitate and glycerol kinetics during brief starvation in normal weight young adult and elderly subjects. *J Clin Invest* 1986; 78:928–933.

28. Jeevandam M, Young DH, Schiller WR: Energy cost of fat-fuel metabolism in

geriatric trauma. *Metabolism* 1990; 39:144–149.

29. Morley JE, Mooradian AD, Rosenthal MJ, et al: Diabetes mellitus in elderly patients: Is it different? *Am J Med* 1987; 83:533–544.

30. Boosalis MG, Ott L, Levine AS, et al: Relationship of visceral proteins to nutritional status in chronic and acute stress. *Crit Care Med* 1989; 17:741–747.

31. Murray MJ, Marsh M, Wochos DN, et al: Nutritional assessment of intensive care unit patients. *Mayo Clin Proc* 1985; 63:1106–1115.

32. Lai ECS, Tam P-C, Paterson IA, et al: Emergency surgery for severe acute cholangitis. *Ann Surg* 1990; 211:55–59.

33. Christou NV, Tellado-Rodriguez J, Chastrano L, et al: Estimating mortality risk in preoperative patients using immunologic, nutritional and acute-phase response variables. *Ann Surg* 1989; 210:69–77.

34. Rich MW, Keller AJ, Schechtman KB, et al: Increased complications and prolonged hospital stay in elderly cardiac surgical patients with low serum albumin. *Am J Cardiol* 1989; 63:714–718.

35. Agarwal N, Acevedo F, Leighton LS, et al: Predictive ability of various nutritional variables in elderly people. *Am J Clin Nutr* 1988; 48:1173–1178.

36. Herrmann FR, Safran C, Levkoff SE, et al: Serum albumin level on admission as a predictor of death, length of stay and readmission. *Arch Intern Med* 1992; 152:125–130.

37. Constans T, Bacq Y, Brechot J-F, et al: Protein-energy malnutrition in elderly medical patients. *J Am Geriatr Soc* 1992; 40:263–268.

38. Foster MR, Heppenstall RB, Friedenberg ZB, et al: A prospective assessment of nutritional status and complications in patients with fractures of the hip. *J Orthop Trauma* 1990; 4:49–57.

39. Patterson BM, Cornell CN, Carbone B, et al: Protein depletion and metabolic stress in elderly patients who have a fracture of the hip. *J Bone Joint Surg* 1992; 74:251–260.

40. Barstow MD, Rawlings J, Allison SP: Undernutrition, hypothermia and injury in elderly women with fractured femur: An injury response to altered metabolism. *Lancet* 1983; 1:143–145.

41. Barstow MD, Rawlings J, Allison SP: Benefits of supplementary tube feeding after fractured neck of femur: A randomized controlled trial. *BMJ* 1983; 287:1589–1592.

42. Delmi M, Rapin CH, Bengoa JM, et al: Dietary supplementation in elderly patients with fractured neck of the femur. *Lancet* 1990; 1:1013–1016.

43. Bonjour J-P, Rapin C-H, Rizzoli R, et al: Hip fracture, femoral bone mineral density and protein supply in elderly patients, in Munro M, Schlierf G (eds): *Nutrition of the Elderly.* New York, Raven Press, 1992, pp 151–159.

44. Dickson LR: Hypoalbuminemia in delirium. *Psychosomatics* 1991; 32:317–323.

45. Levkoff SE, Safron C, Cleary PD, et al: Identification of factors associated with the diagnosis of delirium in elderly hospitalized patients. *J Am Geriatr Soc* 1988; 36:1099–1104.

46. Morley JE, Silver AJ: Anorexia in the elderly. *Neurobiol Aging* 1988; 9:9–16.

47. Morley JE: Anorexia in older patients: Its meaning and management. *Geriatrics* 1990; 45:59–66.

48. Morley JE, Reese SS: Clinical implications of the aging heart. *Am J Med* 1989; 86:77–86.

49. Miller DK, Morley JE, Rubenstein LZ, et al: Abnormal eating attitudes and body image in older undernourished individuals. *J Am Geriatr Soc* 1991; 39:462–486.

50. Morley JE, Slag MF, Elson MK, et al: The interpretation of thyroid function tests in hospitalized patients. *JAMA* 1983; 249:2377–2379.

51. Stenstrom G, Svarchsudd K: Pheochromocytoma in Sweden 1958–1981. *Acta Med Scand* 1986; 220:225–232.

52. Gorbien MJ: Cardiac cachexia, in *Geriatric Nutrition.* New York, Raven Press, 1990, pp 315–324.

53. Evans LK, Strumpf NE: A review of literature on physical restraint. *J Am Geriatr Soc* 1989; 37:65–74.

54. Roubenoff R, Ravich WJ: Pneumothorax due to nasogastric feeding tubes. *Arch Intern Med* 1989; 149:184–188.

55. Mullan H, Roubenoff RA, Roubenoff R: Risk of pulmonary aspiration among patients receiving enteral nutrition

support. *JPEN* 1992; 16:160–164.

56. Kelijman M: Age-related alterations of the growth hormone/insulin like growth factor I axis. *J Am Geriatr Soc* 1991; 39:235–240.

57. Rudman D, Nagraj HS, Mattson DE, et al: Hyposomatomedinemia in the nursing home patient. *J Am Geriatr Soc* 1986; 34:427–430.

58. Rudman D, Feller AG, Nagraj MS, et al: Effects of human growth hormone in men over 60 years old. *N Engl J Med* 1990; 323:1–6.

59. Marcus R, Butterfield G, Holloway L, et al: Effects of short term administration of recombinant growth hormone in elderly people. *J Clin Endocrinol Metab* 1990; 70:519–527.

60. Kaiser FE, Silver AJ, Morley JE: The effect of recombinant human growth hormone on malnourished older individuals. *J Am Geriatr Soc* 1991; 39:235–240.

61. Binnerts A, Wilson JHP, Lamberts SW: The effects of human growth hormone administration in elderly adults with recent weight loss. *J Clin Endocrinol Metab* 1983; 56:1278–1281.

62. Rolls BJ, Phillips PA: Aging and disturbances of thirst and fluid balance. *Nutr Res* 1990; 48:137–144.

63. Silver AJ, Morley JE: The role of the opioid system in the hypodipsia associated with aging. *J Am Geriatr Soc* 1992; 40:556–560.

64. Davis KM, Fish LC, Elashi D, et al: Atrial natriuretic peptide levels in the prediction of congestive heart failure risk in frail elderly. *JAMA* 1992; 267:2625–2629.

65. Morley JE, Gorbien MJ, Mooradian AD, et al: Osteoporosis. *J Am Geriatr Soc* 1988; 36:845–859.

66. Tkatch L, Rapin CH, Rizzoli R, et al: Benefits of oral protein supplementation in elderly patients with fracture of the proximal femur (abstract). *J Am Coll Nutr* 1992; 11: 5.

41

Infant and Pediatric Nutrition

Walter Jakob Chwals, M.D.

A growing understanding of the basic pathophysiologic alterations that accompany acute injury states has led to a heightened awareness of the importance of specialized nutrition in the critical care setting. Reductions in mortality and morbidity following injury have increasingly evolved from advances in the areas of metabolism, nutrition, immunology, and infectious disease that

727

improve management of the acutely ill patient. Implicit in this evolution is a more comprehensive understanding of mechanisms underlying the response of the human body to acute metabolic stress.

It is reasonable to assume that events that characterize this response have a teleologically beneficial purpose in promoting recovery. Adverse consequences may result when the host is unable to meet the metabolic demands imposed by various injury states. Furthermore, it is now apparent that the intensity of the injury insult can disrupt the homeostatic host mechanisms that temper the acute metabolic stress response, thus increasing the toxic effects of injury. Strategies designed to block certain aspects of this response may be effective but must be carried out with care to avoid depriving the host of necessary defense mechanisms to combat injury insult and promote recovery. Most successful therapeutic modifications to date serve to enhance certain aspects of the response mechanism by supplementing host deficiencies.

The principles of nutritional support during critical illness are more in keeping with a general concept of metabolic resuscitation than with maintenance of standard nutritional parameters. The nutritional requirements to meet metabolic demands during injury states are more extensive in scope and quite different from the nutritional needs of healthy subjects. Although many putatively beneficial effects of therapeutic modifications have been described, the most convincing are those that result in improved clinical outcome.

Although much of the data discussed in this chapter have been generated through the study of animal and adult human subjects, they provide an important foundation for ongoing investigations of the injury response in acutely ill infant and pediatric subjects. A substantial effort has been made to include data generated in infants and young children whenever possible, although

much work has yet to be done in these populations.

NUTRITIONAL REQUIREMENTS AND DELIVERY IN HEALTHY CHILD

Nutritional needs can be divided into the general categories of energy, protein, and nonprotein substrate delivery. Amounts differ in children as compared with adults, primarily because of increased requirements for growth and activity in the pediatric population. This is especially true during early infancy, where visceral organ growth is rapid and extensive relative to muscle and fat growth (Fig 40–1).[1] Growth alteration during acute metabolic stress is age dependent and constitutes a major distinguishing factor between the metabolic stress response of infants vs. older children.

Energy Requirements

Energy can be partitioned into maintenance metabolic needs (basal metabolic rate, activity, and heat loss to the environment) and growth. Energy requirements are age related and are three to four times higher for infants than for adults (Table 41–1). In premature infants, daily needs may increase to 150 kcal/kg/day.[2] Although high infant energy needs are partially attributable to

TABLE 41–1.

Age-Adjusted Energy Requirements*

| Age (yr) | Energy Delivery† | |
	kcal/kg/day	kcal/day
0–1	120–90	500–1000
1–7	90–75	1000–1500
7–12	75–60	1500–2000
12–18	60–30	2000
>18	30–25	2000–1300

*Adapted from Wretlind A: Nutr Metab 1972; 14(suppl):1–57.
†The left-sided values in each column indicate requirements at the lowest age of the interval (e.g., 120 kcal/kg/day or 500 kcal/day at the age of 0 years).

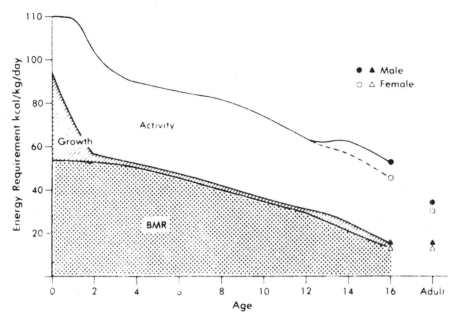

FIG 41–1.
Change in energy requirement per kilogram of body weight during growth. BMR = basal metabolic rate. (From Holliday MA: Body composition and energy needs during growth, in Falkner F, Tanner JM (eds): *Human Growth: A Comprehensive Treatise*, ed 2. *Postnatal Growth Neurobiology*, vol 2. New York, Plenum Publishing Corp, 1986, p 102. Used by permission.)

an accelerated metabolic rate, a substantial portion of energy is also required for growth. Normal healthy infants will utilize approximately 35% to 40% of the daily caloric intake for growth (energy cost of tissue synthesis and energy stored in new tissue) during the first 6 months of life. At 2 years of age, only about 2% to 5% of energy intake is used for this purpose.[1] The basal metabolic rate is approximately 50 to 55 kcal/kg/day in infancy and gradually declines to about 20 to 25 kcal/kg/day during adolescence.[3]

Protein Requirements

Protein requirements correlate with the basal metabolic rate (as assessed by resting energy expenditure) and decrease with age.[4] Protein caloric delivery is therefore relatively constant and should constitute approximately 7% to 10% of the total caloric intake. In hospitalized patients, we generally provide 2.0 to 2.5 g/kg/day to infants up to 2 years of age, 1.5 to 2.0 g/kg/day to chil-

dren 2 to 10 years of age, and 1.0 to 1.5 g/kg/day thereafter.

Nonprotein Requirements

Most infant enteral formulations provide a relatively balanced delivery of nonprotein calories in the range of 45% ± 4% of the total caloric intake each for carbohydrate and fat. In the postnatal period, infant metabolism is characterized by a greater dependence on lipid substrate for energy needs.[5] There is some evidence that premature infants, because of impaired fat absorption by an immature gut, may benefit from increased concentrations of medium-chain triglycerides (MCTs) in enteral formulations.[6] Carbohydrates remain important as a source of energy and are optimally provided in the form of starches such as those found in cereals, vegetables, and flour. Simple sugars such as sucrose should be limited but are generally overused in the American diet.

Noncaloric Requirements

Recommended dietary allowances for vitamins, minerals, and trace elements have been suggested for healthy infants and children.[7] Some special concerns merit brief review because these may be important in the selection of proper formulations for certain populations. Vitamin C and D requirements have been reported to be greater for infants as compared with older children.[8] However, there is growing concern that vitamin needs for premature infants, particularly lipid-soluble vitamins, have been overestimated, and clinical studies are currently under way to reevaluate this issue. Premature infants have higher trace element requirements, especially zinc.[9] Premature infants also require increased supplements of calcium, phosphorus, iron, and folate. The putative value of vitamin E supplementation in preventing retrolental fibroplasia and intraventricular hemorrhage is currently being evaluated in clinical trials, but this remains controversial. Carnitine supplementation in premature infants may improve fat utilization by increasing fatty acid availability for mitochondrial oxidation.[10]

Enteral Feeding

Breast feeding remains the gold standard for nutritional support of the healthy neonate. In addition to fostering the psychosocial bonding between mother and child, breast milk is believed to provide optimal nutrient content to support human growth. It also supplements infant immunocompetence by providing immunoactive substrates. Breast milk feeding is recommended for up to 4 to 6 months after birth but may need to be supplemented or discontinued if maternal production is inadequate or if problems such as breast milk–associated jaundice, hypernatremia (resulting from low milk production), or mastitis occur. Supplemental iron and vitamin D are suggested if breast milk is continued af-

ter 4 months. Primarily because of inadequate calcium deposition, fortified breast milk is recommended for premature infants.

Infant enteral formulations generally mimic breast milk in caloric density but provide more protein, calcium, phosphorus, and iron. Products designed for premature infants contain even higher concentrations of these constituents, and many include a substantial portion of fat substrate as MCT (for reasons previously discussed). Most formulations are within the isoosmolar range. Since gastric emptying is inversely proportional to caloric density and osmolarity, concentrated preparations must be used with caution because they can predispose to aspiration. In premature infants, the initial use of a carefully placed, soft gastric or transpyloric feeding tube for continuous drip feedings may be beneficial until gastric function improves and suck/swallow coordination matures. Neonatal gastrointestinal tract immaturity, characterized by decreased secretion of amylase, pancreatic lipase, disaccharidase, and lactase, has led to enteral product modifications in fat (MCTs) and carbohydrate (lactose-free) substrates to increase nutrient absorption.

Inadequate absorption can result in poor growth or diarrhea. The biochemical products of malabsorption are better than diarrhea for evaluating feeding intolerance.[11] Carbohydrate malabsorption can be documented by a fecal pH less than 5.5 and the presence of greater than 0.25 g/dL of reducing substances in the stool. Fat malabsorption is assessed by the fat content of a 72-hour stool collection. Age-adjusted values have been reported,[12] but after 6 months of age, healthy infants should absorb 90% of ingested fat.

NUTRITIONAL ASSESSMENT

Accurate nutritional and metabolic assessment is particularly difficult in the neonatal and pediatric intensive care settings. This is true because the metabolic events that accompany acute injury states in infants and children are incompletely understood. In addition, they frequently cause changes that render standard techniques based on assumptions derived from the evaluation of nonstressed subjects invalid.

Anthropometry

The gold standard for assessing the adequacy of nutritional delivery in the healthy nonstressed child is growth. Growth may be assessed by body weight norms for age and sex[13] and these have been revised for premature infants.[14] Heel-crown length and head circumference are useful adjuncts to body weight in the infant population, as is height in older children. Malnutrition in the nonstressed pediatric population can more accurately be determined by weight-for-height and height-for-age evaluation.[15] Surveys have indicated that acute and chronic malnutrition may approach 15% and 50% respectively in hospitalized pediatric patients.[16]

Anthropometric techniques of body composition analysis can be based on measurements of skin fold thickness and limb circumferences.[17] These methods rely on the assumption that single or multiple measurements, taken at various anatomic sites, accurately reflect the fat mass and lean body mass of the entire subject, a premise that is controversial.[18]

There are several important problems involved with the use of anthropometric techniques in critically ill pediatric patients, particularly in infant populations. A wide variability in body compartment composition exists because of differences in body habitus in infants.[19] Moreover, infant body composition is known to change rapidly as a function of differential growth and development.[1, 20] The rate of these changes may be significantly different in premature infants[21] or with growth retardation. Even healthy infants and children have a broad range of normal growth for any

given age and sex.[19, 22] It is therefore difficult to assess body composition by using these techniques in children and impossible to evaluate growth unless previous sequential data have been gathered over a longer term. The main problem in the intensive care setting, however, relates to the fact that critically ill subjects tend to increase weight because of third-space fluid gains during acute metabolic stress at the very time when catabolism of endogenous protein, fat, and carbohydrate stores is taking place. This phenomenon can lead to spurious results when using the standard anthropometric techniques discussed above.[23]

Bioelectric Impedance Analysis

This form of body composition analysis is based on the physical principle that fat has low electrical conductivity and high impedance relative to water. A small, imperceptible current (800 μA; frequency, 50 kHz) is passed through electrodes attached to the hands and feet of the subject. Electrical resistance and reactance are measured, and total-body water (TBW) volumes are determined.[24] In studies involving healthy, nonstressed adults, TBW measured with this technique correlated well with TBW measured by using $^2H_2^{18}O$ dilution analysis.[25] This type of comparison was recently carried out in nonstressed, low–birth weight infants with promising results.[26] In this study, the authors were also able to establish a reasonably good correlation between extracellular water determinations obtained by using bioelectric impedance analysis (BIA) as compared with bromide dilution values. Although this method has not yet been investigated in critically ill patients, it is of great potential value because it can be carried out quickly, easily, and safely at the patient's bedside. If validated accuracy is established, such technology could be used to calculate body cell mass changes as they occur in response to acute metabolic stress and would thereby be of considerable value in monitoring the efficacy of therapeutic strategies as they relate to protein, carbohydrate, and fat metabolism during this critical period.

Immunocompetence

Total lymphocyte counts and delayed hypersensitivity testing have been used to assess degrees of protein-calorie malnutrition.[27, 28] Since injury states are known to induce anergy and frequently induce substantial alterations in the white cell population, these methods have limited applicability during acute metabolic stress.

METABOLIC ASSESSMENT

Acute Metabolic Stress: Overview

In response to a variety of local or systemic injury stimuli (such as trauma, sepsis, acute inflammatory conditions), a series of metabolic changes that characterize the acute stress state occur (Fig 41–2). In large part, this response is stereotypical and does not depend as much upon the nature of the insult as its degree. Among the early features of injury response are the release of cytokines followed rapidly by important alterations in the hormonal environment: increased counterregulatory hormone levels associated with insulin and growth hormone resistance. As a result,

a sequence of metabolic events is initiated that includes the catabolism of endogenous stores of protein, carbohydrate, and fat to provide essential substrate intermediates (primarily amino acids) and energy necessary to fuel the ongoing response process. Amino acids from catabolized proteins flow to the liver, where they provide substrate for the synthesis of acute-phase proteins and glucose (gluconeogenesis). The acute metabolic stress response, then, represents a hypermetabolic, hypercatabolic state[29] that results in the loss of endogenous tissue[30] and can lead to poor clinical outcome in the absence of appropriate exogenous support.[31] As the acute response resolves, adaptive anabolic metabolism ensues to restore catabolic losses.[32] In children, this phase is characterized by the resumption of somatic growth. The goal of metabolic and nutritional resuscitation in the critically ill child is to promote the earlier and more complete evolution to growth recovery.

Cytokines and Nonprotein Mediators of Inflammation

Over the past several years, intense interest has focused on a group of peptides that are secreted by a number of cells, including macrophages, monocytes, lymphocytes, and vascular

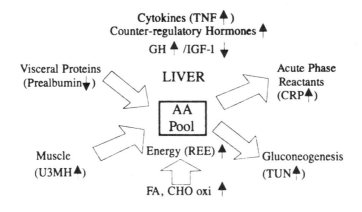

FIG 41–2.

Metabolic response to acute injury. *TNF* = tumor necrosis factor; *GH* = growth hormone; *IGF-I* = insulin-like growth factor I; *AA* = amino acid; *CRP* = C-reactive protein; *TUN* = total urinary nitrogen; *FA, CHO oxi* = fatty acid and carbohydrate oxidation; *U3MH* = urinary 3-methylhistidine; *REE* = resting energy expenditure.

smooth muscle, in response to a variety of metabolic stress stimuli. These peptides, called cytokines, appear to have important regulatory functions in mediating the metabolic and immune responses to injury. Several prominent cytokines (among an ever-growing list) are tumor necrosis factor (TNF), interleukin-1 (IL-1), interleukin-2 (IL-2), interleukin-6 (IL-6), and interferon-γ (IFN-γ). Although these peptides are secreted in small amounts and have relatively short serum half-lives, they appear to individually or synergistically mediate a cascade of events with widespread metabolic and immunologic effects.[33, 34] Cytokines have been shown to play an important role in the host response mechanism to a variety of inflammatory, neoplastic, and acute injury states.[33, 34]

Production of TNF is induced by a number of stimuli, particularly endotoxin.[35–37] This cytokine is thought to play a crucial role in the pathophysiology of endotoxin shock.[34] In fact, many effects of endotoxin are identical to those of TNF.[38, 39] Among many other effects, TNF induces neutrophil release from bone marrow (leukocytosis), regulates neutrophil degranulation and superoxide production,[40] causes increased endothelial permeability,[41] and causes the release of IL-1 and prostaglandin E_2 (PGE$_2$) in vitro and in vivo.[42, 43] TNF may promote muscle catabolism[44] and decrease muscle amino acid uptake[45] while increasing hepatic uptake of amino acids[46] and is associated with elevations in the serum concentrations of acute-phase proteins[47] and adrenocorticotropic hormone (ACTH)[38] levels. Systemic manifestations associated with TNF such as fever and tachycardia are blocked by ibuprofen,[38] thus suggesting that these responses involve cyclooxygenase-mediated intermediates of arachidonic acid such as PGE$_2$.

The systemic and metabolic effects of IL-1 are generally similar to those of TNF.[33] They include fever, neutrophilia, anorexia, lethargy, increased synthesis of hepatic acute-phase proteins, decreased synthesis of hepatic visceral proteins, increased ACTH secretion, increased IL-6 concentrations, hypozincemia, and hypoferremia. At higher levels, IL-1 induces hypotension and leukopenia. In addition, IL-1 stimulates fibroblast proliferation and collagen production,[33] effects that have an impact on wound healing. In contrast, however, are recent data that show an early decrease in serum insulin-like growth factor 1 (IGF-1) levels following the administration of IL-1,[48] an effect that may contribute substantially to infant growth retardation during acute metabolic stress. Like TNF, IL-1 can activate both T and B lymphocytes.[33] In addition, IL-1 may be instrumental in stimulating T-helper cells to produce IL-2.[49]

Interleukin-6 plays a dominant role in inflammation. Its principal effect appears to be the stimulation of hepatic synthesis of acute-phase proteins.[50] Following acute injury, serum IL-6 concentrations increase prior to and correlate well with subsequent increases in serum C-reactive protein (CRP) concentrations in patients with normal liver function.[51] High IL-6 levels are also associated with elevated IgM and IgG serum concentrations[50] and thrombocytosis,[50, 52] thus suggesting strong bone marrow stimulation. Interleukin-6 can act in concert with IL-2 or IFN-γ to stimulate myeloid cell growth and T-cell differentiation.[53]

IL-2 and IFN-γ have important immunomodulatory functions and have elevated concentrations in response to antigen-antibody interactions. The most dominant effect of IL-2 is its tumoricidal activity,[54] but it also induces elevation of counter regulatory hormone levels and is associated with systemic symptoms such as malaise, fever, and tachycardia.[55] IL-2 may also stimulate the release of IFN-γ.[56] This mechanism may be an important determinant of sepsis-related death since anti–IFN-γ improves the survival rate of mice following endotoxin challenge.[57]

Many biological properties are shared by a number of cytokines.[33] In addition, various cytokines may act synergistically to augment toxicity. Negative nitrogen balance, muscle proteolysis, and hemodynamic imbalance are substantially increased by TNF and IL-1 given together rather than separately.[43] IL-1 has also been found to potentiate the lethal effects of TNF.[58]

Cytokines can effect their own elaboration or the elaboration of other cytokines through receptor-specific regulatory mechanisms[59, 60] or through the induction of metabolic products like oxygen scavenger molecules or corticosteroids.[33] PGE_2 has been shown to regulate TNF gene expression. Furthermore, the release of macrophage-derived cytokines caused by endotoxin challenge can be upregulated by PGE_1.[61] Receptor downregulation is thought to be the mechanism responsible for the injury protective effects, such as improved survival following the administration of endotoxin, that are observed when animals have been pretreated with TNF or IL-1.[33, 34] In addition, presumably because excessive or prolonged exposure to cytokines such as TNF or IL-1 can result in exhaustion of host defense functions, the use of monoclonal antibodies or naturally occurring inhibitors of cytokines (or their receptor proteins) can improve survival following endotoxin challenge.[33, 34, 62, 63]

Nonprotein molecules induced by cytokines mediate many of the inflammatory and immunologic events associated with the acute injury response. These molecules include arachidonic acid metabolites synthesized via the cyclooxygenase pathway, of which PGE_2 is the principal immunomodulator (see "Nutritional Immunomodulation" below).[49] IL-1 stimulates macrophage and neutrophil synthesis of leukotrienes from arachidonic acid via the lipooxygenase pathway,[64, 65] and these leukotrienes have important inflammatory functions and also play key roles, along with PGE_2, in T- and B-lymphocyte activation.[49] Cytokines also induce leukocyte production of superoxide radicals,[66] which can contribute significantly to the local inflammatory response to injury. Ischemia, caused by cytokine-induced hypoperfusion, activates microvascular endothelial xanthine oxidase. Resuscitative reperfusion improves oxygen delivery to ischemic tissue and results in the formation of superoxide radicals by endothelial cells, neutrophils, and fixed macrophages, which then injure the endothelium. The use of antioxidant therapy (superoxide dismutase) has been shown to preserve endothelial integrity.[67, 68] Finally, IL-1 has been shown to induce the production of nitric oxide,[69] which mediates vasodilation during sepsis[70] and may regulate the production of cyclooxygenase metabolites.[71] The stimulation by endotoxin, TNF, IL-1, or IFN-γ of a variety of cells (including endothelial cells, macrophages, Kupffer cells, and hepatocytes) results in the release of nitric oxide. This mechanism is thought to play an important role in sepsis-related hypotension. N^G-monomethyl-L-arginine inhibition of nitric oxide production has been shown to decrease endotoxin-induced hypotension but also promotes increased hepatocellular injury.[72]

Hormonal Alterations and the Catabolic Response

Insulin is a potent anabolic hormone responsible for glycogen synthesis and the storage of carbohydrate, lipogenesis and the storage of fat, and new protein synthesis.[73] Insulin and IGF-1 are essential hormones for somatic growth in infants and children. Acute metabolic stress is characterized by substantial increases in serum concentrations of catecholamines, glucagon, and cortisol, referred to as counterregulatory hormones because they counteract, or oppose, the anabolic effects of insulin. Catecholamines cause hyperglycemia by promoting hepatic glycogenolysis, by causing conversion of skeletal muscle glycogen to lactate, which is then transported to the liver for conversion to glucose (Cori cycle), and by suppression of the pancreatic secretion of insulin. Catecholamines also induce lipolysis, which results in the mobilization of free fatty acids (FFAs). Finally, catecholamines induce hypermetabolism, which results in an increase in the basal metabolic rate, an effect that can be blocked by β-adrenergic receptor antagonists. Cortisol promotes gluconeogenesis and induces muscle proteolysis, perhaps in conjunction with TNF.[74] The major amino acid sources for gluconeogenesis are alanine[75] and glutamine[76] from skeletal muscle and gut. Hepatic uptake of these amino acids is accelerated during acute metabolic stress.[77, 78] Cortisol also causes insulin resistance. Although insulin levels may be elevated during acute metabolic stress, its anabolic effects are abrogated. Glucagon induces glycolysis and gluconeogenesis. The administration of these hormones has been shown to result in increased protein catabolism associated with increased whole-body protein turnover in healthy adult subjects.[79] This effect may be due, in part, to net muscle protein catabolism.[80] Increased muscle proteolysis, assessed by elevated levels of 3-methylhistidine (3-MH), an amino acid released as a result of skeletal muscle catabolism, has been noted following TNF administration in rats.[81] We have measured urinary 3-MH levels in surgically stressed infants (see Fig 41–2) and have observed significantly increased postoperative urinary values by postoperative day 3 that return to normal after 7 days as stress resolves (unpublished data).

In health, the major actions of growth hormone (GH) are to decrease protein catabolism and promote protein synthesis, to promote fat mobilization and the conversion of FFA to acetylcoenzyme A, and to decrease glucose oxidation while increasing glycogen deposition.[82] However, the anabolic effects of GH, particularly as they relate to protein metabolism, are mediated principally by IGF-1.[83] During acute metabolic stress, IGF-1 levels fall, and IGF-1 inhibitory binding protein concentrations rise. In this state, the substrate-mobilizing effects of GH prevail and result in increased lipolysis and FFA oxidation.[84]

Both term and premature neonatal infants are capable of generating a counterregulatory response to surgically induced injury.[85, 86] The response is relatively short-lived (24 hours) and can be dampened by fentanyl anesthesia. Recent work in preterm baboons demonstrates a graded counterregulatory hormone response based on injury severity.[87] However, the onset of the response appears to be delayed and of longer duration as compared with the hormonal response reported in more mature stressed infants, thus suggesting the possibility that functional immaturity associated with curtailed gestational development may play a role in this process.

Visceral Protein Status

The liver normally synthesizes a number of proteins that constitute labile pools within the serum compartment. Among others, these proteins include albumin, transferrin, prealbumin, and retinol binding protein. These proteins account for early nitrogen losses resulting from catabolism induced by injury (or starvation).[73] As compared with albumin (half-life [t], 20 days), both prealbumin (t, 2 days) and retinol binding protein (t, 10 hours) have shorter serum half-lives and constitute smaller protein pools. Visceral proteins with shorter half-lives correlate better than albumin with other variables of malnutrition.[88] Although serum albumin[89] and prealbumin[90] concentrations both decrease precipitously in response to surgical trauma, prealbumin concentrations appear to be more significantly depressed.[90] We measured albumin, prealbumin, and retinol binding protein preoperatively and on postoperative days 1 and 5 in ten infants (average age, 7.5 months). Both prealbumin and retinol binding protein were superior to albumin in assessing acute changes resulting from visceral protein catabolism (preoperative to postoperative day 1) and following resumption of visceral protein synthesis (postoperative day 1 to postoperative day 5) as the metabolic stress response resolved (Fig 41–3). Changes were most easily seen with prealbumin, which is the visceral protein marker we prefer.

Total Urinary Nitrogen

Protein and fat catabolism during acute metabolic stress results in increased urinary nitrogen losses. Protein catabolism increases the size of the hepatic free amino acid pool. The liver deaminates a substantial portion of these amino acids to synthesize glucose (gluconeogenesis); this results in increased nitrogen that is excreted in the urine as urea.[73] Fat catabolism (lipolysis) yields increased FFAs, which when oxidized, result in ketone body formation. These ketoacids are buffered by ammonia and excreted in the urine.[91] Because urea nitrogen losses correlate poorly with ammonia nitrogen losses in the urine during injury states, it is pref-

erable to measure 24-hour total urinary nitrogen (TUN).[92] Since serial urinary nitrogen measurements reflect the degree and duration of catabolism resulting from various categories of injury and correlate grossly with hypermetabolism (increased stress-related energy expenditure),[29] this technique can be used to monitor the acute metabolic stress response and may also be valuable in determining injury severity.[93] We have noted a small (0.2 to 0.5 g of N_2) but significant increment in TUN during the first 2 to 4 days following major surgery in infants. These values return to normal levels by postoperative days 7 to 10 (Fig 41–4). Similar changes have been noted by others[94] and may also reflect nutritional repletion as the acute stress response resolves.[95] We have observed higher TUN in septic infants, but interpatient variability precludes estimating these losses from clinical impression alone.

Precise 24-hour urine output measurements are required. Bladder catheterization is often unnecessary since carefully applied urine collection bags can be adequate. Diapers must be weighed so that leakage can be accurately tabulated if it occurs. If 24-hour nitrogen intake (N_1) is calculated (24-hour protein intake [g]/6.25), then daily

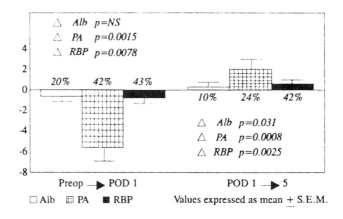

FIG 41–3.
Mean percent change (Δ) of visceral proteins during acute metabolic stress. *Alb* = serum albumin (g/dL); *PA* = serum prealbumin (mg/dL); *RBP* = serum retinol binding protein (mg/dL); *Preop* = within 24 hours prior to surgery; *POD* = postoperative day. Statistical analysis used the paired *t*-test.

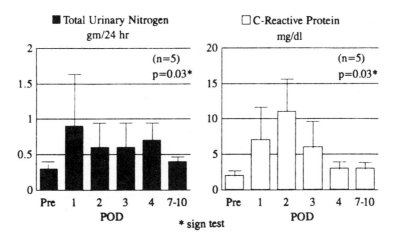

FIG 41–4.
Infant metabolic response to surgical stress. *Pre* = values obtained within 24 hours before surgery; *POD* = postoperative day.

nitrogen balance (NB) can be calculated for infants as follows:

$$NB = N_I - (TUN + 75 \text{ mg/kg N}_2),$$

assuming approximately 50 to 60 mg/kg N_2 daily fecal losses[96] and 15 mg/kg daily cutaneous N_2 losses (Table 41–2). Appropriate modifications can be easily made with minimal or absent fecal excretion. A negative nitrogen balance is generally observed during acute metabolic stress, whereas a positive nitrogen balance is associated with growth (anabolism).

TABLE 41–2.

Guidelines for Infant Metabolic Monitoring During Acute Stress

Parameter	Stress Characteristic Evaluated*
Prealbumin	Visceral protein catabolism Hepatic synthesis
Total urinary nitrogen (TUN)	Protein and fat catabolism Gluconeogenesis $NB = N_I - (TUN + 75 \text{ mg/kg N}_2)$
C-reactive protein	Acute-phase response
Indirect calorimetry	Energy expenditure and RQ $EB = E_I - MEE$ $RQ = \dot{V}_{CO_2}/\dot{V}_{O_2}$

*NB = nitrogen balance; N_I = 24-hour nitrogen intake; EB = energy balance; E_I = energy intake; MEE = measured energy intake; RQ = respiratory quotient

Acute-Phase Response

One of the key features of the acute metabolic stress response is an increase in the hepatic synthesis of certain specialized proteins. These acute-phase proteins, so called because they were found in serum obtained from patients acutely ill with infectious disease, are now known to appear in response to a variety of stimuli such as tissue injury, inflammation, bacterial infection, antigen-antibody interactions, and endotoxin challenge.[97] This process is mediated by cytokines (principally IL-6[51]) that selectively redirect hepatic protein synthesis such that the synthesis of acute-phase proteins is increased while the synthesis of visceral protein is retarded. The reprioritization of hepatic protein synthesis in response to injury has been elegantly demonstrated in a guinea pig burn model[98] and appears to be cytokine induced.[33, 51] These proteins appear to carry out a number of important immunologic and repair functions during the acute stress period.[97] CRP is an acute-phase protein that, among its several known biological functions, is capable of activating the complement pathway in the absence of immunoglobulin. In the presence of activated complement, it can also induce monocyte phagocytosis of bacteria and enhance natural killer (NK) cell activity.[99] After injury, there is a latent period of 6 to 16 hours followed by increased serum levels that generally peak at 24 to 48 hours. Since its serum half-life is 4 to 6 hours, decreases in the hepatic synthesis of CRP (as the acute metabolic stress response resolves) are promptly reflected in decreased serum levels of this acute-phase protein. In children, marked increases in serum CRP concentrations have been observed following a variety of metabolic stress stimuli,[100-102] even in immunosuppressed hosts.[103] In infants, this same effect has been noted in response to bacterial etiologies.[104-106] We investigated the perioperative acute-phase response in infants and observed significant increases in serum CRP concentrations on postoperative day 1 (relative to preoperative values) that returned toward normal values by postoperative day 4.[107] We have noted a similar CRP response pattern in neonates following surgical trauma. These changes in serum acute-phase protein levels appear to coincide with urinary nitrogen excretion, thus demonstrating two important aspects of altered protein metabolism during acute metabolic stress (Fig 41−4). Serum CRP concentrations can be easily and accurately measured by using laser beam nephelometry or rapid turbidimetric methods.[101, 108] Approximately 0.5 cc of venous blood is required. Measurements can be carried out within 10 minutes, and many hospital laboratories now possess this capability.

Indirect Calorimetry

Energy expenditure is a characteristic feature of metabolism that can be measured by the amount of heat released. This is the principle of direct calorimetry[73] in which energy release is quantified by the amount of heat required to raise the temperature of 1 cc of water by 1°C from 15 to 16°C (1 calorie). Since this methodology involves confining the subject in a closed calorimeter for extended time periods. It is impractical for clinical use. In contrast, indirect calorimetry can be carried out at the patient's bedside. It involves the measurement of the differences in O_2 and CO_2 concentrations between a known volume (minute ventilation) of inspired and expired gas. In this way, oxygen consumption ($\dot{V}o_2$) and carbon dioxide production ($\dot{V}co_2$) may be calculated. These calculations[109] are based on known and constant relationships between $\dot{V}o_2$, $\dot{V}co_2$, and heat produced (energy expenditure) for many metabolic processes. These include, among others, the oxidation of various carbohydrates, fats, and proteins as well as lipogenesis.[110] The respiratory quotient (RQ), which may be expressed as $\dot{V}co_2/\dot{V}o_2$ (Table 41−2), is also specific and constant for each of these processes, for instance, the total oxidation of carbohydrate (RQ = 1.0) or fat (RQ = 0.7). For lipogenesis (the synthesis of fat from carbohydrate), the RQ equals 2.75.[111]

The value of indirect calorimetry in the intensive care setting lies in the fact that estimations of energy expenditure based on other clinical criteria are notoriously inaccurate.[112] The actual measured energy expenditure (MEE) is frequently much less than predicted values based on clinical grounds.[113, 114] While average MEE values in large patient series tend to differentiate various degrees of injury,[29] individual subjects can respond to similar injury states with widely diverse MEE values.[115] We studied 20 critically ill infants and found a 3.5-fold difference in MEE (adjusted for age and weight) between the lowest and highest interpatient values.[116] Although an improved understanding of the metabolic stress response in infants may eventually provide other indices that adequately predict energy expenditure, at present the only accurate clinical means of determining daily energy expenditure in the critical care setting is to measure it.

Energy expenditure measurements have been shown to correlate well with weight gain following nutritional repletion of malnourished children.[117] In the critical care setting, indirect calorimetry may be useful in accurately determining caloric needs during acute metabolic stress to avoid overfeeding and promote optimal growth recovery (see "Nutritional Repletion" ahead).

Metabolic cart technology employing pneumotachometers that precisely measure small tidal volumes is available and has been validated in infant populations.[116, 118, 119] Such carts are easily used in the intensive care setting and can measure energy expenditure in mechanically ventilated as well as nonventilated infants. Accurate MEE can be obtained in mechanically ventilated infants with noncuffed endotracheal tubes if no audible air leak is present.[120] An adequate determination of MEE usually requires 20 to 30 minutes and correlates well with 24-hour MEE values in both acutely stressed adult and infant populations.[121, 122]

Therapeutic Inhibition of Acute Metabolic Stress Response

As previous discussion of the factors that mediate the response to acute injury emphasizes, this sequence of metabolic events constitutes a complex and delicately balanced process. Teleologically, the acute metabolic stress response represents the best defense mechanism against insult that the body has been able to generate during millenia of evolutionary selection. While this fact certainly does not imply that the process is faultless or that it cannot be improved through therapeutic modification, it does suggest that such modification be undertaken with caution so as not to disrupt endogenous response homeostasis to the degree that the overall result is counterproductive. It would seem reasonable to assume that the greatest likelihood of success might derive from interventions that fine-tune the response rather than those that cause gross, multifaceted alterations.

It is increasingly apparent that the massive metabolic alterations caused by severe injury states can overwhelm the endogenous regulatory mechanisms that ensure response homeostasis, thus promoting rather than abrogating the toxic effects of injury. This understanding has led to attempts to block certain response pathways known to propagate further harm during critical illness. One such intervention is the use of corticosteroids. As previously discussed, endogenous cortisol release following injury is known to cause a variety of catabolic effects. Additional effects include suppression of immunologic function such as lymphopenia[123] and suppression of inflammation. The exogenous use of corticosteroids has been shown to potentiate many of these endogenous effects. For instance, pretreatment with corticosteroids can decrease TNF elaboration and dampen the clinical symptoms associated with endotoxin challenge.[124] The evaluation of corticosteroid therapy to inhibit acute metabolic stress presents many problems, and a variety of flaws in major investigations that focus on this topic have been pointed out.[125] Early work with patients in septic shock showed a marked survival advantage when corticosteroids were administered vs. placebo.[126] A substantial number of subsequent investigations, however, have failed to demonstrate a survival advantage in large placebo-controlled series of septic patients treated with high-dose corticosteroid therapy.[127–129] It is possible that carefully defined patient subgroups might benefit from corticosteroid therapy, as was the case in a cohort with typhoid fever.[130] However, this was a group of young, otherwise healthy patients who did not require inotropic or ventilatory support. In contrast, a recent report of septic subjects demonstrated a significant increase in mortality among a subgroup of patients with serum creatinine concentrations greater than 2.0 mg/dL who received high-dose methylprednisolone vs. placebo.[131] Another recent report evaluated single-dose perioperative methylprednisolone combined with postoperative indomethacin and bupivacaine/morphine analgesia vs. postoperative morphine/acetaminophen in otherwise healthy well-nourished patients undergoing elective colon resection.[132] Although postoperative pain control was better, wound dehiscence occurred in 2 of 11 patients in the steroid-treated group vs. zero of 9 in the control group. Pneumonia developed in 2 control group patients (vs. none in the steroid-treated group), but this complication might have been prevented by aggressive attention to pulmonary toilet, whereas complications in the study group were likely due to steroid inhibition of wound healing.

Recent evidence has suggested the presence of in vivo mechanisms regulating cytokine activity during acute metabolic stress states.[63] In addition to stress-induced glucocorticoid release, which can downregulate TNF and IL-1 production, naturally occurring proteins that inhibit TNF and IL-1 activity have been identified in the serum and urine of acutely stressed patients. The function of these inhibitory proteins may be to downregulate excessive cytokine activity during the stress response. Isolation and sequence analysis of these proteins have demonstrated that they constitute at least two TNF receptor proteins[133, 134] and one IL-1 receptor protein.[135, 136] They inhibit TNF and IL-1 activity by competitively bonding with (thus blocking) TNF and IL-1 receptors and are now available in recombinant form (monoclonal antibodies). These TNF[137] and IL-1[138] receptor antagonists have been shown to decrease mortality in septic animals and are currently being evaluated in clinical trials.[63] It is important to note, however, that the use of anticytokine therapy has also been shown to increase mortality in several studies using animal infection models.[139-141] Furthermore, low-dose TNF administration has been shown to improve leukocyte function in vitro,[142] and IL-1 administration has been shown to improve survival in septic mice.[143] There are also reports that associate decreased endogenous cytokine activity with poor clinical outcome in critically ill septic patients.[144, 145] While it is apparent that an excessive cytokine response can increase injury to the host, it also seems that an appropriate cytokine response is necessary to promote the beneficial metabolic and immune conditions essential to a successful clinical outcome.

Alternative means of limiting the toxic effects of the acute metabolic stress response have recently been explored. As discussed earlier (see the section on cytokines), the arachidonic acid metabolite PGE_1 is known to mediate macrophage production of cytokines in response to endotoxin. Misoprostol, a PGE_1 analogue, has been shown to downregulate the murine peritoneal macrophage production of TNF, IL-1, and IL-6 following endotoxin challenge in vitro, presumably by interfering with the PGE_1 signal.[146] The N^G-monomethyl-L-arginine inhibition of nitric oxide, a compound released during sepsis that relaxes vascular smooth muscle cells, causes decreased endotoxin-induced hypotension but also results in increased hepatic injury.[72] Antioxidant therapy using oxygen free radical scavengers such as superoxide dismutase may prevent mucosal reperfusion injury by decreasing the levels of toxic oxygen metabolites.[68] Free radical spin trapping has been recently shown to downregulate TNF transcription following endotoxin administration in mice.[147] Fentanyl, known to dampen the counterregulatory response to injury, may improve mortality in a select subgroup of infants undergoing surgical correction of severe cardiac anomalies.[148] Finally, monoclonal and polyclonal antibodies directed against lipopolysaccharide have been shown to protect against the toxic effects of endotoxin and gram-negative bacteria in a variety of animal models.[149] This therapy does not block the stress response but, instead, reduces the injury insult. Initial results from randomized, prospective, placebo-controlled human trials demonstrate decreased mortality in some subsets of patients with gram-negative sepsis, but the value of these agents remains controversial.

In summary, these studies reinforce the view that the acute metabolic stress response is a finely balanced, very complex process. When response homeostasis is disrupted or overwhelmed by excessive mediator release (a condition that may be particularly frequent following severe injury), toxic effects may result. Therapeutic strategies designed to attenuate these effects by blocking the specific pathways that mediate them may provide substantial clinical benefit. However, such intervention must be undertaken with care to not inhibit the salutary effects of the response so that counterproductive outcomes might be avoided. It is clear that a more comprehensive understanding of the homeostatic mechanisms that mediate the acute metabolic stress response as well as a more precise stratification of injury severity is needed to increase the likelihood of success.

ASSESSMENT UTILIZATION

Injury Severity

The value of establishing injury severity lies in the metabolic response to such injury and the ability to predict clinical outcome from that response. This allows for the evaluation of treatment programs on the basis of comparable severity scores. The implication is that when injury response is stratified, then severity-related therapeutic strategies can be developed to supplement or enhance the response and improve the outcome. A number of severity scoring systems have been proposed for critically ill adult patients, and some have greater prognostic value than others in

predicting outcome, depending on the nature of the injury.[150-156] A scoring system relating injury severity (based on multiple physiologic variables) to mortality has been devised for pediatric patients.[157] A recent study has suggested that metabolic response parameters (energy expenditure and nitrogen excretion) may be useful in predicting mortality in the pediatric intensive care setting.[158] Metabolic monitoring has been used to stratify the injury response on the basis of energy expenditure and urinary nitrogen excretion.[29] A metabolic stress scoring system has been devised that uses modified nitrogen balance calculations.[93] Both CRP[101, 159] and prealbumin[160] have reported value in injury stratification and outcome. Serum TNF concentrations have been found to correlate with mortality in critically ill adult and pediatric patients following infection.[37, 161, 162]

Since the metabolic stress response represents an evolving phenomenon, it would seem most appropriate to evaluate the progress of this response in a serial fashion, at least daily, until the acute stress period has resolved. This fact is important because injury severity is a function not only of intensity but also of duration. Metabolic indices that reflect ongoing injury on day 5 certainly have very different prognostic connotations from those showing the same injury status on day 1 following the onset of acute metabolic stress and may have significant therapeutic implications.

In attempting to assess the metabolic response of the infant surgical population to acute injury (see Fig 41–2), we have routinely measured daily energy expenditure (MEE), serum indices (TNF, CRP, and prealbumin), and TUN throughout the perioperative period (preoperatively and on postoperative days 1 to 5, 7, and 10) (see Table 41–2). We stratified these patients by peak postoperative CRP values to high (CRP ≥ 7.0 mg/dL) and low (CRP < 7.0 mg/dL) stress groups. Serum prealbumin levels were lower and remained depressed for a significantly longer time period in the high-stress vs. the low-stress group.[163] These findings are consistent with results in critically ill adults.[160] In addition, when we grouped infants by postoperative mortality (within 30 days of surgery), we observed significant differences in serum prealbumin and peak CRP levels between survivors and nonsurvivors,[164] thus suggesting the potential predictive value of these metabolic indices for serial perioperative evaluation in this patient population (Figs 41–5 and 41–6). The strongest potential predictor appears to be day 5 prealbumin levels (Fig 41–7). Failure of the liver to resume visceral protein synthesis by this time (indicating continued acute metabolic stress) was associated with the most significant increase in infant mortality seen in our critical care population.

Nutritional Repletion During Metabolic Stress and Growth Recovery

For reasons previously discussed, the acute metabolic stress response represents a predominantly catabolic state. Endogenous tissue stores of protein, carbohydrate, and fat are invariably decreased during this period, and growth is impeded. This phenomenon has been clearly demonstrated in acutely ill premature infants[165, 166] (Fig 41–8). Cytokine-induced decreases in IGF-1[48] likely play an important role in stress-related growth retardation. Approximately 35% of predicted energy requirements for healthy infants are needed for growth (see Fig 41–1).[1] In addition, because of the reductions in activity and insensible losses typically observed in sedated infants in a thermoneutral intensive care environment, caloric requirements during acute metabolic stress are reduced to amounts necessary to meet basal metabolic needs alone. Therefore, if caloric repletion based on the predicted requirements for healthy infants is administered during the acute phase of metabolic stress, when the energy required for growth is negli-

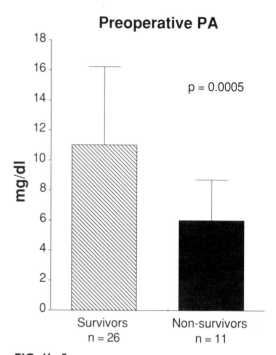

FIG 41–5.
Preoperative serum prealbumin *(PA)* concentrations obtained within 24 hours before surgery, where *n* is the number of patient data points obtained during this time interval.

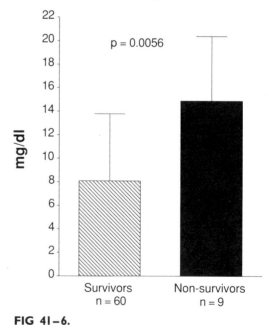

FIG 41–6.
Peak postoperative serum C-reactive protein *(CRP)* concentrations obtained within 48 hours following surgery, where *n* is the number of patient data points obtained during this time interval.

Late Prealbumin (POD 4 - 7)

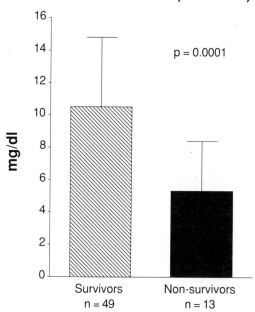

p = 0.0001

Survivors
n = 49

Non-survivors
n = 13

FIG 41–7.
Late postoperative serum prealbumin concentrations obtained from postoperative days *(POD)* 4 to 7 (average values), where *n* is the number of patient data points obtained during this time interval. These prealbumin concentrations in surviving infants represent a substantial increase from POD I levels that was not observed in the nonsurvivors, thus indicating ongoing acute metabolic stress in the latter (nonsurvivor) group.

gible, substantial overfeeding is likely.[116]

Infant energy expenditure following uncomplicated surgical procedures does not increase substantially over expected baseline testing values[167, 168]; in fact it may be lower for the reasons discussed above. In our original study including infants with a wide variety of stress insults,[116] there was substantial interpatient variability in MEE relative to the predicted basal metabolic rate. This variability may be attributable to substantial differences in the acute metabolic demands imposed by the underlying disease process.[29] For instance, an analysis of our current data base of acutely stressed infants demonstrates a trend toward significantly higher energy expenditure in actively septic vs. nonseptic subjects irrespective of surgical intervention, although considerable interpatient variability continues to be present (unpublished data).

As the acute phase of metabolic stress resolves, the adaptive (anabolic) phase ensues and results in resumption of somatic growth. Recovery is characterized by decreasing CRP and TUN values in association with increasing prealbumin, thus indicating that hepatic synthesis has shifted back toward repleting the visceral protein pool. This trend can be establish by the serial postinjury monitoring of these parameters.[116, 164, 169]

To avoid overfeeding infants during the acute metabolic stress period, our practice is to provide adequate protein supplements while limiting calorie repletion to amounts slightly in excess of *basal* metabolic needs.[3] Nutritional delivery during this period consists of protein (2.0 to 2.5 g/kg/day), fat (2 g/kg/day), and carbohydrate (10 g/kg/day) administered at rates necessary to meet maintenance daily fluid requirements (Table 41–3). This provides approximately 65 to 70 kcal/kg/day. Initially, peripheral vein parenteral delivery may constitute the majority of the caloric intake budget; however, in nearly all cases, we are able to provide 2 mL/hr enterally (via a soft, transpyloric feeding tube) in an attempt to avoid gut mucosal atrophy. In fact, we have found that many infants can receive most or all of this basal nutrition delivery (continuous rate, not a bolus) from elemental formulations containing short polypeptides as the major portion of protein substrate. When serial measurements of the metabolic parameters mentioned above demonstrate resolution of the acute stress phase, nutritional supplements are increased, preferably via the enteral route. To avoid premature increments in caloric delivery, daily indirect

TABLE 41–3.

Guidelines for Infant Nutritional Support During Acute Stress

Initial postinjury nutrition (enteral or parenteral at a maintenance volume rate)	Protein (2.5 g/hg/day) Fat (2 g/hg/day) Carbohydrate (10 g/hg/day)
Increase nutrition intake (enteral route preferred)	Respiratory quotient (<1.0 or decreased $\times$ 48 hr)

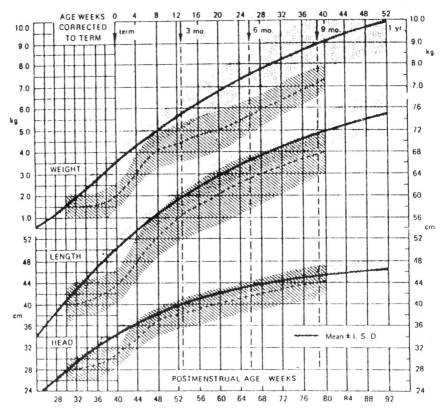

FIG 41–8.
The *diagonal shading* represents longitudinal growth of sick preterm infants, 28 to 32 weeks' gestation (mean ± 1 SD) superimposed on Babson's curve for postnatal growth in well infants. Note the growth cessation during acute illness. (From Maisels MJ, Marks KH: *J Pediatr* 1981; 98:663. Used by permission.)

calorimetric measurements are carried out to assess the RQ. Since RQ equals $\dot{V}_{CO_2}/\dot{V}_{O_2}$ and since overfeeding causes increased lipogenesis (and thus increased $\dot{V}_{CO_2}$ relative to $\dot{V}_{O_2}$[111]), excessive caloric intake (especially excessive carbohydrate intake[170, 171] generally results in a RQ greater than 1.0.

Using indirect calorimetry, we have observed that infants usually have RQ values above 1.0 after nutritional support (as outlined above) has been initiated in the immediate postoperative period.[169] This suggests some overfeeding even at near-basal caloric repletion rates during acute metabolic stress. At constant substrate and caloric delivery rates, the RQ usually falls below 1.0 in conjunction with resolution of the injury response (as confirmed by serum and urine metabolic parameters), usually within 5 days of surgery. This effect

likely occurs, at least in part, because of increased energy needs resulting from the resumption of anabolic metabolism (growth).

To test this hypothesis, we have calculated daily energy balance (EB) during the postoperative period in surgically stressed neonates. Somatic growth is characterized by a positive EB, which for healthy infants is usually greater than 45 to 50 kcal/kg/day.[96] In addition, we have found that a positive EB is associated with recovery of hepatic visceral protein synthesis following surgery in infants.[172] Calculation of EB can be made as follows:

$$EB = E_1 - MEE,$$

where E_1 represents energy intake and MEE represents measured energy expenditure (see Table 41–2).

We compared EB with RQ and CRP values obtained simultaneously and found that RQ was greater than 1.0 associated with EB near zero and high CRP values on postoperative day 1. We maintained constant daily caloric and substrate delivery until the RQ fell below 1.0, at which time caloric delivery was increased (see Table 41–3). By postoperative day 9, positive EB values had risen to levels consistent with normal growth, and these were associated with a RQ less than 1 and low CRP levels.[169] Since it has been shown that infant growth can be inhibited in association with acute illness (see Fig 41–8), we feel that this method provides a potentially useful guide to advance caloric delivery and optimize growth recovery without overfeeding infants recuperating from acute metabolic stress.

It is important to deliver precise protein-calorie support during the acute metabolic stress period. Excessive caloric delivery (overfeeding) can result in liver compromise,[173] which may impede the stress response. In addition, overfeeding (especially with excess carbohydrate) can rapidly increase carbon dioxide production and result in increased ventilatory requirements to avoid hypercapnia.[174] There is evidence that short-term caloric restriction (but not protein restriction) may improve the outcome following acute injury.[175] However, insufficient caloric delivery can increase reliance on endogenous lipid to meet the energy demands of acute stress. Following cardiac surgery in children receiving 10.5 kcal/kg/day (<20% mean energy expenditure), 78% of the total substrate utilization was contributed by oxidation of endogenous fat.[168] Such requirements may be difficult to meet for underfed neonates, especially premature infants, because of their limited fat stores.

Drawbacks of Total Parenteral Nutrition

Following the advent of total parenteral nutrition (TPN) in 1968[176] and the realization that it could save the lives of previously doomed infants with conditions that precluded adequate enteral nutrition such as gastroschisis and short-bowel syndrome, there has been great and often indiscriminate support for the use of this modality for nutritional repletion in pediatric patients. More recently, however, a growing consensus has evolved, particularly among clinicians who work in nutrition and critical care, that the indications for enteral nutrition are much broader than previously thought and that TPN should be used only when enteral nutrition is not possible. There are at least two compelling arguments that support this opinion.

The use of TPN has been associated with hepatobiliary disfunction, the onset of which is particularly rapid in the infant population, especially in preterm infants.[177, 178] Substantial liver compromise (within 2 to 3 weeks following the initiation of this mode of nutrition) characterized by jaundice, hepatomegaly, biochemical alterations including elevated liver enzyme levels and hyperbilirubinemia, and possibly eventual liver failure can develop in infants receiving TPN. Associated histopathologic findings include cholestasis, portal fibrosis, and cirrhosis. Catheter-related sepsis and thrombolic occlusion of the vena cava are common complications. Furthermore, acutely stressed infants, particularly those with sepsis, can have an even more precipitous course, although the effects of critical illness independent of TPN are also likely pathophysiologic factors that have an influence on this process.

The use of TPN vs. enteral nutritional delivery in acutely stressed high-risk patients (including children) has now been evaluated in a substantial number of randomized prospective trials. Recent meta-analysis of eight of these trials (involving high-risk surgical patients) shows a significant reduction in septic complications (18% vs. 35%) in the enterally fed patient group.[179] In addition, a study of 39 patients with greater than 50% total body surface area burns demonstrated significantly increased mortality rates (63% vs. 26%) in the group randomized to receive TPN supplementation of enteral calories vs. enteral calories alone.[180]

These data support the preferential use of enteral nutritional delivery if clinically feasible.

GUT INTEGRITY AND ACUTE METABOLIC STRESS

There is increasing recognition of the supportive role of the gut in acute injury states. The metabolic, immunologic, and infectious pathophysiologies of this important organ system are key factors in determining the metabolic stress response.

Gut Barrier

Because the intestines contain bacteria and endotoxin, maintenance of gut barrier function is essential. The gut barrier includes the intestinal mucosa and submucosa, the lymphatic system of the mesentery, the reticuloendothelial system (RES), and other immunocompetent cells within the splanchnic bed. Recent investigations suggest that physical or functional disruption of this barrier can result in the translocation of gut-derived bacteria and endotoxin. Translocation can lead to systemic bacteremia and/or endotoxemia culminating in increased morbidity and mortality.[181] Three basic mechanisms for translocation are intestinal bacterial overgrowth, especially with gram-negative organisms[182, 183]; impairment of host immune defenses[184]; and physical disruption of the gut mucosal barrier.[185, 186] Groups at high risk for translocation include immunocompromised and malnourished patients, burn and trauma victims, and critically ill patients with multisystem organ failure.[181, 187–191] Studies suggest that

the clinical outcome depends on the balance between injury severity and the adequacy of host defense mechanisms. For instance, translocation is more extensive as injury severity increases.[192] Excessive translocation can lead to impaired systemic immunity,[193] overwhelm RES clearance capacity, and result in injury to postsplanchnic organ systems.[194–196] In contrast, low levels of translocation may cause salutary immune system activation and result in protection against infectious challenge.[197]

Neonatal gut mucosal barrier function may be altered because of immaturity, especially in preterm infants. Newborn piglet gut allows increased transmucosal bacterial passage when compared with the gut of older, weaning piglets.[198] Prolonged endotoxemia has been associated with postoperative bowel dysfunction, wound dehiscence, and sepsis in human neonates.[199]

REINFORCING MUCOSAL BARRIER INTEGRITY

Enteral vs. Parenteral Feeding

Enteral nutritional delivery is critical in preventing bacterial translocation.[200] Parenteral nutrition (without glutamine supplementation) is associated with mucosal atrophy. In contrast, enteral formulations stimulate trophic gut hormone secretion and nourish the mucosa. Enterally fed, stressed humans have been found to have fewer postoperative septic-related complications when compared with those fed parenterally.[201] In guinea pigs, early vs. late enteral feeding has been shown to reduce the hypermetabolic response to burn injury and promote gut mucosal growth.[202] This effect on energy expenditure is likely due to decreased translocation resulting in a decreased metabolic stress response. In rats, immediate postoperative enteral feeding is associated with improved wound strength and less weight loss when compared with late feeding.[203] In all of these studies, better maintenance of intestinal barrier function with early, enteral nutrition is the most probable reason for improved outcome.

Small Polypeptides Vs. Free Amino Acids

Considerable debate has focused on whether short-chain polypeptides (two to five carbon length) diets are absorbed better by intestinal mucosa than formulations consisting primarily of free amino acids. In unstressed animals, polypeptide vs. amino acid diets are associated with decreased translocation,[204] improved bowel growth,[205] improved trophic gut hormone secretion,[206] and improved somatic growth and IGF-1 production.[205] Polypeptide diets also improve early somatic growth recovery[207] and survival[208–211] when compared with amino acid diets in metabolically stressed animals. Finally, polypeptide diets have been shown to be superior to amino acid diets in decreasing diarrhea, improving visceral protein synthesis, and decreasing the hospital stay of trauma patients.[212] These data suggest that polypeptide diets are better than amino acid diets in supporting bowel function during acute injury states.

Glutamine

Glutamine is the most abundant amino acid in plasma and skeletal muscle, but serum levels fall precipitously following acute metabolic stress, primarily because of increased uptake and metabolism by the gut.[213] Glutamine is a major energy source for intestinal mucosa[214] and may stimulate increased protein synthesis in enterocytes during acute injury states such as sepsis.[215] It is also deaminated by the gut to form alanine, which then flows via the splanchnic circulation to the liver. During acute stress, this gut-to-liver pathway provides a major contribution to the he-

patic amino acid pool.[216] Provision of standard parenteral nutrition is associated with atrophy of the intestinal mucosa.[217] In contrast, glutamine-enriched parenteral nutrition has been shown to increase gut mucosal weight and DNA content,[218] stimulate villus growth,[219] and improve gut glutamine utilization.[220] Moreover, glutamine-supplemented TPN decreases bacterial translocation when compared with standard TPN.[221] During acute metabolic stress, gut glutamine uptake is enhanced.[222] Improved survival has been achieved with glutamine-enriched TPN in septic rats.[223] This effect may be due to enhancement of the immunologic rather than the physical gut barrier function.[224] Glutamine has been used safely in infants[225] and appears to be a valuable adjunct to gut nutrition when enteral delivery is contraindicated.

Peptide Growth Factors

Peptide growth factors are naturally occurring proteins that induce cell proliferation. The removal of such growth factors from cell culture causes cessation of proliferation, even in the presence of adequate nutrient substrate. Investigations designed to establish the role of peptide growth factors in gastrointestinal growth and function have focused primarily on epidermal growth factor (EGF), transforming growth factor α (TGF-α), and IGF-1.

Both EGF and TGF-α are synthesized by gut mucosa and are known to stimulate proliferation of intestinal mucosa.[226, 227] The administration of EGF in malnourished rat models has resulted in increased mucosal weight, villus height, and crypt cell production.[228, 229] These effects are enhanced by the addition of glutamine,[228] perhaps because of increased (EGF-induced) glutamine transport by intestinal mucosa.[230] Mucosal EGF levels increase following gastrointestinal ulceration.[231] The administration of EGF[232] and the induction of increased endogenous EGF production (by using GH-releasing factor)[233] have both been associated with improved ulcer healing.

The role of peptide growth factors present in mammalian milk may be especially important in infant gut maturation. In newborn rat models, EGF has a pronounced trophic effect on intestinal mucosa[234] and has also been found to promote hepatic growth.[235] The importance of IGF-1 in gastrointestinal growth and development in the neonate has also been intimated in a porcine model.[236] Intestinal growth, macromolecular transport, and functional maturation in this model were all quantitatively related to variations in IGF-1 protein content and receptor numbers. Furthermore, it is possible that enteral nutrition provided by fetal swallowing of amniotic fluid containing a variety of growth factors, including EGF and IGF-1, supports gut maturation and growth during gestation.[237]

These studies suggest a putatively beneficial role for the adjunctive uses of peptide growth factors during acute metabolic stress to enhance gastrointestinal function and support the gut mucosal barrier.

MODIFICATIONS OF NUTRITIONAL SUPPORT DURING INJURY STATES

Hormonal Supplementation

While the timely provision of nutrient substrates can promote recovery from acute metabolic stress states, it is also clear that aggressive nutritional repletion alone may be insufficient to overcome the catabolic effects caused by more severe injury stimuli, especially in patients with low endogenous substrate reserves.[238, 239] Since this consequence may be at least partially due to compromised hepatic (and skeletal muscle) utilization of available protein substrates, recent investigations have focused on the adjunctive use of GH during acute metabolic stress to promote anabolic

metabolism and blunt endogenous substrate catabolism.[240, 241] The anabolic effects of GH, especially as they affect protein metabolism, are mediated primarily by IGF-1.[242–244] It has been demonstrated that with moderate stress, GH administration can optimize utilization of adjuvant nutritional support and counteract protein catabolic effects of the injury response by increasing protein synthesis and by inducing IGF-1 synthesis and release. Consequently, protein breakdown decreases, and nitrogen retention improves. As a result, body cell mass is preserved and even restored, wound healing is promoted, immunologic function is enhanced, and hospital stay is shortened.[240, 241, 245–247]

However, with increased injury severity (particularly sepsis), the GH-induced IGF-1 response is blunted, and exogenous GH is relatively ineffective in promoting anabolic metabolism.[248–250] To circumvent this type of stress-related GH resistance, the exogenous use of IGF-1 during severe metabolic stress states has recently been proposed.[84] Although its effects in the acute stress setting have yet to be adequately evaluated, IGF-1 administration has been found to promote improved postoperative nitrogen balance, bowel trophic effects, and total-body weight gain in rats undergoing an 80% small-bowel resection.[251] Locally administered IGF-1 in rats has also been shown to reverse corticosteroid inhibition of wound healing.[252] In healthy adult humans, IGF-1 can attenuate nitrogen losses caused by hypocaloric feeding while conserving cellular amino acid stores.[253] Its effects in critically ill human subjects are largely unknown. It was recently reported that a single postoperative dose of IGF-1 (40 μg/kg subcutaneously) was well tolerated and resulted in increased serum IGF-1 concentrations and IGF-1 activity vs. placebo in adult patients following major gastrointestinal surgery.[254]

Adjunctive hormonal therapy of this nature may be of particular benefit in acutely stressed infants. As previously discussed, acute illness in infants is associated with growth retardation that is generally followed by a period of accelerated ("catch-up") growth when the injury response resolves.[165, 166] It is noteworthy, however, that "catch-up" growth following acute metabolic stress may be inadequate to achieve normal anthropometric values for age and sex (see Fig 41–8).[165] The importance of the failure to achieve normal anthropometric standards lies in associated mental retardation and neuromotor functional handicaps.[255, 256] It is certainly possible that shortening the interval of the catabolic response to injury and promoting earlier recovery of anabolic metabolism through the use of adjunctive hormonal therapy could facilitate complete growth recovery and perhaps avoid the long-term consequences of growth retardation. This represents an important area of future clinical investigation.

Branched-Chain Amino Acids

The predominant metabolic effects during acute stress result in catabolism and reduced total-body protein synthesis. The demands placed on the liver are extensive during this period, and hepatic protein synthesis actually increases.[257] Amino acids mobilized from visceral protein pools, muscle, and gut are taken up by the liver and used to synthesize acute-phase proteins and glucose (gluconeogenesis). The failure of the liver to respond to these demands because of the magnitude or duration of the stress insult is associated with increased mortality. While 40% to 100% of most amino acids are metabolized as they pass through the liver, branched-chain amino acids (BCAAs)—leucine, isoleucine, and valine) are thought to undergo minimal hepatic degradation and are therefore available to support muscle. Solutions enriched with BCAAs have been shown to reduce skeletal muscle proteolysis, increase protein synthesis, and decrease the release of aromatic amino acids from muscle.[258] BCAAs, particularly leucine, are also as-

sociated with increased hepatic acute-phase protein synthesis and decreased urea production.[259] In septic rats, enriched BCAA solutions have resulted in significant muscle sparing and improved nitrogen balance.[260] Clinical studies in metabolically stressed humans have shown similar effects.[261, 262] Because of BCAA effects in lowering aromatic amino acid production and decreasing ureagenesis, solutions enriched with BCAAs may be of benefit in treating hepatic encephalopathy and renal failure.[263, 264] Most studies suggest that BCAA enrichment should approach 45% to 50% for optimal effect.

Medium-Chain Triglycerides

MCT preparations contain saturated fatty acids with 6- to 12-carbon chain lengths. They are directly absorbed into the circulatory system from the gut and do not require bile for absorption. They are rapidly cleared from the bloodstream, exhibit rapid mitochondrial uptake, and do not require carnitine for metabolism. In contrast to long-chain triglycerides (LCTs),[265] MCT preparations do not appear to impair RES clearance of bacteria.[266, 267] They are incorporated in several enteral formulations and can improve fat absorption from dysfunctional bowel.

NUTRITIONAL IMMUNOMODULATION

Recent data suggest that several dietary components can exert a variety of effects on the immune system. Since increased metabolic stress severity is associated with substantial immunocompromise, the ability to enhance immunologic function by dietary alterations offers the possibility of improving clinical outcome following injury. Research interest has focused on three major substrate subgroups: ω-3 fatty acids, nucleotides, and arginine.

ω-3 Polyunsaturated Fatty Acids

In addition to providing important substrates for energy, essential fatty acids, fat-soluble vitamins, and cell membrane constituents, lipid metabolism may also modulate immune function via arachidonic acid synthetic pathways.[49] Increased intake of linoleic acid (ω-6 polyunsaturated fatty acid [PUFA]), an important precursor of arachidonic acid, has been shown to inhibit immune function by impeding neutrophil chemotaxis, neutrophil phagocytosis, neutrophil bactericidal activity, macrophage phagocytosis, and lymphocyte proliferation.[268] The metabolism of linoleic acid via the cyclooxygenase pathway yields mono and dienoic prostaglandins (such as PGE_2), which are known to have widespread macrophage and lymphocyte immunosuppressant effects at the high serum concentrations ($>10^{-8}M$) associated with severe metabolic stress conditions such as sepsis and burn trauma.[268]

In contrast, diets high in ω-3 PUFAs (such as fish oil) result in comparatively less arachidonic acid production and yield the less potent trienoic prostaglandins. As a result, PGE_2 production is decreased, and immunosuppression is reduced. Diets rich in ω-3 vs. ω-6 PUFAs have been shown to improve immunologic function in burned animals[269, 270] and have been associated with improved survival in acutely stressed human[271] and animal[272] study populations, although this effect may be model dependent.[273]

Nucleotides

In vitro investigations suggest that the metabolic activities of stimulated lymphocytes are nucleotide dependent.[274] Enhanced immunologic function has been reported when animals were fed nucleotide-supplemented vs. nucleotide-free diets in studies of allograft rejection,[275] bacterial challenge,[276] and delayed hypersensitivity.[277] Immunosuppression resulting from the absence of dietary nucleotides appears to be due primarily to increased helper T-cell suppression and decreased IL-2 production. These findings appear to be uracil dependent.[277]

Arginine

In vitro arginine enhances lymphocyte activation (improves mitogenesis, increases the synthesis of nucleic acids and protein).[278] It has been suggested that arginine becomes an essential amino acid during acute metabolic stress states because of insufficient endogenous production to meet increased demands. Animal studies demonstrate improved survival with arginine-supplemented diets following burn injury and peritonitis,[279, 280] presumably by improving T-lymphocyte–dependent immunocompetence. This concept is supported by investigations in postoperative human subjects that show that the mitogenic response of circulating lymphocytes is increased as a result of arginine supplementation.[278, 281] Arginine-enriched diets have also been associated with improved wound healing[282, 283] and may inhibit the growth and development of malignant tumors because of enhanced immune function.[278]

Of special potential importance from a pediatric prospective, arginine may induce increased pituitary GH secretion[284] and may be necessary for optimal growth in healthy human infants.[278] Further clinical studies are needed to evaluate the immune modulating effects of various nutrients. The clinical utility of these nutrients remains unclear at the present time (see the individual chapters on each nutrient).

SUMMARY

The successful treatment of critically ill infants and children requires an understanding of the acute metabolic stress response. A poor clinical outcome can result when the metabolic demands of acute injury exceed the ability of endogenous host mechanisms to compensate. Appropriate exogenous supplementation may provide the crucial metabolic and nutritional support necessary to ensure recovery. As knowledge in this area grows, more effective treatment strategies are evolving. The potential for further advances, especially in the infant critical care population, offers the hope for substantial progress in the near future.

REFERENCES

1. Holliday MA: Body composition and energy needs during growth, in Falkner F, Tanner JM (eds): *Human Growth: A Comprehensive Treatise,* ed 2, vol 2. New York, Plenum Publishing Corp, 1986.
2. Reichman BL, Chessex P, Putet G: Partition of energy metabolism and energy cost of growth in the very low–birth weight infant. *Pediatrics* 1982; 69:446–451.
3. Talbot FB: Basal metabolism standards for children. *Am J Dis Child* 1938; 55:455–459.
4. Young VR, Steffee WP, Pencharz PB, et al: Total human body protein synthesis in relation to protein requirements at various ages. *Nature* 1975; 253:192–194.
5. Carlson SE, Barness LA: Macronutrient requirements for growth, in Walker AW, Watkins JB (eds): *Nutrition in Pediatrics.* Boston, Little, Brown, 1985.
6. Dupont C, Rocchiccioli F, Bougneres PF: Urinary excretion of dicarboxylic acids in term newborns fed with 5% medium-chain triglycerides–enriched formula. *J Pediatr Gastroenterol Nutr* 1987; 6:313–315.
7. Committee on Dietary Allowances Food and Nutrition Board: *Recommended Dietary Allowances.* Washington, DC, National Academy of Sciences/National Research Council, 1980.
8. Schwarz KB: Vitamins, in Walker WA, Watkins JB (eds): *Nutrition in Pediatrics.* Boston, Little, Brown, 1985.
9. Hambidge KM: Trace elements in human nutrition, in Walker WA, Watkins JB (eds): *Nutrition in Pediatrics.* Boston, Little, Brown, 1985.
10. Brasseur D, Johansson A, Goyens P, et al: Carnitine (C) balance in the parenterally fed premature neonate receiving a new C-containing fat emulsion (abstract 53). *JPEN* 1991; 15(suppl)25.
11. Roberts P, Meredith JW, Black K, et al: Diarrhea does not alter impaired small bowel absorption following trauma. *JPEN* 1993; 17(suppl):34.
12. Shmerling DH, Forrer JCW, Prader A: Fecal fat and nitrogen in healthy children and in children with malabsorption or maldigestion. *Pediatrics* 1970; 46:690–695.
13. Hamill PVV, Drizd TA, Johnson CL: Physical growth: National center for health statistics percentiles. *Am J Clin Nutr* 1979; 32:607–629.
14. American Academy of Pediatrics Committee on Nutrition: Nutritional needs of low birthweight infants. *Pediatrics* 1985; 75:976–1086.
15. Waterlow JC: Classification and definition of protein-calorie malnutrition. *BMJ* 1972; 3:566–569.
16. Merritt RJ, Suskind RM: Nutritional survey of hospitalized pediatric patients. *Am J Clin Nutr* 1979;32:1320–1325.
17. Heymsfield SB, McManus CB, Seitz SB, et al: Anthropometric assessment of adult protein-energy malnutrition, in Wright RA, Heymsfield S (eds): *Nutritional Assessment.* Boston, Blackwell, 1984.
18. Johnston FE: Relationships between body composition and anthropometry. *Hum Biol* 1982; 54:221–245.
19. Huenemann RL: Environmental factors associated with preschool obesity. I. Obesity in six-month old children. *J Am Diet Assoc* 1974; 64:480.
20. Pencharz P: Body composition and growth, in Walker W, Watkins (eds): *Nutrition in Pediatrics; Basic Science and Clinical Application,* ed 1. Boston, Little, Brown, 1985.
21. Reichman B, Chessex P, Putet G, et al: Diet, fat accretion, and growth in premature infants. *N Engl J Med* 1981; 305:1495–1500.
22. Johnson C, Fulwood R, Abraham S,

et al: Basic data on anthropometric measurements and angular measurements of the hip and knee joints for selected age groups 1–74 years of age, United States, 1971–1975. National Center for Health Statistics, Vital and Health Statistics. Series II, No. 219. Department of Health and Human Services Publication No (PHA) 81-1669. Washington, DC, US Government Printing Office, 1981.

23. Pollack MM, Wiley JS, Holbrook PR: Early nutritional depletion in critically ill children. *Crit Care Med* 1981; 9:580–583.

24. Nyboer J, Bogna S, Nimo LF: *The Electrical Impedance Plethysmograph—An Electrical Volume Recorder.* Washington, DC, National Academy Press, 1943, NRC report 149.

25. Schoeller DA, Van Santen E, Peterson DW, et al: Total body water measurement in humans with ^{18}O and ^2H labeled water. *Am J Clin Nutr* 1984; 33:2686–2693.

26. Mayfield RS, Uauy R, Waidelich D: Body composition of low–birth-weight infants determined by using bioelectrical resistance and reactance. *Am J Clin Nutr* 1991; 54:296–303.

27. Miller CL: Immunological assays as measurements of nutritional status: A review. *JPEN* 1978; 2:554–566.

28. Twoney R, Ziegler D, Rombeau J: Utility of skin testing in nutritional assessment: A critical review. *JPEN* 1982; 6:50–58.

29. Long CL, Schaffel N, Geiger JW, et al: Metabolic response to injury and illness: Estimation of energy and protein needs from indirect calorimetry and nitrogen balance. *JPEN* 1979; 3:452–456.

30. Kinney JM, Elwyn DH: Protein metabolism in the traumatized patient. *Acta Chir Scand Suppl* 1984; 522:45–56.

31. Cerra RB: Hypermetabolism, organ failure, and metabolic support. *Surgery* 1987; 101:1–14.

32. Moore FD: Bodily changes in surgical convalescence. I. The normal sequence: Observations and interpretations. *Ann Surg* 1953; 137:289–315.

33. Dinarello CA: Interleukin-1 and interleukin-1 antagonism. *Blood* 1991; 77:1627–1652.

34. Rock CS, Lowry SF: Tumor necrosis factor-α. *J Surg Res* 1991; 51:434–445.

35. Ayala A, Perrin MM, Meldrum DR, et al: Hemorrhage induces an increase in serum TNF which is not associated with elevated levels of endotoxin. *Cytokine* 1990; 2:170–174.

36. Beutler B, Krochin N, Milsark IW, et al: Control of cachectin (tumor necrosis factor) synthesis: Mechanisms of endotoxin resistance. *Science* 1986; 232:977–980.

37. Marano MA, Fong Y, Moldawer LL, et al: Serum cachectin/tumor necrosis factor in critically ill patients with burns correlates with infection and mortality. *Surg Gynecol Obstet* 1990; 170:32–38.

38. Michie HR, Spriggs DR, Manogue KR, et al: Tumor necrosis factor and endotoxin induce similar metabolic responses in human beings. *Surgery* 1988; 104:280–286.

39. Tracey KJ, Lowry SF, Fahey TJ III, et al: Cachectin/tumor necrosis factor induces lethal septic shock and stress hormone responses in the dog. *Surg Gynecol Obstet* 1987; 164:415–422.

40. Figari IS, Mori NA, Palladino MA: Regulation of neutrophil chemotaxis and superoxide production by recombinant tumor necrosis factor α and β: Effects of interferon γ and interleukin 1. *Blood* 1987; 70:979–984.

41. Tracey KJ, Beutler B, Lowry SF, et al: Shock and tissue injury induced by recombinant human cachectin. *Science* 1986; 234:470–474.

42. Ertel W, Morrison MH, Ayala A, et al: Mechanisms responsible for the increase of interleukin-6 synthesis. *Surg Forum* 1992; 43:88–90.

43. Warner SJC, Libby P: Human vascular smooth muscle cells: Target for and source of tumor necrosis factor. *J Immunol* 1989; 142:100–109.

44. Flores EA, Bistrian BR, Pomposelli JJ, et al: Infusion of tumor necrosis factor/cachectin promotes muscle catabolism. A synergistic effect with interleukin 1. *J Clin Invest* 1989; 83:1614–1622.

45. Zamir O, James JH, Hasselgren PO, et al: The effects of endotoxemia and cytokines on amino acid transport in skeletal muscle and the possible role

of glucocorticoids (abstract 101). *Surg Forum* 1991; 42:101–103.

46. Pacitti AJ, Souba WW: Stimulation of hepatic system A amino acid transport by tumor necrosis factor (TNF) (abstract 18). Presented at the 25th Annual Meeting of the Association for Academic Surgery, Colorado Springs, 1991, p 18.

47. Warren RS, Starnes, Jr. HF, Gabrilove JL, et al: The acute metabolic effects of tumor necrosis factor administration in human. *Arch Surg* 1987; 122:1396–1400.

48. Lazarus DD, Lowry SF, Moldawer LL: Cytokines acutely decrease circulating insulin-like growth factor-1 (IGF-1) and IGF binding protein-3 (IGFBP-3). *Surg Forum* 1992; 43:92–94.

49. Kinsella JE, Lokesh B, Broughton S, et al: Dietary polyunsaturated fatty acids and eicosanoids: Potential effects on the modulation of inflammatory and immune cells: An overview. *Nutrition* 1990; 6:25–44.

50. Nijsten MWN, Hack CE, Helle M, et al: Interleukin-6 and its relation to the humoral immune response and clinical parameters in burned patients. *Surgery* 1991; 109:761–767.

51. Ohzato H, Yoshizaki K, Nishimoto N, et al: Interleukin-6 as a new indicator of inflammatory status: Detection of serum levels of interleukin-6 and C-reactive protein after surgery. *Surgery* 1992; 111:201–209.

52. Lotem J, Shabo Y, Sachs L: Regulation of megakaryocyte development by interleukin-6. *Blood* 1989; 74:1545–1551.

53. Koj A: The role of interleukin-6 as the hepatocyte stimulating factor in the network of inflammatory cytokines. *Ann N Y Acad Sci* 1989; 557:1–8.

54. Dinarello CA, Meir JW: Current concepts: Lymphokines. *N Engl J Med* 1987; 317:940–945.

55. Michie HR, Eberlein TJ, Spriggs DR, et al: Interleukin-2 initiates metabolic responses associated with critical illness in humans. *Ann Surg* 1988; 208:493–503.

56. Levi R, Krell RD: Biology of leukotrienes, *Ann N Y Acad Sci* 1988; 524:91.

57. Redmond HP, Chavin KD, Bromberg JS, et al: Inhibition of macrophage-

activating cytokines is beneficial in the acute septic response. *Ann Surg* 1991; 214:502–509.

58. Waage A, Espevik T: Interleukin-1 potentiates the lethal effect of tumor necrosis factor alpha/cachectin in mice. *J Exp Med* 1981; 81:1162–1172.

59. Wallach D, Holtmann H, Engelmann H, et al: Sensitization and desensitization to lethal effects of tumor necrosis factor and IL-1. *J Immunol* 1988; 140:2994–2999.

60. Ye K, Koch CK, Clark BD, et al: Interleukin-1β downregulates gene and surface expression of interleukin-1 receptor type I by destabilizing its mRNA whereas interleukin-2 increases its expression. *Immunology* 1992; 75:427–434.

61. Martin CA, Dorf ME: Differential regulation of interleukin-6, macrophage inflammatory protein-1, and JE/MCP-1 cytokine expression in macrophage cell lines. *Cell Immunol* 1991; 135:245–258.

62. Sheppard BC, Norton JA: Tumor necrosis factor and interleukin-1 protection against the lethal effects of tumor necrosis factor. *Surgery* 1991; 109:698–705.

63. Lowry S: Anticytokine therapies in sepsis. *New Horizons* 1993; 1:120–126.

64. Censini S, Bartalini M, Tagliabue A, et al: Interleukin 1 stimulates production of LTC_4 and other eicosanoids by macrophages. *Lymphokine Res* 1989; 8:107–114.

65. Smith RJ, Epps DE, Justen JM, et al: Human neutrophil activation with interleukin-I. *Biochem Pharm* 1987; 36:3851–3858.

66. Tanaka H, Ogura H, Yokota J, et al: Acceleration of superoxide production from leukocytes in trauma patients. *Ann Surg* 1991; 214:187–191.

67. Lefer AM, Xin-Liang MA: Cytokines and growth factors in endothelial dysfunction. *Crit Care Med* 1993; 21(suppl):9–14.

68. Schiller HJ, Reilly PM, Bulkley GB: Antioxidant therapy. *Crit Care Med* 1993; 21(suppl):92–102.

69. Beasley D, Schwartz JH, Brenner BM: Interleukin 1 induces prolonged L-arginine–dependent cyclic guanosine monophosphate and nitrite pro-

754   Specific Disease States

duction in rat vascular smooth muscle cells. *J Clin Invest* 1991; 87:602–608.

70. Ochoa JB, Udekwu AO, Billiar TR, et al: Nitrogen oxide levels in patients after trauma and during sepsis. *Ann Surg* 1991; 214:621–626.

71. Stadler J, Harbrecht BG, Curran RD, et al: Nitric oxide regulates release of cyclo-oxygenase products of rat Kupffer cells. *Crit Care Med* 1991; 19(suppl):96.

72. Harbrecht BG, Billiar TR, Stadler J, et al: Nitric oxide synthesis serves to reduce hepatic damage during acute murine endotoxemia. *Crit Care Med* 1992; 20:1568–1574.

73. Wilmore DW: In *The Metabolic Management of the Critically Ill*. New York, Plenum Publishing Corp, 1977.

74. Zamir O, Hasselgren PO, Higashiguchi T, et al: Tumor necrosis factor and interleukin-1 induce muscle proteolysis through different mechanisms (abstract 83). Presented at the 25th Annual Meeting of the Association for Academic Surgery, Colorado Springs, 1991, p 83.

75. Consoli A, Nurjhan N, Reilly JJ, et al: Contribution of liver and skeletal muscle to alanine and lactate metabolism in humans. *Am J Physiol* 1990; 259:677–684.

76. Smith RJ, Wilmore DW: Glutamine nutrition and requirements. *JPEN* 1990; 14(suppl):94–99.

77. Pacitti AJ, Austgen TR, Souba WW: Adaptive regulation of alanine transport in hepatic plasma membrane vesicles from the endotoxin-treated rat. *J Surg Res* 1991; 51:46–53.

78. Souba WW, Smith RJ, Wilmore DW: Effects of glucocorticoids on glutamine metabolism in visceral organs. *Metabolism* 1985; 34:450–456.

79. Bessey PQ, Watters JM, Aoki TT, et al: Combined hormonal infusion simulates the metabolic response to injury. *Ann Surg* 1984; 200:264–281.

80. Gore DC, Jahoor F, Herndon DN: Acute response of human muscle protein to catabolic hormones (abstract 60). *Surg Forum* 1991; 42:60–62.

81. Zamir O, Hasselgren PO, Kunkel SL, et al: Evidence that tumor necrosis factor participates in the regulation of muscle proteolysis during sepsis. *Arch Surg* 1992; 127:170–174.

82. Kostyo JL, Reagan CR: The biology of growth hormone. *Pharmacol Ther* 1976; 2:591–604.

83. Daughaday WH, Rotwein P: Insulin-like growth factors I and II. Peptide, messenger ribonucleic acid and gene structures, serum, and tissue concentrations. *Endocr Rev* 1989; 10:68–91.

84. Chwals WJ, Bistrian BR: Role of exogenous growth hormone and insulin-like growth factor I in malnutrition and acute metabolic stress: A hypothesis. *Crit Care Med* 1991; 19:1317–1322.

85. Anand KJS, Brown MJ, Bloom SR, et al: Studies on the hormonal regulation of fuel metabolism in the human newborn infant undergoing anesthesia and surgery. *Horm Res* 1985; 22:115–128.

86. Anand KJS, Hanson DD, Hickey PR: Hormonal-metabolic stress responses in neonates undergoing cardiac surgery. *Anesthesiology* 1990; 73:661–670.

87. Taylor AF, Lally KP, Chwals WJ, et al: Hormonal response of the premature primate to operative stress. *J Pediatr Surg*, in press.

88. Young GA, Chem C, Hill GL: Assessment of protein-calorie malnutrition in surgical patients from plasma proteins and anthropometric measurements. *Am J Clin Nutr* 1978; 31:429–435.

89. Myers MA, Fleck A, Sampson B, et al: Early plasma protein and mineral changes after surgery: A two stage process. *J Clin Pathol* 1984; 37:862–866.

90. Fletcher JP, Little JM, Guest PK: A comparison of serum transferrin and serum prealbumin as nutritional parameters. *JPEN* 1987; 11:144–147.

91. Felig P, Marliss EB, Cahill GF Jr: Metabolic response to human growth hormone during prolonged starvation. *Clin Invest* 1971; 50:411–421.

92. Loder PB, Kee AJ, Horsburgh R, et al: Validity of urinary urea nitrogen as a measure of total urinary nitrogen in adult patients requiring parenteral nutrition. *Crit Care Med* 1989; 17:309–312.

93. Bistrian BR: A simple technique to estimate severity of stress. *Surg Gynecol Obstet* 1979; 148:675–678.

94. Rickham PP: In *The Metabolic Response to Neonatal Surgery.* Cambridge, Mass, Harvard University Press, 1957.

95. Helms RA, Mowatt-Larssen CA, Boehm KA, et al: Urinary nitrogen constituents in the postsurgical preterm neonate receiving parenteral nutrition. *JPEN* 1993; 17:68–72.

96. Catzeflis C, Schutz Y, Mitcheli JL: Whole body protein synthesis and energy expenditure in very low–birth-weight infants. *Pediatr Res* 1985; 19:679–687.

97. Pepys MB, Baltz ML: Acute phase proteins with special reference to C-reactive protein and related proteins (Pentaxins) and serum amyloid A protein. *Adv Immunol* 1983; 34:141–212.

98. Dickson PW, Bannister D, Schreiber G: Minor burns lead to major changes in synthesis rates of plasma proteins in the liver. *J Trauma* 1987; 27:283–286.

99. Gewurz H: Biology of C-reactive protein and the acute phase response. *Hosp Pract* 1982; 17:67–81.

100. Daniels JC, Larson DL, Abston S, et al: Serum protein profiles in thermal burns. *J Trauma* 1974; 14:1553–162.

101. Nudelman R, Kagan BM: C-reactive protein in pediatrics. *Adv Pediatr* 1983; 30:517–547.

102. Peltola H, Ahlqvist J, Rapola J, et al: C-reactive protein compared with white blood cell count and erythrocyte sedimentation rate in the diagnosis of acute appendicitis in children. *Acta Chir Scand* 1986; 152:55–58.

103. Gronn M, Slordahl SH, Skrede S, et al: C-reactive protein as an indicator of infection in the immunosuppressed child. *Eur J Pediatr* 1986; 145:18–21.

104. Forest JC, Lariviere F, Dolce P, et al: C-reactive protein as biochemical indicator of bacterial infection in neonates. *Clin Biochem* 1986; 19:192–194.

105. Philip AGS: The protective effect of acute phase reactants in neonatal sepsis. *Acta Paediatr Scand* 1979; 68:481–483.

106. Sabel KG, Wadsworth C: C-reactive protein (CRP) in early diagnosis of neonatal septicemia. *Acta Paediatr Scand* 1979; 68:825–831.

107. Chwals WJ, Thorne MT, Charles BJ: Assessment of the metabolic response to surgical stress in infants using C-reactive protein (CRP) (abstract). Presented at the 23rd Annual Meeting of Pacific Association of Pediatric Surgery, Kona, Hawaii, 1990, p 31.

108. Peltola H, Holmberg C: Rapidity of C-reactive protein in detecting potential septicemia. *Pediatr Infect Dis* 1983; 2:374–376.

109. Weir JB: New methods for calculating metabolic rate with special reference to protein metabolism. *J Physiol* 1949; 109:1–9.

110. Bursztein S, Elwyn DH, Askanazi J, et al: In Grayson TH (ed): *Energy Metabolism Indirect Calorimetry, and Nutrition.* Baltimore, Williams & Wilkins, 1989.

111. McGilvery RW: In *Biochemistry: A Functional Approach,* ed 2. Philadelphia, WB Saunders, 1979, p 534.

112. Cortes V, Nelson LD: Errors in estimating energy expenditure in critically ill surgical patients. *Arch Surg* 1989; 124:287–290.

113. Baker JP, Detsky AS, Stewart S: Randomized trial of total parenteral nutrition in critically ill patients: Metabolic effects of varying glucose-lipid ratios as an energy source. *Gastroenterology* 1984; 87:53–59.

114. Fredrix EW, Soeters PB, Von Meyenfeldt MF, et al: Resting energy expenditure in cancer patients before and after gastrointestinal surgery. *JPEN* 1991; 15:604–607.

115. Swinamer DL, Phang PT, Jones RL, et al: Twenty-four hour energy expenditure in critically ill patients. *Crit Care Med* 1987; 15:637–643.

116. Chwals WJ, Lally KP, Woolley MM, et al: Measured energy expenditure in critically ill infants and young children. *J Surg Res* 1988; 44:467–472.

117. Salas JS, Dozio E, Goulet OJ, et al: Energy expenditure and substrate utilization in the course of renutrition of malnourished children. *JPEN* 1991; 15:288–293.

118. Alverson D, Isken V, Cohen R: Effect of booster transfusions on oxygen utilization in infants with bronchopulmonary dysplasia. *J Pediatr* 1988; 113:722–726.

119. Mayfield RS, Uauy R: Validation of a computerized indirect calorimeter for use in research studies of mechanically ventilated neonates (abstract). *Pediatr Res* 1986; 20:414.

120. Chwals WJ, Lally KP, Woolley MM: Indirect calorimetry in mechanically-ventilated infants and children: Measurement accuracy with absence of audible airleak. *Crit Care Med* 1992; 20:768–770.

121. Powell K, Albernaz L, Skipper E, et al: Does measurement of 20 minute energy expenditure represent the 24 hours energy expenditure in the critically ill (abstract 125)? *JPEN* 15:37S, 1991; 15(suppl):37.

122. Pierro A, Carnielle V, Filler RM, et al: Partition of energy metabolism in the surgical newborn. *J Pediatr Surg* 1991; 26:581–586.

123. Calvano SE, Barber AE, Hawes AS, et al: Effect of combined cortisol-endotoxin (LPS) administration on peripheral blood leukocyte numbers and phenotype in normal humans. *Arch Surg* 1992; 127:181–186.

124. Barber AE, Coyle SM, Fong Y, et al: Impact of hypercortisolemia on the metabolic and hormonal responses to endotoxin in man. *Surg Forum* 1990; 41:74–77.

125. Sjolin J: High-dose corticosteroid therapy in human septic shock: Has the jury reached a correct verdict? *Circ Shock* 1991; 35:139–151.

126. Schumer W: Steroids in the treatment of clinical septic shock. *Ann Surg* 1976; 184:333–341.

127. Bone RC, Fisher CJ, Clemmer TP, et al: A controlled clinical trial of high-dose methylprednisolone in the treatment of severe sepsis and septic shock. *N Engl J Med* 1987; 317:653–658.

128. Sprung CL, Caralis PV, Marcial EH, et al: The effects of high-dose corticosteroids in patients with septic shock. *N Engl J Med* 1984; 311:1137–1143.

129. The Veterans Administration Systemic Sepsis Cooperative Study Group: Effect of high-dose glucocorticoid therapy on mortality in patients with clinical signs of systemic sepsis. *N Engl J Med* 1987; 317:659–665.

130. Hoffman SL, Punjabi NH, Kumala S, et al: Reduction of mortality in choloramphenicol-treated severe typhoid fever by high-dose dexamethasone. *N Engl J Med* 1984; 310:82–88.

131. Slotman GJ, Fisher CJ, Bone RC, et al: Detrimental effects of high-dose methylprednisolone sodium succinate on serum concentrations of hepatic and renal function indicators in severe sepsis and septic shock. *Crit Care Med* 1993; 21:191–195.

132. Schulze S, Sommer P, Bigler D, et al: Effect of combined prednisolone, epidural analgesia, and indomethacin on the systemic response after colonic surgery. *Arch Surg* 1992; 127:325–331.

133. Engelmann H, Novick D, Wallach D: Two tumor necrosis factor–binding proteins purified from human urine. *J Biol Chem* 1990; 265:1531–1536.

134. Kohno T, Brewer MT, Baker SL, et al: A second tumor necrosis factor receptor gene product can shed a naturally occurring tumor necrosis factor inhibitor. *Proc Natl Acad Sci U S A* 1990; 87:8331–8335.

135. Eisenberg SP, Evans RJ, Arend WP, et al: Primary structure and functional expression from complementary DNA of a human interleukin-1 receptor antagonist. *Nature* 1990; 343:341–345.

136. Hannum CH, Wilcox CJ, Arend WP, et al: Interleukin-1 receptor antagonist activity of a human interleukin-1 inhibitor. *Nature* 1991; 343:336–339.

137. Tracey KJ, Fong Y, Hesse DG, et al: Anti-cachectin/TNF monoclonal antibodies prevent septic shock during lethal bacteremia. *Nature* 1987; 330:662–664.

138. Alexander HR, Doherty GM, Venzon DJ, et al: Recombinant interleukin-1 receptor antagonist (IL-1ra): Effective therapy against gram-negative sepsis in rats. *Surgery* 1992; 112:188–194.

139. Nakane A, Minagawa T, Kato K: Endogenous tumor necrosis factor (cachectin) is essential to host resistance against *Listeria monocytogenes* infection. *Infect Immun* 1988; 56:2563–2569.

140. Havell EA: Evidence that tumor necrosis factor has an important role in antibacterial resistance. *J Immunol* 1989; 143:2894–2899.

141. Echtenacher B, Falk W, Mannel DN, et al: Requirement of endogenous tumor necrosis factor/cachectin for recovery from experimental peritonitis. *J Immunol* 1990; 145:3762–3766.

142. Simms HH, D'Amico R: Endotoxin suppresses matrix protein–induced upregulation of PMN candicidal activity: An effect reversed by low-dose TNF-α. *J Surg Res* 1992; 52:489–498.

143. O'Reilly M, Silver GM, Davis JH, et al: Interleukin 1β improves survival following cecal ligation and puncture. *J Surg Res* 1992; 52:518–522.

144. Luger A, Graf H, Schwarz H-P, et al: Decreased serum interleukin 1 activity and monocyte interleukin 1 production in patients with fatal sepsis. *Crit Care Med* 1986; 14:458–461.

145. Munoz C, Misset B, Fitting C, et al: Dissociation between plasma and monocyte-associated cytokines during sepsis. *Eur J Immunol* 1991; 21:2177–2184.

146. Pogrebniak HW, Prewitt TW, Matthews W, et al: Cytokine downregulation and protection from tumor necrosis factor by a prostaglandin analogue. *Surg Forum* 1992; 43:99–102.

147. Pogrebniak HW, Merino MJ, Hahn SM, et al: Spin trap salvage from endotoxemia: The role of cytokine downregulation. *Surgery* 1992; 112:130–139.

148. Anand KJS, Hickey PR: Halothane-morphine compared with high-dose sufentanil for anesthesia and postoperative analgesia in neonatal cardiac surgery. *N Engl J Med* 1992; 326:1–9.

149. Fink MP: Adoptive immunotherapy of gram-negative sepsis: Use of monoclonal antibodies to lipopolysaccharide. *Crit Care Med* 1993; 21(suppl):32–39.

150. Arregui LM, Moyes DG, Lipman J, et al: Comparison of disease severity scoring systems in septic shock. *Crit Care Med* 1991; 19:1165–1171.

151. Elebute EA, Stoner HB: The grading of sepsis. *Br J Surg* 1983; 70:29–31.

152. Fry DE, Pearlstein L, Fulton RL, et al: Multiple system organ failure. The role of uncontrolled infection. *Arch Surg* 1980; 115:136–140.

153. Goris RJA, te Boekhorst TPA, Nuytinck JKS, et al: Multiple-organ failure: Generalized autodestructive inflammation? *Arch Surg* 1985; 120:1109–1115.

154. Knaus WA, Draper EA, Wagner DP, et al: APACHE II: A severity of disease classification system. *Crit Care Med* 1985; 13:818–829.

155. Knaus WA, Draper EA, Wagner DP, et al: Prognosis in acute organ-system failure. *Ann Surg* 1985; 202:685–693.

156. Lemeshow S, Teres D, Pa: 'des H, et al: A method for predicting survival and mortality of ICU patients using objectively derived weights. *Crit Care Med* 1985; 13:519–525.

157. Pollack MM, Ruttimann UE, Getson PR: Pediatric risk of mortality (PRISM) score. *Crit Care Med* 1988; 16:1110–1116.

158. Steinhorn DM, Green TP: Severity of illness correlates with alterations in energy metabolism in the pediatric intensive care unit. *Crit Care Med* 1991; 19:1503–1509.

159. Mustard RA, Bohnen JMA, Haseeb S, et al: C-reactive protein levels predict postoperative septic complications. *Arch Surg* 1987; 122:69–73.

160. Boosalis MG, Ott L, Levine AS, et al: Relationship of visceral proteins to nutritional status in chronic and acute stress. *Crit Care Med* 1989; 17:741–747.

161. Debets JM, Kampmejer R, van der Linden MP, et al: Plasma tumor necrosis factor and mortality in critically ill septic patients. *Crit Care Med* 1989; 17:489–494.

162. Grau GE, Taylor TE, Trop M, et al: Tumor necrosis factor and disease severity in children with falciparum malaria. *N Engl J Med* 1989; 320:1586–1591.

163. Fernandez ME, Chwals WJ: Increased severity delays recovery of visceral protein synthesis in postoperative neonates. Presented at the 61st Annual Scientific Meeting and Postgraduate Course, Southeastern Surgical Con-

gress, Tarpon Springs, Fla, Feb 7–11, 1993.

164. Chwals WJ, Fernandez MD, Jamie AC, et al: Relationship of metabolic indices to postoperative mortality in surgical infants. *J Pediatr Surg,* 1993; 28:819–822.

165. Marks KH, Maisels MJ, Moore E, et al: Head growth in sick premature infants—a longitudinal study. *J Pediatr* 1979; 94:282–285.

166. Prader A, Tanner JM, Von Harnack GA: Catch-up growth following illness or starvation. *J Pediatr* 1963; 62:646–659.

167. Shanbhogue RL, Lloyd DA: Absence of hypermetabolism after operation in the newborn infant. *JPEN* 1992; 16:333–336.

168. Gebara BM, Gelmini M, Sarnaik A: Oxygen consumption, energy expenditure, and substrate utilization after cardiac surgery in children. *Crit Care Med* 1992; 20:1550–1554.

169. Chwals WJ, Fernandez M, Charles BC: Adjustment of nutritional repletion using bedside indirect calorimetry in infants recovering from surgical stress. *Crit Care Med* 1992; 20(suppl):11.

170. Bresson JL, Bader B, Rocchiccioli, et al: Protein-metabolism kinetics and energy-substrate utilization in infants fed parenteral solutions with different glucose-fat ratios. *Am J Clin Nutr* 1991; 54:370–376.

171. Piedboeuf B, Chessex P, Hazan J, et al: Total parenteral nutritional in the newborn infant: Energy substrates and respiratory gas exchange. *J Pediatr* 1991; 118:97–102.

172. Chwals WJ, Fernandez ME, Charles BJ, et al: Serum visceral protein levels reflect protein-calorie repletion in neonates recovering from major surgery. *J Pediatr Surg* 1992; 27:317–321.

173. Lowry SF, Brennan MF: Abnormal liver function during parenteral nutrition: Relation to infusion excess. *J Surg Res* 1979; 26:300–307.

174. Askanazi J, Rosenbaum S, Hyman R: Respiratory changes induced by the large glucose loads of total parenteral nutrition. *JAMA* 1980; 243:1444–1447.

175. Peck MD, Babcock GF, Alexander JW: The role of protein and calorie restriction in out some from salmonella infection in mice. *JPEN* 1992; 16:561–565.

176. Wilmore DW, Dudrick SJ: Growth and development of an infant receiving all nutrients exclusively by vein. *JAMA* 1968; 203:860–864.

177. Payne-James JJ, Silk DB: Heptobiliary dysfunction associated with total parenteral nutrition. *Dig Dis* 1992; 9:106–124.

178. Fisher RL: Hepatobiliary abnormalities associated with total parenteral nutrition. *Gastroenterol Clin North Am* 1989; 18:645–666.

179. Moore FA, Feliciano DV, Andrassy RJ, et al: Early enteral feeding, compared with parenteral, reduces postoperative septic complications. *Ann Surg* 1992; 216:172–183.

180. Herndon DN, Barrow RE, Stein M, et al: Increased mortality with intravenous supplemental feeding in severely burned patients. *J Burn Care Rehabil* 1989; 10:309–313.

181. Border JR, Hassett J, LaDuca J, et al: The gut origin of septic states in blunt multiple trauma (ISS = 40) in the ICU. *Ann Surg* 1987; 206:427–448.

182. Berg RD: Promotion of the translocation of enteric bacteria from the gastrointestinal tracts of mice by oral treatment with penicillin, clindamycin, or metronidazole. *Infect Immun* 1981; 33:854–861.

183. Maejima K, Deitch EA, Berg R: Promotion by burn stress of the translocation of bacteria from the gastrointestinal tracts of mice. *Arch Surg* 1984; 119:166–172.

184. Berg R, Wommack E, Deitch EA: Immunosuppression and intestinal bacterial overgrowth synergistically promote bacterial translocation from the GI tract. *Arch Surg* 1988; 123:1359–1364.

185. Deitch EA, Berg R, Specian R: Endotoxin promotes the translocation of bacteria from the gut. *Arch Surg* 1987; 122:185–190.

186. Deitch EA, Bridges W, Baker J, et al: Hemorrhagic shock–induced bacterial translocation is reduced by xanthine oxidase inhibition or inactiva-

tion. *Surgery* 1988; 104:191–198.

187. Carrico CJ, Meakins JL, Marshall JC, et al: Multiple organ failure syndrome. *Arch Surg* 1986; 121:196.

188. Deitch EA, Ma WJ, Ma L, et al: Protein malnutrition predisposes to inflammatory-induced gut origin septic states. *Ann Surg* 1990; 211:560–568.

189. Deitch EA, Winterton J, Li M, et al: The gut as a portal of entry for bacteremia: Role of protein malnutrition. *Ann Surg* 1987; 205:681–692.

190. Garrison RN, Fry DE, Berborich S, et al: Enterococcal bacteremia: Clinical implications and determinants of death. *Ann Surg* 1982; 196:43–47.

191. Jarrett F, Balish L, Moylan JA, et al: Clinical experience with prophylactic antibiotic bowel suppression in burn patients. *Surgery* 1978; 83:523–527.

192. Mainous MR, Tso P, Berg RD, et al: Studies of the route, magnitude, and time course of bacterial translocation in a model of systemic inflammation. *Arch Surg* 1991; 126:33–37.

193. Deitch EA, Xu D, Qi L, et al: Bacterial translocation from the gut impairs systemic immunity. *Ann Surg* 1991; 109:269–270.

194. Caty MG, Guice KS, Oldham KT, et al: Evidence for tumor necrosis factor–induced pulmonary microvascular injury after intestinal ischemia-reperfusion injury. *Ann Surg* 1990; 212:694–700.

195. Koike K, Poggetti RS, Moore FA, et al: Endotoxin after gut ischemia/reperfusion (I/R) causes irreversible lung injury. *J Surg Res* 1992; 52:656–662.

196. Yoshioka T, Fahey TJ, Fantini GA: Role of TNF and nitric oxide in the cardiovascular response to endotoxin (abstract 140). Presented at the 25th Annual Meeting of the association for Academic Surgery, Colorado Springs, 1991, p 140.

197. Alexander JW: Nutrition and translocation. *JPEN* 1990; 14(suppl):170–174.

198. Smith SD, Cardona M, Wishnev S, et al: Unique characteristics of the neonatal intestinal mucosal barrier. *J Pediatr Surg* 1992; 27:333–338.

199. Imura K, Funkui Y, Yagi M, et al: Perioperative change of plasma endotoxin levels in early infants. *J Pediatr Surg* 1989; 24:1232–1235.

200. Alverdy JC, Aoys E, Moss GS: Total parenteral nutrition promotes bacterial translocation from the gut. *Surgery* 1988; 104:185–190.

201. Moore F, Feliciano D, Andrassy R, et al: Enteral feeding reduces postoperative septic complications (abstract 32). *JPEN* 1991; 15(suppl):22.

202. Mochizuki H, Trocki O, Dominioni L, et al: Mechanism of prevention of postburn hypermetabolism and catabolism by early enteral feeding. *Ann Surg* 1984; 200:297–310.

203. Bortenschlager L, Zaloga G, Black KW, et al: Immediate post-operative enteral feeding decreases weight loss and improves wound healing following abdominal surgery in rats (abstract). *Crit Care Med* 1992; 20:115–118.

204. Shou J, Ruelaz EA, Redmond HP, et al: Dietary protein prevents bacterial translocation from the gut (abstract 75). *JPEN* 1991; 15(suppl):29.

205. Zaloga GP, Ward KA, Prielipp RC: Effect of enteral diet on whole body and gut growth in unstressed rats. *JPEN* 1991; 15:42–47.

206. Rerat A, Nunes CS, Mendy F, et al: Amino acid absorption and production of pancreatic hormones in non-anaesthetized pigs after duodenal infusions of a milk enzymatic hydrosylate or of free amino acids. *Br J Nutr* 1988; 60:121–130.

207. Imondi AR, Stradley RP: Utilization of enzymatically hydrolyzed soybean protein and crystalline amino acid diets by rats with exocrine pancreatic insufficiency. *J Clin Invest* 1974; 104:793–801.

208. McAnena OJ, Harvey LP, Bonau RA, et al: Alteration of methotrexate toxicity in rats by manipulation of dietary components. *Gastroenterology* 1987; 92:354–360.

209. Stanford JR, King D, Carey L, et al: The adverse effects of elemental diets on tolerance for 5-FU toxicity in the rat. *J Surg Oncol* 1977; 9:493–501.

210. Trocki O, Mochizuki H, Dominioni L, et al: Intact protein versus free amino

acids in the nutritional support of thermally injured animals. *JPEN* 1986; 10:139–145.

211. Zaloga GP, Knowles R, Ward K, et al: Total parenteral nutrition (TPN) increases mortality following hemorrhage. *Crit Care Med* 1991; 19:54–59.

212. Meredith JW, Ditesheim JA, Zaloga GP: Visceral protein levels in trauma patients are greater with peptide diet than intact protein diet. *J Trauma* 1990; 30:825–829.

213. Souba WW, Smith RJ, Wilmore DW: Glutamine metabolism by the intestinal tract. *JPEN* 1985; 9:608–617.

214. Windmueller HG: Glutamine utilization by the small intestine. *Adv Enzymol* 1982; 53:201–237.

215. Higashiguchi T, Frederick JA, Zamir O, et al: Effect of glutamine on protein synthesis in isolated enterocytes from septic rats. *Surg Forum* 1992; 43:26–28.

216. Souba WW, Herskowitz K, Austgen RT, et al: Glutamine nutrition: Theoretical considerations and therapeutic impact. *JPEN* 1990; 14(suppl):237–243.

217. O'Dwyer ST, Smith RJ, Hwang TL, et al: Maintenance of small bowel mucosa with glutamine enriched parenteral nutrition. *JPEN* 1989; 13:579–585.

218. Hwang TL, O'Dwyer ST, Smith RJ, et al: Preservation of small bowel mucosa using glutamine-enriched parenteral nutrition. *Surg Forum* 1987; 38:56.

219. Grant J: Use of L-glutamine in total parenteral nutrition. *J Surg Res* 1988; 44:506–513.

220. Klimberg VS, Souba WW, Sitren H, et al: Glutamine-enriched total parenteral nutrition supports gut metabolism. *Surg Forum* 1989; 40:175–177.

221. Burke D, Alverdy JC, Aoys E, et al: Glutamine supplemented TPN improves gut immune function. *Arch Surg* 1989; 124:1396–1399.

222. Salloum RM, Copeland EM, Souba WW: The early response of the brush border glutamine (GLN) carrier to endotoxemia (abstract 101). Presented at the 25th Annual Meeting of the Association for Academic Surgery, Colorado Springs, 1991, p 101.

223. Inoue Y, Grant JP, Snyder PJ: Effect of glutamine-supplemented intravenous nutrition on survival after *Escherichia coli*–induced peritonitis. *JPEN* 1993; 17(suppl):41–46.

224. Helton S, Scheltinga, Rodrick M, et al: Glumatine-enriched intravenous feedings may enhance immune function following chemotherapy-induced gut barrier dysfunction in rats (abstract 29). Presented at the 11th Annual Meeting of the Surgical Infection Society, Fort Lauderdale, Fla, 1991, p 48.

225. Crouch J, Wilmore D: The use of glutamine-supplemented parenteral nutrition (PN) in very low birth weight infants (abstract 51). *JPEN* 1991; 15(suppl):25.

226. Elder JB, Ganguli PC, Gillespie IE: Effect of urogastrone on gastric secretion and plasma gastrin levels in normal subjects. *Gut* 1975; 16:887–893.

227. Thompson JS, Sharp JG, Saxena SK, et al: Stimulation of neomucosal growth by systemic urogastrone. *J Surg Res* 1987; 42:402–410.

228. Jacobs DO, Evans DA, Mealy K, et al: Combined effects of glutamine and epidermal growth factor on the rat intestine. *Surgery* 1988; 104:358–364.

229. Tsujikawa T, Bamba T, Hosoda S: The trophic effect of epidermal growth factor on morphological changes and polyamine metabolism in the small intestine of rats. *Gastroenterol Jpn* 1990; 25:328–334.

230. Salloum RM, Schultz GS, Souba WW: Epidermal growth factor (EGF) stimulates brush border glutamine transport (abstract 33). *JPEN* 1991; 15(suppl):22.

231. Wright NA, Pike CM, Elia G: Ulceration induces a novel epidermal growth factor–secreting cell lineage in human gastrointestinal mucosa. *Digestion* 1990; 46(suppl 2):125–133.

232. Olsen PS, Poulsen SS, Therkelsen K, et al: Oral administration of synthetic human urogastrone promotes healing of chronic duodenal ulcers in rats. *Gastroenterology* 1986; 90:911–917.

233. Konturek SJ, Brzozowski T, Dembinski A, et al: Interaction of growth hormone–releasing factor and somatostatin on ulcer healing and mu-

cosal growth in rats: Role of gastrin and epidermal growth factor. *Digestion* 1988; 41:121–128.

234. Berseth CL: Enhancement of intestinal growth in neonatal rats by epidermal growth factor in milk. *Am J Physiol* 1987; 253:662–665.

235. Berseth CL, Go VL: Enhancement of neonatal somatic and hepatic growth by orally administered epidermal growth factor in rats. *J Pediatr Gastroenterol Nutr* 1988; 7:889–893.

236. Schober DA, Simmen FA, Hadsell DL, et al: Perinatal expression of type I IGF receptors in porcine small intestine. *Endocrinology* 1990; 126:1125–1132.

237. Trahair JF: Is fetal enteral nutrition important for normal gastrointestinal growth? A discussion. *JPEN* 1993; 17:82–85.

238. Shaw JH, Wildbore M, Wolfe RR: Whole-body protein kinetics in severely septic patients. *Ann Surg* 1987; 205:288–266.

239. Streat SJ, Beddoe AH, Hill GL: Aggressive nutritional support does not prevent protein loss despite fat gain in septic intensive care patients. *J Trauma* 1987; 27:262–266.

240. Jiang ZM, He GZ, Zhang SY, et al: Low-dose growth hormone and hypocaloric nutrition attenuate the protein-catabolic response after major operation. *Ann Surg* 1989; 210:513–525.

241. Ziegler TR, Young LS, Manson JMcK, et al: Metabolic effects of recombinant human growth hormone in patients receiving parenteral nutrition. *Ann Surg* 1988; 208:6–16.

242. Schalch DS, Heinrich UR, Draznin B, et al: Role of the liver in regulating somatomedin activity: Hormonal effects on the synthesis and release of insulin-like growth factor and its carrier protein by the isolated perfused rat liver. *Endocrinology* 1979; 104:1143–1151.

243. Van Neste L, Husman B, Moller C, et al: Cellular distribution of somatogenic receptors and insulin-like growth factor-I mRNA in rat liver. *J Endocrinol* 1988; 119:69–74.

244. Zapf J, Froesch ER: Insulin-like growth factors/somatomedins: Structures, secretion, biological actions

and physiological role. *Horm Res* 1986; 24:121–130.

245. Gore DC, Honeycutt D, Jahoor F, et al: Effect of exogenous growth hormone on whole-body and isolated-limb protein kinetics in burned patients. *Arch Surg* 1991; 126:38–43.

246. Herndon DN, Barrow RE, Kunkel KR, et al: Effects of recombinant human growth hormone on donor-site healing in severely burned children. *Ann Surg* 1990; 12:424–431.

247. Zaizen Y, Ford EG, Costin G, et al: The effect of perioperative exogenous growth hormone and wound bursting strength in normal and malnourished rats. *J Pediatr Surg* 1990; 25:70–74.

248. Dahn MS, Lange MP, Jacobs LA: Insulin-like growth factor 1 production is inhibited in human sepsis. *Arch Surg* 1988; 123:1409–1414.

249. Gottardis M, Benzer A, Koller W, et al: Improvement of septic syndrome after administration of recombinant human growth hormone (rhGH)? *J Trauma* 1991; 31:81–86.

250. Kimbrough TD, Shernan S, Ziegler TR, et al: Insulin-like growth factor-I response is comparable following intravenous and subcutaneous administration of growth hormone. *J Surg Res* 1991; 51:472–476.

251. Lemmey AB, Martin AA, Read LC, et al: IGF-I and the truncated analogue des-(1—3)IGF-I enhance growth in rats after gut resection. *Am J Physiol* 1991; 260:213–219.

252. Suh DY, Hunt TK, Spencer EM: Insulin-like growth factor-I reverses the impairment of wound healing induced by corticosteroids in rats. *Endocrinology* 1992; 131:2399–2403.

253. Thompson WA, Coyle SM, Lazarus D, et al: The metabolic effects of a continuous infusion of insulin-like growth factor (IGF-1) in parenterally fed man (abstract). *Surg Forum* 1991; 42:23–25.

254. Miell JP, Taylor AM, Jones J, et al: Administration of human recombinant insulin-like growth factor-I to patients following major gastrointestinal surgery. *Clin Endocrinol* 1992; 37:542–551.

255. Gross SJ, Oehler JM, Eckerman CO: Head circumference at birth and growth at six weeks as predictors of

developmental outcome in very low birth weight infants (abstract). *Pediatr Res* 1980; 14:343.

256. Hack M, Gordan D, Merkatz I, et al: The prognostic significance of postnatal growth in very now birth weight infants. *Pediatr Res* 1980; 14:434.

257. Birkhahn R, Long C, Fitkin D, et al: Effects of major skeletal trauma on whole body protein turnover in man measured by 1, 14 C leucine. *Surgery* 1980; 88:294–300.

258. Fischer JE: Branched-chain–enriched amino acid solutions in patients with liver failure: An early example of nutritional pharmacology. *JPEN* 1990; 14(suppl):249–256.

259. Bruzzone P, Siegel JH, Chiarla C, et al: Leucine dose response in the reduction of urea production from septic proteolysis and in the stimulation of acute-phase proteins. *Surgery* 1991; 109:768–778.

260. Kawamura I, Yamazaki K, Tsuchiya H, et al: Optimum branched-chain amino acids concentration for improving protein catabolism in severely stressed rats. *JPEN* 1990; 14:398–403.

261. Brennan FM, Cerra F, Daly JM, et al: Report of a research workshop: Branched chain amino acids in stress and injury. *JPEN* 1986; 10:446–452.

262. Desai SP, Bistrian BR, Polombo JR, e al: Branched chain amino acid administration in surgical patients. *Arch Surg* 1987; 127:760–764.

263. Abel RM, Beck CH Jr, Abbott WM, et al: Improved survival from acute renal failure after treatment with intravenous essential L-amino acids and glucose. *N Engl J Med* 1973; 288:695–699.

264. Cerra RB, Cheung NK, Fischer JE, et al: Disease-specific amino acid infusion (FO 80) in hepatic encephalopathy: A prospective, randomized, double-blind, controlled trial. *JPEN* 1985; 9:288–295.

265. Katz S, Plaisier BR, Folkening WJ, et al: Intralipid adversely affects reticuloendothelial bacterial clearance. *J Pediatr Surg* 1991; 26:921–924.

266. Hamawy KJ, Moldawer LL, Georgieff M, et al: Effect of lipid emulsions on the reticuloendothelial system func-

tion in the injured animal. *JPEN* 1985; 9:559–565.

267. Sobrado J, Moldawer LL, Pomposelli JJ, et al: Lipid emulsions and reticuloendothelial system function in healthy and burned guinea pigs, *Am J Clin Nutr* 1985; 42:855–863.

268. Kinsella JE, Lokesh B: Dietary lipids, eicosanoids, and the immune system. *Crit Care Med* 1990; 18(suppl):94–113.

269. Alexander JW, Saito H, Trocki O, et al: The importance of lipid type in the diet after burn injury. *Ann Surg* 1986; 204:1–8.

270. Mochizuki H, Trocki O, Dominioni L, et al: Optimal lipid content for enteral diets following thermal injury. *JPEN* 1984; 8:638–646.

271. Alexander JW, Gottschlich MM: Nutritional immunomodulation in burn patients. *Crit Care Med* 1990; 18(suppl):149–153.

272. Peck MD, Ogle CK, Alexander JW: Composition of fat in enteral diets can influence outcome in experimental peritonitis. *Ann Surg* 1991; 214:74–82.

273. Clouva-Molyvdas P, Peck MD, Alexander JW: Short-term dietary lipid manipulation does not affect survival in two models of murine sepsis. *JPEN* 1992; 16:343–347.

274. Rudolph FB, Kulkarni AD, Fanslow WC, et al: Role of RNA as a dietary source of pyrimidines and purines in immune function. *Nutrition* 1990; 6:45–52.

275. Van Buren CT, Kulkarni AD, Schandle VP, et al: The influence of dietary nucleotides on cell-mediated immunity. *Transplantation* 1983; 36:350–352.

276. Kulkarni AD, Fanslow WC, Rudolph FB, et al: Modulation of delayed hypersensitivity in mice by dietary nucleotide restriction. *Transplantation* 1988; 44:847–849.

277. Kulkarni AD, Fanslow WC, Rudolph FB, et al: Effect of dietary nucleotides on response to bacterial infections. *JPEN* 1986; 10:169–171.

278. Barbul A: Arginine and immune function. *Nutrition* 1990; 6:53–62.

279. Madden HP, Breslin RJ, Wasserkrug HL, et al: Stimulation of T cell immu-

nity enhances survival in peritonitis. *J Surg Res* 1988; 44:658–663.

280. Saito H, Trocki O, Wang S, et al: Metabolic and immune effects of dietary arginine supplementation after burn. *Arch Surg* 1987; 122:784–789.

281. Daly JM, Reynolds JV, Thom A, et al: Immune and metabolic effects of arginine in the surgical patient. *Ann Surg* 1988; 208:512–523.

282. Kirk SJ, Barbul A: Role of arginine in trauma, sepsis, and immunity. *JPEN* 1990; 14(suppl):226–229.

283. Nirgiotis JG, Hennessey PJ, Andrassy RJ: The effects of an arginine-free enteral diet on wound healing and immune function in the postsurgical rat. *J Pediatr Surg* 1991; 26:936–941.

284. Merimee TJ, Rabinowitz D, Riggs L: Plasma growth hormone after arginine infusion: Clinical experiences. *N Engl J Med* 1967; 276:434–439.

42

Refeeding Syndrome

Anita F. Jolly, M.S., R.D., CNSI, LDN

Roy Blank, M.D.

Knowledge of the dangers of refeeding famine victims dates back many centuries. During the time of the siege of Jerusalem it was recognized that the hunger the deserters experienced in captivity was less lethal than the uncontrolled feasting they enjoyed upon fleeing to Rome.[1] Sudden death from refeeding starved individuals was also observed in the mid-1940s. After World War II a number of investigators reported the unexpected death of starved prisoners of war (POW) shortly after reintroduction of high-calorie, high-carbohydrate foods. Autopsies on those individuals did not reveal any obvious cause.[1-5] In the classic Minnesota experiment of Keys et al.[6] 32 volunteers with normal cardiac function underwent 6 months of semistarvation; diminished cardiac reserve developed, in 1 volunteer to the point of cardiac failure, during the refeeding phase. These findings correlated with reports of an increased incidence of hypertension, cardiac insufficiency, and peripheral edema in the population of Leningrad after the postsiege restoration of normal food and fluid intake.[4, 6] Peripheral edema was reported in starved Japanese POWs, with several deaths reported after initiation of treatment.[3] Edema was prevalent in postfamine victims in the Netherlands[2] as well as the Minnesota volunteers.[6]

These potentially life-threatening refeeding complications became apparent once again in the 1970s and 1980s with the widespread use of total parenteral nutrition (TPN) in hospitalized patients who were often malnourished.[7] Silvis and Paragas[8] reported the death of three starved patients in whom severe hypophosphatemia developed within 4 to 7 days of initiating TPN. Weinsier and Krumdieck[5] reported the sudden death of two chronically malnourished, stable patients given aggressive TPN therapy. Within hours of the initiation of TPN, acute cardiopulmonary decompensation resulting in death developed in both patients. Although other abnormalities were found, severe hypophosphatemia induced by refeeding was believed to be the contributing factor for cardiopulmonary failure. More recently, Gustavsson and Eriksson[9] reported the case of a 19-year-old anorexic who sustained acute respiratory failure during TPN with symptomatic hypophosphatemia. Although parenteral nutrition therapy has received the most attention in the literature as a precipitator of the refeeding syndrome, enteral feedings are not without risk. Patrick[10] reported the sudden death of four malnourished children within 6 to 9 days of starting high-calorie enteral feedings.

The refeeding syndrome has typically been thought of as severe hypophosphatemia and its associated complications occurring in malnourished patients receiving parenteral support.[7] Solomon and Kirby[7] have proposed that the refeeding syndrome be redefined to include the changes that occur in phosphorus, potassium, magnesium, and glucose metabolism; vitamin status; and fluid needs. This definition should not be limited to the parenteral route.

Aggressive nutrition support is an integral part of the care of the critically ill patients who often arrive at the intensive care unit (ICU) with manifestations of malnutrition. Nutrition support, when properly managed, can contribute to the patient's recovery from critical illness or injury. However, poorly managed, overzealous nutrition support can be lethal. The critical care specialist must be familiar with the potentially life-threatening complications that may occur during specialized nutrition support. Proper management of nutrition support requires familiarity with nutrition assessment techniques, an understanding of the hormonal and metabolic effects of malnutrition and refeeding on various organ systems, knowledge of how and what to feed, and the ability to identify those patients at risk of the development of refeeding syndrome. Cautious refeeding and close monitoring of laboratory data, weight and fluid status, and the organ system response to substrate can prevent complications and enable intervention in a timely manner, should problems occur.

CLASSIFICATION OF MALNUTRITION

Generally, malnutrition in nonpediatric hospitalized patients can be classified as one of two types: adult marasmus or hypoalbuminemic malnutrition. Semistarvation and stress are the two variables that determine the degree and type of malnutrition.[11] Anorexia or functional impairment of the gastrointestinal tract results in semi-

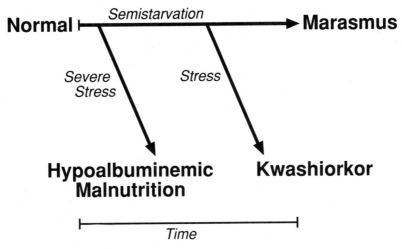

FIG 42–1.

General scheme of the pathophysiology of hospital malnutrition. Semistarvation can lead to marasmus, while the severe stress of major injury or sepsis can result in hypoalbuminemic malnutrition in a well-nourished subject. Less severe stress can lead to a kwashiorkor-like state in a marasmic individual. (From Bistrian BR: Assessment of protein energy malnutrition in surgical patients, in Hill GL (ed): *Nutrition and the Surgical Patient,* vol 2. Edinburgh, Churchill Livingstone, 1981. Used by permission.)

starvation leading to weight loss from fat and muscle. There is a reduction in muscle mass and fat stores, but immune function is usually preserved. This is called adult marasmus when the condition is severe.[11–13] The addition of stress or injury, mediated by hormonal and cytokine responses, causes an increase in protein loss from both skeletal muscle and viscera that leads to hypoalbuminemia and anergy.[11, 14] The moderate stress of routine surgery or infection in a marasmic patient can lead to an adult kwashiorkor-like syndrome (Fig 42–1).[11]

Identification of the chronically ill, marasmic patient is of utmost importance because this type patient is at greatest risk of the development of refeeding complications after initiation of nutrition therapy.

PHYSIOLOGY OF STARVATION

Survival during prolonged periods of inadequate food supply depends upon the body's ability to adapt to substrate deprivation.[15–17] The body adapts to insufficient exogenous energy supply by a voluntary reduction in physical work, thereby reducing energy expenditure, and an involuntary reduction in the basal metabolic rate (BMR), thereby reducing the rate of deterioration of body stores.[16] The reduction in BMR is mediated by decreased protein turnover and decreased levels of thyroid hormones, catecholamines, and somatomedins.[18] When the lowered BMR does not reequate the energy output to the limited intake, endogenous fuels must be used to balance the equation. This is the thermodynamic law of starvation.[19] Major changes in fuel utilization then occur.

The major storage fuel of humans and animals is fat in the form of triglycerides. During fasting, the body's fat supply is the major determinant of the length of survival, which in a nonobese individual coincides roughly with the predicted time of depletion of fat stores, approximately 60[19] to 75 days.[20]

Carbohydrate, in contrast, is quantitatively an insignificant storage fuel. The total caloric value of liver and muscle glycogen and circulating free glucose is approximately 1200 kcal, less than 1 day's resting energy requirement.[15, 19, 21]

Body protein content is approximately 12 kg. Although theoretically protein could supply close to 2 weeks' worth of calories, this depletion would have profound adverse effects since each molecule of protein is reserved for non-fuel functions.[15, 19]

When exogenous fuel is unavailable, hormonal changes develop in response to an early fall in blood sugar levels. There is a prompt decrease in insulin secretion and an increase in glucagon, growth hormone (GH), and catecholamines. Liver glycogenolysis and skeletal muscle proteolysis are enhanced. Circulating triiodothyronine (T_3) levels decline, while reverse T_3 (rT_3) and plasma cortisol levels rise. Hepatic gluconeogenesis is enhanced, and lipolysis is facilitated. At this time, the brain is living primarily off glucose produced from muscle protein breakdown. Alanine and glutamine are the major sources of three-carbon gluconeogenic precursors released by skeletal muscle. About 75 g of muscle protein or 12 g of nitrogen (N) is catabolized during the first 2 to 3 days of a fast. Glycerol from triglyceride breakdown and lactate and pyruvate from the Cori cycle and muscle glycogenolysis also contribute to the precursor pool for hepatic gluconeogenesis.[21] Figure 42–2 illustrates fuel origin and metabolism in an acutely fasted individual.

The breakdown of muscle protein to meet the brain's energy demands is incompatible with survival for more than 2 weeks, if allowed to persist.[21] Therefore, after 10 to 14 days of starvation, the body makes another major adaptation by switching from glucose to fat as the major energy source. Gluconeogenesis is reduced and protein breakdown minimized. Ketone bodies, produced from hepatic oxidation of fatty acids, are utilized by most tissues for energy and essentially replace glucose as brain fuel. Protein breakdown drops to approximately 20 g/day.[16] Figure 42–3 shows the adaptation to fasting that occurs after 5 to 6 weeks.

In early starvation the liver is the primary site of gluconeogenesis. As starvation is prolonged, the kidney plays an

Fasting Man
(24 hours, basal: ~1800 calories)

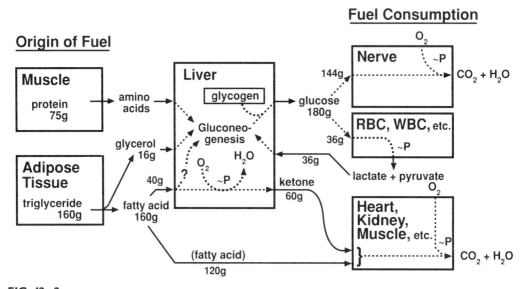

FIG 42–2.
Schematic representation of fuel metabolism in a normal reference male in an acute fasted state. (From Cahill GF: *N Engl J Med* 1970; 282:668. Used by permission.)

Fasting Man, Adapted (5-6 weeks)
(24 hours, basal: -1500 calories)

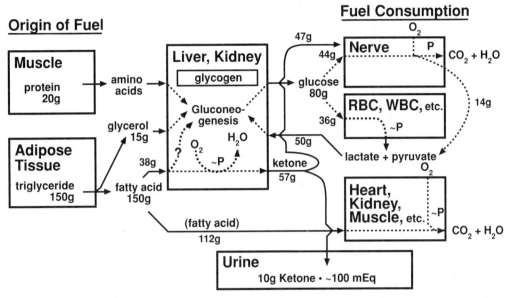

FIG 42–3.
Schematic representation of fuel metabolism after 5 to 6 weeks of starvation. (From Cahill GF: *N Engl J Med* 1970; 282:668. Used by permission.)

increasingly important role as a glucose-producing organ.[15]

BODY COMPOSITION CHANGES

There is a progressive fall in body weight proportional to the decrease in food intake. Weight loss is greatest at the beginning of a fast because of a disproportionate loss of water. The rate of weight loss gradually declines and levels off as a result of reduced physical activity and decreased BMR. Changes in body composition occur. Body fat and lean body mass are reduced. As starvation progresses, fat contributes to a greater percentage of the weight loss, and this reduces the contribution from lean body mass as protein-sparing adaptations take place.[16] There is a relative expansion of extracellular fluid (ECF) space and a decrease in intracellular fluid (ICF) space from the loss of protein and cell water.[16, 22–24] Bone mass is essentially maintained except in pro-longed, severe starvation.[6, 16, 25] Figure 42–4 represents the body composition of a normal 70-kg reference adult and the alterations in body composition after a 15-kg weight loss.

FLUID AND ELECTROLYTE CHANGES IN STARVATION

Changes in the water, electrolyte, and mineral content of the body take place during fasting. A reduction in total-body water (TBW) is most significant during the first 10 days to 2 weeks of fasting.[26, 27] Water losses occur from both the ICF and ECF spaces. As lean body mass is reduced, ICF is lost through cell attrition.[26] As opposed to the changes in fluid space observed in acute starvation, protein-calorie malnutrition (PCM) or prolonged starvation results in a relative expansion in ECF volume. Water and sodium are conserved as inadequate food intake continues over several months and may be manifested as edema.[6, 26]

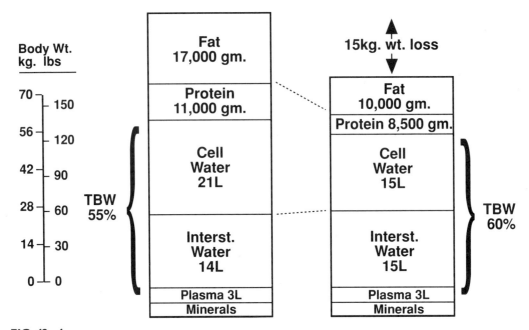

FIG 42–4.

Representative values for the body composition of a normal adult and the changes in composition after a weight loss of 15 kg. There is a relative increase in extracellular space and a disproportionate loss of intracellular components after weight loss. (From Bland J: *Clinical Metabolism of Water and Electrolytes.* Philadelphia, WB Saunders, 1963. Used by permission.)

A brisk natriuresis occurs within 48 hours of the onset of total fasting. By the first to second week of fasting the urinary losses of sodium decrease considerably. The natriuresis of total fasting is prevented by even small amounts of carbohydrates.[28–30] Potassium is lost during fasting in amounts that parallel sodium losses. Catabolism of body cell mass accounts for the majority of potassium losses, although other factors may play a role.[27] Phosphorus is lost in the urine during fasting, and these losses can be suppressed by glucose infusion. Blood levels remain unchanged. Cell attrition accounts for most of these losses. Significant losses of magnesium also occur during prolonged fasting, largely because of cell attrition. However, renal losses also contribute to magnesium losses. Serum magnesium levels usually remain normal.[26] Urinary zinc excretion is enhanced by catabolism but is only a fraction of what would be expected to be released from skeletal muscle breakdown.[31]

METABOLIC RESPONSE TO REFEEDING

The primary factor responsible for the metabolic response to refeeding is a shift from body fat to carbohydrate as the major fuel source. Refeeding with carbohydrates and protein produces a change in circulating insulin levels that plays a key role in the transition from the use of endogenous fuel sources to exogenous ones. The increase in insulin concentration antagonizes the action of glucagon in the liver. Glycogenolysis and gluconeogenesis are reduced, and fatty acid mobilization from adipose tissues is inhibited by insulin.[32] Cellular uptake of glucose, potassium, phosphorus, and magnesium are all enhanced by the action of insulin.[33, 34]

Refeeding with carbohydrate produces an abrupt cessation of urinary sodium excretion in subjects who have fasted for as little as 3 days.[28–30, 35] Insulin release induced by carbohydrate refeeding is believed to be a major factor[28, 33, 36, 37] because of its antinatriuretic effect.[33] There is an expansion of ECF space associated with refeeding that cannot be totally explained by an increase in carbohydrate intake[23, 24] and is independent of the route of substrate administration.[6, 23, 24, 27, 38-44] It may be manifested as refeeding edema. Fluid retention is most pronounced during the first few days of refeeding and again during the first few days after increasing the caloric load above maintenance levels.[42-44]

EFFECTS OF STARVATION/ REFEEDING ON VARIOUS ORGAN SYSTEMS

Cardiovascular System

Starvation Effects

The heart is not spared during prolonged starvation as once erroneously believed.[6, 45-47] Cardiac muscle atrophies in parallel with the loss of lean body mass.[6, 46, 48-50] PCM results in the catabolism of cardiac contractile and sarcoplasmic proteins.[51] Cardiac function is reduced in proportion to declining ventricular mass, with a concomitant reduction in cardiac output and stroke volume.[6, 46, 48, 50-52] Hypotension, bradycardia, and a decreased metabolic rate are associated with uncomplicated starvation.[2, 4, 6, 23, 24, 45, 52] This allows the heart to function in the setting of reduced oxygen consumption[6, 48, 51] and is not to be confused with circulatory failure.[4, 48] Decreased ventricular compliance has been noted in starved animals.[49] Indices of ventricular contractility may be reduced in kwashiorkor-type malnutrition[49] but are usually normal in marasmus.[45, 46, 52]

Refeeding Response

Changes induced by refeeding can have adverse effects on the cardiovascular system. Refeeding reverses the hypometabolic state of starvation.[51] There are increases in heart rate, blood pressure, oxygen consumption,[6, 48] and cardiac output and an expansion of plasma volume.[6, 51, 52] The extent of the cardiovascular response to refeeding is dependent on the amount of calories, protein, and sodium administered. The malnourished heart can easily be faced with a metabolic demand that exceeds its supply capabilities.[6, 52] The consequences of refeeding are even more severe in marasmic patients with underlying cardiac disease.[51] Keys et al.[6, 48] noted that the heart was closer to failure in the early refeeding phase of the Minnesota experiment than during starvation.

Congestive heart failure (CHF) is a common complication of specialized nutrition support. Several factors can predispose the critically ill patient to the development of CHF upon refeeding. The malnourished patient may not be able to increase cardiac output sufficiently to meet the hemodynamic demands imposed by rapid expansion of the plasma volume, increased oxygen consumption, and increases in blood pressure and heart rate.[52] Even minimal volume and calorie infusions can trigger CHF in patients with pre-existing cardiac disease.[50] Furthermore, injury and sepsis in themselves impose metabolic and hemodynamic responses that tax myocardial reserves.[18] Strong antidiuretic tendencies occur when injury is superimposed on simple starvation.[27] CHF has been reported in subjects refed orally,[6, 38, 47] nasoenterically,[42-44, 53] and parenterally.[27, 54]

Respiratory System

Starvation Effects

Malnutrition adversely affects all aspects of the respiratory system.[55] Expiratory and inspiratory muscles are catabolized during prolonged food deprivation.[56] There is a reduction in diaphragmatic mass proportional to the reduction in body weight.[56-59] Respiratory muscle strength,[43] maximum voluntary ventilation, vital capacity, and maximum inspiratory pressure are all reduced in malnutrition.[6, 56, 60, 61] The lowered metabolic rate associated with starvation results in a decreased ventilatory response to hypoxia and hypercapnia.[62, 63] Deterioration in the function of the parenchyma and emphysematous changes have also been reported in starvation.[56] Decreased surfactant synthesis, storage, and secretion associated with malnutrition can lead to serious complications during trauma and sepsis.[64] Air space enlargement resulting from increased surface elastic forces and decreased lung tissue elasticity may also occur in malnutrition.[65] Finally, malnourished patients have increased susceptibility to pulmonary infections from compromised immune function, a reduced ability to clear secretions, and impaired muscle function.[55]

Refeeding Response

Excess carbon dioxide (CO_2) production and increased oxygen (O_2) consumption may result from excess glucose administration and overfeeding. Parenteral glucose infusions beyond 5 mg/kg/min result in an increased respiratory quotient (RQ) as glucose is converted to fat for storage. Energy is required for triglyceride synthesis from carbohydrate, and this results in an increased metabolic rate, increased CO_2 and water production, and increased O_2 consumption.[66] The increase in CO_2 production and possibly other respiratory stimuli associated with carbohydrate loading produces large increases in minute ventilation.[67] This excess CO_2 production and increased minute ventilation can precipitate respiratory distress in patients with compromised pulmonary status from underlying respiratory disease or malnutrition-induced respiratory muscle wasting.[67-71] It may make weaning difficult in mechanically ventilated patients.[72] Overfeeding carbohydrates en-

terally has also been shown to increase minute ventilation, O_2 consumption, CO_2 production, RQ,[53] and $paco_2$.[73] Protein administered either orally[55] or parenterally[55, 56] induces an increase in resting minute ventilation and oxygen consumption and also enhances the ventilatory responses to hypercapnia and hypoxia. Patients with compromised respiratory function may experience dyspnea because of an inability to sustain an increased ventilatory drive.[56] Furthermore, pulmonary edema may develop in some patients because of the increased water load from both the infusion rate and lipogenesis.[69]

Gastrointestinal System

Starvation Effects

Starvation, even of short duration, has a negative impact on gastrointestinal mass and function. In the early stages the formation of enterocytes is decreased, and nutrient absorption is impaired.[74] Levels of brush border disaccharidases and pancreatic enzymes are reduced because of mucosal atrophy and the loss of intraluminal stimulation[75-78] and possibly from generalized protein depletion.[6] As starvation progresses, the gut atrophies with decreased crypt cell proliferation and reduced villus height.[79] The entire wall and the mucosal lining of the gastrointestinal tract are thinner than normal in PCM, and brush border height is reduced.[75] Intestinal mass is reduced,[76] and there is thickening and coarsening of the mucosal folds of the small intestine.[80] Decreased gastric acidity[2, 75] and malabsorption of glucose, D-xylose, fat,[75, 80] and vitamin B_{12}[77] have also been reported. Delayed gastric emptying was reported in the fasted Minnesota volunteers,[6] and decreased intestinal motility has been noted in malnourished children and adults.[75, 80]

Diarrhea is a common problem in starvation.[2, 3, 6, 75, 80] Bacterial overgrowth, unconjugated bile salts, hypoalbuminemia, and bowel wall edema may contribute to the diarrhea of starvation.[2, 6, 75, 80]

Refeeding Response

Reduced enzyme activity appears to be an adaptive response to substrate deprivation.[74-76] The activity of brush border enzymes and pancreatic enzyme secretion return to normal with refeeding. However, this requires a period of readaptation to food so as to minimize gastrointestinal complaints.[6, 74, 75, 78, 81] The Minnesota volunteers[6] and postwar famine victims[2, 3] were able to consume relatively large amounts of food without gastric disturbances. Gastric irritation was noted in subjects who indiscriminately ate unlimited amounts of foods, especially bulky, gas-forming foods.[6] The adaptation to oral refeeding that is seen in starvation does not occur in critically ill malnourished patients receiving enteral feedings. Diarrhea occurs in as many as 50% of critically ill patients.[82] Nausea and vomiting are also frequent complaints in this group of patients.[83] The causes of these disturbances are multifactorial and are exacerbated by the structural and functional changes in the gastrointestinal tract associated with malnutrition.[82]

METABOLIC CONSEQUENCES OF REFEEDING

Excess Glucose

Glucose is an important substrate in specialized nutrition support. As previously discussed, overfeeding carbohydrates (enterally or parenterally) may result in adverse consequences. Hyperglycemia is a common complication of specialized nutrition support. Critically ill patients are often hypermetabolic and insulin resistant because of the metabolic response to stress and infection. Gluconeogenesis continues in the stressed patient because of hormonal mediators in spite of high circulating levels of insulin. Hyperglycemia develops in nondiabetic patients if given large amounts of glucose. This is especially true in the hypercatabolic, stressed state.[66] Uncontrolled hyperglycemia can lead to hyperosmolar nonketotic coma, which has a mortality rate as high as 40%.[84] The deaths usually occur from the complications of dehydration.[85] Hyperglycemia may also place the compromised, critically ill patient at higher risk of the development of sepsis.[37] The expansion of ECF space leading to the edema that is associated with glucose feeding may delay wound healing and result in a higher incidence of postsurgical complications.[39, 41] Serum glucose levels should be kept in the range of 100 to 200 mg/dL.[37]

Phosphorus

Hypophosphatemia is one of the most serious metabolic complications observed in response to specialized nutrition support[5, 85-87] and may occur rapidly and often dramatically after the initiation of nutrition therapy. Plummeting serum phosphorus levels may be seen within 24 to 72 hours after beginning therapy.[5, 8, 87-90] However, it is possible to see a delay in the development of hypophosphatemia of 5 to 10 days in patients who have normal body stores of phosphorus. Hypophosphatemia results from inadequate phosphorus supplementation and/or abnormal phosphorus losses.[1] In response to refeeding, there is a movement of inorganic phosphorus from the extracellular to the intracellular space because of the utilization of phosphorus for the synthesis of phosphorylated compounds.[1] Insulin also promotes the uptake of both phosphorus and glucose in skeletal muscle and liver.[85] Severe hypophosphatemia (below 1.0 mg/dL) is associated with serious life-threatening complications involving all major organ systems.[1, 85, 91] It can lead to respiratory failure,[5, 9, 91-93] cardiac abnormalities,[5, 94, 95] central nervous system (CNS) dysfunction[1, 85, 88] including seizures,[8] red blood cell dysfunction,[85, 96, 97] leukocyte dysfunction,[85] and difficulty in weaning from the respirator.[91, 98]

Table 42–1 lists conditions associated with hypophosphatemia that are exacerbated by refeeding. These conditions include alcoholism, diabetic ketoacidosis, use of phosphorus-binding antacids, the recovery/diuretic phase after severe burns, diuretic therapy, respiratory alkalosis,[85] diarrhea, and nasogastric suctioning.[91]

Potassium

Refeeding causes a shift of potassium into cells and may result in hypokalemia if potassium is not adequately supplied in the diet. Potassium moves into cells along with glucose and other energy substrates. Protein anabolism results in incorporation of potassium into the cell protoplasm.[99]

Symptoms of hypokalemia include muscle weakness, paralysis, paralytic ileus, cardiac arrhythmias, coronary ischemia, rhabdomyolysis, renal dysfunction, abnormal carbohydrate metabolism, decreased insulin release, and negative nitrogen balance.[33]

Hypokalemia resulting from excessive potassium losses commonly occurs secondary to protracted vomiting; prolonged nasogastric suctioning; severe diarrhea; the use of steroids, loop and thiazide-type diuretics, and amphotericin B; and hypomagnesemia (Table 42–2).[33]

TABLE 42–1.

Conditions Associated With Hypophosphatemia

Chronic alcoholism
Diabetic ketoacidosis
Use of phosphorus-binding antacids
Recovery/diuretic phase after severe burns
Respiratory alkalosis
Insulin administration
Diarrhea
Nasogastric suctioning
Malabsorption
Corticosteroid administration

TABLE 42–2.

Primary Causes of Hypokalemia

Insulin administration
Protracted vomiting
Prolonged nasogastric suctioning
Severe diarrhea
Steroids
Loop and thiazide-type diuretics
Amphotericin B
Hypomagnesemia
Mineralocorticoid excess

Magnesium

Magnesium shifts intracellularly with refeeding and new tissue synthesis.[34] Hypomagnesemia is a frequent complication of both enteral[100] and parenteral nutrition support.[34, 101]

Magnesium serves a critical function in intracellular metabolism. It is an important cofactor in many enzyme systems involved in energy storage and utilization and in protein synthesis. It is also important for proper functioning of the CNS, the peripheral neuromuscular system, and the cardiovascular system.[34] Clinical deficiency symptoms are associated with serum levels below 1.0 mEq/L.[34] Hypomagnesemia may lead to cardiac arrhythmias.[101, 102] Release of parathyroid hormone is impaired in hypomagnesemia and may cause hypocal-

TABLE 42–3.

Factors Associated With Hypomagnesemia

Malnutrition
Prolonged nasogastric suctioning
Prolonged severe diarrhea
Extensive bowel resection
Presence of intestinal or biliary fistulas
Pancreatitis
Chronic alcoholism
Hypoparathyroidism
Primary aldosteronism
Medications
  Mannitol
  Urea
  Aminoglycosides
  Cisplatin
  Diuretics
  Cardiac glycosides
  High doses of insulin

cemia as calcium moves from the ECF to bone. Deficiency symptoms include hyperreflexia, stridor, papilledema, seizures, a positive Chvostek or Trousseau sign, muscle tremors, fasciculations, and muscular weakness.[101]

The principal causes of magnesium deficiency are listed in Table 42–3. These include malnutrition, prolonged nasogastric suctioning, diarrhea, extensive bowel resection, the presence of intestinal or biliary fistulas, pancreatitis, alcohol abuse, hypoparathyroidism, and primary aldosteronism.[34, 101] Certain medications may also predispose to increased magnesium losses. These include mannitol, urea, gentamicin, cisplatin, diuretics, and cardiac glycosides.[101]

VITAMIN DEFICIENCY AND REFEEDING

Thiamine

Solomon and Kirby[7] suggest that thiamine deficiency contributes to the refeeding syndrome. It is commonly a consequence of alcoholism and chronic undernutrition and results from reduced tissue stores. Thiamine functions as a cofactor in intermediary carbohydrate metabolism. The requirement for thiamine directly correlates with the amount of carbohydrate ingested or administered.[103] Refeeding carbohydrates to deficient patients, without adequate thiamine supplementation, can lead to deficiency symptoms. Those at highest risk are patients with a history of alcohol abuse, anorexia nervosa, or prolonged fasting or starvation and pregnant women with hyperemesis gravidarum.[7] Thiamine requirements may also be increased after bariatric surgery or prolonged intravenous hydration[7] or in cases of intractable fever and hyperthyroidism.[103] Some degree of thiamine deficiency may exist in patients with CHF because of inadequate caloric and vitamin intake and may exacerbate cardiac failure.[104] Conditions that may

TABLE 42–4.

Conditions Leading to Thiamine Deficiency Symptoms

Refeeding carbohydrates
Alcohol abuse
Anorexia nervosa
Prolonged fasting or starvation
Pregnancy with hyperemesis gravidarum
After bariatric surgery
Prolonged intravenous hydration
Intractable fever
Hyperparathyroidism
Cardiac cachexia/conjestive heart failure

lead to thiamine deficiency are summarized in Table 42–4.

The nervous and cardiovascular systems are primarily affected by thiamine deficiency. The most common symptoms in adults are mental confusion, ataxia, muscle weakness, edema (wet beriberi), muscle wasting (dry beriberi), tachycardia and cardiomegaly.[103] While the most severe neurologic manifestation, Wernicke's encephalopathy, is usually associated with chronic deficiency states, it can be precipitated by carbohydrate refeeding in thiamine-deficient patients.[7] Normally, 0.5 mg/1000 kcal is sufficient to prevent deficiency symptoms.[103] However, the development of Wernicke's encephalopathy has been reported during TPN with the usual recommended daily thiamine dose of 3.2 mg.[105] In our practice, we routinely give high-risk patients 100 mg of thiamine intramuscularly daily for at least 3 to 5 days, in addition to daily maintenance doses, to replete tissue stores and cover possible increased requirements.

PREVENTION OF THE REFEEDING SYNDROME

The key to prevention of the refeeding syndrome is to be aware of it and its consequences. Prevention begins with recognition of those patients at greatest risk of the development of potentially lethal complications from rapid, overzealous feeding. Conditions that may trig-

Conditions Placing Patients at Highest Risk for Refeeding Syndrome

Chronic alcoholism
Anorexia nervosa
Classic marasmus
Classic kwashiorkor
Chronic undernourishment
Morbid obesity with massive weight loss
Prolonged hypocaloric intravenous hydration
Prolonged fasting
Nothing by mouth for greater than 7–10 days
Cardiac and cancer cachexia

ger the syndrome are listed in Table 42–5. These include chronic alcoholism, classic marasmus, anorexia nervosa, chronic PCM, morbid obesity with massive weight loss, prolonged hypocaloric intravenous hydration, prolonged fasting,[7] and cardiac and cancer cachexia.

RECOMMENDATIONS FOR REFEEDING

Calories

Before initiating specialized nutrition support, a comprehensive nutrition assessment, including an evaluation of organ system function, must be performed. Then, calorie and protein requirements should be determined. Apovian and coworkers[106] recommend determining basal energy expenditure (BEE) by using the Harris-Benedict formula based on the patients's actual body weight or by using indirect calorimetry, when available. The goal for the first week of refeeding should be to provide calories at the estimated BEE to no more than 1.2 times BEE. Glucose should be initially restricted to no more than 2 mg/kg/min or approximately 150 to 200 g of dextrose per day.[106] Lipids should provide approximately 20% to 30% of the nonprotein calories. Both parenteral and enteral feedings should be initiated slowly and increased gradually over a period of 5 to 7 days, as tolerated, until the final goal is achieved.[5] The metabolic and cardiovascular responses to refeeding are most signifi-

cant during the first few days of refeeding,[42–44] and it may take 1 week to adapt to the increased O_2 demand.[42] Attempts to achieve weight gain should not be a goal during the first week of refeeding.

Protein

Normally, 1.2 to 1.5 g of protein per kilogram per day can be safely administered to patients with normal hepatic and renal function.[5, 106] In our practice, we use actual body weight in marasmic patients and adjusted ideal body weight in obese individuals. Some clinicians recommend using ideal body weight,[5, 106] but we have found the use of this weight to result in excessive protein loading in very emaciated or elderly patients.

Fluid

Insulin release associated with carbohydrate refeeding results in an expansion of the ECF space. Very thin individuals (40 to 45 kg), the frail elderly, and obese short people are most susceptible to overexpansion of ECF.[41] Fluid must be judiciously administered during the first few days[42–44] to few weeks[106] of refeeding. Weight gain greater than 1 kg (from lean body mass accretion) during the first week represents fluid retention. Fluid may need to be restricted to 800 to 1000 cc/day.[5] Daily weights, accurate intake and output records, close attention to the heart (S3 gallop) and the lungs (rales), and assessment of peripheral tissues for signs of edema can prevent complications from fluid overload.[52] Increases in blood pressure, heart rate, and respiratory rate may be early signs of fluid excess.[10] If edema develops, digoxin and diuretics may be necessary.[10, 51]

Electrolytes

Electrolyte abnormalities should be corrected prior to initiating specialized nutrition support.[5] Serum electrolyte levels including phosphorus and magnesium should be monitored daily until stable and then at least every other day, depending upon clinical circumstances.

Sodium

In the early refeeding period, sodium should be administered cautiously to prevent overexpansion of the ECF space. No more than 30 to 60 mEq/day should be given to malnourished patients especially those with underlying cardiopulmonary diseases.[107, 108] Most enteral feeding products are low in sodium, and parenteral formulations can be tailored to meet individual needs. After the first week, calories, fluid, and sodium intake can be liberalized as the metabolism adjusts to the increased intake.[106]

Phosphorus

Additional phosphorus is required when refeeding starved patients because of decreased body stores and increased demands. TPN supplemented with 13.6 to 15 mM/L of phosphorus may be required initially to prevent plummeting serum levels upon refeeding.[87, 109] If serum levels are low prior to the initiation of therapy, as much as 20 mM/L may be needed to maintain normal serum levels.[87] Patients receiving enteral feeding also require additional supplementation, and this group of patients must be closely monitored. Treatment of serum phosphorus levels below 1.0 mg/dL requires intravenous replacement.[91, 92, 109] Zaloga usually begins phosphorus replacement with 0.2 to 0.8 mM/kg every 12 hours; larger doses are given in cases of multifactorial, prolonged deficiency[91] (i.e., 0.16 mM/kg has been recommended in these cases). Any one dose should not exceed 0.24 mM/kg to minimize the side effects associated with phosphorus administration.[109] In our practice, we routinely administer doses of 15 to 20 mM of phosphorus over a 6- to 8-hour period for levels below 1.2 to 1.5 mg/dL and have not encountered any adverse ef-

fects. Phosphorus levels should be checked shortly after the phosphorus infusion is completed and the dose repeated as needed. Oral phosphorus replacement can be started in patients with functioning gastrointestinal tracts once the serum level is above 2.0 mg/dL. Two hundred fifty to 500 mg/day for 5 to 7 days may be needed to replenish depleted body stores.[91] Patients with renal disease require more careful replacement and closer monitoring.

Potassium

Potassium is utilized in the cellular uptake of glucose, in glycogen synthesis, and in lean tissue anabolism.[34] Carbohydrate refeeding results in as much as 600 g of glycogen synthesis with approximately 1 mEq of potassium required for ever 3 g of glycogen produced. Also, about 3 mEq of potassium per gram of nitrogen is retained during protein synthesis.[106] Repletion of decreased body stores apart from anabolic needs will be necessary in malnourished patients. Initially, at least 80 to 120 mEq/day may be needed to replete potassium stores and meet daily requirements.[108] Grant[34] recommends that 1.2 to 1.5 mEq/kg be given initially in patients with normal renal function. In cases of severe depletion, as much as 2.5 mEq/kg may be needed. Serum values should be kept in the high normal range to ensure optimal metabolic conditions.[34]

Magnesium

Magnesium is retained during anabolism at the rate of 0.5 mEq for each gram of nitrogen used for protein synthesis. Patients receiving TPN require 12 to 15 mEq/day. More may be needed in patients who have depleted stores or increased gastrointestinal or renal losses.[108] Hypomagnesemia is frequently seen in critically ill patients, and prevention is the best therapy. The daily intravenous administration of 8 to 16 mEq (1 to 2 g) of magnesium salt can prevent deficiency. In patients with renal insufficiency, replacement should be guided by serum magnesium levels so as to prevent hypermagnesemia. Magnesium sulfate is routinely used as the replacement salt. Sulfate ions can bind calcium, so magnesium chloride (9.25 mEq Mg/g) may be a better choice for hypocalcemic patients. Replacement can also be given intramuscularly or orally, but the intravenous route is preferred in malnourished, critically ill patients.[101]

Vitamins/Minerals

Vitamins and minerals should be routinely administered during nutritional support. Needs should be individualized according to the disease state, nutritional requirements, and body losses.

Complications of the refeeding syndrome are principally related to the fluid and electrolyte abnormalities that result from the sudden introduction of exogenous glucose in a host whose metabolism has adapted to chronic semistarvation. Awareness of this syndrome combined with careful administration and monitoring of specialized nutritional support allows for safe nutritional therapy in high-risk patients.

REFERENCES

1. Ritz E: Acute hypophosphatemia. *Kidney Int* 1982; 22:84.
2. Burger GCE, Drummond JC, Sandstead HR (eds): *Malnutrition and Starvation in Western Netherlands, September 1944–July 1945*, parts I and II. The Hague, Netherlands, General State Printing Office, 1948.
3. Schnitker MA, Mattman PE, Bliss TL: A clinical study of malnutrition in Japanese prisoners of war. *Ann Intern Med* 1951; 35:69.
4. Brozek J, Chapman CB, Keys A: Drastic food restriction. *JAMA* 1948; 137:1569.
5. Weinsier RL, Krumdieck CL: Death resulting from overzealous total parenteral nutrition: The refeeding syndrome revisited. *Am J Clin Nutr* 1981; 34:393.
6. Keys A, Brozek J, Henschel A, et al: *The Biology of Human Starvation*, vol 1–2. Minneapolis, University of Minnesota Press, 1950.
7. Solomon SM, Kirby DF: The refeeding syndrome: A review. *JPEN* 1990; 14:90.
8. Silvis SE, Paragas PD: Paresthesias, weakness, seizures and hypophosphatemia in patients receiving hyperalimentation. *Gastroenterology* 1972; 62:513.
9. Gustavvson CG, Eriksson L: Acute respiratory failure in anorexia nervosa with hypophosphatemia. *J Intern Med* 1989; 225:63.
10. Patrick J: Death during recovery from severe malnutrition and its possible relationship to sodium pump activity in the leukocyte. *BMJ* 1977; 1:1051.
11. Bistrian BR: Assessment of protein energy malnutrition in surgical patients, in Hill GL (ed): *Nutrition in the Surgical Patient*. Edinburg, Churchill Livingstone, 1981.
12. Blackburn GL, Bistrian BR, Maini BS, et al: Nutritional and metabolic assessment of the hospitalized patient. *JPEN* 1977; 1:11.
13. Bistrian BR, Sherman M, Blackburn GL, et al: Cellular immunity in adult marasmus. *Arch Intern Med* 1977; 137:1408.
14. Bistrian BR, Blackburn GL, Scrimshaw NS, et al: Cellular immunity in semistarved states in hospitalized adults. *Am J Clin Nutr* 1975; 28:1148.
15. Cahill GF: Starvation in man. *N Engl J Med* 1970; 282:668.
16. Levenson SM, Seifter E: Starvation: Metabolic and physiologic responses, in Burke J (ed): *Surgical Physiology*. Philadelphia, WB Saunders, 1983.
17. Torun B, Viteri FE: Protein-energy malnutrition, in Shils ME, Young VR (eds): *Modern Nutrition in Health and Disease*, ed 7. Philadelphia, Lea & Febiger, 1988.
18. Schlichtig R, Ayres SM: *Nutritional Support of the Critically Ill*. St Louis, Mosby–Year Book, 1988.
19. Hoffer LJ: Starvation, in Shils ME, Young VR (eds): *Modern Nutrition in Health and Disease*, ed 7. Philadelphia, Lea & Febiger, 1988.
20. Whittaker JS, Jeejeebhoy KN: Alimentation, in DeGroot LJ (ed): *Endocri-*

nology. vol 1–3. Philadelphia, WB Saunders, 1989.

21. Cahill GF: Starvation: Some biological aspects, in Kinney JM, Jeejeebhoy KN, Owen OE (eds): *Nutrition and Metabolism in Patient Care.* Philadelphia, WB Saunders, 1988.

22. Bland JH: *Clinical Metabolism of Body Water and Electrolytes.* Philadelphia, WB Saunders, 1963.

23. Vaisman N, Corey M, Rossi MF, et al: Changes in body composition during refeeding of patients with anorexia nervosa. *J Pediatr* 1988; 113:925.

24. Vaisman N, Rossi MF, Goldberg E, et al: Energy expenditure and body composition in patients with anorexia nervosa. *J Pediatr* 1988; 113:919.

25. Barac-Nieto M, Spurr GB, Lotero H, et al: Body composition in chronic undernutrition. *Am J Clin Nutr* 1978; 31:23.

26. Hood VL: Fluid and electrolyte disturbances during starvation, in Kokko JP, Tannen RL (eds): *Fluid and Electrolytes.* Philadelphia, WB Saunders, 1986.

27. Albina JE, Melnik G: Fluids, electrolytes, and body composition, in Rombeau JL, Caldwell MD (eds): *Parenteral Nutrition.* Philadelphia, WB Saunders, 1986.

28. Bloom WL: Carbohydrates and water balance. *Am J Clin Nutr* 1967; 20:157.

29. Veverbrants E, Arky RA: Effects of fasting and refeeding. I. Studies on sodium, potassium and water excretion on a constant electrolyte and fluid intake. *J Clin Endocrinol* 1969; 29:55.

30. Katz AI, Hollingsworth DR, Epstein FH: Influence of carbohydrate and protein on sodium excretion during fasting and refeeding. *J Lab Clin Med* 1968; 72:93.

31. Richards MP, Rosebrough RW, Steele NC: Effects of starvation and refeeding on tissue zinc, copper and iron in turkey poults. *J Nutr* 1987; 117: 481.

32. Newsholme EA, Leech AR: *Biochemistry for the Medical Sciences.* Chichester, Great Britain, John Wiley & Sons, 1983.

33. Rose BD: *Clinical Physiology of Acid-Base and Electrolyte Disorders,* ed 3. New York, McGraw-Hill, 1989.

34. Grant JP: *Handbook of Total Parenteral Nutrition,* ed 2. Philadelphia, WB Saunders, 1992.

35. Cooke CR, Turin MD, Whelton A, et al: Studies of marked and persistent sodium retention in previously fasted and sodium-deprived obese subjects. *Metabolism* 1987; 36:609.

36. Affarah HB, Hall WD, Heymsfield SB, et al: High carbohydrate diet: Antinatriuretic and blood pressure response in normal men. *Am J Clin Nutr* 1986; 44:341.

37. McMahon M, Manji N, Driscoll DF, et al: Parenteral nutrition in patients with diabetes mellitus: Theoretical and and practical consideration. *JPEN* 1989; 13:545.

38. Patrick J. Golden M: Leukocyte electrolytes and sodium transport in protein energy malnutrition. *Am J Clin Nutr* 1977; 30:1478.

39. Starker PM, LaSala PA, Forse RA, et al: Response to total parenteral nutrition in the extremely malnourished patient. *JPEN* 1985; 9:300.

40. Franch G, Guirao X, Garcia-Domingo M, et al: The influence of calorie source on water and sodium balances during intravenous refeeding of malnourished rabbits. *Clin Nutr* 1992; 11:59.

41. Sitges-Serra A, Arcas G, Guirao X, et al: Extracellular fluid expansion during parenteral refeeding. *Clin Nutr* 1992; 11:63.

42. Heymsfield SB, Casper K, Funfar J: Physiologic response and clinical implications of nutrition support. *Am J Cardiol* 1987; 60:75.

43. Heymsfield SB, Casper K: Continuous nasoenteric feeding: Bioenergetic and metabolic response during recovery from semistarvation. *Am J Clin Nutr* 1988; 47:900.

44. Casper K, Matthews DE, Heymsfield SB: Overfeeding: Cardiovascular and metabolic response during continuous formula infusion in adult humans. *Am J Clin Nutr* 1990; 52:602.

45. Gottdiener JS, Gross HA, Henry WL, et al: Effects of self-induced starvation on cardiac size and function in anorexia nervosa. *Circulation* 1978; 58:425.

46. Heymsfield SB, Bethel RA, Ansley JD, et al: Cardiac abnormalities in cachectic patients before and during nutri-

tional repletion. *Am Heart J* 1978; 95:584.

47. Garnett ES, Barnard DL, Ford J, et al: Gross fragmentation of cardiac myofibrils after therapeutic starvation for obesity. *Lancet* 1969; 1:914.

48. Keys A, Henschel A, Taylor HL: The size and function of the human heart at rest in semi-starvation and in subsequent rehabilitation. *Am J Physiol* 1947; 150:153.

49. Abel RM, Grimes JB, Alonso D, et al: Adverse hemodynamic and ultrastructural changes in dog hearts subjected to protein-calorie malnutrition. *Am Heart J* 1979; 97:733.

50. Freund HR, Holroyde J: Cardiac function during protein malnutrition and refeeding in the isolated rat heart, *JPEN* 1986; 10:470.

51. Heymsfield SB: Cardiac cachexia. Presented at the Fourth Clinical Congress of The American Society for Parenteral and Enteral Nutrition, January 30, 1979, and at the conference Malnutrition in Hospitalized Patients, Boston, Harvard Medical School, May 13, 1980.

52. Heymsfield SB, Hoff RD, Gray TF, et al: Heart disease. In Kinney JM, Jeejeebhoy KN, Hill GL, et al (eds): *Nutrition and Metabolism in Patient Care*. Philadelphia, WB Saunders, 1988.

53. Heymsfield SB, Head CA, McManus CB, et al: Respiratory, cardiovascular, and metabolic effects of enteral hyperalimentation: Influence of formula dose and composition, *Am J Clin Nutr* 1984; 40:116.

54. Schocken DD, Holloway JD, Powers PS: Weight loss and the heart. *Arch Intern Med* 1989; 149:877.

55. Weissman C, Askanazi J: Parenteral nutrition, malnutrition, and the respiratory system. *Nutr Supp Serv* 1985; 5:46.

56. Askanazi J, Weissman C, Rosenbaum SH, et al: Nutrition and the respiratory system. *Crit Care Med* 1982; 10:163.

57. Arora NS, Rochester DF: Effect of general nutritional and muscular status on the human diaphragm. *Am Rev Respir Dis* 1977; 115:84.

58. Thurlbeck WM: Diaphragm and body weight in emphysema. *Thorax* 1978; 33:483.

59. Dureuil B, Viires N, Veber B, et al: Acute diaphragmatic changes induced by starvation in rats. *Am J Clin Nutr* 1989; 49:738.

60. Arora NS, Rochester DF: Respiratory muscle strength and maximal voluntary ventilation in undernourished patients. *Am Rev Respir Dis* 1982; 126:5.

61. Whittaker JS, Ryan CF, Buckley PA, et al: The effects of refeeding on peripheral and respiratory muscle function in malnourished chronic obstructive pulmonary disease patients. *Am Rev Respir Dis* 1990; 142:283.

62. Doekel RC, Zwillich CW, Scoggin CH, et al: Clinical semistarvation. Depression of hypoxic ventilatory response. *N Engl J Med* 1976; 295:358.

63. Baier H, Somani P: Ventilatory drive in normal man during semistarvation. *Chest* 1984; 85:222.

64. Rubin JW, Clowes GHA, Macnicol MF, et al: Impaired pulmonary surfactant synthesis in starvation and severe nonthoracic sepsis. *Am J Surg* 1972; 123:461.

65. Sahebjami H, Vassallo CL: Effects of starvation and refeeding on lung mechanics and morphometry. *Am Rev Respir Dis* 1979; 119:443.

66. Wolfe RR: Regulation of glucose metabolism, in Burke J (ed): *Surgical Physiology*. Philadelphia, WB Saunders, 1983.

67. Robin AP, Askanazi J, Cooperman A, et al: Influence of hypercaloric glucose infusions on fuel economy in surgical patients: A review. *Crit Care Med* 1981; 9:680.

68. Askanazi J, Elwyn DH, Silverberg PA, et al: Respiratory distress secondary to a high carbohydrate load: A case report. *Surgery* 1980; 87:596.

69. Askanazi J, Rosenbaum SH, Hyman AI, et al: Respiratory changes induced by the large glucose loads of total parenteral nutrition. *JAMA* 1980; 243:1444.

70. Askanazi J, Nordenstrom J, Rosenbaum SH, et al: Nutrition for the patient with respiratory failure: Glucose vs fat. *Anesthesiology* 1981; 54:373.

71. Covelli HD, Black JW, Olsen MS, et al: Respiratory failure precipitated by high carbohydrate loads. *Ann Intern Med* 1981; 95:579.

72. Jenkinson SG: Nutritional problems

during mechanical ventilation in acute respiratory failure. *Respir Care* 1983; 28:641.

73. Martyn PA, Vasquez RM, Golden MAK: Paco$_2$ and enteral overfeeding: Could there be a relationship? *Nutr Supp Serv* 1984; 4:41.

74. Vanderhoof JA: Physiologic effects of protein-calorie malnutrition on the gastrointestinal tract, in *Enteral Feeding: Scientific Basis and Clinical Applications.* Columbus, Ohio, Ross Laboratories, 1988.

75. Viteri FE, Schneider RE: Gastrointestinal alterations in protein-calorie malnutrition. *Med Clin North Am* 1974; 58:1487.

76. Young EA, Ramos RG, Harris MM: Gastrointestinal and cardiac response to low-calorie semistarvation diets. *Am J Clin Nutr* 1988; 47:981.

77. Alvarado J, Vargas W, Diaz N, et al: Vitamin B$_{12}$ absorption in protein-calorie malnourished children and during recovery: Influence of protein depletion and of diarrhea, *Am J Clin Nutr* 1973; 26:595.

78. Holt PR, Kotler DP: Adaptive changes of intestinal enzymes to nutritional intake in the aging rat. *Gastroenterology* 1987; 93:295.

79. Howard L, Michalek AV, Alger SA: Enteral nutrition and gastrointestinal, pancreatic, and liver disease, in Rombeau JL, Caldwell MD (eds): *Enteral and Tube Feeding,* ed 2. Philadelphia, WB Saunders, 1990.

80. Mayoral LG, Tripathy K, Bolanos O, et al: Intestinal, functional, and morphological abnormalities in severely protein-malnourished adults. *Am J Clin Nutr* 1972; 25:1084.

81. Earnest DL: Gastrointestinal mucosal changes from starvation and stress, in *The Gastrointestinal Response to Injury, Starvation, and Enteral Nutrition.* Columbus, Ohio, Ross Laboratories, 1988.

82. Rolandelli RH, DePaula JA, Guenter P, et al: Critical illness and sepsis, in Rombeau JL, Caldwell MD (eds): *Enteral and Tube Feeding,* ed 2. Philadelphia, WB Saunders, 1990.

83. Silk DBA, Payne-James JJ: Complications of enteral nutrition, in Rombeau JL, Caldwell MD (eds): *Enteral and Tube Feeding,* ed 2. Philadelphia, WB Saunders, 1990.

84. Bivins BA, Hyde GL, Sachatello CR, et al: Physiopathology and management of hyperosmolar hyperglycemic nonketotic dehydration. *Surg Gynecol Obstet* 1982; 154:534.

85. Knochel JP: The pathophysiology and clinical characteristics of severe hypophosphatemia. *Arch Intern Med* 1977; 137:203.

86. Hayek ME, Eisenberg PG: Severe hypophosphatemia following institution of enteral feedings. *Arch Surg* 1989; 124:1325.

87. Thompson JS, Hodges RE: Preventing hypophosphatemia during total parenteral nutrition. *JPEN* 1984; 8:137.

88. Furlan AJ, Hanson M, Cooperman A, et al: Acute areflexic paralysis. *Arch Neurol* 1975; 32:706.

89. Mezoff AG, Gremse DA, Farrell MK: Hypophosphatemia in the nutritional recovery syndrome. *Am J Dis Child* 1989; 143:1111.

90. Cumming A, Farquhar JR, Boucher AD: Refeeding hypophosphatemia in anorexia nervosa and alcoholism. *BMJ* 1977; 295:490.

91. Zaloga GP: Hypophosphatemia in COPD: How serious—and what to do? *J Crit Illness* 1992; 7:364.

92. Martin BK, Slingerland AW, Jenks JS: Severe hypophosphatemia associated with nutritional support. *Nutr Supp Serv* 1985; 5:34.

93. Newman JH, Neff TA, Ziporin P: Acute respiratory failure associated with hypophosphatemia. *N Engl J Med* 1977; 296:1101.

94. Darsee JR, Nutter DO: Reversible severe congestive cardiomyopathy in three cases of hypophosphatemia. *Ann Intern Med* 1978; 89:867.

95. Clark WR, Copeland RL, Bonaventura MM, et al: Ventricular tachycardia associated with hypophosphatemia. *Nutr Int* 1985; 1:102.

96. Jacob HS, Amsden T: Acute hemolytic anemia with rigid red cells in hypophosphatemia. *N Engl J Med* 1971; 285:1446.

97. Lichtman MA, Miller DR, Cohen J, et al: Reduced red cell glycolysis, 2,3-diphosphoglycerate and adenosine triphosphate concentration, and increased hemoglobin-oxygen affinity caused by hypophosphatemia. *Ann Intern Med* 1971; 74:562.

98. Augusti AGN, Torres A, Estopa R, et

al: Hypophosphatemia as a cause of failed weaning: The importance of metabolic factors. *Crit Care Med* 1984; 12:142.

99. Shoemaker WC: Fluids and electrolytes in the acutely ill adult, in Shoemaker WC, Ayres MD, Grenvik A, et al (eds): *Textbook of Critical Care*, ed 2. Philadelphia, WB Saunders, 1989.

100. Haynes-Johnson V: Tube feeding complications: Causes, prevention, therapy. *Nutr Supp Serv* 1986; 6:17.

101. Chernow B, Smith J, Rainey, et al: Hypomagnesemia: Implications for the critical care specialist. *Crit Care Med* 1982; 10:193.

102. Iseri LT, Freed J, Bures AR: Magnesium deficiency and cardiac disorders. *Am J Med* 1975; 58:837.

103. McCormick DB: Thiamin, in Shils ME, Young VR (eds): *Modern Nutrition in Health and Disease*, ed 7. Philadelphia, Lea & Febiger, 1988.

104. Pittman JG, Cohen P: The pathogenesis of cardiac cachexia, *N Engl J Med* 1964; 271:403.

105. Mattioli S, Miglioli M, Montagna P, et al: Wernicke's encephalopathy during total parenteral nutrition: Observation in one case. *JPEN* 1988; 12:626.

106. Apovian CM, McMahon MM, Bistrian BR: Guidelines for refeeding the marasmic patient. *Crit Care Med* 1990; 18:1030.

107. Echenique MM, Bistrian BR, Blackburn GL: Theory and techniques of nutritional support in the ICU. *Crit Care Med* 1982; 10:546.

108. Jeejeebhoy KN: Nutrient metabolism. In Kinney JM, Jeejeebhoy KN, Hill GL, et al (eds): *Nutrition and Metabolism in Patient Care*. Philadelphia, WB Saunders, 1988.

109. Lentz RD, Brown DM, Kjellstrand CM: Treatment of severe hypophosphatemia. *Ann Intern Med* 1978; 89:941.

43

Acquired Immunodeficiency Syndrome

Bruce Friedman, M.D.

Nutritional deficiencies in the patient with acquired immunodeficiency syndrome

Wasting syndrome

Mechanism of wasting

Malnutrition and impaired nutrient intake

Intestinal malabsorption

Pharmacotherapeutic nutritional impairment

Deficiency of individual nutrients

Nutritional assessment of human immunodeficiency virus disease

Nutritional management in human immunodeficiency virus disease:

Practical considerations

Enteral and parenteral nutrition support

Indications for enteral and parenteral alimentation

Anorexia and weight loss

Diarrhea/malabsorption

Alternative nutritional therapies

The acquired immunodeficiency syndrome (AIDS) has become a major world health problem. This diverse clinical syndrome, induced by the human immunodeficiency virus (HIV), has infected at least 1.5 million Americans and several times that number globally. The clinical presentation of AIDS is varied, and it can affect organs singly or multiply, depending on its severity. HIV produces profound defects in systemic and mucosal immunity that are associated with a variety of opportunistic infections and malignancies. This chapter will deal specifically with the nutritional alterations in AIDS.

Protein-energy malnutrition is common in patients with AIDS. Nutritional deficiencies may precede overt manifestations of the disease.[1] Clinical manifestations of AIDS include many symptoms or signs that affect nutritional status and intake. Oral and esophageal lesions cause pain during eating; fever, common to HIV disease, increases energy requirements and adversely alter food intake; nausea and vomiting limit nutritional intake; and a multiplicity of opportunistic intestinal infections, lesions, and other conditions contribute to nutritional decline via malabsorption and diarrhea. Additionally, various drug treatments interfere with nutrient absorption or metabolism, and conversely, poor nutrition may compromise drug therapy. These factors contribute to weight loss, undernutrition, failure to thrive, and the wasting syndrome manifested in the debilitated AIDS patient. The deadly outcome of many AIDS victims may be a direct consequence of progressive wasting rather than the infection itself.

This chapter will examine the available information on the nutritional aspects of HIV infection. Through a review of recent scientific literature, recommendations on nutrition practices and support will be proposed. The data presented should provide the health care practitioner with guidelines on how to best integrate nutritional support with other therapeutic interventions required for the AIDS patient.

NUTRITIONAL DEFICIENCIES IN THE PATIENT WITH ACQUIRED IMMUNODEFICIENCY SYNDROME

Malnutrition is a common finding in the AIDS patient, and its etiologies are multifactorial. In order to develop a proper assessment schema and nutritional guidelines, we must first understand the complexities of malnourishment that potentially face the AIDS population.

Wasting Syndrome

Progressive weight loss characterized by loss of lean muscle mass is common in AIDS. Wasting remains a major cause of debilitation and mortality in HIV infection.[2] Studies of body composition, as determined by total-body potassium content, have evaluated the effects of wasting by analyzing the magnitude of lean body mass depletion as a function of time before death.[3, 4] The relationship between malnutrition and survival was explored in 28 patients not receiving nutritional support and dying of

wasting syndrome within 3 months of study.[5] Multiple measurements of body cell mass were obtained over time. The data fit a linear relationship and intercepted at 54% of normal body cell mass at the time of death. Earlier studies had shown that body fat content was not a reliable marker of wasting, since many AIDS patients had decreased body cell mass with a normal to elevated fat content.[3] Chlebowski et al., investigating nutritional status and gastrointestinal dysfunction in the AIDS patient, confirmed that those with the greatest degree of wasting had the shortest survival time.[6]

These data suggest that in certain AIDS patients, the timing of death is related to the magnitude of body cell mass depletion rather than the direct effects of malignancy or infectious processes. This pattern of depletion resembles the stressed or injured state rather than semistarvation. Semistarvation is associated with nitrogen sparing and increased fat utilization. In contrast, body cell mass in the AIDS patient is reduced out of proportion to weight loss. Thus, the timing of death in AIDS wasting illnesses may be more related to the degree of depletion of body cell mass than its underlying cause.

Mechanisms of Wasting

The multifactorial causes of wasting in the AIDS patient can be divided into two broad categories: disturbances in metabolism and decreased nutrient intake. There are several potential underlying mechanisms for each of these categories. It should be emphasized that multiple processes may be active at any one time in the individual patient.

Disturbances in metabolism are thought to contribute to wasting by multiple mechanisms, which include increased energy expenditure and depletion of body constituents, especially protein. The host response to infection alters metabolism. Mediators of host immune response, cytokines, are believed to be responsible for the alterations in metabolism experienced by very ill patients such as those with tumor or infective burdens. Recent studies suggest that cytokines contribute to the process of wasting.[7]

Weight loss and severe hypertriglyceridemia may both accompany infection. Well-defined infectious processes such as HIV disease produce a decrease in the clearance of triglyceride-rich lipoproteins and in levels of lipoprotein lipase.[8] The decreased clearance of triglyceride may lead to fat storage in adipose tissue.[9] In animals, tumor necrosis factor (TNF), a well-documented cytokine, has been shown to cause both weight loss and decreased synthesis and storage of fat.[10] Early studies of TNF in AIDS patients found TNF levels to be elevated and postulated that TNF was responsible for wasting in HIV disease.[11] However, in further studies, no correlation between weight loss and TNF levels was detected.[12] TNF levels have been found to be equally elevated in HIV-negative high-risk groups and patients with frank AIDS, which suggests that these elevations may not be secondary to HIV infection or AIDS alone.[13] Despite the lack of a well-defined role for TNF in AIDS, other cytokines (including interleukin-1 [IL-1] and interferons-α, -β, and -γ) have similar effects to TNF in promoting a catabolic state in fat cells.[13–15] TNF elevates serum triglyceride levels by increasing hepatic lipogenesis and very low-density lipoprotein (VLDL) production.[2] Multiple cytokines such as IL-1, IL-6, and interferon-α also share the ability to increase hepatic fatty acid synthesis.[16, 17] It appears that the critical link between the multiple actions of cytokines in the AIDS patient and their contribution to the wasting syndrome is their ability to stimulate fatty acid synthesis and the process of futile cycling.[4] Cytokines stimulate lipolysis and hepatic lipid synthesis; fatty acids are released from fat, returned to the liver where they are reesterfied into triacylglyceroids, secreted as VLDL, and

returned to the fat cell for breakdown and restorage as triglycerides.[9] The action of TNF and other cytokines on lipid metabolism could explain how fat mass is sustained throughout a period of weight loss during AIDS. However, it should be noted that futile cycling does not necessarily cause wasting. Theoretically, increased caloric intake could compensate for this process.

Clearly, much remains to be learned about the mechanisms underlying the changes in metabolism that accompany cachexia and appear to contribute to wasting in the end stages of HIV infection. From our current fund of knowledge of AIDS and its interaction with cytokines, it is possible to develop a theoretical basis for the wasting syndrome of HIV disease. Increased circulating levels of interferon-α induce hypertriglyceridemia, which is caused by decreased clearance and/or increased production of VLDL.[13] The elevated VLDL levels result from hepatic lipogenesis and/or increased reesterfication of fatty acids in a futile cycle. This can be compensated for by increased nutritional support or lowered total energy expenditure. However, when a secondary infection occurs, new cytokines such as TNF or IL-1 are released. The combination of multiple cytokine release acts synergistically to accelerate energy expenditure, enhance protein breakdown, and produce anorexia.[4] These changes result in decreased nutritional intake leading to fatigue, decreased activity, and ultimately progressive wasting and debilitation.

MALNUTRITION AND IMPAIRED NUTRIENT INTAKE

Intestinal Malabsorption

Gastrointestinal disorders, from mouth to anus, are extremely common in HIV-infected individuals. It is estimated that up to 90% experience symptoms at some point in the course of their disease. The gut compromise

TABLE 43–1.

Gastrointestinal Pathogens in HIV Disease

Bacterial	Viral	Fungal	Protozoan
Salmonella	Cytomegalovirus	Candida sp.	Cryptosporidium
Shigella	Herpes simplex virus	Histoplasma	Microsporida
Campylobacter	Human immunodeficiency	Coccidioides	Isopora belli
Mycobacterium tuberculosis	virus	Sporothrix	Entamoeba
Mycobacterium	Adenovirus	Cryptococcus	Blastocystis
avium-intracellulare	Epstein-Barr virus	Blastomyces	Pneumocystis carinii
Clostridium difficile	Human papillomavirus		Giardia lamblia
Bacillary peliosis	Hepatitis B, C, D		

associated with AIDS plays a substantial role in the diminished nutrient intake that may accelerate the wasting syndrome. The gastrointestinal tract is vulnerable to luminal pathogens because it lacks a strong physical barrier. This problem is accentuated in AIDS because of progressive loss of immune defenses. HIV infection impairs gastrointestinal mucosal immunity in a manner similar to its effects on systemic immunity. T-cell depletion, paralleling the peripheral circulation, is found in the gut mucosa.[18] Gut barrier immune processes such as IgA-secreting plasma cells and luminal IgA have been shown to be diminished, thus suggesting impairment in secretory gut immunity. These defects increase the likelihood of gastrointestinal pathology contributing to a diminution in nutrient intake. Diarrhea and malabsorption are common

gastrointestinal manifestations of AIDS. Nutrient malabsorption accompanies small intestinal disease and is due to a diminution in intestinal surface area, functional defects in cells damaged directly by pathogens, and immaturity of villus epithelial cells related to rapid cell turnover.[19–21] Gastrointestinal complications in HIV infection may be caused by a myriad of enteric pathogens or by systemic disorders that secondarily involve the gut (Table 43–1).

TABLE 43–3.

AIDS Gastrointestinal Tract Complications (Interfering With Food Intake)

Complication	Causal Factor(s)
Diarrhea/malabsorption	Cryptosporidiosis, Isospora, Giardia, Entamoeba, Clostridia difficile, bacterial enteridites, Blastocystis, Strongyloides, adenovirus, MAI
Colitis	CMV and others
HIV enteropathy	HIV and cytokines
Chronic infections	Histoplasmosis, Cryptococcus, Coccidioides
Anorectal disease	HSV2, STDs, anal ulcers, anogenital neoplasms
Hepatitis	Hep B/C/D, M. TB, bacillary peliosis, MAI, immune, drugs
Sclerosing cholangitis	CMV, MAI, KS, Cryptosporidium, lymphoma
Pancreatitis	CMV, MAI, fungals, KS, lymphoma, drugs, 2′, 3′-dideoxyinosine, Pentax, TMP-SMX)

MAI = Mycobacterium avium-intracellulare; CMV = cytomegalovirus; HIV = human immunodeficiency virus; HSV2 = herpes simplex virus 2; STD = sexually transmitted disease; Hep = hepatitis; M. TB = Mycobacterium tuberculosis; KS = Kaposi's sarcoma; TMP-SMX = trimethoprim-sulfamethoxazole.

TABLE 43–2.

Oral/Esophageal HIV Disease (Interfering With Food Intake)

Condition	Symptoms
Candidiasis	Pain, odynophagia, dysphagia, dysgeusia
Herpes simplex virus	
Human papillomavirus	Dysphagia, odynophagia, esophagitis
Herpes zoster	
Cytomegalovirus	Epithelial, hyperplasia
Hairy leukoplakia	Pain, vesicular areas
Cryptosporidiosis	Dysphagia, esophagitis
Peridontitis	Asymptomatic
Gingivitis	Dysphagia
Esophageal ulcers	Bone destruction
Kaposi's sarcoma	Halitosis, gum bleeding
Non-Hodgkin's lymphoma	Odynophagia
	Dysphagia, obstruction
	Dysphagia

A variety of disorders affecting the oral cavity and esophagus are commonly seen in the HIV-infected patient.[22-24] These oral and esophageal manifestations of AIDS may substantially interfere with nutrient intake (Table 43–2). Candidiasis occurs in up to 80% of patients with AIDS and may often be the initial manifestation of the disease.[25] Oral symptoms of *Candida* infection (thrush) include pain, odynophagia, dysphagia, dysgeusia, and obstruction. Neoplasms such as Kaposi's sarcoma,[26] non-Hodgkin's lymphoma,[27] and rare cases of squamous cell carcinoma may also occur. These diseases of the oral cavity interfere with food intake and contribute to the malnutrition of the AIDS patient.

Primary and secondary intestinal complications occur quite frequently in the HIV-infected person[28] (Table 43–3). These may be limited to the small bowel or colon or may involve both simultaneously. Protozoa are the major pathogens, and they cause chronic, refractory diarrhea and malabsorption. Primary infectious processes and organisms include *Cryptosporidium*,[29] *Isospora belli*,[30] microsporidiosis *(Enterocytozoon bieneusi)*,[31] *Giardia lamblia*,[32] *Entamoeba histolytica*,[33] bacterial enteridites (i.e., caused by *Shigella*,[34] *Salmonella*,[35] and *Campylobacter*[36]), *Clostridium difficile*,[37] *Blastocystis hominis*,[24] *Strongyloides stercoralis*,[24] and adenoviruses.[38] These infections are manifested as diarrhea, malabsorption, and/or colitis. Systemic infections such as cytomegalovirus (CMV),[39] mycobacterial disease (i.e., *Mycoplasma tuberculosis* [TB], *Mycoplasma avium-intracellulare* [MAI][40]), HIV-induced enteropathy,[41, 42] and fungal diseases (From *Histoplasma*,[43] *Cryptococcus*,[44] *Coccidioides*[45]) may re-

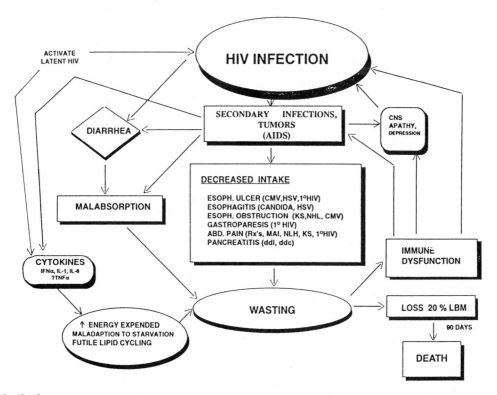

FIG 43–1.

Proposed connection between HIV infection and the mechanisms of the wasting process (*CNS* = central nervous system; *ESOPH* = esophageal; *CMV* = cytomegalovirus; *HSV* = herpes simplex virus; *KS* = Kaposi's sarcoma; NHL= non-Hodgkin's lymphoma; *MAI* = *Mycobacterium avium-intracellulare*; *IFNα* = interferon-α; *IL-I* = interleukin-1; *TNFα* = tumor necrosis factor α; *LBM* = lean body mass).

sult in secondary intestinal complications such as malabsorption, diarrhea, colitis, chronic inflammatory bowel disease, and hepatitis. All of these infections are associated with progressive wasting in the HIV-infected individual.

Anorectal diseases such as herpes simplex virus 2 (HSV-2),[46] neoplasms (i.e., Kaposi's sarcoma,[26] B-cell lymphomas,[47] and anogenital carcinomas), venereal diseases, and idiopathic anal ulcers also occur commonly.[24] Hepatobiliary diseases include granulomatous hepatitis,[48] peliosis hepatitis,[49] and sclerosing cholangitis.[50] The pancreas may be affected by the AIDS virus, CMV, MAI, and neoplasms.[51] Pancreatic disease may also be induced by commonly used medications such as 2', 3'-dideoxyinosine,[52] trimethoprim-sulfamethoxazol (TMP/SMX),[53] and pentamidine.[54] It is clear that these gastrointestinal complications cause a variety of clinical syndromes that alter food intake and nutrient absorption. The resulting malnutrition, in association with the potential for cytokine-mediated wasting phenomenon, correlates with the morbidity and mortality associated with AIDS. The proposed connection between HIV infection and the mechanisms of the wasting process is schematically presented in Figure 43–1.

Pharmacotherapeutic Nutritional Impairment

In order to provide effective treatment for the infectious complications, neoplasms, and/or HIV, an elaborate arsenal of pharmaceutical agents has been employed. Unfortunately, these drug-patient interactions are not without significant impact on nutritional intake. Clearly, the pharmacotherapy utilized in the AIDS population has multiple side effects that contribute to decreased nutrient intake and weight loss. The impact of AIDS pharmacotherapy on nutritional support is outlined in Table 43–4. The most common drug side effects are nausea, vomiting, fatigue, di-

TABLE 43–4.

Nutritional Impact of AIDS Pharmacotherapy

Drug	Side Effects
AZT*	Nausea, fatigue, dysgeusia, mouth ulcers, edema, reduced vitamin B_{12}
Acyclovir	Diarrhea, N/V, fatigue, dysgeusia
Amphotericin B	Anorexia, N/V, wt loss, diarrhea
Bleomycin	N/V, wt loss, anorexia, stomatitis
Bromopirimine	N/V, fatigue, diarrhea
Cyclosporine	Anorexia, N/V
2', 3'-dideoxyinosine	Pancreatitis
Etoposide	Anorexia, N/V, diarrhea
Fluconazole	N/V, hepatitis, Abd pain
Foscarnet	N/V, fatigue, electrolyte imbalance
Ganciclovir	Nausea, anorexia
IL-2	Anorexia
Ketoconazole	N/V, Abd pain
Nystatin	N/V, diarrhea, GI upset
Pentamidine	N/V, pancreatitis, folate deficiency hypo/hyperglycemia, dysgeusia
Rifabutin	Dysgeusia, anorexia, fatigue
Somatostatin	Dry mouth, anorexia, throat discomfort
Spiramycin	N/V, diarrhea, acute colitis
Sulfadiazine	N/V, anorexia, diarrhea
Suramin	GI distress
TMP/SMX	Anorexia, glucose intolerance, stomatitis, pancreatitis, folate deficiency
Trimetrexate	Mucositis
Vidarabine	GI upset
Vinblastine	Anorexia, N/V, diarrhea, mucositis

AZT = azidothymidine (zidovudine); N/V = nausea/vomiting; Abd = abdominal; IL-2 = interleukin-2; GI = gastrointestinal; TMP-SMX = trimethoprim-sulfamethoxazole.

rect weight loss, electrolyte disturbances, diarrhea, and anorexia.

Commonly used drugs such as zidovudine (azidothymidine, AZT), amphotericin B, nystatin, pentamidine, and TMP/SMX figure prominently in these nutritional compromising complications.[55] Pancreatitis can develop as a direct side effect of several drugs. The development of vitamin and mineral deficiencies may cause a further decrease in appetite. Vitamin B_{12} deficiency may occur with AZT. Pentamidine and TMP/SMX may cause folate deficiency.[55] These drug side effects must be recognized and appropriate supplementation, dose reduction, and alternative agents sought. The nutritional impact on food intake, combined with infection, contribute to the malnutrition encountered in the HIV patient.

Deficiency of Individual Nutrients

Single nutrient deficiencies are rare. However, a variety of specific nutrient deficiencies have been documented in HIV infection (Table 43–5). The antioxidants vitamins A, E, and C and selenium may be deficient and contribute to impaired humoral immunity and natural killer cytotoxicity.[56] The exact functional significance of many nutrient deficiencies throughout the course of HIV infection is not well known and requires further study. Serum zinc levels correlate with T-cell function in patients with advanced HIV disease.[57] Proliferation of mononuclear cells is accelerated in the zinc-deficient HIV patient.[57] The clinical impact of zinc on CD4 proliferation and immune function has been evaluated in several studies. Zinc levels decrease progressively with worsening clinical and immunologic condition, and this is manifested by the progression of AIDS-related complex (ARC) to full-blown AIDS.[58] A correlation was also noted with serum zinc levels and CD4-positive lymphocytes when comparing ARC and AIDS patients.[58] Other groups have found less correlation of zinc levels with

TABLE 43–5.

Common Nutrient Deficiencies in HIV Disease

Nutrient	Measurement
Folate	CNS folate
	Serum/RBC Folate
Vitamin B_{12}	Serum cobalamin
Vitamin B_6	Serum B_6
Zinc	Serum zinc
	Zinc-thymulin
Selenium	Plasma/serum selenium
	RBC/cardiac selenium
Copper	Serum copper
Iron	Serum iron/ferritin

T-cell immune function.[59] No single indicator of zinc nutritional status is ideal, since it can be affected by hypoalbuminemia, drugs that alter binding to plasma proteins, infections, as well as nutritional deficiency. We must therefore view zinc measures in AIDS with caution.

Folate and vitamin B_{12} deficiencies are common findings in patients with HIV disease. Deficiencies may result from impaired dietary intake, poor absorption, active infectious processes, or gastrointestinal neoplasm.[58, 60, 61] Circulating antibodies to intrinsic factor were noted in 9 of 100 patients.[60] Investigators also noted a high frequency of elevated gastrin levels, a condition associated with defective vitamin B_{12} absorption.

Vitamin B_6 deficiency is widely prevalent during the early stages of HIV infection.[62] Studies in non-AIDS populations have suggested a significant relationship between vitamin B_6 levels and immune function.[63] In Baum and associates' investigation,[62] asymptomatic HIV-infected patients showed a significant correlation between lowered serum vitamin B_6 levels and in vitro measurements of immune parameters such as lymphocyte proliferation. Interpretation of these data must be cautioned due to the large variability in vitamin B_6 levels and in vitro lymphocyte stimulation tests, the presence of liver dysfunction, poor dietary intake, and the potential toxicity of repleting B_6 in large doses.[58] Overall, few data implicate vitamin B_6 as a major cause of immune deficiency in AIDS. Levels of trace elements such as copper,[64] iron,[65] and selenium[66] may be lowered in the AIDS patient and could also have an impact on overall immune dysfunction. When viewed as a group, studies of nutrient status suggest that deficiencies are common in HIV infection, especially in its advanced stages. The extent of overt or marginal deficiency is less clear. Confounding variables such as chemotherapy, comorbid disease processes, and infectious states must also be considered as a cause of nutrient deficiencies. The immune and functional ramifications of these nutrient deficits are well documented. However, their relevance to HIV disease and nutritional support needs further investigation.

NUTRITIONAL ASSESSMENT IN HUMAN IMMUNODEFICIENCY VIRUS DISEASE

The primary goals of nutritional therapy are the maintenance of normal nutritional indices and positive nitrogen balance and body weight. Difficulty in achieving and maintaining nutritional stores is characteristic of HIV infection and disease. Malnutrition may begin in asymptomatic stages of HIV infection, long before clinical signs and symptoms occur. For these reasons, dietary interventions are important in the overall care of patients with HIV disease.

The nutritional assessment involves an evaluation of key indices, including visceral and somatic proteins, fat reserves, nitrogen balance, and gastrointestinal function and an estimate of daily caloric and protein requirements. Visceral protein reserve is estimated from serum total protein, albumin, prealbumin, and transferrin levels. Somatic protein reserve is calculated by collecting a 24-hour urine specimen and quantitating the total creatinine. This is compared with a non-AIDS, stressed individual of similar weight and height (creatinine/height index).[67] Fat reserve is determined by using anthropometric measurements of the patient's triceps skin fold. These values are categorized into either mild, moderate, or severe malnutrition. Nutritional therapy is indicated when these indices suggest either moderate or severe malnutrition.

The caloric and protein requirements of malnourished HIV-infected patients vary with their clinical situation. Maintenance caloric requirements are usually 30 to 35 kcal/kg/day based on usual weight. However, as the disease

progresses, the daily caloric requirements may increase to 40 to 45 kcal/kg/day.[67] The caloric requirement can be calculated by using the Harris-Benedict equations or estimated by indirect calorimetry. In a recent study, resting energy expenditure (REE) was measured by indirect calorimetry, over a period of 28 days, in patients with HIV infection/AIDS.[68] These investigators found that REE was increased in HIV/AIDS. Weight loss primarily resulted from decreased caloric intake (with REE not declining despite less nutrition), and rapid weight loss or anorexia suggested a secondary infection.[68]

Protein requirements range from 1.0 to 1.5 g/kg/day, with stressed patients needing 2.0 to 2.5 g/kg/day. Hypermetabolism driven by cytokine production and the wasting phenomenon in the AIDS patient usually requires 2.0 to 2.5 g/kg/day to achieve a positive nitrogen balance, maintain nutritional homeostasis, and avoid continued weight loss. The optimal nonprotein calorie-to-nitrogen ratio is 100 to 120 fat-carbohydrate calories per gram of nitrogen. In the hypermetabolic, severely ill patient this ratio may be reduced to 75 to 80:1. Nutritional therapy should be closely monitored and includes weekly 24-hour nitrogen balance determinations, blood chemistries, and visceral protein markers. Prealbumin and somatomedin C may be the most accurate visceral protein markers, although conflicting data in this area demand further study. By monitoring patients in this manner, the nutrition team can modify and determine the most appropriate nutritional support.

NUTRITIONAL MANAGEMENT IN HUMAN IMMUNODEFICIENCY VIRUS DISEASE: PRACTICAL CONSIDERATIONS

Malnutrition weakens the immune system. It is therefore vital to provide adequate nutritional therapy to the

HIV-infected patient. Early intervention, with proper dietary composition, may forestall related complications of AIDS progression. An oral diet is recommended for nutritional maintenance and repletion, if at all possible. A balanced and varied oral intake can preclude problems of nutritional deficiencies and toxicities resulting from single-nutrient emphasis and/or nutrient interactions that would compete for gut absorption.[55] A high-calorie, high-protein, low-fat diet is the initial recommendation for the HIV-infected patient with normal gut function. A variety of nutrient-dense foods should be provided, especially in cases of inadequate caloric intake due to anorexia, chewing difficulties, nausea, or other problems.

If the patient is unable to meet caloric goals, food supplements are indicated. These include Vivonex TEN (amino acid, low-fat formula), Carnation Instant Breakfast, Ensure, Resource, Nutren, or Peptamen (predigested protein). The decision to recommend oral supplementation of nutrients should consider gastrointestinal tract function as well as drug therapy interactions. Multivitamins and/or multimineral combinations should also be supplemented if oral intake is reduced. As noted previously, vitamin B_6, B_{12}, and folate levels can be compromised in the HIV-infected patient. Levels of supplementation to correct deficient serum values and proof of benefit from vitamin supplementation are not well defined. However, intramuscular vitamin B_{12} at 1000 to 1200 μg/mon and 25 to 50 mg of B_6 per day have been shown to normalize serum levels.[55] The provision of adequate oral intake (based on calculated protein-caloric needs), proper vitamin and mineral supplementation, and emphasis on variety of nutrient intake should provide nutritional homeostasis in the HIV-infected patient. As indicated in Table 43–4, AIDS pharmacotherapy makes the HIV-infected person vulnerable to drug-nutrient interactions. These may lead to nutrient deficiencies, compromised nutritional status, and altered drug efficacy. Common deficiencies involving folate (pentamidine, TMP/SMX) and vitamin B_{12} (AZT) should be carefully monitored and properly treated.[58, 61, 69]

A routine pattern of meals should be established for each patient. However, these should match the patient's lifestyle and expected level of physical activity. Overall, flexible nutritional support with appropriate meal patterning can provide for nutritional requirements due to infection or other complications. Food safety must also be emphasized. HIV-infected individuals are vulnerable to food-borne infections, including salmonellosis, listeriosis, and campylobacteriosis. Dining out, preparation and handling of food at home, cooking foods to proper temperatures (165 to 212° F), and storing foods properly must all be addressed. Sanitizing cooking equipment areas, containers, and utensils must also be a priority. It is important that patients and their significant support systems (i.e., friends, family, etc.) be educated to the special nutritional needs of the HIV population.

ENTERAL AND PARENTERAL NUTRITION SUPPORT

Severe wasting that is unresponsive to conventional oral dietary management often accompanies AIDS. These patients may be candidates for parenteral or enteral nutrition support. Of the many complications in AIDS patients, their propensity to the development of infections remains the most concerning. Enteral nutrition via gastrostomies, nasoenteric tubes, or jejunostomies can potentially result in bacterial infection. Similarly, parenteral alimentation administered by intravenous catheter is also a source of infection in this immunocompromised population. Only one small study that investigated percutaneous endoscopically placed gastrostomies (PEG) examined the risk of infection over several months in patients with AIDS.[70] The study looked at eight patients with 850 days of indwelling PEG. Only one case of infection was noted, which is similar to non-AIDS data.[71] The safety of parenteral nutrition revolves around the increased risk of infection from central line placement. Several studies have evaluated these complications by investigating the use of chronic indwelling catheters such as the Hickman.[72] It appears that the complication rate for catheter line bacteremia is higher in HIV-infected patients as compared with those without AIDS. However, most institutions and investigators suggest that with careful attention to aseptic technique and close monitoring, long-term parenteral therapy can be administered with an acceptable risk of infection.

Enteral and parenteral alimentation has been shown to be effective at increasing lean body mass in selected AIDS patients with impaired food intake.[70, 73] There are only a few small studies that have reviewed efficacy in the application of alimentation to the AIDS patient. The results of both enteral and parenteral studies suggest that nutrition support can effectively maintain body composition, reverse the depletion of fat and lean tissue, and improve visceral protein parameters in HIV-infected patients with evidence of cachexia.[70, 73] However, in the severely malnourished AIDS patient, reversal of the hypermetabolic state, if prolonged, has been more difficult. There have been no studies to date that have shown benefits on outcome in this severely nutritionally depleted population. This is consistent with the difficulties in nutritional support encountered in other hospitalized hypermetabolic patients. Alimentation has been shown to improve immune function, as measured by increased total lymphocyte counts. However, although body weight and composition improved, the more sensitive immune markers, CD4 cell numbers, remained unchanged.[58] Establishment of the efficacy of nutritional support also requires the demonstration of improved quality of life, decreased length or frequency of hospitalization, and ultimately prolonged survival; no studies are available in these areas, and they should receive priority in future research efforts.

INDICATIONS FOR ENTERAL AND PARENTERAL ALIMENTATION

Enteral nutrition via feeding tube should be the next nutritional intervention when oral liquid formula supplementation is inadequate in providing appropriate intake. The gut should be used, if at all possible, to maintain mucosal integrity, retain the immunologic barriers and normal flora, and prevent the complication of translocation bacteremia. Oral/esophageal lesions, neurologic dysfunction affecting swallowing, mental status changes compromising airway protection, anorexia, and fatigue are all clear indications for enteral nutrition. Other indications are listed in Table 43–6. Delivery can be accomplished nasoenterically into the stomach or duodenum, via a gastrostomy (surgical or percutaneous), or through a jejunostomy. The choice of feeding method depends on the length and nature of the underlying abnormality, the length of support, and the risk of aspiration. Enteral alimentation should be considered early in the course of HIV disease before significant complications occur.

Mucosal atrophy and gut dysfunction

TABLE 43–6.

Indications for Nutrition Support in HIV Disease

- 20%–30% weight loss
- Mechanical/physiologic gut dysfunction
- Progressive protein/calorie malnutrition
- Significant trace element deficiencies
- Multiple wound healing problems
- Poor recovery from secondary infections
- Slow weaning from mechanical ventilation

are associated with HIV disease. An optimal enteral formula in these patients is isosmolar, requires minimal digestion, is low in fat (medium-chain triglycerides are better absorbed), contains trace elements (selenium, chromium, molybdenum) that are known to be deficient in AIDS patients, is pectin rich and lactose free, and has adequate protein.

Total parenteral nutrition (TPN) should only be initiated when oral or enteral supplementation fails to provide adequate calories or is contraindicated. TPN should be considered for bowel obstruction, severe or refractory diarrhea, intractable vomiting, or malabsorption. With parenteral nutrition, two options are available: peripheral and/or central vein formula infusion. Peripheral parenteral nutrition (PPN) is utilized in patients who can tolerate large-volume loads and require short-term nutrition support (usually less than 10 days). However, with the introduction of peripheral indwelling catheters (PIC lines), PPN may be used for longer periods of time. Central TPN can be delivered for extended periods of time. Line placement can be done with either extended implantable catheters (which are expensive and require an operating room charge) or with serial rotating central line sites, which if dedicated for central TPN, can remain in place for several weeks. Double-lumen extended catheters are recommended to allow for delivery of other medications and/or to prepare for potential clogging/thrombotic complications. TPN formulas are tailored to the individual. It is important to include adequate trace elements and vitamins. Reduced volume can be attained by using high-protein (15% Novamine), D70 formulations. Fat emulsions may be included in the same formula bottle (3-in-1 solution). Monitoring of electrolytes, fluid balance, glucose, central line sites, and triglyceride levels and periodic nutritional assessment should be standard when TPN is utilized.

ANOREXIA AND WEIGHT LOSS

Anorexia is common in AIDS even in the absence of weight loss. It can be caused by many conditions including neuropsychiatric, endocrinologic, and gastrointestinal diseases or as a consequence of HIV pharmacotherapy. The devastating psychosocial impact of AIDS increases its neuropsychiatric manifestations, including clinical depression, anxiety, neurosis, frank psychosis, and organic brain syndromes (including HIV dementia and encephalopathy).[74, 75] The presence of upper alimentary tract pathology and oral manifestations of HIV infection are common causes of weight loss and anorexia resulting in poor caloric intake. Endocrine problems may be manifested by the relatively uncommon adrenal insufficiency of AIDS.[74]

Several specific therapies have been explored to reduce anorexia. Dietary interventions stress small, low-fat meals with clear liquid protein supplementation rather than heavy, high-calorie, fatty foods that usually are not tolerated by the ill AIDS patient.[76] In addition to nutritional management, appetite stimulants have been tried in these patients (Table 43–7). Megestrol acetate (Megace), a progestinal agent, can stimulate appetite and cause weight gain in several groups of patients with cancer anorexia-cachexia.[77] A pilot study has recently reported similar results in AIDS patients treated with Megace at doses ranging from 320 to 640 mg/day.[78, 79] There remains some question as to whether the weight gain found is due partly to fluid retention.[80] Several side effects are of concern, includ-

TABLE 43–7.

Potential Appetite Stimulants in HIV Disease

- Megestrol acetate (Megace)
- Cyproheptadine (Antihistamines)
- Anabolic agents (growth hormone)
- Anticytokines (ω-3 fatty acids)
- Metabolic inhibitors (hydrazine sulfate)
- Cannabinoid derivatives (dronabinol [Marinol])

ing the drug's potential for inducing deep-vein thrombosis and emboli. Exacerbation of diabetes has also been reported with high-dose Megace.[81] Anabolic agents such as growth hormone have been used to reverse catabolism in preliminary studies of HIV-infected patients.[82, 83] Early results indicate the promotion of a positive nitrogen balance and weight gain. However, it remains to be determined whether these effects can be sustained and alter the clinical outcome. Anticytokine therapies would theoretically be beneficial to the nutritionally impaired AIDS patient since these are present in excess and account for many of the complications of the disease. ω-3 fatty acids may decrease cytokine production, especially in the mononuclear cell where HIV replication occurs.[84] Enteral diets with high mixtures of ω-3 fatty acids may be of benefit, but this requires further study.

The metabolic inhibitor hydrazine sulfate may theoretically induce anabolism by blocking catabolic pathways through the inhibition of gluconeogenesis.[85] Recent studies have found improved appetite and caloric intake and increased albumin levels in cancer patients.[86] Current investigations are under way in HIV disease. Cannabinoid derivatives have been used as appetite stimulants in cancer patients. A recent trial using 2.5 mg of dronabinol two to three times a day revealed improvement in mood as well as weight gain.[87] Despite these exciting potential pharmaceutical advances in appetite stimulation, attempts to establish the underlying cause of anorexia should be the primary goal. Removal or reduction of an offending drug or institution of appropriate medical therapy for an indolent infectious process may be all that is required.

DIARRHEA/MALABSORPTION

The gastrointestinal tract is a major organ whose function is altered by HIV infection and subsequent opportunistic disease. Diarrhea develops in the majority of patients and can become severe and debilitating. Fifty percent of patients will not have an identifiable pathogen, and HIV infection alone is felt to be the causative factor. Significant sequelae of diarrhea include fluid and electrolyte losses. Voluminous stool output may result from secretory diseases such as cryptosporidiosis. In patients with identifiable pathogens, specific anti-infective treatment should be initiated along with fluid-electrolyte and supplemental nutritional therapy. In patients without identifiable or treatable pathogens, antimotility agents can be attempted. These include loperamide (Imodium) (8 to 12 doses per day), Lomotil, and deodorized tincture of opium (15 to 45 mg/day). However, in many patients, these are not well tolerated, and secretory diarrhea persists in ranges from 500 mL to 10 L per day. Several studies evaluated the use of the hormonal agent octreotide as adjunctive therapy to reduce stool output, increase appetite and weight gain, and improve the quality of life.[88, 89] Doses of 300 to 1500 μg/day subcutaneously reduce stool output by 35% to 50% over a 2-week period. One study, using intravenous infusions of octreotide at 75 to 100 μg/hr, reported similar results in a single patient.[90] On the basis of these reports and anecdotal clinical data, this somatostatin analogue may have a role in the treatment of refractory diarrhea. Octreotide has also been suggested as an appetite stimulant. Controlled trials will be needed to elucidate the efficacy and safety of this intervention.

Glutamine, administered in a 20-g slurry with juice or lemonade (Crystal Light), may also reduce gut dysfunction and malabsorption in the AIDS patient. Preservation of the integrity of the small bowel via this method may enhance the absorption of nutrients in the HIV-infected patient with malabsorption. When gut dysfunction is suspected, enteral and parenteral diets supplemented with glutamine should be considered.

ALTERNATIVE NUTRITIONAL THERAPIES

AIDS and other patients who have terminal illnesses often seek out alternative treatments that offer them some hope. The prevalence of this practice ranges from 19% to 32% of all patients surveyed in several studies.[58, 91–93] A vast array of medicinal herbs and alternative diet plans have been tried by the HIV-infected population. Many of these are outlined in Table 43–8. Potential adverse effects can occur due to misdosage, mislabeling, contamination, or adulteration of these diets. Gastrointestinal, hematologic, mental status, allergic, and electrolyte disturbances have all been described with many of these remedies.[93] The macrobiotic, yeast-controlled, and Dr. Berger's Immune power diets are examples of regimens that may result in an inadequate

TABLE 43–8.

Alternative Nutritional Therapies in AIDS

Herbals
  Aloe vera
  AL-721
  Astralgus
  Bee pollen
  BHT
  Blue-green manna
  Burdock
  Chaparral
  Comfrey
  Coenzyme Q
  Garlic
  Ginseng
  Lentinen
  Licorice
  Pau d' arco
  Peony
  Primrose oil
  Red clover
  Salvia
  Shitake
  Tang-kuei
  Thymus
  Vitamins/minerals
Diets
  Yeast free
  Macrobiotic
  Dr. Berger's Immune Power
  Max immunity
  Vegetarian
  Fasting

intake of calories, protein, and other nutrients. Some vitamins and minerals have been shown to improve function (i.e., folic acid; vitamins A, B_6, C, and E; zinc, iron, copper, and selenium). However, oversupplementation of these nutrients can result in immunosuppression.[94] A safe recommendation includes a multivitamin/mineral supplement that provides 100% of the recommended daily allowances. Additional nutrient supplements should be based on individual nutritional assessment. The frequency of medicinal herbs and alternative diets and therapies used by AIDS patients underscores the need to become familiar with and informed about the risks and benefits of these controversial therapies so that ongoing medical treatments are not compromised.

Knowledge of nutritional needs in HIV disease arises out of clinical experience with other chronic debilitating diseases. The current evidence indicates that wasting and loss of endogenous nutrients can be diminished by aggressive nutritional intervention and education and counseling in the early stages of HIV infection. Nutritional goals are to maximize protein-calorie support and micronutrient balance throughout progression of the HIV condition. Interventions can be individualized to the clinical and physiologic manifestations of AIDS. They should be revised through serial nutritional assessment. Appropriate nutrition support systems are clearly fundamental to the survival and improved quality of life in this rapidly advancing and fatal disease.

REFERENCES

1. Council of State and Territorial Epidemiologists, AIDS Program, Center for Infectious Diseases, CDC: Revision of the CDC surveillance case definition for AIDS. *MMWR* 1987; 36:35–155.
2. Grunfeld C, Feingold KR: Metabolic disturbances and wasting in the acquired immunodeficiency syndrome. *N Engl J Med* 1992; 327:329–337.
3. Kotler DP, Wang J, Peirson R: Studies

of body composition in patients with AIDS. *Am J Clin Nutr* 1985; 42:1255–1265.

4. Grunfeld C, Kotler DP: The wasting syndrome and nutritional support in AIDS. *Semin Gastroenterol Dis* 1991; 2:25–36.

5. Kotler DP, Teirney AR, Francisco A, et al: The magnitude of body cell mass depletion determines the timing of death from wasting in AIDS. *Am J Clin Nutr* 1989; 50:444–447.

6. Chlebowski RT, Grosvenor MB, Bernhard NH, et al: Nutritional status, gastrointestinal dysfunction, and survival in patients with AIDS. *Am J Gastroenterol* 1989; 84:1288–1293.

7. Grunfeld C, Pang M, Doerrler W, et al: Lipids, lipoproteins, triglyceride clearance, and cytokines in human immunodeficiency virus infection and the acquired immunodeficiency syndrome. *J Clin Endocrinol Metab* 1992; 74:1045–1052.

8. Kaufmann RL, Matson CF, Beisel WR: Hypertriglyceridemia produced by endotoxin: Role of impaired triglyceride disposal mechanisms. *J Infect Dis* 1976; 133:548–555.

9. Grunfeld C, Kotler DP, Hamadeh R, et al: Hypertriglyceridemia in the acquired immunodeficiency syndrome. *Am J Med* 1989; 86: 27–31.

10. Beutler BA, Cerani A: Cachectin: More than tumor necrosis factor. *N Engl J Med* 1987; 316:379–385.

11. Lahdevirta J, Maury CPJ, Teppo AM, et al: Elevated levels of circulating cachectin/tumor necrosis factor in patients with acquired immunodeficiency syndrome. *Am J Med* 1988; 85:289–291.

12. Reddy MM, Sorrell SJ, Lange M, et al: Tumor necrosis factor and HIV P24 antigen in the serum of HIV-infected population. *J Acquir Immune Defic Syndr* 1988; 1:436–440.

13. Grunfeld C, Kotler DP, Shigenaga JK, et al: Circulating interferon-alpha levels and hypertriglyceridemia in AIDS. *Am J Med* 1991; 90:154–162.

14. Patton JS, Shapard HM, Wilking H, et al: Interferons and tumor necrosis factors have similar catabolic effects on 3T3-L1 cells. *Proc Natl Acad Sci U S A* 1986; 83:8313–8317.

15. Beutler BA, Cerami A: Recombinant interleukin-1 suppresses lipoprotein lipase activity in 3T3-L1 cells. *J Immunol* 1986; 135:3969–3971.

16. Feingold KR, Soued M, Serio MK, et al: Multiple cytokines stimulate hepatic lipid synthesis in vivo. *Endocrinology* 1989; 125:267–274.

17. Grunfeld C, Adi S, Soved M, et al: Search for mediators of the lipogenic effects of tumor necrosis factor: Potential role for interleukin-6. *Cancer Res* 1990; 50:4233–4238.

18. Ellakany S, Whiteside TL, Schade RR, et al: Analysis of intestinal lymphocyte subpopulations in patients with AIDS and ARC. *Am J Clin Pathol* 1987; 87:356–364.

19. Dworkin B, Wormser GP, Rosenthal WS, et al: Gastrointestinal manifestations of AIDS: A review of 22 cases. *Am J Gastroenterol* 1985; 80:774–778.

20. Kotler DP: Intestinal and hepatic manifestations of AIDS. *Adv Intern Med* 1989; 34:43–71.

21. Ulrich R, Zeitz M, Heise W, et al: Small intestinal structure and function in patients infected with HIV: Evidence for HIV-induced enteropathy. *Ann Intern Med* 1989; 111:15–21.

22. Raufman JP: Odynophagia/dysphagia in AIDS. *Gastroenterol Clin North Am* 1988; 17:599–614.

23. Wilcox CM: Esophageal disease in the acquired immunodeficiency syndrome: Etiology, diagnosis and management. *Am J Med* 1992; 92:412–421.

24. Edison SA, Kotler DP: How HIV infection and AIDS affect the gastrointestinal tract. *J Crit Ill* 1992; 7:37–55.

25. Banacini M, Young T, Laine L: The causes of esophageal symptoms in HIV infection. *Arch Intern Med* 1991; 151:1567–1572.

26. Tnechman SL, Wright TL, Altman DF: Gastrointestinal Kaposi's sarcoma in patients with AIDS. *Gastroenterology* 1985; 89:102–108.

27. Bernal A, del Junco GW: Endoscopic and pathologic features of esophageal lymphoma: A report of four cases in patients with AIDS. *Gastrointest Endosc* 1986; 82:96–99.

28. Kotler DP (ed): *Gastrointestinal and Nutritional Manifestations of AIDS.* New York, Raven Press, 1991.

29. Soave R: Cryptosporidiosis and isosporiasis in patients with AIDS. *Infect Dis Clin North Am* 1989; 2:485–493.

30. Dehbvitz JA, Pape JW, Buncy M, et al: Clinical manifestations and therapy of *Isospora belli* infections in patients with AIDS. *N Engl J Med* 1986; 315:87–90.

31. Shadduck JA: Human microsporidiosis and AIDS. *Rev Infect Dis* 1989; 11:203–207.

32. Smith PD: Gastrointestinal infections in AIDS. *Ann Intern Med* 1992; 116:63–77.

33. Allason-Jones E, Mindel A, Sargeaunt P, et al: *Entamoeba histolytica* as a commensal intestinal parasite in homosexual men. *N Engl J Med* 1986; 315:353–356.

34. Baskin DH, Lax JD, Barenberg D: *Shigella* bacteremia in patients with AIDS. *Am J Gastroenterol* 1987; 82:338–341.

35. Sperber SJ, Schleupner CJ: Salmonellosis during infection with HIV. *Rev Infect Dis* 1987; 9:925–934.

36. Perlman DM, Ampel NM, Schifman RB, et al: Persistent *Campylobacter jejuni* infections in patients infected with HIV. *Ann Intern Med* 1988; 108:540–546.

37. Tanowitz HB, Simon D, Wittner M: Gastrointestinal manifestations of AIDS. *Med Clin North Am* 1992; 76:45–62.

38. Janoff EV, Orenstein JM, Manischewitz JF, et al: Adenovirus colitis in AIDS. *Gastroenterology* 1991; 100:976–979.

39. Jacobson MA, Mills J: Serious cytomegalovirus disease in AIDS: Clinical findings, diagnosis and treatment. *Ann Intern Med* 1988; 108:585–594.

40. Gray JR, Rabeneck L: Atypical mycobacterial infection of the GI tract in AIDS patients. *Am J Gastroenterol* 1989; 84:1521–1524.

41. Kotler DP, Gaetz HP, Lange M, et al: Enteropathy associated with AIDS. *Ann Intern Med* 1984; 101:421–428.

42. Greensan JK, Belitsos PC, Yardley JH, et al: AIDS enteropathy: Occult enteric infections and duodenal mucosal alterations in chronic diarrhea. *Ann Intern Med* 1991; 114:366–372.

43. Wheat LJ, Kohler RB, Frane PT, et al: *Histoplasma capsulatum* polysaccharide antigen detection in diagnosis and management of disseminated histoplasmosis in patients with AIDS. *Am J Med* 1989; 87:396–400.

44. Chuck SL, Sande MA: Infections with *Cryptococcus neoformans* in AIDS. *N Engl J Med* 1989; 321:794–799.

45. Fish DG, Ampel NM, Galgiani JN, et al: Coccidioidomycosis during HIV infection: A review of 77 patients. *Medicine (Baltimore)* 1990; 69:384–391.

46. Goodell SE, Quinn TC, Mkrtichian E, et al: Herpes simplex virus proctitis in homosexual men. Clinical, sigmoidoscopic, and histopathological features. *N Engl J Med* 1983; 308:868–871.

47. Levine AM: AIDS associated malignancy lymphoma. *Med Clin North Am* 1992; 76:253–268.

48. Banacini M: Hepatobiliary complications in patients with HIV infection. *Am J Med* 1992; 92:404–411.

49. Perkocha LA, Geaghan SM, Benefict Yen TS, et al: Clinical and pathologic features of bacillary peliosis hepatitis in association with HIV infection. *N Engl J Med* 1990; 323:1581–1586.

50. Cello JP: AIDS cholangiopathy: Spectrum of disease. *Am J Med* 1989; 86:539–546.

51. Banacini M: Pancreatic involvement in HIV infection. *J Clin Gastroenterol* 1991; 13:58–64.

52. Maxson E, Greenfield S, Turner J: Acute pancreatitis as a complication of ddI therapy in AIDS. *Am J Gastroenterol* 1990; 85:1254.

53. Antonow DR: Acute pancreatitis associated with TMP/SMX. *Ann Intern Med* 1986; 104:363–365.

54. Pauwels A, Eliaszewicz M, Larrey D, et al: Pentamidine-induced acute pancreatitis in AIDS. *J Clin Gastroenterol* 1990; 12:457–459.

55. Newman CF: Practical dietary recommendations in HIV infection, in Kotler DP (ed): *Gastrointestinal Manifestations of AIDS*. New York, Raven Press, 1991.

56. Beisel WR: Single nutrients and immunity. *Am J Clin Nutr* 1982; 35(suppl):417–468.

57. Falutz J, Tsoukas C, Cardaro T: Serum zinc in homosexual men. *Clin Chem* 1989; 35:704–705.

58. Raiten DJ: Nutrition in HIV infection. *Nutr Clin Pract* 1991; 6(suppl):1–94.

59. Bro S, Buhl M, Jorgensen PJ, et al: Serum zinc in homosexual men with antibodies against HIV. *Clin Chem* 1988; 34:1929–1930.

60. Herbert V, Fong W, Gulle V, et al: Low holotranscobalamin II is the earliest serum marker for subnormal vitamin B_{12} absorption in patients with AIDS. *Am J Hematol* 1990; 34:132–139.

61. Harriman GR, Smith PD, Hone MK, et al: Vitamin B_{12} malabsorption in patients with AIDS. *Arch Intern Med* 1989; 149:2039–2041.

62. Baum MK, Mantero-Atienza E, Shor-Posner G, et al: Association of vitamin B_6 status with parameters of immune function in early HIV-1 infection. *J Acquir Immune Defic Syndr* 1991; 4:1122–1132.

63. Merrill AH, Henderson JM: Diseases associated with defects in vitamin B_6 metabolism and utilization. *Annu Rev Nutr* 1987; 7:137–156.

64. Heise W, Nehmk, L'Age M, et al: Concentrations of magnesium, zinc and copper in serum of patients with AIDS. *J Clin Chem Clin Biochem* 1989; 27:515–517.

65. Blumber BS, Hann HWL, Mildvan D, et al: Iron and iron-binding proteins in persistent generalized lymphadenopathy and AIDS. *Lancet* 1984; 1:347.

66. Dworkin BM, Rosenthal WS, Wormser GP, et al: Selenium deficiency in AIDS. *JPEN* 1986; 10:405–407.

67. Hickey MS, Weaver KE: Nutritional management of patients with ARC or AIDS. *Gastroenterol Clin North Am* 1988; 17:545–561.

68. Grunfeld C, Pang M, Shimzu L, et al: Resting energy expenditure, caloric intake, and short-term weight change in HIV infection and AIDS. *Am J Clin Nutr* 1992; 55:455–460.

69. Baum MK, Javier JJ, Mantero-Atienza E, et al: Zidovudine-associated adverse reactions in a longitudinal study of asymptomatic HIV-1 infected homosexual males. *J Acquir Immune Defic Syndr* 1991; 4:1218–1226.

70. Kotler D, Teirney A, Ferraro R, et al: Effect of enteral alimentation upon body cell mass in patients with AIDS. *Am J Clin Nutr* 1991; 53:149–154.

71. Mamel J: Percutaneous endoscopic gastrostomy: A review. *Nutr Clin Pract* 1987; 12:65–75.

72. Raviglione MO, Battan R, Pablos-Mendez A, et al: Infections associated with Hickman catheters in patients with AIDS. *Am J Med* 1989; 86:780–786.

73. Kotler D, Teirney AR, Culpepper-Morgan JA, et al: Effect of home TPN on body composition in patients with AIDS. *JPEN* 1990; 14:454–458.

74. Greene JB: Clinical approach to weight loss in the patient with HIV infection. *Gastroenterol Clin North Am* 1988; 17:573–586.

75. Weaver KE: Psychosocial aspects pertaining to nutrition, in Kotler DP (ed): *Gastrointestinal Manifestations of AIDS*, New York, Raven Press, 1991.

76. Hellerstein MK, Kahn J, Mudie H, et al: Current approach to the treatment of HIV associated weight loss: Pathophysiologic considerations and emerging management strategies. *Semin Oncol* 1990; 17(suppl 9):17–33.

77. Loprinzi CL, Ellison NM, Schaid DJ, et al: Controlled trial of megestrol acetate for the treatment of cancer anorexia and/or cachexia. *J Natl Cancer Inst* 1990; 82:1127–1132.

78. Von Roenn JH, Murphy RL, Weber KM, et al: Megestrol acetate for treatment of cachexia associated with HIV infection. *Ann Intern Med* 1988; 109:840–841.

79. Von Roenn JH, Murphy RL, Wegener N: Megestrol acetate for treatment of anorexia and cachexia associated with HIV infection. *Semin Oncol* 1990; 17(suppl 9):13–16.

80. Bruera E, Macmillan K, Kuehniv, et al: A controlled trial of megestrol acetate on appetite, caloric intake, nutritional status, and other symptoms in patients with advanced cancer. *Cancer* 1990; 66:1279–1282.

81. Henry K, Rathgober S, Sullivan C, et al: Diabetes mellitus induced by megestrol acetate in a patient with AIDS and cachexia. *Ann Intern Med* 1992; 116:53–54.

82. Krentz AJ, Koster FT, Crist D, et al: Beneficial anthropometric effects of human growth hormone in the treatment of AIDS (abstract). *Clin Res* 1991; 39:220.

83. Mulligan K, Grunfeld C, Hellerstein M, et al: Growth hormone treatment of HIV-associated catabolism (abstract). *FASEB J* 1992; 6:1942.

84. Endress S, Ghorbani R, Kelley VE, et al: The effect of dietary supplementation with N-3 polyunsaturated fatty acids on the synthesis of interleukin-1 and TNF by mononuclear cells. *N Engl J Med* 1989; 320:265–271.

85. Loprinzi CL, Ellison NM, Goldberg RM, et al: Alleviation of cancer anorexia and cachexia: Studies of Mayo Clinic and the North Central Cancer Treatment Group. *Semin Oncol* 1990; 6(suppl 9):8–12.

86. Chlebowski RT, Heber D, Richardson B, et al: Influence of hydrazine sulfate on abnormal carbohydrate metabolism in cancer patients with weight loss. *Cancer Res* 1984; 44:857–861.

87. Gorter R: Management of anorexia-cachexia associated with cancer and HIV infection. *Oncology* 1991; 5:13–17.

88. Cook DJ, Kelton JG, Stanisz AM, et al: Somatostatin treatment for cryptosporidial diarrhea in a patient with AIDS. *Ann Intern Med* 1988; 108:708–709.

89. Cello JP, Grendell JH, Basuk P, et al: Effect of octreotide on refractory AIDS-associated diarrhea: A prospective, multicenter clinical trial. *Ann Intern Med* 1991; 115:705–710.

90. Katz MD, Erstad BL, Rose C: Treatment of severe *Cryptosporidium*-related diarrhea with octreotide in a patient with AIDS. *Drug Intell Clin Pharm* 1988; 22:134–136.

91. Taber-Pike J: Alternative nutritional therapies—Where is the evidence? *AIDS Pt Care* 1988; 31:31–33.

92. Taber J: Nutrition in HIV infection. *Am J Nurs* 1989; 1446–1451.

93. Kassler WJ, Blanc P, Greenblott R: The use of medicinal herbs by HIV infected patients. *Arch Intern Med* 1991; 151:2281–2288.

94. Chandra RK: Immunodeficiency in undernutrition and overnutrition. *Nutr Rev* 1981; 39:225–231.

44

Diabetes Mellitus

M. Molly McMahon, M.D.

Robert A. Rizza, M.D.

Regulation of carbohydrate metabolism	Parenteral and enteral nutrition
Normal physiology	Metabolic effects, indications, and caveats
Effect of diabetes mellitus	Use in patients with diabetes mellitus
Effect of illness	

Diabetes mellitus is caused by an absolute (insulin-dependent diabetes mellitus, type I) or a relative (non-insulin-dependent diabetes mellitus) lack of insulin. Insulin-dependent diabetes mellitus is associated with onset at an early age, a tendency toward ketosis, and an absolute dependency on insulin. Non-insulin-dependent diabetes mellitus, by far the more common type, is associated with onset predominantly after the age of 40 years, a tendency to obesity, and insulin resistance. Because of the prevalence of diabetes mellitus and the comorbidity (e.g., nephropathy, macrovascular disease, gastroparesis, ulcerations) of the disease, all intensive care unit physicians will at some time manage diabetic patients receiving nutritional support. Following a review of the effects of diabetes mellitus, illness, and feeding on carbohydrate metabolism, an approach to the design of a nutritional program for the diabetic patient will be presented.

REGULATION OF CARBOHYDRATE METABOLISM

Normal Physiology

In nondiabetic subjects, the plasma glucose concentration is closely regulated in both the postabsorptive (6 to 14 hours after a meal) and the postprandial periods. In the postabsorptive period, plasma glucose is primarily derived from the liver, since cellular glucose release requires the action of glucose-6-phosphatase, an enzyme present in significant amounts only in the liver and kidney. Endogenous glucose production results both from glycogenolysis (the breakdown of glucose stored as glycogen) and from gluconeogenesis (the formation of glucose from precursors).[1, 2] Euglycemia is maintained because the rate of hepatic glucose release (glucose production) approximates the combined rate of glucose uptake (glucose utilization) by the liver, brain, and peripheral tissues. These rates average 2 mg/kg/

min in a nondiabetic subject in the post-absorptive period, or approximately 200 g/day for a 70-kg subject.

Following meal ingestion (or an infusion of dextrose), the increase in plasma glucose leads to an increase in plasma insulin levels. Both of these variables are key modulators of glucose turnover rates (the rates of glucose release and glucose uptake). The elevation in plasma glucose levels activates glycogen synthetase (the enzyme stimulating glycogen synthesis) and decreases both glycogenolysis and gluconeogenesis.[3, 4] The liver is quite sensitive to changes in insulin concentration. Under euglycemic conditions, an increase in the plasma insulin level from 10 μU/mL (average preprandial concentration) to 25 to 30 μU/mL results in a significant suppression of hepatic glucose release with near-maximal suppression at an insulin concentration of 50 to 60 μU/mL (the average postprandial insulin level is 30 to 100 μU/mL).[5] Lack of suppression of hepatic glucose release in the presence of hyperinsulinemia denotes resistance to the action of insulin at the liver, i.e., hepatic insulin resistance. Hyperglyce-

mia, due to a mass effect, increases the peripheral uptake of glucose.[6, 7] In addition, hyperinsulinemia enhances glucose uptake. A significant increase in glucose uptake occurs at a plasma insulin concentration of 50 to 60 μU/mL, with a near-maximal effect observed at insulin concentrations in excess of 200 μU/mL[5] (Fig 44–1). The lack of appropriate glucose uptake in the presence of hyperinsulinemia denotes resistance to the action of insulin by extrahepatic tissues, i.e., peripheral insulin resistance. The hyperglycemia and hyperinsulinemia of the fed state convert the liver from an organ that produces glucose to one that takes up glucose and stimulates peripheral glucose uptake, thereby preventing the postprandial glucose concentration from exceeding 150 mg/dL. Postprandially, as the plasma glucose and insulin concentrations fall, the rates of glucose release and glucose uptake are restored to preprandial levels. The drop in insulin level permits an increase in hepatic glucose release and a decrease in glucose uptake in insulin-sensitive tissues, namely, liver, muscle, and fat.

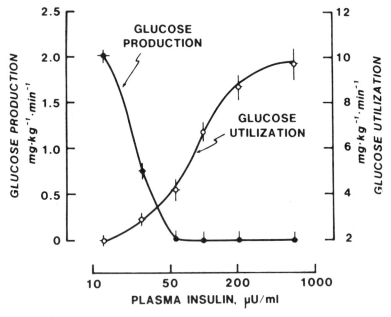

FIG 44–1.
Insulin dose-response curves for glucose production and utilization. (From Rizza R, Mandarino L, Gerich J: *Am J Physiol* 1981; 240:630–639. Used by permission.)

Effect of Diabetes Mellitus

Patients with diabetes mellitus have both preprandial and postprandial hyperglycemia. The hyperglycemia is due to excessive hepatic glucose release, impaired glucose uptake, and decreased insulin secretion.[8-11]

Effect of Illness

Under conditions of severe stress, hyperglycemia may develop in patients without an antecedent diagnosis of diabetes mellitus.[12, 13] "Stress diabetes," included under the category of secondary diabetes,[14] represents an important cause of hyperglycemia in the critically ill patient. Severe stress is accompanied by a marked increase in the plasma concentration of glucagon, epinephrine, and cortisol. These counterregulatory hormones all increase hepatic glucose release. Each stimulates gluconeogenesis[15-17] and glycogenolysis,[16-18] with cortisol also exerting a "permissive" effect. The term "permissive" denotes that glucocorticoids are required for the full hepatic response to the other hormones. As with glucose production, the counterregulatory hormones have opposite effects on glucose uptake from insulin, with the counterregulatory hormones decreasing glucose uptake. Glucagon inhibits hepatic glucose uptake,[19] while epinephrine and cortisol decrease the peripheral uptake of glucose.[20, 21] Animal and human studies have evaluated the role of counterregulatory actions and interactions in the pathogenesis of stress-induced hyperglycemia. The hormones were infused individually and in combination in healthy subjects in doses designed to reproduce the hormonal milieu of stress[22, 23] (Fig 44–2). While single hormonal infusion caused only mild hyperglycemia, combined infusion resulted in plasma glucose levels in excess of 200 mg/dL because of an increase in hepatic glucose release and a decrease in glucose uptake. Cytokines may also have profound effects on carbohydrate metabolism. Interleukin-1 and tumor necrosis factor (TNF) stimulate hepatic glucose output,[24-26] with the former either inhibiting or stimulating insulin secretion, depending on the concentration and length of exposure. Interleukin-1 is capable of creating a stress hormone profile.[27] Finally, endotoxin can cause hyperglycemia by stimulating hepatic glucose production.[28]

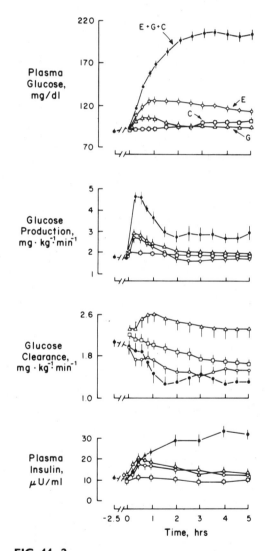

FIG 44–2.

Effect of combined hormonal infusion (epinephrine [E] plus glucagon [G] plus cortisol [C]) on plasma glucose concentration, glucose production, glucose clearance, and plasma insulin concentration in normal subjects. The responses are compared with those during the individual infusion of epinephrine, glucagon, and cortisol. (From Shamoon M, Hendler R, Sherwin R: *J Clin Endocrinol Metab* 1981; 52:1235–1241. Used by permission.)

PARENTERAL AND ENTERAL NUTRITION

Metabolic Effects, Indications, and Caveats

Continuous intravenous feeding differs from enteric feeding in that nutrients immediately enter the systemic circulation and bypass initial entry through the splanchnic circulation. In addition, continuous parenteral or enteral nutrition causes a sustained hyperinsulinemia. In nondiabetic subjects, the plasma insulin concentration increases from the fasting level of 6 to 10 μU/mL to 40 to 100 μU/mL after meal ingestion. However, the hyperinsulinemia subsides within a few hours of eating to basal levels. By contrast, the peripheral insulin concentration in nondiabetic subjects receiving central parenteral nutrition has been reported to be in the 60 to 90-μU/mL range.[29, 30] However, these studies date back to a time when it was common practice to provide more calories and more dextrose calories than is the current practice. During cyclic parenteral nutrition, in which the nutrition is discontinued for a period each day, the peripheral insulin concentration has been reported to drop from 90 μU/mL (termination of the central parenteral nutrition cycle) to 30 μU/mL (termination of the infusion-free period).[30] Hyperinsulinemia is one of the potential causes of the hepatic dysfunction related to central parenteral nutrition and can affect electrolyte levels and salt and water balance.

The beneficial effects of dextrose as a substrate in parenteral nutrition are attributed to the provision of calories with a nitrogen-sparing effect. These effects are believed to result from suppression of hepatic glucose release (decrease in the need for gluconeogenic precursors) and from stimulation of glucose oxidation (decrease in the requirement for amino acid oxidation as an energy source). To determine the "optimal" dextrose infusion rate, Wolfe et al. studied glucose kinetics in five postoperative, nonseptic patients receiving three dextrose infusion rates (4, 7, and 9 mg/kg/min).[31] The respiratory quotient during the two higher dextrose infusion rates was greater than 1, thus suggesting that net lipogenesis was occurring. The authors concluded that not only was there a limit in the ability to derive energy from infused glucose but there was also a detrimental effect from infusing excess dextrose.

Over the short term, the indications for nutritional support and the daily estimate of caloric, protein, and lipid requirements are similar in diabetic and nondiabetic critically ill patients. The percentage of recent (previous 3- to 6-month period) weight loss, the presence or absence of clinical markers of stress, and the anticipated time that the patient will be unable to meet nutritional needs orally all influence the need for nutritional support (Table 44–1).[32, 33] In general, a recent weight loss of less than 10% from usual weight is well tolerated. For the well-nourished and unstressed (afebrile, normal leukocyte count and differential) or mildly stressed patient who is anticipated to be eating in the next 10 days, provision of fluid and electrolytes should be sufficient. Those who have lost 10% to 20% of their usual weight should receive supplemental nutrition if moderately or severely stressed. Prompt nutritional support should generally be provided for severely stressed patients (e.g., after closed-head injury, major burn, multi-

TABLE 44–1.

Indications for Feeding*

Recent Weight Loss (%)	Stress	Intervention
<10	Mild or moderate	Fluid and electrolytes alone for up to 7–10 days
10–20	Mild or moderate	Fluid and electrolytes
	Severe†	Nutrition
>20	Any	Nutrition
Any	Severe	Nutrition

*From McMahon MM, Bistrian BR: *Dis Month* 1990; 36:375–417. Used by permission.
†Closed head injury, multiple trauma, severe burn, or sepsis.

ple trauma, or severe sepsis) since the stress response generally exceeds 7 to 10 days, as well as for those who have recently lost more than 20% of their usual weight.

The daily caloric requirement of a patient can be estimated by the use of nomograms such as the Harris-Benedict equation (using the current weight for patients with a stable weight or for patients who have lost weight or using the "dry weight" estimate in volume-overloaded patients), which is based on the premise that basal caloric needs are related to body cell mass.[34, 35] The variables of height, weight, age, and gender in the equation reflect the relationship between body weight and body cell mass. Direct measurement of daily energy requirements by indirect calorimetry may be useful in selected situations. The previous practice of providing all critically ill patients with additional calories for stress has been challenged by recent work. Studies comparing the measured (indirect calorimetry) and estimated (Harris-Benedict equation) daily caloric expenditure demonstrate that the best group estimate of caloric requirements in intensive care unit patients was the basal Harris-Benedict estimate, or approximately 22 to 25 kcal/kg of body weight.[36, 37] An indirect calorimetric measurement of energy needs may be helpful in the following types of patients: severely malnourished, volume overloaded if a "dry weight" estimate is uncertain, severely stressed (defined above; the measured daily caloric requirement will often exceed the estimated daily caloric requirement), morbidly obese, severely marasmic, or the ventilator-dependent patient experiencing weaning difficulty. In the absence of significant hepatic or renal disease, the stressed patient should generally receive 1.5 g of protein per kilogram of body weight per day. In the obese patient, it is reasonable to base the protein requirement on an estimated lean weight. Parenteral administration of lipid is best limited to 30% of calories and provided continuously at

rates that not exceed 30 to 50 mg/kg/hr. The majority of complications (i.e., impairment of reticuloendothelial system clearance and immune function) related to the use of parenteral lipid have been demonstrated at high infusion rates.[38] Investigators demonstrated that while lipid infusion over a 10-hour period impaired reticuloendothelial system clearance, there was no impairment if the same lipid load was infused continuously over a 24-hour interval.[39]

The use of dextrose as the only source of nonprotein calories is no longer recommended because of potential complications including hepatic lipogenesis, hepatic dysfunction, and hyperglycemia. Provision of a portion of the calories by lipid can minimize the development of hepatic and respiratory complications. A randomized prospective study compared the metabolic effects of a dextrose-and-protein solution with an isocaloric program in which one third of the nonprotein calories were supplied as lipid.[40] Patients receiving the dextrose-based parenteral nutrition had serum insulin levels that were significantly higher (85.8 ± 23.1 vs. 34 ± 17.8 μU/mL; neutral lipid, 0 to 20) on day 7 than did patients on an isocaloric program in which one third of the calories were replaced with lipid. There were similar trends for triglyceride levels (110.5 ± 16.8 vs. 71.5 ± 11.5 mg/dL; neutral lipid, 30 to 160), and serum glutamate pyruvate transaminase (SGPT) (102.9 ± 22.0 vs. 60.3 ± 9.8 units/L; neutral lipid, 7 to 40). It is important to point out that these patients received an average of 41 kcal/kg of body weight per day (i.e., probably excessive for needs). Although it is not known whether the abnormalities would persist or would lead to clinically significant morbidity, it seems prudent to avoid high-dextrose feedings.

Use in Patients With Diabetes Mellitus

A major goal in the care of the hospitalized diabetic patient is to avoid the extremes of hyperglycemia and hypoglycemia. A reasonable approach is to aim to maintain the plasma glucose level between 100 and 200 mg/dL. Once nutritional support is established, more tightly regulated plasma glucose concentrations (i.e., 100 to 150 mg/dL) may be desirable in stable patients. The function of polymorphonuclear leukocytes has been reported to be impaired in poorly controlled diabetic patients. In vitro studies document that abnormalities in granulocyte adherence, chemotaxis, phagocytosis, and microbicidal function in poorly controlled diabetic patients improve with enhanced glycemic control.[41–47] More recent studies have focused on the effect of hyperglycemia on complement function.[48–51] Covalent attachment of the third component of complement (C3) to the microbial surface is a critical determinant of phagocytic recognition. This opsonic process is regulated by the internal thioester bond of C3. Theoretically, attachment of glucose to the opsonic binding site within the C3 thioester bond could divert this protein from the surface of invading bacteria and generate a dysfunctional complement-glucose complex.

Since the majority of diabetic patients will require insulin coverage for dextrose in the parenteral nutrition admixture to avoid excessive increases in blood glucose, we customarily add a basal amount of human regular insulin (Table 44–2) to all parenteral nutrition solutions. The availability of insulin from the parenteral nutrition admixture is variable and appears to depend on the composition of the formulation (the presence of ions, pH, etc.).[52] We initially add approximately 0.1 units of insulin per gram of dextrose (e.g., 15 units/L of 15% dextrose [D_{15}], 20 units/L of 20% dextrose [D_{20}]). In our experience, this ratio of insulin to dextrose is unlikely to be associated with hypoglycemia unless the patient has significant renal disease. Dextrose in the parenteral nutrition solution should be limited to approximately 200 g on the first day of nutrition.[53, 54] While it is preferable that supplemental crystalloid infusions not contain dextrose, the presence of significant hypernatremia may necessitate an infusion of 5% dextrose in water (D_5W). The dextrose content of the parenteral nutrition solution can temporarily be decreased to avoid overfeeding. Plasma glucose levels should be measured at least two to four times daily with adherence to an insulin algorithm for the subcutaneous administration of regular insulin (Table 44–3). Unstable patients may initially require more frequent glucose monitoring. If careful attention is paid to quality control, reflectance meters can be used for glucose monitoring.

Once glycemic control is acceptable, an alteration in the frequency of monitoring is appropriate. At this point, the dextrose (and insulin) load may be increased as necessary to meet caloric requirements.[54] Plasma glucose concen-

TABLE 44–2.

Insulin Preparation Pharmacokinetics (Human)

Preparation	Route	$t_{1/2}$ (min)	Glucose Nadir (hr)	Effects (hr)
Rapid onset				
Regular	SC	60	2–6	4–12
	IV	3–6	0.5	3.5
Intermediate acting				
NPH	SC		6–16	12–18
Lente	SC		6–16	12–18
Long acting				
Ultralente	SC		14–24	16–32

NPH = neutral protamine Hagedorn

TABLE 44–3.

Algorithm for Administration of Regular Insulin

Plasma Glucose (mg/dL)*	Subcutaneous Insulin Dose (Units)†	Intravenous Insulin Dose (Units)‡
200–250	3	3
251–300	6	4
301–350	9	5
351–400	12	6

*Notify the physician if the glucose value is less than 80 mg/dL or greater than 200 mg/dL. The algorithm may need to be modified for certain patients.
†Subcutaneous administration of regular insulin should not be given more often than every 4 hours.
‡An intravenous bolus of regular insulin should not be given more often than every hour.

trations in excess of 200 mg/dL may be managed by an increase in intravenous parenteral nutrition insulin coverage by 0.05-unit increments per gram of dextrose. The insulin algorithm for the subcutaneous administration of insulin may also need to be modified. If the plasma glucose content remains greater than 200 mg/dL with this insulin coverage and adherence to an insulin algorithm for the subcutaneous administration of regular insulin, a further increase in parenteral nutrition insulin coverage or initiation of either an intravenous insulin bolus program (Table 44–3) or a variable insulin infusion (Table 44–4) should be considered. If an intravenous bolus of insulin is given, the plasma glucose level should be checked 1 hour later. If the plasma glucose concentration is lower but not in the target range, the bolus should be repeated and the glucose level rechecked in 1 hour. If there is an inadequate response, the bolus may be increased by 50%. If there is still an inadequate response, one should consider initiation of a variable insulin infusion. This degree of hyperglycemia may be reflective of insulin resistance due to overfeeding, illness, medications, or volume depletion.

Glycemic control during the transition from parenteral to enteral nutrition is often difficult. Enteral calories can generally be delivered with subcutane-

ously administered insulin. The possibility of erratic oral intake by a patient during the first few days of oral intake necessitates conservative use of intermediate-duration insulin and adherence to a regular insulin supplementation algorithm. The use of intermediate-duration insulin should be safe once the daily oral intake approaches 1000 kcal for several days in a row. If the feedings are continuous, twice-daily subcutaneous administration of intermediate-duration insulin may·at times be supplemented with regular insulin. Changes in the enteral nutrition infusion rate should not be made until the longer-acting subcutaneous insulin dose can be appropriately adjusted. In patients with unstable insulin requirements or a changing clinical condition, an intravenous insulin infusion may be necessary.

The recent availability of an enteral formula that is lower in carbohydrate and higher in fat content than standard formulas has prompted studies comparing the glycemic response. One product contains 18% glucose oligosaccharides, 7% fructose, 8% soluble fiber, and 50%

TABLE 44–4.

Insulin Infusion Algorithm: A Suggested Initial Insulin Infusion*

Plasma Glucose (mg/dL)	IV infusion rate (mL/hr)	Insulin Infusion Rate (Units/hr)
>300	8	4.0
250–300	6	3.0
200–249	5	2.5
150–199	4	2.0
120–149	3	1.5
100–119	2	1.0
70–99	1	0.5
<70	0	0.0

*This algorithm is appropriate for the "average healthy 70-kg patient" who generally would require 0.75 to 1.0 units of insulin per hour as a basal rate at a glucose concentration of 80 to 100 mg/dL. Infusion rates may have to be modified proportionately for larger or smaller individuals and for individuals who are insulin resistant due to their medical illness (e.g., sepsis, shock). The infusion rates listed above are intended as a general guideline. They should be modified depending on the clinical situation and the desired glycemic goals. If the glucose level does not fall as desired, progressively increase the infusion rate for all glucose concentrations greater than 200 mg/dL by 1 50% increments until the desired response is observed. However, the infusion rate for glucose levels less than 200 mg/dL should only rarely be modified so as to minimize the risk of hypoglycemia.

fat, while standard formulas contain approximately 50% simple carbohydrate and 30% fat. The glucose response to these products was studied in ten patients with insulin-dependent diabetes mellitus.[55] While an initial report suggested that the glycemic response to the lower-carbohydrate product was blunted in comparison to standard formulas, a follow-up study reported that the glycemic response was very variable in each patient.[56] The clinical significance of these studies is unclear because the subjects ingested very small amounts of the formula over a few hours, a very different pattern from that of continuous tube feeding or gravity administration of the feeding. The avoidance of overfeeding is likely more important than is the use of a specific enteral formula.

Careful monitoring of the diabetic patient receiving nutritional support is essential to safe use of this form of therapy. Accurate recording of daily weight and fluid balance is essential. A daily weight increase in excess of 0.25 kg should be attributed to fluid gain rather than to the accretion of lean tissue. In stressed patients, day-to-day weight changes generally reflect shifts in fluid balance. With an acute increase in plasma insulin levels, renal sodium excretion falls and may lead to salt and water retention. DeFronzo et al. studied the effect of an acute increase in plasma insulin concentration on urinary sodium excretion in six nondiabetic subjects.[57, 58] Insulin administration enhanced the tubular reabsorption of sodium independent of changes in the filtered load of glucose, the glomerular filtration rate, renal blood flow, and plasma aldosterone levels. The effect of chronic hyperinsulinemia on sodium excretion is not known. Hyperinsulinemia may also cause a drop in the plasma levels of potassium and phosphorus if the supplementation is inadequate.[59] Some studies suggest that insulin increases the sodium permeability of skeletal muscle cells. The increased

cytosolic sodium concentration activates Na, K-adenosine triphosphatase (ATPase).[60] As sodium is transported from the cell, electronegativity is generated and promotes the inward movement of potassium from the extracellular fluid. From a nutritional standpoint, hypokalemia can also be due to malnutrition or to anabolism. Total-body potassium is stored almost entirely within lean tissue. Because the amount of lean tissue is decreased in malnutrition, the body stores of potassium may also be decreased. Since 3 mEq of potassium is retained per gram of nitrogen, potassium requirements may increase during anabolism, the accretion of lean tissue.[61] Plasma potassium levels should be interpreted in light of the plasma glucose level. Hyperkalemia, if accompanied by hyperglycemia, may be effectively treated by an increase in insulin supplementation. Phosphorus has an important role in intermediary metabolism. Glucose- and insulin-stimulated glycolysis enhances the cellular uptake and utilization of phosphorus for the phosphorylation of glucose and fructose and for the synthesis of adenosine triphosphate. Thus, insulin infusion may lower phosphorus levels and exacerbate pre-existing hypophosphatemia.

Hyperglycemia may cause a pseudohyponatremia.[62] Because glucose penetrates cells slowly, an increase in the plasma glucose level raises the plasma osmolality and causes water to move from the cells to the extracellular volume. This lowers the plasma sodium concentration by dilution. In general, every 62-mg/dL increment in the plasma glucose level will draw enough water out of the cells to reduce the plasma sodium concentration 1 mEq/L. Hyperglycemia can also cause an osmotic diuresis. As the filtered load of glucose (glomerular filtration rate times the plasma glucose concentration) rises, it may exceed the tubular reabsorptive capacity. As a result, glucose remains in the tubular lumen and acts as an osmotic diuretic by increasing the urinary loss of electrolytes and water. An osmotic diuresis is generally associated with water loss in excess of solute, thereby raising the plasma sodium concentration.

Sudden discontinuation of parenteral nutrition has been reported to have dramatic effects on plasma glucose, insulin, and glucagon levels. An early study reported that symptomatic hypoglycemia could be induced only by increasing the flow rate of parenteral nutrition 30 minutes before its acute discontinuation.[63] The plasma glucose level during the infusion was reported to be in the 400-mg/dL range. In clinical practice it would be uncommon to significantly increase the flow rate of the parenteral nutrition solution shortly before its discontinuation. More recently, Wagman et al. studied the effects of acute cessation of parenteral nutrition (drop in the infusion rate by 50% for 1 hour before cessation) on plasma glucose, insulin, and glucagon concentrations in 48 patients without hepatic or renal disease.[64] Four patients had diabetes mellitus, and 11 patients were receiving insulin for stress hyperglycemia. Only 4 patients had a plasma glucose level less than 70

mg/dL in the first hour after discontinuation of the infusion. These are impressive results in light of the fact that the patients received an average of 2856 kcal (plus an additional 550 kcal three times weekly due to lipid infusion). Although the average body weight was not provided, this caloric provision is very high and would be expected to lead to a significant insulin response. Although a drop in the infusion rate by 50% for 1 hour prior to discontinuation of parenteral nutrition appears safe, the tapering should probably be slower if large amounts of insulin are present in the admixture.

Since peritoneal dialysis (PD) is often used in diabetic patients with renal failure, it is helpful to review certain points. Dextrose in the PD fluid serves as the osmotic gradient for fluid removal. Since high dextrose–containing PD fluid is frequently employed in fluid-overloaded patients to achieve a negative fluid balance, a significant proportion of the dextrose instilled into the peritoneal cavity may be absorbed.[65, 66] Using indirect calorimetry and analyzing the dialysis effluent for dextrose concentration,

TABLE 44-5.

Peritoneal Dialysis*

Metabolic cart studies in patients receiving high dextrose dialysate (mean + SEM)

Patient	$\dot{V}_{CO_2}$ (mL/min)	$\dot{V}_{CO_2}$ (mL/min)	RQ†	Energy Expenditure (kcal/24hr)
1	182 ± 2	239 ± 4	1.30 ± 0.03	1396 ± 15
2	225 ± 6	252 ± 2	1.18 ± 0.03	1396 ± 34
3	196 ± 2	209 ± 2	1.06 ± 0.01	1424 ± 15
4	168 ± 5	193 ± 1	1.15 ± 0.03	1236 ± 27
5	215 ± 3	246 ± 1	1.14 ± 0.01	1592 ± 19

Dextrose absorption during PD†

	PD infused			PD Effluent		
Patient	Volume (L/Day)	Dextrose (g/Day)	Effluent Dextrose Concentration (g/dL)	Volume (L/day)	Dextrose (g/Day)	Estimated Dextrose Absorption (g/Day)
1	21.51	914	1.15	24.03	276	638
2	10.10	429	0.83	11.80	98	331
3	24.00	1020	1.60	29.22	467	553
4	16.00	680	0.71	18.18	98	551
5	40.00	1700	2.22	42.63	946	754

*From Manji N, Shikora S, McMahon M, et al: *Crit Care Med* 1990; 18:29–31. Used by permission.
†RQ = respiratory quotient; PD = peritoneal dialysis.

Manji et al. studied the effects of high dextrose–containing dialysates in five patients with acute renal failure who were undergoing PD (Table 44–5).[67] Despite minimal caloric intake, all five patients had a respiratory quotient in excess of 1, consistent with net lipogenesis due to dextrose absorbed from the peritoneal cavity. Four of the five patients absorbed more than 500 grams of dextrose per day from the peritoneal cavity. These data suggest that in diabetic patients receiving nutritional support and undergoing PD, the caloric (and dextrose) content should be appropriately decreased to avoid overfeeding.

In summary, over short-term hospitalization, the tenets underlying design of a nutritional program for the critically ill diabetic patient are similar to those for feeding a nondiabetic critically ill patient. The finely tuned homeostatic mechanisms regulating carbohydrate metabolism in a healthy subject can be affected by diabetes mellitus, feeding, and stress. It is important to avoid the extremes of hyperglycemia or hypoglycemia. Should there be an unexplained deterioration in glycemic control, one needs to be certain that overfeeding, illness, medication use, or dehydration is not aggravating the hyperglycemia (Table 44–6). Finally, familiarity with the effects of hyperinsulinemia on electrolytes should mitigate the incidence of electrolyte abnormalities.

TABLE 44–6.

Potential Causes of an Acute Increase in Plasma Glucose Levels

Nutritional program
  Excess calories
  Excess dextrose load (nutrition + crystalloid + peritoneal dialysis)
  Insufficient insulin
Infection/inflammation
  Role of counterregulatory hormones
  Role of cytokines
Medications
  Glucocorticoid
  Phenytoin
  Infusion of sympathomimetic agent
Volume depletion

REFERENCES

1. Dietz G, Wicklmayr M, Hepp K, et al: On gluconeogenesis of human liver: Accelerated hepatic glucose formation induced by increased precursor supply. *Diabetologia* 1976; 12:555–561.
2. Wahren J, Felig P, Ahlborg G, et al: Glucose metabolism during leg exercise in man. *J Clin Invest* 1971; 50:2715–2725.
3. Buschiazzo H, Exton J, Park C: Effects of glucose on glycogen synthetase, phosphorylase, and glycogen deposition in the perfused rat liver. *Proc Natl Acad Sci U S A* 1971; 65:383–387.
4. Ruderman N, Herrera M: Glucose regulation of hepatic gluconeogenesis. *Am J Physiol* 1968; 214:1346–1351.
5. Rizza R, Mandarino L, Gerich J: Dose-response characteristics for effects of insulin on production and utilization of glucose in man. *Am J Physiol* 1981; 240:630–639.
6. Verdonk C, Rizza R, Gerich J: Effects of plasma glucose concentration on glucose utilization and glucose clearance in normal man. *Diabetes* 1981; 30:535–537.
7. Cherrington A, Williams P, Harris M: Relationship between the plasma glucose level and glucose uptake in the conscious dog. *Metab Clin Exp* 1978; 27:787–791.
8. Pehling G, Tessari P, Gerich J, et al: Abnormal carbohydrate disposition in insulin-dependent diabetes: Relative contributions of endogenous glucose production and initial splanchnic uptake and effect of intensive insulin therapy. *J Clin Invest* 1984; 74:985–991.
9. Firth R, Bell P, Marsh H, et al: Postprandial hyperglycemia in patients with noninsulin-dependent diabetes mellitus. *J Clin Invest* 1986; 77:1525–1532.
10. McMahon M, Rizza R: The contribution of initial splanchnic glucose clearance and gluconeogenesis to postprandial hyperglycemia in noninsulin-dependent diabetes mellitus, (abstract). *Clin Res* 1987; 35:899.
11. Bell P, Firth R, Rizza R: Assessment of insulin action in insulin-dependent diabetes mellitus using [6-^{14}C] glucose, [3-^{3}H] glucose, and [2-^{3}H] glucose. *J Clin Invest* 1986; 78:1479–1486.

12. Batstone G, Aloberti K, Hinks L, et al: Metabolic studies in subjects following thermal injury. Intermediary metabolites, hormones, and tissue oxygenation. *Burns* 1976; 2:207–225.

13. Willerson J, Hutcheson D, Leshin S, et al: Serum glucagon and insulin levels and their relationship to blood glucose values in patients with acute myocardial infarction and acute coronary insufficiency. *Am J Med* 1974; 57:747–753.

14. Harris M, Cahill G, Bennett P, et al: National Diabetes Data Group. *Diabetes* 1979; 28:1039–1057.

15. Exton J: Gluconeogenesis. *Metabolism* 1972; 21:945–989.

16. Exton J, Park C: The role of cyclic AMP in the control of liver metabolism. *Adv Enzyme Regul* 1968; 6:391–407.

17. Long C, Smith O, Fry E: Actions of cortisol and related compounds on carbohydrate and protein metabolism, in Wolstenholm O, Connor M (eds): *Metabolic Effects of Adrenal Hormone.* London, Churchill, 1960.

18. Shulman G: Glucose disposal during insulinopenia in somatostatin-treated dogs: The roles of glucose and glucagon. *J Clin Invest* 1978; 62:487–492.

19. Hers H: The control of glycogen metabolism in the liver. *Annu Rev Biochem* 1976; 45:167–189.

20. Walaas O, Walaas E: Effect of epinephrine on rat diaphragm. *J Biol Chem* 1950; 187:769–776.

21. Munck A: Studies on the mode of action of glucocorticoids in rats. *Biochim Biophys Acta* 1962; 57:318–326.

22. Shamoon M, Hendler R, Sherwin R: Synergistic interactions among antiinsulin hormones in the pathogenesis of stress hyperglycemia in humans. *J Clin Endocrinol Metab* 1981; 52:1235–1241.

23. Bessey P, Watters J, Aoki T, et al: Combined hormonal infusion stimulates the metabolic response to injury. *Ann Surg* 1984; 200:264–281.

24. Fukushima R, Saito H, Taniwaka K, et al: Different roles of IL-1 and TNF on hemodynamics and interorgan amino acid metabolism in awake dogs. *Am J Physiol* 1992; 262:275–281.

25. Flores EA, Istfan N, Pomposelli JJ, et al: Effect of interleukin 1 and tumor necrosis factor/cachectin on glucose turnover in the rat. *Metabolism* 1990; 39:738–743.

26. Pomposelli JJ, Flores EA, Bistrian BR: Role of biochemical mediators in clinical nutrition and surgical metabolism. *JPEN* 1988; 12:212–218.

27. Besedovsky H, Del Ray A, Sorkin E, et al: Immunoregulatory feedback between interleukin-1 and glucocorticoid hormones. *Science* 1986; 233: 652–654.

28. Fong Y, Marano MA, Moldawer LL, et al: The acute splanchnic and peripheral tissue metabolic response to endotoxin in humans. *J Clin Invest* 1990; 85:1896–1904.

29. Wood R, Bengoa J, Sitrin M, et al: Calciuretic effect of cyclic versus continuous total parenteral nutrition. *Am J Clin Nutr* 1985; 41:614–619.

30. Benotti P, Bothe A, Miller J, et al: Cyclic hyperalimentation. *Compr Ther* 1976; 2:27–36.

31. Wolfe R, O'Donnell T, Stone M, et al: Investigation of factors determining the optimal glucose infusion rate in total parenteral nutrition. *Metabolism* 1980; 29:892–900.

32. Bistrian BR: Nutritional assessment of the hospitalized patient: A practical approach, in Wright RA, Heymsfield S (eds): *Nutritional Assessment.* Boston, Blackwell Scientific, 1984, pp 183–205.

33. McMahon M, Bistrian BR: The physiology of nutritional assessment and therapy in protein-calorie malnutrition. *Dis Mon* 1990; 36:375–417.

34. Harris JA, Benedict FG: *A Biometric Study of Basal Metabolism in Man.* Washington, DC, Carnegie Institute of Washington, Publication No 279, 1919.

35. Roza AM, Shizgal HM: The Harris-Benedict equation re-evaluated: Resting energy requirements and the body cell mass. *Am J Clin Nutr* 1984; 40:168–182.

36. Hunter DC, Jaksic J, Lewis D, et al: Resting energy expenditure in the critically ill. *Crit Care Med* 1985; 13:173–177.

37. Paauw JD, McCamish MA, Dean RE: Assessment of caloric needs in stressed patients. *J Am Coll Nutr* 1984; 3:51–59.

38. Miles JM: Intravenous fat emulsion in

nutrition support. *Curr Opin Gastroenterol* 1991; 7:306–311.

39. Jensen GL, Mascioli EA, Seidner DL, et al: Parenteral infusion of long- and medium-chain triglycerides and reticuloendothelial system function in man. *JPEN* 1990; 14:464–471.

40. Meguid MM, Akahoshi MP, Jeffers S, et al: Amelioration of metabolic complications of conventional total parenteral nutrition. *Arch Surg* 1984; 119:1294–1298.

41. Bagdade J, Stewart M, Walters E: Impaired granulocyte adherence. A reversible defect in host defense in patients with poorly controlled diabetes. *Diabetes* 1978; 27:677–681.

42. Mowat A, Baum J: Chemotaxis of polymorphonuclear leukocytes from patients with diabetes mellitus. *N Engl J Med* 1971; 284:621–627.

43. Bagdade J, Nielson K, Bulger R: Reversible abnormalities in phagocytic function in poorly controlled diabetic patients. *Am J Med Sci* 1972; 263:451–456.

44. Bagdade J, Koot R, Bulger R: Impaired leukocyte function in patients with poorly controlled diabetes. *Diabetes* 1974; 23:9–15.

45. Nolan C, Beaty H, Bagdade J: Impaired granulocyte bactericidal function in patients with poorly controlled diabetes. *Diabetes* 1978; 127:889–894.

46. Repine J, Clawson C, Goetz F: Bactericidal function of neutrophils from patients with acute bacterial infections and from diabetes. *J Infect Dis* 1980; 142:869–875.

47. Karnovsky M: The metabolism of leukocytes. *Semin Hematol* 1968; 5:156–165.

48. Hostetter MK: Handicaps to host defense: Effects of hyperglycemia on C_3 and *Candida albicans*. *Diabetes* 1990; 39:271–275.

49. Gilmore BJ, Retsinas EM, Lorenz JJ, et al: An iC3b receptor on *Candida albicans*: Structure, function, and correlates for pathogenicity. *J Infect Dis* 1988; 157:38–46.

50. Hostetter MK, Krueger RA, Schmeting DJ: The biochemistry of opsonization: Central role of the reactive thioester of the third component of complement. *J Infect Dis* 1984; 150:653–661.

51. Hostetter MK, Lorenz JS, Preus L, et al: The iC3b receptor on *Candida albicans*: Subcellular localization and modulation of receptor expression by glucose. *J Infect Dis* 1990; 161:761–768.

52. Mitrano FP, Newton DW: Factors affecting insulin adherence to type 1 glass bottles. *Am J Hosp Pharm* 1982; 39:1491–1495.

53. Mascioli E, Bistrian B: TPN in the patient with diabetes. *Nutr Support Serv* 1983; 3:12–16.

54. McMahon M, Manji N, Driscoll DF, et al: Parenteral nutrition in patients with diabetes mellitus. Theoretical and practical considerations. *JPEN* 1989; 13:545–553.

55. Peters AL, Davidson MB, Isaac RM: Lack of glucose elevation after simulated tube feeding in patients with type I diabetes. *Am J Med* 1989; 87:178–182.

56. Peters AL, Davidson MB: Effects of various enteral feeding products on postprandial blood glucose response in patients with type I diabetes. *JPEN* 1991; 16:69–74.

57. DeFronzo R, Sherwin R, Dillingham M, et al: Influence of basal insulin and glucagon secretion on potassium and sodium metabolism. *J Clin Invest* 1978; 61:472–479.

58. DeFronzo R, Cooke C, Andres R, et al: The effect of insulin and renal handling of sodium, potassium, calcium, and phosphate in man. *J Clin Invest* 1985; 55:845–855.

59. Knochel JP: Complications of total parenteral nutrition (letter) *Kidney Int* 1985; 27:489–496.

60. Moore RD: Stimulation of NA:H exchange by insulin. *Biophys J* 1981; 33:203–210.

61. Acheson KJ, Flatt JP, Jéquier E: Glycogen synthesis versus lipogenesis after a 500 gram carbohydrate meal in man. *Metabolism* 1982; 31:1234–1240.

62. Rose BD: Hypoosmolal states—Hyponatremia, in Rose BD (ed): *Clinical Physiology of Acid-Base and Electrolyte Disorders*. New York, McGraw-Hill, 1989, pp 601–638.

63. Sanderson I, Deitel M: Insulin response in patients receiving concentrated infusion of glucose and casein hydrolysate for complete parenteral nutrition. *Ann Surg* 1974; 179:387–394.

64. Wagman LD, Miller KB, Thomas RB, et

al: The effect of acute discontinuation of total parenteral nutrition. *Ann Surg* 1986; 204:524–529.

65. Albert A, Takamatsu H, Fonkalsrud E: Absorption of glucose solutions from the peritoneal cavity in rabbits. *Arch Surg* 1984; 119:1247–1251.

66. Schade D, Eaton R, Friedman W, et al: Prolonged peritoneal infusion in a diabetic man. *Diabetes Care* 1980; 3:314–317.

67. Manji N, Shikora S, McMahon M, et al: Peritoneal dialysis for acute renal failure: Overfeeding resulting from dextrose absorbed during dialysis. *Crit Care Med* 1990; 18:29–31.

45

Diarrhea: Diagnosis and Treatment

Mark J. Koruda, M.D.

Gastrointestinal physiology	Fecal impaction
Pathophysiology of diarrhea	Drugs
Osmotic diarrhea	Infections
Secretory diarrhea	Antiobiotics
Motility disorders	Enteral feeding
Causes of diarrhea in the critically ill patient	**Treatment**

Diarrhea is considered a frequent complication of the critically ill patient. Few data are actually available that accurately define the prevalence of diarrhea in this population. In the intensive care unit (ICU), diarrhea and tube feeding are thought to travel "hand in hand." One early prospective study found a 41% incidence of diarrhea in a general ICU.[1] Diarrhea developed in 68% of those patients receiving tube feeding, while it was present in only 29% of those not fed. Additionally, patients with diarrhea experienced a threefold increase in the length of ICU stay.

Part of the problem in ascertaining the prevalance of diarrhea is that its definition varies widely. *Diarrhea* is derived from the Greek *dia* (through) and *rhein* (to flow). Three dimensions of bowel elimination—stool frequency, consistency, and quantity—are commonly used to define diarrhea. As many as 14 definitions of diarrhea found in the literature used one or more of these three characteristics.[2] A common definition of diarrhea is the passage of loose or liquid stools at an increased frequency with the resultant loss of water and electrolytes in the stool.[3] For research purposes diarrhea is most commonly defined as a stool weight greater than 200 g/day.[4] Realistically, it may not be appropriate to apply the definition of diarrhea used for "scientific" studies to everyday clinical practice. In the day-to-day setting it may be most practical to define diarrhea as the passage of too-frequent or too-loose stools that are inconvenient to the patient and/or nursing staff.[5] This definition is particularly pertinent to critically ill patients. It most certainly is an ordeal for the conscious, intubated patient to communicate the need for a bedpan or to suffer the repetitive indignity of incontinence. Fecal incontinence is obviously detrimental to local wound and skin care, and the resultant odor may be quite distressful to staff, visitors, and family members. More practical "costs" associated with diarrhea include increased nursing time, frequent dressing and linen changes, and the expense of the medical workup and treatment.[6]

GASTROINTESTINAL PHYSIOLOGY

In order to better understand the pathophysiology of diarrhea, it is best to review the physiology of normal bowel function. The normal daily volume of gastric contents includes 1 to 2 L of oral intake and 3 L of gastric and salivary secretions. Isotonic chyme readily enters the duodenum, whereas anisotonic material is delayed. Pancreatic, biliary, and intestinal secretions contribute an additional 4 L, such that 9 L of fluid enter the jejunum every 24 hours (Table 45–1).[3, 7]

As a result of the relatively permeable mucosal epithelium within the jejunum, the absorption of nutrients produces hypotonic luminal fluid that in turn forces water to be absorbed with solute. Sodium and potassium are also absorbed passively by solvent drag, as is chloride, the major anion. The jejunum is 45% effective in absorbing water such that approximately 5 L of effluent enters the ileum daily.[3, 8]

Within the ileum, the intercellular mucosal junctions are tighter, which permits active resorption of sodium and chloride, and water is prevented from leaking back into the lumen. Seventy percent of effluent entering the ileum is resorbed, which normally leaves approximately 1.5 L entering the colon.

A healthy colon is very efficient in conserving sodium and water because 90% of the effluent presented to the colon is absorbed. Under normal circumstances only 100 to 200 mL of fecal water is excreted daily. Active colonic sodium absorption reduces its fecal concentration to 30 mmol/L, while potassium accumulates to concentrations of 75 mmol/L to maintain ionic equilibrium. Seventy percent of fecal anions are composed of the short-chain fatty acids (SCFAs) acetate, butyrate, and propionate.

SCFAs are the by-products of bacterial fermentation of unabsorbed carbohydrates and dietary fiber (nonstarch) polysaccharides. Within the colon, the breakdown of starches resistant to digestion and nonstarch polysaccharides is the result of the concerted action of many species of intestinal microflora, predominantly the anaerobes. Initially, the large polymers are hydrolyzed to monomeric units (glucose, galactose, xylose, and uronic acids), and fermentation proceeds via glycolysis. Many intermediate metabolites are produced, but the ultimate end products are volatile SCFAs and the gases hydrogen, carbon dioxide, and methane (Fig 45–1).[9] Bacterial proliferation is also stimulated by the fermentation of polysaccharides. The pattern of fermentation may be substantially modified by the relative proportions of individual microbial species, which may have clinical significance,

TABLE 45–1.

Normal 24-Hour Intestinal Fluid and Electrolyte Transport*

Site	Fluid Received (L)	Amount Absorbed (L)	Efficiency (%)	Electrolyte Absorption		
				Na$^+$	K$^+$	Cl$^-$
Duodenum/ jejunum	9.0	4.0	45	Passive	Passive	Passive
Ileum	5.0	3.5	75	Active	Passive	Active
Colon	1.5	1.35	> 90	Active	Passive	Active

*Adapted from Pietrusko R: *Am J Hosp Pharm* 1979; 36:757–767.

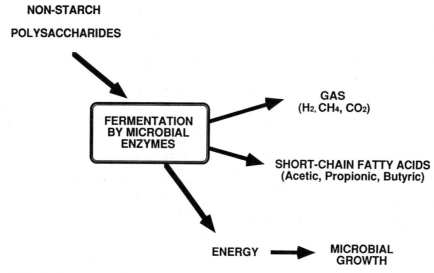

FIG 45–1.

Colonic fermentation of nonstarch, fiber polysaccharides.

particularly for patients exposed to broad-spectrum antibiotics.[9, 10]

SCFAs are the predominant anions in human feces, with concentrations ranging from 60 to 170 mmol/L. Three SC-FAs, acetic, propionic, and butyric acids, represent more than 80% of all SCFAs produced. Small amounts of other SCFAs (isobutyrate, valerate, and isovalerate) are also present (1 to 2

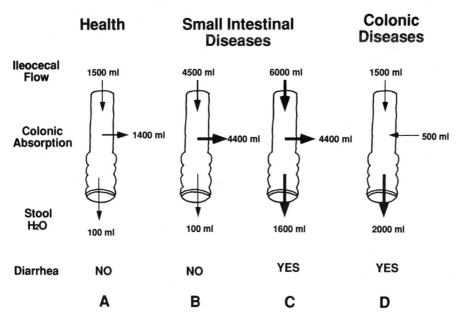

FIG 45–2.

Importance of colonic absorptive capacity in determining stool water (i.e., diarrhea). **A,** normal balance in humans. Significant changes in small intestinal fluid absorption will not produce diarrhea **(B)** so long as colonic absorptive capacity is not exceeded. Diarrhea occurs when the ileocecal flow exceeds the colonic absorptive capacity. **(C).** A decrease in colonic absorption with normal small intestinal function will also result in an increase in stool water secretion **(D).** (Adapted from Binder H: Absorption and secretion of water and electrolytes by small and large intestine, in Fordtran JS, Sleisenger M (eds): *Gastrointestinal Disease: Pathophysiology, Diagnosis, Management.* Philadelphia, WB Saunders, 1989, pp 1022–1040.)

mmol/L). The relative proportions of these three principal SCFAs (60:25:15 acetic:propionic:butyric) show remarkable similarity across various animal species and diets.[9]

SCFAs are intriguing substances. Normally, 200 to 700 mmol of SCFAs are produced per day, which represents 60% to 70% of the potential energy available had the carbohydrates been absorbed intact.[9] This energy constitutes 2% to 7% of the daily caloric intake in low-fiber diets.[11]

SCFAs are primarily metabolized by the colonic mucosa and liver. In fact, butyrate is the preferred oxidative substrate of the colonic epithelium and accounts for 80% of colonocyte oxygen consumption.[12] Acetate and propionate are oxidized to a lesser extent. SCFAs are metabolized by the colonic mucosa to the ketone bodies acetoacetate and β-hydroxybutyrate and to carbon dioxide.[13] Butyrate and the other primary SCFAs are important respiratory fuels for the colonic epithelium, and their production may be important to the maintenance of a healthy local mucosa. SCFAs stimulate colonic mucosal proliferation and the active absorption of sodium and water.[12]

TABLE 45–2.

Causes of Acute Diarrhea in the Critically Ill Patient*

Medications
  Hyperosmolar
    Antacids
    Elixirs/solutions—theophylline solution, potassium chloride slurry
  Cathartics—magnesium, phosphate
  Promotility agents—metaclopramide
  Antibiotics
Iatrogenic infections
  Pseudomembranous colitis
  Bacterial overgrowth: secondary to antibiotic usage or decreased gastric acidity
  Candida albicans overgrowth
  Bacterial contamination of formula
Tube feedings
  Hyperosmolar formula
  Fat content
  Peptide/amino concentration
  Rate
  Lactose
  Bacterial contamination
Patient related
  Ischemic bowel
  Partial bowel obstruction—fecal impaction
  Parasitic infection (rare)
  Idiopathic inflammatory bowel disease (rare)
  Refeeding syndrome—gut atrophy
  Motility disorders
  Malabsorption (mucosal defect, biliary or pancreatic insufficiency)

*Adapted from Hill M: Factors affecting bacterial metabolism, in Hill M (ed): *Microbial Metabolism in the Digestive Tract.* Boca Raton, Fla, CRC Press, 1986, pp 22–29.

TABLE 45–3.

Pathophysiology of Diarrhea*

Type of Diarrhea	Mechanism	Characteristics	Stool Composition
Osmotic	Unabsorbable solute in the alimentary tract	24-hr stool volume < 1 L	Osmotic gap > 100 mOsm/kg
		Stool volume decreases with fasting	Stool [Na] < 60 mmol/L
Secretory	Increased secretory activity of the alimentary tract, with or without absorption of intestinal contents; may also result from inhibition of electrolyte and water absorption	24-hr stool volume > 1 L Stool volume does not decrease with fasting	Osmotic gap < 40 mOsm/kg Stool [Na] > 90 mmol/L
Mixed	Increased rate of transit as in hypermotility states; osmotic effect of ingested solutes may result from rapid transit and decreased net absorption	Variable	Variable

*Adapted from Greenberger N: *Gastrointestinal Disorders: A Pathophysiologic Approach.* St Louis, Mosby–Year Book, 1986, p 191.

The absorptive capacity of the colon is limited. Studies in normal human subjects have determined that the maximum daily absorptive capacity of the colon is approximately 5 to 6 L for water and 800 mEq for sodium.[14] If there is a decrease in small intestinal fluid absorption, diarrhea will not develop until the absorptive capacity of the colon is exceeded (Fig 45–2).[15] On the other hand, relatively small decreases in colonic water absorption can lead to substantial increases in stool water excretion and hence diarrhea.[7]

PATHOPHYSIOLOGY OF DIARRHEA

Diarrhea in the critically ill patient may result from a number of causes (Table 45–2).[16] The treatment of diarrhea most naturally depends on identifying its etiology. This is perhaps the most difficult, yet most important exercise in the management of this problem.

The mechanisms of diarrhea can be divided into three major categories: osmotic diarrhea, secretory diarrhea (deranged water and electrolyte transport), and motility disorders. Not infrequently, more than one mechanism may contribute (Table 45–3).[17]

Osmotic Diarrhea

Osmotically active substances induce excessive water influx into the lumen of the jejunum. Diarrhea will result if the influx of water surpasses the absorptive capacity of the ileum and colon. Additionally, if the solute is a carbohydrate that is able to be metabolized by the colonic bacteria, the osmotic load may be significantly increased because 1 mol of disaccharide is fermented to nearly 4 mol of SCFA. This increased solute load promotes the movement of more fluid into the colon and exacerbates the osmotic effects that occurred in the small bowel. The osmotic effect of a solute is determined by the number of

molecules present in a given volume of solution and their inabilty to pass across the epithelium by which they are confined. Small, low–molecular-weight substances (sugars, amino acids) are osmotically more active than high–molecular-weight polymers (starches, proteins, lipids). Since osmotic diarrheas result from an increased intraluminal fluid flux caused by osmotically active particles, the diarrhea should stop when the offending agent is no longer ingested. Determining fecal sodium and potassium concentrations

TABLE 45–4.

Classification of Osmotic (Malabsorptive) Diarrhea*

Exogenous

Laxatives

Polyethylene glycol/saline (Golytely), $Mg(OH)_2$ (Milk of Magnesia), $MgSO_4$ (Epsom salts), Na_2SO_4 (Glauber's or Carlsbad salt), Na_2PO_4 (neutral phosphate)

Antacids

Those containing MgO or $Mg(OH)_2$

Dietetic foods, candy or chewing gum, and elixirs containing sorbitol, mannitol, or xylitol

Miscellaneous drugs

Chronic ingestion of colchicine, cholestyramine, neomycin, para-aminosalicyclic acid, lactulose

Endogenous

Congenital

Specific malabsorptive diseases

Disaccharidase deficiencies (lactase, sucrase-isomaltase, trehalase)

Glucose-galactose or fructose malabsorption

Generalized malabsorptive diseases

Abetalipoproteinemia and hypobetalipoproteinemia

Congenital lymphangiectasia, microvillus inclusion disease

Enterokinase deficiency

Pancreatic insufficiency (cystic fibrosis or Schwachman's syndrome)

Acquired

Specific malabsorptive diseases

Postenteritis disaccharidase deficiency

Generalized malabsorptive diseases

Pancreatic insufficiency (alcohol), bacterial overgrowth, celiac sprue, rotavirus enteritis, parasitic diseases (*Giardia*, coccidiosis), metabolic diseases (thyrotoxicosis, adrenal insufficiency), inflammatory disease (eosinophilic enteritis, mastocytosis), protein-calorie malnutrition, short-bowel syndrome, jejunoileal bypass

*Adapted from Powell D: Approach to the patient with diarrhea, in Yamada T (ed): *Textbook of Gastroenterology.* Philadelphia, JB Lippincott, 1991, pp 732–778.

and the osmotic gap of the stool (measured stool osmolality minus 2 times the sum of the concentrations of stool sodium and potassium) will confirm the diagnosis. Osmotic gaps greater than 100 mOsm/kg H_2O are associated with osmotic diarrheas (Table 45–3).[4]

TABLE 45–5.

Classification of Secretory Diarrhea*

Exogenous

Laxatives

Phenolphthalein, anthraquinones, bisacodyl, oxyphenisatin, senna, aloe, ricinoleic acid (castor oil), dioctyl sodium sulfosuccinate

Medications

Diuretics (furosemide, thiazides); asthma medication (theophylline)

Cholinergic drugs—glaucoma eye drops and bladder stimulants (acetylcholine analogues or mimetics); myesthenia gravis medication (cholinesterase inhibitors); cardiac drugs (quinidine and quinine); gout medication (colchicine)

Prostaglandins (misoprostol); di-5-aminosalicylic acid (azodisalicylate); gold (may also cause colitis)

Toxins

Metals (arsenic); plants (mushroom, e.g., *Amanita phalloides*); organophosphates (insecticides and nerve poisons); seafood toxins (ciguatera, scombroid poisoning, paralytic or neurotoxic shellfish poisoning); coffee, tea, or cola (caffeine and other methylxanthines); ethanol

Bacterial toxins

Staphylococcus aureus, Clostridium perfringens and *botulinum, Bacillus cereus*

Gut allergy without histologic change

Endogenous

Congenital

Microvillus inclusion disease; congenital chloridorrhea (absence of $Cl:HCO_3$ exchanger); congenital Na diarrhea (absence of Na:H exchanger)

Bacterial enterotoxins

Vibrio cholerae; toxigenic *Escherichia coli; Campylobacter jejuni; Yersinia enterocolitica; Klebsiella pneumoniae; Clostridium difficile; Staphylococcus* aureus (toxic shock syndrome)

Endogenous laxatives

Dihydroxy bile acids and long-chain fatty acids, especially hydroxylated ones

Hormone-producing tumors

Pancreatic cholera syndrome and ganglioneuromas (vasoactive intestinal peptide); medullary carcinoma of the thyroid (calcitonin and prostaglandins); mastocytosis (histamine); villous adenoma (secretagogue unknown).

*Adapted from Powell D: Approach to the patient with diarrhea, in Yamada T (ed): *Textbook of Gastroenterology*. Philadelphia, JB Lippincott, 1991, pp 732–778.

Table 45–4 lists some of the more common causes of osmotic diarrhea encountered in the management of the critically ill patient.

Secretory Diarrhea

Secretory diarrheas result from the failure to absorb or from the active secretion of Na, K, Cl, or HCO_3. In distinction to osmotic diarrhea, in secretory diarrhea, stool output should not be significantly affected by fasting, and no osmotic gap results. Electrolyte secretion may be passive, as caused by inflammatory bowel disease; invasive strains of *Shigella* species, *Salmonella,* and *Escherichia coli;* laxatives; and radiation enteritis. Active electrolyte secretion can result from the presence of toxin-producing bacteria *(Vibrio cholera, Clostridium perfringens, E. coli,* tumors that secrete activating hormones, and bile acids.[3] Table 45–5 summarizes some of the causative factors of secretory diarrhea.

Motility Disorders

The mechanism by which fluid and electrolyte movement is affected by alterations in intestinal motility is not clearly understood. Diarrhea is probably underestimated as a manifestation of multisystem organ failure. Gastric atony and small-bowel ileus frequently accompany critical illness. The hypomotility of the critically ill patient is only compounded by the liberal use of opiate analgesics in this population. Possible causes of diarrhea in this setting include malabsorption caused by diversion of blood flow from the intestinal mucosa during shock or as a result of exogenous catecholamine administration, failure to absorb sodium and water from the colon against high electrochemical and concentration gradients, and perhaps a change in bile acid metabolism.[6]

CAUSES OF DIARRHEA IN THE CRITICALLY ILL PATIENT

Fecal Impaction

Long considered the most common cause of diarrhea in the institutionalized patient, fecal impaction cannot be ignored as a contributing factor in diarrhea in the ICU. The need to perform a digital rectal examination and perhaps even an abdominal radiograph cannot be minimized in the workup of a patient with diarrhea.

Drugs

A plethora of pharmacologic agents have diarrhea as a significant side effect. Antiarrhythmics, particularly quinidine but also lidocaine and procainamide, are commonly associated with diarrhea. The diarrhea may be profuse and correlates with the use of the drug. Most antacids contain magnesium hydroxide, which at moderate to high dosage frequencies readily produces diarrhea. Many chemotherapeutic agents are associated with an enteritis that is characterized by the passage of frequent, watery stools. A host of other diarrhea-associated drugs include antiepileptics, thyroid preparations, warfarin, and H_2-receptor antagonists. The pathophysiology behind the association of diarrhea with these agents is not completely understood but probably involves impaired fluid and electrolyte transport and increased gastrointestinal motility.[18]

Infections

Classic infectious diarrhea caused by organisms such as *Salmonella, Shigella, Campylobacter,* enterotoxigenic *E. coli,* and *Yersinia* are uncommon causes of diarrhea in the ICU. *Clostridium difficile* infection, on the other hand, accounts for the vast majority of pathogen-associated diarrhea in the hospitalized patient.

C. difficile causes pseudomembranous colitis (PC) solely in the presence of exposure to antibiotics. The incidence of PC among outpatient populations varies between 1 and 3 cases per 100,000 patients treated with oral antibiotics. On the other hand, the incidence of PC in antibiotic-treated hospitalized patients may be as high as 1:1000 to 1:100.[19] The presence of *C. difficile* does not always induce symptoms. The *C. difficile* organism or its toxin can be detected in a similar proportion of patients both with and without symptoms.[20] Virtually every antibiotic has been implicated in causing PC, with the most common being clindamycin, ampicillin, and the cephalosporins. Risk factors for PC include advanced age, duration of hospitalization (especially in the ICU), burn injury, and the use of multiple antibiotics.[19, 21, 22]

Symptoms usually appear after 5 to 10 days of antibiotic therapy but can follow a single dose. The diarrhea is usually watery and occurs more than five times per day. Systemic symptoms are common and include leukocytosis, fever, protein-losing enteropathy, abdominal pain, and cramping.

The diagnosis is confirmed by detection of the cytotoxin toxin B in the stool or by visualization of pathognomonic pseudomembranes on endoscopy of the descending and sigmoid colon. When diarrhea is the only symptom, the *C. difficile* toxin is found in only 10% to 25% of patients. With increasing severity of symptoms, toxin detection approaches 95%.[15] Treatment with vancomycin (125 mg orally four times daily or 500 mg orally four times daily), metronidazole (500 mg orally three times daily), or bacitracin (25,000 units orally four times daily) for 10 to 14 days appears to be equally effective. A 5% to 33% relapse rate has been reported with all three drugs.[19]

Another more recently recognized pathogenic cause of diarrhea in the critically ill patient is due to *Candida.* Although *Candida* may be seen in up to 30% of oropharyngeal cultures and 65% of stool cultures from normal subjects, it can proliferate in the gastrointestinal tract because of alterations in gut flora and other host factors and become pathogenic.[23] *Candida*-associated diarrhea (CAD) is predominantly secretory with frequent watery stools but usually without blood, mucous, tenesmus, or abdominal pain. Elderly, malnourished, and critically ill patients being treated with multiple antibiotics or chemotherapeutic drugs are at risk for CAD. The diarrhea is frequently severe enough to lead to dehydration, electrolyte imbalance, and hyperchloremic metabolic acidosis. The diagnosis of CAD is made by culture of *Candida albicans* from the stool, exclusion of other causes of diarrhea, and the persistence of diarrhea while fasting. CAD responds dramatically to oral nystatin (500,000 units orally every 6 hours) within 2 days of therapy.

Antibiotics

Diarrhea occurs in up to 20% of patients who receive antibiotics. Antibiotic-associated diarrhea (AAD) can be mild or debilitating. The pathogenesis of AAD is unknown but may be related to an altered intestinal microflora that allows proliferation of pathogenic species, to altered SCFA profiles, or to increases in unabsorbable carbohydrates.[10, 20] Surawicz et al. performed an extensive clinical review of AAD and found that it was not trivial.[20] The mean number of days of diarrhea was 4.5 ± 2.9 with a range of 2 to 11 days. Significant risk factors for AAD were multiple antibiotic regimens that included clindamycin, cephalosporins, or trimethoprim-sulfamethoxazole, as well as antibiotics combined with tube feeding. The authors found no significant association between the presence of *C. difficile* or its toxin and the development of AAD. Interestingly, the prophylactic administration of the nonpathogenic

yeast *Saccharomyces boulardii* (250 mg twice daily) reduced the incidence of AAD from 22% to 9% ($P = .04$) and the incidence of *C. difficile*–related diarrhea from 31% to 9% ($P = .07$). The mechanism of how *S. boulardii* exhibits this apparent prophylaxsis against AAD is unknown.[20]

Enteral Feeding

Diarrhea is commonly considered a significant problem in the management of the tube-fed critically ill patient, and it is the conception of many that it is the limiting factor in the supply of nutrients via the enteral route. As with many popular notions in medicine, the true prevalence of diarrhea in the tube-fed patient is not clear. The inconsistency in the definition of diarrhea accounts for the great discrepancies in prevalence rates ranging from a low of 2% to as high as 68% in the critically ill patient population.[1, 2, 24]

Diarrhea in the tube-fed patient may result from any of the previously discussed etiologic agents. In many instances, however, multiple factors are present, and it may be impossible to determine the exact cause of diarrhea.

Bacterial contamination of the enteral products and their delivery systems was a commonly recognized cause of diarrhea.[25–28] However, recently improved practices for enteral formula administration have dramatically lowered the incidence of diarrhea caused by diet contamination.

One commonly held misconception is that hyperosmolar feedings are major offenders predisposing to diarrhea. It is common practice in many institutions for diet formulas to be diluted to one-half to one-quarter strength at the outset of diet administration. However, studies have repeatedly demonstrated the safe, efficacious use of full-strength isotonic to hypertonic formulas in a variety of patient populations without the use of starter regimens.[11, 29–33] In fact, starter regimens have been shown to result in greater gastrointestinal complications and poorer nutritional outcome.[30]

As outlined earlier, medication-related causes of diarrhea include the use of antibiotics, hyperosmolar drug solutions, certain antacids, and other medications that have a direct effect on gastrointestinal function. In a recent study, prospective determinations of the causes of diarrhea were performed in a cohort of patients who were enterally fed. Thirty-two episodes of diarrhea occured in 123 tube-fed patients (26%). A single cause was found in 29 cases. The tube feeding formula was responsible for diarrhea in only 21% of these cases. Medications were directly responsible in 61% and *C. difficile* in 17%. The stool osmotic gap correctly distinguished osmotic from nonosmotic diarrhea in all cases.[34] These authors made the eye-opening observation that the elixir medications commonly used in tube-fed patients contain varying amounts of sorbitol. Additionally, these amounts were not listed on package inserts. Theophylline preparations show a particular predilection for producing diarrhea. In a recent review of 20 consecutive patients receiving sorbitol-based theophylline elixir, 15 patients (75%) had diarrhea for 2 or more days.[35] Commonly used medications (acetaminophen, theophylline, cimetidine) contain between 5% and 65% sorbitol in their elixir preparations, certainly enough to cause diarrhea with one dose (Table 45–6).[24]

Liquid formula diets themselves may induce diarrhea, even in subjects with normal gastrointestinal function.[36] Although most patients have other predisposing factors, diarrhea may subside if enteral nutrition is discontinued. This effect is particularly common in patients who have not received oral or enteral nutrients for several days. Intestinal atrophy could be the basis for refeeding diarrhea after periods of little or no enteral nutrient intake.[37] The small bowel loses villus height and ceases the production of brush border enzymes. Support for this concept lies in the widely held observation that enteral feedings are toler-

TABLE 45–6.

Sorbitol Content of Some Commonly Used Liquid Medications*

Product	Manufacturer	Sorbitol (g/5 mL)
Robitussin	AH Robbins	0
Robitussin CF		1.16
Robitussin DM		0
Robitussin PE		0
Reglan syrup		1.75
Elixophyllin	Forest	0
Elixophyllin GG		0
Tegretol suspension	Geigy	0.85
Zantac syrup	Glaxo	0.05
Lasix solution	Hoechst-Roussell	1.22
Phenobarbitol Elixir	Lilly	0
Theolair liquid	3M	0.75
Imodium AD liquid	McNeil	0
Adult Tylenol elixir		<0.67
Children's Tylenol elixir		<1
Dilantin suspension	Parke Davis	0
Theophylline Oral Solution	Roxane	3.25
Lomotil liquid	Searle	1.05
Tagamet liquid	SmithKline Beecham	2.52
Theragram liquid	Squibb	0
Kaopectate concentrate	Upjohn	0

*Sorbitol contents are from the product manufacturers (July 1991).

ated less well the longer enteral nutrition administration is delayed in the critically ill patient.[33, 38, 39]

As the primary site for fecal sodium and water absorption, the colon naturally determines the final stool concentration and composition. It has been suggested that in some instances the diarrhea associated with enteral feeding may result from altered colonic mucosal function. The use of fiber-deficient diets and the prescription of broad-spectrum antibiotics may alter the colonic microflora and hence the production of SCFAs. Diarrhea has also been more prevalent in enterally fed patients receiving antibiotics.[30, 33, 42] The relatively high incidence of diarrhea in patients receiving concomitant antibiotic therapy could be due to the detrimental effect on the colonic microflora. A recent study has, in fact, demonstrated diminished fecal SCFA production in patients prescribed broad-spectrum antibiotics.[10] A reduction in SCFA synthesis or an alteration of their profile may impair sodium/water absorption and predispose to diarrhea. This hypothesis has

been tested in a study of normal subjects who were fed, in a crossover fashion, a fiber-free liquid formula diet with and without supplementation with 1% citrus pectin.[36] Pectin is a soluble fiber polysaccharide that is completely fermented to SCFAs. The pectin-free diet produced liquid stools with low SCFA content. Pectin supplementation normalized fecal SCFA concentration and stool consistency. Applying this concept to the critically ill population has not been as successful. Several studies have not been able to demonstrate improvement of the stool output in ICU patients who are fed "fiber"-containing formulas.[40–43] The lack of a demonstrable effect of these diets may result from the type of fiber present in these formulas. The fiber sources in these studies contained very small amounts of soluble, readily fermentable fiber polysaccharides (Fig 45–3).[44] Hence, with the administration of fiber sources with variable fermentation capacity and the concomitant alteration of the bacterial flora by the use of broad-spectrum antibiotics, it can be hypothesized that

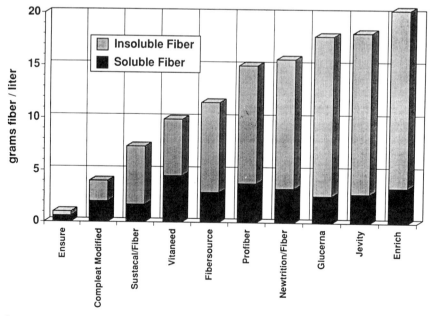

FIG 45–3.

Soluble and insoluble fiber contents of "fiber-supplemented" enteral feeding formulas. Ensure is a non–fiber-supplemented formula included for comparison. (Adapted from Freedstrom S, Baglien K, Lampe J, et al: *JPEN* 1991; 15:450–453.)

SCFA production may not have been significant enough to cause a physiologic effect on stool composition in this critically ill population.

Hypoalbuminemia is frequently implicated as a cause of diarrhea in critically ill patients who receive enteral feedings.[45] Hypoalbuminemia is common in hospitalized patients and usually reflects the degree and duration of hypermetabolism, as well as fluid shifts and plasma losses. The purported mechanism for hypoalbuminemia-induced diarrhea is a decrease in oncotic pressure that produces intestinal edema and either a secretory or malabsorptive state. The transport of fluids across the capillary wall depends on the difference in hydrostatic and oncotic pressures. Plasma oncotic pressure is between 20 and 25 mm Hg, and albumin accounts for approximately 65% of this effect.

Gottschlich and coworkers performed an extensive investigation of the incidence and etiology of diarrhea in tube-fed burn patients. The overall incidence of diarrhea in this patient population was 32%.[33] Hypoalbuminemia (< 2 g/dL) was present in more patients without diarrhea (19) than in patients with diarrhea (10), although this difference did not reach statistical significance. There is some evidence that correcting hypoalbuminemia with exogenous albumin may improve dietary tolerance in the hypoalbuminemic patient.[46] Several studies have demonstrated success in using peptide-based formulas in avoiding diarrhea in the tube-fed, hypoalbuminemic, critically ill patient.[45, 47] However, in a larger, prospective, randomized study conducted on critically ill, hypoalbuminemic patients, no significant tolerance or nutritional advantage was obtained with a peptide-based formula as compared with a standard, polymeric formula.[48] The hypothesis of hypoalbuminemia-induced diarrhea in patients still awaits confirmation.

TREATMENT

The treatment of diarrhea naturally depends on its etiology (Table 45–7). A thorough workup of its possible cause(s) is essential. In the enterally fed patient one should not automatically discon-

TABLE 45–7.
Etiology and Treatment of Diarrhea With Enteral Feeding

Diarrhea Etiology	Therapy
Infectious	Review potential sources of contamination
	Treat gastrointestinal pathogens as confirmed
Dietary	
Hyperosmolar solutions	Dilute solutions or decrease volume infused
Lactose deficiency	Change enteral formula to lactose free
Fat malabsorption	Change enteral formula to low-fat solution
	Give pancreatic enzymes
Osmotic	Change to an oligomeric diet formula
Protein malnutrition	Use isotonic solutions; consider oligomeric formula
	Supplement with parenteral nutrition
	Use antidiarrheal medication loperamide (Imodium), diphenoxylate (Lomotil), paregoric (camphorated opium)
Drugs	Evaluate the need for antibiotics
Antibiotics	Use antidiarrheal medication; *avoid* Imodium, Lomotil, paregoric, and codeine
	Use Kaopectate or cholestyramine
Hyperosmolar electrolyte solutions and medications	Dilute medications; mix with enteral feedings or give parenterally; check for sorbitol-containing elixirs.
Other medications (digoxin, methyldopa [Aldomet], and so on)	Antidiarrheal medications (paregoric, Imodium, Lomotil)
Magnesium-containing antacids	Alternate with magnesium-free antacids

tinue enteral nutrition at its outset. In the majority of cases, enteral feeding itself cannot be identified as the cause of diarrhea in the tube-fed patient. As outlined above, the common agents eliciting diarrhea include sorbitol, magnesium antacids, cimetidine, potassium and phosphorus supplements, lactulose, and laxatives. Fecal cultures for pathogens including *Candida* should be routinely performed and treatment directed appropriately. Nonspecific antibiotic-associated diarrhea may be more common than PC associated with *C. difficile* infection. Malabsorption or even fecal impaction may also be responsible. In patients with severe hypoalbuminemia ($\leq$2.5 g/dL) and no identifiable cause for diarrhea, intravenous albumin supplementation is given to correct their albumin deficit and obtain a serum level $\geq$2.5 g/dL.[49]

In the process of examining for organic causes of diarrhea, I have had some success with initiating treatment with a kaolin-pectin agent given at a dosage of 30 to 45 mL every 4 to 6 hours for 48 hours. If diarrhea continues with this treatment and no cause has been identified, an opiate is added if there is

no contraindication to its use (Table 45−8). It is generally recommended that agents that slow intestinal transit, such as the opiates, are contraindicated with diarrhea of infectious etiology. The effect of the prophylactic or empirical use of yeast administration in the avoidance or treatment of diarrhea has not been critically evaluated in the ICU setting. If the diarrhea continues, then the tube feeding administration rate is slowed or even stopped and consideration given to supplementing the patient with parenteral nutrition.

If the diarrhea subsides upon discontinuing the diet infusion, the diarrhea can be considered osmotic and the formula the causative agent. The measurement of stool electrolytes and osmolality and calculation of the osmotic gap are useful in diagnosing osmotic diarrhea.[34] Diarrhea is considered osmotic if the stool osmotic gap is greater than 100 mmol/L. Barring any medication as the osmotic agent, the diet can then be implicated as the causative factor and feeding restarted with an oligomeric formula.

If the diarrhea continues while the patient is off tube feeding, then the di-

TABLE 45−8.

Antidiarrheal Medications for Diarrhea of Nonspecific Etiology

Medication	Dosage
Opiates	
Natural	
Tincture of opium (10 mg/mL)	0.5−1.5 mL 1−3 ×/day
Paregoric acid (0.4 mg/mL)	4−8 mL 1−2 ×/day
Codeine	16−64 mg 1−2 ×/day
Synthetic	
Diphenoxylate HCl (0.5 mg/mL) + atropine sulfate (0.005 mg/mL) (Lomotil)	Initial: 5 mg 1−2 ×/day
	Maintenance: 2.5 mg 2 ×/day
Loperamide HCl (Imodium)	Initial: 4 mg/ bowel movement
	Maintenance: 2 mg/ bowel movement
Anticholinergics	
Atropine sulfate	0.6−1 mg 3 ×/day
Tincture of belladonna	12−15 drops/day
Propantheline bromide (Pro-Banthine)	15 mg 3 ×/day
Adsorbents	
Kaolin (4.5 g/mL) + pectin (6 mg/mL) (Kaopectate)	45−180 mL/day
Cholestyramine (Questran)	4 g 3 ×/day
Bismuth subsalicylate (Pepto-Bismol)	60 mg/day
Lactobacillus acidophilus	4−8 capsules (1 g)/day

arrhea can be considered secretory and a workup for secretory diarrhea pursued. The tube feeds can then be restarted and continued if the diarrhea does not increase on the feeds. If the tube feeding exacerbates the diarrhea, then consideration should be given to changing the diet to a more oligomeric, peptide-based formula or to a fiber-containing formula. In many instances, optimizing serum albumin, the medication profile, and the diet formula will not improve the patient's diet tolerance. In these cases parenteral nutrition should be relied upon.

The management of diarrhea in the ICU can be a perplexing and frustrating problem. The solutions are as varied as the etiologies. Although enteral feeding is commonly associated with diarrhea, the tube feeding formula itself should not be automatically considered the responsible agent. Early institution of enteral feeding has enhanced the tolerance of enteral formulas. A systematic approach to the problem while paying particular attention to the medications the patient is receiving commonly identifies the cause and, hence, the solution to the problem of controlling diarrhea in the critically ill patient.

REFERENCES

1. Kelly T, Patrick M, Hillman K: Study of diarrhea in critically ill patients. *Crit Care Med* 1983; 11:7–9.
2. Bliss D, Guenter P, Settle R: Defining and reporting diarrhea in tube-fed patients—what a mess! *Am J Clin Nutr* 1992; 55:753–759.
3. Pietrusko R: Drug therapy reviews: Pharmacotherapy of diarrhea. *Am J Hosp Pharm* 1979; 36:757–767.
4. Powell D: Approach to the patient with diarrhea, in Yamada T (ed): in *Textbook of Gastroenterology*. Philadelphia, JB Lippincott, 1991, pp 732–778.
5. Silk D: Fibre and enteral nutrition. *Gut* 1989; 30:246–264.
6. Dobb G: Diarrhoea in the critically ill. *Intensive Care Med* 1986; 12:113–115.
7. Binder H: Pathophysiology of acute diarrhea. *Am J Med* 1990; 88(suppl):2–4.
8. Banwell J: Pathophysiology of diarrhea disorders. *Rev Infect Dis* 1990; 12(suppl):30–35.
9. Cummings J, Branch W: Fermentation and the production of short chain fatty acids in the human large intestine, in Vahouny G, Kritchevsky D (eds): *Dietary Fiber: Basic and Clinical Aspects*. New York, Plenum Publishing Corp, 1986, pp 131–152.
10. Clausen M, Bonnen H, Tvede M, et al: Colonic fermentation to short-chain fatty acids is decreased in antibiotic-associated diarrhea. *Gastroenterology* 1991; 101:1497–1504.
11. Ruppin H, Bar-Meir S, Soergel K: Effects of liquid diets on proximal gastrointestinal function. *Gastroenterology* 1979; 76:1231.
12. Roediger W, Rae D: Trophic effect of short chain fatty acids on mucosal handling of ions by the defunctioned colon. *Br J Surg* 1982; 69:23–25.
13. Roediger W: Utilization of nutrients by isolated epithelial cells of the rat colon. *Gastroenterology* 1982; 83:424–429.
14. Debongie J, Phillips S: Capacity of the human colon to absorb fluid. *Gastroenterology* 1978; 74:698–703.
15. Binder H: Absorption and secretion of water and electrolytes by small and large intestine, in Fordtran JS, Sleisenger M (eds): *Gastrointestinal Disease: Pathophysiology, Diagnosis, Management*. Philadelphia, WB Saunders, 1989, pp 1022–1040.
16. Hill M: Factors affecting bacterial metabolism, in Hill M (ed): *Microbial Metabolism in the Digestive Tract*. Boca Raton, Fla, CRC Press, 1986, pp 22–29.
17. Greenberger N: *Gastrointestinal Disorders: A Pathophysiologic Approach*. St Louis, Mosby–Year Book, 1986, p 191.
18. Tabibian N: Diarrhea in critically ill patients. *Am Fam Physician* 1989; 40:135–140.
19. Andrejak M, Schmit J, Tondriaux A: The clinical significance of antibiotic-associated pseudomembranous colitis in the 1990s. *Drug Saf* 1991; 6:339–349.
20. Surawicz C, Elmer G, Speelman P, et al: Prevention of antibiotic-associated

diarrhea by *Saccharomyces boulardii:* A prospective study. *Gastroenterology* 1989; 96:981–988.

21. Grube B, Heimbach D, Marvin J: *Clostridium difficile* diarrhea in critically ill burned patients. *Arch Surg* 1987; 122:655–661.

22. Gerding D, Olson M, Peterson L, et al: *Clostridium difficile*–associated diarrhea and colitis in adults. *Arch Intern Med* 1986; 146:95–100.

23. Gupta T, Ehrinpreis M: *Candida*-associated diarrhea in hospitalized patients. *Gastroenterology* 1990; 98:780–785.

24. Heimburger D: Diarrhea with enteral feeding: Will the real cause please stand up? *Am J Med* 1990; 88:89–90.

25. Hosteller C, Lipman T, Geraghty M: Bacterial safety of reconstituted continuous drip tube feeding. *JPEN* 1982; 6:232–235.

26. Scheimer R, Fitzer H, Gfell M: Environmental contamination of continuous drip feedings. *Pediatrics* 1979; 63:232–237.

27. Schroeder P, Fisher D, Volz M: Microbial contamination of enteral feeding solutions in a community. *JPEN* 1983; 7:364–367.

28. White W, Acuff T, Sykes T: Bacterial contamination of enteral nutrient solution: A preliminary report. *JPEN* 1979; 3:459–461.

29. Rees R, Keohane P, Grimble G, et al: Tolerance of elemental diet administered without starter regimen. *BMJ* 1985; 290:1869–1870.

30. Keohane P, Attrill H, Love M: Relation between osmolality of diet and gastrointestinal side effects in enteral nutrition. *BMJ* 1984; 288:678–680.

31. Jones B, Lees R, Andrews J: Comparison of an elemental and polymeric enteral diet in patients with normal gastrointestinal function. *Gut* 1983; 24:78–84.

32. Zarling E, Parmer J, Mobarhan S: Effect of enteral formula infusion rate, osmolality, and chemical composition upon clinical tolerance and carbohydrate absorption in normal subjects. *JPEN* 1986; 10:588–590.

33. Gottschlich M, Warden G, Michel M, et al: Diarrhea in tube-fed burn patients: Incidence, etiology, nutritional impact, and prevention. *JPEN* 1988; 12:338–345.

34. Edes T, Walk B, Austin J: Diarrhea in tube-fed patients: Feeding formula not necessarily the cause. *Am J Med* 1990; 88:91–93.

35. Hill D, Henderson L, McClain C: Osmotic diarrhea induced by sugar-free theophylline solution in critically ill patients. *JPEN* 1991; 15:332–336.

36. Zimmaro D, Rolandelli R, Koruda M, et al: Isotonic tube feeding formula induces liquid stool in normal subjects: Reversal by pectin. *JPEN* 1989; 13:117–123.

37. Roediger WEW: Metabolic basis of starvation diarrhoea: Implications for treatment. *Lancet* 1986; 1:1082–1083.

38. Chiarelli A, Enzi G, Casadei A, et al: Very early nutrition supplementation in burned patients. *Am J Clin Nutr* 1990; 51:1035–1039.

39. McDonald W, Sharp C, Deitch E: Immediate enteral feeding in burn patients is safe and effective. *Ann Surg* 1991; 213:177–183.

40. Guenter P, Settle R, Perlmutter S, et al: Tube feeding-related diarrhea in acutely ill patients. *JPEN* 1991; 15:277–280.

41. Hart GK, Dobb GJ: Effect of a fecal bulking agent on diarrhea during enteral feeding in the critically ill. *JPEN* 1988; 12:465–468.

42. Frankenfield D, Beyer P: Soy-polysaccharide fiber: Effect on diarrhea in tube-fed, head-injured patients. *Am J Clin Nutr* 1989; 50:533–538.

43. Dobb G, Towler S: Diarrhoea during enteral feeding in the critically ill: A comparison of feeds with and without fiber. *Intensive Care Med* 1990; 16:252–255.

44. Fredstrom S, Baglien K, Lampe J, et al: Determination of the fiber content of enteral feedings. *JPEN* 1991; 15:450–453.

45. Brinson R, Curtis W, Singh M: Diarrhea in the intensive care unit: The role of hypoalbuminemia and the response to a chemically defined diet (case reports and review of the literature). *J Am Coll Nutr* 1987; 6:517–523.

46. Ford E, Jennings M, Andrassy R: Serum albumin (oncotic pressure) corre-

lates with enteral feeding tolerance in the pediatric surgical patient. *J Pediatr Surg* 1987; 22:597–599.

47. Brinson R, Kolts B: Diarrhea associated with severe hypoalbuminemia: A comparison of a peptide-based chemically defined diet and standard enteral alimentation. *Crit Care Med* 1988; 16:130–136.

48. Mowatt-Larssen C, Brown R, Wojtysiak S, et al: Comparison of tolerance and nutritional outcome between a peptide and a standard enteral formula in critically ill, hypoalbuminemic patients. *JPEN* 1992; 16:20–24.

49. Hardin T, Page C, Schwesinger W: Rapid replacement of serum albumin in patients receiving total parenteral nutrition. *Surg Gynecol Obstet* 1986; 193:359–362.

PART V

Factors and Issues

46

Growth Factors and the Care of the Injured Patient

Yuman Fong, M.D.

Peter W.T. Pisters, M.D.

Homeostasis requires maintenance of normal cell mass at each organ through repletion of those cells lost in normal turnover by adequate cellular proliferation. At most organ sites, disease and injury disrupt homeostasis by increasing cellular loss as well as by decreasing cellular proliferation. The consequent whole-body wasting as reflected in a net loss of skeletal muscle, fat stores, and red cell mass leads to the cachexia that is well known in clinical disease. Particularly in the critical care patient population, skeletal muscle wasting often complicates respiratory failure, anemia confounds cardiovascular management, and leukopenia may significantly compromise survival from infection. Even with supracaloric feedings through enteral or parenteral routes, such whole-body and organ-specific wasting often persists.[1, 2] Therefore, adjunctive mea-

TABLE 46–1.

Partial List of Known Growth Factors

Endocrine growth factors
  Growth hormone
  Insulin-like growth factors
  Insulin
  Thyroid hormones
  Androgenic steroids
  Epidermal growth factors
  Erythropoietin
  Colony-stimulating factors
Paracrine growth factors
  Insulin-like growth factors
  Platelet-derived growth factors
  Epidermal growth factors
  Bone morphogenetic proteins
  Interleukin-1
  Tumor necrosis factor
  Interleukin-6

---

sures to nutritional supplementation have long been sought for treatment of the cellular wasting associated with injury and disease.

Cellular proliferation is intimately dependent upon endogenous growth factors. These growth factors may function in an endocrine fashion by traveling through the bloodstream to their cell targets, or they may act principally in a paracrine fashion by diffusing to neighboring cell targets near the sites of growth factor synthesis (Table 46–1). Growth factors also vary greatly in their scope of action. Some have specific effects on very limited cell targets, for example, erythropoietin and colony-stimulating factors (CSFs) have activities predominantly on hematopoietic stem cells. Others, such as insulin and growth hormone (GH), have rather more pluripotent effects upon diverse tissues within the host. Many strategies have been proposed to capitalize on the growth-potentiating effects of these protein mediators in the treatment of wasting and cachexia.

Recent advances in molecular biology and molecular pharmacology have brought the field of growth factor biology into clinical applicability. Laboratory design and production of analogues of androgenic steroids have created a

class of synthetic growth factors known as anabolic steroids that are potential therapeutic agents for clinical cachexia. Molecular genetic techniques have also allowed insertion of genes for human growth factors into the genome of bacteria or yeast. The human gene that is inserted by such "recombinant" technology may be elaborated by these microorganisms to yield unlimited quantities of human growth factors for potential clinical applications.[3]

The current chapter will concentrate on growth factors that are in or near clinical trials. We will begin with three recombinant growth factors with specific trophic influences that have already reached clinical usage in the injured and critically ill, namely, erythropoietin and two of the CSFs, granulocyte CSF (G-CSF) and granulocyte-macrophage CSF (GM-CSF). Roles for other growth factors in the injured patient are less well defined. Although recombinant hormones such as GH and insulin are clearly indispensable agents in the treatment of patients with congenital deficiencies of these proteins, a role for these pluripotent growth factors in injured or critically ill patients has not been clearly established. A great amount of work is under way to examine the potential for these growth factors, as well as insulin-like growth factor 1 (IGF-1) and anabolic steroids, to preserve body mass and protein reserves in the injured patient. We will discuss the theoretical aspects of using these agents as well as clinical trials to date.

GROWTH FACTORS WITH TROPHIC ACTIVITIES FOR SPECIFIC ORGANS

Erythropoietin

Physical Properties

Erythropoietin is a glycoprotein with a molecular weight of 39,000 kd that acts on erythroid progenitor cells to stimulate the formation of erythroblast colonies and thereby increase red blood cell (RBC) mass. In contrast to most other hematopoietic growth factors, erythropoietin is produced primarily by a single organ, the kidney, and regulation of erythropoietin production is by classic feedback control. The renal juxtatubular cells contain a heme-containing protein that effectively functions as an oxygen sensor.[4] Relative hypoxia stimulates erythropoietin release from the renal juxtatubular cells, thereby expanding red cell mass, while hyperoxia reduces the amount of circulating erythropoietin and consequently decreases RBC production. Thus, erythropoietin continuously adjusts the red cell mass in order to satisfy the oxygen requirements of the body.

Under baseline conditions, erythropoietin levels range from 10 to 20 units/L of plasma. The constitutive production of erythropoietin maintains erythropoiesis at a rate sufficient to replace dying and senescent red cells and maintain the RBC mass at its normal size of 25 to 30 mL/kg. The relationship between the decrease in hemoglobin concentration and increase in endogenous immunoreactive erythropoietin concentration is exponential. Under conditions of severe anemia, reduced oxygen delivery to the kidneys results in logarithmic increases in erythropoietin synthesis such that at a hematocrit of 15% erythropoietin levels of 10,000 units/L may be observed.[5]

Although recombinant human erythropoietin (r-HuEPO) can be administered by intravenous or subcutaneous routes, subcutaneous administration of r-HuEPO results in lower, more sustained levels of erythropoietin as compared with intravenous injection (intravenous half-life, 4 to 9 hours; subcutaneous half-life, >24 hours).[6-8] For this reason, a satisfactory hemoglobin concentration can be maintained with less r-HuEPO when administered subcutaneously than when administered intravenously,[9] and the subcutaneous route is the preferred route for dialysis patients.

Iron is essential for erythropoiesis, and adequate iron stores are required for an optimal response to r-HuEPO. Serum iron, total iron binding capacity, and the percentage of transferrin saturation (serum iron divided by the total iron binding capacity) should be determined at baseline and at regular intervals during therapy. A nomogram is available to aid in determining how much iron is required when starting r-HuEPO therapy.[10] Practical guidelines, however, have suggested that iron be administered (ferrous sulfate orally or iron dextran intravenously) if the serum ferritin level is less than 200 μg/L or the transferrin saturation is less than 15% to 20%.[9, 11]

Erythropoietin therapy has been associated with remarkably few adverse effects. Hypertension has been the most serious side effect noted in early trials of r-HuEPO therapy. In a multicenter study in anemic patients with end-stage renal disease, blood pressure changes required adjustment of antihypertensive medications in 25% of patients.[12] Interestingly, hypertension following r-HuEPO therapy has only been observed in patients being treated for renal anemias. Normal subjects receiving long-term erythropoietin and patients receiving r-HuEPO for nonrenal anemias have not become hypertensive.[13] The mechanism underlying r-HuEPO–associated hypertension in patients with chronic renal failure is not understood.[14] Erythropoietin itself has no known, direct pressor effect.[15] It has been postulated that the worsening of hypertension results primarily from increased peripheral resistance due to increased blood viscosity and loss of hypoxia-induced vasodilatation.[16-20] However, this still does not explain why the hypertension appears to be specific to treatment for renal-based anemias.

Clinical Utility

Although the existence of a circulating factor responsible for control of red cell mass has long been postulated, only within the last decade has erythropoietin been isolated and its genetic sequence determined.[21, 22] r-HuEPO became available in 1985 and over the past 7 years has been investigated in the treatment of a variety of anemic conditions[23-38] (Table 46-2). Erythropoietin is currently approved for treatment of the anemia associated with dialysis-dependent and dialysis-independent chronic renal failure and for the anemia observed with zidovudine therapy in patients with acquired immunodeficiency syndrome (AIDS). In this past year it was employed in 85,000 of 110,000 dialysis patients in the United States.[9]

The anemia of chronic renal failure is due to a classic hormone deficiency state associated with low endogenous production of erythropoietin. When r-HuEPO is administered to anemic long-term dialysis patients at doses between 15 and 500 units/kg three times per week, a dose-dependent increase in hematocrit is observed.[23] This treatment of deficient endogenous hormone with r-HuEPO not only reverses the associated anemia but also has a salutary effect on the quality of life,[40, 41] cognitive function, exercise tolerance, and sexual potency.[42]

To date, few studies have addressed the pathophysiology of anemia in acute renal failure (ARF). This anemia develops rapidly in the first few days of ARF.[43] Erythropoietin concentrations decline within 2 to 3 days of the onset of ARF[43, 44] and remain inappropriately low for the degree of anemia during the course of ARF.[38, 45, 46] This may be due to decreased hormone synthesis as opposed to increased clearance of erythropoietin.[38] Following recovery from ARF, appropriate erythropoietin levels are not seen until 2 to 3 weeks after the serum creatinine level and renal tubular concentrating ability have returned to normal.[43, 44] Two small studies have demonstrated that a significant reticulocytosis and normalization of hemoglobin levels can be observed in ARF

TABLE 46-2.

Clinical Investigations With Recombinant Human Erythropoietin

First Author	Anemic Condition
Eschbach[23] Winearls[24]	Dialysis-dependent chronic renal failure
Eschbach[25]	Dialysis-independent chronic renal failure
Fischl[26]	Zidovudine therapy for AIDS
Halperin[27]	Prematurity
Goodnough[28]	Autologous blood donation prior to elective surgery
James[29]	Cisplatin and carboplatin chemotherapy
Pincus[30]	Rheumatoid arthritis
Abels[31]	Cancer
Ludwig[32]	Multiple myeloma
Stein[33]	Myelodysplastic syndromes
Oster[34]	Non-Hodgkin's lymphoma
Danko[35]	Postpartum state
Nielson[38]	Acute renal failure
Yoshimura[39]	Chronic transplant rejection

patients before the renal failure resolves.[38, 46] Hence, preliminary evidence suggests a possible role for r-HuEPO in ARF. Treatment with r-HuEPO may facilitate a more rapid and complete recovery of RBC mass. Larger randomized trials will be required to more precisely define the role r-HuEPO will have in the treatment of patients with ARF.

In conditions of infection or inflammation, such as surgical trauma,[47] infection,[47] tumor-bearing states,[48] AIDS,[49] and rheumatoid arthritis,[50-52] there is evidence to suggest that anemia-induced release of endogenous erythropoietin from renal juxtatubular cells is impaired or blunted.[9] In addition to blunted erythropoietin production, it also appears that in injured patients there may be a blunted physiologic response to circulating erythropoietin. Patients with the anemia of rheumatoid arthritis have required higher doses of r-HuEPO than have patients with renal failure to produce comparable increases in hematocrit.[53] It has been postulated that these effects are due to alterations in the profile of other circulating or local cytokines that modulate the immune response and hematopoiesis.[54] In particular, tumor necrosis factor α (TNF-

$\alpha)^{55-58}$ and interleukin-1 (IL-1)[59] have been shown to decrease erythropoiesis in humans[56] and animals.[55, 57–59] The role of cytokines in the modulation of the erythropoietin-hemoglobin feedback loop is just beginning to be understood, but at least one clinical implication of this impaired response is clear—stressed and critically ill patients have inadequate erythropoietin. Further investigations are needed to determine whether the administration of high doses of r-HuEPO can overcome the anemia associated with injury and thereby reduce the transfusion requirement and its associated hazards in the injured and critically ill. Future investigations will also need to explore the role of erythropoietin in augmenting preoperative collection of autologous blood prior to elective surgery.

COLONY-STIMULATING FACTORS

Physical Properties

The CSFs are a group of glycoprotein cytokines that have powerful regulatory influences on the production, differentiation, and function of granulocytes and monocytes. They include macrophage CSF (M-CSF), G-CSF, GM-CSF, and interleukin-3 (IL-3 or multi-CSF). These cytokines were originally discovered because of their ability to promote the formation of macrophages and granulocytes in cultures of bone marrow cells.[60, 61] These mediators have since been isolated, had their structures determined, and are available in large amounts through recombinant technology.[62–64] This has permitted their introduction as pharmacologic agents (G-CSF and GM-CSF) and has led to large-scale phase I to III clinical trials.

The CSFs are secreted by multiple cell types, including endothelial cells, fibroblasts, stromal cells, and lymphocytes.[65] Constitutive production of these cytokines is at low levels, and their precise role in normal hematopoietic physiology remains unclear.[66] Endogenous CSF secretion is increased by various infectious stimuli, including endotoxin or foreign antigens.[67] Elevated CSF levels result in the stimulation of hematopoietic cell production (Fig 46–1) either directly or indirectly by induction of IL-1 and other cytokines.[68, 69]

Unique membrane receptors exist for each CSF. Granulocyte-macrophage progenitors simultaneously express specific receptors for all four CSFs.[70, 71] This permits collaborative interactions between the CSFs on individual cells. The CSFs can stimulate both normal and leukemic bone marrow progenitors.[72–74] In addition, these cytokines stimulate mature hematopoietic cells both in vitro and in vivo.[75, 76] Data from a number of in vitro and phase I studies of G-CSF[77–86] and GM-CSF[87–104] are presented in Table 46–3, which serves to summarize the major physiologic effects of these two mediators. In general, in vivo responses reflect the myelostimulatory effects first noted in vitro. G-CSF induces primarily granulocytic responses, with only minor increase in macrophages and no change in eosinophil production. GM-CSF administration results in rises in the numbers of macrophages, eosinophils, and at high concentrations, megakaryocytes.[105]

Current dose recommendations are 1 to 20 µg/kg/day for G-CSF and 0.3 to 10 µg/kg/day for GM-CSF therapies.[66] The subcutaneous route is convenient, well tolerated, and amenable to self-administration. Blood counts should be monitored at least twice weekly during G-CSF and GM-CSF treatment. Twice weekly monitoring of liver and renal function is recommended with GM-CSF administration because of occasional renal insufficiency or elevation in aminotransferase levels.[66] In general, CSF should not be administered prior to or concomitantly with chemotherapy because the CSF may increase the myelotoxicity of the chemotherapy.[106]

Adverse effects associated with the

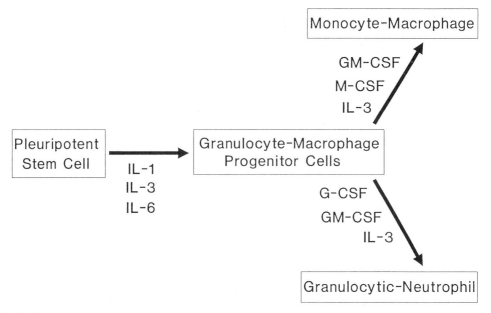

FIG 46–1.
Cytokine regulation of hematopoiesis. (*GM-CSF* = granulocyte-macrophage colony-stimulating factor; *IL-3* = interleukin-3.)

clinical use of these recombinant proteins have been minimal. Bone pain has been the most common side effect noted with G-CSF therapy, especially at doses greater than 30 μg/kg.[79, 80, 82] GM-CSF therapy has resulted in fever, chills, anorexia, weight change, bone pain, lethargy, and tissue reactions at the injection sites in some patients.[100, 101, 107]

After an initial (usually intravenous) dose of GM-CSF (>1 μg/kg), flushing, dyspnea, tachycardia, and hypotension associated with arterial hypoxemia have developed in a small number of patients.[93] GM-CSF should not be given to patients with a history of idiopathic thrombocytopenic purpura because reactivation has been observed.[101]

TABLE 46–3.

Major Hematologic Effects of GM-CSF and G-CSF

Cell Type	GM-CSF	G-CSF
Neutrophil		
↑ Peripheral count	+	+ +
↑ Immature forms	+	+
↑ Marrow production	+	+ + +
↑ Superoxide anion generation (FMLP primed)	+	+
↑ Half-life	+	−
↑ Marrow promyelocytes, myelocytes	+	+
Monocyte/macrophage		
↑ Peripheral count	+ +	+*
↑ Cytotoxicity	+	−
Class II MHC expression	+	−
↑ Phagocytosis	+	−
Eosinophils		
↑ Peripheral count	+	−
↑ Marrow precursors	+	−

FLMP = N-formyl methionyl leucyl phenylalanine; MHC = major histocompatibility complex.
*High doses only.

Clinical Utility

Clinical use of the CSFs has focused on the treatment of different types of neutropenia. Since their introduction into clinical research in 1986, the majority of the clinical efforts have focused on applications in hematologic oncology, particularly on the application of these growth factors as adjuvants to myelotoxic chemotherapy. In this regard, the role of CSF in the treatment of chemotherapy-induced neutropenia may be prophylactic (to prevent infectious complications) or may be therapeutic (to stimulate neutrophil production when fever develops in a neutropenic patient). Detailed reviews of these clinical uses of CSFs have recently been published.[75, 76, 106] Table 46-4 summarizes the major clinical applications of the CSFs to date and is derived from a number of recently published phase II and III studies in humans.[108-142] The weight of evidence thus far supports the concept that pro-

TABLE 46-4.

Clinical Applications of the Colony-Stimulating Factors

Condition	CSF	Reference	Comments
Chemotherapy-induced neutropenia	G-CSF	108, 109	Virtually all studies have demonstrated increased neutrophil counts A randomized prospective, placebo-controlled, double-blind study found decreased febrile neutropenic events, infections, hospitalizations, antibiotic usage, duration of antibiotic usage[108]
Myeloablative chemotherapy with BMT			
Autologous	G-CSF	110, 111	Accelerated recovery of neutrophils Decreased hospitalization and requirement for TPN
	GM-CSF	112-115	Accelerated recovery of neutrophils in ¾ studies A randomized placebo controlled study found decreased time to neutropenic recovery, hospitalization, duration of antibiotic therapy
Allogeneic	G-CSF	116	Accelerated neutrophil recovery
	GM-CSF	117, 118	Possibility of graft-vs.-host disease complicates evaluation of CSF in allogeneic transplantation
Autologous transplantation of peripheral stem cells	GM-CSF G-CSF	119 120	Administered after cyclophosphamide chemotherapy during leukocyte recovery Accelerated recovery of platelets and neutrophils
Congenital neutropenia/idiopathic chronic neutropenia	G-CSF	121-123	Congenital neutropenia is associated with elevated endogenous CSF levels,[121] which suggests relative CSF resistance
Cyclic neutropenia	G-CSF	124, 125	Decreased neutropenic cycle length and reduced frequency of fever, infection, mucositis
Aplastic anemia	G-CSF GM-CSF	126 127-130	Patients with severe marrow hypoplasia are unresponsive to either agent
AIDS	G-CSF	86	Administered during concomitant therapy with erythropoietin and zidovudine
	GM-CSF	131-133	In vitro evidence suggests that GM-CSF may augment the antiviral effects of zidovudine but may also stimulate replication of HIV in monocytes[131]
Myelodysplastic syndromes	G-CSF GM-CSF	134, 135 136-139	Randomized GM-CSF trial[136]: increased neutrophils, eosinophils, reduced no. infections. Development of acute leukemia in four patients in each group
Acute myeloid leukemia	G-CSF GM-CSF	140-142	Accelerated neutrophil recovery

BMT = bone marrow transplantation; TPN = total parenteral nutrition; HIV = human immunodeficiency virus.

phylactic G-CSF treatment reduces the morbidity of cancer chemotherapy and decreases the length of hospital stay in several neutropenic populations.

It should also be noted that the use of CSFs in the treatment of patients with myeloid leukemia is considered experimental. This is because of the well-described potential of cytokines to stimulate acute leukemia.[143-145] Preliminary studies suggest that GM-CSF and G-CSF may significantly reduce the duration of neutropenia in both acute lymphoblastic and acute myelogenous leukemia. Trials are also currently under way that are evaluating the use of CSFs as priming agents to stimulate acute myeloid leukemic blast cells to become more sensitive to cell cycle-specific drugs.

Studies are currently in progress to examine the potential utility of CSFs in the treatment of the leukopenia and leukocyte dysfunction associated with injury or critical illness. Recent investigations have demonstrated that GM-CSF[146] and G-CSF[147] have reversed some of the neutrophil dysfunction seen with thermal injury. Animal studies have suggested that G-CSF may decrease the morbidity of burn wound sepsis,[148] septic shock,[149] and hemorrhagic shock.[150] The CSFs, by reversing or blunting some of the other cytokine-mediated immunosuppressive aspects of sepsis, may have a clinical role in the treatment of infectious diseases.[151, 152] Data from these and future clinical investigations will likely define a role for CSFs in the treatment of the immune defects associated with infection and injury.

GROWTH FACTORS WITH TROPHIC ACTIVITIES FOR DIVERSE ORGANS

Insulin

Physical Properties

Insulin is a 51-amino acid polypeptide produced by the β cells of the pancreatic islets of Langerhans. It is synthesized first as proinsulin. Enzymatic cleavage of this precursor molecule results in the formation of insulin and C peptide, both of which are stored in secretory granules.[153-155] Stimuli for release of insulin include glucose, amino acids, free fatty acids (FFAs), keto acids, gut hormones, and β-adrenergic and vagal signals.[156-158] Approximately 60 units of insulin is released daily by the pancreatic islet cells. After entering the portal circulation, approximately half of the insulin is cleared by the liver on the first pass. Therefore, under normal circumstances approximately 30 units of insulin reaches the systemic circulation each day.[159]

The cellular effects of insulin appear to be mediated through both direct and indirect mechanisms. After binding to cellular receptors, the insulin-receptor complex is internalized and acts at many intracellular organelles, including the Golgi apparatus, endoplasmic reticulum, and nuclei. At these sites, insulin can directly stimulate net protein synthesis both at the transcriptional level in the liver[160, 161] and at the translational level in extrahepatic tissue.[162] Insulin also appears to act through the formation of second messengers, which are the proteolytic products of membrane proteins generated after initial insulin-receptor interaction. These messengers are likely phosphatases that activate or inactivate insulin-sensitive enzymes through phosphorylation or dephosphorylation.[163]

Insulin acts upon a wide variety of tissues. At adipose tissues, this hormone promotes glucose uptake, lipogenesis, and decreased lipolysis.[164] At skeletal muscle, insulin promotes glucose uptake, as well as amino acid uptake[158] and protein synthesis.[165, 166] At the liver, insulin increases glycogen synthesis and inhibits glycogenolysis.[167] These effects are clearly anabolic and result in storage of excess nutrient intake as glycogen, protein, and fat. Certain tissues metabolize glucose in an insulin-independent manner. These include the central nervous system, hematogenous cells, wounds, and the kidney, all tissues vital to the survival of the organism. Insulin-independent glucose uptake in these tissues has great implication during injury.

A variety of alterations in insulin actions occurs during injury, which can be characterized as a generalized insulin-resistant state. Although there is usually increased gluconeogenesis and hyperglycemia, there is decreased glucose uptake by insulin-dependent tissues. The resulting effect is a preservation of glucose for the vital, insulin-independent tissues. Although there is a rise in circulating insulin levels, these are inappropriately low for the circulating glucose levels.

Clinical Utility

Relative hepatic and peripheral tissue resistance to the influence of insulin is a frequent feature of the catabolic patient. Investigators have therefore attempted to overcome this resistance and reverse the disease-associated catabolism by the administration of pharmacologic insulin dosages to such populations.

To date three major studies of insulin administration to nondiabetic injured patients have been reported. The first was that of Hinton and his colleagues,[168] who reported the administration of 200 to 600 units of insulin per day along with a 50% glucose infusion to maintain normoglycemia. Nine patients were treated with a high insulin–glucose regimen, while nine patients served as controls. Insulin administration was associated with a decrease in urine urea, as well as a reduction in urinary potassium excretion. Even though these data would suggest a protein-sparing effect of such insulin therapy, the insulin-treated patients had a significantly higher caloric intake than did the control patients. It was difficult to differentiate the effects of insulin from those of hypercaloric feedings.

In a subsequent update in burn and trauma patients, Woolfson and his colleagues also examined the effects of a continuous infusion of insulin (2 to 20 units of insulin per hour) and glucose on urine urea nitrogen excretion rates.[169] In catabolic patients, such administration of insulin significantly decreased urea production. A subsequent study examined the acute effects of a continuous insulin infusion at a lower dose (5 units/hr) on protein metabolism in trauma patients. A 4-hour insulin infusion produced a decrease in urinary nitrogen, 3-methylhistidine excretion, and forearm amino acid efflux.[170]

The time span between the first and last of these studies was 16 years. So why has high-dose insulin infusion not become a more common modality in clinical nutrition? The answer is twofold. First, life-threatening hypoglycemia is not a trivial complication of insulin administration. In these studies, serum glucose was monitored as frequently as every hour.[168] Second, high-dose insulin and glucose infusions may produce respiratory and hepatic compromise. Although high-dose insulin infusion produces increased tissue glucose uptake, this may not be accompanied by an increase in systemic glucose oxidation. The excess glucose may result in an increase in lipogenesis. Such an increase in lipogenesis is often manifested as increased CO_2 production. In turn, the CO_2 production produces an increased ventilatory demand that can overcome the pulmonary reserve of the critically ill. Increased lipogenesis may also lead to fatty liver formation and hepatic dysfunction.[171] Thus, high-dose insulin alone is unlikely to be a clinically useful adjunct to nutritional supplementation. More recently, combination therapy consisting of GH and insulin has been studied as an adjunct to nutritional supplementation. Preliminary studies in volunteers[172] and cancer patients[173] have shown that daily injections of GH for 3 days followed by a constant infusion of insulin acutely promotes skeletal muscle and whole-body nitrogen retention. The doses of insulin used are a log magnitude less than those used in the previously discussed clinical studies. Whether combinations of insulin with other growth factors will be useful awaits future studies.

GROWTH HORMONE

Physical Properties

GH is a 191−amino acid polypeptide secreted by the anterior pituitary gland. The important role of this hormone in normal growth and development is underscored by the syndrome of hypopituitary dwarfism seen in patients lacking this hormone during puberty. This hormone is important for growth and maturation during childhood. In addition, GH appears to be important for normal homeostasis in the adult. Throughout adult life, this hormone is released in an intermittent pulsatile pattern with a periodicity of 6 to 8 hours in adults and daily peaks between midnight and 3 A.M.[174]

Release of GH is dependent upon the neuroendocrine milieu. GH-releasing hormone stimulates release of GH, while somatostatin, thyroid-stimulating hormone (TSH), and IGF-1 are all potent inhibitors of GH release.[174] Physiologic stimuli for increased release of this hormone include exercise, deep sleep, hypoglycemia, and increased serum levels of certain amino acids such as arginine.[175] Pathophysiologic conditions associated with increased release of this hormone include tumor-bearing states[176, 177] and trauma and injury.[175, 178, 179] GH secretion falls with age.[180] Parenteral nutrition is also associated with a decreased mean pulse amplitude of GH secretion.[181]

At least two circulating GH binding proteins have been identified and have been found to be structurally related to the GH receptor.[182] These proteins consist of a 60- to 85-kd high-affinity species,[182, 183] as well as a 100-kd low-affinity species.[184] The levels and activity of GH binding proteins are influenced by physiologic and pathophysiologic states, including age, sex, and disease conditions.[185] Binding of GH in the circulation by these proteins is thought to regulate the bioavailability of GH at the tissue level.[186, 187]

GH unquestionably affects body nitrogen balance. The effects of this hormone on nitrogen balance appear to be due to an anabolic rather than an anticatabolic influence on skeletal muscle. The positive influence of GH on protein synthesis has been confirmed by numerous experimental studies. Isotope dilution methods examining[15] N enrichment of urinary urea nitrogen[188] as well as plasma ^{14}C-leucine appearance[189] have confirmed that GH increases the protein synthetic rate with no change in protein breakdown. GH administration also decreases the appearance of 3-methylhistidine, a marker of protein breakdown.[161, 188] Finally, increased transcription of mRNA for the myosin heavy chain has been documented after infusions of GH in man.[190]

Data on the effects of GH on carbohydrate metabolism at first glance seem confusing. Depending on the study, GH has been found to increase,[189, 191, 192] decrease,[193–195] or have no effect[191] on hepatic glucose output. GH has also been found to increase,[191, 192] decrease,[193, 194, 196, 197] or have no effect[189] on peripheral glucose uptake. Such confusion stems from two important physiologic phenomena. First, the effects of GH on metabolism are dependent upon substrate availability and the chronicity of administration. Second, GH, in the setting of adequate substrate availability, elicits the release of insulin and alters insulin receptor binding.[193, 198] The relative influences of substrate availability, the overall hormonal milieu, as well as the dose of GH administered on carbohydrate metabolism await further definition. Nevertheless, the effects of GH on carbohydrate metabolism can at present be simplistically summarized. Acutely, pharmacologic doses of GH result in decreases in blood sugar and gluconeogenesis and a decrease in peripheral glucose uptake.[194, 199] However, long-term administration results in hyperglycemia despite hyperinsulinemia secondary to increased splanchnic glucose release[192] and peripheral insulin resistance.

The predominant effect of long-term GH exposure on fat metabolism is increased lipolysis.[200] The role of GH in lipolysis is likely permissive rather than active. Except at high doses, GH alone causes little lipolysis in the absence of other lipolytic agents.[201-203] Preincubation of adipocytes with GH and glucocorticoids synergistically increases glycerol appearance following epinephrine exposure. GH appears to augment the action of counterregulatory hormones on lipolysis by increasing the activities of hormone-sensitive lipase.[204, 205] These actions of GH are dependent upon substrate availability. GH rapidly increases mobilization of peripheral lipid stores when insulin levels are low. By contrast, during conditions of hyperinsulinemia associated with intravenous feedings, no change is noted in peripheral FFA flux.[206] Similarly, in longer-term experiments GH administration during hypocaloric supplementation produces elevated levels of FFA and glycerol and diminishes the respiratory quotient. These findings are suggestive of increased lipolysis.[188, 207] When GH is administered with hyperalimentation, however, no evidence of increased fat mobilization or oxidation is noted.[208, 209]

Clinical Utility

The anabolic properties of GH, complemented by its lipolytic effects and sensitivity to the prevailing substrate background, are all theoretical advantages of this growth factor as a treatment for the catabolic patient. Theoretically, during hypocaloric feedings, GH would selectively stimulate lipolysis as the source of fuel while preserving proteins. During hyperalimentation, GH together with the attendant hyperinsulinemia would enhance utilization of exogenously administered substrates while preserving host substrate stores, including lipids. Despite these clear theoretical advantages, proving the clinical utility of GH in injured patients has been difficult.

GH has long been used in the clinical setting to successfully enhance growth and protein accrual in hypopituitary patients. The thought of using this hormone as a nutritional adjunct for catabolic patients has almost as long a history. In 1941, Cuthbertson et al. first demonstrated in a rodent model of femur fracture that pituitary extracts decreased weight loss and urinary nitrogen loss and suggested that a pituitary factor may be useful for the treatment of catabolic states.[210] Since then many clinical studies examining the efficacy of GH have been performed. These are summarized in Table 46–5. The majority of these studies were performed in burn patients. Historically, the major obstacle to clinical study of this hormone was the limited supply of GH. The earliest studies were performed with bovine GH.[211, 212] Subsequent studies used human GH isolated from cadaveric pituitary glands.[213-216] The two problems with this source of GH were that there was a limited supply that was needed by hypopituitary patients and that transmission of fatal viral infections became a clinical problem. Since the mid-1980s, however, the problem of the shortage of GH has been overcome by recombinant technology. Since then numerous preclinical studies and at least eight clinical studies have been performed[88, 89, 208, 217-221] (Table 46–5). Unfortunately, even though the majority of studies provided evidence for improved nitrogen retention with GH administration, none has as yet provided evidence that this is accompanied by improved clinical outcome.

Additionally, the most convincing

TABLE 46–5.

Clinical Trials of Growth Hormone for Wasting Associated With Disease

First Author	Agent	Patient Population	Feeding Regimen	Findings
Prudden,[211] 1956	bGH	Burn patients (n = 4)	—	Improved N balance
Pearson,[212] 1960	bGH	Burn patients (n = 4)	—	Improved electrolyte balance
Liljedahl,[213] 1961	cGH	Burn patients (n = 5)	1,900–3,200 cal	Weight gain Improved N balance
Roe,[214] 1962	cGH	Surgical/trauma (n = 4)	—	Decreased respiratory quotient
Soroff,[215] 1967	cGH	Burn patients (n = 6)	9 g N, 1,500 cal/m²/day	Improved K and N balance
Wilmore,[216] 1974	cGH	Burn patients (n = 9)	N-calorie ratio = 1:150	Improved K, N retention
Ward,[208] 1987	rhGH	GI surgery patients (n = 7)	5% dextrose (400 kcal/day)	Increased fat oxidation Decrease protein oxidation
Manson,[188] 1988	rhGH	Normal volunteers (n = 8)	TPN (30%–100% of caloric requirements)	Decreased muscle AA efflux
Snyder,[217] 1988	rhGH	Obese volunteers (n = 10)	18 cal/kg, 1.2 g protein/kg	Nitrogen retention despite caloric restriction
Jiang,[218] 1989	rhGH	GI surgery (n = 9)	TPN, 20 cal/kg/day, 1 g protein/kg/day	Increased protein synthesis
Douglas,[189] 1990	rhGH	Septic (n = 25)	TPN (12), enteral (13)	Reduced protein loss
Pape,[219] 1991	rhGH	COPD† (n = 7)	35 kcal/kg, 1 g protein/kg	Weight gain, improved inspiratory force
Hammarqvist,[220] 1992	rhGH	Cholecystectomy (n = 8)	TPN, 0.2 g N/kg/day, 135 kJ/kg/day	Improved N balance
Ziegler,[221] 1992	rhGH	TPN (n = 15)	TPN, 30 cal/kg/day, 1.6 g protein/kg/day	Improved N balance

bGH = bovine growth hormone; cGH = cadaveric GH; rhGH = recombinant human GH; TPN = total parenteral nutrition; AA = amino acid; COPD = chronic obstructive pulmonary disease.

data for improved nitrogen accrual are those from patients with only moderate stress. There is still concern that in severely stressed patients such as those in the intensive care unit, added GH may not be biologically active. In fact, a number of recent studies in the critically ill population have been unable to show a benefit of GH even as measured by urinary nitrogen excretion.[222, 223] These studies offer an interesting mechanistic explanation for the lack of response to GH. It is now clear that a large number of the physiologic actions of GH are mediated at the tissue level by IGFs that are released in response to GH. In studies of the critically ill, a consistent finding is that of a blunted response of IGF to GH.[224] Whether an altered appearance of GH binding proteins or IGF binding proteins may also be at play in the resistance to GH in the critically ill is an area of active research at present.

In the meantime, it can be concluded that GH can promote nitrogen retention in patients under little or moderate stress who are receiving adequate nutrient supplementation. It is less clear whether this hormone is useful in patients under severe stress. No study has documented that short courses of GH improve patient outcome (i.e., the length of hospital stay, the rate of complications, or mortality). Clinical research to date has involved small sample sizes. A priority in studies of anabolic growth factors (i.e., GH) should be the design and execution of a large clinical trial to determine whether these growth factors improve clinical outcome. Lacking such data, it is unlikely that GH will be a routine modality in nutritional medicine.

INSULIN-LIKE GROWTH FACTOR 1

Physical Properties

Experimental and clinical evidence support the conclusion that IGF-1 is an intermediary hormone that mediates many of the actions of GH. Originally isolated and called somatomedin C, IGF-1 has been determined to be a 70-amino acid single-chain protein. This polypeptide shares approximately 43% homology with proinsulin.[225] In addition, the IGF-1 receptor also shares homology with the insulin receptor,[226] and not surprisingly IGF-1 can bind to the insulin receptor and exerts insulin-like metabolic activities.

IGF-1 can be synthesized at numerous tissue sites, but the primary source of this growth factor is thought to be hepatic tissues. Many different hormones can elicit IGF-1 release, including insulin,[227] prolactin,[228] and chorionic somatomammotropin,[229] but clearly the prime stimulus for IGF-1 release is GH.[230] Not surprisingly then, IGF-1 levels generally parallel those of GH. Of note, contrary to GH levels, IGF-1 levels fall during sepsis,[231] severe injury,[232] in malnourished children,[233] and poorly controlled diabetes.[234] The low levels of IGF-1 in these pathophysiologic conditions may contribute to the associated wasting seen in these conditions. IGF-1 levels are decreased by other hormones and pathophysiologic states including glucocorticoid exposure,[235] estrogens,[229] liver disease,[236] and renal failure.[237] Furthermore, as with GH, nutritional status is a major determinant of IGF-1 release and action. Fasting results in a profound fall in plasma IGF-1 levels.[238, 239]

As with GH, in vivo investigations of IGF-1 actions are complicated by the existence of binding proteins for this growth factor. At least three such IGF binding proteins (IGFBP) have been identified for IGF-1, including a 25-kd IGFBP-1, a 55-kd GH-independent IGFBP-2 complex, and a 150-kd GH-dependent IGFBP-3 binding complex.[240] These binding proteins regulate IGF-1 availability. The major binding protein in the circulation is IGFBP-3, whereas IGFBP-2 has a much more prominent role within specific tissues, particularly within the central nervous system.[241] Expression of IGFBP-1 seems to be dependent on the prevailing substrate background. When substrate and insulin are plentiful, IGFBP-1 concentrations decrease, while glucose deprivation results in increased expression of IGFBP-1.[242] The biology of these binding proteins is complex and under active investigation and has recently been reviewed in detail.[243, 244]

As mentioned above, IGF-1 exerts many of the effects of insulin, including hypoglycemia[245, 246] and inhibition of lipolysis.[246] In both regards, this protein is much less potent than insulin. In vitro, IGF-1 stimulates protein synthesis,[247] and in vivo, this protein inhibits proteolysis.[248] With recent synthesis of this molecule by recombinant techniques, unlimited quantities are now available, thus facilitating in vivo studies and making large scale clinical trials possible.

Clinical Utility

Although many catabolic states such as malnutrition and severe injury are often associated with an increased circulating level of GH, the levels of IGF-1 are often found to be inappropriately low. This blunted appearance of IGF-1 is thought to contribute to paradoxical wasting in the setting of high GH levels. The administration of exogenous GH in pharmacologic doses may or may not overcome this IGF-1 deficiency. An attractive strategy, therefore, is to supplement hypercaloric feedings with exogenous IGF-1 during nutritional treatment of these patients. Until recently the limited availability of IGF-1 made even animal experiments difficult. With recent production of the protein by recombinant techniques, animal as well as preclinical studies are under way to examine the utility of this protein in combating cachexia. It is likely that the first clinical trials will be published shortly.

In a recent preclinical study in normal volunteers, a 6-day continuous IGF-1 infusion (25/µg/kg/hr) given in the setting of hypocaloric parenteral nutrition produced nitrogen sparing and gluconeo-genesis without an increase in lipoly-sis.[249] This and previous animal studies certainly encourage clinical studies of this protein growth factor in catabolic patients.

Another intriguing potential use for IGF-1 is as a specific growth factor for intestinal mucosa. As will be discussed at greater length later for epidermal growth factor (EGF), the intestinal mu-cosa is an important barrier to patho-logic organisms that reside in our gas-trointestinal system. Injury and bowel rest are potent stimuli for intestinal atrophy, which in turn is thought to lead to bacterial translocation and con-sequent pathophysiologic sequelae. In addition to its anabolic effects on skele-tal muscle, IGF-1 also appears to be tro-phic for the gastrointestinal tract. In animal studies, this growth factor in-creased intestinal mass when adminis-tered both parenterally[250] and enteral-ly.[251] Whether this or other growth factors will be useful in the maintenance of gastrointestinal barrier function and absorptive function in the critically ill awaits future studies.

ANABOLIC STEROIDS

Physical Properties

Androgenic steroids are produced mainly in the Leydig cells of the testes and the zona reticulosa of the adrenal cortex and have potent anabolic activi-ties.[252] The natural androgens are pro-duced from cholesterol by modifications that include elimination of the C_{20-21} side chain and oxygenation of the C_3 and C_{17} positions.[163] Pharmacologic modifications of the natural androgens have been performed with the aim of re-ducing their androgenic actions, in-creasing the ease of administration, and enhancing their anabolic actions. Such efforts have resulted in the production of synthetic compounds referred to as anabolic steroids.

Three mechanisms for the anabolic

actions of this class of compounds have been proposed. The first two involve ac-tions at the skeletal muscle effector cells, where intracellular actions of ste-roids include both anabolic as well as anticatabolic activities. Within the cell nuclei, androgenic steroids activate DNA-dependent RNA polymerase I and II[253] and result in enhanced synthesis of messenger and ribosomal RNAs and ul-timately enhanced synthesis of myofi-brillar proteins. An anticatabolic effect through inhibition of the cortisone-dependent myofibrillar protease also oc-curs[254] and may be due to a competitive inhibition of glucocorticoid binding to the cytosol receptors.[254, 255] Anabolic steroids also appear to act at the kidneys to decrease amino acid excretion.[256]

Clinical Utility

The anabolic potential of androgenic and other anabolic steroids in un-stressed animals is clear. What remains largely undetermined is whether utiliza-tion of these compounds in the hospital-ized patient improves outcome.

These compounds have been tested in the clinical setting for a long time. As early as 1944, Abels et al. examined the effects of testosterone and testosterone propionate on the nitrogen economy of three patients with gastric cancer and found the administration of these an-drogenic steroids to improve urinary ni-trogen balance.[257] Since then, the clin-ical utility of anabolic steroids has been examined in diverse clinical popula-tions, including lung resections,[258, 259] gastrointestinal surgery,[260] gastrecto-my,[261] and trauma.[256]

The only studies of even moderate size were those of Danylewick et al.[262] and Hansell et al.[263] In the former, 113 patients were separated into "normally nourished" and "malnourished" groups by body composition. Patients in each group were randomized to receive or not receive weekly injections of nandrolone decanoate (Deca-Durabolin) along with total parenteral nutrition (TPN). No ef-

TABLE 46–6.

Clinical Trials of Anabolic Steroids in Treatment of Cachexia

First Author	Agent	Patient Population	Findings
Abels,[257] 1944	Testosterone	Gastric cancer ($n = 3$)	Improved N balance
Kennedy,[259] 1959	Norethandrolone	Lung resection ($n = 7$)	No significant change
Johnston,[260] 1963	Methandienone	GI surgery ($n = 11$)	Improved N balance
Michelsen,[264] 1982	Nandrolone decanoate	Hip replacement ($n = 8$)	Attenuated changes in muscle AA
Young,[265] 1983	Nandrolone decanoate	Perioperative patients ($n = 12$)	Decreased plasma AA
Hansell,[263] 1989	Stanozolol	Colorectal surgery ($n = 30$)	Improved N balance
Danylewick,[262] 1989	Deca-Durabolin	TPN patients ($n = 57$)	Improved body cell mass
Hausmann,[256] 1989	Nandrolone decanoate	Trauma patients ($n = 10$)	Improved N balance
Bonkovsky,[266] 1991	Oxandrolone	Alcoholic hepatitis ($n = 18$)	Improved serum markers

TPN = total parenteral nutrition; AA = amino acid.

fect of this steroid on the "normally nourished" patients was seen, while the malnourished patients benefited from the steroid administration as determined by measurements of body cell mass. Likewise, in the studies of Hansell et al., 60 colorectal surgery patients were randomized to receive or not receive stanozolol along with either a hypocaloric diet or adequate caloric supplementation. Benefit of the steroid was only demonstrated in the group with hypocaloric nutrition.

Table 46–6 summarizes some of the clinical studies that have been performed to date. Several conclusions can be drawn from these studies. First, most of these studies include few patients, which makes it difficult to interpret results. Second, the nutritional regimens and the steroid preparations used varied greatly among studies, which makes this literature difficult to decipher. Finally, even though a number of studies have shown an improvement in serum or urine parameters of nitrogen retention, no study to date has shown an improvement in any clinical outcome parameter. The question of whether anabolic steroids have any role as an adjunct to clinical nutrition therefore demands further study. Certainly, a large trial, possibly in a multicenter fashion, is necessary to evaluate utility by clinical outcome.

It is important to bear in mind that androgenic and anabolic steroids are not without side effects. Virilization is a potential side effect, often manifested by hirsutism, acne, clitoral hypertrophy, voice coarsening, and male pattern baldness that may persist despite discontinuation of therapy.[267] Alternatively, peripheral conversion of testosterone and androstenedione to estradiol and estrone may result in feminizing effects such as gynecomastia.[268] Other potential detrimental effects include hypogonadism,[269] lipoprotein abnormalities including increased low-density lipoproteins (LDLs),[270] sleep apnea,[271] and hepatic complications including the development of hepatocellular carcinoma.[272] These side effects will undoubtedly remain obstacles to the routine use of anabolic steroids in catabolic and malnourished patients.

EPIDERMAL GROWTH FACTOR

Physical Properties

EGF is a soluble peptide of 53 amino acids that was inadvertently discovered over three decades ago when investigators searching for factors that promoted nerve cell growth noted that the snake venom used as a reagent in experiments actually had nerve growth factor–like activity.[273] This factor was subsequently termed EGF because of its capacity to induce cell proliferation in the basal cells of skin.[274] EGF was ultimately purified and isolated from murine salivary gland extracts,[275] and by 1972 the peptide was purified and sequenced.[276] This greatly facilitated the elucidation of EGF biochemistry and physiology. Recombinant EGF is now available for study and clinical usage.

EGF has been identified in many tissues and body fluids,[277–279] including the salivary gland,[275] pancreas,[280] kidney,[281, 282] brain,[283, 284] maternal decidua,[285] blood,[286] saliva,[287] urine,[288, 289] milk,[290, 291] tears,[292] and breast fluid.[293] Some of the highest concentrations of EGF have been found in salivary and pancreatic tissues and secretions. Circulating EGF can be detected in small concentrations both as a free peptide and bound to platelets.[286] Urinary EGF, known also as urogastrone,[289] was thought to arise primarily from the kidney,[281, 282] but recent evidence suggests that urogastrone may originate from renal clearance of circulating EGF.[294]

EGF exerts its effects through a specific cell surface receptor that it shares with a closely related growth factor, transforming growth factor α (TGF-α). TGF-α is a 50–amino acid peptide and shares a 42% sequence homology with EGF.[295] The EGF receptor is a glycoprotein that has generated significant scientific interest with the observation that it bears striking similarity to the V-*erb* B oncogene[296] and the realization that altered EGF receptor–like proteins may provide a stimulus for abnormal cell growth. Concern over a potential relationship between EGF, its receptor, and oncogenesis have limited its introduction as a therapeutic agent.

EGF is involved in a complex array of physiologic and pathophysiologic processes. EGF plays a significant role in embryo and fetal development[297–299] and an incompletely defined role in normal postnatal physiology. The current range of partially characterized biological activity of recombinant EGF or salivary EGF includes (1) stimulation of cell growth and differentiation,[274, 300] (2) wound or cutaneous ulcer healing,[301–304] (3) inhibition of gastric acid secretion,[305, 306] and (4) gastric mucosal cytoprotection.[305, 307] Milk and salivary EGF may be important in promoting neonatal gastrointestinal mucosal development[308, 309] and may possibly have a role in the adaptation to intestinal resection.[310, 311]

Clinical Utility

The role of EGF in clinical medicine has been limited to date. This is in part due to the unanswered question concerning its role in oncogenesis. Topical EGF in silver sulfadiazine applied to skin graft donor sites accelerates the rate of healing of partial-thickness skin wounds.[302] This may facilitate more rapid donor site reharvesting and has some application in patients with extensive burns and limited donor sites.

EGF may also have clinical utility because of its actions on the intestinal mucosa. In hospitalized patients, particularly critically ill patients, a multitude of factors, including loss of luminal trophic factors, altered splanchnic blood flow, and nutritional deprivation, lead to gastrointestinal mucosal atrophy.[312, 313] Such deterioration of the gastrointestinal physical barrier as well as altered gastrointestinal IgA secretion[314] has been associated with the systemic appearance of bacteria normally resident and confined to the gastrointestinal tract.[315, 316] This bacterial translocation is thought to play a detrimental role in altering host immune function and possibly in the initiation of sepsis. In animal studies, EGF stimulates DNA synthesis,[317] promotes intestinal growth, and attenuates structural and functional derangements associated with bowel rest. A continuous infusion of EGF in rodents significantly increased cell proliferation and intestinal weight throughout the gastrointestinal tract.[318] Similar trophic effects of EGF on intestinal cells have also been demonstrated in primates.[319] The role of this growth factor in hospitalized patients, particularly in critically ill patients, awaits further study.

In one part of the gastrointestinal tract, a clinical role for EGF has already been suggested by human studies. Preliminary studies have shown that EGF administration is associated with satisfactory healing of peptic ulcers with 48 weeks of therapy.[320] This study suffers from a lack of control groups receiving conventional therapy. Nevertheless, the data presented encourage future trials of this growth factor as treatment of ulcerating diseases of the gastrointestinal mucosa. Other intriguing possibilities for use of this growth factor include utilization in the treatment of short-bowel syndrome.

GROWTH FACTORS AND CANCER

A major theoretical obstacle to routine usage of growth factors in the clinical setting is the fear that growth factors may stimulate cancer growth. Not only is there concern that growth factors may stimulate cancer growth in existing tumors during treatment of cancer patients, there is also worry that growth factors may stimulate new cancer growth. This is not a trivial issue because of the high prevalence of cachexia in cancer patients, both from the neoplastic process and from iatrogenic causes such as surgery and chemotherapy. Cancer patients are therefore a large population for potential use of growth factors.

Animal and in vitro studies have linked GH to the development of certain lymphoid malignancies.[321] IGF-1 has also been shown to be a stimulus for in vitro growth of breast tumors[322] and lung tumors.[323] IL-3, G-CSF, and GM-CSF have been found to stimulate certain leukemic cell lines in vitro.[143–145] Additionally, platelet-derived growth factor and TGF-α and -β are produced by certain malignancies and may function as autocrine growth factors for these tumors.[324, 325] The EGF receptor has been noted to be remarkably similar to the V-erb B oncongene,[54] and altered EGF receptor–like proteins may provide a stimulus for abnormal cell growth. Data also exist that show that GH administration in rats actually decreased the number of tumor metastases in a transplantable adenocarcinoma model in rodents.[326] The relative influences of the mitogenic effects of growth factors as compared with their beneficial influence on host cancer surveillance through improvements in immunocompetence remain to be determined. Further, if certain growth factors are capable of shifting tumors into the proliferative phase, such action may render tumors more sensitive to radiotherapy or chemotherapy. Therapeutic investigations using this treatment strategy are currently under way in myeloid leukemia where CSFs are being administered as priming agents to stimulate acute myeloid leukemic blast cells to become more sensitive to cell cycle–specific chemotherapy.

No human study to date has shown an effect of growth factors on cancer appearance or growth. Studies in this area will not only be interesting but will also be necessary before accepting growth factor therapy as a routine clinical modality. Trials of growth factors as adjuncts to chemotherapy or radiotherapy will undoubtedly be an area of fruitful future investigations.

CONCLUSION

A marriage of immunology and endocrinology with molecular and pharmacologic technology has made available a host of pluripotent as well as specific growth factors. Although some of these, such as CSFs and erythropoietin, have reached clinical application, clinical roles for most growth factors remain to be fully defined. Enthusiasm for using these proteins in the clinical setting must be tempered by their potential deleterious effects. Perhaps with the exception of erythropoietin, all of these proteins have significant metabolic side effects. The potential of many of these growth factors to enhance tumor growth must be regarded as real until further evidence to the contrary is found. Finally, the costs of these growth factors are not insignificant. Therefore, carefully conducted clinical trials are needed to prove the benefits of these growth factors.

REFERENCES

1. Warnold I, Eden E, Lundholm K: The inefficiency of total parenteral nutrition to stimulate protein synthesis in moderately malnourished patients. *Ann Surg* 1988; 208:143–149.
2. Stein TP, Ang SD: Effect of increasing TPN on protein metabolism. *JPEN* 1983; 7:525–529.
3. Fong Y, Moldawer LL, Lowry SF: Experimental and clinical applications of molecular cell biology in nutrition and metabolism. *JPEN* 1992; 164:477–486.
4. Goldberg MA, Dunning SP, Bunn HF: Regulation of the erythropoietin gene: Evidence that the oxygen sensor is a heme protein. *Science* 1988; 242:1412–1415.
5. Erslev AJ, Caro J, Miller O, et al: Plasma erythropoietin in health and disease. *Ann Clin Lab Sci* 1980; 10:250–257.
6. Egrie JC, Eschbach JW, McGuire T: Pharmacokinetics of recombinant erythropoietin (rHuEPO) administered to hemodialysis (HD) patients (abstract). *Kidney Int* 1988; 33:262.
7. Kindler J, Eckardt KU, Ehmer B: Single-dose pharmacokinetics of recombinant human erythropoietin in patients with various degrees of renal failure. *Nephrol Dial Transplant* 1989; 4:345–349.
8. McMahon FG, Vargas R, Ryan M, et al: Pharmacokinetics and effects of recombinant human erythropoietin after intravenous and subcutaneous injection in healthy volunteers. *Blood* 1990; 76:1718–1722.
9. Eschbach JW: Erythropoietin 1991—An overview. *Am J Kidney Dis* 1991; 18(4 suppl 1):3–9.
10. van Wyck DB, Stivelman JC, Ruiz J, et al: Iron status in patients receiving erythropoietin for dialysis-associated anemia. *Kidney Int* 1989; 35:712–716.
11. Erslev AJ: Erythropoietin. *N Engl J Med* 1992; 324:1339–1344.
12. Eschbach JW, Abdulhadi MH, Browne JK, et al: Recombinant human erythropoietin in anemic patients with end-stage renal disease. Results of a phase III multicenter clinical trial. *Ann Intern Med* 1989; 111:992–1000.
13. Eschbach JW: Erythropoietin-associated hypertension. *N Engl J Med* 1990; 323:999–1000.
14. Haley NR, Davidson RC, Eschbach JW: Patterns of development of hypertension with recombinant human erythropoietin (rHuEPO) therapy: A prospective study (abstract). *Am J Hypertens* 1989; 2(suppl):56.
15. Nissenson AR, Nimer SD, Wolcott DL: Recombinant human erythropoietin and renal anemia: Molecular biology, clinical efficacy, and nervous system effects. *Ann Intern Med* 1991; 114:402–416.
16. Jelkman W: Erythropoietin: Structure, control of production, and function. *Physiol Rev* 1992; 72:449–489.
17. Johnson WT, McCarthy JT, Yanagihara T, et al: Effects of recombinant human erythropoietin on cerebral and cutaneous blood flow and on blood coagulability. *Kidney Int* 1990; 38:919–924.
18. Onoyama K, Kumagai H, Takeda K, et al: Effects of human recombinant erythropoietin on anaemia, systemic haemodynamics and renal function in predialysis renal failure patients. *Nephrol Dial Transplant* 1989; 4:966–970.
19. Raine AEG: Hypertension, blood viscosity, and cardiovascular morbidity in renal failure: Implications of erythropoietin therapy. *Lancet* 1988; 1:97–99.

20. Raine AEG: Seizures and hypertension events. *Semin Nephrol* 1990; 10(suppl 1):40–50.

21. Lin FK, Suggs S, Lin CH: Cloning and expression of the human erthropoietin gene. *Proc Natl Acad Sci U S A* 1985; 92:7580–7585.

22. Jacobs K, Shoemaker C, Rudersdorf R, et al: Isolation and characterization of genomic and cDNA clones of human erythropoietin. *Nature* 1992; 313:806–810.

23. Eschbach JW, Egrie JC, Downing MR, et al: Correction of the anemia of end-stage renal disease with recombinant human erythropoietin: Results of a combined phase I and II clinical trial. *N Engl J Med* 1987; 316:73–78.

24. Winearls CG, Oliver DO, Pippard MJ, et al: Effect of human erythropoietin derived from recombinant DNA on the anaemia of patients maintained by chronic haemodialysis. *Lancet* 1986; 2:1175–1178.

25. Eschbach JW, Kelly MR, Haley NR, et al: Treatment of the anemia of progressive renal failure with recombinant human erythropoietin. *N Engl J Med* 1989; 321:158–163.

26. Fischl M, Galpin JE, Levine JD: Recombinant human erythropoietin for patients with AIDS treated with zidovudine. *N Engl J Med* 1990; 322:1488–1493.

27. Halperin DS, Wacker P, LaCourt G: Effects of recombinant erythropoietin in infants with the anemia of prematurity: A pilot study. *J Pediatr* 1990; 116:779–786.

28. Goodnough LT, Rudnick S, Price TH, et al: Increased preoperative collection of autologous blood with recombinant human erythropoietin therapy. *N Engl J Med* 1989; 321:1163–1168.

29. James RD, Wilkinson PM, Belli F, et al: Recombinant human erythropoietin in patients with ovarian carcinoma and anaemia secondary to cisplatin and carboplatin chemotherapy: Preliminary results. *Acta Hematol* 1992; 87(suppl):12–15.

30. Pincus T, Olsen NJ, Russel J: Multicenter study of recombinant human erythropoietin in correction of anemia in rheumatoid arthritis. *Am J Med* 1990; 89:161–168.

31. Abels RI, Larholt KM, Krantz KD: Recombinant human erythropoietin (r-HuEPO) for the treatment of the anemia of cancer, in Murphy MJ Jr (ed): *Blood Cell Growth Factors: Their Present and Future Use in Hematology and Oncology. Proceedings of the Beijing Symposium.* Dayton, Ohio, AlphaMed Press, 1991, pp 121–141.

32. Ludwig H, Fritz E, Kotzman H: Erythropoietin treatment of anemia associated with multiple myeloma. *N Engl J Med* 1990; 322:1693–1699.

33. Stein RS, Abels RJ, Krantz SB: Pharmacologic doses of recombinant human erythropoietin in the treatment of myelodysplastic syndromes. *Blood* 1991; 78:1658–1663.

34. Oster W, Herman F, Gamm H: Erythropoietin for the treatment of anemia of malignancy associated with neoplastic bone marrow infiltration. *J Clin Oncol* 1990; 8:956–962.

35. Danko J, Huch R, Huch A: Epoietin alfa for treatment of postpartum anaemia. *Lancet* 1990; 1:737–738.

36. Hollowood K, Pease C, Mackay AM, et al: Sarcomatoid tumours of lymph nodes showing follicular dendritic cell differentiation. *J Pathol* 1991; 163:205–216.

37. McDougall A, McGarrity G: Extra-abdominal desmoid tumours. *J Bone Joint Surg [Br]* 1979; 61:373–377.

38. Nielsen OJ, Thaysen JH: Erythropoietin deficiency in acute tubular necrosis. *J Intern Med* 1990; 227:373–380.

39. Yoshimura N, Oka T, Ohmori Y: Effects of recombinant human erythropoietin on the anemia of renal transplant recipients with chronic rejection. *Transplantation* 1989; 48:527–529.

40. Evans RW, Rader B, Manninen DL: Cooperative Multicenter EPO Clinical Trial Group. The quality of life of hemodialysis recipients treated with recombinant human erythropoietin. *JAMA* 1990; 263:825–830.

41. Canadian Erythropoietin Study Group: Association between recombinant human erythropoietin and quality of life and exercise capacity of patients receiving haemodialysis. *BMJ* 1990; 300:573–578.

42. Nissenson AR: Recombinant human erythropoietin: Impact on brain and cognitive function, exercise tolerance, sexual potency, and quality of life. *Semin Nephrol* 1989; 9(suppl 2):25–31.

43. Lipkin GW, Kendall RG, Haggett P, et al: Erythropoietin in acute renal failure (letter). *Lancet* 1989; 1:1029.

44. Lipkin GW, Kendall RG, Russon LJ, et al: Erythropoietin deficiency in acute renal failure. *Nephrol Dial Transplant* 1990; 5:920–922.

45. Nielsen OJ, Thaysen JH: Erythropoietin deficiency in acute renal failure (letter). *Lancet* 1989; 1:624–625.

46. Thaysen JH, Nielsen OJ, Branki L, et al: Erythropoietin deficiency in acute crescentic glomerulonephritis and in total bilateral renal cortical necrosis. *J Intern Med* 1991; 229:363–369.

47. Adamson JW, Eschbach JW: Management of the anaemia of chronic renal failure with recombinant erythropoietin. *Q J Med* 1989; 73:1093–1101.

48. Miller CB, Jones RJ, Piantadosi S, et al: Decreased erythropoietin response in patients with the anemia of cancer. *N Engl J Med* 1990; 322:1689–1692.

49. Spivak JL, Barnes DC, Fuchs E, et al: Serum immunoreactive erythropoietin in HIV-infected patients. *JAMA* 1989; 261:3104–3107.

50. Baer AN, Dessypris EN, Goldwasser E, et al: Blunted erythropoietin response to anaemia in rheumatoid arthritis. *Br J Haematol* 1987; 66:559–564.

51. Hochberg MC, Arnold CM, Hogans BB, et al: Serum immunoreactive erythropoietin in rheumatoid arthritis: Impaired response to anemia. *Arthritis Rheum* 1988; 31:1318–1321.

52. Vreugdenhil G, Wognum AW, Van Eijk HG, et al: Anaemia in rheumatoid arthritis: The role of iron, vitamin B_{12}, and folic acid deficiency, and erythropoietin responsiveness. *Ann Rheum Dis* 1990; 49:93–98.

53. Means RT, Olsen NF, Krantz SB, et al: Treatment of the anemia of rheumatoid arthritis with recombinant human erythropoietin: Clinical and in vitro studies. *Arthritis Rheum* 1989; 32:638–642.

54. Jelkmann W, Wolff M, Fandrey J: Modulation of the production of erythropoietin by cytokines: In vitro studies and their clinical applications.

Contrib Nephrol 1990; 87:68–77.

55. Tracey KJ, Wei H, Manogue KR, et al: Cachectin/tumor necrosis factor induces cachexia, anemia, and inflammation. *J Exp Med* 1988; 167:1211–1227.

56. Blick MS, Sherwin SA, Rosenblum M, et al: Phase I study of recombinant tumor necrosis factor in cancer patients. *Cancer Res* 1987; 47:2986–2989.

57. Johnson CS, Cook CA, Furmanski P: In vivo suppression of erythropoiesis by tumor necrosis factor-α (TNF-α): Reversal with exogenous erythropoietin (EPO). *Exp Hematol* 1990; 18:109–113.

58. Johnson RA, Waddelow TA, Caro J, et al: Chronic exposure to tumor necrosis factor in vivo preferentially inhibits erythropoiesis in nude mice. *Blood* 1989; 74:130–138.

59. Johnson CS, Keckler DJ, Topper MI, et al: In vivo hematopoietic effects of recombinant interleukin-1α in mice: Stimulation of granulocytic, monocytic, megakaryocytic, and early erythroid progenitors, suppression of late-state erythropoiesis, and reversal of erythroid suppression with erythropoietin. *Blood* 1989; 73:678–683.

60. Bradley TR, Metcalf D: The growth of mouse bone marrow cells in vitro. *Aust J Exp Biol Med Sci* 1966; 44:287–299.

61. Ichikawa Y, Pluznik DH, Sachs L: In vitro control of the development of macrophage and granulocyte colonies. *Proc Natl Acad Sci U S A* 1966; 56:488–495.

62. Stanley ER, Chen DM, Linn HS: Induction of macrophage production and proliferation by purified colony-stimulating factor. *Nature* 1978; 274:168–169.

63. Cantrell MA, Anderson D, Cerretti DP, et al: Cloning, sequence, and expression of a human granulocyte/macrophage colony-stimulating factor. *Proc Natl Acad Sci U S A* 1985; 82:6250–6254.

64. Nagata S, Tsuchiya M, Asano S, et al: Molecular cloning and expression of cDNA for human granulocyte colony-stimulating factor. *Nature* 1986; 319:414–418.

65. Groopman JE, Molina JM, Scadden

DT: Hematopoietic growth factors: Biology and clinical applications. *N Engl J Med* 1989; 321:1449–1459.

66. Lieschke GJ, Burgess AW: Granulocyte colony-stimulating factor and granuloctye-macrophage colony stimulating factor. (First of two parts). *N Engl J Med* 1992; 327:28–35.

67. Metcalf D: Haemopoietic growth factors 1. *Lancet* 1989; 1:825–827.

68. Seelentag WK, Mermod JJ, Montesano R, et al: Additive effects of interleukin 1 and tumor necrosis factor-alpha on the accumulation of the three granulocytic and macrophage colony-stimulating factor mRNAs in human endothelial cells. *EMBO J* 1987; 6:2261–2265.

69. Koeffler HP, Gasson J, Tobler A: Transcriptions and post-transcriptional modulation of myeloid colony-stimulating factor expression by tumor necrosis factor and other agents. *Mol Cell Biol* 1988; 8:3432–3438.

70. Gearing DP, King JA, Gough NM, et al: Expression cloning of a receptor for human granulocyte-macrophage colony-stimulating factor. *EMBO J* 1989; 8:3667–3676.

71. Hayashida K, Kitamura T, Forman DM, et al: Molecular cloning of a second subunit of the receptor for human granulocyte-macrophage colony-stimulating factor (GM-CSF): Reconstitution of high-affinity GM-CSF receptor. *Proc Natl Acad Sci U S A* 1990; 87:9655–9659.

72. Metcalf D: The molecular control of cell division, differentiation commitment and maturation in haemopoietic cells. *Lancet* 1989; 1:27–30.

73. Onetto-Pothier N, Aumont N, Hamon A, et al: Characterization of granulocyte-macrophage–colony-stimulating factor receptors on the blast cells of acute myeloblastic leukemia. *Blood* 1990; 75:59–66.

74. Budel LM, Touw IP, Delwel R, et al: Granulocyte colony-stimulating factor receptors in human acute myelocytic leukemia. *Blood* 1989; 74:2668–2673.

75. Rowe JM, Rapoport AP: Hematopoietic growth factors: A review. *J Clin Pharmacol* 1992; 32:486–501.

76. Moore MAS: The clinical use of colony stimulating factors. *Annu Rev Immunol* 1991; 9:159–191.

77. Duhrsen U, Villeval JL, Boyd J, et al: Effects of recombinant human granulocyte colony-stimulating factor on hematopoietic progenitor cells in cancer patients. *Blood* 1988; 72:2074–2081.

78. Lindemann A, Herrmann F, Oster W, et al: Hematologic effects of recombinant human granulocyte colony-stimulating factor in patients with malignancy. *Blood* 1989; 74:2644–2651.

79. Gabrilove JL, Jakubowski A, Scher H, et al: Effect of granulocyte colony-stimulating factor on neutropenia and associated morbidity due to chemotherapy for transitional-cell carcinoma of the urothelium. *N Engl J Med* 1988; 318:1414–1422.

80. Gabrilove JL, Jakubowski A, Fain K, et al: Phase I study of granulocyte colony-stimulating factor in patients with transitional cell carcinoma of the urothelium. *J Clin Invest* 1988; 82:1454–1461.

81. Morstyn G, Campbell L, Lieschke G, et al: Treatment of chemotherapy induced neutropenia by subcutaneously administered granulocyte colony-stimulating factor with optimization of dose and duration of therapy. *J Clin Oncol* 1989; 7:1554–1562.

82. Morstyn G, Campbell L, Souza LM, et al: Effect of granulocyte colony stimulating factor on neutropenia induced by cytotoxic chemotherapy. *Lancet* 1988; 1:667–672.

83. Bronchud MH, Potter MR, Morgenstern G, et al: In vitro and in vivo analysis of the effects of recombinant human granulocyte colony-stimulating factor in patients. *Br J Cancer* 1988; 56:64–69.

84. Bronchud MH, Scarffe JH, Thatcher N, et al: Phase I/II study of recombinant human granulocytic colony-stimulating factor in patients receiving intensive chemotherapy for small cell lung cancer. *Br J Cancer* 1987; 56:809–813.

85. Lord BI, Bronchud MH, Owens S, et al: The kinetics of human granulopoiesis following treatment with granulocyte colony-stimulating factor in vivo. *Proc Natl Acad Sci U S A* 1989; 86:9499–9503.

86. Miles SA, Mitsuyasu RT, Moreno J, et al: Combined therapy with recombinant granulocyte colony-stimulating factor and erythropoietin decreases hematologic toxicity from zidovudine. *Blood* 1991; 77:2109–2117.

87. Kaplan SS, Basford RE, Wing EJ, et al: The effect of recombinant human granulocyte macrophage colony-stimulating factor on neutrophil activation in patients with refractory carcinoma. *Blood* 1989; 73:636–638.

88. Sullivan R, Fredette JP, Socinski M, et al: Enhancement of superoxide anion release by granulocytes harvested from patients receiving granulocyte-macrophage colony-stimulating factor. *Br J Haematol* 1989; 71: 475–479.

89. Wing EJ, Magee DM, Whiteside TL, et al: Recombinant human granulocyte/macrophage colony-stimulating factor enhances monocyte cytotoxicity and secretion of tumor necrosis factor α and interferon in cancer patients. *Blood* 1989; 73:643–646.

90. Addison IE, Johnson B, Devereux S, et al: Granulocyte-macrophage colony-stimulating factor may inhibit neutrophil migration in vivo. *Clin Exp Immunol* 1989; 76:149–153.

91. Devereux S, Bull HA, Campos-Costa D, et al: Granulocyte macrophage colony stimulating factor induces changes in cellular adhesion molecule expression and adhesion to endothelium: In-vitro and in-vivo studies in man. *Br J Haematol* 1989; 71:323–330.

92. Socinski MA, Cannistra SA, Sullivan R, et al: Granulocyte-macrophage colony-stimulating factor induces the expression of the CD11b surface adhesion molecule on human granulocytes in vivo. *Blood* 1988; 72:691–697.

93. Lieschke GJ, Cebon J, Morstyn G: Characterization of the clinical effects after the first dose of bacterially synthesized recombinant human granulocyte-macrophage colony-stimulating factor. *Blood* 1989; 74:2634–2643.

94. Aglietta M, Piacibello W, Sanavio F, et al: Kinetics of human hemopoietic cells after in vivo administration of granulocyte-macrophage colony-stimulating factor. *J Clin Invest* 1989; 83:551–557.

95. Phillips N, Jacobs S, Stoller R, et al: Effect of recombinant human granulocyte-macrophage colony-stimulating factor on myelopoiesis in patients with refractory metastatic carcinoma. *Blood* 1989; 74:26–34.

96. Socinski MA, Cannistra SA, Elias A, et al: Granulocyte-macrophage colony stimulating factor expands the circulating haemopoietic progenitor cell compartment in man. *Lancet* 1988; 1:1194–1198.

97. Antman K, Griffen JD, Elias A, et al: Effect of recombinant human granulocyte-macrophage colony-stimulating factor on chemotherapy-induced myelosuppression. *N Engl J Med* 1988; 319:593–598.

98. Herrmann F, Schulz G, Lindemann A: Hematopoietic responses in patients with advanced malignancy treated with recombinant human granulocyte-macrophage colony-stimulating factor. *J Clin Oncol* 1989; 7:159–167.

99. Steward WP, Scarffe JH, Austin R, et al: Recombinant human granulocyte macrophage colony stimulating factor (rhGM-CSF) given as daily short infusions—a phase I dose-toxicity study. *Br J Cancer* 1989; 59:142–145.

100. Lieschke GJ, Maher D, O'Connor M, et al: Phase I study of intravenously administered bacterially synthesized granulocyte-macrophage colony-stimulating factor and comparison with subcutaneous administration. *Cancer Res* 1990; 50:606–614.

101. Lieschke GJ, Maher D, Cebon J, et al: Effects of bacterially synthesized recombinant human granulocyte-macrophage colony stimulating factor in patients with advanced malignancy. *Ann Intern Med* 1989; 110:357–364.

102. Lord BI, Gurney H, Chang J, et al: Haemopoietic cell kinetics in humans treated with rGM-CSF. *Int J Cancer* 1992; 50:26–31.

103. Coleman DL, Chodakewitz JA, Bartiss AH, et al: Granulocyte-macrophage colony stimulating factor enhances selective effector functions of tissue-derived macrophages. *Blood* 1988; 72:573–578.

104. Fischer HG, Frosch S, Reske K, et al: Granulocyte-macrophage colony-

stimulating factor activates macrophages derived from bone marrow cultures to synthesis of MHC class II molecules and to augmented antigen presentation function. *J Immunol* 1988; 141:3882–3888.

105. Metcalf D, Begley CG, Williamson DJ, et al: Hemopoietic responses in mice injected with purified recombinant murine GM-CSF. *Exp Hematol* 1987; 15:1–9.
106. Lieschke GJ, Burgess AW: Granulocyte colony-stimulating factor and granulocyte-macrophage colony-stimulating factor. (Second of two parts). *N Engl J Med* 1992; 327:99–106.
107. Peters WP, Shogan J, Shapall EJ, et al: Recombinant human granulocyte-macrophage colony stimulating factor produces fever. *Lancet* 1988; 1:950.
108. Crawford J, Ozer H, Stoller R, et al: Reduction by granulocyte colony stimulating factor of fever and neutropenia induced by chemotherapy in patients with small-cell lung cancer. *N Engl J Med* 1991; 325:164–170.
109. Kotake T, Miki T, Akaza H: Effect of recombinant granulocyte colony-stimulating factor (rG-CSF) on chemotherapy-induced neutropenia in patients with urogenital cancer. *Cancer Chemother Pharmacol* 1991; 27:253–257.
110. Taylor KM, Jagannath S, Spitzer G, et al: Recombinant human granulocyte colony-stimulating factor hastens granulocyte recovery after high-dose chemotherapy and autologous bone marrow transplantation in Hodgkin's disease. *J Clin Oncol* 1989; 7:1791–1799.
111. Sheridan WP, Morstyn G, Wolf M, et al: Granulocyte colony-stimulating factor and neutrophil recovery after high-dose chemotherapy and autologous bone marrow transplantation. *Lancet* 1989; 2:891–895.
112. Devereaux S, Linch DC, Gribben JG, et al: GM-CSF accelerates neutrophil recovery after autologous bone marrow transplantation for Hodgkin's disease. *Bone Marrow Transplant* 1989; 4:49–54.
113. Blazer BR, Kersey JH, McGlave PB, et al: In vivo administration of recombinant human granulocyte/macrophage colony-stimulating factor in acute

lymphoblastic leukemia patients receiving purged autografts. *Blood* 1989; 73:849–857.
114. Nemunaitis J, Singer JW, Buckner CD, et al: Use of recombinant human granulocyte-macrophage colony stimulating factor in autologous marrow transplantation for lymphoid malignancies. *Blood* 1988; 72:834–836.
115. Brandt SJ, Peters WP, Atwater SK, et al: Effect of recombinant human granulocyte-macrophage colony-stimulating factor on hematopoietic reconstitution after high-dose chemotherapy and autologous marrow transplantation. *N Engl J Med* 1988; 318:869–876.
116. Masaoka T, Moriyama Y, Kato S: A randomized, placebo-controlled study of KRN8601 (recombinant human granulocyte colony-stimulating factor) in patients receiving allogeneic bone marrow transplantation. *Jpn J Med* 1990; 3:233–239.
117. Nemunaitis J, Buckner CD, Apelbaum FR, et al: Phase I/II trial of recombinant human granulocyte-macrophage colony-stimulating factor following allogeneic bone marrow transplantation. *Blood* 1991; 77:2065–2075.
118. Powles R, Smith C, Milan S, et al: Human recombinant GM-CSF in allogeneic bone-marrow transplantation of leukaemia: Double-blind, placebo-controlled trial. *Lancet* 1990; 1:1417–1420.
119. Gianni AM, Siena S, Bregni M, et al: Granulocyte-macrophage colony-stimulating factor to harvest circulating haemopoietic stem cells for auto-transplantation. *Lancet* 1989; 2:580–585.
120. Sheridan WP, Begley CG, Juttner CA, et al: Effect of peripheral-blood progenitor cells mobilized by filgrastim (G-CSF) on platelet recovery after high-dose chemotherapy. *Lancet* 1992; 1:640–644.
121. Mempel K, Pietsch T, Menzel T, et al: Increased serum levels of granulocyte colony-stimulating factor in patients with severe congenital neutropenia. *Blood* 1991; 77:1919–1922.
122. Jakubowski A, Souza L, Kelly F, et al: Effects of human granulocyte colony-stimulating factor in a patient with idiopathic neutropenia. *N Engl J Med* 1989; 320:38–42.

123. Dale DC, Hammond WP, Gabrilove J: Long term treatment of severe chronic neutropenia with recombinant human granulocyte factor (r-metHuG-CSF), (abstract). *Blood* 1990; 76(suppl 1):139.

124. Migliaccio AR, Migliaccio G, Dale DC, et al: Hematopoietic progenitors in cyclic neutropenia: Effect of granulocyte colony-stimulating factor in vivo. *Blood* 1990; 75:1951–1959.

125. Hammond WPIV, Price TH, Souza LM, et al: Treatment of cyclic neutropenia with granulocyte colony-stimulating factor. *New Engl J Med* 1989; 320:1306–1311.

126. Kojima S, Fukuda M, Miyajima Y, et al: Treatment of aplastic anemia in children with recombinant human granulocyte colony-stimulating factor. *Blood* 1991; 77:937–941.

127. Antin JH, Smith BR, Holmes W, et al: Phase I/II study of recombinant human granulocyte-macrophage colony-stimulating factor in aplastic anemia and myelodysplastic syndrome. *Blood* 1988; 72:705–713.

128. Champlin RE, Nimer SD, Ireland P, et al: Treatment of refractory aplastic anemia with recombinant human granulocyte-macrophage–colony-stimulating factor. *Blood* 1989; 73:694–699.

129. Nissen C, Tichelli A, Gratwohl A, et al: Failure of recombinant human granulocyte-macrophage colony-stimulating factor therapy in aplastic anemia patients with very severe neutropenia. *Blood* 1988; 72:2045–2047.

130. Vadhan-Raj S, Buescher S, Broxmeyer HE, et al: Stimulation of myelosuppression in patients with aplastic anemia by recombinant human granulocyte-macrophage colony-stimulating factor. *N Engl J Med* 1988; 319:1628–1634.

131. Perno CF, Yarchoan R, Cooney DA, et al: Replication of human immunodeficiency virus in monocytes: Granulocyte/macrophage colony-stimulating factor (GM-CSF) potentiates viral production yet enhances the antiviral effect mediated by 3'-azido-2'3'-dideoxythymidine (AZT) and other dideoxynucleoside congeners of thymidine. *J Exp Med* 1989; 169:933–951.

132. Pluda JM, Yarchoan R, Smith PD, et al: Subcutaneous recombinant granulocyte-macrophage colony-stimulating factor used as a single agent and in an alternating regimen with azidothymidine in leukopenic patients with severe immunodeficiency virus infection. *Blood* 1990; 76:463–472.

133. Groopman JE, Mitsuyasu RT, DeLeo MJ, et al: Effect of recombinant human granulocyte-macrophage colony-stimulating factor on myelopoiesis in the acquired immunodeficiency syndrome. *N Engl J Med* 1987; 317:593–598.

134. Negrin RS, Haeuber DH, Nagler A, et al: Treatment of myelodysplastic syndromes with recombinant human granulocyte colony-stimulating factor: A phase I-II trial. *Ann Intern Med* 1989; 110:976–984.

135. Negrin RS, Haeuber DH, Nagler A, et al: Maintenance treatment of patients with myelodysplastic syndromes using recombinant human granulocyte colony-stimulating factor. *Blood* 1990; 76:36–43.

136. Schuster MW, Larson RA, Thompson JA: Granulocyte-macrophage colony-stimulating factor (GM-CSF) for myelodysplastic syndrome (MDS): Results of a multi-center randomized controlled trial (abstract). *Blood* 1990; 76(suppl 1):318.

137. Herrmann F, Lindemann A, Klein H, et al: Effect of recombinant human granulocyte-macrophage colony-stimulating factor in patients with myelodysplastic syndrome with excess blasts. *Leukemia* 1989; 3:335–338.

138. Ganser A, Volkers B, Greher J, et al: Recombinant human granulocyte-macrophage colony-stimulating factor in patients with myelodysplastic syndromes—a phase I/II trial. *Blood* 1989; 73: 31–37.

139. Valdhan-Raj S, Keating M, LeMaistre A, et al: Effects of recombinant human granulocyte-macrophage colony-stimulating factor in patients with myelodysplastic syndromes. *N Engl J Med* 1987; 317:1545–1552.

140. Ohno R, Tomonaga M, Kobayashi T, et al: Effect of granulocyte colony-stimulating factor after intensive induction therapy in relapsed or refrac-

tory acute leukemia. *N Engl J Med* 1990; 323:871–877.

141. Estey EH, Dixon D, Kantarjian HM, et al: Treatment of poor-prognosis, newly diagnosed acute myeloid leukemia with ara-C and recombinant human granulocyte-macrophage colony-stimulating factor. *Blood* 1990; 75:1766–1769.

142. Buchner T, Hiddemann W, Koenigsman M, et al: Recombinant human granulocyte-macrophage colony-stimulating factor after chemotherapy in patients with acute myeloid leukemia at higher age or after relapse. *Blood* 1991; 78:1190–1197.

143. Miyauchi J, Kelleher CA, Yang YC, et al: The effect of three recombinant growth factors, IL-3, GM-CSF and G-CSF, on the blast cells of acute myeloblastic leukemia maintained in short term suspension culture. *Blood* 1987; 70:657–663.

144. Vellenga E, Ostapovicz D, O'Rourke B, et al: Effect of recombinant IL-3, GM-CSF, and G-CSF on proliferation of leukemic clonogenic cells in short term and long term cultures. *Leukemia* 1987; 1:584–589.

145. Griffen JD, Young D, Herrmann F, et al: Effects of recombinant human GM-CSF on proliferation of clonogenic cells in acute myeloblastic leukemia. *Blood* 1986; 67:1488–1453.

146. Cioffi WG, Burleson DG, Jorden BS, et al: Effects of granulocyte-macrophage colony-stimulating factor in burn patients. *Arch Surg* 1991; 126:74–79.

147. Sartorelli KH, Silver GM, Gamelli RL: The effect of granulocyte colony-stimulating factor (G-CSF) upon burn-induced defective neutrophil chemotaxis. *J Trauma* 1991; 31:523–530.

148. Mooney DP, Gamelli RL, O'Reilly M, et al: Recombinant human granulocyte colony-stimulating factor and *Pseudomonas* burn wound sepsis. *Arch Surg* 1988; 123:1353–1357.

149. Gorgen I, Hartung T, Leist M, et al: Granulocyte colony-stimulating factor treatment protects rodents against lipopolysaccharide-induced toxicity via suppression of systemic tumor necrosis factor-alpha. *J Immunol* 1992; 149:918–924.

150. Abraham E, Stevens P: Effects of granulocyte colony-stimulating factor in modifying mortality from *Pseudomonas aeruginosa* pneumonia after hemorrhage. *Crit Care Med* 1992; 20:1127–1133.

151. Rose RM: The role of colony-stimulating factors in infectious disease: Current status, future challenges. *Semin Oncol* 1992; 19:415–421.

152. Nemunaitis J, Meyers JD, Buckner CD, et al: Phase I trial of recombinant human macrophage colony-stimulating factor in patients with invasive fungal infections. *Blood* 1991; 78:907–913.

153. Wold F: In vivo modification of proteins (post-translational modification). *Annu Rev Biochem* 1981; 50:783.

154. Steiner DF, Oyer PE: The biosynthesis of insulin and a probable precursor of insulin by a human islet cell adenoma. *Proc Natl Acad Sci U S A* 1967; 57:473.

155. Steiner DF, Cunningham L, Spigelman L, et al: Insulin biosynthesis: Evidence for a precursor. *Science* 1967; 157:697.

156. Gordon P, Roth J: Plasma insulin: Fluctuations in the "big" insulin component in man after glucose and other stimuli. *J Clin Invest* 1969; 48:2225–2234.

157. Porte DJ, Popo AA: Insulin responses to glucose: Evidence for a two pool system in man. *J Clin Invest* 1969; 48:2309–2319.

158. Hopfer U, Groseclose R: The mechanism of a Na-dependent glucose transport. *J Biol Chem* 1980; 255:4453.

159. Genuth SM: The endocrine system, in Berne RM, Levy MN (eds): *Physiology.* St Louis, Mosby–Year Book, 1983.

160. Noguchi T, Inoue H, Taneka T: Regulation of rat liver L-type pyruvate kinase mRNA by insulin and fructose. *Eur J Biochem* 1982; 128:583–588.

161. Okamura K, Okuma T, Tabira Y, et al: Effect of administered human growth hormone on protein metabolism in septic rats. *JPEN* 1989; 13:450–454.

162. Jefferson LS, Rannels DE, Munger BL, et al: Insulin in the regulation of protein turnover in heart and skeletal muscle. *Fed Proc* 1974; 33:1098–1104.

163. Larner J: Insulin and glycogen synthase. *Diabetes* 1971; 21:428.

164. Geelen MJH, Harris RA, Beynen AC, et al: Short term hormonal control of hepatic lipogenesis. *Diabetes* 1980; 29:1006–1022.

165. Jefferson LS, Li JB, Rannels DE: Regulation by insulin of amino acid release and protein turnover in the perfused rat hemicorpus. *J Biol Chem* 1977; 252:1476–1483.

166. Jefferson LS: Role of insulin in the regulation of protein synthesis. *Diabetes* 1980; 29:487–496.

167. Huijing F: Glycogen metabolism and glycogen storage disease. *Physiol Rev* 1975; 55:609.

168. Hinton P, Allison SP, Littlejohn S, et al: Insulin and glucose to reduce catabolic response to injury in burned patients. *Lancet* 1971; 1:767–769.

169. Woolfson AMJ, Heatley RV, Allison SP: Insulin to inhibit protein catabolism after injury. *N Engl J Med* 1979; 300:14–17.

170. Inculet RI, Finley RJ, Duff JH, et al: Insulin decreases muscle protein loss after operative trauma in man. *Surgery* 1986; 99:752–758.

171. Burke JF, Wolfe RR, Mullany CJ, et al: Glucose requirements following burn injury. *Ann Surg* 1979; 190:274–285.

172. Wolf RF, Heslin MJ, Newman E, et al: Growth hormone and insulin combine to improve whole body and skeletal muscle protein kinetics. *Surgery* 1992; 112:284–291.

173. Wolf RF, Pearlstone DB, Newman E, et al: Growth hormone and insulin reverse net whole body and skeletal protein catabolism in cancer patients. *Ann Surg* 1992; 216:280–290.

174. Reuchlin S: Neuroendocrinology, in Wilson JD, Foster DW (eds): *William's Textbook of Endocrinology.* Philadelphia, WB Saunders, 1991.

175. Wilmore DW, Orcutt TW, Mason AD, et al: Alterations in hypothalamic function following thermal injury. *J Trauma* 1975; 15:697–703.

176. Andrews GS: Growth hormone and malignacy. *J Clin Pathol* 1983; 36:935–937.

177. Solomon N, Copeland EM, MacFayden BV: Intravenous hyperalimentation and growth hormone in cancer patients. *Surg Forum* 1974; 25:59–60.

178. Carey LC, Cloutier CT, Lowery BD: Growth hormone and adrenal cortical response to shock and trauma in the human. *Ann Surg* 1971; 174:451–460.

179. Fischer JE: A teleological view of sepsis. *Clin Nutr* 1991; 10:1–9.

180. Bazzaro TL, Johanson AJ, Huseman CA: *Growth Hormone and Related Peptides.* Amsterdam, Excerpta Medica, 1976, pp 261–270.

181. Barber AE, Marano MA, Fong Y, et al: Circadian rhythms of growth hormone and cortisol in parenterally fed man. *Clin Nutr* 1989; 8(suppl):50.

182. Leung DW, Spencer SA, Cachianes G, et al: Growth hormone receptor and serum binding protein: Purification, cloning, and expression. *Nature* 1987; 330:537–543.

183. Baumann G, Stolar MW, Amburn K, et al: A specific growth hormone–binding protein in human plasma: Initial characterization. *J Clin Endocrinol Metab* 1986; 62:134–141.

184. Baumann G, Shaw MA: A second lower affinity growth hormone binding protein in human plasma. *J Clin Endocrinol Metab* 1990; 70:680–686.

185. Baumann G, Shaw MA, Amburn K: Regulation of plasma growth hormone–binding protein in health and disease. *Metabolism* 1989; 38:683–689.

186. Baumann G, Amburn K, Buchanan TA: The effect of circulating growth hormone binding protein on metabolic clearance, distribution, and degradation of human growth hormone. *J Clin Endocrinol Metab* 1987; 64:657–660.

187. Herrington AC, Ymer S, Stevenson J: Identification and characterization of specific binding protein for growth hormone in normal sera. *J Clin Invest* 1986; 77:1817–1823.

188. Manson JM, Smith RJ, Wilmore DW: Growth hormone stimulates protein synthesis during hypocaloric parenteral nutrition. Role of hormonal-substrate environment. *Ann Surg* 1988; 208:136–142.

189. Douglas RG, Humberstone DA, Haystead A, et al: Metabolic effect of re-

combinant human growth hormone: Isotopic studies in the post absorptive state and during total parenteral nutrition. *Br J Surg* 1990; 77:785–790.

190. Fong Y, Rosenbaum M, Tracey KJ, et al: Recombinant growth hormone enhances muscle myosin heavy-chain mRNA accumulation and amino acid accrual in humans. *Proc Natl Acad Sci U S A* 1989; 86:3371–3374.

191. Bratusch-Marrain PR, Smith D, DeFronzo RA: The effect of growth hormone on splanchnic glucose and substrate metabolism following oral glucose loading in healthy man. *Diabetes* 1984; 33:19–25.

192. Bishop JS, Steele R, Altszuler N, et al: Diminished responsiveness to insulin in the growth hormone treated normal dog. *Am J Physiol* 1967; 212:272–278.

193. Bratusch-Marrain PR, Smith D, DeFronzo RA: The effect of growth hormone on glucose metabolism and insulin secretion in man. *J Clin Endocrinol Metab* 1982; 55:973–982.

194. Adamson U, Wahron J, Cerasi E: Influence of growth hormone on splanchnic glucose production in man. *Acta Endocrinol* 1977; 86:803–812.

195. Cheng JS, Kalent N: Effects of insulin and growth hormone on the flux rates of plasma glucose and free fatty acids in man. *J Clin Endocrinol Metab* 1970; 31:647–653.

196. Rabinowitz D, Klassen G, Zierler KL: Effect of human growth hormone on muscle and adipose tissue metabolism in the forearm of man. *J Clin Invest* 1965; 44:51–61.

197. Galbraith HJB, Ginsberg J, Paton A: Decreased response to intraarterial insulin in acromegaly. *Diabetes* 1960; 9:459–465.

198. Schulman G, Seman V, Tamborlane V, et al: Rapid onset of diabetogenic effect of physiological increments of growth hormone (abstract). *Clin Res* 1980; 28:266.

199. Fineberg SE, Merimee TJ: Acute metabolic effects of human growth hormone. *Diabetes* 1974; 23:499–504.

200. Kostyo JL, Cameron CM, Olsen KC, et al: Biosynthetic 20-kilodalton methionyl–human growth hormone has diabetogenic and insulin-like activities. *Proc Natl Acad Sci U S A* 1985; 82:4250–4253.

201. Goodman HM: Multiple effects of growth hormone on lipolysis. *Endocrinology* 1968; 83:300–308.

202. Fain JN: Effect of dibutyryl-3', 5'-AMP, theophylline, and norepinephrine on lipolytic action of growth hormone and glucocorticoid on white fat cells. *Endocrinology* 1968; 82:825–830.

203. Goodman HM: The effects of epinephrine on glycerol production in segments of adipose tissue preincubated with dexamethasone and growth hormone. *Proc Soc Exp Biol Med* 1969; 130:909–912.

204. Gilman G: G proteins and dual control of adenylate cyclase. *Cell* 1984; 36:577–579.

205. Goodman HM, Gorin E, Honeyman TW: Biochemical basis for the lipolytic activity of growth hormone, in Underwood LE (ed): *Human Growth Hormone.* New York, Marcel Dekker, 1988, pp 75–111

206. Fong Y, Rosenbaum M, Hesse DG, et al: Influence of substrate background on peripheral tissue response to growth hormone. *J Surg Res* 1988; 44:702–708.

207. Manson JM, Wilmore DW: Positive nitrogen balance with growth hormone and hypocaloric intravenous feeding. *Surgery* 1986; 100:188–197.

208. Ward HC, Halliday D, Sim AJW: Protein and energy metabolism with biosynthetic human growth hormone after gastrointestinal surgery. *Ann Surg* 1987; 206:56–61.

209. Ponting GA, Ward HC, Halliday D, et al: Protein and energy metabolism with biosynthetic human growth hormone. *JPEN* 1990; 14:437–441.

210. Cuthbertson DP, Shaw GB, Young FG: The influence of anterior pituitary extract on the metabolic response of the rat to injury. *J Endocrinol* 1941; 2:468–474.

211. Prudden JF, Pearson E, Soroff HS: Studies on growth hormone: The effect on the nitrogen metabolism of severely burned patients. *Surg Gynecol Obstet* 1956; 102:695–701.

212. Pearson E, Soroff HS, Prudden JF, et

al: Studies on growth hormone: V. Effect on the mineral and nitrogen balances of burned patients. *Am J Med Sci* 1960; 239:17–26.

213. Liljedahl S, Gemzell C, Plantin L, et al: Effect of human growth hormone in patients with severe burns. *Acta Chir Scand* 1961; 122:1–14.

214. Roe CF, Kinney JM: The influence of human growth hormone on energy sources in convalescence. *Surg Forum* 1962; 13:369–371.

215. Soroff HS, Rozin RR, Mooty J, et al: Role of human growth hormone in the response to trauma: I. Metabolic effects following burns. *Ann Surg* 1967; 166:739–752.

216. Wilmore DW, Moylan JA, Bristow BF, et al: Anabolic effects of human growth hormone and high caloric feedings following thermal injury. *Surg Gynecol Obstet* 1974; 138:875–884.

217. Snyder DK, Clemmons DR, Underwood LE: Treatment of obese, diet restricted subjects with growth hormone for 11 weeks; effects on anabolism, lipolysis, and body composition. *J Clin Endocrinol Metab* 1988; 67:54–61.

218. Jiang Z, He G, Zhang S, et al: Low dose growth hormone and hypocaloric nutrition attenuate the protein-catabolic response after major operation. *Ann Surg* 1989; 210:513–525.

219. Pape GS, Friedman M, Underwood LE, et al: The effect of growth hormone on weight gain and pulmonary function in patients with chronic obstructive lung disease. *Chest* 1991; 99:1495–1500.

220. Hammarqvist F, Stronberg C, von der Decken A, et al: Biosynthetic human growth hormone preserves both muscle protein synthesis and the decrease in muscle-free glutamine, and improves whole-body nitrogen economy after operation. *Ann Surg* 1992; 216:184–191.

221. Ziegler TR, Rombeau JL, Young LS, et al: Recombinant human growth hormone enhances the metabolic efficacy of parenteral nutrition: A double-blinded, randomized controlled study. *J Clin Endocrinol Metab* 1992; 74:865–873.

222. Belcher HJCR, Mercer D, Judkins KC,

et al: Biosynthetic human growth hormone in burned patients: A pilot study. *Burns* 1989; 15:99–107.

223. Dahn MS, Lange P, Jacobs LA: Insulin-like growth factor 1 production is inhibited in human sepsis. *Arch Surg* 1988; 123:1409–1414.

224. Ross R, Miell J, Freeman E, et al: Critically ill patients have high basal growth hormone levels with attenuated oscillatory activity associated with low levels of insulin-like growth factor-I. *Clin Endocrinol* 1991; 35:47–54.

225. Rinderknecht E, Humbel RE: The amino acid sequence of human insulin-like growth factor 1 and its structural homology to proinsulin. *J Biol Chem* 1971; 253:2769–2776.

226. Ullrich A, Gray A, Tam AW, et al: Insulin-like growth factor I receptor primary structure: Comparison with insulin receptor suggests structural determinants that define functional specificity. *EMBO J* 1986; 5:2503–2512.

227. Saenger P, Levine LS, Wiedemann E, et al: Growth with absent growth hormone by radioimmunoassay. *J Pediatr* 1974; 85:137–138.

228. Kenny FM, Guyda HJ, Wright JC, et al: Prolactin and somatomedin in hypopituitary patients with "catch-up" growth following operations for craniopharyngioma. *J Clin Endocrinol Metab* 1973; 36:378–380.

229. Schwarz E, Wiedemann E, Simon S, et al: Estrogenic antagonism of metabolic effects of administered growth hormone. *J Clin Endocrinol Metab* 1969; 29:1176–1181.

230. Sara V, Hall K: Insulin-like growth factors and their binding proteins. *Physiol Rev* 1990; 70:591–614.

231. Lazarus DD, Marano M, Fisher E, et al: Interleukin-1 causes a decrease in plasma IGF-1 concentrations in baboons. *Clin Nutr* 1990; 9(suppl):5.

232. Coates CL, Burwell RG, Carlin SA, et al: Somatomedin activity in plasma from burned patients with observations on plasma cortisol. *Burns* 1981; 7:425–433.

233. Grant DB, Hambley J, Becker D, et al: Reduced sulphation factor in undernourished children. *Arch Dis Child* 1973; 48:596–600.

234. Winter RJ, Phillips LS, Klein MN, et al: Somatomedin activity and diabetic control in children with insulin-dependent diabetes. *Diabetes* 1979; 28:952–954.

235. Elders MJ, Wingfield BS, McNatt ML, et al: Glucocorticoid therapy in children: Effect on somatomedin secretion. *Am J Dis Child* 1975; 129:1393–1396.

236. Wu A, Grant DB, Hanhley J, et al: Reduced serum somatomedin activity in patients with chronic liver disease. *Cli Sci Mol Med* 1974; 47:359–366.

237. Lewy JE, Van Wyk JJ: Somatomedin and growth retardation in children with chronic renal insufficiency. *Kidney Int* 1978; 14:361–364.

238. Isley W, Underwood LE, Clemmons DR: Changes in plasma somatomedin-C in response to ingestion of diets with variable protein and energy content. *JPEN* 1984; 8:407.

239. Clemmons DR, Seek MM, Underwood LE: Supplemental essential amino acids augment the somatomedin-C/insulin-like growth factor I response to refeeding after fasting. *Metabolism* 1985; 34:391–395.

240. Donovan SM, Hintz RL, Rosenfeld RG: Insulin-like growth factors I and II and their binding proteins in human milk: Effect of heat treatment on IGF and IGF binding protein stability. *J Pediatr Gastroenterol Nutr* 1991; 13:242–253.

241. Zapf J, Schmid C, Guler HP, et al: Regulation of binding proteins for insulin-like growth factors in humans. *J Clin Invest* 1990; 86:952–961.

242. Baxter RC: Physiological roles of the IGF binding proteins. 2nd International Symposium on the Insulin-like Growth Factors/Somatomedins (abstract). 1991; 2:22.

243. Clemmons DR: Insulin-like growth factor binding proteins: Roles in regulating IGF physiology. *J Dev Physiol* 1991; 15:105–110.

244. Clemmons DR, Underwood LE: Nutritional regulation of IGF-1 and IGF binding proteins. *Annu Rev Nutr* 1991; 11:393–412.

245. Moxley RT, Arner P, Moss A, et al: Acute effects of insulin-like growth factor 1 and insulin on glucose metabolism in vivo. *Am J Physiol* 1990; 259:561–567.

246. Guler HP, Zapf J, Froesch ER: Short term metabolic effects on insulin-like growth factor 1 in healthy adults. *N Engl J Med* 1987; 317:137–140.

247. Badesch DB, Lee PDK, Stenmark KR: Insulin-like growth factor stimulates elastin synthesis by bovine pulmonary smooth muscle cells. *Biochem Biophys Res Commun* 1989; 160:382–387.

248. Jacob R, Barret E, Plowe G, et al: Acute effects of insulin-like growth factor 1 on glucose and amino acid metabolism in the awake fasted rat. *J Clin Invest* 1989; 83:1717–1723.

249. Thompson WA, Coyle S, Lazarus D, et al: The metabolic effects of a continuous infusion of insulin-like growth factor-1 (IGF-1) in parenterally fed man. *Surg Forum* 1991; 42:23–25.

250. Lemmey AB, Martin AA, Read LC, et al: IGF-1 and the truncated analogue des-(1-3) IGF-1 enhance growth in rats after gut resection. *Am J Physiol* 1991; 260:213–219.

251. Seidel ER, Chaurasia O, Groblewski GE: Intraluminal IGF-1 and stimulation of gastrointestinal mucosal growth. 2nd International Symposium on the Insulin-like Growth Factors/Somatomedins (abstract). 1991; 2:54.

252. Kruskemper HL: *Anabolic Steroids.* New York, Academic Press, 1968.

253. Rogozkin V: Metabolic effects of anabolic steroid on skeletal muscle. *Med Sci Sports* 1979; 11:160–163.

254. Mayer M, Rosen F: Interaction of anabolic steroids with glucocorticoid receptor sites in rat muscle cytosol. *Am J Physiol* 1975; 229:1381–1386.

255. Seene T, Viru A: The catabolic effect of glucocorticoids on different types of skeletal muscle fibres and its dependence upon muscle activity and interaction with anabolic steroids. *J Steroid Biochem* 1982; 16:349–352.

256. Hausmann DF, Nutz V, Rommelsheim K, et al: Anabolic steroids in polytrauma patients. Influence on renal nitrogen and amino acid losses: A double-blind study. *JPEN* 1990; 14:111–114.

257. Abels JC, Young NF, Taylor HC: Effects of testosterone and of testosterone propionate on protein formation

in man. *J Clin Endocrinol Metab* 1944; 4:198–201.

258. Davies D, Pines A: Effect of methylandrostenediol on post-operative loss of weight. *BMJ* 1955; 1:200–201.

259. Kennedy JH, Peters HA, Serif GS: Observations on the effect of norethandrolone in favoring anabolism in patients undergoing pulmonary resection for tuberculosis. *Surg Forum* 1959; 9:364–367.

260. Johnston IDA, Chenneour R: The effect of methandienone on the metabolic response to surgical operation. *Br J Surg* 1963; 50:924–928.

261. Abbott WE, Levey S, Kreiger H, et al: The effect of 19-nortestosterone cyclopentylpropionate on nitrogen balance and body weight in postoperative patients. *Surg Forum* 1954; 4:80–83.

262. Danylewick RW, Almasi M, Shizgal HM: Effect of an anabolic steroid on the efficacy of total parenteral nutrition. *Surg Forum* 1989; 40:1–4.

263. Hansell DT, Davies JW, Shenkin A, et al: The effects of an anabolic steroid and peripherally administered intravenous nutrition in the early postoperative period. *JPEN* 1989; 13:349–358.

264. Michelsen CB, Askanazi J, Kinney JM, et al: Effect of an anabolic steroid on nitrogen balance and amino acid patterns after total hip replacement. *J Trauma* 1982; 22:410–413.

265. Young GA, Yule AG, Hill GL: Effects of an anabolic steroid on plasma amino acids, proteins, and body composition in patients receiving intravenous hyperalimentation. *JPEN* 1983; 7:221–225.

266. Bonkovsky HL, Fiellin DA, Smith GS, et al: A randomized, controlled trial of treatment of alcoholic hepatitis with parenteral nutrition and oxandrolone. I. Short-term effects on liver function. *Am J Gastroenterol* 191; 86:1200–1208.

267. Damste PH: Voice change in adult women caused by virilizing agents. *J Speech Hear Disord* 1967; 32:126.

268. Wilson JD, Aiman J, MacDonald PC: The pathogenesis of gynecomastia. *Adv Intern Med* 1980; 25:1.

269. Camino-Torres R, Ma L, Snyder PJ: Testosterone induced inhibition of the LH and FSH responses to gonadotropin-releasing hormone oc-

curs slowly. *J Clin Endocrinol Metab* 1977; 44:1142.

270. Haffner SM, Kushwaha RS, Foster DM, et al: Studies on the metabolic mechanism of reduced high density lipoproteins during anabolic steroid therapy. *Metabolism* 1983; 32:413.

271. Sandblom RE, Matsumoto AM, Schoene RB, et al: Obstructive sleep apnea induced by testosterone administration. *N Engl J Med* 1983; 208:508.

272. Turani H, Levi J, Zevin D, et al: Hepatic lesions in patients on anabolic androgenic therapy. *Isr J Med Sci* 1983; 19:332.

273. Levi-Montalcini R, Cohen S: Effects of the extracts of the mouse submaxillary salivary glands on the sympathetic system of mammals. *Ann N Y Acad Sci* 1960; 85:324–341.

274. Cohen S, Elliott GA: The stimulation of epidermal keratinization by a protein isolated from submaxillary gland of the mouse. *J Invest Dermatol* 1963; 40:1–5.

275. Cohen S: Isolation of a mouse submaxillary gland protein accelerating incisor eruption and eyelid opening in the new-born animal. *J Biol Chem* 1962; 237:1555–1562.

276. Savage CR, Inagami T, Cohen S: The primary structure of epidermal growth factor. *J Biol Chem* 1972; 247:7612–7621.

277. Hirata Y, Orth DN: Epidermal growth factor (urogastrone) in human tissues. *J Clin Endocrinol Metab* 1979; 48:667–672.

278. Hirata Y, Orth DN: Epidermal growth factor (urogastrone) in human fluids: Size heterogeneity. *J Clin Endocrinol Metab* 1979; 48:673–679.

279. Konturek JW, Bielanski W, Olesky J, et al: Distribution and release of epidermal growth factor in humans. *Gut* 1989; 30:1189–1200.

280. Jaworek J, Konturek SJ: Distribution, release and secretory activity of epidermal growth factor in the pancreas. *Int J Pancreatol* 1990; 6:189–196.

281. Rall LB, Scott J, Bell GI: Mouse prepro-epidermal growth factor synthesis by the kidney and other tissues. *Nature* 1985; 313:228–231.

282. Olsen PS, Nexo E, Poulsen SS, et al:

Renal origin of rat epidermal growth factor. *Regul Pept* 1985; 10:767–771.

283. Fallon JH, Serogy KB, Loughlin SE: Epidermal growth factor immunoreactive material in the central nervous system: Location and development. *Science* 1984; 224:1107–1109.

284. Plata-Salaman CR: Epidermal growth factor and the nervous system. *Peptides* 1991; 12:653–663.

285. Han VK, Hunter ES III, Pratt RM: Expression of rat transforming growth factor alpha mRNA during development occurs predominantly in the maternal decidua. *Mol Cell Biol* 1987; 7:2335–2343.

286. Oka Y, Orth DN: Human plasma epidermal growth factor urogastrone in association with blood platelets. *J Clin Invest* 1983; 72:249–259.

287. Byyny RL, Orth DN, Cohen S: Radio-immunoassay of epidermal growth factor. *Endocrinology* 1972; 90:1261–1266.

288. Starkey RH, Cohen S, Orth DN: Epidermal growth factor: Identification of a new hormone in human urine. *Science* 1975; 189:800–802.

289. Gregory H: Isolation and structure of urogastrone and its relationship to epidermal growth factor. *Nature* 1975; 257:325–327.

290. Koldovsky O: Is breast-milk epidermal growth factor biologically active in the suckling? *Nutrition* 1989; 5:233–235.

291. McCleary MJ: Epidermal growth factor: An important constituent of human milk. *J Hum Lact* 1991; 7:123–128.

292. van-Setten GB, Tervo T, Viinikka L, et al: Epidermal growth factor in human tear fluid: A minireview. *Int Opthalmol* 1991; 15:359–362.

293. Connolly JM, Rose DP: Epidermal growth factor–like proteins in breast fluid and human milk. *Life Sci* 1988; 42:1751–1756.

294. Konturek SJ, Pawlik W, Mysh W: Comparison of organ uptake and disappearance half-time of human epidermal growth factor and insulin. *Regul Pept* 1990; 30:137–148.

295. Sporn MB, Roberts AB, Wakefield LM, et al: Transforming growth factor beta: Biological function and chemical structure. *Science* 1986; 233:532–534.

296. Downward J, Yarden Y, Mayes E: Close similarity of epidermal growth factor receptor and V-*erb* B oncogene protein sequences. *Nature* 1984; 307:521–527.

297. Miyazawa K: Role of epidermal growth factor in obstetrics and gynecology. *Obstet Gynecol* 1992; 79:1032–1040.

298. Hammerman MR, Rogers SA, Ryan G: Growth factors and metanephrogenesis. *Am J Physiol* 1992; 262:523–532.

299. Leung BS: Perspective: Growth factors in normal and abnormal fetal growth. *In Vivo* 1987; 1:363–368.

300. Brown GL, Curtsinger L III, Brightwell JR, et al: Enhancement of epidermal regeneration by biosynthetic epidermal growth factor. *J Exp Med* 1986; 163:1319–1324.

301. Brown GL, Curtsinger LJ, White M, et al: Acceleration of tensile strength of incisions treated with EGF and TGF-β. *Ann Surg* 1988; 208:788–794.

302. Brown GL, Nanney LB, Griffen J, et al: Enhancement of wound healing by tropical treatment with epidermal growth factor. *N Engl J Med* 1989; 321:76–79.

303. Jijon AJ, Gallup DG, Behzadian MA, et al: Assessment of epidermal growth factor in the healing process of clean full-thickness skin wounds. *Am J Obstet Gynecol* 1989; 161:1658–1662.

304. Pittelkow MR: Growth factors in cutaneous biology and disease. *Adv Dermatol* 1992; 7:55–81.

305. Konturek SJ: Role of growth factors in gastroduodenal protection and healing of peptic ulcers. *Gastroenterol Clin North Am* 1990; 19:41–65.

306. Shaw GP, Halt JF, Anderson NG, et al: Action of epidermal growth factor on acid secretion by rat isolate parietal cells. *Biochem J* 1987; 244:699–704.

307. Konturek JW, Brzozowski T, Konturek SJ: Epidermal growth factor in protection, repair, and healing of gastroduodenal mucosa. *J Clin Gastroenterol* 1991; 13(suppl 1):88–97.

308. Weaver LT, Walker WA: Epidermal growth factor and the developing human gut. *Gastroenterology* 1988; 94:845–847.

309. Lebenthal E, Leung YK: Epidermal

growth factor (EGF) and the ontogeny of the gut. *J Pediatr Gastroenterol Nutr* 1987; 6:1–5.

310. Lentze MJ: Intestinal adaptation in short-bowel syndrome. *Eur J Pediatr* 1989; 148:294–299.

311. Read LC, Ford WD, Filsell OH, et al: Is orally-derived epidermal growth factor beneficial following premature birth or intestinal resection? *Endocrinol Exp* 1986; 20:199–207.

312. Johnson LR, Copeland EM, Dudrick SJ, et al: Structural and hormonal alterations in the gastrointestinal tract of parenterally fed rats. *Gastroenterology* 1975; 68:1177–1183.

313. Hosudo N, Nishi M, Nakagawa M, et al: Structural and functional alterations in the gut of parenterally or enterally fed rats. *J Surg Res* 1989; 47:129–133.

314. Alverdy J, Chi HS, Sheldon GF: The effect of parenteral nutrition on gastrointestinal immunity. *Ann Surg* 1985; 202:681–684.

315. Alverdy JC, Aoys E, Moss GS: Total parenteral nutrition promotes bacterial translocation from the gut. *Surgery* 1988; 104:185–190.

316. Rock CS, Barber AE, Ng E-H, et al: TPN versus oral feeding: Bacterial translocation, cytokine responses, and mortality after *E. coli* LPS administration. *Surg Forum* 1990; 41:14–16.

317. Scheuing LA, Yeh YC, Tsai TH, et al: Circadian phase stimulatory effects of epidermal growth factor on deoxyribonucleic acid synthesis in the duodenum, jejunum, ileum, cecum, colon and rectum of the adult male mouse. *Endocrinology* 1980; 106:1498–1503.

318. Goodlad RA, Wilson TJG, Lenton W, et al: Proliferative effects of urogastrone-EGF on the intestinal epithelium. *Gut* 1987; 28:37–43.

319. Read LC, Tarantal A, George-Nascimento C: Effects of recombinant human epidermal growth factor on the intestinal growth of fetal rhesus monkeys. *Acta Paediatr Scand* 1984; 351:97–103.

320. Itoh M, Joh T, Imai S: Experimental and clinical studies on epidermal growth factor for gastric mucosal protection and healing of gastric ulcers. *J Clin Gastroenterol* 1988; 10(suppl):7.

321. Rogers PC, Kemp D, Rogol A, et al: Possible effects of growth hormone on development of acute lymphoblastic leukemia. *Lancet* 1977; 1:434–435.

322. Lippman ME, Dickson RB, Bates S, et al: Autocrine and paracrine growth regulation of human breast cancer. *Breast Cancer Res Treat* 1986; 7:59–70.

323. Nakanishi Y, Mulshine JL, Kaspryzk PG, et al: Insulin-like growth factor can mediate autocrine proliferation of human small cell lung cancer line in vitro. *J Clin Invest* 1988; 82:354–359.

324. Townsend CM, Beauchamp RD, Singh P, et al: Growth factors and intestinal neoplasm. *Am J Surg* 1988; 155:526–536.

325. Goustin AS, Leof EB, Shipley GD, et al: Growth factors and cancer. *Cancer Res* 1986; 46:1015–1029.

326. Donoway RB, Torosian MH: Growth hormone inhibits tumor metastases. *Surg Forum* 1989; 40:413–415.

47

Issues Involving Nutrition for Critically Ill Patients

Nora Kizer Bell, Ph.D.

New options/difficult choices

The legacy of Nancy Cruzan

Patient Self Determination Act of 1990

Provider-patient relationships

Fallout for nutritional support teams

Preview of future concerns

> (dying is fine) but Death. . . .
> when (instead of stopping to think) you
> begin to feel of it, dying
> 's miraculous
> why? be
> cause dying is
> perfectly natural; perfectly
> putting
> it mildly lively (but
> Death
> is strictly
> scientific
> & artificial &
> evil & legal). . . .
> —e.e. cummings, 1894–1962

NEW OPTIONS/DIFFICULT CHOICES

Until the past three decades, the use of medicine and technology to prolong life was virtually unknown. Prior to the discovery of antibiotics, for example, the onset of acute infection frequently resulted in death. Major-organ failure usually meant the loss of life. Whereas early care providers could offer patients little more than comfort and care, mod-ern medicine and technology offer an incredible array of treatment choices—from cardiopulmonary resuscitation (CPR), to organ transplantation, to mechanical life support, to sophisticated enteral and parenteral nutrition options, to increasingly complex surgical, chemical, and radiologic interventions. Many of these are choices, unfortunately, that sometimes will not heal, restore health, or help recovery. To be sure, advances in medical science and technology now make it possible to keep patients alive long after any meaningful existence has ceased.

Accordingly, in recent years, public debate, court cases, and legislative initiatives have focused attention on the subject of life-sustaining medical treatment for critically ill patients who have little prospect for continued meaningful life. However, in spite of state statutes defining "brain death" and "permanent unconsciousness" and statutes allowing advance directives or the appointing of a proxy for treatment decisions, many of the ethical issues generated by such cases are still not settled. Decision making for care providers, patients, and families in this new medical context has become very complex.

We might agree that several factors are important to note as confounding care choices in modern medicine.

First, the process of medical decision making has evolved and is still evolving from a formerly paternalistic approach to a more patient-centered approach to care that favors individual autonomy and the respecting of patients' wishes. In the 1983 report of the President's Commission for the Study of Ethical Problems in Medicine and Biomedical and Behavioral Research, commission members recommended that life-sustaining choices should and can only be made voluntarily by a competent and informed adult patient or, if the patient is incompetent, by an appropriately informed surrogate.[1] Even so, ensuring that patients' wishes are followed and resolving conflicts between the claims of vulnerable patients, the expectations of fearful families, and the professional judgment of members of the medical team can be daunting to the ethical care provider.

Second, there have clearly been changes in what occurs at death. As Daniel Callahan, director of the Hastings Center, has observed, whereas people used to experience "tame deaths"— that is, deaths that occurred relatively

peacefully, at home, with loved ones around, and in the full conviction that death was an important part of and the natural end to a full life—they now experience "wild deaths." This newer form of death occurs most frequently in hospitals, in intensive care units, in the company of noisy (sometimes painful and frightening) technology, with artificially provided nutrition, and with family members waiting anguishingly in hospital corridors.[2] Death is resisted and fought against, treated as the enemy of modern medical science. This newer "wild" death, Callahan argues, is a consequence of medicine's and society's failure to reflect on the limits of medical progress as well as begin a new discussion of critical illness, death, and their respective places in the life cycle.

In addition, the notion of what counts as a justifiable intervention at the end of life is changing. Those who execute "living wills" or health care powers of attorney, for example, clearly believe that some medical interventions are harmful to the dying person. The very existence of such legal mechanisms reflects a paradox in society's perception of the dying process: persons want to control those technologies designed to help control their dying. As Callahan argued, they feel that their deaths will be out of their control. While persons want their living prolonged, they do not want their dying prolonged. In contrast to what is perceived as the battle being waged by medical practitioners against death—medicine's so-called fight for life—most patients do not want tortured care at the end of life. They are not persuaded by the technological imperative.

And finally, economic factors are playing a crucial role in individual and policy determinations of what counts as appropriate care. While the cost of health care cannot accurately be measured solely in financial terms, economic considerations figure importantly in the decisions of patients and care providers alike. Currently, for example, over $1.3

billion is being spent annually in the United States on the care of persons in a persistent vegetative state.[3] And lest the issues be understood to be issues only of the elderly and aging, one must note that we also spend in excess of $1.5 billion annually on the care of critically ill newborns, many of whom do not survive either physically or neurologically intact and whose care after discharge is also enormously costly.

Like it or not, ready or not, many care providers now have to deal with new bioethical issues for which they were not specifically trained, for which they lack clear guidelines, and which they fear could subject them to legal liability. An increasing number of families now face complex questions of conscience as they attempt to cope with the emotional trauma of a desperate illness or the impending death of a loved one. Institutions and professional organizations are wrestling with articulating policies that reflect their moral commitment to patient well-being, their philosophy of care, as well as the current economic realities.

What does this have to do with nutrition?

After two decades of debate around "death with dignity" issues, the issues surrounding nutritional support in the critically ill remain largely unresolved. For many persons food and mealtimes are symbolically and emotionally significant—evoking strong feelings—and based on the positive experiences that those persons associate with food and eating. On the other hand, discussions of the depriving or withholding of food recall for many ghastly images of wartime concentration camps, emaciated and starving dissidents, or ethnic and racial purges. And in spite of court cases and ethical commentary that suggest that medical nutrition and hydration are *not* distinguishable in any morally relevant way from other life-sustaining medical treatments that may on occasion be withheld or withdrawn, some

persons are still reluctant to count nutrition as medical therapy.* Hence, many of the decisions surrounding questions of nutritional support in the critically ill are intellectually and emotionally complex, not to mention ripe for potential conflict.

THE LEGACY OF NANCY CRUZAN

While the much publicized *Cruzan* case highlighted the importance of "advance directives" for making known one's wishes about the use of lifesustaining therapies in the event of one's becoming incompetent during the course of medical treatment, the *Cruzan* case also spotlighted dilemmas surrounding the withdrawal of care from the irreversibly unconscious/ill patient. Nancy Beth Cruzan's parents, Lester and Joyce Cruzan, sought to terminate her artifically provided nutrition and hydration 7 years after an automobile accident left her in persistent vegetative state. They argued that such a decision was and would be what Nancy wanted. The ensuing debate made the provision of artificial nutrition and hydration a central focus of the ethical and legal struggle.

The issue brought before the Supreme Court in the *Cruzan* case was whether Missouri could demand that Nancy Cruzan's parents not be allowed to discontinue nutritional support without clear evidence that this was Nancy's expressed wish. Important for our pur-

---

*The courts of more than a dozen states have addressed this issue, as have professional societies including the American Medical Association. Each final appellate court has held that artificial feeding is medical treatment that may be rejected. As the New Jersey Supreme Court in the *Conroy* decision stated, "Analytically, artifical feeding by means of a nasogastric tube or intravenous infusion can be seen as equivalent to artificial breathing by means of a respirator. Both prolong life through mechanical means when the body is no longer able to perform a vital bodily function on its own."

poses, therefore, is the fact that the *Cruzan* decision affirmed that states *could* demand "clear and convincing" evidence that the patient herself would have chosen to discontinue life-sustaining treatment—in this case, nutrition and hydration—were she able to do so. The U.S. Supreme Court upheld Missouri's choice of a rigorous standard of proof and said that it was an appropriate standard for ensuring that one's personal choices about one's dying be respected. In addition, the *Cruzan* decision made clear that the U.S. Supreme Court recognized that individuals have a general liberty interest in deciding their own medical treatment, even to the point of permitting competent patients to refuse lifesaving treatment. Put differently, the *Cruzan* decision suggests that an explicit advance directive refusing nutrition and hydration, a wish expressed by a competent patient who later becomes incompetent, should be honored. What is less clear from the Court's decision is exactly what might count as an expressed wish.

Part of what was at stake in the *Cruzan* case was an important distinction between first-person treatment refusal and third-person treatment refusal. In finding that states can demand that surrogates be allowed to make treatment decisions for an incompetent patient only when that patient has herself made her wishes explicitly known, the Court was recommending that judgment on these matters should reside exclusively with the patient. This, of course, is a standard much more rigorous than that imposed by most states. Most states now allow—some by providing the statutory means for persons to designate health care proxies—surrogate decision makers to refuse or discontinue treatment.

Decisions such as that made in the *Cruzan* case are not anomalous, however. Of those values seen as central to discussions of ethics in the critical care setting, none has been more staunchly defended than autonomy. Although it has been argued that the focus on autonomy is particularly Western and perhaps overemphasized, it remains very clear that struggles over autonomy continue to lie at the center of ethical conflict in the clinical setting. For those who champion patients' rights, the *Cruzan* decision was seen as a strong affirmation of the importance of patient autonomy and patient self-determination.

PATIENT SELF DETERMINATION ACT OF 1990

For a variety of reasons, "patient self-determination," "autonomy," and "advance directives" have become the buzzwords in patient care in the 1990s. The Patient Self Determination Act (PSDA) of the 1990 Omnibus Reconciliation Act was enacted in October 1990 and went into effect December 1, 1991—not quite 1 year after a Missouri circuit court judge finally granted Nancy Cruzan's parents the authority to discontinue her nutritional support and not quite 1 year after Nancy Cruzan finally died.

The crux of the PSDA was to ensure that all patients, especially critically ill patients, be provided the opportunity to exercise control over their care through one of the of the currently available legal mechanisms for doing so. In most states, those mechanisms include "living wills" (or some other instructional directive), durable powers of attorney for health care (allowing the appointment of a health care proxy), and health care consent laws (spelling out explicitly the succession of those family members who may act as a surrogate decision maker in the absence of an advance directive).

An important aspect of advance directives is that they provide persons the opportunity to clearly state what they wish to have done as well as what they wish to have withheld if they should become permanently noncognitive. In addition, the PSDA requires that care providers inform patients about such options if they do not understand them and that they inform patients of any institutional policies that might prohibit the provider from following such directives in terminating life-sustaining treatment such as tube feedings.

Important opportunities and challenges are advanced by both the *Cruzan* decision and the PSDA. For example, both affirm the value choices that underlie the use of any type of advance directive:

- That autonomy is a central value in patient care.
- That "quality-of-life" determinations are the patient's to make, not the care provider's.
- That patients be allowed to weigh for themselves the "cost" to themselves and their families of life-sustaining treatment.
- That there should be dignity in death. As the final sentence of an award-winning article written several years ago suggested, "Death is not the enemy, Doctor, inhumanity is. . . ."[4]
- That patients are not bound by the technological imperative.
- That we (society and care givers) respect others' choices about what matters to them.
- That respecting patients' choices commits one to informing and educating patients about their illnesses and their treatment options.

The *Cruzan* decision and the PSDA also underscore the rights of professionals to exercise personal conscience in the provision of care to critically ill patients. Health care professionals are not required to abide by a patient's choices in an advance directive; the provider's choices and values must also be respected if doing so does not harm the patient. When the patient's choices cause a provider ethical discomfort or genuine ethical conflict, a variety of options exists for managing that conflict.

Most health organizations, even individual units within those organizations, now have processes or mechanisms in place for the discussion of ethical dilemmas and value conflicts arising in patient care. For example, most health care organizations now have ethics committees whose primary function is to help address the difficult choices faced by patients and providers in a variety of care-giving settings. Once the care giver's dilemma has been defined and explored and the conflict of values thoroughly discussed, the provider can choose to continue the care—perhaps with a new understanding of his moral accountability—or can withdraw from the case and transfer care of the patient to another provider.

Since informed persons are best able to make autonomous treatment decisions, the PSDA and the *Cruzan* decision also both affirm the importance of education about one's options in the course of one's illness or in dying. In fact, they hold the promise of helping to develop a better informed, more responsible patient population, not to mention healthier, more responsive patient/provider relationships.

Finally, both the *Cruzan* decision and the PSDA have underscored the importance of communication—the importance of making one's wishes known well in advance of any life-threatening illness. Too often, patients' families and care providers alike can only guess what a patient's preferences might have been. The cost of failing to communicate one's wishes can be physically and emotionally devastating to all involved.

PROVIDER-PATIENT RELATIONSHIPS

Paradoxically, the very thing that the PSDA and the *Cruzan* decision are intended to foster—namely, communication—could now also be at greatest risk.

One of the results hoped for in the formalizing of mechanisms for making patient's wishes known is that the use of advance directives will become a standard part of the medical intake process—in physician offices, in emergency rooms, in the admitting offices of hospitals and nursing homes, and in home health agencies. But some worry that the reliance on written advance directives, coupled with the implications of the "clear and convincing" evidence standard upheld in the *Cruzan* decision, will lead those caring for the critically ill to seek to satisfy what they perceive to be a legal or judicial mandate while overlooking the ethical mandate inherent in provider-patient relationships. Communication, trust, and caring are the moral underpinnings of the provider-patient relationship, but the language of a good provider-patient relationship is hardly the language of the law.

In most providers' recent memory, many decisions about foregoing futile treatment in the care of a critically ill patient were made carefully and lovingly by family members and care providers, all of whom were understood as placing the patient's well-being and comfort foremost. Together they decided when to stop. When patients said to their physicians, "I don't want to be a burden any longer," that was taken to mean: "Allow me to die. Please don't engage in futile attempts to keep me going." Such patients' wishes were usually quietly respected.

Now, however, some would say that legislatures and the courts have made it difficult to do what common sense and compassion would suggest. The question lingering after the *Cruzan* decision is how explicit one's expressed wish must be. Although the patient may say, "I don't want to be a burden any longer," the courts seem to be looking for "I don't want to be artificially fed or hydrated if I become permanently noncognitive," or, "If I am permanently unconscious, please discontinue parenteral nutrition and mechanical ventiliation." Clearly, people do not talk like that.[3] Yet, many fear that ordinary oral communication between provider and patient will be replaced by the discussion and signing of legal documents. Some also fear, perhaps rightly so, that the insistence on and preoccupation with the use of such documents will erode rather than enhance provider-patient relationships and replace trust with suspicion and uncertainty as to how one will be treated.

The reliance on legal and judicial solutions to the human problems that occur in the treatment of the critically ill has other negative implications as well. For reasons of ethnicity or because of long-held cultural beliefs, the use of written documents for expressing one's wishes about treatment refusal is unthinkable in some cultures. For these people, "writing it down" is equivalent to bringing it about. Accordingly, while they might wish to discuss their feelings about discontinuing nutritional support or terminating ventilator support should they be about to die, they fear bringing on death by signing anything like a living will.

Will care providers feel so pressured to use statutory options for treatment refusal that they abandon nonstatutory options altogether? Such a decision would clearly disserve many patient populations and disserve care providers as well.

FALLOUT FOR NUTRITIONAL SUPPORT TEAMS

Obviously, not all nutritional decisions revolve around life-and-death matters. In fact, the ethical issues faced by nutritional support teams and their patients are far broader than the issue merely of feeding persistently vegetative patients.

As Alexander Capron argued in his article "The Implications of the *Cruzan* decision for Clinical Nutrition Teams," this case afforded Americans an incredible opportunity to learn about advances made in enteral and parenteral nutrition that can save and sustain patients who would have died 20 years ago.[5] Instead, as Capron described it,[5]

> The trial court characterized nutrition as a "death prolonging procedure," a phrase repeated by the Supreme Court. . . . Thus, the *Cruzan* case shined a spotlight of public attention on artificially provided nutrition as a procedure that prolongs dying in otherwise hopeless patients whose families want to relieve them from the prospect of being maintained in an unconscious state for months or years. . . ."

To focus purely on the life-and-death decision-making dimension of nutritional support is, as Capron[5] notes, something that must have been terribly disappointing and frustrating to nutrition providers. They were denied an important forum for discussing the "virtues and accomplishments" of artificial feeding, and instead, nutritional support came to be referred to as a "death-prolonging" intervention.

A final issue for nutrition providers comes as a direct result of strides made in the field. Because of the advances made in nutritional support, nutrition providers sometimes also succumb to the power of their technology. Even in persistently vegetative patients, nutritional support has an observable—some think, positive—impact. Hence, in spite of the commitment of all care providers to patient self-determination, it is not uncommon for nutrition providers to feel disappointed or angry when patients or their families decide to discontinue feeding. In fact, in Nancy Cruzan's case, although the hospital director ultimately complied with her parents' instructions to discontinue feeding, many of the nurses who had cared for her over 7 years could not participate in caring for her as she died.

PREVIEW OF FUTURE CONCERNS

As the pressure for health care reform mounts regionally and nationally, the impetus for discussions of proposals for rationing care becomes greater. The pressure to address fundamental questions surrounding the grounds proposed for rationing is also mounting. Should we ration by disease, by prognosis, by cost, or according to futility of treatment, life-style choices, or certain minimum presumptions we have about human rights?

Although most persons would agree that we need to have an open and public discussion of rationing, such discussions are not yet proceeding in a careful and organized way. Rather, proposals for rationing care seem to be offered for our consideration piecemeal. Former Governor Lamm and Daniel Callahan (among others) have suggested, for example, that age be a criterion for rationing care, that we simply choose an age beyond which certain health services simply will not be provided.

Others have argued that persons with acquired immunodeficiency syndrome (AIDS) or human immunodeficiency syndrome (HIV) be excluded from government-funded health services (other than screening for presence of the virus) on the grounds that treatment of HIV disease is too costly—approximately $300 per day for medication alone—that the ultimate prognosis is uniformly futile, and that infection follows inappropriate life-style choices.

Still others have looked at plans for health care reform, such as Oregon's, and viewed rationing as something that should occur only within the context of Medicaid-funded health services. Their view reflects the sentiment that persons should have access to whatever they can afford.

Still others have encouraged consideration of purely economic data in deciding what medical interventions ought to be provided to patients. They point to discharge data for neonatal intensive care units, for example, to argue that care should be withheld from newborns weighing less than 500 g.

Even technology is playing a part in rationing proposals. Although only 15 hospitals nationwide currently have it,

APACHE III (Acute, Physiology, Age, and Chronic Health Evaluation), a computer program that predicts the mortality of individual patients by comparing their medical status with that of nearly 18,000 other patients in its data base, is increasingly being used to assist treatment decisions in critical care medicine. In an era where the cost of care and rationing are inextricably linked, critics of APACHE fear that its predictions could unduly influence care providers, patients, and their families as they wrestle with the difficult questions of whether to discontinue treatment. They worry that the factors given weight in the APACHE equation already militate against certain kinds of patients—the aged, those with AIDS, and those with little pyschosocial support, for example. Interestingly, those who support the use of APACHE III see that as an advantage, not a drawback. They view entitlement to care as one's ability to respond to treatment.

As the debate over rationing takes shape, nutrition providers can expect to be at the center of those discussions inasmuch as nutrition and hydration are considered by many—providers and patients alike—to be basic to the provision of quality health care.

Of course, many of the issues described above are those around which the greatest controversy swirls. For many nutrition providers there are other, less dramatic, ethical struggles such as the struggle to demonstrate daily in the practice of their profession the high value they place on other human beings. The provision of nutritional support, like other care giving, is, at root, a moral endeavor—one that leads nutrition providers to seek to ensure human dignity by enhancing patient well-being throughout the course of illness and treatment.

REFERENCES

1. *Deciding to Forego Life Sustaining Treatment: Ethical, Medical and Legal Issues in Treatment.* President's Commission for the Study of Ethical Problems in Medicine and Biomedical and Behavioral Research, Washington, DC, 1983.
2. Callahan D: The euthanasia debate: Where are we going? Presented at Ending Human Life: A Symposium on the Ethical Issues Surrounding Death and Dying, Newberry, SC, The Center for Ethical Development, Newberry College, Feb 4, 1992.
3. American Hospital Association: Forum on final care. Chicago, Oct 4, 1990. (Videotape of proceedings, 1991.)
4. Caroline NL: Dying in academe. *New Physician* 1972; 655–657.
5. Capron AM: The implications of the Cruzan decision for clinical nutrition teams. *Nutr Clin Pract* 1991; 6:89–94.

Index

A

Abdominal abscess after trauma surgery, route of nutritional support and, 580

Abdominal surgery, perioperative total parenteral nutrition in, 310–311

Abdominal trauma, clinical trials of enteral nutritional support, 291

Abdominal Trauma Index (ATI), 573

Abdominal wall
  infection, in operative gastrostomy, 346
  necrosis, with percutaneously placed tubes, 354

Accupep HPF
  nutrient sources and composition, 450–455
  peptide lengths, 441
  trace elements, 277

Acetate
  as gut-specific nutrient, 552
  in total parenteral nutrition formulations, 387

Acetone, for skin antisepsis, 412

Acidosis
  lactic, endotoxin-induced, 200
  metabolic, glutamine supplementation in, 127
  in peritoneal dialysis, 430–431

Acquired immunodeficiency syndrome (AIDS), 783–799 (see also Human immunodeficiency virus)
  anorexia and weight loss, 793–794
  assessment in HIV disease, 790
  cost of treatment, 871
  diarrhea and malabsorption, 794
  malnutrition and impaired nutrient intake
    deficiency of individual nutrients, 789–790
    intestinal malabsorption, 785–788
    pharmacotherapeutic nutritional impairment, 788–789
  management in HIV disease, 790–791
  nutritional effects, 783–785
  nutritional support, 791–792
    alternative therapies, 795
    indications, 792–793
  wasting, 784–785, 787

Activity factors, in estimating energy needs, 374, 375

Acute, Physiology, Age, and Chronic Health Evaluation (APACHE III), 872

Acute renal failure (see Renal failure, acute)

Adenosine triphosphate, in energy transfer, 35, 36

Adult respiratory distress syndrome (ARDS)
  fish oil and, 200
  intra-abdominal sepsis and, therapy, 177
  lipid feeding and, 175–176

Aging (see also Geriatric nutrition)
  energy balance, 717–719
  hypernatremia, 249
  hypodipsia, 723
  hyponatremia, 248–249
  insulin growth factor 1, 722–723
  macronutrient metabolism, 719

AIDS (see Acquired immunodeficiency syndrome)

Alanine, in muscle, 86

Albumin
  diarrhea and, 342, 825
  in elderly, 719–720
  in head injury, 694–695
  in nutritional assessment, 19, 21
    pediatric, 735–736
  as nutritional index, 20, 143–144
  in spinal cord injury, 697
  supplementation, 143–156
    administration and enteral feeding tolerance, 150
    based on empirical formula, 148
    in cirrhosis, 150
    for intravascular expansion, 147–148
    in open heart surgery, 149
    in pulmonary insufficiency, 148
    Starling's law as guide, 145–147
    in thermal injury, 149–150
    titration by hemodynamic stabilization, 148
    in total parenteral nutrition, 150–152

Alcohol, for skin antisepsis, 412

AlitraQ
  nutrient sources and composition, 450–455, 610, 611
  peptide lengths, 441
  trace elements, 277

Cardiopulmonary reserve, branched-chain
amino acids and, 98–100
Cardiovascular system, starvation and
refeeding effects, 771
Carnation Diet Instant Breakfast, trace
elements in, 279
Carnation Instant Breakfast, trace elements
in, 279
Carnitine
in enteral nutrition products, 455, 461,
467
in peritoneal dialysis, 428
requirements in peritoneal dialysis
adults, 432
children, 434
β-Carotene, 219–221
Casec, nutrient composition, 446
β-Casomorphin, 64–65, 69
Catabolic index, 23
Catabolic response, hormone alterations
and, 734–735
Catabolism, in renal failure, 662
Catecholamines, 734–735
Catheters
care and maintenance, 407–415
care protocols
catheter dressing materials, 413
ethanol, 415
flushes, 414
hub contamination, 413–414
hydrochloric acid, 415
occlusion, 414
skin antisepsis, 411–413
thrombolytic therapy, 414–415
infection
catheter materials, 409–410
culture methods, 408–409
definitions, 11, 407–408
duration of catheterization, 411
insertion site, 409
multiple-lumen catheters, 411
rates, 407
occlusion
in jejunostomy, 341, 342
with percutaneously placed tubes, 355
for parenteral nutrition
insertion, 381–382, 383
location, 381–382
selection, 379–384
sepsis, 384–385, 580, 581
Cefamandole, 488
Cefotetan, 488
Cefoxitin, 488
Ceftizoxime, 488
Celiac disease, amino acid and peptide
absorption in, 62, 67
Cellular immunity, in nutritional
assessment, 27
Cellulose, 184
Central nervous system
amino acid effects, 158–159
disorders from thiamine deficiency, 229

Central venous catheters (*see* Catheters)
Cephadrine, 488
Chemical analysis, in nutritional
assessment, 25–26
Chemotherapy
colony-stimulating factors and, 839
diarrhea from, 821
parenteral nutrition and, 286–287,
711–712
Children, nutrition for (*see* Pediatric
nutrition)
Chlorhexidine gluconate, for skin
antisepsis, 412–413
Chloride
in enteral nutrition products, 453, 459,
465
in peritoneal dialysis, 425
in total parenteral nutrition
formulations, 387
Cholecalciferol, 222
Cholecystokinin (CCK), 551
Cholesterol, aging and, 719
Choline, 241–242
in enteral nutrition products, 453, 459,
465
Chromium, 262
deficiency states, 262–263
in enteral nutrition products, 277–279,
455, 461, 467
metabolism, 262
Chronic obstructive pulmonary disease
(COPD)
energy needs, 650–651
geriatric malnutrition, 721
liver damage and, therapy, 177
malnutrition effects, 648
refeeding, 650
mortality, 647–648
theophylline in, 495, 499
weight loss, 158
Chronic renal failure (*see* Renal failure,
chronic)
Cimetidine, for stress gastritis, 624
Ciprofloxacin, in enteral feeding,
496
Circadian rhythms, tube feedings and,
363–364
Cirrhosis (*see also* Liver disease), albumin
in, 150
Cisplatin, 488, 491
Citrotein, trace elements in, 279
Clinical trials, prospective randomized
controlled (PRCTs), of nutritional
support, 285, 286–292
Clostridium difficile, diarrhea from, 821,
822
Cobalamin, 233
Cobalt, 273
Cola, for feeding tube patency, 404
Colitis, ulcerative (*see also* Inflammatory
bowel disease), total parenteral
nutrition in, 315